GEORGE L. PORTER, M. D.
224 DOCTORS BUILDING
3707 GASTON AVENUE
DALLAS, TEXAS 75246

George Porter M.D.

224 Doctors Bldg

3707 Gaston Ave

Dallas Texas 75246

Aug 14, 1979

GEORGE L. PORTER, M.D.
3707 GASTON, SUITE 224
DALLAS, TEXAS 75246
(214) 824-2559

1979
CURRENT THERAPY
1979

CONSULTING EDITORS:

FREDERIC C. BARTTER
WALTER A. BONNEY
GEORGE E. BURCH
BENJAMIN BURROWS
JAMES B. FIELD
WILLARD E. GOODWIN
LAWRENCE C. KOLB
CLARENCE S. LIVINGOOD
DANIEL J. McCARTY
FRED PLUM
CHARLES H. RAMMELKAMP
JAMES L. A. ROTH
R. WAYNE RUNDLES
THOMAS E. VAN METRE, Jr.

W. B. SAUNDERS COMPANY / PHILADELPHIA / LONDON / TORONTO

1979

CURRENT THERAPY

LATEST APPROVED METHODS OF TREATMENT FOR THE PRACTICING PHYSICIAN

EDITED BY HOWARD F. CONN, M.D.

W. B. Saunders Company:	West Washington Square
Philadelphia, PA 19105

1 St. Anne's Road
Eastbourne, East Sussex BN21 3UN, England

1 Goldthorne Avenue
Toronto, Ontario M8Z 5T9, Canada

Current Therapy	ISBN 0–7216–2664–5

© 1979 by W. B. Saunders Company.   Copyright under the International Copyright Union.   All rights reserved.   This book is protected by copyright.   No part of it may be reproduced, stored in a retrieval system, or transmitted in any form or by any means, electronic, mechanical, photocopying, recording, or otherwise, without written permission from the publisher.   Made in the United States of America.   Press of W. B. Saunders Company.   Library of Congress catalog card number 49–8328.

Last digit is the print number:	9	8	7	6	5	4	3	2	1

Consulting Editors

THE ENDOCRINE SYSTEM
FREDERIC C. BARTTER, M.D.

Clinical Professor of Medicine, Georgetown University Medical School. Chief, Hypertension-Endocrine Branch, Clinical Center, National Institutes of Health, Bethesda, Maryland.

OBSTETRICS AND GYNECOLOGY
WALTER A. BONNEY, M.D.

Clinical Professor, Obstetrics and Gynecology, West Virginia University School of Medicine, Morgantown, West Virginia.

THE CARDIOVASCULAR SYSTEM
GEORGE E. BURCH, M.D., F.A.C.P.

Emeritus Professor of Medicine, Tulane University School of Medicine, New Orleans, Louisiana.

THE RESPIRATORY SYSTEM
BENJAMIN BURROWS, M.D.

Professor of Internal Medicine, University of Arizona College of Medicine. Staff, Arizona Health Sciences Center; Consultant, Veterans Administration Hospital, Tucson, Arizona.

METABOLIC DISORDERS
JAMES B. FIELD, M.D.

Rutherford Professor of Medicine and Head, Division of Endocrinology and Metabolism, Baylor College of Medicine, Houston, Texas.

THE UROGENITAL TRACT
WILLARD E. GOODWIN, M.D., F.A.C.S., F.A.A.P.

Professor of Surgery/Urology (Pediatric Urology), University of California School of Medicine, Los Angeles. Staff Urologist, University of California Medical Center, Los Angeles; Senior Consultant in Urology, Wadsworth Veterans Administration Hospital, Los Angeles; Consultant in Urology, Los Angeles County Harbor General Hospital, Torrance; Consultant, St. Francis Hospital, Lynwood; Consulting Staff, Hollywood Presbyterian Hospital, Los Angeles; Honorary Consulting Staff, Santa Monica Hospital, Santa Monica; Courtesy Staff, St. John's Hospital, Santa Monica, and Hospital of the Good Samaritan, Los Angeles; Consulting Staff, The Cedars of Lebanon Hospital and Mount Sinai Hospital, Los Angeles, California.

PSYCHIATRY
LAWRENCE C. KOLB, M.D.

Emeritus Professor of Psychiatry, College of Physicians and Surgeons, Columbia University. Consultant in Psychiatry and Honorary Member, Medical Board, The Presbyterian Hospital in the City of New York, New York.

DISEASES OF THE SKIN AND THE VENEREAL DISEASES
CLARENCE S. LIVINGOOD, M.D.

Chairman Emeritus, Department of Dermatology, Henry Ford Hospital. Clinical Professor of Dermatology, University of Michigan Medical School. Staff Physician, Department of Dermatology, Henry Ford Hospital, Detroit, Michigan.

THE LOCOMOTOR SYSTEM
DANIEL J. McCARTY, M.D.

Professor of Medicine, The Medical College of Wisconsin. Senior Attending Physician and Director of Medical Service, Milwaukee County General Hospital, Milwaukee, Wisconsin.

THE NERVOUS SYSTEM
FRED PLUM, M.D.

Anne Parrish Titzell Professor and Chairman, Department of Neurology, Cornell University Medical College, New York, New York.

THE INFECTIOUS DISEASES
CHARLES H. RAMMELKAMP, M.D., D.Sc.

Professor of Medicine and Professor of Preventive Medicine, Case Western Reserve University Medical School. Director of Medicine, Cleveland Metropolitan General Hospital, Cleveland, Ohio.

THE DIGESTIVE SYSTEM
JAMES L. A. ROTH, M.D., Ph.D., D.Sc. (Hon.), F.A.C.P.

Professor of Clinical Medicine, School of Medicine, University of Pennsylvania. Director, Institute of Gastroenterology, and Chief, Gastroenterology Service, Presbyterian–University of Pennsylvania Medical Center; Consulting Gastroenterologist, U. S. Naval Medical Center, Bethesda, Maryland, and U. S. Naval Hospital, Lankenau Hospital, and Roxborough Memorial Hospital, Philadelphia, Pennsylvania.

THE BLOOD AND SPLEEN
R. WAYNE RUNDLES, Ph.D., M.D.

Professor of Medicine, Duke University Medical School. Hematology-Oncology Staff, Member of Comprehensive Cancer Center, Durham, North Carolina.

DISEASES OF ALLERGY
THOMAS E. VAN METRE, Jr., M.D.

Associate Professor of Medicine, The Johns Hopkins University School of Medicine. Physician-in-Charge, Allergy Clinic, The Johns Hopkins Hospital, Baltimore, Maryland.

NOTICE

Extraordinary efforts have been made by the authors, the editors, and the publisher of this book to insure that dosage recommendations are precise and in agreement with standards officially accepted at the time of publication.

It does happen, however, that dosage schedules are changed from time to time in the light of accumulating clinical experience and continuing laboratory studies. This is most likely to occur in the case of recently introduced products.

It is urged, therefore, that you check the manufacturer's recommendations for dosage, *especially if the drug to be administered or prescribed is one that you use only infrequently or have not used for some time.*

THE PUBLISHER

Preface

This edition of *Current Therapy,* the thirty-first of an annual series, continues the original purpose of bringing to the physician authoritative, current methods of therapy in a convenient form for reference. The articles have been written specifically to give concise, accurate, and sufficiently detailed information unhampered by material not directly related to the therapy proposed. Careful planning is constantly in effect to ensure that the book continues to carry out its intended purpose as a quick, adequate reference volume. The space limitation of a single volume prohibits discussions of diagnosis if the aim of the book is to be maintained, and the authors have assumed that a correct diagnosis has been made before the book is consulted.

This policy has met with enthusiastic approval in the preceding editions, and it is gratifying to learn that *Current Therapy* has been of great help to the practicing physician in the care of his patients.

The term "method" refers to the regimen in current use by the author-clinician; it does not necessarily imply that the named author was the originator of the regimen. Present-day treatment is by and large a summation of the work of many clinicians over the years, and no attempt has been made to confine coverage to recent advances only. Traditional therapy, if an author considers it still to be the best available, is included along with modern advances; the result is a well-balanced treatise on the management of each disease.

It will be noted that obsolete procedures are not mentioned and that methods or agents not fully tested are so designated. Certain procedures or drugs currently under investigation may not be advised for general use until it can be stated definitely that they have been accepted as standards in treatment.

This is a new edition rather than a revision of the old. Many topics have been rotated among authors from several countries, and many of the authors of this edition are contributing to *Current Therapy* for the first time. A few articles from the previous edition dealing with disease entities in which there has been little or no change in therapy have been revised or approved by their authors for this edition. In keeping with variations in the importance of certain diseases, and with the world-wide distribution of the book, certain deletions and additions of topics have been made.

The effectiveness and success of *Current Therapy* have been due in greatest measure to the Contributors and Consultants, to whom the Editor is deeply grateful. This book would not have been possible without their wholehearted cooperation. The Editor also wishes to express his appreciation to Mr. C. F. Robinson and Mrs. Franklin Cole for their valuable assistance and to the staff of the W. B. Saunders Company for their thoughtful help and guidance in the preparation of the book.

HOWARD F. CONN, M.D., F.A.C.P.
Uniontown, Pennsylvania

Contributors

ELIZABETH A. ABEL, M.D.

Clinical Assistant Professor of Dermatology, Stanford University School of Medicine; Clinical Assistant Professor of Dermatology, Stanford University Medical Center, Palo Alto, California
Psoriasis

KEDAR K. ADOUR, M.D.

Chief, Cranial Nerve Research Clinic, Department of Otolaryngology, Kaiser-Permanente Medical Center, Oakland, California
Acute Peripheral Facial Paralysis

JOHN ADRIANI, M.D.

Professor of Pharmacology, Anesthesiology, and Clinical Surgery, Louisiana State University School of Medicine; Consultant in Pharmacology and Anesthesiology, Louisiana, Health, and Human Resources, New Orleans, Louisiana
Narcotic Poisoning

JAMES W. ANDERSON, M.D.

Professor of Medicine, University of Kentucky College of Medicine; Chief, Endocrine-Metabolic Section, Veterans Administration Hospital, Lexington, Kentucky
Reactive Hypoglycemia

PHILIP C. ANDERSON, M.D.

Professor, University of Missouri School of Medicine; Chairman, University of Missouri Medical Center, Columbia, Missouri
Spider Bites and Scorpion Stings

LON S. ANNEST, M.D.

Assistant Professor, University of Washington School of Medicine, Seattle, Washington
Intestinal Obstruction

MICHAEL ANTHONY, M.D., F.R.C.P., F.R.A.C.P.

Clinical Lecturer in Medicine, University of New South Wales; Neurologist, Prince Henry Hospital, Sydney, Australia
Headache

DJAVAD T. ARANI, M.D.

Clinical Assistant Professor of Medicine, State University of New York at Buffalo; Attending Physician, Buffalo General Hospital, Buffalo, New York
Tachycardia

GORDON LEE ARCHER, M.D.

Assistant Professor of Internal Medicine, Virginia Commonwealth University–Medical College of Virginia; Consultant in Infectious Diseases, Medical College of Virginia Hospitals, Richmond, Virginia
Infective Endocarditis

JAY MORRIS ARENA, M.D., B.S.M.

Professor of Pediatrics, Professor of Community Health Sciences, Duke University School of Medicine; Director, Poison Control Center, Duke Medical Center, Durham, North Carolina
Acute Miscellaneous Poisoning

JOHN ASSINI, M.D.

Senior Fellow, University of Colorado School of Medicine; Rheumatologist, Colorado General Hospital, Denver General Hospital and Veterans Administration Hospital, Denver, Colorado
Lupus Erythematosus

G. WILLIAM ATKINSON, M.D.

Associate Professor of Medicine, Director, Division of Pulmonary Diseases, Department of Medicine, Jefferson Medical College, Thomas Jefferson University, Philadelphia, Pennsylvania
Pulmonary Embolism

ROBERT L. BAEHNER, M.D.

Professor of Pediatrics and Clinical Pathology, Indiana University School of Medicine; Director, Pediatric Hematology-Oncology, James Whitcomb Riley Hospital for Children, Indianapolis, Indiana
Childhood Acute Leukemia

ROBERT A. BARBEE, M.D.

Associate Professor of Medicine, University of Arizona College of Medicine; Director, Pulmonary Clinic, Arizona Health Sciences Center, Tucson, Arizona
Chronic Bronchitis and Bronchiectasis

ANN B. BARNES, M.D.

Assistant Clinical Professor, Department of Obstetrics and Gynecology, Harvard Medical School; Assistant Obstetrician-Gynecologist, Massachusetts General Hospital; Obstetrician-Gynecologist, Boston Hospital for Women, Boston, Massachusetts
Dysmenorrhea

RICHARD D. BAUGHMAN, M.D.

Associate Professor of Clinical Medicine (Dermatology), Dartmouth Medical School; Chairman and Program Director, Section of Dermatology, Dartmouth-Hitchcock Medical Center, Hanover, New Hampshire
Neurodermatitis

RICHARD S. BAUM, M.D.

Director, Neonatal Pediatrics, Methodist Hospital of Indiana, Indianapolis, Indiana
Care of the Low–Birth-Weight Infant

SAMUEL F. BEAN, M.D.

Assistant Professor of Dermatology, Baylor College of Medicine; Clinical Assistant Professor of Dermatology, University of Texas Medical School; Dermatologist, Diagnostic Clinic of Houston, Houston, Texas
Pemphigus and Bullous Pemphigoid

WILLIAM BENNETT BEAN, M.D.

Harris Kempner Professor of Medical Humanities, Professor of Internal Medicine, Director, Institute for the Medical Humanities, University of Texas Medical Branch, Galveston, Texas; Sir William Osler Professor of Medicine, University of Iowa College of Medicine, Iowa City, Iowa
Pellagra

ROBERT B. BELSHE, M.D.

Associate Professor of Medicine and Chief, Section of Infectious Diseases, Marshall University School of Medicine; Head of Infectious Diseases, Huntington Veterans Administration Hospital; Attending Physician, Cabell Huntington Hospital; Attending Physician, St. Mary's Hospital, Huntington, West Virginia
Viral Respiratory Infections

ARTHUR A. BERENBAUM, B.S., M.D.

Emeritus Associate Professor of Medicine, University of Pennsylvania; Attending Cardiologist, Graduate Hospital, Philadelphia, Pennsylvania
Cardiac Arrest

JOHN R. BERTRAM, M.D.

Assistant Clinical Instructor, Department of Medicine—Dermatology, University Hospitals, University of Wisconsin; Attending Physician, Dean Clinic, St. Mary's Hospital, and Madison General Hospital, Madison, Wisconsin
Pruritus

MARGARET JOHNSON BIA, M.D.

Assistant Professor of Medicine, Yale University School of Medicine; Attending Physician in Medicine and Nephrology, Yale–New Haven Hospital; Assistant Director of Dialysis and Transplant Program, Yale–New Haven Hospital, New Haven, Connecticut
Diabetes Insipidus

ROBERT P. BIGGANS, M.D.

Clinical Associate Professor of Medicine, University of Pennsylvania; Attending Cardiologist, Graduate Hospital, Philadelphia, Pennsylvania
Cardiac Arrest

D. MONTGOMERY BISSELL, M.D.

Assistant Professor of Medicine, University of California, San Francisco; Attending Physician, University of California Hospitals and San Francisco General Hospital, San Francisco, California
Porphyria

LILLIAN R. BLACKMON, M.D.

Associate Professor of Pediatrics, Associate Professor of Obstetrics and Gynecology, Kenan McBryde Scholar in Neonatology, Co-Director, Division of Perinatal Medicine, Duke University School of Medicine, Durham, North Carolina
Hemolytic Disease of the Newborn

MANUEL G. BLOOM, M.D.

Clinical Associate Professor of Dermatology, Baylor College of Medicine; Clinical Professor of Oral Diagnosis, University of Texas, Dental Branch; Senior Attending Physician, Dermatology, Methodist Hospital; Consultant in Dermatology, St. Luke's Episcopal Hospital and Texas Children's Hospital, Houston, Texas
Disorders of the Mouth (Benign)

JOHN R. BONAME, M.D., J.D.

Associate Professor of Anesthesia, Samford University; Chairman, Anesthesia Department, Baptist Medical Center–Montclair, Birmingham, Alabama
Disturbances Due to Heat

JOHN H. BOND, M.D.

Associate Professor of Medicine, University of Minnesota School of Medicine; Chief, Gastroenterology Section, Minneapolis Veterans Administration Hospital, Minneapolis, Minnesota
Gaseousness

JAMES R. BONNER, M.D.

Assistant Professor of Medicine, University of South Alabama College of Medicine; Active Staff, University of South Alabama Medical Center; Associate Staff, Springhill, Mobile Infirmary and Providence Hospitals, Mobile, Alabama
Bacterial Pneumonia

P. C. BORNMAN, M.B., M.MED. (SURG.), F.R.C.S.ED.

Senior Lecturer, Department of Surgery, University of Cape Town; Senior Specialist, Groote Schuur Hospital, Cape Town, Republic of South Africa
Chronic Pancreatitis

H. WORTH BOYCE, JR., M.D.

Professor of Medicine; Chief, Section of Gastroenterology, University of South Florida College of Medicine, Tampa, Florida
Dysphagia and Esophageal Obstruction

R. RANDOLPH BRADHAM, M.D.

Clinical Professor of Thoracic Surgery, Medical University of South Carolina; Chief of Surgery, Roper Hospital; Section Chairman, Thoracic Surgery, St. Francis Xavier Hospital, Charleston, South Carolina
Empyema Thoracic

PAUL F. BRENNER, M.D.

Associate Professor, Department of Obstetrics and Gynecology, University of Southern California School of Medicine; Attending Physician, Women's Hospital, Los Angeles County–University of Southern California Medical Center, Los Angeles, California
Abortion

JEROME S. BRODY, M.D.

Professor of Medicine and Associate Professor of Biochemistry, Boston University School of Medicine; Associate Director, Pulmonary Division, Boston University School of Medicine; Chief, Pulmonary Sections, Boston City Hospital and University Hospital, Boston, Massachusetts
Acute Respiratory Failure

STANLEY BROSMAN, M.D.

Associate Professor of Surgery/Urology, University of California, Los Angeles, School of Medicine, Los Angeles, California; Chief of Urology, Harbor General Hospital, Torrance, California
Trauma of the Genitourinary System

JOHN F. BROWN, JR., M.D.

Assistant Professor of Medicine, University of Southern California, School of Medicine; Assistant Chief Physician, Pulmonary Disease Service, Los Angeles County–University of Southern California Medical Center, Los Angeles, California
Coccidioidomycosis

DEREK A. BRUCE, M.B., CH.B.

Assistant Professor of Neurosurgery, University of Pennsylvania School of Medicine; Associate Neurosurgeon, Children's Hospital of Philadelphia, Philadelphia, Pennsylvania
Head Injuries in Children

HOWARD A. BUECHNER, M.D., F.A.C.P., F.C.C.P.

Professor of Internal Medicine, Louisiana State University School of Medicine; Senior Visiting Physician, Charity Hospital of Louisiana, New Orleans, Louisiana
Silicosis; Bagassosis, Farmer's Lung and Other Forms of Hypersensitivity Pneumonitis

B. HUGH BUFF, M.D., F.A.C.P.

Department of Internal Medicine, Mercy Hospital and Medical Center, San Diego, California
Rabies

PAUL A. BUNN, JR., M.D.

Assistant Professor of Medicine, Georgetown University Medical Center; Senior Investigator, NCI-VA Medical Oncology Branch, Veterans Administration Hospital, Washington, D.C.
Mycosis Fungoides and the Sezary Syndrome

KENNETH D. BURMAN, M.D.

Assistant Professor of Medicine, Uniformed Services University of the Health Sciences, Bethesda, Maryland; Assistant Chief, Endocrine-Metabolic Service, Walter Reed Army Medical Center, Washington, D.C.
Hypothyroidism

JOSEPH W. BURNETT, M.D.

Professor and Head, Division of Dermatology, University of Maryland School of Medicine, Baltimore, Maryland
Bacterial Infections of the Skin

JOHN F. BUSEY, M.D.

Clinical Professor of Medicine, University of Mississippi School of Medicine; Director, Medical Education, Mississippi Baptist Medical Center, Jackson, Mississippi
North American Blastomycosis

HENRY K. BUTLER, JR., M.D.

Dermatologist, Rutherford Hospital, Murfreesboro, Tennessee
Miliaria

THOMAS BUTLER, M.D.

Assistant Professor of Medicine, Case Western Reserve University; Assistant Physician, University Hospitals, Cleveland, Ohio
Plague

DAVID ALLEN BYRNE, M.D.

Clinical Assistant Professor of Dermatology, Indiana University School of Medicine; Bloomington Hospital, Bloomington, Indiana
Pityriasis Rosea

JEFFREY P. CALLEN, M.D.

Assistant Clinical Professor, Department of Medicine (Dermatology), University of Louisville School of Medicine; Attending Physician, Louisville General Hospital, Veterans Administration Hospital, Louisville, Kentucky
Drug Eruptions

DONALD B. CALNE, D.M., F.R.C.P.

Clinical Director and Chief, Experimental Therapeutics Branch, IRP National Institute of Neurological and Communicative Disorders and Stroke, National Institutes of Health, Department of Health, Education, and Welfare, Bethesda, Maryland
Parkinson's Disease

JOHN J. CANARY, M.D.

Professor of Medicine and Director, Division of Endocrinology, Georgetown University School of Medicine and The University Hospital, Washington, D.C.
Cushing's Syndrome

JAMES T. CASSIDY, M.D.

Professor of Medicine and Pediatrics, University of Michigan Medical School, Ann Arbor, Michigan
Juvenile Rheumatoid Arthritis

FRED F. CASTROW II, M.D.

Clinical Associate Professor, University of Texas Medical School, Houston, Texas
Hidradenitis Suppurativa

NEIL S. CHERNIACK, M.D.

Professor of Medicine, Case Western Reserve University; Veterans Administration and University Hospitals, Cleveland, Ohio
Chronic Bronchitis and Emphysema

PAUL A. CHERVENICK, M.D.

Professor, Internal Medicine, University of Pittsburgh School of Medicine; Attending Physician, Presbyterian-University Hospital, Pittsburgh, Pennsylvania
Neutropenia

FREDRIC L. COE, M.D.

Professor, University of Chicago Pritzker School of Medicine; Director, Renal Division, Michael Reese Hospital and Medical Center, Chicago, Illinois
Renal Calculi

MIGUEL COLON-MORALES, M.D.

Associate Professor of Clinical Anesthesiology, University of Puerto Rico School of Medicine; Director, Department of Anesthesiology and Respiratory Therapy, Teacher's Hospital, San Juan, Puerto Rico
Obstetric Analgesia and Anesthesia

CHARLES A. COLTMAN, JR., M.D.

Professor of Medicine, University of Texas Health Science Center at San Antonio; Director, Clinical Medical Oncology Section, Department of Medicine, University of Texas Health Science Center at San Antonio; Medical Director, Cancer Therapy and Research Center, San Antonio, Texas
Hodgkin's Disease: Chemotherapy

REX B. CONN, M.D.

Professor of Pathology and Laboratory Medicine, Emory University School of Medicine; Director, Clinical Pathology Laboratories, Emory University Hospital, Atlanta, Georgia
Laboratory Reference Values of Clinical Importance

ELIZABETH B. CONNELL, M.D.

Associate Professor, Northwestern University School of Medicine; Northwestern Memorial Hospital, Chicago, Illinois
Contraception

WILLIS I. COTTEL, M.D.

Associate Professor, Department of Internal Medicine, University of Texas Health and Science Center; Associate Attending Physician, Baylor University Medical Center, Dallas, Texas
Cancer of the Skin

PHILIP C. CRAVEN, M.D.

Assistant Professor of Medicine, University of Texas Health Science Center; Attending Physician, Infectious Diseases, Audie L. Murphy Veterans Administration Hospital and Bexar County Hospital, San Antonio, Texas
Bacterial Meningitis

WERNER CREUTZFELDT, M.D., F.R.C.P.

Professor of Internal Medicine, Department of Medicine, University of Göttingen, Göttingen, Federal Republic of Germany
Acute Pancreatitis

TAKEY CRIST, M.D., F.A.C.O.G., F.A.C.S., I.C.S.

Clinical Assistant Professor, University of North Carolina Medical School; Attending Physician, Onslow Memorial Hospital, Jacksonville, North Carolina
Postpartum Care

MARIA DA COSTA, M.D.

Associate Professor of Medicine, New York Medical College; Attending Physician, Metropolitan Hospital, New York, New York
Macrocytic (Megaloblastic) Anemia (Other than Pernicious Anemia)

JOHN G. DALEY, M.D.

Associate Professor of Obstetrics and Gynecology, University of North Carolina School of Medicine; Attending Obstetrician-Gynecologist and Gynecologic Endocrinologist, New Hanover Memorial Hospital, Wilmington, North Carolina
Menopause

MORRIS DAVIDMAN, M.D.

Assistant Professor of Medicine, University of Minnesota School of Medicine; Attending Nephrologist, Hennepin County Medical Center, Minneapolis, Minnesota
Chronic Renal Failure

THOMAS P. DAVIN, M.D.

Assistant Professor, University of Minnesota School of Medicine; Attending Nephrologist, University Hospital, Minneapolis, Minnesota
Acute Renal Failure

MICHAEL E. DeBAKEY, M.D.

Professor, Department of Surgery, Baylor College of Medicine; Director, National Heart and Blood Vessel Research and Demonstration Center, Baylor College of Medicine, Houston, Texas
Acquired Diseases of the Aorta

ALBERT DEL NEGRO, M.D.

Assistant Professor of Medicine, Georgetown University School of Medicine; Chief of Catheterization Laboratory, Georgetown University Medical Center, Washington, D.C.
Atrial Fibrillation

GERALD F. DiBONA, M.D.

Professor and Vice Chairman, Department of Internal Medicine, University of Iowa College of Medicine; Staff Physician, University of Iowa Hospitals and Clinics; Chief, Medical Service, Veterans Administration Hospital, Iowa City, Iowa
Glomerular Disorders

ROBERT G. DLUHY, M.D.

Associate Professor of Medicine, Harvard Medical School; Senior Associate in Medicine, Peter Bent Brigham Hospital, Boston, Massachusetts
Pheochromocytoma

JERRY DOLOVICH, M.D., F.R.C.P.(C.)

Professor of Pediatrics, McMaster University; Active Staff, Department of Pediatrics, McMaster University Medical Center, Hamilton, Ontario, Canada
Allergic Rhinitis Due to Inhalant Factors

JAMES A. DONALDSON, M.D.

Professor of Otolaryngology, University of Washington School of Medicine; Attending Otolaryngologist, University of Washington–University Hospital, Harborview Medical Center, United States Public Health Service Hospital, Veterans Administration Hospital, Children's Orthopedic Hospital and Medical Center, Seattle, Washington
Acute Otitis Media

RICHARD JOSEPH DUMA, M.D., Ph.D.

Professor of Medicine, Microbiology, and Pathology, Medical College of Virginia, Virginia Commonwealth University; Chairman, Division of Infectious Diseases, Medical College of Virginia and McGuire Veterans Administration Hospitals, Richmond, Virginia
Rocky Mountain Spotted Fever

JARL E. DYRUD, M.D.

Professor of Psychiatry, University of Chicago; Attending Psychiatrist, University of Chicago Hospitals and Clinics, Chicago, Illinois
Schizophrenia

J. DONALD EASTON, M.D.

Professor and Chairman, Department of Neurology, University of Missouri–Columbia; Neurologist-in-Chief, University of Missouri Medical Center, Columbia, Missouri
Rehabilitation of the Patient with Hemiplegia

EDWARD R. EICHNER, M.D.

Professor of Medicine, University of Oklahoma School of Medicine; Attending Hematologist-Oncologist, University Hospital and Clinics, Veterans Administration Hospital, and The Presbyterian Hospital, Oklahoma City, Oklahoma
Anemia Due to Iron Deficiency

ERVIN EPSTEIN, M.D.

Associate Clinical Professor (Emeritus) of Dermatology, University of California, San Francisco, Medical School, San Francisco; Veterans Administration Hospital, Martinez, California; Peralta, Merritt, Providence and Children's Hospitals, Oakland, California
Keloids

CHARLES D. ERICSSON, M.D.

Assistant Professor of Medicine, University of Texas Medical School at Houston; Consultant in Infectious Diseases, University of Texas, Hermann Hospital, Houston, Texas
Rat-Bite Fever

EUGENE M. FARBER, M.D.

Professor and Chairman, Department of Dermatology, Stanford University School of Medicine; Physician-in-Chief, Department of Dermatology, Stanford University Medical Center, Palo Alto, California
Psoriasis

ZOHEIR FARID, M.D., D.T.M.&H.(ENGLAND)

Head, Clinical Tropical Medicine Department, United States Naval Medical Research Unit No. 3; Consultant Physician, Abbassia Fever Hospital, Ministry of Health, Cairo, Egypt
Amebiasis

MURRAY J. FAVUS, M.D.

Assistant Professor, University of Chicago, Pritzker School of Medicine; Attending Physician, Division of Endocrinology and Metabolism, Department of Medicine, Michael Reese Hospital and Medical Center, Chicago, Illinois
Renal Calculi

ALWYCE BETTY FISCHMANN, M.B., B.S., M.R.C.P.ED.

Assistant Professor of Medicine, Georgetown University School of Medicine; Chief, Dermatology Section, Veterans Administration Hospital, Washington, D.C.
Mycosis Fungoides and the Sezary Syndrome

ALEXANDER A. FISHER, M.D.

Clinical Professor, Department of Dermatology, New York University Post-Graduate Medical School; Associate Attending Physician in Dermatology, University Hospital, New York University Medical Center, New York, New York
Poison Ivy Dermatitis

MICHAEL FISHER, M.D.

Associate Professor of Medicine, Albert Einstein College of Medicine; Director, Dermatology Division, Bronx Municipal Hospital Center, Hospital of Albert Einstein College of Medicine, Bronx, New York
Herpes Gestationis; Papular Dermatitis of Pregnancy

EUGENE S. FLAMM, M.D.

Associate Professor of Neurosurgery, New York University School of Medicine; Associate Attending Physician in Neurosurgery, University Hospital (New York University Medical Center) and Bellevue Hospital; Attending Physician in Neurosurgery and Chief of Service, New York, New York
Intracerebral Hemorrhage

ROY FLEISCHMANN, M.D.

Clinical Instructor in Medicine, University of Texas Southwestern Medical School; Chief, Division of Rheumatology, St. Paul Hospital, Dallas, Texas
Rheumatoid Arthritis

ROSS D. FLETCHER, M.D.

Associate Professor of Medicine, Georgetown University Medical School; Chief of Cardiology, Veterans Administration Hospital, Washington, D.C.
Atrial Fibrillation

FREDERICK J. FLEURY, M.D.

Clinical Assistant Professor, Southern Illinois University School of Medicine, Springfield, Illinois
Ectopic Pregnancy

SANDRA C. FOOTE, M.D.

Fellow, National Institutes of Health, Bethesda, Maryland
Typhoid Fever

BOY FRAME, M.D.

Clinical Professor of Medicine, University of Michigan Medical School, Ann Arbor, Michigan; Physician in Charge, Henry Ford Hospital, Detroit, Michigan
Rickets and Osteomalacia

SAMUEL O. FREEDMAN, M.D.

Dean and Professor of Medicine, McGill University; Senior Physician, Division of Clinical Immunology and Allergy, Department of Medicine, Montreal General Hospital, Montreal, Quebec, Canada
Anaphylaxis and Serum Sickness

JOEL B. FREEMAN, M.D.

Associate Professor of Surgery, University of Ottowa School of Medicine; Head, Department of General Surgery, Ottowa General Hospital, Ottowa, Ontario, Canada
Thyroid Gland Malignancies

ARTHUR B. FRENCH, M.D.

Professor, Internal Medicine, University of Michigan Medical School; Staff, University Hospital; Consultant, Ann Arbor Veterans Administration Hospital, Ann Arbor, Michigan
Gastritis

EMANUEL A. FRIEDMAN, M.D., Sc.D.

Professor of Obstetrics and Gynecology, Harvard Medical School; Obstetrician–Gynecologist-in-Chief, Beth Israel Hospital, Boston, Massachusetts
Hemorrhage in Late Pregnancy

ALVIN E. FRIEDMAN-KIEN, M.D.

Associate Professor of Dermatology and Microbiology, New York University Medical Center; Attending Physician, University Hospital and Bellevue Hospital; Chief of Dermatology, Goldwater Memorial Hospital, New York, New York
Herpes Simplex

EDUARD G. FRIEDRICH, JR., M.D.

Associate Professor of Gynecology and Obstetrics, Medical College of Wisconsin; Staff Obstetrician-Gynecologist,

Milwaukee County Medical Complex, Milwaukee, Wisconsin
Vulvovaginitis

JAMES F. FRIES, M.D.

Associate Professor of Medicine, Stanford University School of Medicine, Palo Alto, California
Scleroderma

IRVING G. FROHMAN, M.D.

Emeritus Attending Physician, Associate Pathologist, Peninsula Hospital Center; Attending Physician, St. Johns Hospital, Far Rockaway, New York
Portuguese Man-of-War Stings

VINCENT A. FULGINITI, M.D.

Professor and Head, Department of Pediatrics, University of Arizona College of Medicine; Director, Clinical Pediatrics, University Hospital; Consultant, Tucson Medical Center, Kino Community Hospital, Davis Monthan Air Force Base Hospital, Tucson General Hospital, Tucson, Arizona
Active Immunization for Infectious Diseases

PAUL GABOS, M.D.

Clinical Assistant Professor, Obstetrics and Gynecology, University of Pittsburgh School of Medicine; Active Staff, West Penn Hospital and Magee Women's Hospital, Pittsburgh, Pennsylvania
Amenorrhea

RICHARD A. GAMS, M.D.

Professor of Medicine, University of Alabama School of Medicine; Attending Hematologist-Oncologist, University Hospital and Veterans Administration Hospital, Birmingham, Alabama
Non-Hodgkin Lymphoma

RICHARD C. GIBBS, M.D.

Clinical Professor of Dermatology, New York University Medical Center; Attending Physician in Dermatology, University Hospital and Bellevue Hospital Center, New York, New York
Warts

DONALD H. GILDEN, M.D.

Associate Professor of Neurology, University of Pennsylvania School of Medicine, Philadelphia, Pennsylvania
Viral Meningoencephalitis

BRUCE C. GILLILAND, M.D.

Professor, Medicine and Laboratory Medicine, University of Washington; Medical Director, Providence Medical Center, Seattle, Washington
Hemolytic Anemia—Immune

ALLAN GOLDBLATT, M.D.

Associate Professor of Pediatrics, Harvard Medical School; Chief, Pediatric Cardiology, Massachusetts General Hospital, Boston, Massachusetts
Rheumatic Fever

FRANZ GOLDSTEIN, M.D.

Professor of Medicine, Jefferson Medical College, Thomas Jefferson University; Chief, Division of Gastroenterology, Lankenau Hospital, Philadelphia, Pennsylvania
Constipation

NORMAN D. GRACE, M.D.

Associate Clinical Professor of Medicine, Tufts University School of Medicine; Chief of Gastroenterology, Faulkner Hospital and Lemuel Shattuck Hospital, Boston, Massachusetts
Cirrhosis

J. ANDREW GRANT, M.D.

Associate Professor of Internal Medicine and Human Biological Chemistry and Genetics, University of Texas Medical Branch; Attending Physician, University of Texas Medical Branch Hospitals, Galveston, Texas
Allergic Reactions to Insect Stings

JOSEPH GREENBAUM, M.D., F.R.C.P.(C.)

Assistant Clinical Professor of Medicine, McMaster University; Active Staff, St. Joseph's Hospital, Hamilton, Ontario, Canada
Allergic Rhinitis Due to Inhalant Factors

DAVID G. GREENE, M.D.

Professor of Medicine, Associate Professor of Physiology, Medical School of the State University of New York at Buffalo; Attending Physician, Buffalo General Hospital; Consultant in Cardiology, Veterans Administration Hospital, Buffalo, New York
Tachycardia

KENNETH E. GREER, M.D.

Associate Professor of Dermatology, University of Virginia School of Medicine, Charlottesville, Virginia
Dermatomyositis-Polymyositis

JOHN P. GRIFFIN, M.D., F.A.C.P., F.C.C.P.

Clinical Professor of Pulmonary Medicine, University of Tennessee Center for Health Sciences; Chief, Pulmonary Disease Section, Veterans Administration Hospital; Staff, Pulmonary Medicine, Baptist Memorial Hospital, Memphis, Tennessee
Viral and Mycoplasmal Pneumonias

W. LEROY GRIFFING, M.D.

Trainee in Rheumatology, Mayo Medical School, Mayo Foundation, Mayo Clinic, Rochester, Minnesota
Polyarteritis

WILLIAM J. GRIFFITHS, M.D., Ph.D.

Assistant Professor, Department of Medicine, The University of Oklahoma College of Medicine, Oklahoma City, Oklahoma
Peptic Ulcer

THOMAS R. GRIGGS, M.D.

Assistant Professor of Medicine and Pathology, University of North Carolina School of Medicine; Director, Coronary Care Unit, North Carolina Memorial Hospital, Chapel Hill, North Carolina
Acute Myocardial Infarction

ROLF M. GUNNAR, M.D.

Professor of Medicine, Chief, Section of Cardiology, Loyola University Stritch School of Medicine, Maywood, Illinois
Heart Block

W. DAVID HAGER, M.D.

Clinical Instructor, Department of Obstetrics and Gynecology, University of Kentucky School of Medicine; University of Kentucky Medical Center, Central Baptist Hospital, Lexington, Kentucky
Gonorrhea

JAMES A. HALL, M.D.

Assistant Professor, Obstetrics and Gynecology, Indiana University School of Medicine, Indianapolis, Indiana; Memorial Hospital, Logansport, Indiana
Preoperative and Postoperative Care for Elective Gynecologic Surgery

THOMAS C. HALL, M.D.

Clinical Professor of Medicine, University of California, Irvine, California; Attending Internist, Huntington Memorial Hospital and St. Luke's Hospital, Pasadena, California; Hollywood Presbyterian Hospital, Los Angeles, California
The Chronic Leukemias

PAUL E. HAMMERSCHLAG, M.D.

Assistant Professor of Otolaryngology, University of Washington School of Medicine; Attending Otolaryngologist, University of Washington–University Hospital, Harborview Medical Center, United States Public Health Service Hospital, Veterans Administration Hospital, Children's Orthopedic Hospital and Medical Center, Seattle, Washington
Acute Otitis Media

BRUCE H. HAMORY, M.D.

Assistant Professor of Internal Medicine, University of Missouri School of Medicine–Columbia; Attending Physician, University of Missouri Medical Center and Harry S. Truman Memorial Veterans Administration Hospital, Columbia, Missouri
Typhus Fever

JAMES BARRY HANSHAW, M.D.

Professor and Chairman, Department of Pediatrics, University of Massachusetts School of Medicine; Pediatrician-in-Chief, University of Massachusetts Medical Center, and St. Vincent Hospital, Worcester, Massachusetts
Measles

JOSEPH HARASZTI, M.D.

Consultant in Psychiatry, University of Chicago; Attending Psychiatrist, University of Chicago Hospitals and Clinics, Chicago, Illinois
Schizophrenia

F. E. HARGREAVE, M.D.

Associate Professor of Medicine, McMaster University; Active Staff, Department of Medicine, St. Joseph's Hospital, Hamilton, Ontario, Canada
Allergic Rhinitis Due to Inhalant Factors

H. SUMMERS HARRISON, M.D.

Clinical Professor of Pediatrics, West Virginia University School of Medicine; Monongalia General Hospital, Morgantown, West Virginia
Normal Infant Feeding

GAVIN HART, M.D.

Senior Medical Officer, Community and Child Health Services, Public Health Service, West Perth, Australia
Donovanosis; Lymphogranuloma Venereum

IAN RITCHIE HART, M.B., Ch.B., M.Sc., F.R.C.P.(C.), F.A.C.P.

Associate Professor of Internal Medicine, University of Ottawa; Attending Physician, Ottawa Civic Hospital; Consulting Physician, Children's Hospital of Eastern Ontario, Ottawa, Ontario, Canada
Thyroiditis

WILLIAM K. HASS, M.D.

Professor of Neurology, New York University School of Medicine; Associate Director, Neurology Service, Bellevue Hospital, New York, New York
Acute Ischemic Cerebrovascular Disease

ROBERT C. HASTINGS, M.D., Ph.D.

Adjunct Associate Professor of Pharmacology, Clinical Associate, Professor of Internal Medicine, Tulane University School of Medicine, New Orleans, Louisiana; Chief, Pharmacology Research Department, United States Public Health Service Hospital, Carville, Louisiana
Leprosy

DAVID MILLER HAWKINS, M.D.

Associate Professor of Psychiatry, Duke University School of Medicine, Durham, North Carolina
Psychoneurosis

RALPH E. HAYNES, M.D.

Professor and Vice Chairman, Wright State University School of Medicine; Director of Infectious Diseases, The Children's Medical Center, Columbus, Ohio
Mumps (Epidemic Parotitis)

CARL E. HELTNE, M.D.

Fellow, Division of Cardiology, West Virginia University School of Medicine, Morgantown, West Virginia
Congestive Heart Failure

VICTOR HERBERT, M.D., J.D.

Professor of Medicine, State University of New York Downstate Medical Center, Brooklyn, New York; Chief, Hematology and Nutrition Laboratory, Bronx Veterans Administration Hospital, Bronx, New York
Scurvy

ALFRED D. HERNANDEZ, M.D.

Assistant Professor of Medicine, Division of Dermatology, University of Maryland School of Medicine; Research Scientist, National Institutes of Health, National Institute of Allergy and Infectious Disease, Laboratory of Clinical Investigation, Bethesda, Maryland
Bacterial Infections of the Skin

CHRISTIAN HERRMANN, JR., M.D.

Professor, University of California at Los Angeles; Attending Neurologist, University of California Hospitals, Los Angeles, California
Myasthenia Gravis

JEANE PORTER HESTER, M.D.

Assistant Professor of Medicine, Associate Internist, Chief, Supportive Therapy, The University of Texas System Cancer Center, M. D. Anderson Hospital and Tumor Institute, Department of Developmental Therapeutics; Assistant Professor of Medicine, Associate Internist, Chief, Supportive Therapy, M. D. Anderson Hospital and Tumor Institute; Assistant Professor of Medicine, Division of Hematology, Department of Medicine, University of Texas Medical School, Houston, Texas
Bleeding Disorders Secondary to Platelet Abnormalities

CRAIG G. HINMAN, M.D.

Major, U.S.A.F., M.C., Chief Resident, Division of Urologic Surgery, Duke University Medical Center, Durham, North Carolina
Prostatitis

DANIEL ROBERT HINTHORN, M.D.

Associate Professor of Medicine, University of Kansas Medical Center, Kansas City, Kansas
Relapsing Fever

AXEL W. HOKE, M.D.

Associate Clinical Professor of Dermatology, University of California, San Francisco, School of Medicine; Chief of Dermatology Section, United States Public Health Service Hospital, San Francisco, California
Chancroid

EDWARD W. HOLMES, JR., M.D.

Associate Professor of Medicine, Division of Rheumatic and Genetic Diseases, Duke University Medical School, Durham, North Carolina
Gout

DAVID HOOVER, M.D.

Instructor in Medicine, Division of Infectious Diseases, West Virginia University Medical Center, Morgantown, West Virginia
Tularemia

GILBERT HORTON MUDGE, JR., M.D.

Instructor, Harvard Medical School; Associate in Medicine, Peter Bent Brigham Hospital, Boston, Massachusetts
Angina Pectoris

GENE G. HUNDER, M.D.

Professor of Medicine, Mayo Medical School, Mayo Foundation, Mayo Clinic, Rochester, Minnesota
Polyarteritis

DONALD B. HUNNINGHAKE, M.D.

Associate Professor of Medicine and Pharmacology, University of Minnesota, Minneapolis, Minnesota
Xanthoma

ALA E. IMAM, M.D.

Assistant Professor, St. Louis University School of Medicine, St. Louis, Missouri
Acute and Chronic Viral Hepatitis

HAROLD L. ISRAEL, M.D.

Professor of Medicine, Jefferson Medical College, Thomas Jefferson University, Philadelphia, Pennsylvania
Pulmonary Embolism

NORMAN F. JACOBS, JR., M.D.

Clinical Assistant Professor of Medicine, Department of Internal Medicine, Division of Infectious Diseases; Attending Physician, Grady Memorial Hospital and DeKalb General Hospital, Atlanta, Georgia
Gonorrhea

PAUL JOHN JAKUBEC, M.D.

Associate Clinical Professor of Pediatrics, West Virginia University School of Medicine; Monongalia General Hospital, Morgantown, West Virginia
Normal Infant Feeding

C. CONRAD JOHNSTON, JR., M.D.

Professor of Medicine, Director, Division of Endocrinology and Metabolism, Indiana University School of Medicine, Indianapolis, Indiana
Osteoporosis

RALPH E. JOHNSON, M.D.

Director, Gulfcoast Oncology Center, and Director, Department of Radiation Oncology, Bayfront Medical Center, St. Petersburg, Florida
Hodgkin's Disease: Radiation Therapy

HENRY W. JOLLY, JR., M.D.

Professor and Head, Department of Dermatology, Louisiana State University School of Medicine; Senior Visiting Physician, Charity Hospital of Louisiana, New Orleans; Active Staff, Our Lady of the Lake Hospital, Baton Rouge; Consulting Staff, Baton Rouge General Hospital; Staff, Earl K. Long Memorial Hospital, Woman's Hospital and Doctors Memorial Hospital, Baton Rouge, Louisiana
Pruritus Ani and Vulvae

PHILIP C. JOLLY, M.D.

Assistant Professor, University of Washington School of Medicine; Surgeon, The Mason Clinic, Seattle, Washington
Intestinal Obstruction

THOMAS C. JONES, M.D.

Associate Professor of Medicine and Public Health, Cornell University Medical College; Associate Attending Physician, The New York Hospital, New York, New York
Toxoplasmosis

LAWRENCE J. KAGEN, M.D.

Associate Professor of Medicine, Cornell University Medical College; Associate Attending Physician, Hospital for Special Surgery and The New York Hospital, New York, New York
Osteoarthritis

HAROLD S. KAPLAN, M.D.

Associate Professor of Pathology, New York University Medical Center; Director, Blood Bank, University Hospital, New York University Medical Center, New York, New York
Untoward Reactions to Blood Transfusions

DARWIN KARYADI, M.D., Ph.D.

Director, Nutrition Research and Development Center, Ministry of Health, Bogor, Indonesia
Hypo- and Hypervitaminosis A

J. E. KASIK, M.D., Ph.D.

Professor of Internal Medicine, University of Iowa College of Medicine; Attending Physician, University Hospital and Veterans Administration Hospital, Iowa City, Iowa
Tuberculosis and Other Mycobacterial Diseases

JOHN S. KAUFMANN, M.D., Ph.D.

Associate Professor of Medicine and Pharmacology, Bowman Gray School of Medicine of Wake Forest University; North Carolina Baptist Hospital, Winston-Salem, North Carolina
Malignant Carcinoid Syndrome

A. PAUL KELLY, M.D.

Associate Professor of Medicine (Dermatology and Syphilogy), Charles R. Drew Postgraduate Medical School; Staff Physician and Chief, Division of Dermatology, Los Angeles County–Martin Luther King, Jr. General Hospital, Los Angeles, California
Pseudofolliculitis Barbae

ROBERT C. KELSCH, M.D.

Professor of Pediatric Nephrology, University of Michigan School of Medicine; Chief, Section of Pediatric Nephrology, University of Michigan Medical Center, University Hospitals, Ann Arbor, Michigan
Parenteral Fluid Therapy in Children

STEVEN C. KELSON, M.D.

Assistant Professor of Medicine, Case Western Reserve University; Staff, Veterans Administration Hospital and University Hospital, Cleveland, Ohio
Chronic Bronchitis and Emphysema

RAYMOND N. KJELLBERG, M.D.

Associate Clinical Professor of Surgery, Harvard Medical School; Visiting Neurosurgeon, Massachusetts General Hospital, Boston, Massachusetts
Acromegaly

CARL M. KJELLSTRAND, M.D.

Professor of Medicine and Surgery, University of Minnesota Medical School; Chief, Division of Nephrology, University Hospital, Minneapolis, Minnesota
Acute Renal Failure

HAROLD L. KLAWANS, M.D.

Associate Chairman, Department of Neurological Sciences, Rush-Presbyterian-St. Luke's Medical Center, Chicago, Illinois
Parkinson's Disease

MICHAEL KLEEREKOPER, M.D.

Assistant Clinical Professor of Medicine, University of Michigan Medical School, Ann Arbor, Michigan; Staff Physician, Henry Ford Hospital, Detroit, Michigan
Rickets and Osteomalacia

RICHARD J. KLEIN, M.D., D.Sc.

Research Associate Professor, Department of Microbiology, New York University School of Medicine, New York, New York
Herpes Simplex

BERNARD KLIMAN, M.D.

Associate Professor of Medicine, Harvard Medical School, at the Massachusetts General Hospital; Associate Physician, Massachusetts General Hospital, Boston, Massachusetts
Acromegaly

WILLIAM A. KNIGHT, JR., M.D.

Associate Professor of Medicine and Director, Division of Gastroenterology, St. Louis University School of Medicine; Director, Department of Internal Medicine, Saint Mary's Health Center, St. Louis, Missouri
Acute and Chronic Viral Hepatitis

STEVE T. KOEFF, M.D.

Associate Professor of Pediatrics, University of Michigan School of Medicine; Associate Director of Pediatrics and Director, Newborn Nursery, Wayne County General Hospital, Eloise, Michigan; University of Michigan Medical Center, University Hospitals, Ann Arbor, Michigan
Parenteral Fluid Therapy in Children

WARREN WOODSON KOONTZ, JR., M.D.

Professor and Chairman, Division of Urology, Medical College of Virginia, Richmond, Virginia
Bacterial Infections of the Urinary Tract (Male)

BURTON I. KORELITZ, M.D.

Chief, Section of Gastroenterology, Lenox Hill Hospital, New York, New York
Ulcerative Colitis

LAWRENCE R. KRAKOFF, M.D.

Associate Professor of Medicine, Chief, Hypertension Division, Mount Sinai School of Medicine, New York, New York; Consultant Physician, The Bronx Veterans Hospital, Bronx, New York
Hypertension

GUY L. KRATZER, M.D., M.S.

Clinical Professor of Surgery, Hershey Medical Center, Pennsylvania State University; Chief, Division of Colon and Rectal Surgery, Sacred Heart Hospital, and Director, Residency Program, Allentown and Sacred Heart Hospitals, Allentown, Pennsylvania
Hemorrhoids, Anal Fissure, and Anal Fistula

STEPHEN J. KRAUS, M.D.

Clinical Research Investigator, Venereal Disease Control Division, Center for Disease Control, Atlanta, Georgia
Gonorrhea

LARRY E. KUN, M.D.

Assistant Professor of Radiology, Medical College of Wisconsin; Milwaukee County Medical Complex and Milwaukee Children's Hospital, Milwaukee, Wisconsin
Brain Tumors

AHMED C. KUTTY, M.D., F.R.C.P.(C.)

Associate Professor of Medicine, University of Pennsylvania; Attending Cardiologist, Graduate Hospital, Philadelphia, Pennsylvania
Cardiac Arrest

ROBERT A. KYLE, M.D. (M.S. IN MEDICINE)

Professor of Medicine, Mayo Medical School; Consultant, Division of Hematology and Internal Medicine, Mayo Clinic and Mayo Foundation, Rochester, Minnesota
Multiple Myeloma

JOHN C. LAIDLAW, M.A., M.D., PH.D., F.R.C.P.(C.), F.R.S.C.

Professor and Chairman, Department of Medicine, Faculty of Health Sciences, McMaster University; Head, Section of Medicine, McMaster University Medical Center, Hamilton, Ontario, Canada
Adrenocortical Insufficiency

VERNE C. LANIER, JR., M.D.

Clinical Associate Professor of Plastic Surgery, Duke University Medical Center; Attending Plastic Surgeon, Durham Veterans Hospital, Durham, North Carolina
Disorders of the Mouth (Malignant)

P. G. LANKISCH, M.D.

University of Göttingen, Göttingen, Federal Republic of Germany
Acute Pancreatitis

THEODORE HENRY LEHMAN, M.D.

Associate Clinical Professor of Urology, University of Oregon; Emanuel Hospital, Holliday Park Hospital, Good Samaritan Hospital, Meridian Park Hospital, Portland, Oregon
Benign Prostatic Hyperplasia

MARGUERITE RUSH LERNER, M.D.

Professor of Dermatology, Yale University School of Medicine; Yale–New Haven Hospital, New Haven, Connecticut
Pigmentary Disturbances

NORMAN E. LEVAN, M.D.

Professor of Medicine, University of Southern California School of Medicine; Chairman, Dermatology Section, Los Angeles County–University of Southern California Medical Center, Los Angeles, California
Sarcoidosis

JOE U. LEVI, M.D.

Associate Professor of Surgery, University of Miami School of Medicine; Staff Surgeon, Jackson Memorial Hospital; Attending Surgeon, Veterans Administration Hospital, Miami, Florida
Bleeding Esophageal Varices

MYRON M. LEVINE, M.D., D.T.P.H.

Associate Professor, Infectious Diseases, Associate Professor, Preventive Medicine, University of Maryland School of Medicine; Attending Physician, University of Maryland Hospital, Baltimore, Maryland
Bacillary Dysentery

PETER H. LEVINE, M.D.

Professor of Medicine, University of Massachusetts Medical School; Chief of Medicine and Director, New England Area Hemophilia Center, The Memorial Hospital, Worcester, Massachusetts
Hemophilia and Allied Conditions

CHIEN LIU, M.D.

Professor of Medicine and of Pediatrics, University of Kansas Medical Center, Kansas City, Kansas
Relapsing Fever

VIRGIL LOEB, JR., M.D.

Professor of Clinical Medicine, Washington University School of Medicine; Physician and Consultant in Hematology/Oncology, Barnes Hospital, Jewish Hospital, St. Luke's Hospital, St. John's Hospital, St. Anthony's Hospital, Lutheran Hospital, Compton Hill Medical Center, Veterans Administration Hospitals, St. Louis, Missouri
Bone Marrow Failure

JERE W. LORD, JR., M.D.

Professor of Clinical Surgery, New York University School of Medicine; Chief, Vascular Surgery, Cabrini Health Care Center, New York, New York
Primary Varicose Veins

HENRY C. MAGUIRE, JR., M.D.

Professor of Medicine (Dermatology), Hahnemann Medical College; Attending Dermatologist, Hahnemann Hospital, Philadelphia, Pennsylvania
Alopecia

DILIP MAHALANABIS, M.B.B.S., M.R.C.P.

Chief of Pediatric Gastroenterology, Kothari Centre of Gastroenterology and Consultant Physician (Pediatrics), Calcutta Hospital and Medical Research Institute, Calcutta, India
Cholera

CHARLES S. MAHAN, M.D.

Associate Professor of Obstetrics-Gynecology, University of Florida College of Medicine; Director, Division of Ambulatory Services for Women, Shands Teaching Hospital, Gainesville, Florida
Antepartum Care

BARRY MAKE, M.D.

Assistant Professor, Boston University School of Medicine; Director, Clinical Services, Pulmonary Section, Director, Medical Intensive Care Unit, Boston City Hospital, Boston, Massachusetts
Acute Respiratory Failure

GERALD L. MANDELL, M.D.

Professor of Medicine, Director, Division of Infectious Disease, University of Virginia School of Medicine, Charlottesville, Virginia
Typhoid Fever

GEORGE O. MANN, Sc.D., M.D.

Associate Professor of Biochemistry and Medicine, Vanderbilt University School of Medicine, Nashville, Tennessee
Obesity

I. N. MARKS, B.Sc., M.B., F.R.C.P.Ed., F.A.C.G.

Head of Gastroenterology, Groote Schuur Hospital; Senior Lecturer in Department of Medicine, University of Cape Town, Cape Town, Republic of South Africa
Chronic Pancreatitis

PHILIP D. MARSDEN, M.D.

Professor of Medicine, University of Brasilia; Consultant Physician, Sobradinho Hospital D.F., Brasilia, Brazil
Trichinellosis (Trichinosis)

ORLANDO J. MARTELO, M.D.

Professor of Medicine and Director, Hematology-Oncology Division, University of Cincinnati College of Medicine; Attending Physician, C. R. Holmes Hospital, Cincinnati General Hospital; Consultant, Hematology-Oncology, The Jewish Hospital, Veterans Administration Hospital, Cincinnati, Ohio
Hemolytic Anemia—Nonimmune

MANUEL MARTINEZ-MALDONADO, M.D.

Professor of Medicine and Physiology, University of Puerto Rico School of Medicine; Chief, Medical Service, Veterans Administration Hospital, San Juan, Puerto Rico
Parenteral Nutrition in Adults

DENIS G. McDEVITT, D.Sc., M.D., F.R.C.P., F.R.C.P.I.

Professor of Clinical Pharmacology, The Queen's University of Belfast; Consultant Physician, Belfast City Hospital and Royal Victoria Hospital, Belfast, Northern Ireland
Brucellosis

HENRY C. McDUFF, JR., M.D.

Associate Clinical Professor, Obstetrics and Gynecology, Tufts University Medical School, Brown University Program in Medicine; Chief Emeritus, Department of Gynecology, Rhode Island Hospital; Consultant, Gynecology, Women and Infants Hospital of Rhode Island, Providence, Rhode Island
Uterine Cancer

J. MAXWELL McKENZIE, M.D.

Professor of Medicine, McGill University; Director, Division of Endocrinology and Metabolism, Royal Victoria Hospital, Montreal, Quebec, Canada
Hyperthyroidism

DAN G. McNAMARA, M.D.

Professor of Pediatrics, Baylor College of Medicine; Chief, The Lillie Frank Abercrombie Section of Cardiology, Texas Children's Hospital, Houston, Texas
Congenital Heart Disease

PHILIP B. MEAD, M.D.

Associate Professor of Obstetrics and Gynecology, University of Vermont College of Medicine; Attending Obstetrician and Gynecologist, Medical Center Hospital of Vermont, Burlington, Vermont
Pelvic Inflammatory Disease

EDWIN M. MEARES, JR., M.D.

Whitney Professor of Urology, Chairman, Division of Urology, Tufts University School of Medicine; Chairman, Department of Urology, New England Medical Center Hospital, Boston, Massachusetts
Bacterial Infections of the Urinary Tract (Female)

CLAUDE E. MERRIN, M.D.

Chief, Department of Urologic Oncology, Roswell Park Memorial Institute, Buffalo, New York
Tumors of the Genitourinary Tract

JACK METZ, M.D., F.R.C.(PATH.)

Honorary Professor of Clinical Pathology, Chairman of The School of Pathology, University of the Witwatersrand; Director, The South African Institute for Medical Research, Johannesburg, South Africa
Pernicious Anemia and Other Forms of Vitamin B_{12} Deficiency

GLENN A. MEYER, M.D.

Associate Professor of Neurosurgery, The Medical College of Wisconsin, Milwaukee; Staff Neurosurgeon, Milwaukee County General Hospital, Milwaukee; Neurosurgical Consultant, Wood Veterans Administration Hospital; Associate Staff, Milwaukee Children's Hospital, Milwaukee; Associate Staff, Elmbrook Memorial Hospital, Brookfield; and Neurosurgical Consultant, Community Memorial Hospital, Menomonee Falls, Wisconsin
Brain Tumors

RICHARD D. MEYER, M.D.

Assistant Professor of Medicine, University of California, Los Angeles, School of Medicine; Assistant Chief, Infectious Disease Section, Wadsworth Veterans Administration Hospital; Assistant Visiting Internist, University of California, Los Angeles, Center for the Health Sciences, Los Angeles, California
Bacteremia

WILLIAM OBED MILLER, M.D.

Clinical Instructor, University of Tennessee Memorial and Research Hospital, University of Tennessee; St. Mary's Memorial Hospital, Memphis, Tennessee
Urethral Strictures

WILLIAM V. MILLER, M.D.

Director, Missouri-Illinois Regional Red Cross Blood Program; Associate Pathologist, Burnes Hospital and St. Louis University Hospitals, St. Louis, Missouri
Therapeutic Use of Blood Components

LARRY E. MILLIKAN, M.D.

Associate Professor, University of Missouri School of Medicine, Columbia, Missouri
Diseases of the Nails

DANIEL R. MISHELL, JR., M.D.

Professor and Chairman, Department of Obstetrics and Gynecology, University of Southern California School of Medicine; Women's Hospital, Los Angeles County–University of Southern California Medical Center, Los Angeles, California
Abortion

ROBERT C. MOELLERING, JR., M.D.

Associate Professor of Medicine, Harvard Medical School; Associate Physician, Consultant in Bacteriology, Massachusetts General Hospital, Boston, Massachusetts
Salmonellosis (Other than Typhoid Fever)

LEE S. MONROE, M.D.

Clinical Professor of Medicine, University of California, San Diego; Senior Consultant, Gastroenterology, Scripps Clinic, San Diego, California
Intestinal Parasites

JOHN F. MORAN, M.D.

Associate Professor of Medicine, Section of Cardiology, Loyola University Stritch School of Medicine, Maywood, Illinois
Heart Block

HUGO D. MONTENEGRO, M.D.

Assistant Professor of Medicine, Case Western Reserve University, Veterans Administration and University Hospitals, Cleveland, Ohio
Chronic Bronchitis and Emphysema

DAVID Z. MORGAN, M.D.

Professor of Internal Medicine, West Virginia University School of Medicine, Morgantown, West Virginia
Congestive Heart Failure

JILL H. MARRISS, M.D.

Assistant Professor of Pediatrics, Baylor College of Medicine; Associate in Pediatric Cardiology, Texas Children's Hospital, Houston, Texas
Congenital Heart Disease

ARTHUR J. MOSS, M.D.

Clinical Associate Professor of Medicine, University of Rochester School of Medicine and Dentistry; Senior

Associate Physician, Strong Memorial Hospital, Rochester, New York
Premature Beats

STEVEN R. MOSTOW, M.D.

Associate Professor of Medicine, University of Colorado School of Medicine; Chief, Infectious Diseases, Denver Veterans Administration Hospital, Denver, Colorado
Epidemic Influenza

HAROLD G. MUCHMORE, M.D.

Carl Puckett Professor of Pulmonary Diseases, University of Oklahoma College of Medicine; Chief of Tuberculosis Section, Veterans Administration Hospital; Staff Physician, University Hospital and Clinics, Oklahoma City, Oklahoma
Histoplasmosis

LUIZ NASCIMENTO, M.D.

Assistant Professor of Medicine, University of Puerto Rico School of Medicine; Associate Investigator, Veterans Administration Hospital, San Juan, Puerto Rico
Parenteral Nutrition in Adults

HAROLD S. NELSON, M.D.

Associate Clinical Professor of Medicine (Immunology), University of Colorado Medical Center; Chief, Allergy-Immunology Service, Fitzsimons Army Medical Center, Denver, Colorado
Adverse Reactions to Drugs: Hypersensitivity

RALPH A. NELSON, M.D.

Instructor, Department of Otolaryngology, University of Southern California; Attending Otologist, St. Vincent's Medical Center, and the Ear Research Institute of Los Angeles, Los Angeles, California
Meniere's Disease

ROBERT S. NELSON, M.D.

Professor of Medicine, University of Texas, M. D. Anderson Hospital and Tumor Institute, Gastroenterology Service, Medicine Department; Internist, Medicine Department, Gastroenterology Service, M. D. Anderson Hospital and Tumor Institute, University of Texas at Houston, Houston, Texas
Tumors of the Colon and Rectum

JAMES C. NIEDERMAN, M.D.

Clinical Professor of Epidemiology and Medicine, Yale University School of Medicine; Staff Member, Department of Medicine, Yale–New Haven Medical Center, New Haven, Connecticut
Infectious Mononucleosis

H. JUERGEN NORD, M.D.

Associate Professor of Medicine, University of South Florida College of Medicine; Chief, U.S.F. Gastroenterology Service, Tampa General Hospital; Attending Physician, Veterans Administration Hospital, Tampa, Florida
Dysphagia and Esophageal Obstruction

WILLIAM J. OLIVER, M.D.

Professor, University of Michigan School of Medicine; Chairman, Department of Pediatrics, University of Michigan Medical Center, University Hospitals, Ann Arbor, Michigan
Parenteral Fluid Therapy in Children

THOMAS N. PAIGE, M.D.

Clinical Instructor in Dermatology, University of California, San Francisco Medical School; Attending Dermatologist, University of San Francisco Hospital, San Francisco, California, and Kaiser Foundation Hospital, Walnut Creek, California
Pediculosis

LOUIS N. PANGARO, M.D.

Instructor in Medicine, Fellow, Division of Endocrinology, Georgetown University School of Medicine and The University Hospital, Washington, D.C.
Cushing's Syndrome

JOHN A. PARRISH, M.D.

Associate Professor of Dermatology, Harvard Medical School; Assistant Dermatologist, Massachusetts General Hospital, Boston, Massachusetts
Photosensitivity and Sunburn

BRUCE C. PATON, M.D.

Professor of Surgery, University of Colorado School of Medicine; Attending Staff, Colorado General Hospital, Denver Veterans Administration Hospital, Denver General Hospital, Denver Children's Hospital (Courtesy), Fitzsimons Army Hospital (Consultant), Denver, Colorado
Disturbances Due to Cold

DAVID F. PAULSON, M.D., F.A.C.S.

Associate Professor of Urologic Surgery, Director of Urologic Research, Duke University Medical Center, Durham, North Carolina
Prostatitis

DONALD L. PAULSON, M.D.

Clinical Professor, University of Texas Health Science Center; Attending Thoracic Surgeon, Baylor University Medical Center, Houston, Texas; Senior Consulting Thoracic Surgeon, Parkland Memorial Hospital, Dallas, Texas
Primary Lung Cancer

DAVID E. PAYNE, M.D.

Instructor, University of Missouri School of Medicine; Staff, Boone County and Columbia Regional Hospitals, Columbia, Missouri
Contact Dermatitis

RICHARD M. PETERS, M.D.

Professor of Surgery and Bioengineering, University of California Medical Center, San Diego; Co-Head, Division of Cardio-Thoracic Surgery, University Hospital, San Diego, California
Atelectasis

JOHN C. PETERSON, M.D.

Professor of Pediatrics Emeritus, Medical College of Wisconsin; Attending Pediatrician, Milwaukee Children's Hospital, Milwaukee, Wisconsin
Whooping Cough (Pertussis)

JONATHAN H. PINCUS, M.D.

Professor of Neurology, Yale University School of Medicine; Attending Physician, Yale–New Haven Hospital; Consultant in Neurology, West Haven Veterans Administration Hospital; Yale University Health Service, New Haven, Connecticut
Epilepsy in Adolescents and Adults

HIRAM C. POLK, JR., M.D.

Professor and Chairman, Department of Surgery, University of Louisville School of Medicine; Consultant Staff, Jewish Hospital, Norton-Children's Hospital, Louisville General Hospital, Veterans Administration Hospital; Courtesy Staff, St. Anthony Hospital and St. Joseph Infirmary, Louisville, Kentucky
Gas Gangrene and Similar Soft Tissue Anaerobic Infections

PAUL S. PORTER, M.D.

Assistant Professor of Dermatology, University of Pittsburgh School of Medicine, Pittsburgh, Pennsylvania
Atopic Dermatitis

SURAWUT PRICHANOND, M.D.

Formerly Fellow, Section of Rheumatology, Department of Medicine, Abraham Lincoln School of Medicine, University of Illinois; Attending Rheumatologist, Mennonite Hospital, Bloomington, Illinois
Ankylosing Spondylitis

RICHARD DAVID PROPPER, M.D.

Instructor in Pediatrics, Harvard Medical School; Assistant in Medicine, Children's Hospital Medical Center; Senior Clinical Associate, Sidney Farber Cancer Institute, Boston, Massachusetts
Thalassemia

MEL PROSEN, M.D.

Associate Professor, Director of Psychiatric Education, Rush Medical College; Rush-Presbyterian-St. Luke's Medical Center, Michael Reese Hospital, Chicago, Illinois
Affective Disorders

E. J. QUILLIGAN, M.D.

Professor of Obstetrics and Gynecology, University of Southern California; Los Angeles County–University of Southern California Medical Center, Los Angeles, California
Toxemia of Pregnancy

JAMES M. RABB, M.D.

Fellow in Gastroenterology, University of Chicago Hospitals and Clinics; Director, Nutrition Support Unit, University of Chicago Hospitals and Clinics, Chicago, Illinois
The Malabsorption Syndrome

MARTIN FRANCIS RANDOLPH, M.D.

Assistant Clinical Professor, University of Connecticut; Yale Medical Center, University of Connecticut Health Center, Danbury Hospital, Danbury, Connecticut
Streptococcal Pharyngitis

JAMES E. RASMUSSEN, M.D.

Associate Professor of Dermatology and Pediatrics, Department of Dermatology, State University of New York at Buffalo; Dermatologist, The Children's Hospital of Buffalo, E. J. Meyer Memorial Hospital, The Buffalo General Hospital, Deaconess Hospital and the Veterans Administration Hospital, Buffalo, New York
Inflammatory Eruptions of the Hands and Feet

JOHN R. RAYE, M.D.

Associate Professor of Pediatrics, The University of Connecticut School of Medicine; Director, Division of Neonatology, John Dempsey Hospital, Farmington, Connecticut
Resuscitation of the Newborn

JAMES C. REED, M.D.

Dermatologist, Elkhart Clinic, Elkhart, Indiana
Urticaria and Angioedema

L. BARTH RELLER, M.D.

Associate Professor of Medicine, University of Colorado School of Medicine; Attending Physician, Colorado General, Veterans Administration, and Denver General Hospitals, Denver, Colorado
Psittacosis

MARGARET B. RENNELS, M.D.

Fellow in Infectious Diseases, University of Maryland School of Medicine; University of Maryland Hospital, Baltimore, Maryland
Bacillary Dysentery

FRANK SCORGIE RHAME, M.D.

Clinical Assistant Professor, Division of Infectious Diseases, Department of Medicine, Stanford University School of Medicine; Staff Physician, Spinal Cord Injury Service, Palo Alto Veterans Administration Hospital, Palo Alto, California
Q Fever

EDWIN S. ROBBINS, M.D.

Clinical Professor, New York University Medical Center; Assistant Director, Department of Psychiatry, Bellvue Medical Center; Attending Psychiatrist, University, Bellvue, and Cabrini Hospitals, New York, New York
Delerium

GRANT V. RODKEY, M.D.

Associate Clinical Professor of Surgery, Harvard Medical School; Visiting Surgeon, Massachusetts General Hospital, Boston, Massachusetts
Diverticula of the Alimentary Canal

HENRY H. ROENIGK, JR., M.D.

Professor and Chairman, Department of Dermatology, Northwestern University; Chairman of Dermatology, Northwestern Memorial Hospitals, Chicago, Illinois
Stasis Dermatitis and Stasis Ulcers

ARVEY I. ROGERS, M.D.

Professor of Medicine, University of Miami School of Medicine; Chief, Gastroenterology Section, Staff Physician, Veterans Administration Hospital; Co-Director, Gastroenterology Division, University of Miami; Attending Physician, Jackson Memorial Hospital and UMHC-NCCH, Miami, Florida
Acute Viral and Bacterial Dysenteries

ROBERT E. ROGERS, M.D.

Professor, Obstetrics and Gynecology, Indiana University School of Medicine; Chief, Gynecology, Indiana University Hospital, William Wishard Memorial Hospital, Indianapolis, Indiana
Preoperative and Postoperative Care for Elective Gynecologic Surgery

RANDOLPH W. ROLLER, M.D.

Chief Resident, Southern Illinois University School of Medicine, Springfield, Illinois
Ectopic Pregnancy

IRWIN H. ROSENBERG, M.D.

Professor of Medicine, University of Chicago Hospitals and Clinics and the Pritzker School of Medicine; Chief, Section of Gastroenterology, University of Chicago Hospitals and Clinics, Chicago, Illinois
The Malabsorption Syndrome

ROBERT ROSS, JR., M.D.

Urologist, The Venice Hospital, Venice, Florida
Balanitis and Balanoposthitis

WENDELL F. ROSSE, M.D.

Chief Director, Hematology-Oncology, Department of Medicine, Duke University School of Medicine, Durham, North Carolina
Hemolytic Disease of the Newborn

SHELDON P. ROTHENBERG, M.D.

Professor of Medicine, New York Medical College; Attending Physician, Metropolitan Hospital, New York, New York
Macrocytic (Megaloblastic) Anemia (Other than Pernicious Anemia)

JOSEPH J. ROVINSKY, M.D.

Professor of Obstetrics and Gynecology, School of Medicine, Health Sciences Center, State University of New York at Stony Brook; Chairman, Department of Obstetrics and Gynecology, Long Island Jewish–Hillside Medical Center, New Hyde Park, New York
Thrombophlebitis

WILLIAM J. SAHL, JR., M.D.

Clinical Instructor, University of Oklahoma Health Science Center; Attending Dermatologist (Dermatopathologist and Chemosurgeon), Presbyterian Hospital, University Hospital, and Children's Hospital, Oklahoma City, Oklahoma
Dermatitis Herpetiformes

ITAMAR SALAMON, M.D.

Associate Professor of Psychiatry, Albert Einstein College of Medicine; Director, Soundview–Throgs Neck Community Mental Health Center, Bronx, New York
Alcoholism

DEEB N. SALEM, M.D., F.A.C.C.

Assistant Professor of Internal Medicine, Tufts University School of Medicine; Attending Cardiologist, Tufts University, New England Medical Center Hospital, Boston, Massachusetts
Pericarditis

ROSEMARIE SALERNI, M.D.

Assistant Professor of Medicine, University of Pittsburgh School of Medicine; Director, Coronary Care Unit, Presbyterian–University Hospital, Pittsburgh, Pennsylvania
Care and Rehabilitation After Myocardial Infarction

RICHARD J. SANTEN, M.D.

Associate Professor of Medicine, Division of Endocrinology, The Milton S. Hershey Medical Center of The Pennsylvania State University, Hershey, Pennsylvania
Hypopituitarism

WALTER G. SAUNDERS, M.D.

Memorial Hospital of Sheridan County, Sheridan, Wyoming; Consultant, United States Public Health Service Hospital, Crow Agency, Montana
Uterine Myomas

EUGENE R. SCHIFF, M.D.

Professor of Medicine, University of Miami School of Medicine; Chief, Division of Hepatology, University of Miami; Chief, Hepatology Section, Veteran's Administration Hospital, Miami, Florida
Bleeding Esophageal Varices

GILBERT M. SCHIFF, M.D.

Professor of Internal Medicine, Director, CHIMR University of Cincinnati; Attending Physician at Cincinnati General Hospital, Veterans Hospital, Children's Hospital, Jewish Hospital, and Christ Hospital, Cincinnati, Ohio
Rubella

J. DAVID SCHNATZ, M.D.

Professor of Medicine, University of Connecticut School of Medicine, Farmington, Connecticut; Director of Medi-

cine, Saint Francis Hospital and Medical Center, Hartford, Connecticut
Hyperlipoproteinemia

MARY LOUISE SCHOLL, M.D.

Associate Clinical Professor of Neurosciences and Psychiatry, University of California, San Diego; Staff, University Hospital, Children's Hospital, and Veterans Hospital, San Diego, California
Epilepsy in Children

EDWARD SCHOTLAND, M.D.

Assistant Clinical Professor, Department of Medicine (Dermatology), University of Kansas Medical Center; Consulting Dermatologist, Providence–St. Margaret's Medical Center; Lecturer, Kansas City College of Osteopathic Medicine and Bethany Medical Center, Kansas City, Kansas
Herpes Zoster

LUIS SCHUT, M.D.

Associate Professor of Neurosurgery, University of Pennsylvania School of Medicine; Chief, Neurosurgical Services, Children's Hospital of Philadelphia, Philadelphia, Pennsylvania
Head Injuries in Children

ANDREW R. SCHWARTZ, M.D.

Professor of Medicine, Director, Division of Infectious Diseases, Hahnemann Medical College; Attending Physician, West Jersey Hospital System, Hahnemann Hospital and St. Agnes Hospital, Philadelphia, Pennsylvania
Foodborne Illness

RUTH ANDREA SEELER, M.D.

Professor of Pediatrics, Abraham Lincoln School of Medicine, University of Illinois; Chairman, Pediatric Hematology-Oncology, Cook County Hospital, Chicago, Illinois
Vitamin K Deficiency

ALAN R. SHALITA, M.D.

Associate Professor, State University of New York Downstate Medical Center; Chief of Dermatology, State University Hospital, Kings County Hospital Center, Brookdale Hospital Medical Center; Consultant, Veterans Administration Hospital, Brooklyn, New York
Acne Vulgaris

FARID SHAMJI, M.D.

Resident in Surgery, Ottowa General Hospital, Ottowa, Ontario, Canada
Thyroid Gland Malignancies

FRED L. SHAPIRO, M.D.

Professor of Medicine, University of Minnesota School of Medicine; Chief, Division of Nephrology, Hennepin County Medical Center, Minneapolis, Minnesota
Chronic Renal Failure

OM P. SHARMA, M.D.

Associate Professor of Medicine, University of Southern California School of Medicine; Physician, Los Angeles County–University of Southern California Medical Center, Los Angeles, California
Sarcoidosis

JOHN FRANCIS SHEA, M.D.

Assistant Professor of Neurological Surgery, St. Louis University School of Medicine; Staff Neurosurgeon, St. Louis University Hospitals and Cardinal Glennon Memorial Hospital for Children, St. Louis, Missouri
Acute Head Injuries in the Adult

THOMAS W. SHEEHY, M.D.

Professor of Internal Medicine, University of Alabama School of Medicine; Chief of Medicine, University Hospital, Birmingham, Alabama
Malaria

LAURENCE ALAN SHERMAN, M.D.

Professor of Pathology and Medicine, Washington University School of Medicine; Director, Blood Bank, Barnes Hospital, St. Louis, Missouri
Disseminated Intravascular Coagulation (DIC)

JOSEPH C. SHIPP, M.D.

Professor and Chairman, Department of Internal Medicine, University of Nebraska College of Medicine; University of Nebraska Hospital, Bishop Clarkson Hospital, Nebraska Methodist Hospital, Omaha Veterans Administration Hospital, Immanuel Medical Center, Omaha, Nebraska
Diabetes Mellitus in the Adult

WILLIAM A. SHUCART, M.D.

Professor and Chairman, Department of Neurosurgery, State University of New York Downstate Medical Center; Chief of Neurosurgery, State University Hospital and Kings County Hospital, Brooklyn, New York
Brain Abscess

WILLIAM A. SIBLEY, M.D.

Professor and Head, Department of Neurology, University of Arizona Health Sciences Center; Physician-in-Charge, Neurology, University of Arizona Health Sciences Center; Consultant Neurologist, Veterans Administration Hospital, Tucson, Arizona
Peripheral Neuropathy

CHESTER M. SIDELL, M.D.

Valley Presbyterian Hospital, Sherman Oaks Community Hospital, Sherman Oaks, California
Nevi

OTTO F. SIEBER, JR., M.D.

Associate Professor of Pediatrics, University of Arizona Health Sciences Center; Consultant Staff, Tucson Medical Center, and St. Joseph's Hospital, Tucson, Arizona
Diphtheria

DONALD SILVER, M.D.

Professor and Chairman, Department of Surgery, University of Missouri, Columbia; University of Missouri Medical Center, Harry S. Truman Veterans Administration Hospital, Ellis Fischel State Cancer Hospital, Columbia, Missouri
Massive Deep Venous Thrombosis of the Lower Extremities

MICHAEL SILVERMAN, M.D.

Senior Fellow, University of Colorado School of Medicine; Rheumatologist, Colorado General Hospital, Denver General Hospital and Veteran's Administration Hospital, Denver, Colorado
Lupus Erythematosus

FREDERICK R. SINGER, M.D.

Professor of Medicine, University of Southern California School of Medicine, Los Angeles, California
Hyper- and Hypoparathyroidism

JOHN L. SKOSEY, M.D., Ph.D.

Associate Professor of Medicine, Chief, Section of Rheumatology, Department of Medicine, Abraham Lincoln School of Medicine, University of Illinois; Attending Physician, University of Illinois Hospital, Veterans Administration West Side Hospital, and Cook County Hospital, Chicago, Illinois
Ankylosing Spondylitis

R. MICHAEL SLY, M.D.

Professor of Child Health and Development, The George Washington University School of Medicine and Health Sciences; Director of Allergy and Immunology, Children's Hospital National Medical Center, Washington, D.C.
Asthma in Childhood

J. DONALD SMILEY, M.D.

Professor of Medicine, University of Texas Southwestern Medical School; Chief, Division of Rheumatology, Presbyterian Hospital, Dallas, Texas
Rheumatoid Arthritis

EDGAR B. SMITH, M.D.

Professor of Dermatology, University of Texas Medical Branch, Galveston, Texas
Superficial Fungus Infections of the Skin

JEANNE A. SMITH, M.D.

Assistant Professor of Clinical Medicine, Columbia University College of Physicians and Surgeons; Associate Visiting Physician, Harlem Hospital Center, New York, New York
Sickle Cell Disease

KENNETH RUPERT SMITH, JR., M.D.

Professor and Chairman, Section of Neurological Surgery, St. Louis University School of Medicine; Staff Neurosurgeon, St. Louis University Hospitals and Cardinal Glennon Memorial Hospital for Children, St. Louis, Missouri
Acute Head Injuries in the Adult

WILLIAM H. SMOOT, M.D.

Assistant Clinical Professor, University of Washington, Seattle, Washington; Billings Clinic, Billings, Montana
Scabies

MARK STEPHEN SOLOWAY, M.D.

Associate Professor, Department of Urology, University of Tennessee Center for the Health Sciences; Attending Urologist, Baptist Memorial Hospital, Veterans Administration Hospital and the University of Tennessee Hospital, Memphis, Tennessee
Epididymitis

ALFRED SOMMER, M.D.

Ophthalmologist and Research Scientist, Helen Keller International, Inc.
Hypo- and Hypervitaminosis A

SHELDON L. SPECTOR, M.D.

Associate Professor of Medicine, University of Colorado Medical Center; Head, Section of Allergy and Clinical Immunology, National Jewish Hospital and Research Center, Denver, Colorado
Asthma in Adults

MARK A. SPERLING, M.D.

Professor of Pediatrics, Associate Professor of Medicine, University of Cincinnati School of Medicine; Director, Pediatric Endocrinology, Children's Hospital; Attending Endocrinologist, Cincinnati General Hospital, Cincinnati, Ohio
Diabetes Mellitus in Childhood and Adolescence

WILLARD D. STECK, M.D.

Department of Dermatology, The Cleveland Clinic Foundation, Cleveland, Ohio
Decubitus Ulcer

A. DEAN STEELE, M.D.

Chief, Division of Rheumatology, Scott & White Clinic and Hospital, Temple, Texas
Bursitis and Calcific Tendinitis

JAMES C. STEIGERWALD, M.D.

Associate Professor of Medicine, University of Colorado School of Medicine; Attending Rheumatologist, Colorado General Hospital, Veterans Administration Hospital and Denver General Hospital; Rheumatology Consultant, Fitzsimons Army Medical Center, Denver, Colorado
Lupus Erythematosus

ALAN D. STEINFELD, M.D.

Assistant Professor, Radiation Medicine, Brown University Program in Medicine; Assistant Radiotherapist, Department of Radiation Oncology, Rhode Island Hospital; Consultant in Radiation Medicine, Roger Williams General Hospital, Veterans Hospital, Davis Park, Women and Infants Hospital of Rhode Island, Providence, Rhode Island
Uterine Cancer

MARVIN STERN, M.D.

Professor, New York University Medical Center; Executive Chairman, Department of Psychiatry, New York University Medical Center; Attending Psychiatrist, University Hospital and Bellvue Hospital, New York, New York

Delirium

STEPHEN P. STONE, M.D.

Clinical Assistant Professor, Southern Illinois University School of Medicine; Memorial Medical Center, St. John's Hospital, Springfield, Illinois

Rosacea

ROBERT W. SUMMERS, M.D.

Associate Professor, University of Iowa College of Medicine; University of Iowa Hospitals and Clinics, Veterans Administration Hospital, Iowa City, Iowa

Crohn's Disease

MARTIN I. SURKS, M.D.

Professor of Medicine, Albert Einstein College of Medicine; Head, Division of Endocrinology and Metabolism, Attending Physician, Montefiore Hospital and Medical Center and North Central Bronx Hospital, Bronx, New York

Simple Goiter

JOHN O. SUSAC, M.D.

Associate Professor of Neurology, Uniformed Services of Health Sciences, Bethesda, Maryland; Neuroophthalmologist, Winter Haven Regional Hospital, Winter Haven, Florida

Optic Neuritis

STEPHEN L. SWARTZ, M.D.

Research Fellow, Harvard Medical School; Research Fellow, Department of Medicine, Peter Bent Brigham Hospital, Boston, Massachusetts

Pheochromocytoma

CHARLES F. TATE, JR., M.D.

Professor of Medicine, Pulmonary Division, University of Miami Hospital; Attending Physician, Jackson Memorial Hospital and University of Miami Hospital, Miami, Florida

Primary Lung Abscess

JAMES S. TAYLOR, M.D.

Head, Section of Industrial Dermatology, Cleveland Clinic Foundation, Cleveland, Ohio

Occupational Dermatoses

MARVIN J. TENENBAUM, M.D.

Instructor of Internal Medicine, Virginia Commonwealth University, Medical College of Virginia; Fellow in Infectious Diseases, Medical College of Virginia Hospitals, Richmond, Virginia

Infective Endocarditis

JOHN McLELLAN TEW, JR., M.D.

Director, Neurosurgical Training Program, The Good Samaritan and Christ Hospitals; Adjunct Professor of Anatomy, University of Cincinnati Medical Center; Chief, Section of Neurosurgery, Good Samaritan and Deaconess Hospitals, Cincinnati, Ohio

Trigeminal Neuralgia

R. NICOL THIN, M.D., F.R.C.P.E.

Physician in Charge, Department of Genital Medicine, St. Bartholomew's Hospital, West Smithfield; Consultant Venereologist, Eastern Hospital and St. Paul's Hospital, London, England

Nongonococcal Urethritis

JAMES H. THOMAS, M.D.

Assistant Professor of Surgery, University of Kansas Medical Center and Veterans Administration Hospital; Staff Physician, University of Kansas Medical Center and Veterans Administration Hospital, Kansas City, Kansas

Diseases of the Breast

DAVID O. THUESON, PH.D.

Assistant Professor of Internal Medicine and Pharmacology and Toxicology, University of Texas Medical Branch, Galveston, Texas

Allergic Reactions to Insect Stings

RONALD K. TOMPKINS, M.D., M.Sc.

Associate Professor of Surgery, University of California, Los Angeles, School of Medicine; Attending Surgeon, University of California, Los Angeles, Hospital and Wadsworth Veterans Administration Hospital; Consultant Surgeon, Sepulveda Veterans Administration Hospital, Los Angeles, California

Cholecystitis and Cholelithiasis

JONATHAN B. TOWNE, M.D.

Assistant Professor of Surgery, Medical College of Wisconsin; Attending Surgeon, Milwaukee County Hospital; Chief, Vascular Surgery, Wood Veterans Administration Hospital, Milwaukee, Wisconsin

Degenerative Arterial Disease

BISHARA TRABOLSI, M.D.

Senior Physician, Abbassia Fever Hospital, Ministry of Health; Consultant Physician, U.S. Naval Medical Research Unit No. 3, Cairo, Egypt

Amebiasis

B. TODD TROOST, M.D.

Associate Professor of Neurology and Ophthalmology, University of Pittsburgh School of Medicine; Attending Neurologist, Presbyterian–University Hospital, Veterans Medical Center, and Eye and Ear Hospital, Pittsburgh, Pennsylvania

Episodic Vertigo

CHARLES C. TSAI, M.D., F.A.C.O.G.

Associate Professor of Obstetrics and Gynecology, Medical University of South Carolina; Attending Obstetrician/Gynecologist, Medical University Hospital, Charleston County Hospital, and Veterans Administration Hospital, Charleston, South Carolina
Dysfunctional Uterine Bleeding

EDUARDO H. TSCHEN, M.D.

Resident in Dermatology, University of New Mexico School of Medicine, Albuquerque, New Mexico
Superficial Fungus Infections of the Skin

BRUCE A. TUCKER, M.D.

Fellow, Division of Infectious Diseases, University of Alabama Medical Center, Birmingham, Alabama
Chickenpox

MAURAY J. TYE, M.D.

Clinical Professor of Dermatology, Tufts School of Medicine and Boston University School of Medicine; Attending Dermatologist, Haverhill Municipal Hospital, Lawrence General, Boston City, Veterans Administration Hospital, and Lemuel Shattuck Hospital, Boston, Massachusetts
The Erythemas

PAUL BENJAMIN UNDERWOOD, JR., M.D.

Professor, Obstetrics and Gynecology, Medical University of South Carolina; Director, Gynecologic Oncology, Medical University of South Carolina, Charleston, South Carolina
Carcinoma of the Vulva

BARRY H. USOW, M.D.

Instructor, Medical College of Wisconsin; Chief, Section of Urology, Mount Sinai Hospital and St. Luke's Hospital; Attending Physician, St. Francis Hospital, Milwaukee Children's Hospital, and Deaconess Hospital, Milwaukee, Wisconsin
Genitourinary Tuberculosis

BHUPENDRA J. VAKIL, M.D., F.A.C.G.

Professor of Medicine, Grant Medical College; Director, Clinical Pharmacology Unit, Grant Medical College; Physician, J. J. Group of Hospitals and Sir Hurkisondas Hospital, Bombay, India
Tetanus

JOHN VAN DE ERVE, B.S., M.D.

Emeritus Professor of Dermatology, Medical University of South Carolina; Roper Hospital, Medical University Hospital, St. Francis Xavier Baker Hospital, Charleston, South Carolina
Creeping Eruption

JOHANNES D. VELDHUIS, M.D.

Endocrinology Fellow, The Milton S. Hershey Medical Center of The Pennsylvania State University, Hershey, Pennsylvania
Hypopituitarism

RICHARD W. VILTER, M.D.

Gordon and Helen Hughes Taylor Professor of Medicine, Director, Department of Internal Medicine, University of Cincinnati College of Medicine; Director, Department of Medicine, Cincinnati General Hospital and Holmes Hospital; Consultant, Christ Hospital, Deaconess Hospital, Jewish Hospital, and Veterans Administration Hospital, Cincinnati, Ohio
Beriberi

WILLIAM RALPH VOGLER, M.D.

Professor of Medicine, Emory University School of Medicine; Attending Hematologist/Oncologist, Emory University Hospital, Atlanta, Georgia
Acute Leukemia in Adults

R. DIXON WALKER, M.D.

Professor, University of Florida; Co-Director, Pediatric Renal-Urology, Pediatric Urologist, Shands Teaching Hospital; Renal Advisory Committee, Childrens Medical Services, Chairman, Medical Admissions Committee, University of Florida, Gainesville, Florida
Bacterial Infections of the Urinary Tract (Female Children)

BETTI JO WARREN, M.D.

Associate Professor of Pediatrics, Charles R. Drew Postgraduate Medical School; Attending, Division Ambulatory Pediatrics, Martin Luther King, Jr., General Hospital; Director, Regional Pediatric Programs, Southeast Region Los Angeles County, Los Angeles, California
Childhood Enuresis

LEONARD WARTOFSKY, M.D.

Associate Professor of Medicine, Uniformed Services University of the Health Sciences, Bethesda, Maryland; Chief, Endocrine-Metabolic Service, Walter Reed Army Medical Center, Washington, D.C.
Hypothyroidism

RAYMOND HENRY WATTEN, M.D.

Director, U.S. Naval Medical Research Unit Number 3, Cairo, Egypt
Amebiasis

HARRY L. WECHSLER, M.D.

Clinical Associate Professor of Medicine (Dermatology) and Acting Director, Division of Dermatology, University of Pittsburgh School of Medicine; Attending Dermatologist, Presbyterian Hospital and Western Pennsylvania Hospital; McKeesport Hospital, McKeesport, Pennsylvania
Lichen Planus

ROBERT M. WEETMAN, M.D.

Associate Professor of Pediatrics, Indiana University School of Medicine; Staff Hematologist-Oncologist, James Whitcomb Riley Hospital for Children, Indianapolis, Indiana
Childhood Acute Leukemia

ALEKSANDER U. WEINFELD, M.D.

Associate Professor of Internal Medicine, University of Göteborg; Chief, Division of Oncological Hematology, Department of Medicine 11, Sahlgrens Hospital, University of Göteborg, Göteborg, Sweden
Polycythemia Vera

EDWARD I. WEINSHELBAUM, M.D.

Clinical Associate Professor, University of Florida; Consultant in Surgery, Gainesville Veterans Administration Hospital; Staff Surgeon, North Florida Regional Hospital, and Alachua General Hospital, Gainesville, Florida
Tumors of the Stomach

JACK D. WELSH, M.D.

Professor of Medicine, University of Oklahoma College of Medicine; Chief, Digestive Diseases and Nutrition Section, University of Oklahoma Health Sciences Center, Oklahoma City, Oklahoma
Peptic Ulcer

JOHN N. WETTLAUFER, M.D.

Associate Professor of Surgery, Division of Urology, University of Colorado Medical Center, Denver, Colorado
Pyelonephritis

RICHARD J. WHITLEY, M.D.

Assistant Professor of Pediatrics, University of Alabama Medical Center, Birmingham, Alabama
Chickenpox

TIFFANY J. WILLIAMS, M.D.

Professor of Obstetrics and Gynecology, Mayo Medical School; Consultant in Gynecologic Surgery, Mayo Clinic and St. Mary's Hospital, Rochester, Minnesota
Endometriosis

H. OLIVER WILLIAMSON, M.D.

Director, Section on Reproductive Endocrinology, Professor of Obstetrics and Gynecology, Medical University of South Carolina; Staff, Medical University Hospital and Charleston County Hospital; Consultant, Veterans Administration Hospital; Affiliate, Roper Hospital, Charleston, South Carolina
Dysfunctional Uterine Bleeding

C. H. WINGERT, M.D.

Attending Dermatologist, Centre Community Hospital, State College, Pennsylvania; Consulting Dermatologist, Lewistown Hospital, Lewistown, Pennsylvania
Seborrheic Dermatitis

GERALD F. WINKLER, M.D., M.Sc.

Assistant Clinical Professor of Neurology, Harvard Medical School; Associate Neurologist, Massachusetts General Hospital, Boston, Massachusetts
Multiple Sclerosis

STEPHEN C. WRIGHT, M.D.

Associate Clinical Professor of Medicine, Tufts University School of Medicine; Faulkner Hospital, Lemuel Shattuck Hospital, Boston, Massachusetts
Cirrhosis

DAVID J. WYLER, M.D.

Senior Investigator, Laboratory of Parasitic Diseases, National Institutes of Health; Senior Consultant in Infectious Diseases, The Clinical Center, National Institutes of Health; Consultant in Infectious Diseases, National Naval Medical Center, Bethesda, Maryland
Leishmaniasis

DABNEY R. YARBROUGH, III, M.D.

Associate Professor of Surgery, Medical University Hospital of South Carolina, Charleston, South Carolina
Burns

C. THOMAS YARINGTON, JR., M.D., F.A.C.S.

Clinical Professor of Otolaryngology, University of Washington School of Medicine; Chief, Otolaryngology and Facial Plastic Surgery, Mason Clinic and Virginia Mason Hospital, Seattle, Washington
Sinusitis

PHILIP C. YOUNG, M.D.

Clinical Associate Professor of Medicine, Tulane University School of Medicine; Staff Member in Gastroenterology, Ochsner Clinic and Ochsner Foundation Hospital, New Orleans, Louisiana
Hemochromatosis and Hemosiderosis

JANICE W. YUSK, M.D.

Clinical Instructor, University of Louisville School of Medicine; Clinical Assistant Professor in Pediatrics, Norton-Children's Hospital, Louisville, Kentucky
Precancerous Lesions of the Skin and Mucous Membranes

Contents

SECTION 2.   THE RESPIRATORY SYSTEM

SECTION 3.   THE CARDIOVASCULAR SYSTEM

SECTION 4.   THE BLOOD AND SPLEEN

SECTION 5. THE DIGESTIVE SYSTEM

SECTION 6.   METABOLIC DISORDERS

SECTION 7.   THE ENDOCRINE SYSTEM

SECTION 8.   THE UROGENITAL TRACT

SECTION 9.   THE VENEREAL DISEASES

SECTION 10.   DISEASES OF ALLERGY

SECTION 11. DISEASES OF THE SKIN

SECTION 12. THE NERVOUS SYSTEM

SECTION 13.   THE LOCOMOTOR SYSTEM

SECTION 14.   OBSTETRICS AND GYNECOLOGY

The Infectious Diseases

AMEBIASIS

method of
ZOHEIR FARID, M.D.,
BISHARA TRABOLSI, M.D.,
and RAYMOND H. WATTEN, M.D.
Cairo, Egypt

Amebiasis is defined as the state of harboring *Entamoeba histolytica;* this includes patients in whom the parasite dwells as a commensal (asymptomatic cyst passers), and those who suffer tissue invasion by the amebae. Amebae may be located in the bowel lumen, in the intestinal wall, or extraintestinally mainly in the liver. Treatment of all forms is most satisfactory, and failure to achieve cure is usually due to erroneous diagnosis, misuse of amebicides, or inadequate therapy. The introduction of metronidazole (Flagyl) has greatly facilitated the treatment of amebiasis; it is the only safe, well-tolerated, direct-acting amebicide, which is effective in all forms of invasive amebiasis. There is a wide selection of amebicides, but none of them is equally effective in the different forms of amebiasis and the choice of therapy is therefore governed by the different manifestations of the infection. A list of the more commonly available amebicides, their mode of action, and the dose used for different forms of amebic infection follows.

Amebicides

Metronidazole (Flagyl) is effective in luminal (asymptomatic cyst passers), intestinal, and hepatic forms. It is devoid of serious toxicity and is well tolerated. Unfortunately, it cannot be given parenterally. At present it is the drug of choice for all forms of amebiasis whenever oral administration can be used. It may sometimes cause severe headache, nausea, and vomiting, and patients should be cautioned to stop drinking alcohol during therapy. A dose of 750 mg. (3 tablets) three times daily for 10 days is effective in all forms of amebiasis.

Diiodohydroxyquin is effective in luminal infections. It is not absorbed from the intestines and has few side effects (idiosyncrasy to iodine may be one). It is used for the treatment of the asymptomatic cyst passers in a dose of 650 mg. (1 tablet) given orally three times daily for 3 weeks.

Diloxanide furoate (Furamide)* after metronidazole is probably now the drug of choice for treatment of luminal asymptomatic cyst passers. A dose of 500 mg. (1 tablet) given orally three times daily for 10 days is usually effective. It is nontoxic but may occasionally cause excessive flatulence.

Tetracycline probably works in amebic dysentery by modifying bowel flora necessary for growth of *Entamoeba histolytica*. It is very effective in amebic dysentery but has to be combined with a second tissue amebicide to prevent liver disease. It is given in a dose of 250 mg. four times daily for 10 days.

Chloroquine (Aralen) is of value in the treatment of hepatic amebiasis. It is given orally and is rapidly absorbed and concentrated in the liver. It may cause nausea and vomiting. It is given in a dose of 600 mg. base first dose, followed 6 hours later by 300 mg. and then 150 mg. twice daily for 4 weeks. Chloroquine is used in combination with emetine or dehydroemetine in the treatment of hepatic amebiasis. It should be combined with tetracycline 250 mg. four times daily to control dysentery, and diiodohydroxyquin or diloxanide should be added to control luminal infection.

Emetine and dehydroemetine* have similar

---

*In the United States, these drugs are available from the Parasitic Diseases Division, Center for Disease Control, Atlanta, Georgia 30333.

pharmacologic properties, but dehydroemetine is less toxic and, when available, should be preferred to emetine. They are administered subcutaneously or intramuscularly in a dose of 1 to 1.5 mg. per kg. daily for 10 days not to exceed 65 mg. of emetine or 100 mg. of dehydroemetine in a single dose. The elderly, malnourished, and young are given proportionally smaller doses. Both drugs are cardiotoxic and may cause vomiting through a central mechanism. Patients should be kept in bed while on treatment but allowed toilet privileges. When possible, these drugs should be avoided during pregnancy and the presence of heart disease is usually a contraindication. Their greatest use is for the treatment of hepatic amebiasis and other tissue lesions (ameboma). When used for intestinal amebiasis they should be combined with tetracycline and diiodohydroxyquin or diloxanide.

Treatment

Asymptomatic Cyst Passers (Luminal Infections). 1. Metronidazole, 750 mg. three times daily for 10 days, is effective.

In resistant cases repeat treatment or use:

2. Diloxanide,* 500 mg. three times daily for 10 days, or

3. Diiodohydroxyquin, 650 mg. three times daily for 3 weeks.

Intestinal Amebiasis (Amebic Dysentery, Trophozoite Passers). Metronidazole, 750 mg. three times daily for 10 days, is quite effective. If there is severe diarrhea add tetracycline, 250 mg. four times daily for 10 days. In resistant cases or in patients who do not tolerate metronidazole, a combination of drugs has to be used. To be effective, treatment must aim at killing the ameba in the lumen and wall of the bowel and, in addition, liver involvement must be prevented. Either of the following regimens is effective:

1. Emetine or dehydroemetine,* 1 to 1.5 mg. per kg. daily, subcutaneously or intramuscularly plus tetracycline, 250 mg. four times daily for 10 days; plus either diiodohydroxyquin, 650 mg. three times daily for 3 weeks, or diloxanide,* 500 mg. three times daily for 10 days.

2. Chloroquine, 150 mg. base twice daily for 2 weeks, is substituted for emetine or dehydroemetine; tetracycline plus diiodohydroxyquin or diloxanide is given as above along with chloroquine.

In severe amebic dysentery, when oral administration may be impossible, the first regimen should be used. Patients should be kept in bed during treatment but allowed toilet privileges. Dehydration and electrolyte balance, particularly in the elderly, must be corrected by intravenous fluids. Codeine sulfate, 30 mg. three times daily, may help to control severe diarrhea.

Ameboma usually responds rapidly to emetine or dehydroemetine* plus tetracycline and diiodohydroxyquin or diloxanide.* Patients who have suffered an attack of amebic dysentery should have their stools examined repeatedly for at least 3 months after apparent cure.

Hepatic Amebiasis. The introduction of amebic serologic tests, particularly the simple counterimmunoelectrophoresis test, have greatly helped in the rapid diagnosis of hepatic amebiasis. In addition ^{99m}Tc-sulfur colloid liver scans enable the physician to define the size and location of the abscess.

1. Metronidazole, 750 mg. three times daily for 10 days, is usually very effective in hepatic amebiasis and in small abscesses may be the only drug necessary. If there is severe dysentery or a markedly elevated white blood cell count (indicating secondary bacterial infection), tetracycline, 250 mg. four times daily for 10 days is added. If radioisotope scanning of liver shows that the abscess is large and near the surface, or if clinical examination demonstrates severe intercostal tenderness with obvious swelling over the liver, then aspiration of the abscess should be done. This may have to be repeated. A combination of metronidazole, tetracycline, and aspiration of the pus is usually effective in curing the majority of amebic liver abscesses.

2. In patients who cannot take drugs orally, emetine or dehydroemetine,* 1 to 1.5 mg. per kg. daily for 10 days, given subcutaneously or intramuscularly must be immediately started and once oral therapy is possible, chloroquine is added. Chloroquine is given in a 600 mg. base first dose, followed 6 hours later by 300 mg. then 150 mg. twice daily for 4 weeks; the combination of these two drugs is very effective in hepatic amebiasis. Tetracycline, however, should be given to control severe dysentery and diiodohydroxyquin or diloxanide* added to eliminate luminal infection.

Occasionally, an abscess may rupture in the lungs, pericardium, or peritoneum. Amebic lung abscesses usually drain through a bronchus; specific therapy with metronidazole and tetracycline or with emetine or dehydroemetine* plus chloroquine should be given. If empyema develops, repeated aspiration may be necessary and in resistant cases surgical drainage through an intercostal tube may be necessary. Amebic pericarditis with effusion should be treated with emetine

---

*In the United States, these drugs are available from the Parasitic Diseases Division, Center for Disease Control, Atlanta, Georgia 30333.

*In the United States, these drugs are available from the Parasitic Diseases Division, Center for Disease Control, Atlanta, Georgia 30333.

or dehydroemetine* plus chloroquine and aspiration if necessary. Amebic peritonitis is usually treated by surgical drainage of the pus and with emetine or dehydroemetine* and chloroquine.

BACTEREMIA†

method of
RICHARD D. MEYER, M.D.
Los Angeles, California

Introduction and Approach

Appropriate therapy of bacteremia (septicemia) requires knowledge of host defenses, nature and severity of underlying disease, primary site or sites of the infection, specific bacterium(a) responsible, and pharmacologic principles of antimicrobial agents. Survival depends upon the pathogen, underlying disease, adjunctive measures, and proper use of an antimicrobial agent to which the pathogen is susceptible.

People may have transient bacteremia, which is generally unrecognized, of no consequence, and requires no therapy. Mild, intermittent episodes of bacteremia are usually controlled by host defenses. Host factors that influence the development or course of bacteremia include defects in cellular and humoral immunity (e.g., neutropenia, use of cytotoxic or immunosuppressive drugs such as corticosteroids), burns, alcoholism, diabetes mellitus, neoplastic disease, procedures (e.g., surgical procedures, urinary tract manipulation, vascular grafts, indwelling bladder or intravenous catheters, inhalation equipment), and advanced age. Nosocomial acquisition and previous antibiotic therapy are additional factors.

Although isolation of bacteria from blood culture is necessary for diagnosis, clinical manifestations of bacteremia should suggest the diagnosis and the need for obtaining proper cultures and institution of therapy. There is considerable individual variation in signs and symptoms. Shaking chills, high fever, tachycardia, tachypnea, prostration, and, less commonly, nausea and vomiting are early features. Hypotension may ensue within several hours. Delirium or varying degrees of decreased levels of consciousness are seen less frequently. Changes in mental status are more common in elderly people. Fever may be absent in the elderly, in patients receiving corticosteroids, and in uremic patients. Respiratory alkalosis, metabolic acidosis, oliguria, anuria or thrombocytopenia, and disseminated intravascular coagulation should also suggest the diagnosis. Fever in a neutropenic patient may be the only sign of bacteremia which will, if untreated, have a fulminant course. Bacteremia in neonates may be noted only by lethargy, irritability and decreased feeding. Signs and symptoms are similar regardless of the causative agent.

Knowledge of any predisposing conditions and possible nosocomial sources is essential. A review of the history and course, physical examination, and assessment of the gravity of the situation must be rapidly performed. The site or cause of infection may be noted on physical examination (e.g., septic phlebitis, pneumonia, or wound infection). Microscopic examination including Gram stain of urine, respiratory tract secretions, bacteremic skin lesions, pleural effusions, purulent exudates, or cerebrospinal fluid may indicate the likely source of the infection or an accompanying process. Review of previous results from cultures may be useful, particularly in neutropenic patients.

Cultures and smears of the aforementioned sites as indicated and blood cultures must be obtained before administration of antimicrobial therapy. Two blood cultures from different sites (five if endocarditis is suspected) should be made. If the patient is stable, as in many cases of subacute bacterial endocarditis, therapy may be withheld, pending the results of cultures. Supportive measures and the administration of antimicrobial agents, however, are frequently required. Drainage of primary sites or relief of obstruction are important facets of therapy and may be themselves curative with good host defenses. Yet one aim of therapy is prevention of metastatic suppurative complications. Antibiotic therapy alone will fail, however, without drainage.

Selection of Therapeutic Agents

Specific Therapy. The physician must determine if an organism isolated from blood culture is a pathogen or a contaminant. Common contaminants such as *Staphylococcus epidermidis* and *Propionibacterium* sp. may also be pathogens in patients with prosthetic valves, prosthetic grafts, or ventriculoatrial shunts.

Antimicrobial agents of choice and alternatives based upon isolation and in vitro susceptibility of the causative agent are outlined in Table 1 for patients with no allergies. Generally the agent used should have the most narrow and specific antibacterial spectrum in vitro as well as pharmacologic suitability. The intravenous route

---

*In the United States, these drugs are available from the Parasitic Diseases Division, Center for Disease Control, Atlanta, Georgia 30333.

†Supported by the Medical Research Service of the Veterans Administration.

TABLE 1. **Antimicrobial Agents for the Treatment of Bacteremia Caused by Susceptible Pathogens***

ORGANISM	DRUGS OF CHOICE	ALTERNATIVES (IN ORDER OF PREFERENCE)
Gram-positive cocci		
Staphylococcus aureus	Penicillin G	Cephalosporin, vancomycin, clindamycin
Staphylococcus aureus (penicillin-resistant)	Oxacillin, methicillin, or nafcillin	Cephalosporin, vancomycin, clindamycin
Staphylococcus aureus (methicillin-resistant)	Vancomycin	Gentamicin plus cephalosporin
*Staphylococcus epidermidis**	Penicillin G	Cephalosporin, vancomycin
*Staphylococcus epidermidis** (penicillin-resistant)	Vancomycin	Cephalosporin
Streptococcus pyogenes (Group A)	Penicillin G	Cephalosporin, erythromycin, clindamycin
Streptococcus, Groups B, C, G	Penicillin G	Cephalosporin, erythromycin, clindamycin
Streptococcus, Group D	Penicillin G or ampicillin plus strepto- mycin or gentamicin or kanamycin	Vancomycin plus streptomycin or genta- micin
Streptococcus bovis, Group D	Penicillin G plus or minus streptomycin	Cephalosporin, vancomycin
Streptococcus viridans	Penicillin G plus or minus streptomycin or gentamicin	Cephalosporin, vancomycin, clindamycin
Peptostreptococcus sp. (Anaerobic streptococci)	Penicillin G	Cephalosporin, vancomycin, erythromy- cin, clindamycin, chloramphenicol
Streptococcus pneumoniae (pneumococcus)	Penicillin G	Erythromycin, cephalosporin, clindamycin
Gram-negative cocci		
Neisseria gonorrhoeae (gonococcus)	Penicillin G	Ampicillin, tetracycline, erythromycin
Neisseria meningitidis (meningococcus)	Penicillin G	Ampicillin, chloramphenicol, sulfonamide†
Gram-positive bacilli		
Clostridium perfringens	Penicillin G	Chloramphenicol, tetracycline, erythromycin
Listeria monocytogenes	Ampicillin plus or minus gentamicin	Penicillin, tetracycline, erythromycin
Gram-negative bacilli		
Escherichia coli	Ampicillin‡, cephalosporin, gentamicin	Carbenicillin or ticarcillin, tobramycin, chloramphenicol, amikacin§
Klebsiella pneumoniae	Gentamicin plus or minus cephalosporin‡	Chloramphenicol, tetracycline, amikacin§
Enterobacter species	Gentamicin	Carbenicillin or ticarcillin, chloramphenicol, tobramycin, kanamycin, amikacin§
Proteus mirabilis	Ampicillin	Cephalosporin, gentamicin, chloramphenicol, tobramycin, amikacin§
Proteus species (indole-positive) (*P. morganii, P. vulgatus, P. rettgeri*)	Gentamicin	Chloramphenicol, carbenicillin or ticarcillin, amikacin§
Pseudomonas aeruginosa	Tobramycin or gentamicin plus or minus carbenicillin or ticarcillin	Amikacin§
Providencia stuartii	Kanamycin or amikacin§	Carbenicillin or ticarcillin, cefoxitin (investigational)
Providencia alcaligenes	Gentamicin	Carbenicillin or ticarcillin, kanamycin, amikacin§
Salmonella typhi	Chloramphenicol	Ampicillin, sulfamethoxazole- trimethoprim
Salmonella sp. other than *typhi*	Ampicillin	Chloramphenicol, sulfamethoxazole- trimethoprim
Brucella sp.	Tetracycline plus streptomycin	Chloramphenicol plus streptomycin, sulfamethoxazole-trimethoprim
Bacteroides fragilis	Chloramphenicol	Clindamycin, cefoxitin (investigational), metronidazole (investigational), car- benicillin†
Bacteroides species other than *B. fragilis* (head and neck source)	Penicillin G	Clindamycin, chloramphenicol, tetracycline
Serratia marcescens or *S. liquefaciens*	Gentamicin	Chloramphenicol, carbenicillin or ticarcillin, amikacin,§ cefoxitin (investigational)
Shigella species	Ampicillin	Chloramphenicol, trimethoprim- sulfamethoxazole

TABLE 1. **Antimicrobial Agents for the Treatment of Bacteremia Caused by Susceptible Pathogens*** (Continued)

ORGANISM	DRUGS OF CHOICE	ALTERNATIVES (IN ORDER OF PREFERENCE)
Hemophilus influenzae	Chloramphenicol	Ampicillin, trimethoprim-sulfamethoxazole, erythromycin Chloramphenicol, kanamycin, tobramycin
Citrobacter sp.	Gentamicin	Chloramphenicol, kanamycin, amikacin§

*Cidal drugs alone or in combination recommended for endocarditis; unless local epidemiologic factors indicate otherwise therapy for the nonallergic patient is based on same drugs before susceptibility tests are available

†Susceptibility testing results required

‡Hospital-acquired strains frequently resistant

§For enteric gram-negative rod or *Pseudomonas aeruginosa* bacteremia, amikacin may be used if organisms are resistant to gentamicin but susceptible to amikacin. Empiric use is based upon level of resistance to gentamicin and tobramycin among hospital isolates

should generally be employed initially, although follow-up therapy with intramuscular and less frequently with certain oral preparations is occasionally suitable. Intravenous therapy is recommended for the entire course of therapy for endocarditis whenever possible. A penicillin or an aminoglycoside is generally preferred over cephalosporins. A cephalosporin may be given to patients with penicillin allergy other than immediate reactions.

Table 2 lists some of the side effects and the recommended doses of antimicrobial agents for patients with normal renal or hepatic function. The most common adjustment is related to renal function. Nomograms for modification of doses are available in product circulars and in available publications. Estimated creatinine clearances dependent upon age are generally reliable in selection of initial doses. Urinalyses and determinations of serum creatinine level should be done at least thrice weekly and, when possible, creatinine clearances should be performed during and then after therapy with gentamicin, tobramycin, kanamycin, or amikacin. Determination of peak (1 hour after intramuscular or 1/2 hour after a 30 minutes intravenous infusion) and trough (just before next dose) levels of antibiotics help maintain therapeutic levels while avoiding toxicity. Concurrent use of vancomycin, furosemide, ethacrynic acid, or mannitol should be avoided. Patients who receive aminoglycosides should be examined daily for signs of vestibular toxicity and questioned about tinnitus. Audiograms should be performed whenever possible. Aminoglycoside nephrotoxicity may occur in the week following therapy.

Ampicillin, penicillin G, cephalosporins, trimethoprim-sulfamethoxazole, and cefoxitin require moderate adjustments for renal insufficiency. The semisynthetic penicillinase-resistant penicillins require little adjustment for renal failure. Carbenicillin and ticarcillin require modifica-

tion in renal failure and further reduction with accompanying hepatic failure. The doses of clindamycin, chloramphenicol, and erythromycin are not changed in renal failure but chloramphenicol dosage is decreased in hepatic insufficiency. Tetracyclines other than doxycycline are avoided in renal failure.

Pharmacologic principles must be followed for therapy of primary or secondary sites. Aminoglycosides may not achieve adequate urinary levels in the face of renal insufficiency to treat urinary tract infection. Doxycycline and chloramphenicol are routinely of no value in this situation. Cephalosporins or clindamycin should not be given to patients as therapy for suspected or documented meningitis because of inadequate levels of active drug in the cerebrospinal fluid. Aminoglycosides likewise penetrate cerebrospinal fluid poorly; they may require intrathecal administration. Chloramphenicol is excreted predominantly in the bile as the inactive glucoronide and is ineffective with incomplete biliary obstruction, although it penetrates liver tissue well. Aminoglycosides and clindamycin enter bile poorly; aminoglycoside use in biliary sepsis is treatment of bacteremia. Cefazolin and ampicillin, however, are usually concentrated in bile.

Empiric Therapy. Selection of an agent or agents before a bacteriologic diagnosis is confirmed is based upon pharmacologic properties, clinical data, results of microscopic examinations and earlier cultures, presumed site of infection, pathogens known to cause infection there, and their probable in vitro susceptibilities. Local epidemiologic factors in nosocomial isolates are very important if the patient has been hospitalized for more than a few days and has underlying predisposing factors. It is invariably more sensible to administer one or more agents to treat the most likely pathogens than it is to attempt to treat all pathogens. Therapy should be tailored as soon as the diagnosis is clear.

TABLE 2. **Recommended Doses and Potential Toxicity of Antimicrobial Agents Used in Treatment of Bacteremia***

ANTIMICROBIAL AGENT	USUAL TOTAL DAILY DOSE	USUAL INTERVAL BETWEEN DOSES	MAJOR SIDE EFFECTS
Amikacin	15 mg./kg./day	q 8–12 h	Ototoxicity (primarily hearing loss), nephrotoxicity, neuromuscular blockade
Ampicillin	100–200 mg./kg./day	q 6 h	Hypersensitivity, rash, diarrhea
Carbenicillin	500 mg./kg. (*P. aeruginosa*) 200 mg./kg. (non *P. aeruginosa* infections)	q 4 h	Hypersensitivity, sodium overload, hypokalemia, alkalosis, leukopenia, CNS toxicity in uremia, bleeding disorder, interstitial nephritis (rare)
Cefazolin	50–80 mg./kg./day (2–6 grams/day)	q 6 h	Hypersensitivity, CNS toxicity in uremia, thrombophlebitis, possible nephrotoxicity with aminoglycosides
Cephalothin	100–200 mg./kg./day	q 4–6 h	Hypersensitivity, thrombophlebitis, nephrotoxicity with aminoglycosides, leukopenia, hemolytic anemia
Cephapirin	100–200 mg./kg./day	q 4–6 h	Hypersensitivity, thrombophlebitis, probable nephrotoxicity with aminoglycosides
Chloramphenicol	40–100 mg./kg./day	q 6 h	Hematopoietic toxicity (dose related; aplasia rare), gray-baby syndrome
Clindamycin	30–40 mg./kg./day	q 6 h	Diarrhea, pseudomembranous colitis
Colistimethate†	2.5–5.0 mg./kg./day	q 8 h	Nephrotoxicity, circumoral and acral paresthesias
Erythromycin	30–60 mg./kg./day (2–4 grams/day)	q 6 h	Diarrhea, nausea and vomiting, transient deafness (rare), thrombophlebitis
Gentamicin	3–5 mg./kg./day	q 8 h	Nephrotoxicity, ototoxicity (primarily vestibular) neuromuscular blockade
Kanamycin	15 mg./kg./day	q 8–12 h	Ototoxicity (primarily hearing loss), nephrotoxicity, neuromuscular blockade
Methicillin	100–200 mg./kg./day	q 4–6 h	Hypersensitivity, interstitial nephritis
Nafcillin	100–200 mg./kg./day	q 4–6 h	Hypersensitivity, leukopenia, interstitial nephritis (rare)
Oxacillin	100–200 mg./kg./day	q 4–6 h	Hypersensitivity, hepatotoxicity, leukopenia, interstitial nephritis (rare)
Penicillin G	150,000–300,000 units/kg./day	q 4 h	Hypersensitivity, CNS toxicity in uremia, leukopenia
Polymyxin B†	1.5–2.5 mg./kg./day	q 8 h	Nephrotoxicity, neuromuscular blockade
Streptomycin	15–30 mg./kg./day (1–2 grams/day)	q 12 h	Vestibular toxicity, fever, eosinophilia
Sulfonamides	100 mg./kg./day	q 6 h	Rash, nephrotoxicity, anemia, neutropenia, Stevens-Johnson syndrome
Tetracycline	15–30 mg./kg./day (1–2 grams/day)	q 6 h	Diarrhea, nausea and vomiting, nephrotoxicity, hepatotoxicity
Ticarcillin	300 mg./kg./day (*P. aeruginosa*)	q 4 h	Hypersensitivity, anemia, leukopenia, thrombocytopenia, CNS toxicity in uremia
Tobramycin	3–5 mg./kg./day	q 8 h	Nephrotoxicity, ototoxicity (vestibular and cochlear)
Trimethoprim-sulfamethoxazole‡	—	q 12 h	Pancytopenia (trimethoprim) rash, nephrotoxicity, anemia, neutropenia Stevens-Johnson syndrome (sulfa)
Vancomycin	30 mg./kg./day (2 grams/day)	q 6–12 h	Thrombophlebitis, ototoxicity (hearing loss), nausea, hypersensitivity and tinnitus

*Certain doses in this table may be higher than that listed in the manufacturer's official directive
†Rarely indicated in bacteremia
‡Intravenous preparation investigational. This use of this combination is not listed in the manufacturer's official directive.

Urinary tract infections are frequently caused by gram-negative bacilli and less commonly by Group D streptococci. *Escherichia coli* susceptible to ampicillin is common in the community but *E. coli*, other *Enterobacteriaceae*, and *Pseudomonas aeruginosa* which are resistant to ampicillin and cephalosporins are more common in chronic or nosocomially acquired infections. Thus an aminoglycoside should be part of therapy in these cases.

Peritonitis from intestinal perforation is a polymicrobial infection with *Enterobacteriaceae*, aerobic streptococci, peptococci, peptostreptococci, *Bacteroides* sp., *Clostridium* sp., and, if from the colon, *Bacteroides fragilis*. Surgical and supportive therapy and administration of gentamicin and chloramphenicol (or clindamycin) are recommended. Penicillin G is also given if clostridial cellulitis, myonecrosis, or bacteremia is suspected. Use of polyvalent gas gangrene antitoxin is recommended for the syndrome of gas gangrene. Polymicrobial infections are also seen in the female genitourinary tract (e.g., tubal or uterine) although *Neisseria gonorrhea* may also be found in pelvic inflammatory disease.

Cellulitis is caused frequently by aerobic streptococci and *Staphylococcus aureus,* although anaerobic streptococci, and *Clostridia* sp. are also found. Necrotizing fasciitis is polymicrobial and related to fecal flora. Gram-negative bacilli cause cellulitis in neutropenic patients. Burn wounds are commonly infected with *Streptococcus pyogenes* or *S. aureus* unless therapy selects out the gram-negative bacilli, particularly *P. aeruginosa*. A Gram stain of joint fluid from arthritis with a septic course may suggest a diagnosis, but gonococcal septicemia should be suspected with fever, tenosynovitis, polyarthralgias, and skin lesions. Penicillin G given intravenously at 10 million units a day for three days with follow-up oral ampicillin therapy is suitable for uncomplicated disease. Arthritis and a septic course in an intravenous drug addict should suggest staphylococcal, *P. aeruginosa*, or *Candida albicans* infection. The most common community-acquired pneumonias with bacteremia include *Streptococcus pneumoniae; S. aureus, Haemophilus influenzae*, and *S. pyogenes* are less common but also follow influenza. Examination of Gram stain of transtracheal aspiration specimen, pleural fluid, or sputum may yield the diagnosis. Penicillin G is the initial therapy unless *H. influenzae* or *S. aureus* is suspected. Alcoholics are prone to *S. pneumoniae, H. influenzae*, and *Klebsiella pneumoniae* infections. Community-acquired aspiration pneumonias are uncommonly associated with bacteremia; penicillin G is the drug of choice. Nosocomial pneumonias more frequently involve *S. aureus* and gram-negative bacilli; initial therapy should include a semisynthetic penicillin and an aminoglycoside and, if aspiration has occurred,

either penicillin, chloramphenicol, or clindamycin.

Therapy for acute bacterial endocarditis with an unstable clinical situation should be directed against *S. aureus* and *S. pneumoniae*, and, in older persons, group D streptococcus. Oxacillin with penicillin and gentamicin is one suitable empiric regimen. In intravenous drug addicts, oxacillin, carbenicillin and gentamicin (or tobramycin) will treat *S. aureus* and many gram-negative bacilli. Shunt and graft infections in chronic hemodialysis patients suggest *S. aureus* infections. Vancomycin or oxacillin are suitable unless Gram stain shows gram-negative bacilli; then an aminoglycoside should be given.

Immunosuppressed or neutropenic patients, or both, should be treated empirically for staphylococcal and gram-negative bacillary infections (Table 3). Therapy should be given even if fever is the only sign and the patient is otherwise stable.

Neonates and young infants are susceptible to varied pathogens, including the gram-negative enteric bacilli, Group B streptococci, *S. aureus*, and *Listeria monocytogenes*. Ampicillin and gentamicin are recommended unless staphylococcal infection is suspected.

Monitoring of Therapy. Toxicity should be watched for clinically and with appropriate laboratory tests (Table 2). Blood cultures should be repeated during and after therapy. Serum antibiotic determinations are valuable with aminoglycosides. Minimal inhibitory concentrations and minimal bactericidal concentrations are useful in endocarditis and frequently with neutropenic patients. Synergy studies are also useful with endocarditis.

Duration of Therapy. Generally therapy should be given for 2 weeks including at least 5 to 7 days of afebrile state with other signs of infection absent but there is considerable variability. Frequently, longer courses are necessary with surgical

TABLE 3. **Empiric Therapy of Presumed Bacteremia**

Oxacillin or methicillin or nafcillin and gentamicin* (penicillin optional)

or

Cephalosporin* and gentamicin

With severe neutropenia:

Oxacillin or methicillin or nafcillin plus gentamicin† and carbenicillin‡

With gastrointestinal or female genital tract source:

Chloramphenicol or clindamycin plus gentamicin† (plus penicillin if clostridia are suspected)

---

*Generally considered for use in suspected Klebsiella infection or allergy to penicillins

†Amikacin may be substituted for gentamicin if resistance to gentamicin is prevalent in nosocomial setting

‡Cephalosporin and gentamicin should be considered in patients allergic to penicillins

wounds. Endocarditis should be treated 4 to 6 weeks and 6 to 8 weeks for *S. aureus.* Neutropenic patients who respond clinically but have negative initial blood cultures should receive 5 to 7 days of therapy. Failure of therapy usually is due to undrained infection, use of an inappropriate agent, suboptimal levels of an agent, or neutropenia.

Adjunctive Measures

Drainage of suppuration from wounds, empyema, or surgical removal of necrotic tissue are mainstays in therapy. Relief of urinary or biliary obstruction or removal of infected vascular cannulas or shunts are also of paramount importance.

An adequate urinary output must be maintained. The pulse, arterial pressure, central venous or left atrial (pulmonary capillary wedge) pressure, urinary output, and fluid and electrolyte balance must be carefully monitored in the hypotensive patient. A Swan-Ganz catheter is recommended for patients with evidence of congestive heart failure or other cardiac disease. The plasma volume should be expanded with plasma, albumin, blood, or saline to restore blood pressure and maintain a urine output of 50 to 75 ml. per hour and a central venous pressure (CVP) of 13 to 15 cm. H_2O or pulmonary capillary wedge pressure (PCWP) of 15 to 18 mm. H_2O.

Tissue perfusion is more important than an arbitrary blood pressure. Pressors should be given to increase perfusion if plasma expansion is unsuccessful. They are not primary therapy. Dopamine is usually the agent of choice. It increases renal perfusion and has a positive inotropic effect at usual initial doses. It is given intravenously at 2 to 8 micrograms per kg. per minute and increased to 20 to 30 micrograms per kg. per minute if there is no effect. It is recommended for a volume replete patient who is oliguric (urine <20 ml. per hour) even if blood pressure is maintained. The beta-stimulator isoproterenol at an initial dose of 1 to 2 micrograms per minute is another choice; tachycardia and ventricular arrhythmias are relatively common. Metaraminol and levarterenol are of less value. Metabolic acidosis may require bicarbonate therapy. Reversal of disseminated intravascular coagulation documented by fibrin split product determinations is usually accomplished with control of the underlying disease; use of heparin, 5000 to 8000 units every 6 hours, is of controversial value. The use of high dose corticosteroids such as dexamethasone, 3 mg. per kg. intravenously, or methylprednisolone sodium succinate, 300 mg. per kg. and then repeated in 4 hours, is of unproved efficacy. Daily granulocyte transfusions may be of some value in neutropenic patients.

The overall mortality rate is probably 25 to 40 per cent, although it is 75 per cent or greater in some groups.

BRUCELLOSIS

method of
DENIS G. McDEVITT, M.D.
Belfast, Northern Ireland

Brucellosis is an infectious disease caused by microorganisms of the genus *Brucella* that is transmitted to man from lower animals. The three species primarily involved are *B. melitensis* (goats), *B. abortus* (cattle) and *B. suis* (swine). *B. canis* (dogs) has also been isolated occasionally. Eradication programs in the domestic animals concerned and pasteurization of milk and milk products have not only markedly reduced the incidence of human infection—in the United States, from 6300 cases in 1947 to less than 200 cases in 1976—but have also changed the pattern of disease. It is now primarily diagnosed in people whose occupations bring them into contact with infected animals: meat-packing plant employees, who contract infections due to *B. suis* from pork or *B. abortus* from beef, veterinarians, farmers, other livestock producers, and bacteriologists. In the United States, the most commonly isolated organism is *B. suis;* in Britain it is *B. abortus.* Milk products are seldom implicated, except for goat's milk cheese, which may be found locally in the United States or is imported into Britain from Europe. It contains *B. melitensis,* the organism most commonly producing brucellosis on a worldwide basis.

General Measures

Bed rest may be helpful in the early acute phase when the patients are febrile; it may improve weariness and pains, and aches may subside. If not, acetylsalicylic acid (aspirin), 600 mg., or acetaminophen, 1 gram four times daily, may be used to give relief of headache and generalized aches and pains, and either of these drugs can be continued as long as symptomatically necessary. Attention should be paid to the patient's hydration by encouraging adequate fluid intake orally or by the use of intravenous electrolyte or glucose solutions when dehydration is a problem. If troublesome insomnia occurs as part of the illness, a benzodiazepine may be given occasionally at night as a hypnotic—diazepam 2 or 5 mg. or flurazepam 15 mg. are suitable.

Antimicrobial Therapy

The course of acute brucellosis can be shortened and complications prevented by the early use of specific antimicrobial drugs. For patients with uncomplicated disease, tetracycline hydrochloride 0.5 gram orally should be given four times daily for 3 to 4 weeks. It should be taken on an empty stomach and the simultaneous use of iron tablets, antacids, or milk products should be avoided. Tetracycline should be avoided in young children and pregnant females; patients with renal insufficiency should be given oxytetracycline in preference. In some patients, the exhibition of tetracycline may precipitate a Herxheimer-like reaction in the first few hours, with fever, weakness, and hypotension. These symptoms may clear spontaneously but, if not, adrenocorticosteroids should be given (see below). In more severe cases of brucellosis or those with abscesses, streptomycin 0.5 gram intramuscularly twice daily may be given concurrently with the first 2 or 3 weeks of tetracycline therapy: it should not be given alone. When renal insufficiency exists, modification of streptomycin dosage may be required and plasma levels of streptomycin should be monitored if possible. A combination of trimethoprim, 80 mg., and sulfamethoxazole, 400 mg., has also been successfully used in the treatment of brucellosis. Suggested total daily dosage is six or eight tablets, divided for 8- or 12-hourly administration, and it is recommended that treatment be continued for 6 weeks to prevent relapse (this use of trimethoprim-sulfamethoxazole is not listed in the manufacturer's official directive). Trimethoprim-sulfamethoxazole should be used only in patients who are intolerant to or have not responded to the antimicrobials mentioned previously.

Relapse

Relapse of symptoms may occur in up to half the patients treated initially, and in some of these bacteremia will be found to have persisted or recurred. In other patients the pattern of symptoms becomes chronic, accompanied by persistently elevated agglutination titers. In the first instance, a second course of tetracycline should be tried and is often successful. Tetracycline, 0.5 gram four times daily, should be given for a further 4 weeks. If long-term use of broad-spectrum antibiotics results in overgrowth of the gastrointestinal tract with *Candida albicans,* treatment should be instituted with nystatin tablets 500,000 units orally every 8 hours until it clears. Further relapses or chronic symptoms should be treated by increasing the dose of tetracycline to 1 gram four times daily for 4 weeks or by adding streptomycin to the tetracycline therapy. Persistent illness can be treated with courses of antibiotics for 4 weeks every other month for several months. When all these measures fail, symptomatic remission has been induced in patients with chronic brucellosis with levamisole (still under investigation in the United States), a drug which reactivates cellular immune responses.

Corticosteroids

Corticosteroids may be required to prevent or attenuate Herxheimer-like reactions caused by antibiotic therapy. In addition, steroids may help to relieve the prostration of severely ill patients, including fever, toxemia, anorexia, and mental symptoms. When used, hydrocortisone, 100 mg. parenterally every 8 hours, may be given for 1 or 2 days, but at the same time prednisone, 40 mg. orally as a single daily dose, should also be commenced and continued for 4 to 7 days. In all but the most severe cases, oral prednisone will be sufficient on its own.

Complications

Where possible, abscesses should be drained surgically. Bone involvement—for example, spondylitis—can be treated conservatively by bed rest, antibiotic therapy, and appropriate joint support. Brucella endocarditis is an occasional but life-threatening complication; antimicrobial therapy alone is usually insufficient, and early replacement of the diseased valve or valves should be considered. Epididymo-orchitis responds to rest, antibiotics, adequate scrotal support, and analgesics.

Prevention

Effective vaccines are unavailable. Prevention should be directed at pasteurization of all milk and milk products and the use of adequate safety precautions and protective equipment in persons working in occupations involving potential contact with infection. Ultimately, eradication of the disease from animals by properly implemented slaughter programs is the only certain way of eliminating human brucellosis.

CHICKENPOX

method of
BRUCE A. TUCKER, M.D.,
and RICHARD J. WHITLEY, M.D.
Birmingham, Alabama

Introduction

Varicella-zoster virus (VZV), a DNA virus, is responsible for both chickenpox (varicella) and shingles (herpes zoster). Chickenpox, a primary infection, is a highly contagious disease of childhood characterized by fever and intensely pruritic, widespread crops of cutaneous vesicles. Shingles, however, results from reactivation of latent VZV and is characterized clinically by a painful, unilateral vesicular eruption most often localized to clearly demarcated dermatomes. Herpes zoster occurs as a sporadic disease, usually in elderly adults at an annual rate of 3.4 cases per 1000 persons. This chapter will deal specifically with current thoughts on therapy of chickenpox.

Varicella in the Normal Host

Clinical Manifestations.   Chickenpox in childhood is a mild exanthem and is quite contagious with a secondary attack rate of approximately 90 per cent. In adults the illness may be more severe, causing protracted vesicle formation and visceral complications such as pneumonitis and encephalitis. Chickenpox can occur in the neonatal period as a consequence of infection acquired antenatally in utero or at birth if the mother has active disease at the time of delivery. Chickenpox in normal children almost never causes serious illness. In contrast, chickenpox of the newborn and adult-acquired illness may be more severe and even lethal. In the northern hemisphere chickenpox is a disease of winter and spring. The incubation period averages 14 days with a range of 10 to 23 days. More than 90 per cent of cases occur in children between the ages of 2 and 8 years. Virus is transmitted by direct contact as early as two days prior to the onset of vesicular eruption. Low-grade fever and malaise may precede the rash by 48 hours in adults; in children rash is usually the first sign of disease. The rash begins on the trunk and scalp, spreading rapidly centripetally to involve the face and extremities. Crops of vesicular lesions are the hallmark of the disease. Typically lesions appear in all stages of development in a given patient, ranging from clear vesicles, which are most recent, to pustules and crusted or scabbed lesions. New lesions generally do not appear after 2 to 4 days and most will be crusted and noninfectious by the seventh day of illness.

Routine Management of Uncomplicated Cases. Prevention of chickenpox in a normal host is unnecessary and, therefore, no attempt at prophylaxis is indicated for this large patient population. Similarly, contacts need not be quarantined nor isolation procedures applied in the home unless there is an immunocompromised person in the family (see Compromised Host below).

Uncomplicated varicella is a benign illness, and routine medical care is for the most part supportive. Fingernails should be maintained short and clean to prevent the complication of secondary bacterial infection (see Complications below). Clean linens and clothing as well as good skin hygiene will also reduce the risk of secondary infection. Pruritus can be controlled with topical application of calamine lotion, cooling compresses, or soothing baths. Fever is usually not a major problem with chickenpox, but when present it can be managed with acetaminophen or salicylates at dosages appropriate for age. Should pruritus become intense, oral antihistamines are useful. Care should be employed in the utilization of oral antihistamines so as not to mask severe complications such as the development of encephalitis.

Complications in the Normal Host

Skin Infections.   Impetigo and pyoderma result from superinfection of vesicles with bacterial organisms, most commonly group A beta hemolytic streptococci or *Staphylococcus aureus*. Secondary skin infections should be treated with an appropriate systemic antibiotic as determined by cultures of the lesions and antimicrobial sensitivity assays. Bacteremia occurs rarely.

Hemorrhagic Varicella.   Hemorrhagic varicella is very rare but may be serious. It is characterized by generalized hemorrhage into the vesicles, petechiae, and ecchymoses. This particular form of varicella has been most frequently associated with underlying diseases that require cytolytic or cytotoxic drugs for therapy but also occurs in the normal host, particularly adults. No specific therapy of hemorrhagic varicella is indicated unless there is an underlying coagulopathy.

Varicella Pneumonia.   This complication primarily occurs in adults, as frequently as 10 to 15 per cent, and among the immunocompromised. Typically, 2 to 6 days after the appearance of rash and while vesicles continue to form, elevated temperature, cough, dyspnea, and even cyanosis and pleuritic chest pain herald the onset of varicella pneumonitis. Chest roentgenogram reveals bilateral, symmetrical lower and middle lobe infiltrates with hilar involvement that are usually "fluffy" in appearance. The clinical illness ranges from the very mildest and asymptomatic to fatal disease. Diagnosis can sometimes be confirmed by performing cytologic examinations of cells obtained by a deep tracheal aspirate with observation of intranuclear inclusions on histopathologic examination or by isolation of virus, not routinely available at most hospitals. Spontaneous improvement should parallel the resolution of cutaneous disease; however, bacterial superinfection and adult respiratory distress syndrome (ARDS) may complicate the patient's management.

There is no specific therapy for varicella pneumonitis. The usual measures for management of patients with respiratory infections should be implemented, namely, intensive nursing care, fluid management, and oxygen, if necessary. Treatment of ARDS with assisted ventilation and positive end expiratory pressure may be required. If assisted ventilation is required, or in the face of progressive lobar consolidation, surveillance for bacterial superinfection should be initiated and appropriate antimicrobial therapy instituted with a high index of suspicion. Presently, there is no proven benefit of corticosteroids for the management of this complication.

Encephalitis. Varicella encephalitis is reported to occur as frequently as once per 400 to 1000 cases of chickenpox. Encephalitis generally occurs at the end of vesicular eruption but may precede the rash. Characterized initially by confusion, vomiting, and altered consciousness, frequent cerebellar involvement results in ataxia and nystagmus. Central nervous system involvement may also be manifested as an aseptic meningitis characterized by cerebrospinal fluid lymphocytosis and usually normal protein and glucose values.

Asymptomatic cerebrospinal fluid pleocytosis requires only supportive care. In this situation, follow-up lumbar puncture is not indicated. For patients with encephalitis, the usual measures of maintenance—excellent supportive and nursing care—during a period of altered mental state are indicated. The airway must be maintained and, if necessary, intubation or tracheostomy performed in order to assist ventilation and manage secretions. Vital signs must be carefully monitored and intravenous fluids restricted in the event of increased intracranial pressure. Vigilance must be maintained for the appearance of bacterial pulmonary infection in critically ill patients. In the presence of cerebral edema and resultant increased intracranial pressure, dexamethasone has proved useful. The initial dosage of dexamethasone is 8 mg. intravenously followed by 4 mg. every 6 hours for 3 to 5 days or less if the edema is resolved. Corticosteroids should be discontinued promptly after the cerebral edema subsides. In the absence of cerebral edema and increased intracranial pressure, the use of steroids should be avoided. An additional drug useful for the control of cerebral edema is mannitol. A dosage of 1 to 2 grams per kg. can be given over 30 minutes followed by decreasing dosages to be administered as 6 hour continuous infusions. When mannitol is employed, careful attention to fluid intake and output is mandatory. Although fatalities do occur, the ultimate prognosis is favorable.

Although not discussed in detail, additional neurologic complications of varicella infection have been reported. These include transverse myelitis, Reye's syndrome, and Guillain-Barré syndrome.

Varicella Involvement of the Eye. Rarely in the course of chickenpox, vesicular lesions appear on the conjunctivae. They may be unilateral or bilateral, erupting along the lid margins or at the limbus. These vesicular lesions can either resolve spontaneously or evolve to umbilicated ulcers, resulting in secondary corneal involvement. Progression to keratitis, iridocyclitis, or optic neuritis has been described.

To manage eye complications, ophthalmology consultation should be obtained and slit lamp examination requested, searching for evidence of progressive disease. Mydriatics are useful for iritis and keratitis. Although the licensed antivirals idoxuridine (Stoxil) and adenine arabinoside (Vidarabine ophthalmic) have not been established as useful, they may be helpful, and their use is advised. Steroids are contraindicated except for late interstitial keratitis and only after cutaneous disease has resolved.

Chickenpox in the Immunocompromised Host

General Considerations. Susceptible children and adults who are either immunocompromised by disease (leukemia, lymphoma, etc.) or immunosuppressed by receiving medication (high dose steroids, etc.) for control of primary diseases (nephritis, lupus erythematosus, etc.) are at risk of developing progressive varicella, which may result in visceral disease and become life-threatening in a significant number of patients. Similarly, herpes zoster is a major problem for these patients; disseminated skin disease is not uncommon. Moreover, hepatic and pulmonary disease occurs, however, less frequently than with chickenpox. All the complications of varicella described here occur with increased frequency, are typically more severe and may be lethal in the immunocompromised host. Risk for developing varicella in this patient population can be assessed by humoral antibody studies to determine whether or not an individual patient has had prior infection with VZV. Immunocompromised adults and parents of children susceptible to chickenpox should avoid contact with active cases. Should exposure occur, the child's or adult's personal physician should be contacted immediately so that decisions regarding immunoprophylaxis can be made.

Prophylaxis. Susceptible patients who fulfill the criteria listed below should be given zoster immune globulin (ZIG). These criteria, as published in Morbidity and Mortality Weekly Report of October 28, 1977, are:
1. One of the following underlying illnesses or conditions
   A. Leukemia or lymphoma
   B. Congenital or acquired immunodeficiency
   C. Under immunosuppression medication
   D. Newly-born of mother with varicella
2. One of the following types of exposure to varicella or zoster patient
   A. Household contact
   B. Playmate contact (>1 hour indoor play)
   C. Hospital contact (same room or adjacent beds)
   D. Newborn contact (newborn whose mother contacted varicella within 4 days before delivery or within 48 hours after delivery)

3. Negative or unknown prior disease history
4. Age of less than 15 years
5. Request for treatment must be instituted within 72 hours of exposure

Passive immunization with ZIG,* currently an investigational drug, has been shown to prevent disease or at least ameliorate disease when appropriately administered. The drug has no effect once disease is present. The recommended prophylactic dosage is 1.25 ml. per 10 kg. of body weight. Former ZIG consultants and officials from the CDC Immunization Division, although no longer responsible for drug distribution, are available for consultation regarding alternative modes of therapy.

Therapy. Therapeutic measures listed here for complications in the normal host are all applicable to the immunocompromised patient. Because the disease in these patients is associated with both increased mortality and morbidity, numerous therapeutic investigations with experimental antiviral agents have been conducted or are currently underway. Adenine arabinoside and interferon have provided promising results in preliminary studies, but have not been approved by the Food and Drug Administration for routine therapy. Both of these compounds remain under investigation in national collaborative studies.

Other Considerations

Hospital Acquisition. Routine admission of patients with chickenpox should be discouraged. Such a policy only jeopardizes those patients at high risk who require hospitalization. Nevertheless, chickenpox patients do require hospitalization when severe complications occur. Isolation procedures should be instituted until the patient is over the infectious stages of disease (lesions scabbed). In that the major route of transmission is airborne, appropriate precautions should be undertaken to prevent secondary cases, as well as possible.

Chickenpox of the Newborn. Chickenpox in the newborn, developing as a consequence of disease late in gestation or at birth, has been reported to be of increased severity and may be lethal. Late maternal gestational infection does not allow sufficient time for the appearance of maternal antibody and, therefore, little if any, is available for transplacental passage. Mortality rates as high as 35 per cent have been reported in neonatal disease.

As noted under the indications above, ZIG has been approved for the investigational use in

---

*Available from: Division of Clinical Microbiology, Sidney Farber Cancer Institute, 44 Binney Street, Boston, Massachusetts; 617-732–3121

infants whose mothers develop chickenpox within 4 days of delivery or for the newborn who comes in contact with the infected mother within 24 hours of delivery. ZIG is available through the same central system as noted above.

CHOLERA

method of
DILIP MAHALANABIS, M.R.C.P.
Calcutta, India

General Considerations

The symptoms and signs of cholera are due to acute losses of a large volume of isotonic electrolyte solution relatively rich in bicarbonate. The diarrhea due to cholera is self-limiting and stops spontaneously in 2 to 6 days time, provided the patient can be kept alive by concurrent replacement of the lost fluid and salts. If untreated, a patient with severe cholera may die from hypovolemic shock within 24 hours of its onset.

No drug is known to influence the increased small bowel secretory process once the diarrheagenic exotoxin elaborated by the multiplying *Vibrio cholerae* attaches to specific receptor sites on the epithelial cells of the small bowel mucosa. Adenyl cyclase, a cell membrane associated enzyme, is stimulated by this toxin, leading to increased levels of cyclic AMP in the epithelial cells, which in turn triggers this irreversible process of increased secretory state. When this increased secretion exceeds the absorptive capacity of the small and large bowel, diarrhea ensues. A single exposure of this toxin for as short a period as 2 minutes leads to increased secretory state lasting about 24 hours.

In spite of the marked increase in small intestinal secretion, the mechanism of glucose-stimulated sodium and water absorption remains intact during the acute phase of the disease. This has led to the development of a simple and effective method of hydration through oral route by means of a suitable oral glucose electrolyte solution.

Suitable oral antibiotics (e.g., tetracycline) eliminate the cholera vibrio, prevent further production of diarrheagenic toxin, and reduce the duration and magnitude of diarrhea.

Similar clinical disease due to exotoxin-mediated secretory diarrhea indistinguishable from that due to *V. cholerae* may be produced by enterotoxigenic *Escherichia coli* and some noncholera vibrios. Diarrhea, however, is of smaller magnitude and of shorter duration. The principles of treatment remain the same and management of the patient does not depend upon correct bacteriologic diagnosis.

With high rates of fecal losses (more than 200 ml. per hour) the sodium concentration of stool is that of plasma, but the bicarbonate concentration is a good deal higher. As the rate of fecal losses diminishes, its sodium concentration also falls, but the potassium concentration rises. However, the feces remains isosmotic irrespective of its sodium concentration. Thus rehydration fluids should contain adequate base and potassium to prevent complications of acidosis and hypokalemia.

Principles of Treatment

1. *Rapid correction of hypovolemic shock* with intravenous fluids in a patient who has already developed signs of extensive fluid and electrolyte losses. Correction of acidosis and potassium loss concurrently, by a suitable intravenous solution.

2. *Oral glucose electrolyte solution therapy early in the disease* and before hypovolemic shock has developed, whenever possible.

3. *Maintenance of hydration by quantitative replacement of the continued losses* of fluid and electrolytes due to diarrhea by an oral glucose electrolyte solution as well as by judicious use of intravenous fluids to supplement oral therapy wherever necessary. Close supervision of all patients by trained personnel during the acute phase (first 24 hours) of the disease is mandatory.

4. *Use of a suitable antibiotic* to reduce the magnitude and duration of diarrhea. Tetracycline remains the drug of choice.

5. *Early introduction of a normal diet* to maintain nutrition. Occasional hypoglycemia in children is avoided by optimum use of oral glucose electrolyte solution in the general scheme of rehydration therapy.

Evaluation of Patients and Estimation of Volume Deficit

A rapid bedside evaluation is important and should be completed within a minute or two. It should include (1) a quick check on the history of diarrhea, vomiting, muscle cramps, and thirst; and (2) examination of the patient for skin turgor, sunken eyes with soft eyeballs, wrinkled fingers and toes, cold sweaty extremities, rate and volume of the radial pulse, blood pressure, state of the neck veins, the rate and depth of respiration, and weight of the patient. The latter is particularly important in children. These clinical features are of help in evaluating the degree of dehydration.

Clinically, the magnitude of fluid deficit can be assessed as follows:

1. Severe dehydration (approximate fluid deficit of 10 to 11 per cent of body weight) presents with marked thirst, muscle cramps, impalpable or barely palpable radial pulse, and a blood pressure which is often unrecordable. The patients have cold, clammy, and often cyanosed extremities and a marked loss of skin turgor with soft, sunken eyeballs. Stupor or coma may be observed in children. This degree of severity represents an approximate volume deficit equivalent to 100 to 110 ml. per kg. body weight, or 5 to 5.5 liters in a 50 kg. (110 lb.) adult.

2. Moderate dehydration (approximate fluid deficit of 5 to 9 per cent of body weight) presents with decreased skin turgor, postural hypotension, tachycardia, a weak pulse, and an increased thirst. This represents a volume deficit of about 50 to 90 ml. per kg. body weight, or about 4 liters in a 50 kg. (110 lb.) adult.

3. Mild dehydration (approximate fluid deficit up to 5 per cent of body weight) presents with a history of acute watery diarrhea only with slight or no clinical features of dehydration except for the increased thirst. The patient may already have a deficit of 40 to 50 ml. per kg. body weight or 2 to 2.5 liters in a 50 kg. (110 lb.) adult.

Errors in Diagnosis

During epidemics patients in shock with variable history of diarrhea due to other serious illnesses are sometimes brought to treatment centers with a presumed diagnosis of 'cholera.' These may include enteric fever; gram-negative bacteremia; meningitis; fulminant amebic colitis; myocardial infarction; certain neoplasms such as pancreatic adenoma, medullary carcinoma of the thyroid, and neural tumors of the gut; partial intestinal obstruction or other surgical conditions causing marked fluid deficit; and excessive use of laxatives. Such errors in diagnosis are largely avoided by a general awareness of these possibilities.

Electrolyte Replacement Solution

Fluid and electrolyte replacement in cholera has been simplified by the use of a single parenteral solution as well as a single oral glucose electrolyte solution suitable for both adults and children. Intravenous fluids should be used until correction of hypovolemic shock, when oral hydration may be resumed to replace the remaining deficit and further losses due to diarrhea. Nearly all patients who are not in shock and whose stool output after initiation of treatment does not exceed 12 ml. per kg. body weight per hour can be treated with an oral hydration solution alone. Early recognition and use of oral replacement solutions may save many lives in areas where treatment facilities are inadequate.

Intravenous Solutions. Replacement fluids should be designed to correct the volume deficit, by an isotonic salt solution that is rich in bicarbonate and potassium. The approximate composition of cholera stool in mM. per liter is: (1) in adults: sodium, 135; potassium, 15; bicarbonate, 45; and chloride, 100; and (2) in children: sodium, 105; potassium, 25; bicarbonate, 30; and chloride, 90. A suitable intravenous solution should contain a base (25 to 50 mM. per liter as bicarbonate, acetate, or lactate), potassium (10 to 15 mM. per liter), and possibly glucose (about 50 mM. per liter), in addition to sodium (about 110 to 130 mM. per liter). In practice the choice of fluid depends largely on availability and they are:

1. *Ringer's lactate* (Hartmann's solution for injection, BPC and USP) having a composition (in mEq. per liter): sodium, 130; potassium, 4; lactate, 28; chloride, 109; and calcium, 4. This solution has been extensively used both in adults as well as in children with success.

2. *A combination of isotonic sodium chloride solution two parts and one part of 1/6 M sodium lactate solution:* Sets of 3 bottles in a 2:1 ratio are repeated throughout the course of intravenous replacement. This combination provides (mEq. per liter): sodium, 154; lactate, 51; chloride, 103. It is poorly suited for children as there is a risk of producing hypernatremia. Both these solutions can be improved by adding potassium chloride 10 mEq. per liter. Additional glucose may need to be administered, particularly in children, if hypoglycemia is suspected.

3. *Isotonic sodium chloride solution* should be used only when no other suitable solution is available. Although it will correct initial hypovolemia and shock, prompt introduction of oral hydration is essential to replace base and potassium.

4. *An optimum intravenous solution called Diarrhoea Treatment Solution (DTS)* can be specially prepared as follows (in grams per liter): sodium chloride, 4; sodium acetate, 6.5; potassium chloride, 1; and glucose, 8; containing (in mM. per liter) sodium, 118; potassium, 13; chlorine, 83; HCO_3 (as acetate), 48; and glucose, 50. Although not commercially available and hence of no immediate practical value to individual clinicians, DTS is the solution of choice for optimum intravenous replacement and hence for stockpiling intravenous fluids for large scale use. In addition, acetate-containing solutions have a long shelf life.

Oral Glucose Electrolyte Solution. COMPOSITION. A universal oral hydration fluid, as advocated by WHO/UNICEF, has the following composition (in mM. per liter): sodium, 90; potassium, 20; chlorine, 80; HCO_3, 30; glucose, 111; and (in grams per liter) sodium chloride, 3.5; sodium bicarbonate, 2.5; potassium chloride, 1.5; and glucose, 20. Glucose facilitates absorption of sodium and water and as such is an essential ingredient. It can be substituted by sucrose, however, when glucose is not available, the quantity of sucrose required being double that of glucose.

HOW TO PREPARE. It is prepared using ordinary common salt, baking soda, potassium chloride, and glucose, by adding the requisite quantities to drinking water. Hot water should not be used, and the solution should never be autoclaved. It should be prepared daily to avoid bacterial growth. Dry ingredients can be preweighed into polyethylene bags and heat sealed for use when needed. For longer shelf life the salts and glucose should be packaged separately.

A well-tried, practical way of preparing the solution at bedside is to use the empty barrel of a 5-ml. syringe and measure the equivalent volumes of the ingredients (as fine dry powders). The measures by volume with the syringe barrel are: sodium chloride, 3 ml.; sodium bicarbonate, 3 ml.; potassium chloride, 1.5 ml. and glucose, 30 ml., for 1 liter of drinking water. These volume measures of the ingredients correspond to their respective weights for the standard oral solution. When sucrose is substituted for glucose, 40 grams of sucrose are used for 1 liter of fluid and its equivalent volume by syringe barrel is 50 ml.

The oral solution can be given by mouth or nasogastric tube. The latter is especially convenient in children and permits the patient to rest. The solution has slightly salty taste but is well tolerated and accepted by the patient and flavoring is not needed. A nasogastric drip rate of 10 to 15 ml. per kg. per hour (i.e., 500 to 750 ml. per hour in a 50 kg. adult) is well tolerated by adults and children as well.

Vomiting is equally common in both parenterally treated and orally treated patients during the first 4 to 6 hours of treatment. It does not usually interfere with oral hydration, provided it is given in small amounts, frequently. Alternatively, nasogastric drip can obviate the problem of vomiting. If vomiting is severe, intravenous fluids should be given to achieve complete hydration, after which oral fluids may be resumed to replace ongoing losses.

In 10 to 15 per cent of severely affected patients oral fluid may not be adequate to maintain hydration and intravenous fluids are needed to supplement oral therapy, the reasons being (1) rate of fecal losses are too high for oral fluids to keep up with; a patient with a fluid loss of 10 to 20 ml. per kg. per hour (i.e., 10 to 20 liters per day in a

40 kg. adult) or greater is not usually able to maintain fluid balance with oral fluids alone; (2) stool output may increase up to 20 per cent due to oral hydration alone; (3) temporary glucose malabsorption is known to occur in about 2 per cent of patients, as evidenced by lack of clinical response and persistence of profuse watery diarrhea; and (4) a large unabsorbed intestinal or gastric pool or both of fluid may accumulate, leading to the persistence of clinical signs of dehydration. In view of these factors, continued close supervision by trained personnel is important, so that infusion of intravenous solutions to supplement oral fluids may be undertaken whenever necessary.

Initial Replacement

During this phase, fluid is replaced rapidly to correct the deficit already present at the time of admission. Patients admitted with hypovolemic shock must be treated immediately with intravenous fluids. After a quick clinical evaluation, such a patient is preferably put on a "cholera cot" to facilitate stool collection. This is an ordinary cot altered to provide a hole 23 cm. (9 inches) in diameter beneath the patients' buttocks. A rubber sheet with a central sleeve passing through the hole covers the bed. Feces are easily passed through this hole and collected for measurement in a bucket beneath the bed. All fluid output and intake are recorded on a bedside chart.

Adults. A large intravenous needle (18 or 19 gauge) is placed into an arm or leg vein. In a very ill patient two infusions in different sites may be started at the same time and fluids given as fast as possible until blood pressure is restored. If an infusion cannot be established quickly, a femoral vein drip is established as follows: the skin is cleaned with iodine and alcohol, a needle on a syringe is passed vertically into the femoral vein (just medial to the pulsation of femoral artery in the femoral triangle) and a gentle negative suction is kept on the piston until dark nonpulsating venous blood flows into it; the syringe is detached and the infusion started; the needle must be held upright until enough infusion is given to restore blood pressure and a peripheral vein infusion can be started. This procedure avoids the time-consuming venous cutdown. In a severely ill patient, the aim should be to infuse approximately 2 liters in 30 minutes. The total estimated deficit should be given within 2 to 3 hours of starting the treatment.

Children. Use of a scalp vein needle is of practical value in starting an intravenous drip. Any arm or leg vein as well as the jugular vein can be used for this purpose. In case of difficulty, femoral vein infusion can be established to combat the hypovolemic shock. A child in hypovolemic shock should receive 40 to 50 ml. per kg. of body weight of intravenous fluid over a period of 1 hour; this is generally adequate to restore the radial pulse and blood pressure. The same intravenous fluid as used in adults can be used, provided water is given freely by mouth after completing the initial hydration.

Once hypovolemic shock has been corrected by intravenous fluids, the remaining deficit can be made up either by continuing intravenous therapy or by oral rehydration solution. The decision will be guided by the alertness of the patient and the severity of vomiting. The remaining deficit should be corrected over the next 2 to 3 hours in adults and 6 to 8 hours in children. Further fecal losses are quantitatively replaced in addition to the calculated deficit.

Response to rehydration therapy is assessed by absence of the signs of dehydration; weight gain (patients with severe dehydration should gain 8 to 10 per cent of the body weight after adequate hydration, a particularly useful sign in small children) and restoration of urine output to normal (usually takes 12 to 20 hours).

Plasma specific gravity (GP) (normal 1.024 to 1.027) is a useful additional aid and can be measured at the bed side with a temperature-compensated hand refractometer (T.S. Meter, American Optical Co.). In case of severe dehydration plasma specific gravity (GP) may be as high as 1.045 in adults and 1.035 in small children. It is also helpful in patients with shock due to other causes, as the GP may be normal in them.

Maintenance Therapy

During this phase continued stool losses are replaced, as they occur, until diarrhea ceases. As the deficit on admission has already been corrected, the patient is no longer in serious acidosis or shock. Maintenance therapy may be accomplished by oral glucose electrolyte solution alone in the majority of patients. Occasionally, intravenous fluids may need to be given in addition. When adequately treated with antibiotics, this period does not usually last beyond 48 hours, and most of the fecal losses occur during the first 24 hours. Marked increase in the rate of stool output may often be noticed after hypovolemic shock has been corrected by initial hydration.

Amount and Rate of Oral Fluid

The amount of oral fluids to be given is guided by the stool output. Initially, when the output is not known, an approximate rate of 15 ml. per kg. per hour is given. The patient is evaluated every 2 to 4 hours, and an amount equal to 1.5 times the stool output of the previous 4 hours should be given over the next 4 hours. This will replace the fecal losses as well as furnish adequate free water to the adults. Children under 5 years would require additional free water by mouth and efforts should be made to administer water, about 80 to 120 ml. per kg. in 24 hours. With small children when fecal output cannot be measured, repeated clinical examination and weighing will be necessary. An increase in heart rate and a decrease in skin turgor, associated with a rise in plasma specific gravity and hematocrit values indicate inadequate fluid balance, and intravenous supplementation is needed. Restlessness and thirst are useful signs in children to indicate inadequate replacement.

Diet

Normal diet for age should be resumed as soon as the patient is hungry and one should not wait for the diarrhea to cease. Breast-feeding should be resumed after correction of the initial dehydration in breast-fed children. Older children should take their usual solid food as soon as they are well enough to eat. This is important in preventing malnutrition.

Antibiotics

Oral tetracycline is the drug of choice in cholera. It should be given in a dose of 500 mg. every 6 hours for 48 hours in adults, and 12.5 mg. per kg. per dose every 6 hours for 48 hours in children. The drug is started 3 to 6 hours after initiation of treatment. When tetracycline is not available, other useful antibacterial agents are furazolidone and chloramphenicol. The former is given in a 100 mg. dose every 6 hours to adults, and 5 mg. per kg. per day divided into four doses in children. Chloramphenicol is given in a dosage of 500 mg. every 6 hours in adults and 75 mg. per kg. per day divided into four doses in children. Either agent should be given for a period of 72 hours.

Termination of Treatment

Fluid replacement should continue until diarrhea ceases. A full course of tetracycline should be given even though diarrhea stops sooner. The patient may be discharged within 24 hours of the cessation of diarrhea and the completion of antibiotic therapy.

Complications

Pyrogen reaction, a common complication in many cholera-affeced areas of the world, is largely due to the use of unsatisfactory parenteral fluids and administration sets. This is largely eliminated by the use of approved quality intravenous solutions and disposable administration sets.

Serious complications of cholera are largely prevented by appropriate replacement therapy. The following complications may arise due to inadequate treatment: (1) Persistent or recurrent dehydration, leading to hypovolemia and shock is usually due to inadequate volume replacement. When a patient is not responding adequately to therapy, a careful assessment of the fluid replacement should be made. Rarely, a cardiac infarct or infarction of other vital organs may supervene. (2) Persistence of nausea and vomiting is mostly due to inadequate correction of acidosis or hypovolemia or both. (3) Acute renal failure sometimes occurs. Patients with renal failure reported to be caused by cholera were brought to the treatment centers several days after the onset of the disease and had received inadequate replacement therapy associated with prolonged and repeated episodes of hypotension. By instituting prompt and adequate replacement therapy this complication has been largely eliminated. (4) Hypokalemia in adults is rarely symptomatic. In children it may lead to abdominal distention, paralytic ileus, cardiac arrhythmias, and muscular weakness. Routine use of oral hydration fluids containing potassium largely prevents this complication. Potassium replacement can safely be started from the onset of therapy without waiting for urine to flow unless there is a history of preexisting renal disease. (5) Overhydration is a common complication in children manifested by puffiness of the eyes, slow pulse, full neck veins, and ultimately frank cardiac failure. Hypernatremia is an occasional complication of salt overload. Frank pulmonary edema is an occasional complication in patients overhydrated with salt solutions without correction of acidosis. (6) Hypoglycemia is an occasional complication in children who do not receive glucose and can lead to coma and convulsion. Rarely, prolonged coma of uncertain origin is known to occur in children. Adequately managed, they should recover completely. (7) Abortion often occurs in the third trimester of pregnancy when dehydration is severe.

Useless Measures

Some casually employed useless or even harmful measures include: (1) vasopressors (cholera patients with hypovolemic shock are already maximally vasoconstricted), (2) steroids, (3) so-called cardiac stimulants, (4) oxygen, (5) blood or plasma transfusions, and (6) various antidiarrhea medicines.

DIPHTHERIA

method of
OTTO F. SIEBER, JR., M.D.
Tucson, Arizona

Diphtheria is an acute infectious disease caused by *Corynebacterium diphtheriae*. It is characterized by growth of the organism on respiratory mucous membranes or skin and after an incubation period of 1 to 7 days, may be associated with production of an exotoxin leading to systemic disease.

Therapy

The aims of therapy in patients with diphtheria are (1) to neutralize *C. diphtheriae* toxin, (2) to eradicate organisms from the host, (3) to anticipate, to prevent, and to treat complications, (4) to prevent spread of the organisms to other susceptible persons, and (5) to prevent recurrence of infection in treated patients.

The successful therapy of diphtheria is coupled with the decision to institute therapy, which is based upon (1) the skills and awareness of the clinician in considering and diagnosing the disease early; (2) the epidemiology of *C. diphtheriae* in the community (immunization level, socioeconomic status, previous cases in the community, season of the year); (3) the need for treatment prior to proliferation and tissue fixation of large or excessive amounts of antitoxin; and (4) the hazards of available specific therapy (horse-serum).

Uncomplicated Diphtheria

When diphtherial disease is localized to the skin or the mucous membranes of the nose, tonsils, or pharynx without manifest complications, the primary treatment aims are to neutralize free toxin, to eliminate organisms from the primary or local sites of infection which are producing toxin and to prevent complications. The measures that follow are maximally effective only in this phase of the disease, but should be utilized whenever a diagnosis of diphtheria is made.

Hospitalization. Hospitalization is indicated for all patients in whom acute diphtheria is suspected. Because fewer cases of diphtheria are being seen, the uncertainty of the diagnosis may result in a delay. Under such circumstances, an increase in complications should be expected, which warrants therapy and monitoring of the disease course in an hospital setting.

Isolation. Isolation is indicated for all patients in whom diphtheria is considered a clinical diagnostic possibility. Spread of the organism is mainly by droplets but also by contact from patients and carriers. Droplets commonly enter the respiratory tract but occasionally are spread to other mucous membranes such as the conjunctivae. Direct contact or fomite contact may occur from the skin of patients or carriers. The risk of spread to family members or health professionals caring for such patients is great.

Isolation requires a *private room* for each new diphtheria patient. However, patients may be placed together if they are in the same phase of therapy of their disease. This procedure will minimize the possibility of a partially treated patient becoming a carrier if another patient, untreated and fully contagious, is placed in the same room.

Both respiratory and skin isolation techniques must be utilized and must include gown, mask, and, if possible, gloves. Careful handwashing techniques are mandatory.

Isolation may be discontinued when cultures of the nose, throat, or other primary site of infection obtained on 3 consecutive days have been negative. Although organisms may be eliminated from a host as early as the fourth day of a course of antibiotic therapy, cultures to determine the end of the isolation period should be obtained no earlier than 2 days after a full course of antibiotic therapy has been completed (see Duration of Antibiotic Therapy below).

Antitoxin. DIPHTHERIA ANTITOXIN (U.S.P.). This is essential and is indicated in all situations in which the diagnosis of diphtheria is entertained. Its use is based upon clinical indications alone. Untimely delay in its administration, such as awaiting definitive microbiologic diagnosis, is associated with an increase in mortality from 0 per cent (if antitoxin is used within 24 hours of onset of disease) to 16 per cent (if use is delayed as little as 4 days from onset of disease).

PREPARATION OF PATIENTS FOR ADMINISTRATION OF HORSE-SERUM DERIVED ANTITOXIN. As the diphtheria antitoxin is available only as a horse-serum derived bacterial antitoxin, its use requires precautions, including the testing of all patients for sensitivity to horse serum prior to administration. In preparation for sensitivity testing or treatment with antitoxin, a syringe with 1:1000 aqueous epinephrine chloride should be available. Doses of 0.01 ml. per kg. of body weight of the epinephrine solution may be administered subcutaneously or intravenously (maximum 0.5 ml.) if reactions occur.

TEST FOR SENSITIVITY TO HORSE SERUM. Selection of the initial test for determining if sensitivity to horse serum exists is dependent upon the patient's history of prior receipt of or reaction to horse serum. With a positive history of exposure or reaction, a *scratch test* should be performed, followed by an *intradermal test*. A conjunctival test has also been utilized, but has disadvantages (1) in interpretation if used in children or (2) in safety, for the patient who has a positive reaction and is unable to eliminate the antigen from the eye.

The *scratch test* should be performed as the initial test for horse serum hypersensitivity in sensitive persons. A drop of a 1:1000 dilution of antitoxin in isotonic saline solution is placed on the skin, with a drop of diluent placed on a second site as a control. A scratch is made in the skin through both solutions; the testing material removed after 30 seconds; and the test read after 20 minutes. A positive reaction is one in which erythema exceeds 1 cm. size, with induration or pseudopod formation or both. The test may be repeated with a 1:100 dilution of antitoxin if the reaction is negative or doubtful.

An *intradermal skin test* should be employed to test for sensitivity to horse serum prior to its therapeutic administration in any patient. Intradermal testing utilizes 0.1 ml. of a 1:1000 dilution of diphtheria antitoxin in isotonic saline solution. A positive reaction is determined at 20 minutes and is one in which erythema exceeds 1 cm. in size, with induration or pseudopod formation or both. If there is doubt as to the quality of this initial reaction, a second test may be performed using a 1:100 dilution of antitoxin. A control injection of an equal amount of isotonic saline diluent should be utilized in another site.

Desensitization to Horse Serum. If either of the tests for sensitivity to horse serum is positive in a patient, desensitization to the antitoxin is required prior to antitoxin administration for therapeutic purposes. Intramuscular diphenhydramine hydrochloride has been utilized by some to minimize allergic reaction. It is administered prior to the beginning of desensitization (25 mg. for infants and children 2 to 5 years of age; 50 mg., 6 to 14 years of age; 50 to 100 mg., if 15 years of age or over).

Progressively larger amounts of increasingly concentrated dilutions of antitoxin should be utilized by each of three routes of administration beginning with subcutaneous administration of antitoxin, then intramuscular, and finally intravenous administration. The initial injection should be no more than 0.05 ml. of a 1:20 dilution of antitoxin, subcutaneously. At 20 minute intervals, the dose is doubled, until 0.8 ml. is accepted. The same schedule is then followed for the intramuscular route of administration. When this is tolerated, 0.1 ml. of the 1:20 dilution may be given intravenously, followed by careful intravenous administration of 0.1 ml. of undiluted antitoxin.

Dosage of Antitoxin. Dosage is determined by (1) site and localization or extent of disease, (2) severity of symptoms, and (3) time interval from onset of symptoms. Each milliliter of antitoxin contains not less than 500 antitoxic units.

For nasal, tonsillar, or pharyngeal diphtheria that is mild and localized without crossing adjacent anatomical areas, 40,000 units of antitoxin should be used; with increasing severity, as seen with progression to pharyngeal diphtheria, 80,000 units of antitoxin should be given. When treatment is delayed (disease over 48 hours' duration), pharyngeal disease is severe or associated with cervical edema ("bull neck"); with laryngeal disease or involvement of multiple disease sites in the respiratory tract (naso-tonsillo-pharyngo-laryngeal diphtheria), 120,000 units of antitoxin should be administered.

Route of Administration. The dose of antitoxin should be diluted in isotonic saline solution to a 1:10 dilution, but the amount to be administered should not exceed 200 ml. of solution. The total amount of antitoxin and diluent should be administered intravenously over a 30 minute period.

Allergic Reactions to Antitoxin. Two types of reactions may occur after the administration of horse serum antitoxin: immediate (early) and delayed (serum sickness). Some physicians have recommended the use of antagonists of vasoactive amines (cyproheptadine or hydroxyzine hydrochloride) to attempt to modify the course of serum sickness. Both drugs have been described as being efficacious, if given in a prophylactic manner for a 12 day period, beginning on the fourth day after the antitoxin has been administered.

Antibiotics. Antibiotic usage is indicated in all patients with diphtheria. However, antibiotics are only an adjunct, not a substitute for antitoxin administration. An inexperienced physician may inappropriately consider that antibiotics may be used in lieu of antitoxin in an attempt to avoid the administration of horse serum and the patient's possible reaction to it. Clinical diphtheria results from available circulating and fixed toxin, which is not directly affected by antibiotic administration. However, antibiotics effectively eliminate *C. diphtheriae* from the respiratory tract or skin of the host and can eliminate possible secondary bacterial infection from agents such as the group A beta hemolytic streptococcus.

Selection of Antibiotics. penicillin. Penicillin is the drug of choice for treatment of acute diphtheria and may be administered orally if tolerated, or parenterally. In infants and children 25,000 to 50,000 units per kg. per day should be utilized (maximum 1 gram per day); 250 mg. of phenoxymethyl penicillin should be used four times daily for adults. If parenteral therapy is necessary, intravenous aqueous penicillin G (300,000 to 600,000 units per day divided into four doses for infants and children; 2 to 4 million units per day divided into four doses for adults); or intramuscular procaine penicillin G (600,000 units every 12 hours) may be used.

ERYTHROMYCIN. Erythromycin should be used only when penicillin therapy is contraindicated (e.g., penicillin allergy). It may be given orally as 25 to 50 mg. per kg. per day divided into four doses. The intravenous administration of erythromycin is associated with a high incidence of phlebitis, and if the intravenous route of administration is necessary in a penicillin-allergic patient, clindamycin may be used instead.

CLINDAMYCIN. Clindamycin dosage is 25 to 40 mg. per kg. per day divided into four doses, which may be administered orally or intravenously every 6 hours.

DURATION OF ANTIMICROBIAL THERAPY. Antibiotic therapy should be maintained for 7 to 10 days, depending upon the severity of infection. Although most sites of infection are negative for *C. diphtheriae* within 1 to 7 days of the time of initiation of antibiotic therapy, therapy is not completed until a daily culture on each of 3 consecutive days is negative for *C. diphtheriae*. The first culture should be obtained 2 days after antibiotics have been discontinued.

Bed Rest. The cardiac complication rate in diphtheria appears to be related to the level of physical activity permitted during the early stages of the disease. Bed rest should be complete and maintained for a period of 10 to 14 days for all patients with uncomplicated diphtheria. Physical activity should be restricted for an additional 2 weeks after release from the hospital.

Diet. Adequate nutritional support should be maintained throughout the illness. No special diets are necessary if food can be easily swallowed.

Symptomatic Therapy. Codeine (3 mg. per kg. per 24 hours) may be necessary for relief of pain. Isotonic saline solution irrigations of the pharynx will produce relief of pain as well as assist in mechanical removal of the membrane.

Diagnostic Studies. Cardiac complications should be anticipated in all patients with diphtheria. A baseline electrocardiogram, echocardiogram if available, and serum glutamic oxaloacetic transaminase determination should be obtained in all patients, even in the absence of cardiac findings, to provide a comparison of cardiac rhythm and left ventricular function should cardiac complications occur. Daily electrocardiograms (ECGs) should be obtained until the patient is discharged.

Complications of Diphtheria

Complications of diphtheria develop in patients with acute diphtheria if the infection is caused by strains of *C. diphtheriae* that have elaborated large amounts of toxin, if the diagnosis and specific antitoxin therapy has been delayed, if bed rest is not maintained, or if reinfection occurs during the convalescent phase of the acute illness. Complications that may occur include respiratory failure from laryngeal-tracheal obstruction, pneumonia, myocarditis, and cardiac arrhythmia, shock, neuritis, and thrombocytopenia.

Respiratory Failure. Respiratory failure results from proliferation of the diphtheritic membrane in the larynx and trachea leading to obstruction in the respiratory tract with resultant asphyxiation. It should be anticipated in all patients in whom a pharyngeal membrane can be observed, as this identifies the patient with the potential for inferior progression of the membrane to the larynx and trachea. Direct laryngoscopy or bronchoscopy may be useful in determining the extent of the membrane, but should be performed only by a competent physician.

AIRWAY. An airway must be provided in anticipation of or in immediate response to airway embarrassment. It is most successful if provided prior to evidence of frank respiratory failure (cyanosis), with its inherent risk of anoxia and cardiac arrest. Restlessness and use of accessory respiratory muscles are the most reliable clinical indicators for an airway. Indirect insertion of an airway, tracheostomy, laryngoscopy, or bronchoscopy with removal of any dislodged pieces of membrane may be necessary.

OXYGEN. Oxygen is indicated in all instances of respiratory failure. Blood gases should be monitored.

CORTICOSTEROIDS. The efficacy of steroids is unknown. If disease is found to be limited to the larynx (acute laryngeal diphtheria), hydrocortisone sodium acetate, 5 mg. per kg. per day divided into three doses, has been given intravenously or intramuscularly for 1 to 2 days.

Pneumonia. Bronchopneumonia due to *C. diphtheriae* or pneumonia secondary to opportunistic gram-negative hospital-acquired organisms may occur in patients with moderate to severe diphtheria. Antibiotic therapy may be modified to cover gram-negative organisms prevalent in the local hospital environment, such as *Escherichia coli*, *Pseudomonas aeruginosa*, and *Klebsiella pneumoniae*.

Myocarditis. Up to 65 per cent of patients

with diphtheria develop myocarditis. Although signs and symptoms may be present as early as 48 hours after onset of disease, most cardiac manifestations do not occur for 1 to 2 weeks, and, rarely, may be delayed for up to 6 weeks. However, patients with severe diphtheria can be expected to manifest myocardial disease early. Myocarditis may also develop in those patients who have received antitoxin early because of the unusual affinity of diphtheria toxin for myocardial tissue. If severe, myocarditis is manifest by a rapid, thready pulse, distant and poor quality heart sounds, cardiac arrhythmias, and cardiac dilatation with congestive failure and hepatomegaly and edema.

Referral. If myocarditis is manifested, continuous cardiac evaluation is mandatory. If appropriate intensive and continued evaluation and care cannot be provided, transfer to a referral center is indicated.

Monitoring of Cardiac Status. Cardiac monitoring is indicated in all patients with diphtheria. This may be accomplished by obtaining daily ECGs or, preferably, by continuous external cardiac monitoring. Echocardiograms are also indicated.

Conduction defects are common. Left hemianterior block frequently occurs. Complete heart block is an ominous prognostic sign.

1. Strict bed rest is mandatory. Sudden death may occur following arrhythmias induced by physical exertion. Bed rest should be maintained for at least 4 weeks followed by a gradual increase in activity.

2. Transvenous electrical pacing for minor to complete heart block associated with diphtheritic myocarditis has been successful in some patients.

3. Steroids may be useful in the treatment of myocarditis. One to 2 mg. per kg. per day of prednisone for 2 weeks, may lessen the severity of myocarditis.

Heart failure is difficult to treat. It occurs most frequently during the second week of illness and the usual cardiac measures should be used with caution.

1. Central venous pressure should be monitored.

2. Salt and fluid intake should be restricted.

3. Furosemide is preferred as a diuretic.

4. Digoxin should be used for digitalization (limit digitalization dosage to one-half the usual dose and maintenance dosage to one-fifth the usual daily dose).

Shock may occur from myocarditis or with overwhelming toxemia. Shock should be treated with isoproterenol, 0.1 to 0.2 micrograms per kg. per minute, as a continuous intravenous infusion.

Ventricular tachycardia/fibrillation may be a terminal event in severe diphtheritic myocarditis. Lidocaine hydrochloride, 1 mg. per kg. (maximum 50 mg.), may be given by rapid infusion.

Neurologic Complications. Neurologic effects of diphtheritic toxin may occur early (palatal paralysis) or as late as 6 to 8 weeks (respiratory muscle paralysis).

Cranial nerve paralysis may involve cranial nerves III, V, IX, or X, either singly or in combination. The most common paralysis is palatal. Nutritional supportive care should be emphasized when this type of paralysis develops. Nasogastric feedings or hyperalimentation is necessary if paralysis is severe enough.

Respiratory muscle paralysis may require ventilation by mechanical means until return of normal respiratory function.

Thrombocytopenia. Thrombocytopenia may occur in severe diphtheria and is a poor prognostic sign. If present in patients requiring invasive procedures such as tracheostomy, platelet transfusions may be of benefit.

Carrier State

The carrier state occurs when a patient with diphtheria continues to harbor *C. diphtheriae* after being inadequately treated with antibiotics or when the patient has been reexposed to toxigenic organisms during convalescence from the acute illness. It may also occur when contact with a patient with diphtheria leads to carriage of the toxigenic organism by another person who does not develop symptoms. Carriage may result in organisms either on the skin or in the respiratory tract.

The carrier state is treated by confining the carrier to the hospital or home until appropriate administration of an antibiotic has been completed.

1. Oral erythromycin, 20 to 50 mg. per kg. per day in four divided doses (maximum 2 grams per day), is preferred, for a period of 10 days.

2. Clindamycin, 20 mg. per kg. per day orally in four divided doses (maximum 600 mg. per day) for 10 days, may also be effective.

3. When compliance is a problem, or in an epidemic situation, intramuscular penicillin should be given. Benzathine penicillin G may be given intramuscularly (600,000 units for patients 1 to 5 years of age; 1.2 million units for those over 5 years of age).

The carrier state is ended if two nose and throat cultures, taken 24 hours apart and at a time when antibiotic therapy has been ended for 24 hours, are negative for toxigenic *C. diphtheriae*.

Use of diphtheria antitoxin is contraindicated in treating the carrier state because of the risk of development of sensitivity to horse serum and because antimicrobial therapy is so highly successful.

Prevention of Disease in Exposed Persons

Diphtheria is preventable or can be modified extensively by active immunization if a basic series has been completed. Persons exposed to patients with diphtheria may not be completely immunized. They may require an approach in prevention that utilizes both immunization and antibiotic therapy.

For asymptomatic unimmunized contacts (household or health professional):

1. Culture the nasopharynx and throat for toxigenic *C. diphtheriae*.

2. Utilize chemoprophylaxis with erythromycin 20 to 50 mg. per kg. per day in four doses orally for 10 days, or benzathine penicillin G, 600,000 to 1,200,000 units intramuscularly. Either antibiotic may be given at the time contact with a patient with diphtheria has occurred and should not await the results of culture.

3. Begin diphtheria toxoid immunization. As diphtheria toxoid for adults is available only in combination with tetanus toxoid (Td), Td is the only preparation that can be administered. For the child under 8 years of age, pediatric DT may be used; for the child under 6 years of age, DPT may be used.

4. Schick testing is no longer indicated prior to administration of Td.

5. Daily surveillance for symptoms of diphtheria should be provided each contact. This will require close coordination with the local health department.

6. At the present time, the decision to use diphtheria antitoxin for the person who has had contact with a patient with diphtheria must balance the risk of serum reaction to horse serum with the risk of diphtheria. In a recent large outbreak of diphtheria, antimicrobial therapy was utilized in lieu of administration of diphtheria antitoxin with excellent benefit.

Immunization is best accomplished prior to exposure in a schedule such as that recommended by the Report of the Committee on Infectious Diseases, American Academy of Pediatrics, 1977.

All patients with acute diphtheria should be immunized after recovery, because early use of antitoxin interferes with natural immunity.

BACILLARY DYSENTERY

method of
MYRON M. LEVINE, M.D.,
and MARGARET B. RENNELS, M.D.
Baltimore, Maryland

Strictly-speaking, dysentery refers to the presence of blood and mucus in stools of which *Shigella* infection is a major cause. However, bacillary dysentery has become synonymous with shigellosis in any of its clinical presentations. Organisms of the genus *Shigella* are responsible for a spectrum of clinical illness, including asymptomatic infection, diarrhea without fever, and severe dysentery manifested by high fever, toxemia, chills, convulsions (in children), tenesmus, and bloody mucoid stools.

Familiarization with several aspects of the pathogenesis and epidemiology of *Shigella* infection is important for understanding appropriate therapy. Virulent organisms possess the ability to invade mucosal epithelial cells of the ileocecal region and length of the colon; proliferation within epithelial cells results in mucosal destruction and elicitation of intense polymorphonuclear leukocyte infiltration (which may be seen in stool mucus when stained with methylene blue). Man and certain primates are the only natural hosts and reservoirs of *Shigella*. As few as 10 to 200 virulent organisms can result in acute bacillary dysentery in healthy, well-nourished adults; this represents an inoculum size 100- to 10,000-fold smaller than that believed to be required to contract illness with other bacterial enteropathogens such as *Vibrio cholerae, Salmonella typhi* and enterotoxigenic *Escherichia coli*. As a consequence of the extremely small infective inoculum, shigellosis (bacillary dysentery) is typically spread by contact transmission with infected hands, although transmission by contaminated food and water also does occur. Thus, shigellosis spreads easily wherever personal hygiene is primitive, as in day-care nurseries and institutions for mentally-retarded and psychotic persons. In the crowded inner-city ecology, person-to-person transmission of *Shigella* often follows introduction into the household by a young school-age or day-care–age child.

Although any serotype of *Shigella* can cause either mild diarrhea or fulminating dysentery, *S. sonnei* tends to be associated with milder disease than *S. flexneri* or *S. dysenteriae* serotypes. *S. dysenteriae* 1, the Shiga bacillus, is unique among *Shigella* because of its clinical virulence and pandemic potential. Shiga bacillus is commonly associated with fulminant clinical illness, marked by high fever, abdominal pain, toxemia, tenesmus, severe dysentery, vomiting, and convulsions (in children). Leukemoid reactions, marked hypoproteinemia and hemolytic-uremic syndrome have been reported with Shiga dysentery infections in Bangladesh and Central America in recent years.

Therapy

The therapy of acute bacillary dysentery may be divided into four categories including: emergency treatment of life-endangering complications, supportive measures, specific antibacterial drugs, and health education.

Potentially Life-Endangering Emergencies. *Shock,* secondary to diarrheal dehydration, can occur in the course of acute shigellosis, particularly in infants. Severe dehydration, shock, and acidosis must be vigorously treated with an intravenous "push" of 20 to 30 ml. per kg. of Ringer's lactate, isotonic saline, or similar isotonic solution given rapidly over 1 hour. This bolus of fluid rapidly expands the intravascular volume and usually results in disappearance of signs of shock or preshock. Continued repair of dehydration can then proceed with intravenous hypotonic electrolyte solutions or oral glucose/electrolyte solution. The accompanying acidosis usually corrects itself in the course of rehydration.

Convulsions are a well-recognized complication of shigellosis in infants and children. As with convulsions of any cause, aspiration, airway obstruction, and head trauma can occur as a consequence of loss of consciousness. Thus, convulsions should be vigorously treated with intravenous diazepam (up to 10 mg.) or phenobarbital (5 mg. per kg.). If an intravenous line cannot be rapidly established, paraldehyde (0.3 ml. per kg. per dose) mixed 1:1 with mineral oil should be given rectally. The high fever usually associated with *Shigella* convulsions in children should be diminished with tepid water sponge baths and administration of aspirin or acetaminophen.

Supportive Measures. REHYDRATION. Significant dehydration can occur as a consequence of shigellosis, particularly in infants and young children. This can be treated by standard intravenous rehydration regimens. Recently, it has been found that infants with diarrheal dehydration (including that due to *Shigella* diarrhea) of 5 to 10 per cent of body weight can be completely rehydrated with use of oral glucose/electrolyte solution. The formula used was that recommended by the World Health Organization containing (in grams per liter): glucose 20; NaCl 3.5; $NaHCO_3$ 2.5; KCl 1.5. A volume of fluid is given over 6 hours equivalent to twice the calculated fluid deficit; two thirds of the calculated volume is administered as glucose/electrolyte solution and one third is given as free water. For travelers going abroad, a local pharmacy can prepare packets of these ingredients that can be kept in water-tight plastic vials and reconstituted in one liter of water, as necessary.

ANTIMOTILITY AGENTS. Agents that decrease intestinal motility, such as tincture of opium, paregoric, and diphenoxylate, are contraindicated in the treatment of shigellosis or other invasive bacterial diarrheas. There is evidence in humans that duration of fever and excretion of *Shigellae* are prolonged by such agents. Furthermore, administration of such agents converts small animals such as guinea pigs, which are normally quite resistant to shigellosis, into receptive hosts.

OTHER AGENTS. There is no evidence that common antidiarrheal preparations such as kaolin-pectin formulas, bismuth/salicylate preparations, lactobacilli, sour-milk or yogurt have beneficial effects on the clinical or bacteriologic course of shigellosis.

Antimicrobial Therapy. Numerous clinical studies have shown that appropriate antibiotic therapy decreases the duration of fever, diarrhea, and excretion of the pathogen in *Shigella* infections. This experience, coupled with the observation that man is the natural host and reservoir of this contact-transmitted infection offers strong impetus for antibiotic treatment of all patients with shigellosis. However, this must be reconciled with the observations that only a few antibiotics have clinical efficacy in patients (despite the fact that many antimicrobials are effective in vitro) and emergence of resistant strains has repeatedly occurred with *Shigella*. Sulfonamides, the drugs of choice in the 1940s, were of little practical import by the 1950s when, because of resistance, tetracycline became the drug of choice. Widespread resistance to tetracycline led to ampicillin's role as drug of first choice in the 1960s. Prevalence of resistance to ampicillin is now as high as 80 to 90 per cent among *Shigella* strains in many areas.

In deciding whether or not to treat an individual patient, one must consider: (1) the clinical severity, (2) the epidemiologic setting (crowded inner-city family unit, institution, etc.) with regard to likelihood of secondary spread, and (3) the antibiotic sensitivity of the strain.

Sporadic, mild shigella infections in adults or older children, particularly those due to *S. sonnei,* need not be treated with antibiotics. The illness is self-limited and excretion of the organism ceases after one week in approximately 60 per cent of patients. The risk of secondary spread can be minimized with health education by urging careful hand-washing following use of toilet.

If illness is severe or the likelihood of secondary transmission is great, antibiotics should be given. If the isolate is known to be sensitive to tetracycline or ampicillin or if resistance to these antibiotics among *Shigellae* in the community is known to be uncommon, these should be considered the antibiotics of choice. Tetracycline should be reserved for use in nonpregnant adults and children above 8 years of age (because of adverse effects involving drug accumulation in developing bone and teeth). Adults may receive orally either a single one-dose bolus of 2.5 grams or 500 mg. four times daily for 5 days. Since the regimens are equivalent in efficacy, we prefer to use the single bolus method because of lesser expense and ease of administration.

AMPICILLIN. Adults should receive 500 mg. orally four times daily for 5 days. Single bolus therapy has not been shown to be effective for ampicillin. Infants and children should be given 100 mg. per kg. per day in four divided doses for 5 days. If oral medication cannot be given, parenteral ampicillin and tetracycline are highly effective and are given at the same dosage. Amoxicillin is notably ineffective in treatment of shigellosis and should not be prescribed.

If a decision has been made to use antibiotics and the patient's isolate or other *Shigella* strains in the community are commonly resistant to ampicillin or tetracycline, therapy should be started with trimethoprim and sulfamethoxazole, nalidixic acid, or oxolinic acid. If the patient requires antimicrobial therapy and the antibiotic sensitivity of the isolate is not known, one of these three antibiotics should also be used.

TRIMETHOPRIM AND SULFAMETHOXAZOLE.* Adults should receive one tablet (80 mg. trimethoprim and 400 mg. sulfamethoxazole) every 12 hours for 5 days. Children may be given trimethoprim 10 mg. per kg. per day and sulfamethoxazole 50 mg. per kg. per day in two divided doses for 5 days.

NALIDIXIC ACID.* Adults should take 1 gram orally four times daily for five days. Children may receive 55 mg. per kg. per day in four divided doses for 5 days.

OXOLINIC ACID.* Adults may take 750 mg. twice daily for 5 days. Oxolinic acid should not be given to children.

Health Education. Since *Shigella* infection is primarily transmitted by contact, transmission is largely preventable by simple attention to proper personal hygiene. Anyone with known or suspected shigella infection should be instructed to carefully wash their hands after defecation. Professional food handlers should not be allowed to return to work until 3 consecutive negative stool cultures have been recorded.

Commentary. Certain *Escherichia coli* strains have the same ability as *Shigellae* to invade intestinal mucosa. They cause a clinical syndrome identi-

---

*This use of this antibiotic is not yet listed in the manufacturer's official directive, although successful clinical trials have been carried out.

cal to that of *Shigella* bacillary dysentery. While specific therapy of such *E. coli* infections has not been well-studied, we recommend following the same guidelines for treatment of shigellosis as outlined here.

GAS GANGRENE AND SIMILAR SOFT TISSUE ANAEROBIC INFECTIONS

method of
HIRAM C. POLK, JR., M.D.
Louisville, Kentucky

Gas-forming infections occurring in any body part warrant *immediate* measures since in their most virulent form they represent threats to the viability of body parts and the organism itself. However, definitive measures must be tempered by the fact that the majority of gas-forming infections are *not* caused by the "gas bacillus," or Clostridia (Table 1). We will discuss in sequence the preventive treatment of the wound prone to develop such an infection, as well as definitive diagnostic studies and the direct and supportive care of the patient ill of a gas-forming infection.

Management of the Suspect Wound

Two types of wounds are especially prone to invasive infection: first is the fairly contaminated wound, in which several tissue planes are opened; second is the relatively cleaner wound, which has not received initial care and debridement or in which such treatment has been inadequate. The latter case often reflects that the physician initially caring for the wound underestimated its severity or potential for invasive infection or both. Reasonable examples are the penetration of a rusty nail into the sole of the foot and a "simple compound fracture."

Surgical Wound Care. The first step in the management of any wound is appropriate tetanus prophylaxis—including, as indicated, the administration of absorbed tetanus toxoid or human tetanus immune globulin or both. Both passive (immediate protection) and active (later protection) immunization must be considered as discussed elsewhere in this volume.

The surgical treatment of the wound itself embodies several principles and ordinarily requires the skills of a trained surgeon:

1. Meticulous examination of the wound, which may involve additional incisions as for puncture wounds.

TABLE 1. **Microorganisms Which May Produce Gas in Human Tissues**

GRAM STAIN RESULT	AEROBES	ANAEROBES
Gram-positive microorganisms		
Cocci	*Staphylococcus aureus*	Peptostreptococcus (anaerobic Streptococcus)
	Group A Streptococcus (beta-hemolytic Streptococcus)	
Bacilli		Clostridium species which may be responsible for gas gangrene
Gram-negative microorganisms		
Bacilli	*Escherichia coli* *Klebsiella pneumoniae* Enterobacter species	*Bacteroides fragilis*

2. Excision (debridement) of all tissue thought to be devitalized or potentially so and of tissue with embedded dirt and/or other foreign material.

3. Irrigation of the wound with several liters (2 or more depending upon wound size) of isotonic saline or Ringer's lactate solution.

4. In many cases, the wound itself should be left open for delayed primary closure when the wound is clinically free of infection. An open coarse mesh cotton gauze dressing moistened with an isotonic saline solution should be applied. The patient or physician should change the dressing daily, or more often, depending upon the degree of suspicion concerning development of invasive infection. Ultimate closure may be accomplished with tape, simple suture, or even formal reoperation if the geography of the wound so demands.

5. Follow-up care should include daily physician-patient contact—by telephone if convenient. The presence of increased pain in the wound at any time during the first week of care warrants immediate examination of the patient and the wound in minute detail by the physician.

6. For the extensive wound or the lesion at otherwise high risk [e.g., pain without adequate cause disclosed on reexamination (5 above)], formal reexploration of the wound may be warranted. Reexploration should include opening of the wound throughout its extent and a search for residual foreign body or areas of necrosis or both. Postoperative care is as outlined here and may, in the case of certain severe wounds or wounds in areas of decreased accessibility (e.g., perineum), warrant additional formal scheduled reexploration.

Antibiotics. Antimicrobial agents represent reasonable adjuncts to definitive mechanical wound care. In the absence of proper surgical wound care, antibiotic therapy will uniformly fail. The patient with a highly suspect wound should receive 1 to 3 million units of intravenous penicillin every 4 to 6 hours for prevention of classic gas gangrene. In my opinion, extensive soft tissue wounds warrant special treatment because of possible anaerobic infection: either clindamycin (600 mg. administered intravenously every 6 to 8 hours) or chloramphenicol (1 gram administered intravenously every 6 hours).

Other Adjuncts. Gas gangrene antitoxin and hyperbaric oxygen therapy are not warranted for the prevention of gas-forming infections.

Clinical Picture. True gas gangrene has four clinical manifestations, each often coexisting with the other.

1. Crepitant type with gross extensive crepitus; other signs of illness often are scant.

2. Edematous, noncrepitant type in which edema and pain predominate.

3. Profound toxemia in which total body illness may overshadow the local wound signs.

4. Mixed type with any combination of the above.

Gas gangrene typically represents necrosis of striated muscle with initial lesser effects upon connective tissue. This characteristic often helps to segregate it from synergistic, gas-producing infections that involve fascial planes primarily. Three distinct zones of injury are associated with gas gangrene. The central zone is composed of tissue that is overtly dead secondary to initial injury, local ischemia, or bacterial invasion. The second, intermediate zone includes muscles dying from the invasive infection. This zone often appears deceptively normal with some edema surrounding seemingly viable muscle. The third, or peripheral, zone is normal muscle tissue responding secondarily to impinging invasive infection.

The incubation period for gas gangrene varies from as little as a few hours after injury to several days following injury.

Microbiologic Definition. Clinical signs are important but can be misleading. Bacteriologic study is essential to allow application of the correct definitive and adjunctive treatments for the several illnesses presenting as gas forming infections.

The most serious error is failure to make the diagnosis; therefore exploratory incisions through skin, fat, fascia, and into muscle are often warranted to assay the nature of the illness as well as to obtain material for smear and culture.

An immediate Gram stain of tissue exudate is the first data available to the clinician (Table 2). The results of Gram stain can be used to initiate appropriate antibiotic therapy and to orient the operating surgeon to the likely cause and to proper initial therapy. In every case, Gram stains should be confirmed by formal culture and sensitivity testing. One of the unquestioned blessings of the recent era of "anaerobe consciousness" has been the wide dissemination of acceptable techniques for culture of strict and facultative anaerobic bacteria. The physician may want to have the microbiology technician present when such a wound is explored. In every case, obtaining an anaerobic specimen for culture should be the first maneuver following exposure of tissue planes or exudate or both. One should remember that faulty technique is the most common cause of false-negative anaerobic cultures.

Treatment of Existent Infection

Radical Surgical Therapy.   The principles of such care are easily stated but require good judgment in their application:

1. Define the extent of the destructive process.

2. Contain the spread of the disease.

3. Consider preservation of bodily parts or function ONLY when patient survival is assured.

The timing for such treatment is immediate because the patient never improves until definitive operation has been accomplished. One should never "wait until the patient is in better shape." Clostridial myonecrosis requires exploratory incisions, decompression of fascial compartments, and debridement of nonviable tissue. When this disease process is limited in extent and systemic toxicity, one may consider decompression and debridement as primary therapy and observe the patient's response before considering further therapy. More often than not, radical excision (amputation) is warranted. Such wounds should never be closed.

When to utilize amputation properly during the course of clostridial myonecrosis often requires the judgment of the most skilled and experienced surgeon.

Certain problems occur when special organs are involved. For example, extirpation of large segments of the abdominal wall may be required to control spreading infection. Paradoxically, in such cases, containing viscera with Marlex mesh, which is dressed several times daily, may protect the small bowel and allow safe wound closure when the infection is controlled and the prosthesis partially or completely extruded. Uterine infection, most commonly that following illegal abortions, always requires hysterectomy and open drainage.

Necrotizing fasciitis is usually due to mixed gram-negative and gram-positive organisms, which are often facultatively anaerobic. Fascial planes are especially prone to infection and are very slightly resistant to control of infection by virtue of their very limited blood supply. Progressive fascial infection can be controlled only by excision of all fascia involved with a margin well beyond apparent involvement.

Antibiotics.   Selective application of appropriate drugs is an essential adjunct to definitive wound care. The initial choice of drugs should be confirmed by subsequent sensitivity testing of responsible organisms and revised accordingly. Once the infection appears to be controlled and the patient's recovery begins, all antibiotic treatment should be terminated. Superinfection and fungal sepsis are primarily determined by extensive use and random rotations of antibiotic combinations. Drug choices are outlined in Table 2. The watchword of therapy is large, frequent intravenous doses of drugs selected as noted. The utilization of each agent must, of course, be monitored by associated side effects and known toxicities. For mixed infections, which may include anaerobes, penicillin and chloramphenicol constitute a useful combination.

Antitoxin.   Commercially available antitoxin includes products for the toxins of several clostridial strains. The suggested dose is 50,000 units

TABLE 2.   **Antibiotic Treatment of Gas Infections Based on Gram Stain, Cultures, and Sensitivity Tests**

GRAM STAIN RESULT	PRESUMPTIVE MICROORGANISM	ANTIBIOTICS
Gram-positive cocci	Anaerobic Streptococcus	Penicillin Cephalosporins Clindamycin Chloramphenicol
Gram-positive bacilli	Clostridium species	Penicillin Cephalosporins Clindamycin Chloramphenicol
Gram-negative bacilli	Bacteroides species	Chloramphenicol Clindamycin Tetracycline
	Coliforms	Cephalosporins Tobramycin Gentamicin Amikacin Chloramphenicol

administered intravenously every 6 hours for 1 or 2 days. Antitoxin use is controversial and, at best, is warranted only for patients with systemic toxicity manifested by shock and hemolytic anemia, which is often caused by the circulating alpha-toxin. Even then its use is tempered by reactions produced by the heterologous antitoxin.

Hyperbaric Oxygen. The use of hyperbaric oxygen also is controversial. Dispute exists because of testimonial reports of its efficacy and lack of clinically similar trials that indicate its effectiveness, provide evidence of genuine illness in all treated patients, and define adverse effects. Indeed, it is my opinion that if the efforts often expended attempting to achieve patient transfer for hyperbaric therapy had been expended as outlined earlier, there would be no need for such transfer. Delay in standard therapy while attempting to achieve the questionable benefits of hyperbaric oxygen is unconscionable. One real advantage of hyperbaric oxygen appears to be its helpfulness in demarcating nonviable tissue.

Other Adjuncts. The toxic patient ill of gas gangrene or other invasive soft tissue infection requires a full range of supportive care. Because many of these requirements are defined in clinical and laboratory terms and are discussed in detail elsewhere in this volume, I will discuss only those particularly applicable to invasive infections. Toxin-induced hemolysis justifies two additional modes of therapy: packed red cell transfusions to maintain hemoglobin concentrations in excess of 11 grams per dl. (100 ml.) and vigorous fluid therapy to ensure renal tubular lavage and diminish the likelihood of pigment-induced oligemic renal failure. Appropriate tetanus prophylaxis will ordinarily have been given with the initial wound. If this has not been done or if the invasive infection arises as a complication of an elective operative procedure, tetanus immunization is essential.

Exchange transfusion, steroids, and induced hypothermia are additional modalities that have been alleged to be of value in treatment of gas gangrene and related soft tissue gas-forming infections. The data are virtually all testimonial and there appears no sound basis for any of the three methods.

Concluding Comments

The roles of a high index of suspicion, precise surgical wound care, and definitive microbiologic diagnosis have been stressed repeatedly. The validity of adjunctive therapy with carefully chosen antibiotics has also been affirmed. Appropriate actions are the result of good judgment and, as such, consultation should often be undertaken. Due to the litigious atmosphere related to accidents, trauma, and medical complications, every physician involved in the care of such patients should uniformly document carefully in writing all observations and decisions concerning the development and course of each illness.

FOODBORNE ILLNESS
method of
ANDREW R. SCHWARTZ, M.D.
Philadelphia, Pennsylvania

Illness arising from the ingestion of tainted or contaminated food or beverage is a worldwide problem of undefined magnitude. In the United States, foodborne illness is a reportable disease, so some statistical information is available. Although clearly underreported, the most recent figures (released in October, 1977, by the Center for Disease Control) revealed that 438 outbreaks of food- or waterborne illness involving 12,463 persons, occurred during 1976. A specific cause was established in only about one third of these outbreaks.

Foodborne disease may be of either infectious or toxic origin. The physician may approach the diagnosis by establishing the probable interval from ingestion to the onset of symptoms, by the symptom complex presented, or on epidemiologic grounds. When considered by incubation period some useful generalizations are possible. For example (1) *Short* incubation periods: Less than 1 hour—suggest a chemical intoxication; from 1 to 7 hours—probably staphylococcal, or another preformed toxin or chemical; (2) *Intermediate* incubation periods: 8 to 14 hours—associated with bacterial proliferation and toxin production such as *Clostridium perfringens* and *Bacillus cereus;* 14 to 96 hours suggests the presence of an infectious agent such as *Escherichia coli,* Salmonella, Shigella, *Vibrio parahemolyticus, V. cholera, Yersinia enterocolitica, Reovirus*-like agents, etc.; (3) *Prolonged* incubation periods: varying from a few days to many weeks suggest the possible presence of a protozoan (Giardia, amebae) or other parasite (Trichinella) or longer incubating microbe such as Brucella or viruses such as hepatitis virus A and B.

Mortality due to food-transmitted illness is most likely to occur among those who are very young or old or otherwise debilitated. Such events are infrequently reported except for outbreaks of botulism. In 1976, 12.5 per cent (5 of 40) patients died. Among 32 patients in a 1978 outbreak, there were no deaths.

TABLE 1.   **Foodborne Bacterial Diseases Unaccompanied by Fever**

AGENT	INCUBATION PERIOD (RANGE)	CLINICAL PRESENTATION	DIAGNOSIS	THERAPY
Staphylococcus aureus	2–4 (½–8) hours	Nausea, vomiting, prostration, cramps, diarrhea	Isolation of organism from stool or suspected food. Detection of enterotoxin in food	Symptomatic
Clostridium perfringens	9–15 (8–22) hours	Nausea, cramps, diarrhea (little vomiting)	Detection of organism in food and stool	Symptomatic
Bacillus cereus	8–16 (2–20) hours	Nausea, vomiting, cramps, diarrhea	Isolation of organism in stool and food	Symptomatic
Escherichia coli (*enterotoxigenic*)	6–36 (6–96) hours	Watery diarrhea often profuse	Isolation of organism in food and stool (serologic dx)	Symptomatic, may require IV fluids if diarrhea is severe.
Clostridium botulinum	12–48 hours (2 hrs–8 days)	Nausea, vomiting, weakness, dizziness, visual disturbance, cranial nerve palsies, dysarthria, dysphagia	Detection of toxin in serum, stool, or food. Isolation of organism from food	1. Induce vomiting or gastric lavage 2. Cathartic (epsom salts) or high colonic enemas 3. *C. botulinum* antitoxin (obtain from CDC—see text) 4. Guanidine hydrochloride 14–50 mg./kg. po/day (Investigational)

General Therapy of Foodborne Illness

Most cases of food poisoning and infectious gastroenteritis are mild and self-limited. Only those with more severe or prolonged symptoms or those that are part of a local outbreak usually contact the medical community. All such cases should be reported to the local public health authorities.

In general, symptomatic and supportive measures suffice to tide patients over these episodes. Thus, bed rest and gastric rest are most useful in controlling nausea and vomiting. If these symptoms become more pronounced then the use of a parenteral or rectal antiemetic agent (e.g., trimethobenzamide or prochlorperazine) may be helpful. If dehydration develops, parenteral fluid and electrolyte replacement is indicated.

Diarrhea can usually be diminished with kaolin-pectin, paregoric, or diphenoxylate hydrochloride plus atropine, but some caution is indicated. In the presence of overt dysentery or among those with fever and diarrhea, antimotility agents may prove disadvantageous. In patients with febrile diarrheal disease, a stool examination (with a methylene-blue stain) for fecal leukocytes should be carried out. If the stool contains many leukocytes, this suggests the presence of disruption of the mucosal integrity of the distal bowel and if the history suggests an infectious cause, then the agent is most likely to be Shigella, enteropathogenic *E. coli,* Salmonella, Entamoeba, or *Yersinia enterocolitica.* The use of antidiarrheal drugs in these circumstances is likely to enhance the severity of the illness, and thus they should be avoided. The administration of bismuth subsalicylate (Pepto-Bismol), 1 to 2 tablespoonfuls every half-hour for 8 doses, might prove beneficial because of its antagonism to prostaglandin activity in the bowel.

In patients whose diarrhea persists, the administration of oral electrolyte and glucose containing solutions will assist in preventing dehydration and electrolyte imbalance. If not sufficient then intravenous fluid and crystalloid replacement will be necessary.

Botulism

In suspected cases of botulism, serum and stool should be obtained for toxin assay. If any of the implicated food is available this too should be forwarded to the local public health authorities for testing. The physician may contact the Center for Disease Control (Day: 404-633-3311; Night and weekend: 404-633-2176) for consultation and advice on obtaining polyvalent botulinal antitoxin for administration to more seriously afflicted patients.

TABLE 2. **Foodborne Bacterial Illness Accompanied by Fever**

AGENT	INCUBATION PERIOD (RANGE)	CLINICAL PRESENTATION	DIAGNOSIS	THERAPY
Salmonella Gastroenteritis	8–24 (6–48) hours	Diarrhea, cramps, nausea, some vomiting	Isolation of organism in stool and food. Positive fecal leukocyte prep	Symptomatic If clinically septicemic then treat with ampicillin 100–200 mg./kg./day IV in four divided doses, or chloramphenicol 50–60 mg./kg./day IV in four divided doses, or trimethoprim (160 mg.)* plus sulfamethoxazole (800 mg.) twice daily for two weeks
Enteric fever	6–14 days	Headache, fever, cramps, constipation	Isolation of organism from blood, stool, urine, (serology), + fecal leukocytes	Treat with ampicillin, or chloramphenicol, or trimethoprim-sulfamethoxazole,* as indicated above
Shigella	12–50 (7–120) hours	Diarrhea, cramps, fever, tenesmus, urgency, dysentery	Isolation of organism in stool, + fecal leukocytes	*Children:* Ampicillin, 100 mg./kg./day in four doses for five days or trimethoprim (10 mg.). sulfamethoxazole 50 mg./kg./day for five days* *Adults:* Tetracycline, 2.5 grams po as a single oral dose or trimethoprim 160 mg./sulfamethoxazole 800 mg., BID for five days*
Escherichia coli enteropathogenic	8–24 hours	Diarrhea, cramps, fever, tenesmus, urgency (dysentery in some)	Isolation of organism from stool or food, + fecal leukocytes	Symptomatic if severely ill, then treat as for Shigella
Vibrio parahemolyticus	12–24 hours	Diarrhea, occasionally bloody or mucoid stools	Isolation of organism from stool or food, outbreak related to seafood	Symptomatic
Yersinia enterocolitica	? (probably up to 72 hours)	Fever, diarrhea, severe abdominal pain, vomiting, headache, pharyngitis mimes, appendicitis, and mesenteric adenitis	Isolation of organism from stool, blood, appendix, mesenteric lymph nodes, serology, + fecal leukocytes	? Symptomatic

*This use of this drug combination is not listed in the manufacturer's official directive.

TABLE 3. **Foodborne Chemical and Toxic Illness**

AGENT	ASSOCIATED FOODS	INCUBATION PERIOD	CLINICAL PRESENTATION	DIAGNOSIS	THERAPY
Heavy Metals (Tin, copper, lead, zinc, etc.)	Characteristic container and acid foods	3 minutes–3 hours	Metallic taste, nausea, vomiting, cramps, abdominal pain	Detection of metal in food	Symptomatic Penicillamine BAL
Organic Mercury	Fish, meat, and treated grains	few hours	Paresthesias of lips, mouth, tongue, hands, weakness, dysarthria	Detect in serum, urine, or suspected food	Symptomatic BAL Penicillamine
Chinese Restaurant Syndrome (monosodium glutamate)	MSG treated	5–30 minutes	Burning sensation in chest, back, neck, abdomen, palpitations, sweating, flushing	Large amounts of MSG in food	Symptomatic
Mushroom Poisoning	*Amanita muscaria*	1–3 hours	Nausea, vomiting, abdominal pain, diarrhea, liver and kidney dysfunction, salivation, sweating	Detect toxin in mushroom or identify mushroom	Induce vomiting or gastric lavage Atropine for muscarinic effects
	Amanita phalloides	1–18 hours	Nausea, vomiting, abdominal pain, diarrhea, confusion-delirium, visual disturbance	Same	Symptomatic Gastric lavage
Scombroid Poisoning (Histamine-like substances produced by bacterial action on fish)	Tuna, mackerel, albacore, etc.	5 minutes–1 hour	Nausea, vomiting, headache, dizziness, abdominal pain, thirst, pruritus	Increased histamine in fish	Antihistamines
Paralytic Shellfish Poisoning	Clams, muscles, scallops	10–60 minutes	Paresthesias of lips, mouth, face, extremities, dizziness, ataxia, GI symptoms	Detection of toxin	Symptomatic
Ciguatera Poisoning	Fish, oysters, clams	30 minutes–24 hours	Facial paresthesia, dry mouth, GI symptoms	Detection of toxin	Symptomatic

EPIDEMIC INFLUENZA

method of
STEVEN R. MOSTOW, M.D.
Denver, Colorado

Introduction

Outbreaks of influenza have become an annual phenomenon, and epidemics of influenza cause excess mortality every 2 to 3 years. Although there are three immunologic types of influenza virus (A, B, and C), large epidemics and world-wide pandemics are caused primarily by type A. The most recent outbreaks have been caused by A/Victoria, A/Texas and A/USSR. Why this virus is constantly changing, how much change is necessary (antigenic drift) to cause outbreaks, what forces are operative when major changes (antigenic shift) in the hemagglutinin and neuraminidase occur and lead to pandemics, and what happens to the virus between outbreaks are all questions that continue to remain unanswered.

Treatment

Although influenza virus is characterized as a respiratory virus, the illness usually includes severe systemic symptoms. A nonproductive cough is frequent and half the patients have a mild to moderate sore throat. Fever, myalgia, headache, and insomnia, however, are the chief complaints that force the patient to seek medical advice. The basic therapy is directed against these symptoms.

Uncomplicated Cases

1. Analgesics for fever, sore throat, myalgia, and headache. For adults the dose of aspirin (acetylsalicylic acid) is 0.6 grams (10 grains) every 4 hours, but 0.9 gram (15 grains) may be necessary to control severe myalgia or very high temperature $>40°C.$ ($>104°F.$). The patient should be warned that the aspirin may cause drenching sweats. For children (5 to 12 years old) the dose of aspirin is 0.3 to 0.6 gram (5 to 10 grains) every 4 hours. Aspirin suppositories can be used if oral administration is not feasible. If aspirin is contraindicated, 650 mg. of acetaminophen may be given every 4 hours. For children (6 to 12 years old) the dose is 325 mg. every 4 to 6 hours.

2. Cough suppressants such as codeine phosphate or various elixirs containing codeine are useful, if necessary, to permit the patient some uninterrupted sleep. If insomnia is a troublesome problem, promethazine hydrochloride (Phenergan) with codeine may be a helpful combination, since one of the beneficial side effects of this mild antihistamine is drowsiness.

3. Humidification of room air may help to relieve the dry, hacking cough associated with the disease. A cold-water vaporizer is preferred, as steam vaporizers introduce the risk of scalding burns and should not be used for young children or senile adults.

4. Bed rest should be encouraged, especially while the patient is febrile. If tolerated, early ambulation is recommended.

5. Diet should be very light. Soups and liquids should be emphasized to maintain adequate hydration until the patient can tolerate more substantial meals.

6. Reassurance that although the patient may not feel up to par for 2 or 3 weeks he will get better. A gradual rather than an abrupt return to full pre-illness activity is recommended.

7. Smoking should be forbidden for the duration of the illness. An explanation that smoking further paralyzes the already damaged (by virus) ciliated lining of the airways is usually sufficient.

8. Antibiotics should not be used prophylactically, especially as their use may selectively encourage superinfection by drug-resistant bacteria. There are no data to support the claim that prophylactic antibiotics prevent the more serious complications of influenza such as bronchitis and pneumonia.

Complicated Cases

Most complications occur in the elderly, and especially in those with significant chronic illness such as heart and pulmonary disease. Therefore, any patient with influenza, a fever, and an underlying disease needs to be examined periodically for the onset of lower respiratory tract disease.

Lower Respiratory Tract Complications. BRONCHITIS. A negative chest film in the presence of rales and purulent sputum, with or without fever, usually signifies the onset of bronchitis, which may require treatment. Prior to therapy, a sputum smear and culture should be carried out, especially since staphylococcal infection must be recognized as early as possible. Ordinary bronchitis in adults is best treated with an oral dose of 2 grams per day of tetracycline or ampicillin given for 5 to 7 days. If the smear or culture reveals only pneumococci, penicillin alone is adequate. In children, the dose of ampicillin is 50 to 100 mg. per kg. per day. Tetracycline should be avoided in young children because of discoloration of developing teeth.

BRONCHIOLITIS. Hyperinflated lungs, wheezing, and hypoxia in the absence of pneumonia signify the onset of bronchiolitis, which can be of primary influenzal cause. This disease can be devastating, usually because of gas exchange problems. Therefore, determination of arterial blood gas levels and judicious use of oxygen based on arterial gas results are important.

The role of antibiotics is less clear. If the sputum is not purulent, antibiotics need not be given, as this primarily is a viral disease. If the sputum is purulent, however, antibiotics should be given as outlined.

PNEUMONIA. The incidence of staphylococcal pneumonia is significantly higher following influenza epidemics and the patient with staphylococcal pneumonia is at the risk of death. Therefore, it is recommended that all patients with suspected or confirmed pneumonia during an influenza epidemic be hospitalized. Patients with influenza virus should probably be separated from other patients with other diseases, although patients with influenza can be boarded together. Because it is so vitally important to rule out staphylococcal pneumonia, the following procedures should be carried out immediately after the admission of a patient with clinical evidence of pneumonia:

1. Baseline chest x-ray.
2. Sputum smear to rule out staphylococcus infection (large round gram-positive cocci in clusters).
3. Pretreatment sputum and blood cultures (3 times).
4. Antibiotic treatment based on results of Gram stain:

a. If the sputum smear reveals many polymorphonuclear leukocytes (PMNs) and staphylococcus, therapy should be started immediately with a penicillinase-resistant antibiotic (cephalothin or cephapirin, 12 grams per day; methicillin, 12 to 18 grams per day; oxacillin or nafcillin, 6 to 9 grams per day). These large doses should be given intravenously on a 4-hour basis (assuming normal renal function), because of this life-threatening situation.

b. If PMNs and pneumococci (gram-positive diplococci) predominate, low doses of intravenous penicillin (3 million units per day) should be given on a 4-hour basis.

c. If there are many PMNs and *Hemophilus influenzae* (gram-negative pleomorphic rods) or a mixed flora predominates, ampicillin (2 to 4 grams per day) should be given intravenously on a 4-hour basis.

As the patient improves, especially after he becomes afebrile, other routes of administration, including oral, should be considered.

5. Arterial blood gas measurements should be determined if the patient is in severe respiratory distress or if the patient has a history of severe chronic obstructive lung disease.

Upper Respiratory Tract Complications. There is usually an increased incidence of otitis media and sinusitis following influenza. The therapy involves drainage (medically with decongestants or surgically if indicated) and antibiotics. In children under 4 years of age, ampicillin is indicated because of the high incidence of *Hemophilus influenzae* as the causative agent. Be sure to confirm the *H. influenzae* as susceptible to ampicillin.

Cardiovascular Complications. Myocarditis is a rare complication of influenza and usually presents with the sudden onset of congestive heart failure or an arrhythmia or both. Judicious use of digitalis, diuretics, rest, and salt restriction forms the keystone of therapy.

CONGESTIVE HEART FAILURE. Any patient with preexisting heart disease is prone to develop congestive heart failure secondary to the increased metabolic demands associated with fever. Therefore, control of temperature as outlined above is important in patients with severe heart disease.

Neurologic Complications. Reye's syndrome (children) and encephalitis (adults) are uncommon complications of influenza. Consultation with a neurologist or neurosurgeon should allow a rational plan of monitoring and supporting measures to be formulated. Steroids should be avoided on theoretical grounds in any acute viral infection of the brain, but there is no evidence to contraindicate using such preparations in a patient who is rapidly deteriorating because of progressing cerebral edema.

Prevention of Disease

Vaccine Approach. Although influenza vaccines have been in existence for 30 years, effectiveness varies considerably. Well-controlled studies revealed that the vaccine is about 70 per cent effective in preventing disease. However, vaccine is also effective in modifying disease, with the usual dose levels being 80 to 90 per cent effective in preventing fever. All new vaccines are prepared in a purified form. However, vaccines are not effective unless the vaccine is made from current influenza viruses. The physician should confirm that the vaccine he has is up to date, both with regard to the shelf life and the antigenic composition.

Vaccine is available in two forms. The whole virus vaccine is more immunogenic, but causes more adverse reactions. The split virus vaccine is less immunogenic and causes fewer adverse reactions. Only split virus vaccine should be used for children, even though a second dose may be necessary to provide immunity. Neither the whole nor split vaccine should be administered to persons with a history of a severe reaction to influenza vaccine in the past.

Influenza vaccine is recommended yearly in the fall for all of those at risk of death from influenza—these include persons of any age with chronic or debilitating illness and all those over 65 years of age. Vaccine is also recommended for persons whose community functions are essential. Health care personnel should also receive vaccine in order to decrease the chances of spreading the virus to patients and to keep health care facilities operational during an epidemic.

Chemoprophylaxis and Chemotherapy. Amantadine hydrochloride, when taken orally (100 mg. twice daily), will reduce the incidence of epidemic influenza by about 50 per cent. It has been shown to be more effective in the presence of serum antibody if the antibody is relevant for the influenza strain causing disease. The drug is active at several points in the virus reproductive cycle, but the complete details of its action are yet to be reported. It is not effective against influenza B infections or outbreaks.

Amantadine has also been shown effective in reducing the total duration of fever in cases of influenza. In other words, its net therapeutic effect is much like aspirin, but its routine use for this effect of the drug is not encouraged. Amantadine has been shown to decrease the peripheral airway resistance caused by influenza A virus. In patients with severe hypoxia secondary to influenza infection, amantadine should be considered.

The side effects (drowsiness, inability to concentrate, feeling of detachment, depression, and dizziness) are not often seen at normal doses, but occur more frequently in elderly persons. Amantadine should be used with extreme caution in patients with compromised renal function, since it is not easily dialyzed.

The administration of amantadine should be reserved for those chronically ill patients, both vaccinated and unvaccinated, who are at risk of death from influenza. It is especially important for those who are more likely to be exposed, such as senile patients with cardiac or respiratory disease living in homes where there are school children or adults with widespread outside contacts. It should be remembered that to be maximally effective the drug should be given prior to and for the duration of the exposure to the influenza A virus.

LEPROSY

method of
ROBERT C. HASTINGS, M.D.
Carville, Louisiana

Introduction

Leprosy is a chronic infectious disease of man caused by *Mycobacterium leprae* that affects some 12 million persons worldwide. The principal clinical manifestations leading to a diagnosis in the United States are (1) dermatologic lesions of various sorts, (2) neurologic deficits, particularly skin anesthesia either coinciding with skin lesions or in a more general temperature-linked pattern with anesthesia or hypesthesia in cooler parts of the skin, and (3) acute inflammatory manifestations of hypersensitivity to antigens of *M. leprae,* the so-called lepra reactions.

Host-parasite relationships in leprosy are complex and dynamic. The clinical manifestations, bacteriologic load, histopathologic picture, and prognosis, both with and without therapy, are all dependent upon the relative balance between the parasite, *M. leprae,* and the host's cell-mediated immunity to *M. leprae.* These host-parasite relationships are formalized in classification of leprosy. Fundamentally, well-localized leprosy with competent cell-mediated immunity and very few *M. leprae* is called tuberculoid disease. Widely disseminated, anergic disease is called lepromatous leprosy. Forms of leprosy between these two extremes are called borderline types, and the very early form of the disease before full definition of the relative balance between bacterial proliferation and cell-mediated immunity is called indeterminate leprosy. Rational therapy begins with accurate diagnosis of both leprosy itself and the position of a given patient within the leprosy spectrum, i.e., that patient's classification.

In any given patient, successful treatment amounts to (1) rehabilitation of any existing deformities, (2) prevention of further physical deformities, and (3) control of bacterial proliferation.

Existing deformity, frequently the most distressing social and vocational manifestation of leprosy, demands knowledgeable, compassionate, and thorough evaluation and correction or circumvention. Essential components of total patient care in leprosy include rehabilitation in the fields of ophthalmology, plastic surgery, orthopedic surgery (e.g., tendon transplants), prosthetics, occupational therapy, physical therapy, and specialized footwear.

Deformities in leprosy are almost all avoided by (a) early diagnosis and treatment, (b) thorough life-long patient education and motivation as to the care of denervated extremities, (c) halting neural, ocular, and nasal damage caused by bacterial proliferation by means of proper chemotherapy, and (d) prompt recognition and control of lepra reactions.

The principal drawbacks to successful control of bacterial proliferation in leprosy are (a) patient noncompliance, (b) inadequate follow-up, (c) improper treatment by well-intentioned but misinformed physicians, and (d) drug resistant disease.

The medical therapy of leprosy is designed to render *M. leprae* incapable of multiplication, essentially eliminating the patient's infectivity on the one hand, and allowing the body to clear the bacilli on the other, and to control hypersensitivity reactions to antigens of *M. leprae,* i.e., lepra reactions.

Antibacterial Therapy

Antibacterial therapy is given from the time of diagnosis until various periods after the patient's disease has become inactive. Inactivity is defined as a 12-month period in which (a) the disease shows no clinical evidence of activity, (b) no acid-fast bacilli are demonstrated by slit-and-scrape samplings from skin sites, and (c) skin biopsies show no activity (no acid-fast bacilli).

Indeterminate Leprosy.   Dapsone is given in a dosage of 50 mg. daily until 2 years after the disease has become inactive. Inactivity can be expected in 1 to 2 years with therapy. The patient is then skin tested with lepromin (or tested by an in vitro equivalent for delayed type hypersensitivity to *M. leprae* such as lymphocyte blast transformation or leukocyte inhibitory factor assays). If the lepromin skin test is positive, then dapsone may be discontinued. If the lepromin skin test is negative, the patient is treated with dapsone 50 mg. daily for life. Lepromin is not generally available in the United States.

Tuberculoid Leprosy.   Dapsone is given in a dosage of 50 mg. daily until 2 years after the disease has become inactive which can be expected within 1 to 2 years with therapy. Tuberculoid patients have cell-mediated immunity toward *M. leprae* as measured by lepromin skin testing or in vitro equivalents; therefore, dapsone may be discontinued 2 years after the patient's disease has become inactive.

Borderline Leprosy.   Dapsone, 100 mg. daily, is recommended. Within 2 to 6 years such cases can be expected to become inactive. Dapsone, 100 mg. daily, should be continued for an additional 10 years after the patient's disease has become inactive. At that point lepromin skin testing (or in vitro equivalents) is performed and positive cases may discontinue dapsone. Lepromin negative cases should continue dapsone, 100 mg. daily, for life. Again, it should be noted that lepromin is not generally available in the United States.

Borderline-lepromatous and Lepromatous Leprosy.   These patients should receive 100 mg. dapsone daily for life. In over 90 per cent of such patients, the disease will become inactive within 5 to 10 years. In any case cell-mediated immunity to *M. leprae* remains absent, and such patients are continually at risk for relapse or reinfection and should therefore remain on treatment for the rest of their lives. In less than 10 per cent of such patients the disease fails to become inactive. Such patients (1) usually are taking dapsone in low doses or irregularly or both, (2) have developed secondary sulfone-resistant *M. leprae,* or (3) may have been originally infected with sulfone-resistant bacilli, i.e., they may have primary sulfone-resistant disease.

Antireaction Therapy

The most common complications of leprosy are the so-called lepra reactions. These reactions occur in approximately 25 per cent of untreated patients and in approximately 50 per cent of the patients taking chemotherapy. They are fundamentally hypersensitivity reactions to antigens of dead *M. leprae*. There are two major types of lepra reactions, (1) the so-called reversal reactions, or Type I lepra reactions, occurring in borderline to tuberculoid cases and (2) erythema nodosum leprosum (ENL), or Type II lepra reactions, occurring in borderline-lepromatous to lepromatous patients. In contrast to the slow clinical manifestations of bacterial progression in leprosy, these reactions are frequently abrupt in onset and may rapidly create irreversible peripheral neuropathies, ocular damage, etc. Lepra reactions probably account for the majority of deformities in leprosy and their management is of utmost importance in the successful management of leprosy patients. In all but the mildest reactions, it is prudent for a relatively inexperienced clinician to refer such patients to centers where more experienced specialists in leprosy can evaluate the patient and where experimental drugs are available for the management of these reactional episodes.

Reversal Reactions.   These reactions occur in borderline to tuberculoid cases and are manifestations of delayed type hypersensitivity to antigens of *M. leprae*. In their severe form, the ultimate result of these reactions is caseation necrosis of *M. leprae* antigen-containing tissues. The management of these reactions depends on the areas of skin and the peripheral nerves that are involved. Reversal reactions involving significant areas of the skin likely to ulcerate, e.g., facial lesions in females, and those involving nerves causing an acute "significant" neural deficit, namely (a) a sensory loss involving the palms, soles, or cornea or (b) any motor loss, demand immediate steroid therapy (within hours after onset of the neural deficit) in order to reverse the neural deficit. Usually, 80 mg. of prednisone or its equivalent is sufficient for such emergencies and return of peripheral nerve function may be expected within 24 hours if therapy is initiated early enough. The steroid dose and frequency must then be individualized to preserve nerve function. In general, attempts should be made to maintain such patients on single doses of oral steroids every other morning in order to minimize endogenous pituitary-adrenal suppression, e.g., prednisone, 40 mg. orally, every other day in the morning. Dapsone chemotherapy is continued in full doses throughout these reversal reactions. Usually, reversal reactions in such patients will subside within a few weeks to months as efficient cell-mediated immunity clears leprosy bacilli and therefore reduces the antigenic stimulus for the reaction. In the event that reversal reactions become chronic and more than a few months of steroids are required, or in the event that significant steroid side effects are encountered, consideration should be given to the use of an experimental drug, clofazimine, in doses of 200 to 300 mg. daily, for its anti-inflammatory activity. Clofazimine is available to qualified investigators in various centers specializing in leprosy throughout the country.

Erythema Nodosum Leprosum (ENL) Reactions. These reactions occur in patients with borderline-lepromatous and lepromatous leprosy and, in the great majority of these patients, are manifestations of multifocal Arthus reactions to antigens of *M. leprae.* In severe ENL there is evidence of circulating immune complexes with renal damage. In contrast to reversal reactions, which are usually relatively short-lived, ENL reactions tend to be recurrent and chronic. As in reversal reactions, full doses of dapsone are continued throughout ENL reactions. If "significant" acute neuritis is present with ENL, steroids in the doses indicated for reversal reactions are necessary to reverse the acute neural damage. In chronic or recurrent ENL, steroids are not advisable for long-term use and the drug of choice is thalidomide. Thalidomide in doses of 100 mg. four times daily will control ENL within 48 hours in virtually all lepromatous cases. Thalidomide, like clofazimine, is available to qualified investigators at various centers specializing in leprosy throughout the country.

Ocular manifestations of ENL, e.g., acute leprous anterior uveitis or iridocyclitis, are major problems with ENL patients, are frequently difficult to recognize, and can readily result in blindness. Proper recognition and management of these complications frequently require the care of specialists. Frequently, ocular manifestations of ENL can be managed with topical steroids.

In females of child-bearing potential in whom thalidomide is contraindicated because of its well-known teratogenicity, or in ENL occurring in borderline-lepromatous disease in which thalidomide is curiously frequently ineffective or in patients who can not be managed by qualified investigators to whom thalidomide can be made available, clofazimine in doses of 200 to 300 mg. daily will control the majority of manifestations of ENL, through its anti-inflammatory action. If neither thalidomide or clofazimine can be utilized, steroids are necessary in ENL patients to control "significant" neuritis and other problems. Attempts at long-term control of ENL with steroids are fraught with danger because of the side effects of long-term steroids, even in single-dose-every-other-day regimens. Consideration should be given in such patients to referring them to centers specializing in leprosy where they may be followed and treated with experimental drugs as required.

Sulfone Resistant Leprosy

Primary Sulfone Resistant Leprosy. Recently, a small number of patients with primary sulfone resistant leprosy have been reported from two different centers. These previously untreated patients harbored bacilli that multiplied in the footpads of mice fed diets containing low concentrations of dapsone. In 11 such patients detected at Carville, most have shown only partial resistance by mouse footpad testing and all have responded clinically to dapsone in dosages of 100 mg. daily. At present, the only means of detecting such patients is with baseline drug sensitivity testing utilizing the mouse footpad system prior to the initiation of chemotherapy. Such studies currently represent the optimum in patient care and may become routinely advisable in the future. For the present, it should be emphasized that the majority of newly diagnosed patients harbor bacilli that are fully sensitive to dapsone.

Secondary Sulfone Resistance. In an analysis of more than 100 cases of secondary sulfone resistance at Carville, relapse occurred on an average 17 years after the start of sulfone therapy with a range of from 5 to well over 20 years. Two factors were found to be important in the development of secondary sulfone resistance: (1) prolonged low dose treatment (1 year or longer with a dose of sulfone less than 100 mg. per week of dapsone or its equivalent), and (2) irregular treatment (multiple breaks of 1 month or more in taking sulfones). By serial mouse footpad studies it can be shown that the development of sulfone resistance is a step-wise phenomenon and that 1 to 7 years are required from the initial development of partial sulfone resistance (lack of inhibition of bacterial multiplication in mice receiving 0.0001 per cent w/w dietary dapsone, equivalent to approximately 1 mg. daily human dose) until the patient's bacilli show full sulfone resistance (lack of inhibition of bacterial multiplication in mice receiving 0.01 per cent w/w dietary dapsone, equivalent to approximately 100 mg. daily human doses). These considerations make it clear that dapsone should be used in maximum subtoxic doses in all multibacillary cases (100 mg. daily) and that sulfone therapy should be continued without interruption, e.g., for lepra reactions, for as long as it is indicated. When the sulfones are used in this fashion, the risk of an individual patient developing secondary sulfone resistance is small with dapsone monotherapy.

Combination Chemotherapy of Leprosy. All newly diagnosed patients in whom baseline mouse footpad drug sensitivity studies are not performed have potential drug resistant disease (primary sulfone resistance) and all patients, even with baseline mouse footpad drug sensitivity studies, are at some risk for the development of secondary sulfone resistant disease. This has led a number of authorities to take the position that, as in tuberculosis, combination chemotherapy is mandatory in multibacillary leprosy. Certainly it is difficult to argue against such a position from a theoretical point of view. On the other hand, on a practical level, one must admit that (1) no one knows the optimum combination of drugs to employ or for what duration, (2) 20 years or more will be needed to prove that any new regimen (either a new monotherapy or a new combination therapy) is superior to dapsone monotherapy, (3) the great majority of patients treated with regular dapsone monotherapy in the past have had, and continue to have, excellent control over bacterial proliferation, (4) the demands of chronicity and regularity of patient compliance in therapy, as well as the possibility of side effects, are compounded as the number of drugs is increased in the treatment of leprosy, and (5) the advantages of dapsone are enormous compared to the next most efficacious drugs available for leprosy. These considerations lead us to the recommendation that dapsone monotherapy remains the antibacterial treatment of choice for all newly diagnosed leprosy patients.

Therapy of Sulfone Resistant Leprosy. Sulfone resistance must be suspected in any patient who is not responding to prescribed dapsone chemotherapy. It is diagnosed when the patient's disease is shown to be progressive bacteriologically over a 6-month period despite intake of full doses of dapsone, verified either by the patient's receiving an injectable sulfone (not available in the United States) or by periodic monitoring of blood or urine for sulfone levels. The diagnosis is confirmed by mouse footpad multiplication of the patient's bacilli in animals fed dapsone.

The treatment of choice for sulfone resistant leprosy is clofazimine in a dosage of 100 mg. daily. To date, no cases of clofazimine resistance have been described despite fairly extensive use since 1965.

Individual Antileprosy Drugs

Dapsone (4,4′-diaminodiphenyl sulfone, DDS, Alvosulfone). This is the only drug approved for general use for the treatment of leprosy in the United States. As indicated, it is the antibacterial drug of choice in leprosy. In doses of 100 mg. daily, side effects are rare. Hemolytic anemias occur particularly in patients with glucose-6-phosphate dehydrogenase (G-6-PD) deficiencies. Cutaneous allergies have been observed, and the sulfones are cross-allergenic with sulfonamides. Of major significance in underdeveloped countries is the fact that the drug is extraordinarily inexpensive. It currently costs $2.00 to $2.50 per year to treat a patient with 100 mg. daily of dapsone.

Clofazimine (B663, Lamprene) (Experimental). This is the antibacterial drug of choice for sulfone resistant leprosy in doses of 100 mg. daily, and it has additionally useful anti-inflammatory activity in doses of 200 to 300 mg. daily for chronic reversal reactions and chronic ENL reactions. Major side effects include (1) reversible, blotchy, reddish to reddish-black skin pigmentation, which is frequently cosmetically unacceptable, and (2) deposition of the drug in the small bowel with larger doses that can interfere with small bowel motility and can lead to symptoms of small bowel obstruction. Clofazimine is relatively expensive by the standards of underdeveloped countries, costing approximately $30.00 per year to treat a patient with 100 mg. daily.

Thalidomide (Experimental). This is the drug of choice for ENL occurring in lepromatous cases except for females of child-bearing potential in whom it is contraindicated except under extraordinary circumstances. It has no effect on *M. leprae* and is used only for its anti-inflammatory–immunosuppressive activity. Side effects other than teratogenicity and sedation are rare.

Rifampin (Rifadin, Rimactane). This well-known antituberculosis drug is bactericidal for *M. leprae*. Morbidity in leprosy is not immediately related to viability of *M. leprae;* therefore, this characteristic of the drug has not proved a major advantage clinically. The dose in leprosy is 600 mg. daily (this use of rifampin is not listed in the manufacturer's official directive). A major drawback to rifampin, particularly in underdeveloped countries, is its cost, $500 to $600 per year to treat a patient with 600 mg. daily. Resistance has been noted after 3 to 4 years of monotherapy with rifampin, and appears to develop as a single-step mutant. If used in leprosy, rifampin should be given only in combination with another effective antileprosy drug. The principal side effects are hepatotoxicity and a flulike syndrome. Sensitization can occur to rifampin, and discontinuing the drug and its subsequent reinstitution can result in severe thrombocytopenia and renal failure.

Ethionamide (Trecator). This antituberculosis drug is active against *M. leprae* in doses of 250 to 750 mg. daily (this use of ethionamide is not listed in the manufacturer's official directive). Resistance develops after 3 to 4 years of monotherapy and, if used in leprosy, ethionamide, like rifampin, should be used only in combination with another effective antileprosy drug. The principal side effects are gastrointestinal intolerance and hepatotoxicity.

Streptomycin. This well-known drug is active

against *M. leprae* in a dosage of 1.0 gram intramuscularly three times weekly (this use of streptomycin is not listed in the manufacturer's official directive). Resistance develops in 2 to 3 years when the drug is given alone, and like rifampin and ethionamide, if streptomycin is to be used, it should only be given in combination with another effective antileprosy drug. The principal drawbacks of streptomycin are the necessity to administer it intramuscularly and its well-known eighth nerve toxicities.

Thioureas. Thiambutosine (Ciba 1906), in a dosage of 500 mg. three times daily, and thiacetazone (amithiozone, TB 1/698), in a dosage of 150 mg. daily, are relatively inexpensive drugs used primarily in underdeveloped countries against leprosy. They are not available in the United States. Resistance develops within 2 to 3 years when either is given as monotherapy for multibacillary disease and there is cross-resistance between the two compounds and between these two compounds and ethionamide. Their principal use would be in combination with other antileprosy drugs in underdeveloped countries in which their low costs would make them reasonable alternatives to more active compounds.

Additional information regarding the management of leprosy or its complications is available from the National Leprosarium, the United States Public Health Service Hospital, Carville, Louisiana 70721.

LEISHMANIASIS
method of
DAVID J. WYLER, M.D.
Bethesda, Maryland

Leishmaniasis is caused by various species of the protozoan parasite *Leishmania,* which grow within macrophages of susceptible mammalian hosts and is transmitted by the bites of infected sand flies (*Phlebotomus* species). Leishmania infecting man cause cutaneous disease (due to *L. tropica, L. mexicana,* and *L. brasiliensis*) and mucocutaneous disease (due to *L. brasiliensis*), or visceral disease (kala-azar, due to *L. donovani*). The diagnosis is established by a history of exposure to sand flies in an endemic area (although rare autochthonous infections have been reported in the United States and central Europe), a compatible clinical presentation, demonstration of organisms on tissue smears or biopsy, and the in vitro isolation of leishmania using specialized culture medium (e.g., N.N.N medium). A delayed hypersensitivity skin test response to leishmanial antigens (Montenegro test) may be a useful adjunct in the diagnosis of cutaneous and mucocutaneous leishmaniasis; the Montenegro test is negative in active kala-azar. The diagnostic value of serologic tests for leishmaniasis is uncertain at present. The therapeutic approach to leishmaniasis is based upon the form of the disease and the area of the world in which it was acquired. Response to therapy is monitored by clinical assessment. Host factors (e.g., immune response) and parasite strain characteristics are important determinants in the response to chemotherapy.

Chemotherapy

The mainstay of antileishmanial chemotherapy is the use of pentavalent antimonial compounds sodium stibogluconate (Pentostam) and N-methylglucamine antimonate (Glucantime). There are no known clinically important differences between these compounds in terms of efficacy or toxicity. Only Pentostam is available in the United States as an investigational drug (from the Parasitic Diseases Drug Service, Center for Disease Control, Atlanta, Georgia); Glucantime is used primarily in Latin America and in francophonic countries. Pentostam is supplied in vials of 100 ml. (100 mg. antimony per ml.) and is administered intravenously or intramuscularly in a dose of 0.1 ml. per kg. body weight per day (maximum 6 ml.). Injections are given daily for a 6 to 10 day course and a total of three courses can be administered, each separated by an interval of at least 10 days. The pentavalent antimonials are relatively nontoxic and adverse reactions are rare and generally mild when they occur. They include gastrointestinal upset, cough, skin rash, fever, and nonspecific ECG changes.

Old World cutaneous leishmaniasis (due to *L. tropica*) usually heals spontaneously and may not always require chemotherapy. Lesions which could be cosmetically disfiguring because of the scars they might leave, and lesions which are progressive or fail to heal in 3 to 5 months should be treated with pentavalent antimonials. One course is usually sufficient. In contrast, *New World cutaneous leishmaniasis* (due to *L. mexicana* and *L. brasiliensis*) acquired in Central and South America infrequently heal spontaneously and may require pentavalent antimonial therapy. Some patients with cutaneous lesions due to *L. brasiliensis* may subsequently develop oral or nasal involvement. Therefore, in countries in which mucocutaneous leishmaniasis is prevalent, primary cutaneous lesions are often treated vigorously with multiple courses of antimony (as well as amphotericin B in antimony failures) in the hope of preventing the subsequent development of mucocutaneous disease.

Local measures such as intralesional injection of antimonials, application of heat, excision, or cryosurgery have proved efficacious in some cases, but their efficacy relative to therapy with parenteral antimonials is uncertain. A repository antimalarial agent, cycloguanil pamoate (Camolar) can be administered as a single deep intramuscular injection (350 mg.) and repeated in 1 month, in patients who cannot be given pentavalent antimonials (cycloguanil pamoate is not available in the United States). This alternative drug is probably not as efficacious as antimony and response to therapy may be very slow (e.g., 2 to 3 months). Ulcerated cutaneous lesions are frequently superinfected with bacteria and may require debridement and appropriate antibiotic therapy.

Mucocutaneous leishmaniasis (due to *L. brasiliensis*) occurs in Central and South America. Nasal and oral lesions may develop months to years after the primary cutaneous lesion and can be markedly disfiguring and difficult to treat. In many instances, patients fail to respond to repeated courses of pentavalent antimony. In such patients amphotericin B should be administered in the same regimen as for deep mycoses, up to a total dose of 1.5 to 2.0 grams, if tolerated.

Kala-azar acquired in India, China, the Mediterranean, and Latin America responds favorably to a single course of pentavalent antimony, whereas disease acquired in the Sudan and East Africa is often unresponsive to even repeated courses. In cases of kala-azar that prove to be resistant to antimony, pentamidine isethionate (2 to 4 mg. per kg. per day intramuscularly for up to 15 doses; available from the Center for Disease Control) is recommended. This drug is moderately toxic and must be used with caution. Hydroxystilbamidine isethionate has also been successfully used as a second-line drug in this condition.

Patients traveling in endemic areas should avoid contact with sand flies by wearing protective clothing and using insect repellents. Antileishmanial agents are not used for chemoprophylaxis. No vaccine for the prevention of leishmaniasis is presently available, although trials have been carried out in Israel and Russia using live attenuated strains of *L. tropica*.

MALARIA

method of
THOMAS W. SHEEHY, M.D.
Birmingham, Alabama

In dealing with suspected malaria, the first objective is to confirm the diagnosis and to identify the plasmodia. *P. falciparum* causes a rapidly progressive infection in nonimmune persons and is known for its tendency to kill, if untreated. In contrast, *P. vivax, P. ovale,* and *P. malariae* are prone to chronicity and relapse. Infections persist for years, if untreated or treated improperly, but they are relatively benign and seldom kill.

Once the diagnosis of malaria is confirmed, the next objective is to achieve a clinical cure quickly and safely. Since the overt attack is due to continued maturation and release of blood schizonts (asexual erythrocytic forms), cure demands their partial or complete elimination. Drugs used for this purpose are known as "blood" schizonticides to differentiate them from "tissue" schizonticides, which exert their chemotherapeutic action against tissue (exoerythrocytic) forms.

The most commonly used blood schizonticides include: (1) the 4-aminoquinolines, chloroquine and amodiaquine; (2) the cinchona alkaloid, quinine; (3) the diaminopyrimidine, pyrimethamine (Daraprim); (4) the aminoacridine, quinacrine (Atabrine); and (5) the biguanides, proquanil and chloroproquanil.

The biguanides and pyrimethamine are never used alone to treat acute malaria because of their slow chemotherapeutic action; however, in combination with more rapidly acting blood schizonticides, such as quinine, they are extremely effective.

The tissue schizonticides used for therapy include the 8-aminoquinolines, pamaquine, pentaquine, isopentaquine, and primaquine. Primaquine is the most effective and the least toxic of this group. It may be given concurrently with any of the blood schizonticides except quinacrine.

Radical Cure—P. vivax, P. malariae, P. ovale

Radical cure and prevention of relapse requires destruction of both the erythrocytic and tissue forms. Usually, a *total* dose of 1.5 grams of chloroquine base given over 3 days and 210 mg. of primaquine base given over a 14-day period is sufficient for this purpose. Each 500 mg. tablet of chloroquine diphosphate contains 300 mg. of base. Each 26.5 mg. tablet of primaquine diphosphate contains 15 mg. of base.

Chloroquine and primaquine are given orally as follows:

Day 1: 600 mg. of chloroquine base, initially; 300 mg. 6 hours later.

Days 2 and 3: 300 mg. of chloroquine base daily. For children, the total dosage of chloroquine base should never exceed 20 mg. per kg. of body weight.

Days 1 to 14: 15 mg. primaquine base, daily. Primaquine may be given during the acute attack or after overt symptoms have subsided.

Chloroquine and primaquine are given with meals to reduce their irritating effect on the gastrointestinal tract. Both drugs can cause abdominal cramps, nausea, vomiting, and diarrhea. Occasionally, primaquine, in weekly suppressant doses of 45 mg. gives rise to a 24 to 48 hour "flulike syndrome." It may also induce acute hemolysis in patients with glucose-6-phosphate dehydrogenase deficiency.

If vomiting or other conditions preclude its oral use, chloroquine base, 200 mg. in 5.0 ml. of unbuffered sterile distilled water, is given intramuscularly every 6 hours. The total intramuscular dose for adults should never exceed 800 mg. of base per 24 hours. Oral therapy is started as soon as possible.

When amodiaquine dihydrochloride is prescribed, 600 mg. base orally is given initially, followed by 400 mg. daily for the next 2 days; primaquine is administered as above.

These blood schizonticides usually reduce the fever and symptoms of malarial patients within 24 to 48 hours and eliminate asexual (ring) forms within 4 to 5 days. The persistence of either clinical symptoms or schizonts (ring forms) in the peripheral blood following treatment suggests 4-aminoquinoline resistant infection. In this situation, ascertain the degree of parasitemia, make certain that schizonts, not gametocytes, are present in the peripheral blood, and start treatment for drug-resistant malaria. Gametocytes or sexual forms may persist in the peripheral blood for some time after effective clinical treatment and are harmless to the patient but are infective for mosquitos.

Chloroquine Sensitive P. falciparum Malaria

Chloroquine sensitive strains of *P. falciparum* are found in Africa, western Asia, and Central America, with the exception of Panama. Both chloroquine and amodiaquine are effective therapeutically against these strains. Primaquine therapy is not necessary, for there are no tissue forms of *P. falciparum.*

Drug Resistant Strains

Drug resistant *P. falciparum* malaria has spread throughout Southeast Asia and parts of Central and South America. These strains have the ability to survive and multiply in normally lethal concentrations of chloroquine and amodiaquine. Some also show variable responses to quinacrine, pyrimethamine, and even quinine.

Over the past decade, several combined drug regimens have proven effective against drug resistant strains. The most commonly used regimen consists of:

Day 1 to 10: quinine sulfate, 650 mg. orally, every 8 hours.

Day 1 to 3: pyrimethamine, 25 mg., twice daily.

Day 1 to 5: sulfadiazine or sulfisoxazole, 0.5 grams every 6 hours.

Two recently described regimens combine a short course of quinine therapy, 650 mg. (2 tablets) every 12 hours for a total of 4 or 6 doses with other antimalarial agents. One prescribes six doses of quinine, followed by a single (3 tablets) dose of Fansidar. Fansidar tablets contain 25 mg. of pyrimethamine and 500 mg. of sulfadoxine. The other consists of four doses of quinine, followed by a single dose (1.5 grams) (6 tablets) of Mefloquine. Mefloquine, a new quinoline-methanol agent, has been termed the most effective single dose agent for chloroquine resistant strains. At present, this drug is not available commercially in the United States.

Until others verify the effectiveness of the short course regimens described, the three-drug regimen outlined above is the treatment of choice.

Treatment of Severe or Complicated Falciparum Malaria

Severe malaria and its complications are almost invariably due to a high degree of parasitemia, i.e., greater than 100,000 parasites per cu. mm. For this reason, the degree of parasitemia should be ascertained initially and twice daily thereafter. Equally important are the patient's daily weight, fluid intake and output, and hematocrit. These four measures help to predict impending complications:

1. Sudden weight gain signals fluid retention. Pulmonary edema may occur secondary to overhydration. In this instance, fluid restriction is necessary even in the presence of fever, perspiration, and thirst. Occasionally, patients develop acute respiratory distress (ARD). They require intensive pulmonary care, including ventilatory support.

2. A sudden fall in urinary output heralds impending renal failure or dehydration. The sooner oliguria is detected, the better the chances for preventing renal failure through use of mannitol or diuretic therapy and careful fluid management. Acute renal failure is a rare complication and when it occurs, dialysis is mandatory.

3. A sudden drop in hematocrit or change in plasma color suggests an acute hemolytic reaction. This is usually associated with marked parasitemia and occasionally results from disseminated intravascular coagulation.

4. Scrutiny of the patient's behavior and mental status every 6 hours allows early recognition of cerebral malaria. This complication may present with coma, delusions, stupor, convulsions, aphasia, and psychosis. Dexamethasone sodium phosphate, 300 mg. every 8 hours may be helpful.

Intravenous quinine is unsurpassed for the treatment of severe falciparum malaria and complications, such as acute respiratory distress (ARD), renal failure, cerebral malaria, and blackwater fever. The objective of parenteral quinine therapy is to decrease the parasitemia as rapidly as possible and thereby eliminate the base for complications. Quinine dihydrochloride 650 mg., dissolved in 500 ml. of isotonic saline solution is given slowly over 8 hours. Slow administration is necessary to prevent hypotension. The total dose of parenteral quinine per 24 hours should never exceed 1950 mg. Parenteral administration is continued as long as necessary. Oral therapy with quinine sulfate is resumed as soon as possible. Serious toxic side effects are seldom encountered with parenteral quinine. Occasionally, however, premature beats or arrhythmias develop and prolonged use may cause cinchonism.

Patients with renal failure require less quinine; their daily dose is reduced to 600 mg. per 24 hours.

Prophylaxis

Residents or travelers to endemic malaria areas are advised to take 300 mg. of chloroquine base or 400 mg. of amodiaquine base weekly. Prophylactic treatment is started 1 week before entry into endemic areas and is continued for 6 weeks after leaving. Returnees should also be given either 15 mg. of primaquine base for 14 days or 45 mg. weekly for 8 weeks, to eliminate tissue forms of *P. vivax* and *P. malariae* and thus prevent a clinical relapse.

Prophylaxis for drug resistant falciparum malaria is far from ideal. Fansidar, 1 tablet per week, has been used successfully for prevention of chloroquine resistant falciparum malaria in certain areas. However, Fansidar contains pyrimethamine as its major schizonticide and some strains of *P. vivax* and *P. falciparum* are resistant to pyrimethamine.

MEASLES
(Rubeola)

method of
JAMES B. HANSHAW, M.D.
Worcester, Massachusetts

Although measles is far less common than it was prior to 1963, there were approximately 33,000 cases reported in 1976 and 60,000 cases in 1977. It is therefore, a disease of continued importance in spite of the successful development of a measles vaccine. Outside the United States, especially in some countries in Africa, measles continues to be a common epidemic disease.

The failure to control this disease can be attributed to inadequate utilization or misuse of the vaccine. Immunization given prior to 12 months of age is associated with an estimated 37 per cent susceptibility versus 9 per cent for infants vaccinated after one year of age. Other factors resulting in vaccine failure include simultaneous administration of immune serum globin, the use of inactivated measles vaccine (no longer available), inadequate refrigeration, or excessive exposure of the vaccine to light and heat.

Active Immunization

Live measles virus vaccine is prepared from a more attenuated line (Moraten) of measles virus derived from Ender's Edmonston strain and grown in cell cultures of chick embryo free of avian leukosis. The virus may be mixed with rubella or rubella and mumps before lyophilization. Vaccination singly or in combination results in a mild or inapparent infection that induces active immunity in 95 per cent of recipients. Occasionally, fever, mild malaise, and a faint rash may occur one week after immunization. The antibody and protection induced is long lasting in the great majority of persons immunized after 15 months of age. If an epidemic is in progress, children 6 months or older should receive the vaccine. They should then be revaccinated at some time prior to school entry.

Precautions and Contraindications to Active Immunization. Children with a positive tuberculin skin test should not be given measles vaccination unless they receive antituberculous chemotherapy for a period of at least 2 months following vaccination. Infection with another virus or a fever of undetermined origin is an additional contraindication to measles vaccination. There is the strong probability that a preexisting viral infection may preclude successful immunizations with a second live virus. This could be due to the production of interferon by the first agent. Similarly, the administration of any blood product containing measles antibody may interfere with successful vaccination. The importance of humoral antibody is demonstrated in the protective efficacy of immune serum globulin and in the vaccine failure rate in infants under one year of age who continue to have low levels of maternal antibody present.

Other contraindications are those common to all live virus vaccines, i.e., preexisting lymphoreticular disease, leukemia, immunodeficiency diseases of cell-mediated immunity, primary immunologic disorders, and patients who are receiving corticosteroids, alkylating agents, antimetabolites, or radiation. Pregnant women are apparently not at great risk, but should not receive any live virus as a matter of general principle.

Booster Doses. Long-term studies of persons vaccinated against measles suggest that booster doses are not necessary unless the infant was immunized prior to 12 months of age. If vaccination took place at one year or before 15 months of age, it is probably not necessary to revaccinate. In addition, revaccination should be carried out on children who received simultaneous immune serum globulin or a killed measles vaccine.

Passive Immunization—Immune Serum Globulin (ISG)

If a known susceptible child or adult is exposed to measles, immune serum globulin should be administered at a dose of 0.25 ml. per kg. In order to be effective, this must be given within 5 days of exposure. Complete protection is largely dependent upon the rapidity in which the ISG is given following exposure. A modification of the disease may occur if the ISG is given after 5 days, but it is unlikely that inapparent illness will result. The protective effect of ISG lasts for 4 to 6 weeks after administration.

Treatment

The treatment of measles is symptomatic. Cough, perhaps the most distressing symptom, can be improved but not eliminated with one of a variety of preparations such as promethazine with codeine (Phenergan expectorant with codeine). Aspirin (75 mg. per year of age) every 4 to 6 hours, not to exceed 2.4 grams per day, is of value in controlling fever.

Complications

Otitis Media. This is perhaps the most frequent complication of measles. It should be managed as it is in patients without the underlying disease because the cause is the same. Thus, ampicillin, 75 mg. per kg. per day orally, in four divided doses would be appropriate. Amoxicillin may also be used. For children over 5 years of age, penicillin V, 75,000 units per kg. per day orally should be given. Children allergic to penicillin may be given trimethoprim-sulfamethoxazole (8 mg. per kg. per day trimethoprim plus 40 mg. per kg. per day sulfamethoxazole) (this use of trimethoprim-sulfamethoxazole is not listed in the manufacturer's official directive) or erythromycin (30 mg. per kg. per day) in four doses.

Croup. Acute laryngotracheobronchitis may occur as a complication of measles and should be treated in the same way croup caused by parainfluenza virus is treated. This involves a humid environment, either at home or in a croup tent in the hospital. Antibiotics are usually not indicated and corticosteroids are contraindicated. In some patients racemic epinephrine may improve breathing for a limited period. Sedatives are contraindicated. An artificial airway (endotracheal tube or tracheostomy) is usually not indicated.

Pneumonia. Pneumonia associated with measles may be due to the measles virus itself or to secondary bacterial pathogens such as the *Streptococcus pneumoniae*, *Streptococcus pyogenes*, or *Hemophilus influenzae*. *Staphylococcus aureus*, once a common complication of measles, is seen less frequently at the present time. The antibiotic chosen should reflect the list of possible pathogens. It should be noted that *Hemophilus influenzae* is very uncommon in school age children and staphylococcal pneumonia rarely fails to produce a pleural effusion when left untreated for more than 24 to 48 hours. Children under 5 years of age should be given ampicillin (100 mg. per kg. per day in six divided doses). Oxacillin (or nafcillin) should be given if staphylococcal infection is suspected. The dose is 150 mg. per kg. per day.

Other complications of measles include encephalitis, which is treated symptomatically with special attention to seizure control and cerebral edema. The treatment of encephalitis, now extremely rare in measles, is considered elsewhere.

BACTERIAL MENINGITIS *

method of
PHILIP C. CRAVEN, M.D.
San Antonio, Texas

Bacterial meningitis is a true medical emergency in which inappropriate or delayed treatment may markedly increase the already high mortality. Presumptive treatment must begin immediately after a brief examination, long before identification of the pathogen can be accomplished by the microbiology laboratory. The physician must make an estimation of the pathogens likely to be present based upon information at hand the moment the diagnosis is entertained; this estimation will determine the initial presump-

---

*The dose recommendations for some drugs in this article may be higher than those stated in the manufacturers' official directives but these higher doses are considered to be necessary for proper treatment of this life-threatening illness.

tive therapy, which can be modified by subsequent findings.

Predictors of Likely Pathogens

The *age* of the patient strongly affects which bacteria are likely to cause meningitis. Approximately 70 per cent of all cases are caused by only three bacteria: the pneumococcus *(S. pneumoniae),* the meningococcus *(N. meningitidis),* and hemophilus *(H. influenzae). Hemophilus influenzae* is the predominant pathogen in children through three years of age; the meningococcus is common from three months through 20 years of age; and the pneumococcus occurs commonly in young children and adults. Additional pathogens predominate in newborn children (see Table 1). These generalizations based upon age apply chiefly to patients without underlying or associated conditions.

Associated findings or illnesses strongly affect the clinician's prediction of the pathogen, so they must be sought rapidly but carefully in the initial evaluation. *Congenital abnormalities,* such as meningomyelocoele or midline dermal sinus, are frequently associated with meningitis due to *S. aureus,* group A streptococci, and enteric bacilli (*E. coli,* proteus species, etc.). *Nonpenetrating trauma* to the head, which may result in inapparent fracture of the skull or cribriform plate, or a dural tear, can cause pneumococcal meningitis, either shortly after the trauma or years later, and possibly in recurrent episodes. *Penetrating skull trauma* (including neurosurgery) can result in staphylococcal or enteric bacillary meningitis, often with strains of klebsiella, serratia, proteus, or pseudomonas that are hospital-transmitted and resistant to multiple antibiotics; clues to the identity of these strains often lie in infections at other sites, such as urinary tract infections induced by indwelling bladder catheters. Infections associated with *bacteremia,* especially *endocarditis,* may present as meningitis; in addition to the viridans streptococcus often associated with endocarditis, one must consider enterococcal meningitis (which requires different therapy) and, in narcotic addicts, endocarditis due to staphylococcus, pseudomonas, and serratia. Upper respiratory infections, particularly otitis, mastoiditis, and sinusitis, serve as foci for meningeal spread of hemophilus, pneumococcus, and occasionally staphylococcus (as in frontal sinusitis with osteomyelitis); these foci often require surgical drainage. Particularly in old or debilitated persons (including alcoholics), pneumococcal pneumonia may be accompanied by meningitis, which is often initially overlooked. Intracranial foreign bodies, especially ventriculoatrial or ventriculoperitoneal shunts, often cause meningitis due to *Staphylococcus epidermidis, S. aureus,* and diphtheroids, all of which are often penicillin resistant. *Immunocompromised hosts,* particularly with cancer, leukemia, or recent renal transplantation, are host to a variety of bacterial meningitis pathogens, including listeria, pneumococcus, staphylococcus, pseudomonas, and *E. coli*; nonbacterial meningitis or encephalitis (especially due to cryptococcus, varicella, *Herpes simplex,* and *Toxoplasma gondii*) may mimic bacterial meningitis in these patients.

Other infections mimicking bacterial meningitis must be considered in the evaluation of a patient with fever and spinal fluid pleocytosis, as the presumptive therapy would be different. *Brain abscess* usually causes signs of a mass but can present with fever, headache, no focal signs, and spinal fluid pleocytosis with increased protein; low spinal fluid glucose (less than 50 per cent of serum glucose) implies rupture or leak of the abscess; treatment is penicillin, chloramphenicol, and surgical drainage. A *parameningeal focus* of infection can cause pain, fever, and spinal fluid pleocytosis or actual meningitis; examples include vertebral osteomyelitis, subdural empyema, spinal epidural abscess, and retropharyngeal abscess, all of which would normally require prompt surgical drainage for bacteriologic diagnosis and cure.

Tuberculous meningitis can cause a fulminant clinical course with a predominance of polymorphonuclear leukocytes and low glucose in the spinal fluid; apical cavities or a miliary pattern may be evident on the chest radiograph with a positive sputum fluorochrome or Kinyoun smear; however, if no organisms are seen and the chest radiograph is normal, biopsy of the liver and bone marrow for acid-fast stains may be necessary before initiating therapy with isoniazid, ethambutol, and rifampin. *Fungal meningitis,* particularly cryptococcal, candidal, and coccidioidal, may also present with acute meningitis and difficulty

TABLE 1.   **Meningitis Pathogens in Different Age Groups of Normal Hosts**

AGE	COMMON PATHOGENS	LESS LIKELY, BUT POSSIBLE
0 to 30 days	Enteric bacilli Group B streptococcus Listeria	Pneumococcus Staphylococcus *H. influenzae* Group A streptococcus
31 to 60 days	Group B streptococcus Meningococcus *H. influenzae*	Enteric bacilli Pneumococcus Staphylococcus
60 days to 10 years	*H. influenzae* Meningococcus Pneumococcus	
Over 10 years	Meningococcus Pneumococcus	

finding organisms in the spinal fluid itself. Therapy for tuberculous and for fungal meningitis *may* have to be presumptive pending results of cultures and stains. So-called *aseptic meningitis* is clinically benign meningitis with spinal fluid lymphocytosis, normal glucose and modest protein elevation; often this is due to enteroviral infection, occurring in summer and fall months. However, several causes of an "aseptic meningitis" syndrome, such as leptospirosis and syphilis, require specific therapy. Conversely, nontreatable viral meningitis may initially cause predominance of polymorphonuclear cells in the spinal fluid and, occasionally with mumps, low spinal fluid glucose. Leukemia and *H. simplex* meningitis may also cause low CSF glucose. Finally, the unusual entity of *amebic meningoencephalitis* (due to fresh water, free-living Hartmanella and Naeglaria species) can be diagnosed by finding large amebae in spinal fluid or brain biopsy and may respond to amphotericin B therapy.

Approach to the Patient With Possible Bacterial Meningitis

Altered mentation or coma in a patient with fever and signs of meningeal irritation indicate that the prognosis is already poor; prompt administration of presumptive, but appropriate, antibiotic therapy may be lifesaving. Infants may manifest only nonspecific signs, such as poor feeding and irritability; a bulging fontanelle may be detected. A very brief history should include duration of symptoms, antecedent illness or trauma, seizures in the past, use of ethanol or intravenous drugs, and recent administration of antimicrobial agents. A brief examination should search for sinusitis, otitis, mastoiditis, tympanic membrane or retroauricular hematoma, cardiac murmurs and signs of endocarditis, pulmonary consolidation, skin rashes, and equality of tendon reflexes. Blood should be drawn for culture, glucose, white cell count, ethanol level and toxic screen; then 50 ml. of 50 per cent glucose and, in adults, 50 to 100 mg. thiamine should be given. Unless there is papilledema or clear evidence of a mass lesion, lumbar puncture (LP) should be performed immediately and the physician himself should examine unspun cerebrospinal fluid (CSF) for cells and Gram stain of spun CSF for organisms:

1. No penetrating trauma or endocarditis, CSF has polymorphonuclear cells (PMNs):

Patient over 10 years old: definite gram-positive or gram-negative diplococci seen: supervise administration of penicillin immediately; no organisms seen: immediate penicillin administration; gram-negative bacilli: treat for enteric bacillary meningitis (see Table 2).

Patient 60 days to 10 years old: gram-negative pleomorphic coccobacilli definitely seen: initiate ampicillin and chloramphenicol (ampicillin dose should precede chloramphenicol dose); definite gram-positive or gram-negative diplococci: initiate penicillin for pneumococcal or meningococcal meningitis; no organisms seen: ampicillin and chloramphenicol.

Patient less than 60 days old: should receive ampicillin with gentamicin intravenously; if Gram stain (large gram-positive cocci in clumps) or clinical setting suggests staphylococci: add oxacillin or nafcillin; if a prompt response is not noted (24 to 36 hours), or, if the patient is moribund, add gentamicin intrathecally. (This use of intrathecal gentamicin is not listed in the manufacturer's official directive.)

2. Signs of endocarditis, CSF has polymorphonuclear cells (PMNs), patient any age: administer penicillin with oxacillin and intravenous gentamicin; if endocarditis may be enterococcal (arising from urinary or genital source) or enteric bacillary, intrathecal gentamicin should be instilled. (This use of gentamicin intrathecally is not listed in the manufacturer's official directive.)

3. Penetrating head trauma is present, CSF has PMNs, patient any age: initiate therapy with oxacillin, intravenous gentamicin, intrathecal gentamicin (this use of gentamicin intrathecally is not listed in the manufacturer's official directive); if abscess may be present, add chloramphenicol.

4. Non-penetrating head trauma has occurred, with PMNs in CSF: treat with penicillin for pneumococci unless Gram stain suggests other organisms (Hemophilus, staphylococci, and meningococci less commonly follow trauma).

5. Immunosuppressed host (cancer, leukemia, renal transplant) with PMNs in CSF: initial CSF examination *must* include careful India ink preparation for cryptococci; initial treatment for bacterial meningitis should cover listeria, pseudomonas, and staphylococci: carbenicillin, oxacillin, intravenous gentamicin, and intrathecal gentamicin. (This use of gentamicin intrathecally is not listed in the manufacturer's official directive.) Gram stain may help narrow regimen.

6. Patient, any age, seriously ill, but CSF contains predominantly lymphocytes: bacterial cause unlikely, seriously consider viral, fungal, or tuberculous cause.

In mildly ill patients with headache and meningismus who have no organisms on Gram stain and no suggestion of a focus for bacterial meningitis, it is reasonable to await results of glucose and protein determinations and repeat lumbar puncture in 6 hours before deciding about initiating antibiotic therapy. In viral meningitis, the initial PMN predominance will shift to a lymphocyte predominance in 6 to 12 hours in most patients and the glucose and protein will remain very close to normal (except that in mumps and

TABLE 2. **Meningitis Pathogen, Antibiotic Therapy, and Duration of Treatment**

PATHOGEN	PREFERRED ANTIBIOTIC	ANTIBIOTIC FOR PENICILLIN-ALLERGIC PATIENT	DURATION OF THERAPY
Pneumococcus	Penicillin	Chloramphenicol	10–14 days
Meningococcus	Penicillin	Chloramphenicol	7–10 days
H. influenzae	Ampicillin or chloramphenicol	Chloramphenicol	10–14 days
S. aureus	Oxacillin, nafcillin, (methicillin)*	Vancomycin	21–28 days
Group B streptococcus	Penicillin or ampicillin		10–14 days
Listeria			
Normal host	Penicillin	See text	14 days
Immunosuppressed or relapse	Penicillin or ampicillin plus gentamicin IV (and IT† if necessary)		4 weeks
Enteric bacilli			
Unknown susceptibility	Gentamicin IV *and* IT†	—	10–14 days after cultures are negative and fever gone
Known to be susceptible to chloramphenicol	Chloramphenicol	—	10–14 days after cultures are negative and fever gone
Resistant to gentamicin or likely to be so‡	Amikacin IV and IT†	—	10–14 days after cultures are negative and fever gone
Pseudomonas	Carbenicillin with gentamicin IV *and* IT†	—	10–14 days after cultures are negative and fever gone
S. epidermidis	Penicillin or oxacillin or vancomycin (depending on susceptibility)	Vancomycin	14 days after removal of shunt
Enterococcus	Penicillin with gentamicin IV *and* IT†	Vancomycin with gentamicin	10–14 days

*May be more likely to cause interstitial nephritis
†IT = intrathecal (lumbar or ventricular). The intrathecal use of gentamicin or amikacin is not listed in the manufacturers' official directive
‡Based upon susceptibilities of bacterial flora in the hospital

Herpes simplex meningoencephalitis, hypoglycorrhachia may occur).

After deciding upon initial presumptive therapy, additional procedures may help modify therapy before bacterial culture results are known, such as: sinus and mastoid radiographs and aspirates for evidence of a pneumococcal or hemophilus primary source; Gram stain of blood buffy coat, joint fluid, or skin lesion aspirate for meningococci; limulus lysate assay of CSF for evidence of gram-negative endotoxin; counterimmunoelectrophoresis for specific bacterial antigens in CSF (*N. meningitidis, H. influenzae,* and *S. pneumoniae*); India ink preparation and latex cryptococcal agglutination test of CSF for *C. neoformans;* sputum acid-fast stain and chest radiograph for evidence of tuberculosis; brain scan and EEG for brain abscess; bone films, sinus films, and bone scans for a parameningeal focus of infection; and arteriography for subdural abscess.

Specific Therapy (see Tables 2 and 3)

Pneumococcal Meningitis. Penicillin G in high dosage for 10 to 14 days is the preferred treatment; history of immediate skin rash, bronchospasm, or anaphylaxis after penicillin should prompt the use of chloramphenicol. A prompt, thorough search for an otic, sinus, or pulmonary focus should be undertaken to allow surgical drainage if necessary. Recurrent pneumococcal meningitis strongly suggests a cerebrospinal fluid leak or abnormal communication.

Meningococcal Meningitis. Penicillin G for 7 to 10 days is optimal therapy, with alternate chloramphenicol for patients with a history of serious hypersensitivity to penicillin. If hypotension, petechiae, or purpura occur, high dose corticosteroid therapy may be of benefit and the early use of heparin may counteract intravascular clotting. Persons who have had (1) recent (10 days before onset), prolonged or repetitive household contact with a patient or (2) *direct* contact with oral secretions of a patient (mouth to mouth resuscitation) should receive 600 mg. oral rifampin twice daily for two days for adults, 10 mg. per kg. twice daily for children 1 to 12 years of age, and 5 mg. per kg. twice daily for children less than one year old. This prophylaxis should begin immediately for contacts; nasopharyngeal cultures play no role. Hospital contacts of patients are not generally at increased risk; patients need be isolated only for the first 24 hours of antibiotic treatment. Serotype A and C vaccine is very effective in closed military

TABLE 3. **Intravenous Dosage Regimens for Antibiotics Used in Bacterial Meningitis***

ANTIBIOTIC	DAILY ADULT DOSAGE	DAILY PEDIATRIC DOSAGE	NEONATES < 7 DAYS
Penicillin G	12–24 million units (12 doses)	100,000–300,000 units per kg. (6 doses)	50,000–100,000 units per kg. (2–3 doses)
Ampicillin	300–400 mg. per kg. (6 doses)	200–300 mg. per kg. (4 doses)	100 mg. per kg. (4 doses)
Chloramphenicol	4–6 grams (4 doses); after 3 days can decrease to 2–3 grams	100 mg. per kg. (4 doses)	Rarely used
Oxacillin, nafcillin, methicillin	10–12 grams (6 doses)	100–200 mg. per kg. (4 doses)	100–200 mg. per kg. (4 doses)
Gentamicin			
intravenous	3–5 mg. per kg. (3 doses)	6–7.5 mg. per kg. (3 doses)	5 mg. per kg. (2 doses)
intrathecal†	6 mg. every 24 hours	1–4 mg. every 24 hours	1–4 mg. every 24 hours
Amikacin			
intravenous	15 mg. per kg. (2 doses)	15 mg. per kg. (2 doses)	Loading dose of 10 mg. per kg. then 7.5 mg. per kg. every 12 hours
intrathecal†	15 mg. every 24 hours†	4–10 mg. every 24 hours‡	4–10 mg. every 24 hours‡
Vancomycin	2 grams (2–4 doses)	40 mg. per kg. (4 doses)	
Carbenicillin	24–30 grams (6 doses)	300–500 mg. per kg. (6 doses)	

*Doses listed in this table may be higher than usual dose.

†Administer in 1 to 3 ml. saline over 5 to 10 minutes after withdrawing equal volume of spinal fluid; periodically withdraw CSF during administration to confirm location of needle. The intrathecal use of gentamicin or amikacin is not listed in the manufacturers' official directives.

‡Data on appropriate doses are very limited; CSF obtained prior to each dose should be assayed for antibiotic and bactericidal levels

populations, should be used in outbreaks, and may help prevent disease in contacts of less than 5 days if given with rifampin.

Hemophilus Meningitis. Because of recent reports of ampicillin resistance and the rare occurrence of resistance to chloramphenicol, therapy should consist of chloramphenicol and ampicillin until antimicrobial susceptibility has been determined. If susceptibility exists, ampicillin should be used for 10 to 14 days. In truly penicillin-allergic patients, chloramphenicol should be used. If hemophilus meningitis occurs in a patient over 10 years of age, immunoglobulin deficiency or a parameningeal focus should be sought.

Staphylococcal Meningitis. A penicillinase-resistant semisynthetic penicillin (oxacillin, nafcillin, methicillin) should be used for 21 to 28 days. In patients with potentially life-threatening penicillin allergy, vancomycin is indicated, but nephrotoxicity, fever, and rash occur frequently. The currently available cephalosporins do not achieve adequate concentrations in CSF, even across inflamed meninges; they should never be used for meningitis. Except in neonates, patients should have an identifiable reason for the occurrence of staphylococcal meningitis, usually trauma, which may require surgical therapy; if the reason is endocarditis, potentially repairable brain abscesses or arterial aneurysms should be sought

and, of course, antibiotic treatment should be continued for six weeks.

Meningitis Due to Enteric Gram-Negative Bacteria. Because up to 25 per cent of these organisms are resistant to chloramphenicol, initial therapy pending identification and susceptibility determination will usually consist of parenteral gentamicin *in addition to* intrathecal gentamicin (the use of gentamicin intrathecally is not listed in the manufacturer's official directive), administered initially by the lumbar route. (None of the aminoglycosides administered parenterally achieve consistently adequate spinal fluid concentration.) It is best to avoid combining chloramphenicol and aminoglycoside therapy, if possible, to avoid antibiotic antagonism. If response is poor in 24 to 36 hours or if there is reason to suspect impairment of spinal fluid circulation from the lumbar area, gentamicin should be given by cisternal tap or into the ventricles *via* an Ommaya reservoir (this use of gentamicin is not listed in the manufacturer's official directive). Prior cultures may suggest modification of this initial regimen, e.g., if a prior urinary tract isolate is resistant to gentamicin, amikacin should be substituted, or, if pseudomonas is suspected, parenteral carbenicillin should be added. Susceptibilities of the spinal fluid isolate will determine subsequent therapy; chloramphenicol should be used if susceptibility is demonstrated. Therapy should continue *at least* 10 to 14 days after the cultures have become negative. Delayed recovery and relapse are frequent. Surgical repair of dural defects or leaks can be considered after cultures are negative. (The high frequency of resistance to kanamycin among these bacteria in most hospitals dictates against using it in initial therapy.)

Group B Streptococcal Meningitis. This infection of neonatal infants should be treated with high doses of penicillin or ampicillin for 10 to 14 days.

Listeria Meningitis. *Listeria monocytogenes* is often confused with diphtheroids or corynebacteria, and streptococci; the distinction is important because some patients will relapse after treatment for 14 days with recommended doses of penicillin or ampicillin, which are only bacteriostatic against listeria. If the patient has impaired host defenses or has relapsed after initial penicillin therapy, eradication of the infection may require penicillin for 4 to 6 weeks with the addition of gentamicin intravenously and intrathecally for part of that period. (The use of gentamicin intrathecally is not listed in the manufacturer's official directive.) In a truly penicillin-allergic patient, tetracycline (15 mg. per kg. daily, in four doses intravenously) probably should be used, although spinal fluid levels may be erratic; chloramphenicol may also be effective.

Staphylococcus Epidermidis Meningitis. This infection occurs in patients with indwelling spinal fluid shunts or reservoirs, which must be removed or replaced to achieve successful treatment. Because of frequent resistance to penicillin and semisynthetic penicillins, initial therapy pending susceptibility results must consist of intravenous vancomycin or intravenous and intrathecal gentamicin. (The use of gentamicin intrathecally is not listed in the manufacturer's official directive.) Subsequent treatment, preferably with penicillin or a semisynthetic penicillin, should endure 14 days after shunt removal.

Enterococcal Meningitis. This infection, which usually occurs in patients with endocarditis or an evident genitourinary focus, requires parenteral penicillin and gentamicin along with intrathecal gentamicin (the use of gentamicin intrathecally is not listed in the manufacturer's official directive) for 10 to 14 days. Penicillin hypersensitivity requires its substitution by vancomycin; some cures have been achieved by using parenteral vancomycin without gentamicin.

General Measures

Antibiotics. Antibiotics should be administered by the intravenous route during the entire course of therapy, for certainty of dosing and higher serum levels; as inflammation of the meninges diminishes with successful therapy, penetrance of most antibiotics into the spinal fluid also is reduced. The initially high doses of chloramphenicol (4 to 6 grams in adults) may induce a degree of reversible, dose-related marrow suppression; after 2 to 3 days of treatment and a clinical response has been achieved, the dose can be reduced, avoiding serious marrow failure. (The much rarer, idiosyncratic, irreversible aplastic anemia is not dose-related and will already have been risked.)

A history of urticaria, immediate skin rash, or bronchospasm after penicillin implies a higher risk of potentially fatal anaphylaxis and should prompt the use of an alternate drug, *if* a suitable one exists; if the only alternates are distinctly inferior therapeutically (such as cephalosporins, erythromycin, etc.), the physician may elect to proceed with a "desensitization" regimen of increasing doses, then continuous penicillin therapy (Green, G. R. et al.: *Ann. Intern. Med.* 67:235, 1967), in the intensive care unit. Inadequate therapy probably carries a higher risk than penicillin under these circumstances.

Patient Care. Most patients should be admitted to the intensive care unit initially, with at least 2-hourly monitoring by nurses of vital signs and neurologic function (alertness and focal weakness in face, arms, legs). Nothing should be given by mouth until the patient is clearly alert and stable. Maintenance fluid and electrolytes should be administered and any plastic intravenous catheter changed every 2 to 3 days to prevent catheter sepsis. Fluid intake and output should be monitored, as excess fluid intake may contribute to cerebral edema. An indwelling bladder catheter should not be used to assist output determination unless the patient is hypotensive. The possibility of seizures and potential need for respiratory support should be made clear to those caring for the patient. No sedatives, tranquilizers, or sleep medication should be administered. Antipyretics should not be given—as monitoring the temperature response to treatment is very helpful—unless the fever may result in seizures (in children) or hyperthermic brain damage (greater than 104°F. [40°C.]) or cardiac compromise. Under these circumstances, regular doses of antipyretics will provide better control than irregular doses (PRN) and may allow observation of the residual fever.

The physician should examine the patient at least twice daily for changes in mental status, the appearance of rash or focal neurologic signs, evidence of associated disease (such as endocarditis, sinusitis, etc.), and the occurrence of complications such as hospital-acquired infections. Daily measurement of head circumference in young infants will detect the development of hydrocephalus.

Three times weekly the following laboratory studies should be performed: hematocrit, white cell count, platelet count and examination of the peripheral smear, urinalysis, serum electrolytes and urea nitrogen or creatinine. Prothrombin time (PT), partial thromboplastin time (PTT), liver function tests, and chest radiograph should also be monitored 1 to 3 times weekly, depending upon the clinical situation. Conditions to keep in mind when reviewing these results are electrolyte imbalance from inappropriate ADH secretion (hyponatremia) or from inappropriate fluid and electrolyte administration, aminoglycoside nephrotoxicity, chloramphenicol marrow suppression, and nosocomial pneumonia or urinary infection.

Monitoring Therapy. It is important to monitor the efficacy of therapy by repeating the lumbar puncture 1 to 2 days after initiating or changing therapy and again 1 to 2 days after stopping therapy, for glucose, protein, cell count, Gram stain, and culture. Glucose should return to normal (more than 50 per cent of simultaneous serum glucose) after 2 to 4 days of appropriate treatment; both the absolute white cell count and the percentage of polymorphonuclear leukocytes should fall in the same period; protein concentration is slower to return to normal. One to 2 days after a successful course of treatment, the CSF will contain no stainable or culturable organisms, normal glucose concentration, few to no polymorphonuclear cells and the protein concentration at least falling.

Complications

Disseminated Intravascular Coagulation (DIC). DIC may accompany severe gram-negative infections or occasionally gram-positive infections; its presence is suggested by abnormal bleeding, anemia with abnormal red cell forms, low platelet count, prolonged PT and PTT, and diminished fibrinogen or increased fibrin split products. Treatment of DIC includes blood replacement, vigorous treatment of sepsis and drainage of any loculated infection, and the use of full doses of heparin (5000 to 10,000 units intravenously every 4 hours), preferably via a continuous intravenous infusion pump, to achieve an activated partial thromboplastin time (PTT) that is 1.5 to 2.5 times longer than the control value.

Hypotension. Hypotension or shock may accompany meningitis, particularly in meningococcal disease with meningococcemia. Early clues may be the appearance of petechiae or purpura, diminishing urine output, or unexplained hyperventilation. Treatment consists of vigorous fluid replacement (isotonic saline) as rapidly as possible via large intravenous catheters until urine output occurs, the pressure rises, or signs of fluid overload occur (S_3 gallop or pulmonary rales). An indwelling bladder catheter should be placed until urine output is established and, unless the pressure responds promptly, a central venous pressure line or pulmonary wedge pressure catheter should be inserted. If the central venous pressure remains persistently above 15 cm. saline or the mean wedge pressure above 15 cm. after vigorous fluid therapy, without a return to adequate arterial pressure or urine output, vasoactive drugs should be administered (isoproterenol, 5 to 10 micrograms per minute, or dopamine, 2 to 10 micrograms per kg. per minute) until urine output or other evidence of adequate organ perfusion occurs.

Increased Intracranial Pressure. The risk of precipitating temporal lobe or cerebellar herniation in patients with increased intracranial pressure by removing lumbar fluid must be borne in mind. Increased pressure can accompany meningitis without papilledema. The initial diagnostic lumbar puncture, of course, must be done; the risk of herniation can be reduced by using a small needle (20 to 22 gauge) and removing a small volume of fluid; if significantly increased pressure (i.e., more than 300 to 400 mm. water) is documented, the use of steroids (dexamethasone sodium phosphate, 10 mg. intravenously followed by 4 mg. intramuscularly every 6 hours) or osmotic diuretics (mannitol, 1 to 2 grams per kg. intravenously over 30 to 60 minutes every 12 hours) *may* help prevent catastrophe. Although of unproven value, removal of ventricular spinal fluid also may prevent herniation. Repeat lumbar punctures should be avoided in anyone suspected of having an intracranial abscess, until drainage is achieved.

Seizures. Seizures accompanying meningitis usually occur in infants, may be "febrile" seizures, and do not necessarily imply the existence of a focal intracranial process. Seizures should be treated aggressively medically: initial interruption with slow intravenous doses of diazepam (5 to 10 mg. in adults and older children, 0.04 to 0.2 mg. per kg. in younger children, over 2 to 3 minutes), then suppression with phenytoin (diphenylhydantoin) and phenobarbital parenterally. Respiratory and cardiac depression may occur, so resuscitation and ventilatory support equipment should be at hand. Until seizures are controlled, the patient should be positioned on his side or abdomen with head down to prevent aspiration. If seizures are difficult to control, persist after improvement in the meningitis, or occur in adults, specific treatable causes should be sought, such as hyponatremia from inappropriate secretion of antidiuretic hormone, brain abscess, subdural empyema or hematomas, and other focal lesions.

Focal neurologic signs, particularly transient ones, may accompany or follow seizures occurring with meningitis and may have no specific anatomic basis. However, prominent or persistent focal signs indicate the presence of a significant pathologic process other than or in addition to meningitis: (a) increased intracranial pressure may affect function of the third or sixth cranial nerves (for treatment, see above); (b) meningitis may only be one part of a process with a focal lesion, such as a brain abscess "leaking" into the CSF; endocarditis with arterial aneurysm, abscess, or embolism; subdural empyema; or malignant otitis externa; (c) venous thrombosis may complicate meningitis, causing focal signs or seizures; (d) some nonbacterial processes may mimic meningitis with focal signs, such as *Herpes simplex* encephalitis, producing temporal lobe signs and CSF pleocytosis with red cells.

Renal Failure. This may occur during the course of meningitis for a number of reasons. High doses of penicillin in the face of renal failure can cause myoclonic muscle twitching and generalized seizures; hence, with severe oliguria or serum creatinine greater than 3.0 mg. per dl. (100 ml.), the doses of penicillin and the penicillinase-resistant penicillins should be halved; the dose of carbenicillin should be reduced to 4 to 6 grams per day to prevent platelet dysfunction and bleeding. Reductions in the parenteral maintenance doses of all aminoglycosides and vancomycin must accompany *any* diminution in renal function, guided by the package insert recommendations. Chloramphenicol dosage need not be altered in renal failure.

Continued Fever. If unchanged after 24 to 48 hours of therapy, continued fever suggests that: (1) the meningitis is not bacterial—viral, fungal, and tuberculous causes should be reconsidered; (2) the bacteria are not susceptible to the antibiotic regimen chosen (very unlikely for pneumococcal or meningococcal meningitis treated with penicillin or chloramphenicol; more likely for enteric bacillary meningitis); (3) the antibiotics are not being administered properly (i.e., orally or irregularly); (4) there is localized, undrained infection, particularly in paranasal sinuses, middle ear, intracranial abscess, parameningeal osteomyelitis of the cranium or vertebrae, or subdural abscess; the choice of brain scan, bone scan, sinus films, cerebral arteriogram, or direct exploration as means of diagnosis will depend upon how quickly each can be accomplished: very prompt drainage can be lifesaving; (5) in enteric bacillary meningitis being treated by parenteral and lumbar intrathecal aminoglycosides, ventriculitis may not be reached by either route of drug administration; in this case, intraventricular aminoglycoside must be given *via* an indwelling Ommaya reservoir; or

(6) drug fever may be present, which should be the last cause to be considered, as the only definitive diagnosis is accomplished by changing antibiotics, and there are often only 1 to 2 adequate choices.

Fever Relapse. Relapse of fever after an initial response to treatment may be due to any of the above reasons or to the occurrence of nosocomial infection, most commonly urinary tract (if a catheter has been present), pulmonary (if intubation or aspiration has occurred), or thrombophlebitis (from indwelling plastic venous catheter).

INFECTIOUS MONONUCLEOSIS

method of
JAMES C. NIEDERMAN, M.D.
New Haven, Connecticut

Infectious mononucleosis is an acute disease caused by the Epstein-Barr virus (EBV), a member of the herpes group. Classic clinical features of this infection include (1) fever, sore throat, lymphadenopathy and splenomegaly; (2) an absolute increase in the number of lymphocytes, which usually exceed 50 per cent of peripheral leukocytes and include more than 10 per cent atypical lymphocytes; (3) the transient appearance of elevated sheep cell agglutinins (heterophile antibodies) and beef cell hemolysins; (4) development of persistent Epstein-Barr virus antibodies; (5) abnormalities of liver function.

Infectious mononucleosis and EBV infections occur throughout the world and no annual or seasonal variations have been observed in the general population. The age at which infection is acquired is related to economic and hygienic conditions. In developing countries infection occurs early in life and is usually subclinical or inapparent; in areas in which exposure and infection are delayed until late adolescence or young adulthood, EBV infections are expressed as clinical infectious mononucleosis in about 50 per cent of cases. Studies of contact infections suggest an incubation period of 30 to 50 days in the adult. EBV is regularly present in saliva of infectious mononucleosis patients and demonstration of the extracellular location of EBV in saliva explains some of the epidemiologic features of infectious mononucleosis. Prolonged excretion of small amounts of infectious EBV accounts for the moderate contagiousness of this agent. The high rates of transmission of the virus in preschool children and young adults are associated with the greater degree of salivary exchange characteristic of these groups.

Treatment

Most cases of infectious mononucleosis are mild or moderately severe in nature. During a 3 to 5 days' prodromal period, fatigue, headache, and malaise are common. Frank clinical features include fever, sore throat, and cervical adenopathy in more than 80 per cent of patients. An irregular fever may persist for 1 or 2 weeks and subjective symptoms usually continue for 2 or 3 weeks. During the acute febrile period, rest in bed is advisable and limited activity is recommended as long as sore throat, headache, anorexia, and malaise are present. Isolation procedures are not a necessary requirement. Fever is usually controlled by salicylates, and also headache and pharyngeal discomfort are relieved by use of aspirin, 60 mg. (1 grain) per year of age, per dose, up to 0.6 gram (10 grains) every 4 hours. Occasionally, codeine or meperidine (Demerol) may be necessary for management of these symptoms.

Gargling and irrigation of the throat with warm saline or glucose solutions are useful for symptomatic relief of pharyngitis and membranous tonsillitis. In toxic patients, who have severe exudative pharyngotonsillitis with marked dysphagia or potential airway obstruction, corticosteroid therapy should be employed and a tracheostomy set readily available for emergency use. Prednisone or its equivalent in other corticosteroid preparations may be used. An initial prednisone dosage of 10 to 15 mg. four times daily, may be decreased after the first 24 to 48 hours of therapy and discontinued after a period of 7 to 10 days. Corticosteroids in full doses are used in the treatment of other severe complications of this infection which include central nervous system involvement, thrombocytopenic purpura, hemolytic anemia, myocarditis, and pericarditis. However, corticosteroid therapy is not recommended for the treatment of uncomplicated infectious mononucleosis.

Antibiotics have no effect on this virus infection, and gamma globulin does not prevent or modify illness. However, approximately 20 per cent of infectious mononucleosis patients have a concurrent beta hemolytic streptococcal tonsillitis and should receive antibiotic therapy for this. A full 10-day course of oral penicillin, 200,000 to 400,000 units four times daily, or an equivalent amount of erythromycin or parenteral penicillin should be administered. Ampicillin usage should be avoided because of the high frequency of associated hypersensitivity skin rashes with use of this drug in infectious mononucleosis patients.

Roughly 50 per cent of the patients develop splenomegaly. These patients should avoid heavy lifting, vigorous athletics, and any abdominal trauma until splenic enlargement has subsided. Although rare, rupture of the spleen is a potentially fatal complication of this disease. Severe abdominal pain is unusual in infectious mononucleosis except in the presence of splenic rupture, which necessitates emergency surgery; transfusions, treatment of shock, and immediate splenectomy are required.

Hepatic enlargement is detectable in approximately 10 per cent of patients, but in more than 90 per cent liver function tests are abnormal, with persistence for several weeks. Transient, mild jaundice is present in about 5 per cent of patients and requires only bed rest therapy until the serum bilirubin level returns to normal. No special dietary restrictions are indicated.

After acute symptoms subside, most infectious mononucleosis patients recover promptly and resume normal activities within 4 to 6 weeks. Rarely, symptoms may persist for several months and laboratory abnormalities, including liver function tests, resolve slowly. During this time only symptomatic therapy is indicated.

MUMPS
(Epidemic Parotitis)

method of
RALPH E. HAYNES, M.D.
Dayton, Ohio

In children, uncomplicated mumps is usually a benign disease, and in the vast majority, no treatment is indicated. When treatment is required, therapy is directed to the relief of symptoms, which include pain in the region of the parotid gland or other affected salivary glands, fever, and malaise. Symptomatic relief can usually be accomplished by the administration of acetylsalicylic acid (aspirin) in doses of 40 to 80 mg. per kg. per 24 hours in six divided doses. Some patients complain of increased pain on ingestion of sour or tart foods such as lemons or vinegar. For this reason, a bland diet is recommended. Cold applications may afford some relief of local pain. Bed rest has always been recommended, but there are no data to document its value for the primary disease or for the prevention of complications. I generally permit the patient moderate activity according to his individual circumstances and desires. In any case, the period of disability in the absence of complication is about 7 days, even though virus may be excreted for longer periods of time. The period of contagion extends from 1 day prior to onset of parotid swelling to its termination.

Complications of mumps are common and the management of each complication will be discussed.

Mumps Meningoencephalitis

Acute meningoencephalitis is the most common complication, and may be symptomatic or asymptomatic. The complication is symptomatic in 10 to 20 per cent of patients, while abnormalities of the cerebrospinal fluid (CSF) may occur in as many as 65 per cent of patients. The complication may occur before, during, or as long as 3 weeks after parotitis, or may occur in the absence of parotitis. In the majority of patients the major symptoms are fever, headache, and vomiting in association with meningismus. Treatment is symptomatic, and the duration of the illness is usually 5 to 7 days. It is of particular interest that some children with mumps meningoencephalitis (MME) may appear to be quite ill and toxic, and will show dramatic improvement immediately after lumbar puncture. Recovery from meningoencephalitis is usually complete, but unilateral deafness is a rare sequela. The physician should be aware of the variations seen with this complication. A small number of patients may have seizures, and rarely the level of consciousness is markedly altered. The cerebrospinal fluid findings are those characteristic of viral central nervous system infections, but on occasion it is entirely normal. In some patients the initial specimen of cerebrospinal fluid may be normal, though examination of serial specimens usually shows abnormalities. Rarely, the content of glucose is lower than 40 mg. per dl. (100 ml.). The protein content is usually normal or slightly elevated, but in some patients the protein content may be markedly elevated and this abnormality may persist for several months even in the absence of abnormal neurologic signs.

The treatment of meningoencephalitis is symptomatic. Analgesics, as previously mentioned, may be used to relieve headache. Intravenous fluids may be required to maintain hydration. Seizures should be controlled with major anticonvulsant drugs.

Epididymo-Orchitis

The most dreaded complication of mumps is epididymo-orchitis, which is restricted to the adolescent or adult male. The factors which predispose to the complication are unknown, but it occurs in 20 to 35 per cent, and is bilateral in 10 per cent. The onset is usually within 3 to 4 days after the development of parotitis and is characterized by fever, nausea, vomiting, and testicular pain in association with enlargement and acute tenderness of the testicle. The scrotum is swollen, hot, and erythematous. The entire illness is aggravated by the anxiety suffered by most patients. Bed rest is necessitated by the severe pain. Many patients feel better if the scrotum is supported by a crushed towel, along with the continuous application of an ice bag. Aspirin may be tried for the relief of pain, but most often, codeine, in the dose of 3.0 mg. per kg. per 24 hours for children and 3 to 6 mg. per kg. per 24 hours for adults is required. It may be given orally or subcutaneously in six divided doses. In severe cases, meperidine hydrochloride in the dose of 1 mg. per kg. for children and 1.0 mg. to 1.4 mg. per kg. for adults may be given intramuscularly as a single dose. This dose may be repeated at intervals of 4 to 6 hours in the absence of respiratory depression. Hydration may be maintained by the infusion of appropriate fluids intravenously if nausea or vomiting preclude adequate oral intake.

This complication usually lasts for about 3 to 4 days, though swelling and pain may persist for as long as 3 weeks. The infiltration of the spermatic cord with 5 to 10 ml. of 1 per cent lidocaine or procaine hydrochloride results in the immediate relief of pain and a decrease in the duration of systemic manifestations. Anesthetic block of the lumbar sympathetic nerves is also said to be effective.

Surgical incision of the tunica albuginea or the tunica vaginalis should not be performed. Diethylstilbestrol does not appear to be of value.

Corticosteroids have been recommended for control of the inflammatory reaction. Prednisone, in a dose of 40 mg. per square meter of body surface area per day, or its equivalent may be given until the acute reaction has subsided.

Short-term therapy, with tapering of the dose as rapidly as possible without precipitating a relapse, is less likely to result in toxic reactions. The administration of steroids in the presence of an active viral infection should be approached with caution, as there are no controlled studies that support claims of efficacy. Uncontrolled clinical studies have resulted in equivocal results.

A fundamental part of treatment is reassurance. Sterility or impotence or both almost never follow mumps orchitis, even when it is bilateral. Some degree of testicular atrophy, however, occurs in about 30 per cent of patients with long-term follow-up. The wise physician will continue to offer his patient reassurance in an attempt to relieve anxiety.

Pancreatitis

This is an unusual complication, although it is diagnosed rather commonly. Misdiagnosis is related to the frequency of nausea, vomiting, and abdominal pain in mumps, and to the misinterpretation of the marked elevation of the serum amylase levels secondary to inflammation of the salivary glands. Pancreatitis is a clinical diagnosis. Patients with severe disease may require fluids, nasogastric suction, and analgesics for the relief of pain. The acute symptoms persist for 2 to 3 days, and gradually subside. The patient usually recovers without complications.

Presternal Edema

Presternal edema occurs in 5 to 10 per cent of children with mumps. The edema usually extends down over the sternum and parasternal areas to about the level of the third interspace, and rarely to the xiphoid. The swelling is symmetrical and usually soft. Mild erythema and induration are uncommon but do occur. No treatment is required, and swelling subsides in 3 to 5 days. This complication is often mistaken for cellulitis in association with mediastinitis, and awareness of it may prevent unnecessary hospitalization and treatment with antibiotics.

Other complications such as arthritis, ocular complications, myocarditis, thrombocytopenia, oophoritis, and thyroiditis are rare and require symptomatic treatment only. Viruria is common, but nephritis with alterations of renal function is rare and self-limiting.

Prevention

Subclinical infections with mumps virus are common, occurring in about 40 per cent. For this reason, a negative history for mumps parotitis does not indicate susceptibility. Conversely, a positive history of parotitis is a reliable indicator of immunity, and unilateral involvement induces as satisfactory an antibody response as does bilateral disease.

Determination of susceptibility may be accomplished serologically. Skin testing is less reliable. The skin test antigen is a suspension of killed mumps virus prepared from the extraembryonic fluid of the virus-infected chick embryo. The testing procedure involves the intradermal injection of 0.1 ml. of antigen into the volar surface of the forearm. A zone of erythema 1.5 cm. or greater, with or without induration, at 48 hours indicates immunity. No biologic control material is available, and foreign protein reactions may produce false positive reactions. False negative reactions occur also, and therefore the skin test is not a reliable method of determining susceptibility.

The most commonly used serologic test is complement-fixing antibodies to the "V" viral antigen of mumps virus. These antibodies persist and reliably predict immunity.

In the adolescent or adult male who is susceptible to mumps, the administration of 4.5 ml. of hyperimmune globulin early in the incubation period may prevent mumps. It is not effective late in the incubation period, nor does it affect the clinical course or complications of mumps after onset of the disease.

A live attenuated strain of mumps virus is used for immunization. It may be given after 1 year of age, and is indicated in the mumps suceptible adolescent or adult male. The wisdom of administering mumps vaccine to all children after 1 year of age is in question because the duration of immunity has not been determined, and the antibody titers induced by attenuated vaccine virus are lower than those following natural infections. The product most commonly used combines live attenuated virus vaccines against rubella, measles, and mumps, and when used, this product should be given when the child is at or older than 15 months of age.

Mumps vaccine is contraindicated in all persons with sensitivity to eggs or neomycin, during pregnancy, and in all immunocompromised hosts. This includes all persons with defects of humoral or cellular immunity secondary to disease or drugs.

PLAGUE

method of
THOMAS BUTLER, M.D.
Cleveland, Ohio

Introduction

Plague is an acute bacterial infection of man and animals caused by *Yersinia pestis*. The disease has a worldwide distribution, with the countries of Brazil, Burma, and Vietnam reporting several thousand cases in recent years. In the United States, about 20 cases occur annually in Arizona, California, Colorado, New Mexico, and Utah. The natural reservoirs of the organism are urban and wild rodents, and it is transmitted among animals and occasionally to man by bites of infected fleas. *Y. pestis* has caused devastating pandemics, in which pneumonic man-to-man transmission has occurred in addition to the usual flea-to-man spread. In the United States, a significant proportion of plague cases occurs as a result of hunters handling infected animal tissues.

The most common clinical form of *Y. pestis* infection is an acute lymphadenitis called bubonic plague. Typically, there is sudden onset of fever and chills with headache and prostration. The development of the bubo is heralded by painful swelling in the femoral, inguinal, axillary, or cervical region. The buboes are tender, oval swellings, ranging from about 1 to 10 cm. in length, which may produce elevation and erythema of the overlying skin. Most patients have a single bubo, which is commonly located in the femoral area, but some patients may have them in multiple sites.

Less common clinical presentations of plague include the septicemic, pneumonic, and meningeal forms.

Septicemic plague is a rare variant, in which there is no obvious bubo while bacteria are in the blood stream. Primary pneumonic plague is an inhalation pneumonia resulting from man-to-man transmission. It presents as cough productive of purulent or bloody sputum and can be highly contagious and rapidly fatal. Meningeal plague is rare and usually occurs a week or more after inadequately treated bubonic plague.

A bacteriologic diagnosis is readily made in most patients by smear and culture of bubo aspirate. For definitive identification, cultures should be mailed in double containers to the Center for Disease Control, Plague Branch, P.O. Box 2087, Fort Collins, CO 80522 (Tel. 303-482-0213). At this same laboratory, a serologic test, the passive hemagglutination test utilizing Fraction I of *Y. pestis,* can be performed on acute and convalescent serum.

Antibiotics

Untreated plague has an estimated mortality rate of greater than 50 per cent and can evolve into a fulminant course of septic shock. Therefore, the early institution of effective antibiotic therapy is mandatory immediately after appropriate cultures have been taken. In 1948, streptomycin was shown to be the drug of choice for the treatment of plague by reducing mortality to less than 5 per cent. No other drug has been demonstrated to be better or less toxic. Streptomycin should be administered intramuscularly in two divided doses daily totalling 30 mg. per kg. of body weight per day for 10 days. Most patients show improvement rapidly and become afebrile in about 3 days. The 10-day course of streptomycin is recommended to prevent relapses because viable bacteria have been isolated from buboes of patients during convalescence. The risk of vestibular damage and hearing loss caused by streptomycin is minimal during a 10-day course. It should be used cautiously, however, in pregnancy, in older patients who would have trouble adapting to vestibular damage, and in patients who already have hearing difficulty. In these patients, the course of streptomycin can be reasonably shortened to 3 days after the patient becomes afebrile. Renal injury as a result of streptomycin therapy is rare with the usual clinical dosages, but renal function should be monitored. If the serum creatinine rises significantly, the dose of streptomycin should be reduced. In mild renal failure the recommended dose is 1.5 grams a day and, in advanced renal failure, 0.5 gram every 3 days. Most preparations of streptomycin available in the United States are in an oil base and can be administered only intramuscularly.

For patients allergic to streptomycin or in whom an oral drug is strongly preferred, tetracycline is a satisfactory alternative to streptomycin. Tetracycline is administered orally in a dose of 2 to 4 grams a day in four divided doses for 10 days. Tetracycline is contraindicated in children younger than 7 years and pregnant women in order to avoid staining of developing teeth. It is also contraindicated in renal failure.

For patients with meningitis, who will require a drug that penetrates well into the cerebrospinal fluid, and for patients with profound hypotension, in whom an intramuscular injection may not be well absorbed, chloramphenicol should be adminstered intravenously with a loading dose of 25 mg. per kg. of body weight followed by 60 mg. per kg. per day in four divided doses. After clinical improvement, chloramphenicol should be continued orally to complete a total course of 10 days and the dosage may be reduced to 30 mg. per kg. per day to reduce the magnitude of bone marrow suppression, which is reversible after completion of therapy. The irreversible bone marrow aplasia associated with chloramphenicol is so rare (estimated as 1 in 40,000 patients) that its consideration should not deter the use of chloramphenicol for patients seriously ill with plague infection.

Other antimicrobial drugs have been used in plague with varying success. These include sulfonamides, trimethoprim-sulfamethoxazole, kanamycin, and ampicillin. These drugs, however, all appear to be either less effective or more toxic than streptomycin and should, therefore, not be chosen for the treatment of plague.

Antibiotic resistance in human isolates of *Y. pestis* has never been reported, nor has resistance emerged during antibiotic therapy. The three antibiotics streptomycin, tetracycline, and chloramphenicol given alone are clinically very effective and relapses are exceedingly rare. Therefore, there is no rationale for using multiple antibiotics to treat plague.

Supportive Therapy

Most patients with plague are febrile, with constitutional symptoms including nausea and vomiting. Hypotension and dehydration are common. Therefore, intravenous 0.9 per cent saline solution should be given to most patients for the first few days and until clinical improvement occurs. Patients in shock will require additional quantities of fluid with hemodynamic monitoring and the judicious use of epinephrine or dopamine. There is no evidence that corticosteroids are beneficial. Although disseminated intravascular coagulation is commonly present and purpura occasionally develops in severely ill patients, therapy with heparin has no proven benefit in plague infections.

The buboes usually recede without need of local therapy. Occasionally, they enlarge or become fluctuant during the first week of treatment, requiring incision and drainage. The fluid should be cultured to look for evidence of superinfection with other bacteria, but this material is usually sterile.

Prevention

All patients with suspected plague must be reported to the Health Department. Patients with uncomplicated bubonic plague who are promptly treated present no health hazards to other persons. Those with cough or other signs of pneumonia, however, must be placed on strict respiratory isolation for at least 48 hours after the start of antibiotic therapy or until the sputum culture is negative. The handling of the bubo aspirate and blood must be done with gloves and with care to avoid aerosolization of these infected fluids. Laboratory workers who process the cultures should be alerted to exercise precautions; however, standard bacteriologic techniques that safeguard against skin contact with and aerosolization of cultures should be adequate to protect the workers.

A formalin killed vaccine, Plague Vaccine U.S.P. (Cutter Laboratories, Berkeley, CA 94710), is available for travelers to epidemic or hyperendemic areas who must live and work in close contact with rodents. A primary series of two injections is recommended with a 1- to 3-month interval between them. Booster injections are given every 6 months for as long as exposure continues.

The control of plague requires knowledge of the epidemiology of infected rodents, fleas, and the contact of man with these rodents in any particular area. In the United States the Plague Branch of Center for Disease Control in Fort Collins, Colorado, has a field team of entomologists, mammalogists, and epidemiologists to investigate cases. A specific approach to each case should be chosen and usually consists of insecticide use around homes, trapping of animals, and educating people to avoid contact with certain animals.

PSITTACOSIS

method of
L. BARTH RELLER, M.D.
Denver, Colorado

Introduction

Psittacosis (ornithosis) is an infectious disease of birds that occasionally is transmitted to man. It is caused by *Chlamydia psittaci,* an obligate intracellular microorganism that, like bacteria, contains muramic acid in its cell wall and has both RNA and DNA as nucleic acids.

More than 100 types of birds have been shown to harbor *C. psittaci;* these include psittacines (cockatoos, parakeets, and parrots), finches (canaries, goldfinches, and sparrows), poultry (chickens, ducks, and turkeys), and many others from pheasants to pigeons. Sporadic outbreaks have occurred in turkey-processing plants; however, most human cases in the United States are acquired from parrots, pigeons, or parakeets.

Man almost always becomes infected by inhalation of aerosolized particles from the respiratory and cloacal discharges of sick birds. The disease in man usually is mild and often is undiagnosed. The most common clinical picture is that of an influenza-like illness characterized by chills, fever, severe headache, myalgia, and irritating cough with scanty sputum. Radiographs may show more extensive patchy areas of consolidation scattered over both lungs than physical signs would suggest.

To enable timely treatment, the diagnosis of psittacosis must be presumptive based on the clinical findings and a history of contact with birds in the month before illness. Confirmation of the diagnosis depends upon a 4-fold rise in titer of complement-fixing antibodies, since attempts at isolation of *C. psittaci* are hazardous.

Supportive Therapy

Most patients with mild illness can be treated at home. Some patients are much more ill, with involvement of the respiratory, cardiovascular, and central nervous systems; they should be treated in the hospital. Debilitating high fevers of 39 to 40°C. (102 to 104°F.) can be suppressed with aspirin (600 mg.) or acetaminophen (650 mg.) every 4 hours. Once started, antipyretics should be given regularly until the patient is better. Cough or headache or both may be controlled with codeine (15 to 30 mg. every 4 to 6 hours).

Serious complications are unusual in patients treated with effective antibiotics. Rarely, patients may require oxygen and mechanical ventilation for respiratory failure caused by an overwhelming inflammatory response in the lungs.

Specific Therapy

Tetracycline is the best drug for treating psittacosis; the dosage for adults is 500 mg. orally four times a day for 10 to 14 days. In critically ill patients the same dose of tetracycline can be given intravenously until oral medication is possible. Fever and symptoms usually subside within 2 or 3 days after starting antibiotics. Patients with impaired renal function should be treated with doxycycline (100 mg. orally every 12 hours) rather than tetracycline. Young children, pregnant women, and other patients in whom tetracyclines are contraindicated can be treated with chloramphenicol (50 mg. per kg. a day in four divided doses).

The incidence of psittacosis in the United States declined markedly following restrictions on importation of birds. Now all commercial birds imported into the United States are quarantined for a minimum of 30 days in facilities approved by the United States Department of Agriculture. The quarantined birds are fed with medicated feed that contains a specified amount of chlortetracycline. Contraband birds are a health hazard.

Patients acutely ill with psittacosis should be in strict respiratory isolation until the cough subsides. Person-to-person transmission is rare, but it has resulted in serious illnesses and deaths.

Lastly, all cases should be reported to local health departments to enable appropriate epidemiologic investigations aimed at preventing additional cases.

Q FEVER

method of
FRANK S. RHAME, M.D.
Palo Alto, California

Q fever is ordinarily a self-limited disease, ranging in severity from inapparent infection to a severe, influenzalike acute febrile illness with prominent systemic and pulmonary manifestations. It occurs throughout the world and in all seasons. Patients with severe acute infections have the sudden onset of malaise, temperatures ranging from 38 to 40.5°C., (100° to 105°F.) profuse sweating, myalgias, headache, photophobia, and retro-orbital pain. Many patients have a cough which is nonproductive initially but which sometimes progresses to moderate sputum production. A minority of cases progress to chronic disease, manifesting as endocarditis, chronic granulomatous hepatitis, or both.

Treatment

Supportive Therapy. Antipyretics and analgesics may be indicated according to the severity of the infection and the presence of underlying illness. Antipyretics should be administered continuously to avoid extremes of temperatures and fever lysis. Patients with severe disease may require hospitalization and careful fluid and electrolyte management. Severe Q fever pneumonia in debilitated patients may require intensive pulmonary support. No special diet is indicated as long as adequate nutrition is maintained. Forced inactivity is not needed.

Specific Therapy. Considerable clinical evidence is available indicating that tetracyclines and chloramphenicol are beneficial and satisfactory antibiotics in the treatment of acute Q fever. Penicillins, erythromycin, and the aminoglycoside antibodies have no effect in vivo or in vitro. Human volunteer experiments have indicated that tetracycline therapy late in the incubation period will prevent symptomatic Q fever infection. Since Q fever is ordinarily self-limited, antibiotic therapy has less effect when instituted late in the course of disease. However, antibiotic therapy is indicated for patients with known or suspect Q fever as long as symptoms persist. Therapy should be continued until the patient has been afebrile and asymptomatic for a week. This will usually mean 1 to 3 weeks' duration of therapy. Therapy may prevent chronic forms of the disease and it is important in patients with preexisting abnormal heart valves to prevent endocarditis.

In most cases, tetracycline, 500 mg. orally every 6 hours, is the therapy of choice. Severely ill patients may require intravenous administration initially. The intravenous dosage for tetracycline is 250 mg. every 6 hours. Intravenous or oral dosage for doxycycline, which is probably less phlebitogenic, is 100 mg. every 12 hours for 1 day followed by 50 mg. every 12 hours. Doxycycline in this dose should be used orally in patients with moderate-to-severe renal dysfunction. Pregnant women and children under 8 years should receive chloramphenicol rather than tetracycline to avoid dental staining. Chloramphenicol therapy may need to be interrupted at term. Dosages should be 500 mg. orally every 6 hours in adults and 50 mg. per kg. per day in 4 doses in children. Infants under 1 month should receive reduced doses. Complete blood count (CBC) and reticulocyte and platelet counts should be monitored 2 to 3 times a week during chloramphenicol therapy. Therapy should be discontinued if abnormally low values are obtained.

Chronic Q fever infections require prolonged therapy. Endocarditis should probably be treated for at least one year. Surgical valve replacement may be needed for cure.

Coxiella burnetii is widespread among farm animals, where it causes asymptomatic infection, is maintained in many wild animal populations and has no economic impact in the farm industry. For these reasons, elimination of human exposure is not practical at this time. Fetal membranes of infected farm animals have a heavy organism load and should be handled as little as possible. Raw milk should be avoided. A satisfactory vaccine, which would be indicated for high-risk occupations, is not commercially available. In epidemic situations, tetracycline prophylaxis is indicated. When given for short periods at the time of exposure, disease may simply be postponed rather than prevented. Therefore, 7 to 10 days of therapy should be given for prophylaxis.

Hospitalized patients should be provided with a private room. Patients' secretions and urine should be considered hazardous. Clothes and linen should be autoclaved before reuse. Autopsies of fatal cases are particularly hazardous. Cases of Q fever should be reported to local health department for epidemiologic investigation.

RABIES

method of
B. HUGH BUFF, M.D.
San Diego, California

The incidence of human rabies in the United States since 1960 has been one to three cases per year; yet each year over 1 million persons are bitten by animals. The physician is thus confronted with the problem of whether or not to give prophylaxis, since prevention of the infection is the primary means of treatment. Once the disease develops, the outcome is almost invariably fatal. The decision, therefore, is vital, and involves weighing the discomfort and side effects of the treatment against the chances of developing the disease.

Prevention

Avoiding potentially rabid animals is the best prevention. Children and adults should be warned to avoid contact with sick animals, bat-infested areas, and all wild animals. The family dog and cat should be immunized.

Pre-exposure Immunization

Members of high-risk groups should consider immunization prior to exposure. Such groups include veterinarians and their assistants, animal handlers, workers in animal laboratories, and others whose vocations or avocations bring them into contact with potentially rabid dogs, cats, foxes, skunks, or bats.

Pre-exposure immunization comprises two 1.0 ml. doses of duck embryo vaccine (DEV) given 1 month apart in separate sites in the deltoid region, with a third dose 6 to 7 months later.

Neutralizing antibodies should be produced in 80 to 90 per cent of those treated. DEV is a killed vaccine prepared from embryonated duck eggs infected with a fixed virus and then inactivated. It is supplied in 1 ml. single-dose vials of lyophilized vaccine with diluent ampule.

Three to four weeks after the last injection, the treated person's serum should be tested for rabies-neutralizing antibodies. State Health Department Laboratories can perform this test. If the course fails to produce antibody response, consult the State Department of Health regarding further immunization.

Rarely, a person will suddenly be placed in an environment in which rabies exposure is highly likely. In such an instance, accelerated pre-exposure immunization has been suggested, with use of 4 to 5 doses of DEV in a two-week course. Antibody response should be determined before and 30 days after the first injection.

If a person whose antibody titer has been proved responsive is exposed to rabies by bite, five daily doses of 1.0 ml. DEV plus a 1.0 ml. booster dose 20 days later should be given. If the exposure is nonbite (wound or mucous membrane contamination by saliva), a single booster of 1.0 ml. is recommended. No passive immunization should be given.

Postexposure Treatment

Each possible exposure to rabies infection must be individually evaluated.

The Animal.   Carnivorous animals (especially skunks, foxes, coyotes, raccoons, dogs, and cats) and bats are the most likely to be rabies-infected. Cattle, and sometimes horses and mules, can be rabid. Rodents such as squirrels, chipmunks, rats, mice, hamsters, rabbits, and guinea pigs develop rabies so rarely that antirabies prophylaxis is almost never necessary.

In the United States, a properly immunized animal has only a minimal chance of contracting rabies and transmitting the virus. Prevalence in the wild animal population varies in different states; the local Health Department can supply regional epizootiology statistics for the last several years.

Bite Circumstances.   An unprovoked attack, especially from an animal showing erratic behavior, increases the likelihood that the animal is rabid. For example, skunks generally retreat from humans. A rabid skunk will directly attack humans.

Exposure Route.   Only saliva can infect. Thus, a claw scratch not contaminated with animal saliva is a nonexposure. Exposure occurs either when a bite penetrates the skin or when there is contamination of an open wound or mucous membrane with saliva. Occasionally, exposure to aerosolized rabies virus in a poorly-ventilated area (such as a cave) has been associated with clinical disease.

Animal Management. A healthy domestic biting dog or cat, if located, should be confined for 10 days and observed by a competent veterinarian. Any illness in the animal should be reported; if rabies is suspected, the head should be sent to the proper laboratory for testing for rabies fluorescent antibodies (FA test). The head should be shipped under refrigeration. A stray or unwanted pet should be killed immediately and the head examined. If possible, any attacking wild animal should be killed at once for examination by the FA test. If the FA test is negative, the saliva of the animal did not contain rabies virus at the time of the bite.

Sometimes the inability of a child to communicate the source of a bite or contamination when there is known rabies in the region forces the decision to treat without full information.

Local Treatment of Wound. The wound should first be thoroughly and copiously cleaned with a 20 per cent soap solution; this should be followed by thorough cleansing with saline solution, to remove any soap residual. A 1 per cent quaternary ammonium compound such as benzalkonium chloride should then be applied. Primary closure of the wound should be avoided if possible. When indicated, tetanus immunization and antibiotics should be given.

Immunization Therapy. The incubation period for rabies is 10 days to one year, the average time being 20 to 40 days. The decision as to whether or not to treat should usually be made immediately after exposure, and treatment, if indicated, started immediately. However, some authorities feel that if the offending animal exhibited no signs suggestive of rabies, therapy may be delayed for up to 36 to 48 hours while an attempt is made to capture the animal. This should rarely be permitted, as the search is often futile and valuable time is lost. Delay until the FA test report is obtained may also be considered, but only if the test time is short. Occasionally the FA test will take over 48 hours; consequently, while it is being performed, treatment can be started. Even though antirabies therapy has been started, it can be discontinued if the animal is found to be rabies-free (see Table 1).

As soon as the decision has been made to start therapy, the appropriate public health authorities should be notified. The necessity of treatment should be explained to the patient or family members, possible side effects of therapy should be mentioned, and the need for a complete course should be stressed. A consent form signed by the patient or responsible person is recommended.

TABLE 1. **Postexposure Antirabies Treatment Guide**

These recommendations are only a guide. They should be applied in conjunction with knowledge of the animal species involved, circumstances of the bite or other exposure, vaccination status of the animal and presence of rabies in the region.

SPECIES OF ANIMAL	CONDITION OF ANIMAL AT TIME OF ATTACK	TREATMENT OF EXPOSED HUMAN
Wild		
Skunk		
Fox		
Coyote	Regard as rabid	RIG + DEV*
Raccoon		
Bat		
Domestic		
Dog	Healthy	None†
	Unknown (escaped)	RIG + DEV
Cat	Rabid or suspected rabid	RIG + DEV*
Other	Consider individually	

*Discontinue vaccine if fluorescent antibody (FA) tests of animal killed at time of attack are negative.

†Begin RIG + DEV at first sign of rabies in biting dog or cat during holding period (10 days).

Definitions: RIG = rabies immune globulin, human; DEV = duck embryo vaccine.

From Public Health Service Advisory Committee on Immunization Practices. Public Health Service, United States Department of Health, Education, and Welfare, Atlanta, Georgia.

Therapy involves both passive immunization, using hyperimmune rabies globulin (RIG) obtained from human volunteers and available commercially, and active immunization with DEV. Both active and passive immunization is advised for all exposures requiring treatment.

The recommended dose of RIG is 20 IU per kg. of body weight. Fifty per cent of the dosage should be thoroughly infiltrated around the wound, and the rest administered intramuscularly into the buttocks. RIG is given only once. It should not be injected into mucous membranes.

RIG is the drug of choice; however, if it cannot be obtained within 24 hours, antirabies serum obtained from hyperimmunized horses should be given in its stead. The recommended dose is 40 IU per kg., given in the same manner as the RIG. Prior to use of antirabies horse serum, the patient should be skin tested (note that this rarely may itself cause an anaphylactic reaction).

Active immunization using DEV comprises 23 doses, beginning on the day passive immunization is given. Each dose is 1.0 ml. The first 21 doses may be given either as 21 daily doses or as 14 doses in the first seven days (two doses each day) and then seven daily doses. A booster dose should be given 10 days after the twenty-first dose, and a second booster 10 days later. Vaccine should be injected into the subcutaneous tissues of the abdomen, lower back, or lateral aspect of the thigh, avoiding areas near joints. As many sites as feasible should be used; no two consecutive doses should be given into the same site.

The recommended dose schedule for RIG, antirabies horse serum, and DEV is the same for children as for adults. A complete course should be given in all cases (except, as noted in Table 1, if testing or observation of the animal excludes rabies). At the time of the second DEV booster, serum should be collected from the patient and tested by a competent laboratory for rabies-neutralizing antibodies. This can be arranged by State Health Department Laboratories. If no response is noted, additional booster doses should be given and the patient's serum tested 2 to 3 weeks after each booster.

Up to 20 per cent of patients fail to develop antibodies. If the two additional booster doses do not result in demonstrable antibodies, authorities at the State Department of Health or the Center for Disease Control should be consulted for consideration of the use of experimental vaccines. Currently, vaccines are being tested that appear to be more uniformly effective in antibody production; the most promising is human diploid cell rabies vaccines. These vaccines are not yet available for general use.

Complications of Therapy. Reactions to RIG are sometimes noted; these consist of local pain and febrile response. Serum sickness occurs in at least 40 per cent of adult recipients of horse serum, and anaphylactic reactions can occur.

Local reaction to DEV is common, and may include pain, pruritus, induration, and regional lymphadenopathy. The course of treatment should nevertheless be continued. Antihistamines may help relieve the symptoms. In patients with known hypersensitivity to avian tissue, antihistamines may be given with the vaccine. Anaphylactic reactions to DEV have been reported, especially in persons with avian allergic histories. However, the incidence is less than 1 per cent. In such cases, epinephrine should be given. Corticosteroids should be avoided if at all possible, since they interfere with active immunization. Their use is warranted only in the presence of life-threatening complications, when the possibility of active rabies infection as the cause has been excluded. Fatal neuroparalytic reactions have been rare (approximately 1:300,000).

Treatment of Clinical Rabies

Once rabies develops in humans, it is nearly always fatal. The virus is not susceptible to any known antimicrobial agent. One case of survival by a 6-year-old child from what was probably rabies has been reported in the United States. In that case, intensive life-support measures were used. Problems encountered included hypoxia, intracranial hypertension (necessitating craniotomy with placement of an intraventricular catheter), cardiac arrhythmias, seizures, and superinfection. Ultimately, recovery was complete. Another case of prolonged survival (133 days), but with a fatal termination, has also been reported.

RAT-BITE FEVER
method of
CHARLES D. ERICSSON, M.D.
Houston, Texas

Rat-bite fever is an acute illness caused by *Streptobacillus moniliformis* or *Spirillum minus*. The majority of infections in the United States are caused by *S. moniliformis* and occur in children; however, streptobacillary fever is also a recognized hazard among laboratory workers, farmers, urban poor, and persons with frequent exposure to rats. Other animals such as the mouse, cat, and squirrel may transmit the disease.

Characteristically, the incubation period of streptobacillary fever is between 2 and 10 days. Illness is heralded by fever, chills, headache, and upper respiratory symptoms but little or no inflammation at the site of bite. Shortly thereafter, a morbilliform or petechial rash appears and frequently involves the palms and soles. A nonsuppurative migratory polyarthritis is common. In contrast, the incubation period of spirillar fever is usually longer, and illness begins with fever, chills, myalgias, and local reaction and lymphadenitis at the site of bite. The rash is typically macular and deep red-brown in color. Arthritis is uncommon.

Treatment

Prophylaxis. The wound should be cleansed with a povidone-iodine solution. Since the incidence of streptobacillary fever following rat bite is approximately 10 per cent, the immediate administration of phenoxymethyl penicillin, 500 mg. orally four times a day for 3 days, may be recommended, but the value of prophylaxis is unproved.

General Measures. The symptomatic patient should be hospitalized to obtain cultures and to exclude other diseases, particularly Rocky Mountain spotted fever. Antipyretics may be used for symptomatic relief.

Antibiotics. Penicillin is the drug of choice in all age groups for streptobacillary or spirillar fever. Aqueous penicillin G may be used intravenously in doses of 15 mg. (24,000 units) per kg. per day in six divided doses. Procaine penicillin G in doses of 600,000 units intramuscularly every 12 hours is also effective. Therapy with phenoxymethyl penicillin in doses of 500 mg. four times a day may be started once the patient has become afebrile. Therapy should be continued for a minimum of 10 days. Maximal doses of tetracycline (2 grams per day in four divided doses) or streptomycin (15 mg. per kg. per day in two divided doses) is used to treat the adult who is allergic to penicillin. Tetracycline is contraindicated in the penicillin-allergic child who is less than 8 years old; instead, streptomycin, 20 mg. per kg. per day in two divided doses, is recommended. Definitive and least toxic therapy for streptobacillary fever is based on antibiotic sensitivity testing. When Rocky Mountain spotted fever is a differential consideration, then initial therapy must include tetracycline or chloramphenicol.

Complicated Infection. Pneumonia, septic arthritis, meningitis, or endocarditis may develop. Particularly in the case of endocarditis or meningitis, the dose of aqueous penicillin G is increased to 12 to 20 million units daily and given in six divided doses. Endocarditis is treated for 4 weeks.

Clinical Course. In uncomplicated rat-bite fever a marked symptomatic response to antimicrobials generally occurs within 48 hours. If rat-bite fever does not respond to recommended doses of penicillin, then the organism may not be sensitive to penicillin, a septic joint or other locus may need drainage, or L-forms may have emerged. Maximal doses of tetracycline or streptomycin may be substituted for penicillin to treat L-forms.

Prevention. Control of rat-bite fever depends on measures to reduce the rodent population and to reduce occupational exposures. Isolation of a patient is not necessary, as human-to-human transmission has not been reported.

RELAPSING FEVER

method of
DANIEL R. HINTHORN, M.D.,
and CHIEN LIU, M.D.
Kansas City, Kansas

Relapsing fever is an acute systemic infection with intermittent or remittent (relapsing) fevers caused by one of several strains of spirochetes in the genus *Borrelia*. In the western United States relapsing fever is acquired by the painless bite of a predominantly night feeding soft tick of rodents belonging to the genus *Ornithodoros*. In other parts of the world, it may be transmitted by either tick or louse bite. Persons exposed to the wilderness environment are at risk: campers, hunters, fishermen. Clinical manifestations range from mild to fulminating disease, typically including headache, shaking chills, fever, myalgia, diaphoresis, anorexia, and nausea. After the first acute febrile course lasting 3 to 6 days, the patient usually becomes afebrile for about 1 week. Several relapses may occur, and the diagnosis may be confirmed by finding spirochetes in Wright's stained peripheral blood smears taken during the febrile episode. Agglutinins to Proteus OX-K in the majority of patients aid in diagnosis.

Treatment

Management should be directed towards the following goals: (1) supportive care of the acute illness, (2) therapy directed against causative *Borrelia,* (3) management of complications of therapy including the Jarisch-Herxheimer reaction, (4) prevention and treatment of complications of the disease, (5) protection against nosocomial transmission, and (6) prevention of future exposure.

Supportive Care. Bed rest, adequate hydration, fluid and electrolyte balance with close observations for complications are needed in these acutely ill patients, especially for signs of peripheral vascular collapse, splenic rupture, or disseminated intravascular coagulation.

Fever may exceed 40°C. (104°F.) and should be controlled with tepid sponge baths, acetaminophen, 650 mg. orally every 3 to 4 hours, and the use of a hypothermic blanket if needed. *Nausea* and *vomiting* are controlled by antiemetics as chlorpromazine, 25 mg., or thiethylperazine, 10 mg. intramuscularly at 4 to 6 hour intervals. Intravenous fluids may be necessary giving attention to appropriate electrolyte solutions as serum electrolyte values indicate. Adequacy of hydration is monitored by observing clinical appearance, heart rate, blood pressure, intake and urinary output, and daily total body weight. Central venous pressure and pulmonary capillary wedge pressure may be needed to prevent overhydration in patients having underlying cardiac decompensation.

Antimicrobial Therapy

Tetracycline is the drug of choice for treating relapsing fever. For the average adult, the oral dose (30 mg. per kg. per day) is 2 grams daily divided into four equal doses. Duration of therapy is usually 10 days or until the patient becomes afebrile for 7 days. For those who cannot tolerate oral antibiotic due to nausea and vomiting, tetracycline, 10 mg. per kg. per day, is given intravenously in equally divided doses at 8 hour intervals. Chloramphenicol in similar doses is likewise effective but is not generally used because of the potential for bone marrow aplasia. Penicillin has also been used successfully but it is not effective against some strains of *Borrelia,* especially in those transmitted by ticks.

Therapy of the Jarisch-Herxheimer Reaction

A common complication of therapy in relapsing fever is the Jarisch-Herxheimer reaction (JHR). This is caused by endotoxemia resulting from destruction of large numbers of *Borrelia* after the first dose of antimicrobial. After initiation of therapy, there is a delay of about 1 hour before the JHR occurs. Chilling begins and is associated with increased heart rate, blood pressure, and cardiac output. Rigors are severe for as long as 30 minutes, resulting in temperatures from 38.3 to 41.1°C. (101 to 106°F.). Hyperpyrexia as high as 43.3°C. (110°F.) has been observed. Central nervous system manifestations of fever, including confusion, delirium, and convulsions may occur. The transient lactic acidosis is treated with oxygen inhalation although alveolar to arterial diffusion is restricted. After the chill, vasodilatation results in flushing and hypotension. Intravenous fluid therapy may be sufficient to support blood pressure and maintain renal output, but on occasion vasopressors must be used. We favor the use of dopamine (200 mg. ampule diluted in 500 ml. of 5 per cent dextrose solution) infused at 20 to 50 micrograms per kg. per minute (0.25 to 1.0 ml. per minute for adults of average weight). Heart failure requiring digitalization may occur in the elderly. The JHR lasts 6 to 12 hours and subsides completely in 18 hours.

Prevention of the JHR has not yet been possible, although several therapeutic modifications directed at this complication have been attempted. Lowering the antimicrobial dose or using corticosteroids has not proved effective. Thus, expecting and preparing to treat the manifestations of the JHR is most important.

Therapy of Complications of the Disease

The most common causes of death in relapsing fever are cardiac failure, hepatic insufficiency, hyperpyrexic convulsions, and hemorrhagic complications, particularly disseminated intravascular coagulation (DIC). *Cardiac failure* is best managed by strict attention to fluid balance, monitoring of pulmonary wedge pressure or central venous pressure, digitalization, and judicious use of diuretics. *Hepatic insufficiency* is due to hepatocellular necrosis in the central lobular and midzonal areas. Icterus and prolonged prothrombin times are observed. In the absence of DIC, the prolonged prothrombin time may be reversed with vitamin K, 10 to 20 mg. given intramuscularly. *Hyperpyrexic convulsions* are best treated by close attention to fever

patterns with therapy as described previously. *Hemorrhagic complications* include rupture of the spleen and DIC. Splenic rupture is usually a result of necrosis of small infarcts of the spleen. Intense abdominal pain suggests splenic rupture, and emergency splenectomy should be considered. *DIC* is suggested by the development of thrombocytopenia, decreased fibrinogen levels, increased prothrombin (PT) and partial thromboplastin time (PTT). Fibrin split products may also be found. Therapy should be instituted as soon as possible when there is evidence of disseminated intravascular coagulation: (1) intravenous antimicrobial therapy, (2) anticoagulation with heparin using 50 to 100 USP units per kg. body weight administered at once followed by 10 to 15 units per kg. each hour by continuous intravenous infusion, (3) transfusion with platelet concentrates or platelet-rich plasma is not indicated unless there is life-threatening hemorrhage such as intracranial bleeding.

Prevention

Control of the tick and louse population or avoiding contact with them are the means of prevention. All buildings suspected of harboring ticks with *Borrelia* should be sprayed with insecticides as 1.1 per cent Baygon. Visitors in endemic areas such as the North Rim of the Grand Canyon should use an insecticide such as diethyl-m-toluamide (Off) during their stay in these infected areas.

Relapsing fever patients do not require isolation while in the hospital. However, great care should be taken to prevent accidental inoculation of patient's blood into a member of the hospital staff.

RHEUMATIC FEVER

method of
ALLAN GOLDBLATT, M.D.
Boston, Massachusetts

The past 50 years have seen a major decline in the incidence and severity of rheumatic fever. Despite this change in the epidemiology of the disease, it behooves us to be alert to this antigen-antibody reaction and its clinical manifestations. The diagnosis must be established by clinical judgment based on the medical history, abnormal physical findings, and appropriate laboratory studies. The long-term implications and the often unfortunate social stigma associated with this disease require each physician to be secure in his diagnosis before so labeling the patient.

The goals of therapy include eradication of the group A streptococcal infection; suppression of the inflammatory symptoms of the disease; control of the cardiac manifestations, especially congestive heart failure; prevention of recurrences of rheumatic fever; and preservation of the emotional and physical integrity of the patient.

Eradication of the Group A Streptococcal Infection

Prior to initiating antibiotic therapy for the streptococcal infection, a throat culture should be obtained. It must be remembered that the culture may be negative either because of the previous administration of antimicrobial agents or because of the spontaneous disappearance of the streptococci during the latent period between the antecedent pharyngitis and the onset of rheumatic symptoms. The absence of a positive culture does not preclude the diagnosis, and the patient should receive penicillin in amounts to maintain therapeutic levels for 10 days. For older children and adults, a single intramuscular injection of 1.2 million units of long-acting benzathine penicillin G is appropriate. Children under 6 years of age should receive 600,000 units of benzathine penicillin G intramuscularly.

Those patients for whom oral penicillin may be appropriate should receive an initial dose of 800,000 units, to be followed by 400,000 units four times per day for 10 days. Patients sensitive to penicillin may use erythromycin in a dosage of 250 mg. four times per day for 10 days.

Immediately upon completion of the 10 day course of antibiotics, a program of antibiotic prophylaxis should be instituted (see Prevention of Recurrences of Rheumatic Fever).

Suppression of the Inflammatory Symptoms

The drugs most commonly utilized in suppression of the inflammatory symptoms of rheumatic fever are salicylates and steroids. Neither is curative, and there is no convincing evidence that they shorten the course of the illness. In fact, there is no scientific evidence that cardiac damage is prevented or minimized by either salicylates or steroids. Their benefits are palliative in reducing the acute inflammatory manifestations of the disease process. Clinical observation, however, suggests that steroid administration may in fact reduce the acute changes more rapidly in those patients in whom carditis is associated with the rheumatic fever process.

Patients With Polyarthritis Without Carditis

Salicylates are the treatment of choice. If, as has been suggested, administration of aspirin does not affect the long-term sequelae of the disease process, a dosage adequate to relieve the symptoms of arthritis, fever, and malaise is appropriate. A dosage of 50 mg. of aspirin per pound (110 mg. per kg.) of body weight administered in six divided doses per day is usually adequate to accomplish relief of symptoms. Within 48 to 72 hours this can be reduced to four divided doses per day in order to avoid awakening the patient during the night hours. The duration of aspirin therapy is 1 week after all clinical signs have subsided, usually resulting in a 2 to 4 week course of treatment. Blood levels are not routinely necessary except in those instances in which there are either toxic reactions (i.e., vomiting, tinnitus, hyperpnea, or bleeding) or inadequate relief of inflammatory symptoms.

Patients usually tolerate aspirin well, and it may be taken after meals or with milk to reduce gastric acidity.

Patients With Carditis With or Without Congestive Heart Failure

Steroids, specifically prednisone, are the drugs of choice, at least initially. In those patients without overt congestive heart failure, prednisone is administered orally in a dosage ranging from 40 to 80 mg. per day in four divided doses. An adequate response will usually occur in 1 to 2 weeks, at which time the steroid can be tapered rapidly. Aspirin should be instituted several days prior to discontinuation of prednisone and should be continued until all clinical and laboratory signs of rheumatic activity have returned to normal. The average duration of this combined therapy is 6 to 8 weeks. A persistent elevation of the sedimentation rate in the absence of other evidence of rheumatic activity is, in itself, not always an indication to continue therapy.

For those patients with associated congestive heart failure, prednisone will have to be continued for 2 to 4 weeks before substitution with salicylates is begun. The weaning process should be more gradual. The duration of the combined therapy in these patients is usually 12 to 16 weeks.

In addition to the use of suppressive medication, anticongestive measures should be instituted to treat the heart failure. These include bed rest, oxygen, digoxin, fluid and sodium restriction, and diuretics. Dietary potassium intake should be increased in those patients receiving diuretics.

Rebound Phenomena

Occasionally when suppression therapy is reduced or discontinued, clinical or laboratory signs of rheumatic activity will reappear. Mild rebounds usually subside spontaneously within a few days and need no further medication. If, however, the rebound is significant and reinstitution of therapy is required, salicylates should be used rather than steroids.

Bed Rest and Physical Activity

In the past, strict bed rest and restriction of physical activities were considered mandatory for the care of children with rheumatic fever. That need has been questioned more recently, especially in those children without carditis. The patient should be placed at rest during the initial phase of treatment. Within 7 days, with abolition of acute symptoms and laboratory evidence of decreasing inflammatory activity, a program of gradual increase in physical activities may be instituted. If no rebound occurs within 2 weeks, the child may return to school. However, full physical activity, especially competitive sports, should be restricted for approximately 1 month.

For those patients with carditis, bed rest should be prolonged until there is no longer any evidence of progressive cardiac dysfunction. Here the duration of bed rest may last for 6 to 8 weeks, rarely longer. During this period of convalescence, a coordinated program of recreational therapy and school instruction should be carried out in an effort to minimize the often associated emotional and intellectual trauma. Physical activities should be introduced gradually dependent upon the patient's cardiac reserve. The majority of these children will recover completely and be able to lead unrestricted lives.

Chorea

Sydenham's chorea (St. Vitus' dance) is an uncommon but major manifestation of rheumatic fever. It may occur alone or be accompanied by other rheumatic fever signs and symptoms. The condition is self-limiting, with recovery of the neuromuscular and emotional abnormalities usually within 2 to 3 months. Treatment is therefore directed primarily at the physical discomfort and psychologic stress imposed upon the patient and his family. Emotional support to the patient and family is extremely important. Rest and a protective environment are beneficial, and removal from school is usually required. In the more severe cases of chorea, precautions must be taken to avoid injury to the patient. Sedatives, tranquilizers, and steroids have all been tried with varying results. No one drug has been shown consistently to be more effective than another. Every patient with chorea should receive a 10 day course of penicillin, followed by institution of an antibiotic prophylactic regimen to prevent subsequent streptococcal infections.

Prevention of Recurrences of Rheumatic Fever

The ability to prevent recurrences of rheumatic fever is based upon appropriate antibiotic prophylaxis to eradicate repeated streptococcal infections in those patients at risk. Prophylactic therapy should be initiated immediately following treatment for the primary streptococcal infection. The drug of choice is penicillin. The most consistently reliable results are obtained with the intramuscular administration of 1.2 million units of benzathine penicillin G every 4 weeks. For those who prefer oral medication, and most do, success will depend upon patient understanding and cooperation. Oral penicillin in the form of buffered penicillin G, 250,000 units twice a day, is adequate for prevention of recurrences. In those patients with a penicillin sensitivity, either oral sulfadiazine, 1 gram once a day for patients over 60 pounds and 0.5 gram per day for those under 60 pounds, *or* erythromycin, 250 mg. twice a day, should be utilized.

When streptococcal infections occur despite the prophylactic regimen, they should be treated promptly and vigorously (see Eradication of Group A Streptococcal Infection).

The duration of antibiotic prophylaxis is a subject of continuing discussion. All agree that those patients with cardiac involvement should continue their prophylaxis indefinitely. The same can be said of those with chorea because of the significant incidence of associated rheumatic mitral valve disease appearing later in life. Patients with rheumatic fever and no cardiac involvement or chorea should be treated with antibiotic prophylaxis through those years of greatest risk—namely, the first 2 decades of life. In the absence of recurrences, prophylaxis may be discontinued but reinstated during periods of increased risk (e.g., for those in military service or boarding schools, mothers of young children, and school teachers).

Special antibiotic prophylaxis to prevent bacterial endocarditis is recommended for those rheumatic patients with cardiac involvement. Transitory bacteremia may result from dental manipulation, oral surgical procedures, tonsillectomy, adenoidectomy, bronchoscopy, incision and drainage of abscesses, dilatation and curettage, and instrumentation of the genitourinary tract. Thus, appropriate antibiotic coverage must be instituted at the time of those procedures to decrease, if not completely prevent, the occurrence of bacterial endocarditis.

The drug of choice is penicillin. Procaine penicillin G, 600,000 units, plus 600,000 units of crystalline penicillin G intramuscularly 1 to 2 hours before the procedure and once daily for 2 days following the procedure, is recommended. If oral penicillin is to be used, at least 250 mg. of alpha-phenoxymethyl penicillin (penicillin V) four times each day should be administered. This should commence preferably the day before and continue for 2 days after the procedure, for a total of 4 days.

For those patients with a sensitivity to penicillin, erythromycin should be used in a dose of 250 mg. four times a day by mouth for older children and adults. Small children's dosage is 20 mg. per pound not to exceed 1 gram per day. Duration of treatment is again 4 days.

Preservation of the Emotional and Physical Integrity of the Patient

Rheumatic fever is a chronic disease prone to recurrences, and thus ongoing education of the natural history of the disease and emotional support are the cornerstones for fulfillment of the patient's potential as a total person. Society in its uncertainty will often place physical and intellectual limitations on these patients, and it is our duty to work wherever possible for the removal of such restrictions.

ROCKY MOUNTAIN SPOTTED FEVER

method of
RICHARD DUMA, M.D.
Richmond, Virginia

Introduction

Rocky Mountain spotted fever (RMSF) is a systemic infectious disease, principally involving the small vessels (endangiitis), due to a small, obligate, intracellular bacterium, *Rickettsia rickettsii*. The vector is a hard tick, principally the wood *(Dermacentor andersoni)*, dog *(D. variabilis)*, or Lone Star tick *(Amblyomma americanum)*; the reservoir is both the tick itself and the small animal or bird populations upon which it feeds. Man becomes infected following intrusion into this cycle, during which inoculation of the bacterium by an infected feeding tick may occur. On a rare occasion following a laboratory accident, man may become infected via inhalation of aerosolized organisms.

Reported cases of RMSF have been increasing almost yearly. Over the past two decades and in 1977, they were at an all time high. Although cases have been reported from almost every state, the majority have occurred in the southeastern United States. Fewer than 5 per cent of the cases have been reported from the Rocky Mountain states, indicative of the misnomer applied to the disease. Nearly two thirds of cases have been in persons less than 15 years of age. The overall mortality rate has been generally between 5 and 10 per cent and has been highest in the male, the nonwhite, the elderly, inhabitants of rural areas, and in those without a history of tick bites. The single most important factors contributing to mortality have been delay in diagnosis and lack of early institution of correct chemotherapy.

Treatment

If diagnosed and treated promptly, RMSF is eminently curable. Since there are no satisfactory laboratory tests available to *diagnose RMSF in its early stages,* the decision to institute treatment must be based on clinical impressions. Although immunofluorescent techniques have been applied successfully to specimens of skin obtained from patients with rashes, the widespread practical value of such a test remains to be established. In addition, the appearance of a rash often occurs late or occasionally not at all. The attending physician *must not await* laboratory confirmation of his suspicions, but instead must begin therapy promptly based on clinical impressions.

The most common differential diagnoses that should be considered are meningococcemia, enteroviral infections (particularly those due to ECHO viruses), measles (particularly rubeola), scarlet fever, drug reactions, and connective tissue disorders. The first three are by far the most commonly encountered differentials, and the correct diagnosis is not always readily apparent until days after therapy has been instituted.

Treatment consists of instituting either one of two antibiotics: *tetracycline* or *chloramphenicol* (Chloromycetin). Penicillins and cephalosporins are *not* effective and are of *no* value; sulfonamide preparations are *contraindicated,* as they may worsen the condition.

If the disease is diagnosed early and is mild or moderate in severity, tetracycline hydrochloride may be administered orally or parenterally. The recommended oral dose for both children and adults is 25 to 40 mg. per kg. body weight daily, generally given in four divided doses. Caution should be exercised in the selection or use of tetracycline in children who are less than 8 years of age or in women who are pregnant, as this antibiotic or its analogues may produce permanent staining of the teeth or may result in acute hepatocellular necrosis, respectively. Daily doses, particularly when given parenterally, should not exceed 2 grams in adults or 10 mg. per kg. body weight every 12 hours in children. Further caution should be exercised in those patients with renal failure (a frequent complication of RMSF), since the kidneys are principally involved in the excretion of tetracycline hydrochloride. If given orally, the antibiotic should not be taken with meals, milk, or antacids. A wide variety of other complications or adverse side effects from the tetracyclines may occur, and the physician should consult the manufacturer's official directive before usage.

Chloramphenicol may be given either orally or intravenously (but *not* intramuscularly) at 50 mg. per kg. body weight daily divided into four equal doses. Generally, chloramphenicol is reserved for the most serious or the most progressed forms of the disease. The drug is highly diffusible, and this may be an advantage in achieving inhibitory concentrations of the antibiotic in areas of decreased blood supply (due to endangiitis, occlusion of small blood vessels, and infarction of tissues). In addition, chloramphenicol is often used to treat RMSF in which meningococcemia is a strong consideration. Frequent checks on all hematologic parameters are necessary, and the patient should best be in the hospital if this drug is to be administered.

It is important that the physician realize that two types of hematologic suppression may follow therapy with chloramphenicol. The first is related to a direct toxic effect of the antibiotic on the marrow; it is dose-related, reversible, and occurs commonly. The second type of marrow suppression is not dose-related (idiosyncratic), is irreversible, and fortunately is rare.

With prompt administration of either tetracycline or chloramphenicol, the patient improves considerably by 48 to 96 hours, depending on which areas of the body (e.g., brain vs. skin) are most severely involved. Therapy should be administered at least 24 to 48 hours after the patient has become afebrile or generally for 10 days. In patients treated late antibiotics have little effect, since they cannot directly alter the pathology of the condition.

A number of serious complications may occur in RMSF, including renal failure, hyponatremia, hyperkalemia, inappropriate antidiuretic hormone (IADH) secretion, vascular collapse, heart failure, arrhythmia, coma, stupor, hemorrhage, thrombocytopenia, and occlusion of small vessels with resulting multiple infarcts. The most serious complication is the occurrence of a disseminated intravascular coagulopathy syndrome (DIC), which when fully developed is usually irreversible and often results in death of the patient. The DIC syndrome is probably the most common cause of mortality in RMSF; the efficacy of heparin in treating this syndrome of this disease is still unproved. Secondary complications, such as infection (pneumonia or urinary tract) may occur with RMSF, as may gangrene of an extremity due to infarction of tissues from small vessel occlusion.

Prevention

Vector control of insects is of little value, since ticks are not insects and are generally not affected by most insecticides commonly used today. In addition, because the reservoir is sizable, it is impractical to consider effecting significant changes in this area. Man is infected incidentally in this cycle.

Since a period of time (generally about 1 hour) has to pass from the time of attachment of the tick before RMSF may be transmitted, it is worthwhile to inspect children at least twice daily, especially during the tick season (spring through summer). Care should be exercised in removing ticks so as not to leave the heads imbedded; for, in such instances the disease may still be transmitted. Also, if ticks are crushed between the fingers, infected material may eventually find its way into vulnerable surfaces or portals of entry such as the conjunctiva.

Currently available RMSF vaccines are of only limited value and are recommended only for high-risk groups such as foresters, laboratory technicians working with rickettsia, veterinarians, and others. Although the course may be attenuated in vaccinated persons, deaths from RMSF have still occurred in persons who have received the vaccine, so it is not completely protective. The vaccine is prepared from infected embryonated egg yolk sacs; it is given weekly for 3 weeks at a dose of 1.0 ml. subcutaneously; and a booster dose is needed in 6 to 12 months. Efforts are currently under way to find an improved vaccine.

RUBELLA

method of
GILBERT M. SCHIFF, M.D.
Cincinnati, Ohio

Rubella (German measles, 3-day measles) is a mild childhood virus infection highlighted by posterior auricular and occipital lymphadenopathy, absent to low fever, and a generalized maculopapular rash usually lasting 3 days. The disease has serious implications when it occurs in a pregnant woman during the first trimester of gestation. Although the woman may have subclinical or mild illness, the spread of the virus to the products of conception can result in spontaneous abortion, fetal death, or a variety of birth defects. Because of this teratogenic potential of the rubella virus, the development of live, attenuated rubella vaccines has been most welcomed. Widespread use of rubella vaccines in prepubertal children has altered the usual epidemiology of the disease. What was primarily a disease of young school-age children has become a disease of teenagers and young adults.

Treatment

Persons having rubella should avoid contact with a known pregnant woman for 10 days after onset of the rash. Treatment consists of aspirin for the fever and arthralgia/arthritis. The use of steroids for the arthralgia is unnecessary, but they are given frequently because of a misdiagnosis of rheumatoid arthritis. Steroids may be used in the treatment of the rare thrombocytopenia which may occur. There has been no documentation of benefit from the steroid therapy for rubella-associated encephalitis.

Prevention of Rubella

The real target of rubella prevention programs is the susceptible pregnant woman. Although effective live, attenuated rubella vaccines have been developed, they should not be administered to pregnant women because of their theoretical teratogenic potential. To protect the pregnant woman, widespread immunization of prepubertal children should be conducted to achieve a high level of community immunity. Thus, rubella vaccination is recommended as part of the "well-baby routine": immunization at 15 months of age. Vaccine-induced immunity appears long-lasting but continuous surveillance of vaccines is crucial. At present, there is no need for revaccination.

Recent surveys have indicated that 25 to 30 per cent of women in the child-bearing age are susceptible to rubella. Vaccination of a child-bearing age woman should be strongly considered, but only if she (1) has been shown to be susceptible (lacks detectable hemagglutination-inhibition serum antibody), (2) is not pregnant, and (3) will not become pregnant for 3 months postvaccination.

Mass testing of postpubertal women should be encouraged, and should include the testing of high school girls (who are near the end of the period when natural immunity is most likely to be acquired and are still a "captive" population), premarital testing, and prenatal testing. Identification of susceptibles can be followed with careful immunization, if the requirements listed above can be met. Those women found to be immune can be reassured that they are protected against rubella.

The attending physician of any pregnant woman should have an hemagglutination-inhibition test performed at the time of the first prenatal visit. For those found to be immune, it is important to rule out recent infection. If there is a suggestive history of recent infection or exposure in early pregnancy, a repeat hemagglutination-inhibition titer 3 weeks later should be performed to determine if there is a significant rise (4-fold or greater in antibody). If there is a rise in titer, a test to determine the presence of specific IgM antibody should be done. Pregnant women found to be susceptible should be instructed to avoid contact with any person suspected of having rubella, and to be retested for hemagglutination-inhibition antibody monthly during the first 4 months of gestation. A good time for vaccination of the susceptible pregnant woman is during the postpartum period.

If a known susceptible woman in early pregnancy is exposed to a person suspected of having rubella, or, indeed develops a clinical syndrome suggestive of rubella, proper laboratory tests to isolate the virus and to make a serologic diagnosis should be performed. Efforts to make a laboratory diagnosis of rubella should also be done on the contact suspected of having rubella. In my experience, unless a rubella epidemic is present, most clinical diagnoses of rubella prove not to be rubella but enteroviral infections.

If laboratory tests indicate that active infection (either clinical or subclinical) with rubella has occurred during the first 16 weeks of pregnancy, the implications of such a situation should be fully explained to both parents. The chances for birth defects in the fetus due to maternal rubella are generally accepted as being 50, 20, 10 and 5 per cent if the infection occurred during the first, second, third, or fourth month of pregnancy, respectively. Any decision to terminate the pregnancy must be made by both parents and should be based on laboratory confirmation of active rubella infection.

Studies have shown that the vaccine strains of rubella virus can cross the placenta. However, in the few instances that known susceptible pregnant women who were vaccinated went to term, no anomalies were found in the offspring. In the event a woman is vaccinated and discovers she is pregnant and whose immune status to rubella is unknown or known to be susceptible, the theoretical risk of her having an abnormal infant must be considered as great as if she endured a natural infection.

The use of immune globulin after exposure to rubella remains controversial. The immune globulin may prevent infection (and viremia), may modify clinical symptoms (without preventing viremia) or may have no effect. Since persons with clinical rubella are actively shedding virus 7 to 10 days *before* the rash, frequently the exposed person has actually been exposed longer than realized. Studies have indicated that the time from inoculation of virus (intranasally) to first appearance of viremia is 6 days. Therefore, for immune globulin to prevent viremia, it must be given within 6 days of *first* exposure. Twenty ml. of immune globulin intramuscularly is recommended.

There is no controlled data to indicate that immune globulin reduces fetal wastage due to rubella. If immune globulin is administered to a susceptible woman, follow-up hemagglutination-inhibition testing must be done to rule out subclinical rubella infection. If an exposed pregnant woman will not consider termination of pregnancy under any circumstances immune globulin may be given in hopes of having a positive effect.

Treatment of Congenital Rubella

If rubella infection was suspected during early pregnancy and the pregnancy permitted to go to term, the offspring should be tested for evidence of intrauterine infection, even if none of the clinical stigmata of congenital rubella are present. Most congenital rubella infants have "subclinical" infection, and appear normal in a neonatal examination. The congenital rubella baby sheds great quantities of virus in the pharynx for up to 2 years. In addition, a diagnosis of congenital rubella may be made by detection of elevated specific IgM.

Because of the shedding of virus, the child with congenital rubella should be identified and isolated to prevent spread in the nursery and obstetric service and to personnel. The child should be kept out of contact with pregnant women until tests show that shedding has ceased.

There is no specific treatment for congenital rubella. Amantadine hydrochloride has been shown to be effective against rubella virus in vitro, but the few studies conducted in vivo have shown no persistent effect on the clinical features or the viral shedding.

It is important to identify disabilities in these children. Follow-up evaluation of all children suspected or confirmed (including subclinical cases) of having congenital rubella should be instituted. Many of the cardiac and ocular findings may be corrected by surgery. Some of the "temporary" abnormalities (e.g., thrombocytopenia, anemia, myocarditis) may respond to appropriate treatment.

A common defect is hearing loss (partial, complete; unilateral or bilateral) and appropriate testing for such loss should be conducted so that proper measures may be taken (hearing aid, speech therapy) as early as possible. The same may be said for psychomotor defects.

SALMONELLOSIS (OTHER THAN TYPHOID FEVER)

method of
ROBERT C. MOELLERING, JR., M.D.
Boston, Massachusetts

In recent years, the classification of *Salmonellae* has been revised. As a result, the present scheme lists three primary species: *S. typhi*, *S. choleraesuis* (each with only a single serotype), and *S. enteritidis* (which contains more than 1400 antigenically distinct serotypes). We will discuss here infections due to the latter two (nontyphoidal) species. Nontyphoidal salmonellae are commonly recovered from a large number of both wild and domestic animals; in the United States, the latter serve as the largest reservoir for the dissemination of salmonellosis to humans. Man acquires infection through contact with animals and animal-derived food stuffs. Improper preparation, cooking, and handling of food, especially poultry, egg, and dairy products, or beef and pork may result in extensive outbreaks of salmonellosis. In addition, person-to-person spread may amplify outbreaks of salmonellosis, especially in families with young children, in institutions for the mentally retarded, and among groups living under poor socioeconomic conditions. It has been estimated that at least 2 million persons a year are infected with *Salmonellae* in the United States alone, and among these, 99 per cent of the infections are due to nontyphoidal strains.

Infection with *Salmonellae* in man usually results in one of four syndromes: gastroenteritis, bacteremia with or without focal extraintestinal infection, enteric fever, or an asymptomatic carrier state. The management of each of these syndromes demands a different therapeutic approach.

Management

In situations in which antimicrobial therapy is indicated for infections due to *Salmonella* species, susceptibility testing is important, since the past 10 years have seen the emergence of increasing numbers of organisms resistant to ampicillin and even chloramphenicol, the standard effective antibiotics. In most instances, this resistance has been due to the acquisition of plasmids (R-factors) that mediate antibiotic resistance in these organisms. The choice of antimicrobial therapy for salmonella infections on the basis of standard in vitro susceptibility testing, however, is fraught with pitfalls, because the correlation between in vitro and in vivo effectiveness is not complete for all antibiotics against salmonellae. As a general rule, if a strain of salmonella appears resistant to an antibiotic by proper susceptibility testing, that antibiotic will not be effective in vivo. This is especially true in the case of organisms that have acquired R-factors. The converse is not true, however. There are a number of antimicrobials (such as the presently available cephalosporins, oxolinic acid and others) that may appear effective in vitro but are not effective agents for the treatment of salmonella infections. In practice, only four agents (ampicillin and its close relative amoxicillin, chloramphenicol, and trimethoprim-sulfamethoxazole) are likely to be clinically effective. Ampicillin may be administered parenterally (intravenously or intramuscularly) or orally. Chloramphenicol may be administered intravenously or orally but is *not* effectively absorbed when given intramuscularly. At present, only oral forms of amoxicillin and trimethoprim-sulfamethoxazole are available in the United States.

Gastroenteritis

Gastroenteritis is the most common syndrome caused by nontyphoidal *Salmonellae*. Following an incubation period of 12 to 48 hours after oral ingestion of a sufficient number of organisms, initial symptoms of nausea and vomiting ensue. These subside in a few hours and are followed by abdominal cramps and diarrhea which usually last for 3 to 5 days before spontaneously subsiding. The symptoms may be very mild, with only a few loose stools, or may be severe, with marked abdominal pain and up to 20 to 40 loose stools per day, leading to severe dehydration. In 1 to 4 per cent of healthy persons, a positive blood culture for salmonella may be obtained during the course of gastroenteritis, but the bacteremia in uncomplicated gastroenteritis due to nontyphoidal salmonellae is neither high grade nor prolonged in such patients. In persons with profound illness, underlying inflammatory bowel disease, and disorders associated with immunosuppression, however, the rate of bacteremia may be higher.

Management. Patients with mild disease often require little or no specific therapy. However, for those patients who are moderately or severely ill with cramps, severe diarrhea, and dehydration, the following should be considered:

1. The patient should be placed at limited activity or bed rest. In patients who are severely ill, vital signs should be determined frequently, and intake, output, and body weight should be carefully monitored.

2. Fluid and electrolyte imbalances should be corrected, and adequate hydration and electrolyte balance maintained. If vomiting has been unusually severe, the patient may have developed a hypokalemic hypochloremic alkalosis; in this situation, cautious administration of intravenous potassium chloride may be indicated. More commonly, however, the patient's diarrhea results in hypokalemia hyperchloremic acidosis; in this case, sodium bicarbonate may be added to the intravenous fluids to correct the electrolyte abnormality. In selected patients, oral correction of volume and electrolyte deficits may be accomplished using glucose-rich electrolyte solutions, which are reasonably well absorbed by the gastrointestinal tract in salmonella gastroenteritis.

3. Symptomatic relief of nausea and vomiting may be accomplished, when necessary, with prochlorperazine (Compazine) or trimethobenzamide hydrochloride (Tigan). Suggested doses for adults are as follows: prochlorperazine, 5 to 10 mg. orally or intramuscularly every 6 hours, or a 25 mg. rectal suppository every 12 hours; trimethobenzamide hydrochloride, 200 to 250 mg. intramuscularly, orally, or rectally, every 6 to 8 hours. In children, parenteral trimethobenzamide is not recommended, but suppositories (100 mg. for children weighing less than 30 pounds and 100 to 200 mg. for those 30 to 90 pounds) can be used every 8 hours.

4. Severe diarrhea in adults may be controlled by diphenoxylate dihydrochloride with atropine (Lomotil). One or two tablets every 6 hours as needed is usually effective. Alternative drugs include camphorated tincture of opium (paregoric) 1 or 2 teaspoons after each liquid stool up to 3 times per 12 hours in adults or deodorized tincture of opium (DTO) 4 to 8 drops in water every 3 to 6 hours in adults. In children, paregoric 0.5 to 0.75 ml. per kg. per day divided in four doses may be used. The use of agents to suppress diarrhea should be limited to cases in which the patient experiences major discomfort from his symptoms. Recent studies have suggested that the diarrhea may be a protective mechanism, ridding the gastrointestinal tract of pathogenic organisms and toxins. Thus complete suppression of diarrhea may result in bacterial overgrowth, with enhanced incidence of toxicity and bacteremia, and should be avoided.

5. Antibiotic therapy is contraindicated in the majority of patients with nontyphoidal salmonella gastroenteritis. Indeed, a number of studies have shown that neither local nor systemic antibiotic therapy hastens the rate of clinical recovery. Moreover, in some studies, antibiotic administration has been shown to prolong the carrier rate following recovery from symptomatic gastroenteritis. Only in patients with severe underlying disease are the risks of antibiotic therapy outweighed by their potential benefits in minimizing the possibility of high grade bacteremia and

metastatic infection. Patients in whom such therapy might be considered include patients with lymphoproliferative disease and other disorders associated with immunosuppression, patients with intravascular prosthetic material or known aneurysms, and patients with sickle cell disease or other hemolytic anemias. In such patients, antibiotic regimens similar to those used for bacteremia (see below) may be employed.

6. Enteric precautions should be instituted for as long as the patient is excreting salmonellae. These precautions should emphasize careful hand-washing, appropriate disposal of fecally contaminated materials, and removal of the patients from contact with other patients and from food-handling facilities. Precautions should be maintained until the patient has had a minimum of three consecutive negative stool cultures taken at weekly intervals.

Bacteremia and Focal Infection

As noted previously, transient bacteremia may occur in a small percentage of normal patients with gastroenteritis. However prolonged, high-grade bacteremia due to nontyphoidal strains of salmonella occasionally occurs as a consequence of gastrointestinal infection. This syndrome is most likely to be seen in patients with underlying abnormalities of host defense mechanisms or in patients infected with particularly invasive serotypes or species of salmonella such as *S. choleraesuis.* In such patients, the major serious consequence of their bacteremia is the possibility of localized metastatic infection. Abscesses may form at almost any site; bronchopneumonia, empyema, endocarditis, endarteritis (or infected arteriosclerotic aneurysms), pericarditis, pyelonephritis, osteomyelitis, meningitis, or arthritis may develop. There is a striking tendency for *Salmonellae* to localize at sites of preexisting disease. In patients with sustained, high-grade bacteremia (more than 50 per cent of multiple blood cultures positive), the possibility of direct infection of the cardiovascular system (endocarditis or endarteritis) must be strongly considered.

Management. 1. Supportive measures such as those described for gastroenteritis should be employed where indicated.

2. The level of bacteremia should be documented with multiple (at least four to six) blood cultures. In patients without defects in host defense mechanisms in whom sustained bacteremia is demonstrated, careful evaluation of the cardiovascular system for evidence of focal disease is indicated. Meticulous physical examination, and the use of ultrasonic, radionucleotide, and phonocardiographic techniques may be helpful. In addition, particularly in older patients, angiography may be indicated to rule out the presence of an infected arterial aneurysm.

3. In patients with an infected aneurysm, surgical removal (usually after the infection has been controlled with antibiotic therapy) is invariably indicated. Patients with endocarditis may likewise require valve replacement if therapy with antimicrobial agents alone does not result in cure of infection.

4. Metastatic abscesses usually require surgical drainage in addition to antibiotic therapy.

5. Antimicrobial therapy for patients with documented sustained bacteremia with or without localized abscesses should be given by the parenteral route for prolonged periods of time. This usually means 4 to 6 weeks of intravenous therapy, although in patients without evidence of localized infection, 2 weeks of therapy may be adequate. Ampicillin and chloramphenicol are probably equally effective in this situation, but the author prefers ampicillin except in the case of meningitis because it is bactericidal and because of the lesser potential for serious side effects with this drug. The dose of ampicillin in adults is 8 to 12 grams (150 to 200 mg. per kg.) per 24 hours, given intravenously in divided doses every 4 hours. In children, a dose of 200 to 400 mg. per kg. per day may be employed. The dose of chloramphenicol is 50 to 75 mg. per kg. per day in adults and children over the age of 1 month. This is usually given intravenously in divided doses every 6 hours. In children less than 1 month of age, lower doses of chloramphenicol should be employed to prevent the gray syndrome. Hematologic parameters should be monitored carefully in all patients receiving chloramphenicol. Oral therapy with trimethoprim-sulfamethoxazole (80 mg./400 mg. per tablet) 4 to 8 tablets two or three times per day should be used only as second line therapy for this type of salmonella infection. It is best reserved for patients who have infections due to organisms resistant to ampicillin and chloramphenicol or who can tolerate therapy with neither ampicillin nor chloramphenicol. (This use of trimethoprim-sulfamethoxazole is not listed in the manufacturer's official directive.)

Enteric Fever

Enteric fever is characterized by fever, headache, apathy, prostration, cough, splenomegaly, rash, and leukopenia. It usually follows a prolonged course, with fever lasting several weeks if not treated. In general, the enteric fevers caused by nontyphoidal salmonella are less severe than typhoid fever caused by *S. typhi,* but individual patients with nontyphoidal enteric fever may be very ill. Sustained bacteremia with hyperplasia and hypertrophy of the reticuloendothelial system but without endovascular or endocardial involvement characterizes this form of salmonella infection. The nontyphoidal serotypes most often responsible for this syndrome in the United States at the present time are *S. schottmülleri, S. paratyphi,* and *S. hirschfeldi.*

Management. 1. General supportive measures such as those described for gastroenteritis are often indicated in enteric fever. Enteric precautions should be enforced.

2. Antimicrobials are of major importance in the therapy of enteric fever. For patients who are moderately or severely ill, parenteral therapy is preferable. Oral therapy is usually reserved for persons with mild disease, for use under adverse geographical conditions, or for persons who require treatment with trimethoprim-sulfamethoxazole because of resistant infecting organisms or intolerance of ampicillin and chloramphenicol. The following drug regimens are useful for enteric fever:

Chloramphenicol 50 to 60 mg. per kg. per 24 hours in divided doses intravenously every 6 hours. The dose of chloramphenicol must be reduced in children less than 1 month of age.

Ampicillin, 150 to 200 mg. per kg. per 24 hours in divided doses intravenously every 4 hours.

Trimethoprim-sulfamethoxazole (80 mg./400 mg. per tablet), 2 to 4 tablets two or three times daily. (This use of trimethoprim-sulfamethoxazole is not listed in the manufacturer's official directive.)

If parenteral therapy is impossible, one may consider the use of oral chloramphenicol, 0.5 to 1.0 gram orally every 6 hours, or ampicillin, 1.0 gram orally every 6 hours, or amoxicillin, 1.0 gram orally every 6 hours (this use of amoxicillin is not listed in the manufacturer's official directive). Hematologic parameters should be monitored carefully in all patients receiving chloramphenicol.

Antimicrobial therapy should be continued for 10 to 14 days after the patient's temperature has returned to normal.

3. Although some authorities recommend corticosteroids for patients who have severe systemic toxicity or who do not respond after 5 to 6 days of antibiotic treatment, such therapy remains controversial and is not recommended.

Chronic Carrier State

Following symptomatic or asymptomatic infection with nontyphoidal salmonellae, these organisms are excreted in the stool for a varying length of time, despite subsidence of symptoms. Two weeks after an acute episode of nontyphoidal salmonella gastroenteritis, 90 per cent of patients have stool cultures positive for salmonellae. The number declines so that after 20 weeks, only 5 per cent of patients have positive stool cultures and after a year, less than 1 per cent are chronic carriers. In the United States, the site of infection in the chronic carrier is usually the biliary tract. A patient is considered no longer a carrier after three consecutive stool cultures taken at weekly intervals have been negative.

Management. 1. For most patients, no therapy is indicated. Spread of infection by the chronic carrier can be controlled by good hygiene.

2. In patients in whom continued persistence of the carrier state prohibits gainful employment (as a nurse or foodhandler, for example), or whose poor personal hygiene places others at risk, eradicative therapy may be indicated. In such instances high dose ampicillin (4 to 6 grams orally in divided doses four times daily) or amoxicillin (similar dose) (this use of amoxicillin is not listed in the manufacturer's official directive) for 30 to 90 days will result in the cure of the chronic carrier state in the majority of patients. Trimethoprim-sulfamethoxazole (80 mg./400 mg./tablet), 2 to 4 tablets twice daily for a similar period of time, may also be effective. (This use of trimethoprim-sulfamethoxazole is not listed in the manufacturer's official directive.)

3. In patients with gallbladder disease or cholelithiasis, cholecystectomy (under antibiotic coverage with "bacteremic doses" of ampicillin or chloramphenicol for 10 to 14 days) may be necessary.

TETANUS

method of
B. J. VAKIL, M.D.
Bombay, India

Although a completely preventable disease, tetanus takes a toll of as many as half a million people in the world every year. Tetanus is listed by the World Health Organization, among the first 10 causes of death in many tropical countries. The disease is characterized by local or generalized spasms of voluntary muscles resulting from the action of an exotoxin produced by the anaerobic spore-bearing gram-positive bacillus *Clostridium tetani.* The main natural habitat of the tetanus bacilli is soil. Spores are ubiquitous. In the majority of cases tetanus follows some injury. Spores germinate when local anaerobic conditions are produced at the site of infection, by the presence of necrotic tissue, soil, foreign body, or sepsis. The growing bacilli produce a neurotoxin that reaches the central nervous system by spreading along the interstitial spaces of peripheral nerves to spinal cord and via blood. The clinical effects are produced by the fixation of neurotoxin to neurones of the spinal cord and brain stem.

Tetanus is a significant health problem with a mortality of 30 to 50 per cent. Neonatal tetanus carries a mortality of 80 to 95 per cent. The disease can be prevented easily by immunization and prevention of wound contamination. Treatment of the disease is complicated and not always successful.

Tetanus Prophylaxis

The high mortality of tetanus makes prophylaxis an important consideration. Tetanus can be prevented by a number of prophylactic measures.

1. Prevention of wounds. Tetanus commonly follows an injury, incidence of which can be reduced by taking measures that decrease the frequency of injuries, e.g., wearing of shoes.

2. Maintaining strict asepsis during all surgical procedures, particularly minor procedures such as cutting the umbilical cord or piercing ear lobules.

3. Surgical prophylaxis. All wounds should be considered potential portals for tetanus infection and should be properly cleaned and dressed with antiseptics. Surgical prophylaxis alone is not sufficient if the local cleansing of the wound is carried out later than 6 hours after injury or the wound is tetanus-prone (deep wounds, septic wounds, wounds contaminated with soil, or wounds having necrotic tissue).

4. Chemoprophylaxis. Chemoprophylaxis aims at killing or preventing multiplication of tetanus organisms. This method of prophylaxis will work only when the lethal dose of toxin is not already produced. As the incubation period can be very short, it may be wise not to rely on chemoprophylaxis alone in patients seen later than 6 hours after an injury or in those having tetanus-prone wounds. The chemoprophylaxis should be continued until the wound has healed. The organisms are highly sensitive to penicillin. Long-acting penicillin such as mixture of benzathine penicillin, 600,000 units fortified with 300,000 units of benzyl penicillin and 300,000 units of procaine penicillin, is suitable, as it would provide high initial blood concentration followed by adequate blood levels for 2 to 4 weeks. Tetanus bacilli are also sensitive to many other antibiotics including erythromycin and the tetracyclines; strains resistant to penicillin have been reported. The role of chemotherapeutic drugs in prophylaxis should be considered uncertain at present.

5. Prophylaxis by immunization. Tetanus can be prevented by neutralization of the toxin liberated by the organisms from the site of infection before it can reach the central nervous system. This can be achieved either by active or passive immunization.

Passive Immunization. Passive immunization is generally achieved by the subcutaneous or intramuscular administration of 250 units of tetanus immunoglobulin (Human) (TIG [H]) or if unavailable 1500 units of purified horse or bovine antitoxic serum (ATS). In severe or neglected wounds, 500 units of TIG(H) or 3000 units of heterologous antitoxin is advisable. Protection achieved is rapid but transient. The half-life of horse serum antitoxin is about 7 days. Use of animal antitoxin has two main disadvantages: (1) chances of hypersensitivity reactions and (2) sensitizing the individual. Antitoxin serum (ATS) should be given only after a hypersensitivity test by injecting 0.05 ml. of antitoxin subcutaneously. The patient should be observed for one half hour for local and general reactions. Tetanus immune globulin (human), TIG(H), is devoid of these disadvantages and has a half-life of 20 to 40 days.

Active Immunization. Active immunization is achieved by injection of tetanus toxoid. Absorbed toxoid gives a better and longer lasting immune response. Active immunization is achieved with the basic immunizing course consisting of 3 injections suitably spaced. The first dose conditions the antibody-forming tissues of the host so that when a second injection is given antibody response occurs. The second injection is usually given 4 to 6 weeks after the first. The third injection, reinforcing dose, is given 6 to 12 months after the second and produces even greater antibody response. Adequate antitoxin is detected in the blood for 10 years after the basic immunization with adsorbed toxoid, at the end of which a booster dose of toxoid should be given which will then provide immunity for life. The United States Public Health Service Advisory Committee on Immunization Practice recommends a booster every 10 years.

After active immunization the serum antitoxin concentration slowly declines with time. A booster dose of toxoid is given to stimulate a rise in serum antitoxin concentration after an injury. Such a booster dose is not required within 1 year of basic immunization or within 3 years after a previous booster dose unless patient has a severe tetanus-prone wound.

The first injection of toxoid does not provide any prophylactic effect. The response starts 2 weeks after the second injection.

The disadvantages associated with passive prophylaxis are not encountered with active immunization. Tetanus occurring in persons who have been properly immunized is very rare. Hypersensitivity reactions to toxoid are uncommon.

Simultaneous Active and Passive Immunization. Simultaneous active and passive immunization is practicable. The adsorbed toxoid and tetanus immune globulin (Human), TIG(H), or horse serum should be given in separate arms. The second injection of the toxoid can then be given after 4 to 6 weeks and the third injection after 6 months. The simultaneous immunization offers immediate protection to the nonimmunized persons and initiates the basic immunization course.

Based on the foregoing discussion, the following scheme is practiced in our unit.

1. As active immunization is the most effective prophylactic measure and the only way of preventing tetanus following trivial injuries, it should be our endeavor to immunize all who have not been previously immunized.

2. For patients with injury, the following schedule is recommended.

Surgical toilet of the wound with removal of foreign bodies and dead or dying tissues.

For patients with clean wounds of less than 6 hours duration:

In immunized persons: Nothing within 1 year of last toxoid injection; booster toxoid, if last dose of toxoid was more than 1 year ago; add chemoprophylaxis if last toxoid dose was received more than 10 years ago.

In nonimmunized persons: Initiate basic immunization course (no advantage to patient for immediate injury); chemoprophylaxis until wound is healed.

For patients with clean wounds of more than 6 hours duration:

In immunized persons: Booster toxoid plus chemoprophylaxis.

In nonimmunized persons: Initiate basic immunization course; chemoprophylaxis until wound is healed; 250 units TIG(H) *or* 1500 units antitoxin serum (ATS).

For tetanus-prone wounds (i.e., wounds which are severe and contaminated with soil and there is presence of foreign body or dead tissue): TIG(H) 500 units *or* (ATS) 3000 units; chemoprophylaxis until wound is healed; toxoid booster or, in nonimmunized, initiate toxoid course.

Treatment

Treatment is aimed at supporting life and preventing complications until the disease process has worn itself out. The principles of treatment are as follows:

1. General management including maintenance of fluid, calories, and electrolytes.

2. Prevention of further absorption of toxin by surgical toilet of the wound or by neutralizing free circulating toxin.

3. Control of reflex spasms and tonic rigidity.

4. Prevention of complications.

General Management

The patient needs constant supervision and careful management, as even a patient with an apparently mild case may become severely ill and die. Hence, patients can be properly managed only in a hospital in specialized units. Patients need not be kept in dark rooms. Visual and auditory stimuli do not play a significant part in aggravating the symptoms. Manipulation of the patient should be kept to a minimum, as touching increases muscle tone and provokes reflex spasm. Vigilance should be kept to prevent tongue bite or other physical injury during convulsive seizures.

Decubitus. Patients are allowed any comfortable position they want. It is preferable to keep the head in a low position to allow tracheobronchial secretions to drain from the throat. Patients should be encouraged to turn often to change sides.

Feeding. Patients with mild lockjaw are able to take fluids and soft food orally. A nasogastric tube should be passed in those patients who have severe lockjaw or difficulty in swallowing. In severe cases attempts to pass the tube may induce reflex spasms and occasionally death from laryngeal spasm. In such patients administration of diazepam or mephenesin or both intravenously immediately prior to passing the tube is often helpful (mephenesin is not available in the United States). As it is difficult to forecast the progress of the disease, it is our practice to pass a nasogastric tube in all patients on admission. Food must be semisolid and nutritious. Fluid intake should be equal to the previous day's output plus 600 ml. for insensible fluid loss. For patients perspiring copiously, an extra allowance should be made. Adequate calories should be provided.

For those patients in whom a nasogastric tube cannot be passed, intravenous feeding will have to be resorted to until the tube can be passed without danger of provoking laryngeal spasm.

Relief of Apprehension. Many patients are apprehensive and restless. Mild sedation with 2 to 5 mg. of diazepam every 8 hours is helpful in relieving their apprehension and they are able to cooperate better for examination and treatment. Baseline sedation is helpful, as one can easily increase the dose when spasms appear and quickly bring them under control.

Care of Bowels and Bladder. Constipation is commonly encountered and should be relieved with a glycerin or bisacodyl suppository. About 5 per cent of patients develop retention of urine. In some patients penile stimulation is helpful to initiate micturition, but others may require catheterization. Utmost care should be taken to prevent urinary infection.

Relief of Pain. Many patients with severe tonic rigidity complain of pain in the jaw, neck, and chest. Mild pain may be relieved with hot water fomentations or occasional use of analgesics such as aspirin. Morphine and meperidine (pethidine), or other agents that depress respiration should be avoided. Control of rigidity and spasms also relieves the pain.

Pyrexia. The treatment of fever has to be based on its cause. When fever is due to medullary intoxication, it will subside only when the disease subsides. Mild pyrexia calls for no symptomatic therapy, but hyperpyrexia may need symptomatic therapy such as ice-water enema, tepid sponging, or use of antipyretics.

Care of Wound. As tetanus bacilli multiply at the site of the wound and liberate toxin, wounds must be properly attended to. Foreign bodies and dead and dying tissues should be removed and dressing done as per accepted surgical principles. It is recommended that wound surgery be performed after administration of antitoxin. When surgery is indicated for the basic condition, it should be deferred until the patient recovers from tetanus unless emergency operation is necessary. Systemic administration of penicillin or broad-spectrum antibiotics is helpful in preventing multiplication and in the eradication of *Clostridium tetani.*

Prevention of Further Production and Neutralization of Free Toxin

Prevention of Toxin Production. Prevention of further production of toxin is achieved by eradicating the focus of *Clostridium tetani* infection by proper surgical toilet of the wound and by administering suitable antibiotics (see Care of the Wound). Local infiltration of antitoxin in and around the wound used to be practiced in the past. However, this has now been given up, as there is hardly any advantage from such practice.

Neutralizing Free Toxin. Antitoxin has no effect on toxin that has penetrated into the central nervous system. It neutralizes toxin that is passing from the wound to the nervous system and for this human or animal antitoxin should be equally effective. In addition, toxin formed in the wound after the antitoxin has been given will also be neutralized. Although some trials have shown no significant difference in mortality in cases of tetanus with and without use of antitoxin, others have shown that patients given antitoxin fare better than those given none. It is logical to try to neutralize the toxin, which is not fixed and circulating; otherwise, this will ultimately reach the nervous system and worsen the disease. In the United States of America, tetanus immune globulin (Human) is recommended for neutralization of the toxin instead of bovine or equine antitoxin unless tetanus immune globulin (Human) is unavailable. Dose recommendations range from 3000 to 10,000 units, but a dose of 5000 units has been suggested. Tetanus immune globulin must be given intramuscularly, as there is no preparation suitable for intravenous use.

Antitoxin should be given intravenously for quick action as peak blood levels are not achieved for 48 hours after intramuscular injection. On the basis of a series of controlled trials in Bombay, we recommend a single intravenous dose of 10,000 units of horse antitoxin. It is quite likely that a small dose of 500 units may be equally effective, but this remains to be proved.

Some of the toxin that has passed the blood/central nervous system (CNS) barrier may be susceptible to neutralization if it can be reached by antitoxin. Experiments in animals suggest that this may be achieved by a relatively small dose of antitoxin given intrathecally. Administration of animal antitoxin intrathecally may produce severe side effects. The value of tetanus immune globulin (Human) (TIG[H]) intrathecally is at present under investigation.

Owing to its freedom from allergic side effects and from risk of immune reaction, TIG(H) should be preferred over animal antitoxin. As adequate blood levels are maintained for 3 to 24 weeks after a therapeutic dose of antitoxin, repeated administration of antitoxin is not required. Sensitivity testing prior to administration of equine or bovine antitoxin is essential (see Prophylaxis), and those patients who show a positive skin test should ideally be given TIG(H), but if this is not available, desensitization should be carried out by giving gradually increasing doses of diluted antitoxin every half hour under cover of antihistaminics.

Control of Tonic Rigidity and Reflex Spasms

Sedatives, hypnotics and tranquilizers provide basal sedation and help to prevent or minimize the painful and life-threatening muscular spasms. Considerable doubt exists if the drugs are able to reduce death rate. Nevertheless, these drugs afford symptomatic relief to patients and facilitate nursing. Anticonvulsant drugs therefore are used in the treatment of tetanus. These drugs relieve anxiety, induce sleep, and reduce the incidence of reflex spasms. They also have mild muscle relaxant properties. In severe cases larger doses are required and in such doses they depress respiration.

Barbiturates. Phenobarbital (phenobarbitone) and amobarbital (amylobarbitone) are generally used in doses of 30 to 60 mg. for adults (proportionately less for children) every four to six hours. When used alone, they are rarely able to control spasms completely, particularly in severe cases unless very large doses are used. Such large doses lead to undue depression of consciousness and hypoxia. The drugs are cumulative in their action.

Paraldehyde. Paraldehyde is effective in controlling spasms and causes relatively little respiratory depression. Its chief disadvantage is that it has to be given parenterally and may produce induration and abscess at the site of injection. We use it occasionally in addition to phenobarbitone and diazepam to overcome severe spasms.

Chlorpromazine. This is a useful drug in the management of tetanus. It relaxes the rigidity and minimizes the frequency of spasms without troublesome side-effects. It is also used for emergencies such as laryngeal spasm, severe repeated spasms, and before passing a nasogastric tube. The drug can be given intramuscularly in a dose of 50 mg. every four to six hours. For emergencies, the drug may be given intravenously in a dose of 100 mg., as a bolus, or in the drip (see manufacturer's official directive before using intravenously). Hypotension and jaundice are very rarely seen with this dosage schedule. For the neonate a 6 to 12.5 mg. dose is adequate. Larger doses must be avoided, as they may activate muscle spasms. An interval of less than 4 hours between the 2 doses may produce tachyphylaxis.

Diazepam. In our opinion diazepam is the drug of choice. It is more potent as a tranquilizer, muscle-relaxant, and anticonvulsant. It can be given intravenously or intramuscularly in a dose of 5 to 10 mg. every 4 to 6 hours. When used intravenously it should be increased gradually to titrate its effect. It is irritating to veins and when given by this route it is preferable to inject it into a freely running intravenous drip. It should not be diluted in the drip, as it is precipitated.

Chlordiazepoxide and meprobamate have also been in use but are relatively less effective than chlorpromazine or diazepam.

Mephenesin. This drug (not available in the United States) can be given orally or by intramuscular and intravenous injection. It produces muscle relaxation without respiratory depression. Its action is transient and in high doses it may produce hemolysis. The recommended dose is 1 to 3 grams every four to six hours. When given alone it is unable to control the manifestations of tetanus. Hence, it is better used in combination with barbiturates or phenothiazines.

Methocarbamol. This drug produces relaxation of voluntary muscles without causing loss of consciousness. It may be given orally or intravenously in doses of 1 to 3 grams every four to six hours, up to a total dose of 8 to 12 grams per day. (This dose is higher than that listed in the manufacturer's official directive.) Children should receive proportionately smaller doses.

Choice of Drugs. Combination of two sedatives such as diazepam and phenobarbital (phenobarbitone) or chlorpromazine and phenobarbital (phenobarbitone) are found to be better than single drugs. The action is potentiated and toxicity reduced because of smaller doses of individual drugs. Similar combinations of mephenesin with barbiturates or chlorpromazine have also been recommended. We have found combination of diazepam and phenobarbital (phenobarbitone) very satisfactory. We use the combination in such a manner that the 2 agents are given alternately, and the dosage is tailored so that patients are just adequately sedated. The sedation level must be such that when left alone the patient sleeps but can be aroused with a light touch when necessary.

Neuromuscular Blocking Agents. Neuromuscular blocking agents have been used in two ways: first, controlling convulsions while sparing respirations, and second, paralyzing the patient completely and using artificial respiration. Drugs such as curare may be used to control the spasms of tetanus. However, it is difficult to achieve adequate control of convulsions with curare without paralyzing respiration.

Gallamine (Flaxedil). This drug has a greater margin between therapeutic and respiratory paralytic effects than curare, yet its safety margin is too low to be used without facilities for artificial respiration.

Hyperbaric Oxygen. Beneficial results have been claimed with this therapy. Two or three hyperbaric oxygen treatments using oxygen up to 3 atmospheres pressure for periods of between 15 and 90 minutes have been advocated. Rapid regression of symptoms and signs has been reported, but there is no improvement in mortality with this form of therapy. The effect of hyperbaric oxygen is only on the organisms and not on the tetanus toxin. Since tetanus toxin is fixed to the nerve cells by the time clinical manifestations appear, the use of hyperbaric oxygen has a doubtful basis.

Adrenocortical Steroids. Steroids have been reported to improve results when used with sedatives. Animal experiments did not bring out their value. We have not been impressed by their use.

Total Paralysis with Intermittent Positive-Pressure Respiration (IPPR). Some patients with severe tetanus are not controlled with a conservative regimen of antitoxin and anticonvulsants. Such patients continue to have severe, life-threatening spasms. In such patients, it would be reasonable to paralyze them completely and maintain respiration artificially with a respirator. Patients who suffer from respiratory insufficiency or failure also benefit by this regimen. Reports suggest that the method represents a major advance in the treatment of tetanus. A significant reduction in mortality in neonates and adults suffering from severe tetanus has been claimed.

METHOD. After intubation, tracheostomy is performed. Total paralysis is induced with *d*-tubocurarine by intramuscular injection. The tracheostomy tube is connected to a mechanical ventilator. The dose of curare for adults should be 20 to 30 mg. and the drug should be repeated when jerking movements of the limbs are noted. Regular aspiration of secretions is mandatory. The machine should be correctly set so as to maintain adequate pulmonary ventilation. Continuous vigilance is necessary. Pco_2 and Po_2 should be maintained within normal limits. In general, this regimen may have to be continued for 8 to 10 days but in an occasional patient it may be required for longer periods.

HAZARDS. The IPPR regimen is associated with many hazards. Tracheal ulceration, bleeding, infection, and incorrect ventilation may prove disastrous and even fatal. Machine failure may cost life unless a spare machine and trained staff are available around the clock.

INDICATIONS. The IPPR regimen should be reserved only for patients with severe tetanus who are having frequent severe spasms or respiratory failure or both.

Prevention and Treatment of Complications

Respiratory Complications. As already stated respiratory complications are particularly dangerous and difficult to recognize. Constant vigil must be maintained for signs in the chest.

Respiratory complications can be prevented by observing the following principles:

MAINTENANCE OF CLEAR AIRWAY. (a) The oropharyngeal airway should be kept clear by repeated aspiration of the secretions collecting in the pharynx. (b) Tracheostomy may be required when patient develops laryngeal spasms or has secretions that are copious or tenacious and difficult to bring out. It eliminates the danger of further fatal laryngeal spasms and facilitates the removal of secretion.

PREVENTION OF OBSTRUCTIVE PULMONARY COMPLICATIONS. The most common complication is atelectasis due to mucus blocking a bronchus. It is preventable. The patient should be turned from side to side. Physiotherapy to chest should be given twice a day from the beginning.

PREVENTION OF SECONDARY INFECTION. Broad-spectrum antibiotics should be used pro-phylactically when pulmonary complications are imminent.

Treatment of Respiratory Complications. (a) Atelectasis is treated by drainage and aspiration through tracheostomy. (b) Pulmonary infections should be treated with suitable antibiotics. (c) Patients with respiratory failure may need the help of a mechanical respirator.

Protocol of the Treatment of Tetanus

The following is the method of treatment followed in our unit at J. J. Hospital.

1. Detailed examination of the patient to confirm the diagnosis.

2. History of previous immunization.

3. Inspect the wound. Clean and dress the wound. Remove all foreign bodies and dead and dying tissues from the wound.

4. Sensitivity test: put one drop of undiluted equine serum on the skin and make an oblique prick through the thickness of the epidermis but not sufficiently to draw blood. Use the same procedure with saline on the other forearm. Wait 15 to 30 minutes. Look for local erythema or swelling.

5. Inject antitoxin as follows: If there is no skin reaction, inject 10,000 units of horse antitoxin diluted in 500 ml. of 5 per cent glucose intravenously by drip. If patient is sensitive, desensitize as follows: give an antihistaminic, e.g., antazoline, 100 mg. intramuscularly before the first dose; give 0.05 unit of antitoxin intramuscularly as first dose; double the dose every half hour. For example, first dose, 0.05 unit; second dose, 0.1 unit; third dose, 0.2 unit; fourth dose, 0.4 unit.

Note: If at any stage there is reaction, further therapy should be discontinued.

6. Antibiotics: carry out culture and sensitivity of organisms from the wound. Inject procaine penicillin, 400,000 units intramuscularly daily until wound is healed or for 4 days if there is no wound.

Tetracycline or another antibiotic, depending on sensitivity report, should be used if there is secondary sepsis. Antibiotics should be continued further if there is septic complication, e.g., pulmonary infection.

7. Feeding: if the patient has severe lockjaw or is in a poor prognostic group (period of onset less than 36 hours), pass a nasogastric tube on admission. If the patient is already having spasms, give 25 mg. chlorpromazine or 5 mg. diazepam intravenously before passing the tube. Do not force tube if attempt to pass it induces spasms.

In patients in whom oral or tube feeding is not possible, give parenteral fluids, 2 liters of 10 per cent glucose plus 1 liter of glucose in isotonic saline solution fortified with vitamin supplements daily until oral feeding is possible.

8. Physiotherapy: encourage patient to take

deep breaths 10 times every hour. Change the position of the patient every 2 hours. Encourage patient to cough. When secretions are a problem put the patient in head low position. Consider tracheostomy if there is any laryngeal spasm or evidence of respiratory insufficiency owing to collection of secretions in the respiratory tract.

9. Sedatives: to all patients give baseline sedation—diazepam, 5 mg. twice a day. When spasms appear, increase the dose of diazepam. Add barbiturates to alternate with diazepam in a dose of 30 to 60 mg. every 4 to 6 hours. The dose of diazepam and barbiturate is so adjusted that when left alone the patient sleeps comfortably but can be easily aroused. Reduce the dose as spasms diminish.

10. Watch for the retention of urine and stools.

11. At the time of discharge give the first dose of tetanus toxoid and instruct patient to come for the second injection after 6 weeks and the third injection after 6 months.

TOXOPLASMOSIS

method of
THOMAS C. JONES, M.D.
New York, New York

Toxoplasmosis is an infection caused by the protozoa *Toxoplasma gondii,* an obligate intracellular parasite of tissues of all mammals. The disease is maintained in nature by a life cycle primarily between cats, where the sexual cycle occurs, and rodents. Oocysts are formed in intestinal mucosal cells of cats during the sexual cycle. Oocysts in the cat feces are ingested by rodents and an asexual cycle in muscle and brain tissue develops. The cycle is complete when a cat ingests muscle of the infected rodent. Other mammals such as cows, sheep, and pigs become infected by exposure to cat feces, or if they are carnivores, by ingestion of other infected mammals. Man then becomes infected by ingesting rare meat of these infected animals or, less commonly, by ingesting oocysts in cat feces. Infection with this organism is very common; approximately 1 per cent of adults are infected each year of life; thus 35 to 40 per cent of those aged 40 have been infected. The infection is most often asymptomatic (80 per cent). However, because the frequency of infection is high, toxoplasmosis is a common cause of lymphadenopathy and malaise, congenital infection occurs in 1 per 500 to 1000 pregnancies, and it is a common cause of recurrent retinochoroiditis.

Toxoplasmosis should particularly be suspected in patients with painless cervical lymphadenopathy and in patients with an infectious mononucleosis syndrome but a negative heterophil antibody test. *Toxoplasma gondii* has been implicated as a cause of polymyositis, cardiomyopathy, and undifferentiated febrile illnesses. The diagnosis is made by showing a rising toxoplasma antibody titer using the immunofluorescent test (IFA and IgMIFA), Sabin-Feldman dye test (SF), or complement fixation test (CF). The hemagglutination titer (HIA) rises later and is therefore of less value in diagnosis. After the initial infection and illness, the organism lives encysted in muscle and nervous tissue throughout the remainder of the patient's life without causing disease. Antibodies persist in the patient's serum in low titer in response to the continued infection. The titer of serum antibody of patients long after infection is usually 1:256 or less for immunofluorescent or Sabin-Feldman dye tests, the complement fixation test is usually positive in low titer or negative, and the IFA-IgM is negative.

Management

Toxoplasmosis, therefore, is a common infection of humans that usually does not require treatment. Since important disease occurs only during initial exposure to the parasite, with two exceptions to be mentioned, and since infection confers subsequent immunity, treatment of "antibody titers" should be completely discouraged. Since acquiring infection during pregnancy can have the most devastating effects, women should be managed as follows:

1. Pregnant women should be advised to avoid raw or poorly cooked meat products, to avoid contact with scavenger cats, and to avoid potential areas of fecal contamination by such cats.

2. Women with antibodies against *Toxoplasma* prior to conception are immune from transmitting infection to the placenta and fetus and treatment should not be given.

3. Positive antibody titers detected during pregnancy are only significant if recent infection (during that gestation) can be documented by rising titers over a period of 3 to 6 weeks—stable titers indicate distant infection and therefore immunity.

4. If rising antibody titers provide good evidence for intragestational infection, the patient should be advised that the fetus has a 1:4 chance of infection and 1:6 chance of clinical disease detectable at birth.

5. This information should be obtained before the twentieth week of gestation, while the option of therapeutic abortion is available.

The two groups of patients that are exceptions to the recommendation that treatment be given only when recent onset of infection can be documented are those with recurrent retinochoroiditis caused by toxoplasmosis and those patients with antibody titers to *Toxoplasma* who demonstrate evidence of impaired cellular immunity. These patients should be treated during the period of immune suppression, such as while receiving corticosteroids during treatment of retinochoroiditis, or when an illness consistent with toxoplasmosis is seen in a patient with underlying malignancy such as Hodgkin's disease. There is no good evidence that treating patients who have had recurrent abortions is effective. Treatment of immunologically normal persons with symptomatic toxoplasmosis has been of value in hastening recovery from the illness.

Treatment

T. gondii cannot utilize host folic or folinic acid. Therefore, to synthesize purines, pyrimidines, and certain amino acids, it must make its own, starting with *p*-aminobenzoic acid (PABA). Drug combinations that block the biosynthesis of PABA and folinic acid effectively inhibit toxoplasma multiplication.

Pyrimethamine plus sulfadiazine is the most effective drug combination for inhibiting toxoplasma multiplication.

Pyrimethamine, a folic acid antagonist, is given to nonpregnant patients in a loading dose (75 mg. orally for adults, 1 mg. per kg. for infants) for 1 to 3 days, followed by 25 mg. (one tablet) per day for the duration of required therapy. Sulfadiazine is given in divided doses (4 grams per day for adults, 100 mg. per kg. for infants).

Since pyrimethamine is excreted slowly, exact levels in the serum are not easily determined, and severe signs of hematologic toxicity can occur. Therefore, the patient requiring relatively prolonged therapy is usually treated for 3 to 4 weeks, after which therapy is withheld for several weeks; treatment is repeated for another course, then withheld; and so on. In addition, 3 to 6 mg. of folinic acid intramuscularly given as frequently as convenient for the patient (usually twice per week during and for a week after antifolate therapy) provides increased protection against the bone marrow–depressing effects of pyrimethamine without interfering with inhibition of the parasite. Even while folinic acid is being used, it is appropriate to check the patient's hematologic parameters (platelet, white blood cells [WBC], and red blood cells [RBC] counts) once or twice weekly. If there is allergy to sulfadiazine or toxic effects from pyrimethamine, therapy can be continued using only one of the two drugs; however, *Toxoplasma* multiplication is less completely inhibited.

Europeans have relied upon a macrolide antibiotic, spiramycin, for treatment of toxoplasmosis. At present, this drug is unavailable in the United States. In animal studies, spiramycin is less effective than pyrimethamine and sulfadiazine; however, it may be a reasonable alternative for patients exhibiting allergic or toxic reactions to the more effective drugs. Spiramycin is a safe drug for use during pregnancy, since it does not cross the placenta, and, for the same reason, it may well be ineffective in controlling fetal infection. Recent animal studies with clindamycin have been sufficiently encouraging in therapy of toxoplasmosis to consider using this drug (300 to 600 mg. orally or intravenously every 6 hours) in patients with symptomatic toxoplasmosis not involving the central nervous system (CNS) (this use of clindamycin is not listed in the manufacturer's official directive). Since the drug does not readily cross the blood-brain barrier, it is likely to be ineffective in CNS toxoplasmosis. One might still consider it for use in a patient who cannot tolerate first-line drugs even if CNS disease is present, until the drug's efficacy or ineffectiveness is established.

The combination of trimethoprim and sulfamethoxazole has been suggested by some to control signs and symptoms of toxoplasmosis. In animal studies of toxoplasmosis, however, trimethoprim is less effective than pyrimethamine. It is easy to administer (2 tablets twice daily), and induces hematopoietic toxicity less often than pyrimethamine and sulfadiazine. If further studies confirm the effectiveness of this combination, it might be useful in immunosuppressed patients to maintain the antitoxoplasma effect after therapy with pyrimethamine and sulfadiazine.

Glucocorticosteroids are indicated in treatment of toxoplasma retinochoroiditis, since the main damage (inflammation) results from the vigorous delayed hypersensitivity response. Concomitant antitoxoplasma therapy is used to prevent a possible recurrence associated with renewed multiplication of the organism.

TRICHINELLOSIS
(Trichinosis)

method of
PHILIP MARSDEN, M.D.
Brasilia, Brasil

Mature adults of *Trichinella spiralis* are produced within 48 to 72 hours of ingestion of pork containing encysted infective larvae. After copulation, the gravid females burrow into the submucosa of the small intestine and begin to produce larvae. The mild enteritis produced by the adults is rarely identified. It is the progressive cumulative invasion of the body tissues, particularly of the skeletal muscles, that produces symptoms.

The most commonly affected muscles are the limb muscles, diaphragm, intercostals, and tongue. A progressive build-up of larval load occurs and, consequently, symptoms present from 1 to 6 weeks after infection. Apart from malaise and fever, the appearance of muscle tenderness, edema (especially periorbital), petechial hemorrhages, and marked eosinophilia are suggestive. The epidemiologic history is often helpful. Diagnosis is established by finding larvae in muscle biopsy, and by serologic tests. These tests are usually positive 3 weeks after the onset of symptoms.

In the majority of diagnosed patients, symptomatic treatment is all that is required, although muscle aches, malaise, and low fever may persist for several weeks. When symptoms are severe, thiabendazole is still the treatment of choice. Other benzimidazoles have been shown effective in animal models but have not replaced thiabendazole for treating human infections. Thiabendazole is given in an oral dose of 25 mg. per kg. body weight twice daily for 7 days. Subjective improvement, with disappearance of edema, hemorrhage, and muscle pains usually occurs within 2 to 3 days. Probably many encysted larvae are killed, although living larvae have been recovered from follow-up muscle biopsies after longer courses of therapy. In addition, the drug sterilizes or kills the adults in the intestine and has a mild anti-inflammatory reaction. Common side effects are headache, asthenia, gastrointestinal symptoms, skin rash, dizziness, and agitation. Such side effects occur in about half the patients treated but are rarely severe enough to necessitate stopping the administration of the drug.

In a small number of patients, signs of myocarditis or central nervous system involvement occur. In these patients a marked allergic reaction to invading larvae may develop in the third or fourth week of the illness. Although migrating larvae do not invade cardiac muscle fibers, the heart is the site of an active myocarditis with a chronic inflammatory infiltrate. Focal granulomatous lesions in the brain have also been described. Rapid improvement in the electrocardiographic changes and in neurologic signs has been reported following the use of corticosteroids.

A daily dose of 60 mg. of methylprednisolone or 12 mg. of dexamethasone is suitable. Thiabendazole therapy should be given concurrently to prevent further larval invasion.

If material from the infecting pork meal is still available (e.g., sausage), living infective larvae can sometimes be demonstrated in it by digesting the meat overnight in artificial gastric juice in a Baermann funnel apparatus. Over the last 20 years, the incidence of trichinosis in man in the United States has been declining. In studies carried out from 1966 to 1970, the average adjusted human prevalence rate was 2 per cent. The prevalence in farm-raised swine was 0.125 per cent and in garbage-fed swine 0.5 per cent. The meat of game animals such as bear, walrus, and wild pig is particularly dangerous. In 1976, 96 cases of trichinosis were reported to the Center for Disease Control in Atlanta, Georgia. There were no deaths. Jones estimated in 1978 that only 1 in 1000 of human infections is reported.

TULAREMIA

method of
DAVID L. HOOVER, M.D.
Baltimore, Maryland

Tularemia usually results from direct or indirect contact of man with animals or insects infected with *Francisella tularensis.* Infection also occurs commonly in laboratory personnel working with the organism. The diagnosis should be considered in persons with pneumonia, nonspecific febrile illness, or lymphadenopathy with or without cutaneous ulcerations. Although most reported epidemics in this country have been related to contact with muskrats, wild rabbits, ticks, or deerflies, no source may be identifiable in the individual case. Prompt therapy reduces the case fatality rate to less than 1 per cent, compared to the 7 to 50 per cent rates observed before effective antibiotics were available. To achieve this result, treatment must often be based on clinical grounds before serologic or microbiologic confirmation of the diagnosis is obtained.

General Measures

Patients with pneumonia or marked prostration should be admitted to the hospital. Isolation is not necessary. Cutaneous lesions require only application of sterile dressings. Buboes usually resolve spontaneously with antibiotic therapy. Aspiration or surgical drainage is best avoided unless the nodes are about to rupture, since draining sinuses may occur following these procedures and necessitate further excision of the sinus tract. Other general supportive care depends on the disease manifestations.

Antibiotics

Patients who appear severely ill or who have pneumonic tularemia should receive a 10-day course of either streptomycin, 0.5 to 1.0 gram intramuscularly twice daily in adults (10 to 15 mg. per kg. intramuscularly twice daily in children), or gentamicin, 1 mg. per kg. intravenously every 8 hours in adults and children. These antibiotics, because of their bactericidal nature, are not associated with disease relapse. They do, however, require parenteral administration and carry a risk of oto- and nephrotoxicity. Dosage of these agents should be reduced in the presence of renal insufficiency. If vestibular or auditory impairment develops during therapy, the drug should be discontinued.

Less markedly ill patients (e.g., those with ulceroglandular tularemia) may be treated with tetracycline, 500 mg. orally 4 times daily in adults (8 to 10 mg. per kg. 4 times daily in children over 8 years) for 14 days. Relapse of tularemia may occur as long as 6 months after a course of treatment with tetracycline. Retreatment with the same antibiotic, however, is usually curative, since resistance to the drug is not known to occur. Tetracycline should be avoided in children under 8 years of age, in pregnant women, and in persons with renal or hepatic insufficiency. A regimen employing chloramphenicol, 50 mg. per kg. per day in four divided doses daily for 14 days, is also effective, although relapse may occur. The hematologic toxicity of this antibiotic, however, makes it a less attractive agent than the first two mentioned.

Follow-up

A recurrence of fever, especially in the first few weeks after therapy with tetracycline or chloramphenicol, may indicate a relapse. Patients should be advised to report such an event promptly. If fever persists for several days of observation and no source other than tularemia is found, one of the previously mentioned regimens should be employed for retreatment.

Prevention

Clothing with wrist and ankle closures may reduce exposure to ticks. Persons engaged in skinning or other handling of wild rabbits or muskrats should wear rubber gloves. Meat should be adequately cooked.

Significant reduction in the incidence of systemic forms of tularemia and some amelioration of the course of the ulceroglandular form have been associated with the use of a live vaccine in laboratory workers. This investigational product, for vaccination of high-risk persons, may be obtained from the Biological Products Division, Immunobiologics Branch, Center for Disease Control, Atlanta, Georgia 30333.

TYPHOID FEVER

method of
SANDRA C. FOOTE, M.D.,
and GERALD L. MANDELL, M.D.
Charlottesville, Virginia

Introduction

The incidence of typhoid fever has markedly diminished in the United States during the last 80 years. The Center for Disease Control reported only 500 to 700 isolations of *Salmonella typhi* per year for the years 1970 to 1976. The present mortality in typhoid fever patients is less than 5 per cent worldwide and less than 1 per cent in the United States. Much of the diminished incidence can be attributed to improvements in sanitation and in identification, treatment, and surveillance of carriers of *Salmonella typhi*. Reduction in mortality undoubtedly reflects the availability of effective antimicrobial therapy and advances in supportive care during an illness in which fluid and electrolyte replacement and nutritional maintenance are crucial.

The diminished incidence of typhoid fever, however, may act to increase morbidity, mortality, and spread because the rarity of the disease and the increasing unfamiliarity of physicians with it lead to delay in diagnosis, appropriate isolation, and therapy. Approximately one third of patients in the United States acquire the disease during travel to areas in which typhoid fever is endemic, e.g., Mexico, India, and Italy. However, the disease is most frequently acquired in the United States. Institutional clusters account for slightly more than 25 per cent of outbreaks and 13 per cent of cases. Acute care units, neonatal nurseries, and pediatric wards are frequently involved. Case fatality rate is highest in institutionalized patients.

Antimicrobial Therapy

Therapy of typhoid fever may be examined from three aspects: specific antimicrobial therapy, supportive therapy, and therapy of complications. Specific antimicrobial therapy was fairly simple from 1948, when Dr. Theodore Woodward first used chloramphenicol in typhoid fever, until 1974 when an epidemic of typhoid fever caused by an organism resistant to chloramphenicol and several other antibiotics occurred in Mexico.

The introduction of chloramphenicol provided a drug that was highly effective in treating the disease. Chloramphenicol decreased the incidence of complications of typhoid fever, including intestinal perforation and hemorrhage. By decreasing the duration of toxemia, some of the complications of inanition, including bedsores and secondary pneumonia, were reduced. However, the incidence of development of the chronic carrier state was not reduced. In addition, administration of chloramphenicol has been associated with induction of "toxic crises"—toxemic episodes perhaps related to liberation of large amounts of endotoxin by the first or first few doses of drug and with, rarely, development of aplastic anemia (approximately 1 case per 25,000 courses of chloramphenicol therapy).

Since 1948, many bactericidal antibiotics have been tested in typhoid fever in the hope that eradication of the organisms would decrease both immediate complications of the disease and the development of the chronic carrier state. Ampicillin and its more well absorbed congener, amoxicillin, are bactericidal against most strains of *Salmonella typhi* in vitro. Although successful in the majority of patients with typhoid fever, approximately 10 per cent of patients fail to respond to these semisynthetic penicillins. Average response times, as measured by days to resolution of fever, are several days longer than in chloramphenicol-treated patients. Ampicillin-resistant organisms have also developed. Side effects include hypersensitivity reactions with a high incidence of rashes. Gastrointestinal intolerance to the drugs manifested as nausea, vomiting, and, in some patients, diarrhea progressing to pseudomembranous colitis also occurs.

The broad-spectrum combination antimicrobial trimethoprim-sulfamethoxazole (Bactrim, Septra) has been utilized in typhoid fever with varying degrees of success. Initial reports showed complete response with, in many patients, a more rapid resolution of symptoms of toxemia than with chloramphenicol. Fever, however, took as long or longer to resolve with trimethoprim-sulfamethoxazole therapy. Several subsequent reports demonstrated unsatisfactory responses, especially in children in South Africa. An explanation for this difference in response rate is unclear but has been attributed to inadequate drug dosage, differences in strains of *Salmonella typhi,* and differences in "herd" immunity in different geographic areas. (This use of trimethoprim-sulfamethoxazole is not listed in the manufacturers' official directives.)

New, still experimental drugs including cephamandole and mecillinam have demonstrated activity against *Salmonella typhi* both in vitro and in vivo.

The emergence of drug resistance, most commonly mediated by transferable genetic material (R-factors), is a factor in therapy of typhoid fever. The most common R-factor found in *Salmonella typhi* at the present time carries resistance to chloramphenicol, sulfonamides, tetracycline, and streptomycin, but this is fortunately rarely encountered. In addition, strains also resistant to ampicillin have been isolated in various endemic areas.

Therapy of Choice

The best current choice for antimicrobial therapy of typhoid fever is still chloramphenicol, 50 mg. per kg. of body weight per day given in four divided doses by mouth or if necessary via the intravenous route. Parenteral therapy should be changed to oral therapy as soon as possible. Intramuscular chloramphenicol is less effective and should not be given. Total duration of therapy should be at least 2 weeks. If the patient with typhoid fever has acquired the disease in a part of the world where chloramphenicol-resistant strains are presently endemic, ampicillin, 100 mg. per kg. of body weight per day in four divided doses administered intravenously or intramuscularly, may be used in combination with chloramphenicol or alone as initial therapy. Once in vitro sensitivities have been determined, a single antibiotic can be given. For oral therapy, amoxicillin is preferred because of its better gastrointestinal absorption and fewer gastrointestinal side effects. Trimethoprim-sulfamethoxazole, 2 to 4 tablets by mouth twice daily (320 to 640 mg. of trimethoprim and 1600 to 3200 mg. of sulfamethoxazole per day in two divided doses by mouth), may also be used as a secondary choice. (This use of trimethoprim-sulfamethoxazole is not listed in the manufacturers' official directives.) It is the drug of choice for the rare strain resistant to both ampicillin and chloramphenicol. However, one must remember that chloramphenicol-resistant strains of *Salmonella typhi* are resistant to sulfonamides as well, so the only active part of the combination against resistant strains is trimethoprim.

Supportive Therapy

Good general supportive care must be given during the acute phase of typhoid fever. Nausea and anorexia may prevent adequate nutrition and, if prolonged, may call for nasogastric tube or parenteral hyperalimentation. Dehydration from inadequate oral intake or, more rarely, from vomiting or diarrhea requires replacement of fluids and electrolytes. Diarrhea, however, should not be treated with antimotility agents on the theoretical grounds that induction of constipation or impaction might precipitate intestinal perforation or hemorrhage. Antipyretics may be used for fever but can mask treatment failures. Aspirin should not be used because patients may develop hypothermia and hypotension.

Corticosteroids have been used in extremely toxic patients with amelioration of symptoms. However, controlled trials as to efficiency have not been performed. Side effects of administration and masking of abdominal complications such as intestinal perforation would seem to interdict the use of corticosteroids in most situations.

Abnormalities in clotting studies consistent with disseminated intravascular coagulation (prolonged prothrombin time, prolonged partial thromboplastin time, thrombocytopenia, hypofibrinogenemia, or elevated fibrin degradation products) may be seen in up to 50 per cent of patients with typhoid fever. There is no evidence that heparin therapy is beneficial.

Complications

Vigilance for complications of typhoid fever is necessary. Fever or toxemia or both lasting longer than 5 to 7 days should raise the question of antibiotic failure, localization of infection (e.g., heart valves, meninges, or bone), or development of intestinal perforation. Recurrence of fever after resolution of initial fever should suggest relapse, localization of infection, or perforation.

Relapse is retreated with chloramphenicol, 50 mg. per kg. of body weight per day for 14 days, unless the organism is demonstrated to be resistant to chloramphenicol. Second choices for antimicrobial therapy would be ampicillin or trimethoprim-sulfamethoxazole. Localization of infection requires longer courses of the appropriate antimicrobial agent.

Perforation of the intestine should be treated to include coverage of anaerobic flora from the gastrointestinal tract, e.g., aqueous penicillin G, 10 to 20 million units per day, gentamicin, 3 to 5 mg. per kg. per day (with normal renal function), and chloramphenicol, 50 mg. per kg. per day in four divided doses. In the past, surgery has been thought to be contraindicated because of high peri- and intraoperative mortality. Better techniques in anesthesia and fluid and electrolyte replacement have improved operative mortality. Intestinal perforation and massive intestinal hemorrhage are now indications for operative intervention, although some favor nonoperative management in the patient with severe typhoid fever.

Carrier State

Many patients with typhoid fever continue to excrete *Salmonella typhi* in stools for variable periods of time after acquisition of typhoid fever. Approximately 3 per cent continue to excrete the organism for longer than a year after typhoid fever symptoms and are classified as chronic carriers. Interestingly, many chronic carriers cannot give a history of any illness consistent with typhoid fever. As opposed to the acute episode, first choice treatment of the carrier state is amoxicillin in dosages of 4 to 6 grams per day in four divided doses for 3 to 6 weeks. Prior to initiating therapy, cholecystography should be performed to rule out biliary tract disease, since present cure rates with antibiotics alone are less than 25 per cent. Cholecystectomy is the treatment of choice in the chronic carrier with biliary tract disease.

Prevention

Typhoid vaccine is only partially effective. It should be given to persons traveling to endemic areas, to contacts of known carriers, and during institutional or community outbreaks. Dose is two injections of 0.5 ml., 4 weeks apart.

TYPHUS FEVER

method of
BRUCE H. HAMORY, M.D.
Columbia, Missouri

Organisms responsible for the clinical syndromes of typhus fever include *Rickettsia prowazekii* (epidemic or louse-borne typhus), *R. typhi* (endemic, murine, or flea-borne typhus), and *R. tsutsugamushi* (scrub or mite-borne typhus). These agents have distinct clinical manifestations, geographic distributions, and ecologies. They account for the great majority of typhus group infections. Recrudescence of epidemic typhus (*R. prowazekii*) is called Brill-Zinsser disease. *R. canada,* an organism related serologically to *R. prowazekii* and *R. typhi,* may cause a spotted fever–like disease in man.

All these organisms produce diffuse inflammation of the small blood vessels, which probably accounts for most of the physiologic derangements occurring in these illnesses. Rickettsia are intracellular parasites, and current evidence suggests that available antibiotics suppress their growth, but do not kill them. Therefore, general principles of patient management are based on: (1) prompt and appropriate antimicrobial therapy to control the infection until immunity develops; (2) general supportive measures to correct the physiologic derangements which may occur; and (3) prevention or treatment of complications.

Therapy

Louse-borne typhus will be used as the therapeutic model for all these diseases because it is the most severe, it tends to occur in isolated parts of the world, and it is the classic infection of this group. The other typhus fevers are managed using the same principles, unless otherwise stated.

Clinical Classification of Severity

Upon admission, the patient is evaluated in terms of the duration and severity of his disease. Particular attention should be paid to his neurologic state as evidenced by state of consciousness, ability to cooperate, and ability to swallow. Physiologic abnormalities (hypotension or shock, diminished renal or hepatic function, clotting abnormalities), nutritional state, degree of hydration, and evidence of any complications are also evaluated. Duration of illness is important because the length of antibiotic therapy is influenced by this (see below), and complications tend to occur during the second week of clinical disease.

Cooperative patients with mild uncomplicated disease can be given oral antimicrobials and fluids. Even patients with severe disease can usually be managed with oral therapy, as long as they are alert and able to swallow. Patients who are uncooperative, unable to swallow, or who have severe complications require additional methods of treatment.

Antirickettsial Therapy

Prompt administration of adequate doses of antirickettsial drugs is the most important factor in successful treatment. It shortens the course of the clinical disease and reduces mortality.

The drugs of choice are the tetracyclines and chloramphenicol. Tetracyclines are the preferred drugs because they do not cause the marrow depression or aplastic anemia reported with chloramphenicol. *All other antibiotics,* with the possible exception of rifampin, are ineffective against rickettsia. Penicillin, streptomycin, and sulfonamides have been shown to be clinically ineffective. In vitro susceptibility testing of several aminoglycosides, semisynthetic penicillins (including ampicillin), and cephalosporins disclosed no growth inhibition of *R. prowazekii* with clinically achievable concentrations. *Note*: Except for chloramphenicol, none of the drugs used for the treatment of typhoid fever gives either clinical or in vitro evidence of activity in typhus fever. This is important to consider in those parts of the world where both typhus and typhoid fevers occur with some frequency.

Clinical response to either tetracycline or chloramphenicol is rapid, with defervescence occurring by 36 to 72 hours in epidemic or murine typhus and sooner in scrub typhus. Reports of presumed *R. canada* infections also indicate rapid response to both tetracycline and chloramphenicol. Failure of the patient to repond to therapy indicates: (1) mistaken diagnosis, (2) a complication, or (3) a concomitant infection.

1. *Doxycycline,* a tetracycline derivative available for oral and intravenous use is the treatment of choice for louse-borne typhus. A single 100 mg. oral dose routinely cures epidemic typhus fever infections at all stages of disease in adults. A single 50 mg. oral dose for children up to age 10 is also curative. There is no reported experience with the use of this drug for infants with typhus.

Limited evidence suggests that a single 200 mg. oral dose of doxycycline will cure scrub typhus with occasional relapses. However, murine typhus tends to relapse if only 1 dose is given, so daily doses should be given as discussed below. *Note*: Rocky Mountain spotted fever is not cured by single-dose therapy and requires daily therapy with doxycycline or another drug.

2. *Tetracycline HCl* is given orally in 4 to 6 divided doses for a daily dose of 25 to 50 mg. per kg. body weight. Two grams per day given in divided doses (every 4 to 6 hours) suffices for adults. This drug is poorly absorbed if taken with oral medications that contain divalent cations (such as aluminum or magnesium). Decreased dosage in patients with renal or hepatic dysfunction (not necessary in single-dose doxycycline therapy) is necessary. Superinfections may occur due to changes in microbial flora; long-term therapy of children under age 6 should be avoided to prevent staining of developing teeth.

3. *Chloramphenicol* is given in divided oral doses every 4 to 6 hours for a total daily dose of 50 to 75 mg. per kg. body weight. Two grams per day in divided doses suffices for adults. *Caution:* Doses over 25 mg. per kg. body weight may be toxic for infants less than 2 weeks of age. Dosages may have to be lowered in the presence of hepatic impairment to prevent the accumulation of toxic drug levels.

Patients unable to take oral medications (those who are comatose, delirious, unable to swallow, or vomiting) require special management. Intravenous therapy with tetracycline, 0.5 gram every 12 hours, diluted in 100 ml. of 5 per cent dextrose in water or isotonic saline solution and administered over one-half hour; or chloramphenicol sodium succinate 1.0 gram every 8 to 12 hours (diluted to a 10 per cent solution) may be given until the patient is alert and able to swallow. At that time, a single 100 mg. oral dose of doxycycline usually suffices to complete therapy. If intravenous medications or fluids are not available, the oral drugs may be given via nasogastric tube.

Duration of Chemotherapy. As already noted, drugs used for the treatment of rickettsial infections are rickettsiostatic, providing suppression of the infection until host immune responses can control it. Therefore, optimal duration of chemotherapy is related to: (1) the point in the course of the illness at which therapy is started and (2) the length of drug effect upon the particular organism. If therapy is started very early in the course of the disease, it must be continued longer than treatment begun late in the course. A reasonable rule of thumb for administering either chloramphenicol or tetracycline therapy is to administer the drug for at least 48 hours after the patient becomes afebrile. The drug should then be continued until the total time from onset of *clinical* disease is 12 to 14 days, which is roughly the time required for an adequate immune response. This is not the *minimum* necessary regimen, but is used to provide automatic compensation for treatment begun at any stage during the disease.

If drugs are discontinued too soon, the patient may experience a febrile "relapse." This may occur within 12 hours in murine typhus or as long as 6 days after the last dose of therapy in scrub typhus. "Relapses" respond to retreatment with the same drug and should be treated for at least 48 hours after defervescence. Drug resistance, which is inducible in the laboratory, has not been noted in patients.

Steroids.   Use of steroids should be reserved for those instances of neurologic impairment that affect the patient's ability to feed himself or otherwise endanger his health. Examples of this include: (1) inability to swallow, (2) coma, and (3) delirium or agitation. Uncontrolled studies indicate that in outpatient settings, corticosteroids *in conjunction with* appropriate antibiotic therapy may cause rapid reversal of neurologic impairment, enabling faster institution of oral therapy, as well as improvement in the state of well-being and more rapid defervescence. There was no evidence that such therapy adversely affected the course of the infection, when antibiotics were also used. The regimen used was hydrocortisone, 100 mg. intravenously, followed by an intramuscular injection of 200 to 300 mg. cortisone acetate, in addition to 500 mg. tetracycline intramuscularly. This was given to comatose or severely ill "uncooperative" patients on admission. Within 24 to 36 hours the patient was usually able to take oral fluids and food, swallow the last antibiotic dose (100 mg. doxycycline), and had regained bowel and bladder control as well as spontaneous movement. *Note:* Falciparum malaria must be excluded by blood smear before steroid treatment in areas where patients are at risk to both diseases.

Supportive Therapy.   In hospital settings in which intravenous fluids and constant nursing supervision are available, the patient can be supported until his neurologic status improves. The need for hospitalization is determined by the patient's requirements for supportive therapy and nursing care, or the presence of any complications. Mild to moderately severe infections, such as

murine typhus and Brill-Zinsser disease, can usually be managed at home if the patient is able to take oral fluids. Mild to moderately severe cases of epidemic typhus and scrub typhus will also respond well to oral chemotherapy, and simple supportive measures such as bed rest, adequate protein and caloric intake, rehydration, and analgesia for myalgias and headache. These patients may be deloused, given chemotherapy, and followed as out-patients. Patients with altered consciousness, or who are unable to take and retain oral medications, and those who are so debilitated as to be unable to control their bowel and bladder functions need to be hospitalized. They should be deloused on admission (see below) to prevent spread of disease to other patients and the staff. Severe rickettsial disease of all types may display a range of physiologic disturbances requiring special supportive or corrective measures. In the absence of serious underlying disease or concomitant infections, mortality in patients treated early should be essentially zero. When therapy is begun late in the course, deaths still occur despite the most sophisticated supportive therapy.

Nursing Care.   Close observation of patients for changes in mental status is warranted to prevent self-inflicted injury. Some patients may be irrational or agitated to the point of attempting self-destruction, and physical restraint may be required. It should be noted that patients may become irrational after antibiotic therapy has been instituted and even a day or two after defervescence. Comatose patients should be turned frequently to prevent the development of pressure sores and aspiration pneumonitis. The legs should be elevated or placed in support hose to prevent venous stasis and thrombosis. Good oral hygiene is essential.

The patient should be given a diet high in protein and calories. This is important to prevent negative nitrogen balance with attendant muscle loss and hypoproteinemia. In the presence of diminished renal function with azotemia, excessive protein intake should be avoided until renal function improves. Oral fluids sufficient to ensure a urinary flow of 1500 ml. per day should be given. If the patient cannot take oral liquids within a day or two of instituting therapy, fluids should be given via nasogastric tube or by vein. Comatose or uncooperative patients will require intravenous fluids to maintain adequate renal output. These intravenous fluids should be given slowly, and the proper concentrations of electrolytes will be based on urinary output and laboratory determinations. Frequent examinations for signs of congestive heart failure are warranted to avoid overtaxing the cardiovascular system.

Therapy of Complications

Hepatic and Renal Systems. Abnormalities of liver and renal functions are usually transient, responding to antibiotic therapy of the infection, and disappearing in convalescence. Acute renal failure resulting from massive intravascular hemolysis has been reported in glucose-6-phosphate dehydrogenase deficient individuals infected with murine or scrub typhus and can be managed with peritoneal dialysis or hemodialysis.

Blood and Cardiovascular System. Typhus group rickettsia cause widespread focal lesions in the small blood vessels. These lesions are presumed to account for the increased vascular permeability, vascular collapse, and clotting abnormalities (from disseminated intravascular clotting, thrombocytopenia, and diminished hepatic synthesis of clotting factors) which are recognized in several of these infections. Appropriate laboratory tests that pinpoint the specific abnormality present may allow more rational prevention and management of the reported complications of hemorrhage, arterial occlusion (gangrene), or thrombophlebitis.

Specific blood component therapy (i.e., packed red blood cells [RBC] for significant anemia, and albumin for severe hypoproteinemia) is preferred over whole blood or plasma administration. Heparin has been reported as a treatment for intravascular clotting in a single rickettsial infection.

The management of peripheral vascular collapse (usually in the second week of untreated clinical disease) is empirical. It includes: (1) nasal oxygen; (2) use of plasma expanders such as salt-poor albumin; (3) vasopressor drugs such as levarterenol bitartrate (Levophed); and (4) corticosteroids.

Pulmonary edema and congestive heart failure are attributed to hypoproteinemia, increased vascular permeability, and myocarditis. After correcting the hypoproteinemia, they can be managed with digitalis. Use of diuretics must be based on the presence of adequate renal function.

Other Complications. Secondary bacterial pneumonias and other bacterial infections are treated with appropriate antibiotics, based on isolation and antibiotic-sensitivity testing of the causative organism. Gangrene, decubitus ulcers, and thrombophlebitis are treated by the usual surgical and medical methods. As noted, neurologic deficits usually resolve during convalescence, although personality changes and deafness have been reported to persist in certain patients for months. Those deficits caused by large vessel disease (hemorrhage or thrombosis) may not resolve.

Prevention and Control Measures

General control measures for epidemic typhus rest upon louse control with residual insecticides, isolation and chemotherapy of patients, and attempts to improve personal hygiene, such as bathing and washing clothes. These things may or may not be possible in a given area with limited resources.

All patients with epidemic typhus should be deloused with a residual insecticide when first seen in the clinic. Body lice in different parts of the world are developing resistance to various insecticides, so a knowledge of local resistance patterns is important in making the proper selection. Widely used insecticides include: 10 per cent DDT powder, malathion, 1 per cent lindane (gamma hexachlorohexane), and a carbamate (Mobam).

Clothing should be removed from hospitalized patients and autoclaved—heat sterilization will kill the lice, their eggs, and the rickettsia in the louse feces. The patient should be bathed (some hospitals also shave the hair if infestation is heavy), deloused, and retreated at the appropriate intervals with insecticides. If proper delousing and decontamination is performed before admission to the ward and the ward is kept louse-free, physicians and nurses need not take special precautions with epidemic typhus patients. During the delousing, however, gowns, gloves, and masks should be worn to protect the operator from the infected lice and their feces. All these articles should be subjected to heat sterilization after use. Isolation of the patient is not necessary if lice are killed and not present on the ward.

Murine (endemic) typhus is controlled by *first eliminating* rat fleas with insecticides, then controlling rats. If rats are killed before fleas are eliminated, the infected fleas will seek a new host, i.e., man. Personal preventive measures must often suffice for control of scrub and tick typhus. These include (1) avoidance of known habitats of the insect, if possible, or (2) application of repellants to the clothing (benzyl benzoate) and skin (desthyltoluamide, M-1960) if the area must be entered.

Currently available commercial killed vaccines for epidemic typhus are variable in potency but do reduce the severity of clinical disease. An experimental live, attenuated vaccine (Madrid E) shows promise in epidemic situations, but is not yet commercially available. No vaccines are commercially available for preventing murine typhus, scrub typhus, or *R. canada* infections.

WHOOPING COUGH
(Pertussis)

method of
JOHN C. PETERSON, M.D.
Milwaukee, Wisconsin

Whooping cough is an acute contagious disease primarily of infants and children but possible in all age groups. Its occurrence is a community disgrace that should be prevented by proper immunization. It is generally diagnosed by clinical finding, as most laboratories are not equipped to grow and identify the causative organisms, *Bordetella pertussis*. It may be confused with infections caused by *Bordetella parapertussis* or *Bordetella bronchosepticus* and by infections by viruses, primarily adenoviruses. However, there seems no proof that these agents are common factors in clinical pertussis.

The frequency of pertussis has been greatly diminished by routine vaccination with killed vaccine prepared from phase 1 cultures of *B. pertussis* but still occurs with sporadic cases and at times as minor epidemics. Pertussis is a highly contagious infection with attack rates of 80 to 90 per cent among intimately exposed susceptible household contacts and rates of 30 to 80 per cent among susceptibles with lesser exposure. Recovery from an attack of the natural disease provides a high degree of immunity to reinfection but secondary attacks are not unknown, especially at long intervals after the primary infection. Attacks may also occur after vaccination with currently available vaccines that do not engender significant levels of secretory IgA, especially with the waning of antibody level due to time. In such cases, the disease is generally mild.

Serious morbidity and mortality from pertussis occurs almost entirely in infants and young children who have not been immunized. Passive immunity from the mother does not protect the infant from infection. More than two thirds of deaths from pertussis occur in the first year of life and are much more commonly seen in children of families of the poor or in those with poor resistance from other causes.

Treatment

General. Patients should be isolated from the onset of catarrhal symptoms until 3 weeks after the onset of paroxysmal coughing. The isolation should protect the patient from contact with other infectious agents and susceptibles from contact with the patient. Intimately exposed nonimmune children should also be segregated from susceptibles for a period of 2 weeks. Children can be presumed immune if they have had three or more injections of standard vaccine, particularly if the last injection has been made within a period of 2 years.

The patient should be kept in an environment with good ventilation, even temperature, and humidity of 40 to 50 per cent. Factors which excite paroxysms such as anxiety, excitement, odors, inhalant irritants, and vigorous activity should be avoided. Bed rest is indicated if there is fever. Cough suppressants should be avoided. Vomiting may be reduced by more frequent small feedings given immediately after a paroxysm. Choking attacks should be relieved by gentle pharyngeal suctioning. Oxygen should be used for respiratory distress and for convulsions.

Hospitalization is desirable when the patient has frequent severe paroxysms with cyanosis, apnea, frequent severe vomiting, or convulsions. It should also be considered when the home is unable to provide nursing skill and attention or where proper isolation either for the patient's protection or for the protection of other susceptibles, especially small or debilitated children is unavailable.

Specific. Traditionally, human pertussis immune globulin has been used when the disease is diagnosed early in infants in an attempt to ameliorate the disease or to passively immunize exposed infants or children debilitated by other circumstances. It is difficult to evaluate either of these practices, but controlled studies have shown little or no value to this approach; neither can be recommended.

A number of antibiotics have been shown to have in vitro effect against *B. pertussis* but in clinical practice none has been shown to have significant effect in modifying the severity or duration of the clinical course of the disease. Erythromycin has been shown to shorten the time that *B. pertussis* can be recovered from the respiratory tract. This supports the use of erythromycin to shorten the period of transmissibility. This can be accomplished by the early administration of 10 mg. per kg. of erythromycin four times daily for 5 days.

The lack of any effective specific therapy for pertussis makes control by immunization early in infancy imperative for control of the disease.

Complications

Respiratory Tract. The most common complication is the development of pneumonia. It is commonly a bronchopneumonia and shows a fairly typical x-ray picture of perihilar infiltration. It may be caused by *B. pertussis* but more commonly is caused by secondary invaders, influenza, pneumococci, streptococci, and occasionally staphylococci. Attempts should be made to identify the causative agent, but erythromycin, ampicillin, or amoxicillin may be used as initial therapy until a specific antibiotic can be selected.

Atelectasis is also a common complication and, if persistent, may require bronchoscopy and suction for relief.

Children with these complications should not be released from care until all evidence of pulmonary complication has subsided.

Otitis media is also a common complication, especially in infants, and should be suspected in any patient with fever.

Central Nervous System. Encephalopathy with or without convulsions may occur with pertussis. The pathogenesis is complex, being due to such varying factors as cerebral hemorrhage, intoxication from *B. pertussis,* or anoxia from severe paroxysms. Oxygen therapy for the patient with respiratory distress may be a significant preventive measure. Convulsions should be controlled with sedatives. Care should be exercised to avoid cough suppression. Phenobarbital (3 to 5 mg. per kg.) should be initial therapy as this will not depress the cough.

Other Complications. Hemorrhages other than those in the central nervous system may also occur from paroxysmal stress, particularly into the subconjunctivae and as epistaxis.

Herniae may appear or become worse from the stress of coughing and from poor nutrition. Repeated vomiting may interfere not only with nutrition but also with fluid balance, requiring parenteral fluid and electrolyte therapy. Alkalosis from continuing loss of gastric contents can be countered by the administration of calcium gluconate.

Management of Contacts

As mentioned, the use of human immune globulin for prophylaxis can not be recommended even though there is anecdotal and traditional support for its use for passive immunization of high risk infants and children chronically ill with other illnesses. Chemoprophylaxis with erythromycin (10 mg. per kg. four times daily) may be given to those contacts who have not been immunized. This should be continued for a minimum period of 5 days after the contact is broken. Children less than 7 years of age who have been immunized should be given a single booster injection of pertussis vaccine 0.5 ml. especially if their last vaccine injection was more than 2 years past. Children not immune who have not developed pertussis by 14 days after last exposure should be immunized by three injections of vaccine at 1 to 2 month intervals.

Acknowledgments: I am indebted to Julia Hoover Peterson and Karen Montgomery Worsham for typing.

ACTIVE IMMUNIZATION FOR INFECTIOUS DISEASES

method of
VINCENT A. FULGINITI, M.D.
Tucson, Arizona

GENERAL FEATURES OF IMMUNIZATION PRACTICE

Theoretical immunology offers the practitioner an opportunity to place a new vaccine or gamma globulin preparation into scientific perspective. Knowing that antibody cannot abort an established infectious disease will prevent the misuse of gamma globulin.

If one is aware of the cause of a specific infectious disease and its expected course in nature, then use of a vaccine designed to prevent that disease will be intelligent. For example, knowing that rabies is not endemic in rodents and the virus is not transmitted by bites from this species will prevent the use of rabies vaccine in rat, squirrel, and other rodent bites.

Not enough can be said in support of specific knowledge of the biologic products used by any physician. One useful habit to cultivate is the reading, in detail, of the brochure (package insert) available for each product.

One should never administer a vaccine or gamma globulin preparation to a single patient prior to careful examination of the brochure accompanying that product. Specific information as to *all* the contents of the product, of its unique antibiotic or preservative, of its exact infectious or antigen nature, of contraindications and adverse effects and other important information is contained within the brochure by law. It is foolish to fail to read it before applying the product widely across your practice.

Practical Considerations

The *dose* of vaccine must be adequate. Following the manufacturer's recommendation is a prerequisite. Most viral vaccines contain a sufficient dose to ensure injection of a single recipient. It is false economy to split a single dose for multiple recipients, for example several children in a family, only to save the parents money and ensure that *none* of the children are protected.

Bacterial vaccines are calibrated to provide sufficient antigenic mass to invoke the desired response. Reduction in dosage is occasionally desired to avoid or minimize reactions, but the total mass administered usually must remain the same; this usually means additional doses must be administered.

The *route* of vaccine administration may be a critical determinant of both effectiveness and safety. Oral or intramuscular administration of a vaccine given subcutaneously may negate effective immunization. In general, strict adherence to recommended administration method is the safest and most effective practice.

Timing of immunization is crucial. In a disease prevalent in infants, e.g., pertussis, immunization must be administered early enough in life to be effective and preventive yet not so early as to produce inadequate responses nor so late as to miss the period of risk. For each vaccine, the epidemiologic factors of the disease to be prevented determine the timing of vaccine administration.

Some vaccines require *booster doses* due to their failure to invoke long-term immunity. The precise timing of these additional doses is determined by both theory and experience. Some vaccines require multiple, frequent doses over the life-span of an individual; others may be given infrequently, at long intervals. In general, inactivated vaccines require repetitive administration, whereas live ones do not.

Administration of a vaccine is designed to deliver as specific an antigen as possible to the host. Obviously, extraneous organisms are unwanted and undesired. In this regard, bacteria from the environment, especially the skin of the recipient, and hepatitis virus are the greatest risks. To prevent introduction of such agents, aseptic precautions in the manufacture, transport, storage, and administration of biologicals are warranted. In most instances the physician can only assume sterility of the products used. His responsibility begins with receipt of the biological: he must ensure that strict attention is given to the appropriate, recommended storage requirements. This allows adverse conditions for growth of extraneous bacteria and preserves the potency of the desired antigens. He must use sterile administration apparatus to avoid introduction of bacteria and hepatitis virus. Most physicians prefer individualized, sterile plastic syringes and needles. He must use aseptic technique in treating the surface of the vaccine vial *and* the skin of the recipient.

Specific recommendations include the following practices:

1. If a glass syringe is used, it must be adequately sterilized before administering vaccine to another patient. The American Academy of Pediatrics recommends autoclaving at 121°C. for 15 minutes at 15 pounds per square inch (psi). Dry heat for 2 hours at 170°C. or boiling for 30 minutes also is an acceptable procedure, but one must be certain that the time and temperature requirements are met.

2. For most procedures it is sufficient to cleanse the intended injection site and the surface of the immunization container with a 70 per cent solution of alcohol. Some prefer 2 per cent tincture of iodine followed by 70 per cent alcohol. Iodine burns have occurred when the tincture was not removed or was allowed to pool in contact with the skin. Our feeling is that *no* preparation, or at most *gentle* washing with soap and water, is indicated preceding smallpox vaccination.

Another practical consideration is the procedure designed to minimize the risks associated with depot antigens. These products contain substances designed to "hold" the antigens in place and release them slowly for maximal effect (alum, aluminum hydroxide, aluminum phosphate, mineral oil and other organic oils, and other substances under consideration). All such products must be placed deep in a large muscle mass, with care taken to avoid leakage into subcutaneous or dermal tissues. (These substances are irritating and can produce necrosis or irritative foci, the so-called sterile abscess or cyst.) Most experts recommend the Z method of injection (by drawing the skin over the injection site laterally, the tract of administration springs aside when the skin is released at the end of injection). Also, a small amount of air, enough to eject all of the product into the tissue, can prevent deposit of adjuvant along the injection tract.

The site of intramuscular injections is the anterolateral thigh (vastus lateralis), in order to avoid sciatic nerve damage which may follow intragluteal injections, or the deltoid or triceps muscle mass (in older children and adults). One should always aspirate prior to injection to avoid intravenous administration. Aqueous vaccines can be given intramuscularly, subcutaneously, or, on occasion, intracutaneously.

Contraindications to vaccine administration are seldom absolute. Certain disease states are associated with high risk for replication of viruses: all immunodeficiency states and those acquired because of disease (e.g., lymphatic and other malignancies, collagen vascular diseases) or drug administration (e.g., steroids, antimetabolites, cell poisons) are associated with such risks.

Allergic diseases pose special problems for immunization. Since many vaccines are prepared in tissues that potentially share antigens with substances commonly involved in human allergy, great care must be taken to elicit the appropriate sensitivity and to avoid exposure. The physician must be knowledgeable of the specific potential allergenic components of each vaccine. These are amply emphasized in the product brochures, in advertising, and in the description accompanying expert recommendations.

COMMONLY USED BACTERIAL VACCINES

Diphtheria

Active Immunization. Diphtheria toxin, chemically altered, is used as the major immunizing antigen. This product is referred to as diphtheria toxoid. It is prepared in two strengths: a pediatric strength (7 to 25 Lf units) and an adult strength (2 Lf units). Since persons older than 7 years of age may react adversely to large amounts of diphtheria toxoid, only the adult preparation should be given.

There is no indication for the use of fluid toxoid. Since toxoid is alum-adsorbed it should be administered deeply into a substantial muscle mass.

Immunization with diphtheria toxoid does not provide 100 per cent protection among recipients. The best experimental data suggest a five-fold to ten-fold protection against diphtheria in the immunized as contrasted to the unimmunized. Further, severe cases are fewer and deaths are rarely observed in fully immunized individuals.

The basis for immunity is the presence of or potential for circulating diphtheria antitoxin.

Persistence of immunity to diphtheria is longer lasting than previously thought. Reinforcing, booster doses were recommended every 4 to 6 years; it is now suggested that a 10-year interval between doses is adequate. Immunity to diphtheria is related to (1) the retention of serum antitoxin and (2) the ability to produce additional antitoxin promptly.

Schedules.   Rarely used as a single antigen, diphtheria toxoid is most often combined with tetanus and pertussis.

PRIMARY IMMUNIZATION IN INFANCY.   This is accomplished with three doses of DPT at 2-month intervals, beginning at 2 months of age (Table 1), and a booster dose 1 year later. All are in 0.5 ml. doses and administered intramuscularly.

PRIMARY IMMUNIZATION AT 7 YEARS OF AGE OR OLDER.   This is accomplished with Td, containing the lower dose, 2 Lf or less, of diphtheria toxoid in two doses at least 4 weeks apart, and a booster dose 1 year later.

LAPSED IMMUNIZATION.   If doses are missed in the primary series the regimen is continued regardless of the interval, until a primary series of four or three doses is completed. For example, doses may be given at ages 2 months, 6 months, and 8 months, with a booster 1 year later.

RECALL IMMUNIZATION.   This is every 10 years, usually as Td.

SPECIAL CIRCUMSTANCES.   If Td is not available, hypersensitivity to toxoid is determined by the Zeller-Moloney test. If results are positive, immunity is assumed and toxoid is not administered. If results are negative, susceptibility is assumed and either diphtheria toxoid or pediatric DT is administered.

TABLE 1.   **Schedules for Routine Primary Immunization of Infants and Children**

AGE	VACCINES
2 months	DPT,* TOPV†
4 months	DPT, TOPV
6 months	DPT, (TOPV)‡
15 months	Measles§¶
	(Rubella§)
	(Mumps§)
18 months	DPT–TOPV
4 to 6 years	DPT–TOPV
14 to 16 years	Td** (every 10 years)

*DPT: diphtheria-pertussis-tetanus

†TOPV: trivalent oral poliovirus—types 1, 2, 3

‡Optional for those areas at risk from importation

§Combined viral vaccines available include: measles-mumps-rubella, measles-rubella, and mumps-rubella. If administered singly, allow at least 1 month between vaccines

¶A tuberculin test prior to measles vaccine is desirable

**Td: adult tetanus-diphtheria, contains less diphtheria toxin

For children with CNS lesions or with a history of CNS symptoms to previous DPT, DT is administered in fractional doses, 0.05 to 0.1 ml., extending the series to five or more doses.

If a patient survives diphtheria, no immunity is conferred. Therefore, a primary series of immunization should be administered. If a fully immunized person is exposed to diphtheria, 0.5 ml. of toxoid is administered as DT or Td, depending on age.

Adverse Effects of Immunization.   Sensitivity or toxic reactions to diphtheria toxoid are rare in infants and children. However, increasing age and exposure to toxoid can result in a hypersensitive state. Severe local reactions can occur with further doses of full-strength (7 to 25 Lf) toxoid. Adult Td containing 2 Lf of toxoid or less should be utilized in persons without a history of reaction. With history of reaction to diphtheria toxoid–containing products, the Zeller-Moloney test should be conducted or no further toxoid given.

Rare systemic reactions, including anaphylaxis, have been reported.

Passive Immunization.   Diphtheria antitoxin is prepared in horses. It is available in vials containing 1000, 10,000, 20,000, and 40,000 units. It is used both in prophylaxis and therapy of diphtheria.

Prophylaxis.   Ten thousand units are administered to unimmunized, exposed susceptibles who cannot be kept under surveillance. It is preferred to avoid administration of antitoxin; daily examination, throat cultures for *Corynebacterium diphtheriae* with penicillin administered to positives, and toxoid administration should be employed.

Tetanus

Active Immunization.   Tetanospasmin, the *Clostridium tetani* toxin, is modified by chemical treatment to provide a toxoid for immunization. A potent antigen with minimal toxicity, tetanus toxoid is used alone or in combination with diphtheria (DT, Td) and pertussis (DPT). It is one of the most effective antigens used in immunization, virtually assuring protection to a person who receives a complete primary series.

Antitoxin appears to be the sole factor in protection from the disease. In an adequately immunized person, as little as 0.01 I.U. per ml. of antitoxin is protective.

Theoretically, it may be unnecessary to employ booster doses in someone who receives a full primary series. Practically, 10-year interval boosters are recommended to ensure protective levels of antitoxin in the circulation.

Schedules for Immunization. PRIMARY IM-
MUNIZATION IN INFANCY.   Three doses of tetanus
toxoid, usually as DPT, are administered intramuscularly at 2-month intervals, beginning at
age 2 months (see Table 1). To complete the primary series a booster dose is administered 1 year
later. A fifth dose is given just prior to entry into
school.

PRIMARY IMMUNIZATION AT 7 YEARS OF AGE
OR OLDER.   Two doses of either tetanus toxoid
alone (0.5 ml.) or as Td are administered 2 months
apart, with a booster dose 6 months to 1 year later
to complete primary immunization.

LAPSED IMMUNIZATION.   If doses are missed,
the next dose in the series is administered regardless of interval. It is not necessary to begin the
series anew.

RECALL IMMUNIZATION.   Tetanus or Td toxoid should be given every 10 years to maintain
immunity. It is usual to give a booster dose on
school entry (3 to 7 years of age) and every 10 years
thereafter. If an injury occurs that is "tetanus
prone," booster doses (0.5 ml.) should be given if a
5 year interval has elapsed since the last booster.

SPECIAL CIRCUMSTANCES.   In patients who
survive tetanus, full primary immunization, utilizing a schedule appropriate for age, should be administered, since the natural disease does not confer immunity.

Adverse Effects of Immunization. Tetanus
toxoid is an extremely safe biological, associated
with few local or systemic reactions if used according to recommended schedules. A severe, local,
necrotizing Arthus reaction can occur in the person who receives too many doses at too frequent
intervals. High levels of serum antitoxin result,
with local vascular necrosis secondary to toxoid-
antitoxin complexes.

Passive Immunization. Tetanus antitoxin is
now administered as specific immune human
globulin. Horse serum is no longer necessary. The
tetanus immune globulin (TIG) is supplied in vials
containing 250 units and is identical in all respects
to all human gamma globulin except in its measured tetanus antitoxin content.

Pertussis

Active Immunization. Pertussis vaccines are
among the least well defined of immunizing
biologicals. The current vaccine consists of killed
pertussis organisms and fragments of organisms.

Potency of pertussis vaccine has been a critical
issue in its use and in judgment of its efficacy. The
standard test employed is a mouse-protective
model developed in the 1940s. This test correlates
with human protection to a high degree. Vaccines
used in England and elsewhere prior to 1968 were
of low potency as measured by this test. They gave

correspondingly poor results in Britain, to the
point that critics felt that pertussis vaccine use
should be abandoned, especially in view of inherent toxic properties. Potent vaccine, as judged by
mouse-protective units, is capable of providing 85
to 90 per cent protection to the immunized.

Pertussis vaccine can be administered alone or
in combination with diphtheria and tetanus tox-
oids. It is prepared as both a "plain" preparation
and one adsorbed to alum. The adjuvant vaccine
contains 4 protective units per 0.5 ml. dose,
whereas the plain vaccine contains slightly more
antigen. There is little practical use for plain pertussis vaccine; it offers no advantages immunologically and does not improve safety.

Virtually complete immunity follows an attack of the natural disease; rarely, second cases of
bacteriologically proved disease have occurred in
the same patient. Protection following vaccine is
relatively short-lived; booster doses are required
to maintain immunity.

Complicating assessment of immunity is the
occurrence of the pertussis syndrome caused by
agents other than *Bordetella pertussis.* Parapertussis
has been estimated to account for as many as 2 per
cent of clinical cases attributed to pertussis. There
is no cross immunity between these organisms.
Adenoviruses and other viral agents have been
identified in pertussislike syndromes. The occurrence of such infections confuses evaluation of
efficacy of pertussis vaccine unless precise and
definitive laboratory diagnosis is undertaken.

Schedules for Immunization. Pertussis vaccine is most often administered in combination,
viz., DPT. Each dose of DPT contains 4 protective
units of pertussis vaccine.

PRIMARY IMMUNIZATION IN INFANCY.   This
usually is accomplished with DPT. Three doses (a
total of 12 protective units) are given intramuscularly at 2-month intervals, beginning at 2 months
of age. In areas of high endemicity or during
epidemics, it may be desirable to initiate immunization earlier. Often the vaccine (DPT or pertussis,
adsorbed) is begun at 4 to 6 weeks of age, and the
older regimen of three doses 1 month apart is
employed. Rarely, in severe epidemics affecting
very young infants, pertussis immunization can be
initiated in the first few days or weeks of life, but
this is not recommended as a routine procedure.

Completion of primary immunization is accomplished with a booster dose approximately 1
year after the initial series is finished (see Table 1).

RECALL IMMUNIZATION. Routine recall
booster doses are suggested when the child enters
school, and, if pertussis is prevalent in adolescents,
one half the dose should be given to children older
than age 7 (commonly at 12 years of age).

SPECIAL CIRCUMSTANCES. Intimate exposure to pertussis or an epidemic may warrant addi-

tional DPT or pertussis adsorbed vaccine. For children 7 years of age or under, the full 0.5 ml. dose should be employed. For those older than 7 years, one may wish to use 0.25 ml. of either vaccine.

Long thought to contradict pertussis immunization, central nervous system conditions no longer represent a reason for avoidance. In fact, pertussis immunization may be desirable in persons with static central nervous system (CNS) lesions in order to prevent the natural disease and its adverse CNS effects. Seizure disorders are still held by many to be a contraindication. The World Health Organization has even recommended avoidance of pertussis vaccine in children with a family history of convulsion. American experts, and this author, disagree with this view and believe pertussis vaccine should be administered to children with seizure disorders to protect them against the natural disease. However, pertussis vaccine should not be given to children with an evolving CNS disorder. This recommendation stems from a wish to avoid both complication of the vaccine and confusion of the disease's natural progression with vaccine effect.

Local or systemic reactions *without* CNS symptoms to a previous dose of pertussis vaccine do *not* contraindicate its use again. Some physicians prefer separation of pertussis from DT and lower dosage in an extended schedule (for example, 0.25 ml. doses could be given six times), but little data exist to support this practice.

If any CNS symptoms or signs follow pertussis vaccine administration, no further doses should be administered.

Adverse Effects of Immunization. Both local and systemic adverse effects have been noted with administration of pertussis vaccine. Local reactions, consisting of pain, induration, heat, and redness in any combination, are frequent; as many as 70 per cent of recipients in some series have experienced local toxicity. In the rare instance, tissue damage is severe enough to result in development of a "cyst" or local nodule that may drain, the so-called sterile abscess.

Systemic reactions occur with a variable frequency. Fever is common but often unrecorded. The most feared consequence, postpertussis vaccine CNS complications, has occurred. Unfortunately, the true incidence of these complications is clouded by the changes made in the formulation of the vaccine and by the variability in recognition and reporting of such incidents. Many experts believe CNS complications are rare, at least in the United States. Others have reported higher frequencies. One of the major difficulties is the setting in which such complications occur. The population being immunized is subject to a host of infec-

tious agents that produce CNS symptoms. Temporal association with pertussis immunization may lead to mistaken attribution of the CNS symptoms to the vaccine. Also, in true postpertussis vaccine encephalopathy, an interval of hours to days may supervene between administration of the vaccine and the onset of the symptoms. This interval may result in failure to link the two events. The true incidence is unknown, but most experts guess it to be 1:50,000 doses of vaccine, or even less frequent.

There is little evidence to suggest that either anticonvulsants or antipyretics reduce or ameliorate complications. Many experienced clinicians claim infants obtain relief from these medications, but objective data are lacking.

Other adverse reactions reported in association with pertussis immunization include (1) sudden death, (2) angioneurotic edema, (3) gastrointestinal symptoms, (4) various rashes, (5) persistent, uncontrollable screaming, (6) collapse and pallor, and (7) hypersensitivity angiitis. The difficulty in ascribing these reactions with certainty to pertussis immunization is obvious. All these syndromes are seen in infants without reference to prior immunization. Although temporal association is a powerful argument for causation, particularly with collapse or irritability, it does not necessarily link the vaccine and the symptom complex. All experts agree that pertussis vaccine is among the most toxic of products used in immunization; they disagree on extent and frequency of toxicity and on specific etiologic association.

Passive Immunization. A hyperimmune pertussis globulin is available through commercial outlets. There is no convincing evidence that indicates it is effective in either prophylaxis or therapy. The author cannot recommend its use.

Prophylaxis may be more readily achieved with antimicrobial therapy, using either erythromycin or ampicillin. Controlled data are lacking.

Once pertussis is established in the paroxysmal stage there is no specific therapy, although antimicrobials may reduce environmental contamination with the organisms.

COMMONLY USED VIRAL VACCINES

Poliovirus Vaccines

Active Immunization. Inactivated Poliovirus Vaccine. Difficult to obtain currently in the United States, inactivated poliovirus vaccine (IPV) is prepared by the careful formalin inactivation of potent poliovirus, types 1, 2, and 3, grown in monkey kidney tissue culture. The one disaster, in which live poliovirus remained in certain batches of IPV, has not recurred. Precautions in the manufacture of IPV preclude such accidents. IPV contains inactivated poliovirus of the three types, formalin, preservatives, and, possibly, trace amounts of tissue-culture fluid proteins and antibiotics.

One preparation, formerly utilized but not now available in the United States, combined IPV with DPT.

ATTENUATED, LIVE POLIOVIRUS VACCINE. Oral poliovirus vaccine (OPV) consists of a mixture of the three polioviruses, types 1, 2, and 3, grown either in monkey kidney tissue culture or human-fetal-diploid tissue culture. The vaccine contains some elements of the tissue culture system, albeit greatly diluted.

Monovalent OPV containing the single types alone is usually reserved for use in epidemics and is stockpiled nationally for this purpose.

Immunity to Polioviruses. There are two known phases of poliovirus immunity: a topical, mucosal phase and a systemic one. It appears that the secretory IgA antipoliovirus antibody is a significant factor in topical, mucosal immunity. The presence of this antibody in the pharynx, and possibly in the intestinal mucosa as well, serves to neutralize poliovirus and either prevent or limit infection. Other factors may also be involved; the presence of serum antibody correlates directly with immunity and is probably solely responsible for protection from systemic disease.

Systemic immunity is conferred on recipients of both IPV and OPV and also follows recovery from the natural disease. Local immunity has been demonstrated only following successful OPV immunization. Thus, it is possible for wild poliovirus to establish and replicate in the gastrointestinal tract of IPV recipients, despite the presence of serum antibody and the lack of symptoms.

In countries with immunization policies that have resulted solely in the use of IPV, wild poliovirus appears to have been eliminated from circulation in the population. These countries have achieved IPV rates of 95 per cent or more, resulting in elimination of the disease as well as freedom from the virus.

Poliovirus immunity is type specific. Following the natural disease it is lifelong. Thus far OPV seems associated with prolonged immunity (greater than 10 years), perhaps for a lifetime. IPV results in limited immunity. Some disagreement exists concerning the exact duration of IPV immunity, but many experts accept repeat immunizations every 2 to 4 years.

Salk has presented evidence which he believes to demonstrate long-term immunity from a primary series of IPV. He does not accept the need for repetitive booster doses of IPV.

Schedules for Immunization. IPV is currently available in the United States. It is distributed by Elkins-Sinn of Cherry Hill, N.J., for Connaught Laboratories, Canada.

PRIMARY IMMUNIZATION OF INFANTS WITH TRIVALENT OPV (TOPV). Three doses of OPV are given, each containing all three types of poliovirus, at 2 month intervals in the usual sequence, beginning at 2 months of age. The usual routine practice is to administer TOPV orally at the same visit that DPT is given intramuscularly.

For physicians wishing to give OPV separately the following procedures should be followed: (1) begin at 6 to 12 weeks of age or later, if desired; (2) allow at least 6 weeks, preferably 8 weeks, to elapse between doses of TOPV in the primary series; (3) administer at least two doses of TOPV in the primary series; and (4) administer another dose 8 to 12 months later.

True recall immunization is not necessary with OPV. Often a single dose confers immunity against all three types. However, more persons will develop immunity against all three types if multiple doses are given. Any one dose may fail to "take" against one, two, or all three types. Accordingly, the routine to permit maximal responsiveness of as many persons as possible (usually in excess of 95 per cent) to all three types is to give additional doses of TOPV at 18 months of age and prior to entry into school.

PRIMARY IMMUNIZATION OF CHILDREN THROUGH ADOLESCENCE WITH TOPV. Two doses of TOPV given orally 6 to 8 weeks apart and a third dose 8 to 12 months later constitute primary immunization for the unimmunized.

PRIMARY IMMUNIZATION OF ADULTS WITH TOPV. For adults (over 18 years of age) who are unimmunized and unlikely to be exposed to polio, no routine immunization with TOPV can be recommended. The very slight risk of paralytic disease resulting from the vaccine is unacceptable in the unexposed adult. Formerly, IPV was recommended.

If exposure risk is high (in epidemics or contemplated travel to endemic areas), adults should receive OPV, as the risk from the vaccine is infinitely less than that from natural exposure. Many medical personnel are included in this group. The dosage schedule is identical to that for children through adolescence.

PRIMARY IMMUNIZATION WITH MONOVALENT OPV. For physicians preferring OPV containing the single types of polioviruses, monovalent OPV can be substituted for trivalent in the above schedules. Although any order can be chosen, some experts advise type 3 first, type 1 second, and type 2 last. Others have suggested the order 2, 1, 3 is preferable.

LAPSED IMMUNIZATION. If OPV schedules are interrupted for any reason, the doses should be administered as if no interruption occurred.

The suggested intervals are the minimum criteria to ensure routine immunization. Longer intervals do not affect the immunizing potential of OPV.

SPECIAL CIRCUMSTANCES. Breast-feeding, once thought to inhibit OPV immunization, is no longer considered in scheduling. If one wishes to be overly cautious, breast-feeding may be suspended for 6 hours prior to and 6 hours after OPV administration.

Pregnancy does not contraindicate OPV administration, but OPV should be given during pregnancy only if the exposure risk is present. Otherwise it is best to administer OPV after delivery.

In epidemics, monovalent vaccine of the type causing the epidemic should be administered to all persons at risk, regardless of their immunization status.

If a fully immunized person is traveling to an area endemic for polio or is otherwise subject to increased exposure, a single dose of OPV should be administered.

Any individual suspected of immunodeficiency should not receive poliovirus vaccine containing live virus.

For persons who have an uncertain polio immunization history, who have been partially immunized with OPV, or who have received only IPV, a single dose of OPV or two doses 8 weeks apart may be indicated.

In epidemic regions it may be desirable to immunize newborns to ensure early protection. The American Academy of Pediatrics advises use of type 1 vaccine in the newborn, as this is the prevalent epidemic type. Of course, if other types predominate, epidemic-specific vaccine should be used. This use of monovalent vaccine should not be substituted for full trivalent schedules.

Adverse Effects of Vaccines. The major adverse effect of live, attenuated poliovirus vaccine is its capacity for reversion to neurovirulence. Poliomyelitis due to attenuated poliovirus vaccine, either in vaccinees or in their contacts, has been the major cause of paralytic disease in the United States in recent years. To advocates of attenuated vaccine the incidence of paralytic disease, although regrettable, is sufficiently low to be acceptable. Advocates of IPV decry any incidence of paralytic disease, since IPV is unassociated with this risk. The best incidence figures place the risk at 0.06 instances of paralysis per million doses distributed for recipients of OPV, and at 0.14 per million doses of contacts. Some argue that this method of representing risks is inadequate, since "doses distributed" reflect neither actual doses administered nor the fact that one child may receive five or more doses. They contend the actual incidence per children immunized is much higher than the figures indicate. To some the risk is unacceptable.

Other adverse effects have not been consistently noted. OPV is administered during an age period when the recipients are exposed to many infections and other processes. The temporal coincidence of OPV administration and occurrence of specific diseases does not establish a relationship.

Persons with immunodeficiency are at increased risk of attenuated poliovirus-associated disease. A number of instances of severe infection have been recorded in such persons. Therefore, oral poliovirus vaccine (OPV) should *not* be administered to a person with immunodeficiency.

Measles (Rubeola)

Immunizing Antigens. INACTIVATED (KILLED) MEASLES VIRUS (KMV). KMV is no longer available or used, but as hundreds of thousands have received it, a description is included here. KMV was prepared by inactivating live virus grown in tissues derived from monkeys or from chick eggs. Adjuvant was added to the final formulation. It was administered alone or prior to attenuated (live) measles virus vaccine (LMV). The usual series consisted of two or three doses with subsequent boosters of KMV or a dose of LMV.

Inactivated vaccine resulted in antibody production in recipients, with short-lived immunity. After a variable period, usually 6 months or longer, recipients of KMV became susceptible to atypical reactions to either attenuated or wild virus. LMV administration was associated with local reactions (heat, induration, pain, and rash at the site of inoculation) and, occasionally, with systemic reactions (fever, regional adenopathy, headache, malaise). Exposure to wild virus could result in a bizarre disease with an atypical eruption (atypical distribution with peripheral accentuation and onset of the rash, vesicles, petechiae, and purpura) and severe systemic symptoms (fever, headache, serositis, and pleural, peritoneal, and CNS symptoms). Extremely high antibody titers and a skin reaction thought to be either a CMI (delayed hypersensitivity type) or an Arthus (antibody-antigen complex type) reaction were noted. This syndrome is termed "atypical measles."

ATTENUATED (LIVE) MEASLES VIRUS VACCINE (LMV). Two major types of LMV have been developed. The original LMV was developed from the Edmonston strain of measles virus isolated by Enders. An attenuated virus was obtained after many passages in chick embryo tissue culture. This agent (Edmonston B) produced minimal symptoms and reliable immunity. However, the 15 per cent incidence of rash and 80 per cent incidence of fever were judged too severe. Simultaneous but separate administration of measles immune globulin (MIG) reduced the incidence of fever and rash to more acceptable levels without significantly sacrificing immunity.

A second source of attenuated virus was developed by Schwarz initially by additional passage in chick embryo tissue culture. This further attenuated measles virus (FAMV) produced fewer febrile or exanthematous reactions but resulted in lower levels of antibody, which decreased more rapidly and to a greater degree than did the antibody induced by Edmonston B immunization. Despite this decline, vaccinees appear to be equally protected against natural exposure in subsequent years. FAMV vaccine does not require the simultaneous administration of MIG.

Both types of LMV are supplied in lyophilized form for reconstitution just prior to immunization, thus avoiding many of the potency-reducing factors associated with a liquid vaccine that must be stored in the frozen state. The manufacturers' directions should be followed explicitly in the storage, reconstitution, and administration of LMV. The virus is fragile and may be rendered inactive if any of these steps is omitted or changed. Heating the vaccine, adding improper diluent, using glass syringes, and mixing with immune globulin have all been encountered and result in inactivation of the virus, and, hence, no immunization and a susceptible patient.

Measles immune globulin (MIG) is supplied for use only with Edmonston B vaccine. It must be injected at a site separate from that used for LMV, utilizing a separate syringe and needle. If mixed with vaccine or injected at the same site, the live virus can be neutralized and immunization will fail.

LMV has been added to other viruses in a variety of combined vaccines.

Recovery from measles virus infection is probably independent of antibody synthesis. Hypogammaglobulinemic patients with intact cell-mediated immunity have a normal course of measles virus infection.

Active Immunity. Immunity to measles on subsequent exposure is directly correlated with the presence of antibody. Other factors, notably cell-mediated immunity, may be important, but antibody alone seems sufficient. Administration of antibody can totally protect an individual on exposure to wild virus.

Natural measles immunity is lifelong. Experience with isolated populations, which have been exposed at intervals as long as 65 years apart, indicates that a single attack of measles confers immunity and is correlated with the presence of serum antibody.

Immunity following LMV immunization is believed to be equal to that seen after the natural disease. Of course, observation of LMV recipients has only been possible for 16 years. During that time, persons with demonstrable antibody after LMV have been protected against wild virus exposure. The FAMV vaccine has a shorter history: only 13 years have elapsed since its first use. However, immunity has been sustained during this period.

Measles has occurred in vaccine recipients and is usually due to one of the following factors:

1. Administration of LMV prior to 15 months of age. When first licensed, LMV was recommended for persons 9 months of age or older. It soon became apparent that a substantial number of vaccine recipients at 9, 10, or 11 months of age were not successfully immunized. Many believe this failure is linked with undetectable but persistent maternal antibody. Subsequently, 12 months of age was recommended as the earliest age for LMV. In 1975, Yeager and others discovered that up to 15 to 20 per cent of LMV recipients at 12 or 13 months of age also failed to be immunized. Although some dispute these data, it has led to a recommendation that LMV be delayed until 15 months of age to ensure maximal opportunity for 95+ per cent of recipients to be successfully immunized.

In a given miniepidemic of measles, children who were immunized prior to 15 months may develop measles on exposure. This occurrence should not lead to loss of faith in the vaccine, since the majority, if not the bulk, of all children immunized prior to 15 months will be protected. As a rough guide, 65 per cent will be protected at 9 months of age, increasing to 95 to 97 per cent at 15 months of age.

2. Use of impotent vaccine. For a host of reasons (improper storage, dilution, or administration), LMV may be inactivated prior to administration.

3. The natural failure rate. LMV does not successfully immunize all recipients; 3 to 5 per cent may not respond despite adequate vaccine and administration technique. If subsequently exposed to wild virus, these persons may develop measles.

A single report from St. Louis by Cherry and associates is disturbing. Some vaccine failures could not be attributed to the above causes. Full-blown, modified, or atypical measles was noted in a few children who had received LMV. If this report is confirmed or extended, the solidity of measles immunity following LMV immunization might be challenged.

Schedules for Active Immunization. Certain precautions are advisable in LMV use. First, whenever feasible, a negative tuberculin test should be obtained prior to LMV administration. There is a theoretic risk of exacerbating silent tuberculosis. If prior tuberculin testing is not feasible, simultaneous testing can be substituted. In community campaigns or in clinical circumstances in which only a single opportunity for contact exists, the prior tuberculin test may have to be eliminated for practical reasons. Second, illnesses, particularly febrile illnesses, contraindicate LMV administration. Third, any defect in cell-mediated immunity is a contraindication to LMV administration. Fourth, pregnancy contraindicates LMV use. Fifth, LMV should not be given for 2 or 3 months following immune serum globulin (ISG) administration. Measles neutralizing antibody in ISG can counteract effective immunization. Sixth, LMV prepared in egg-derived culture should be used cautiously, if at all, in egg-sensitive persons.

PRIMARY IMMUNIZATION WITH LMV (EDMONSTON B). This vaccine is no longer available.

PRIMARY IMMUNIZATION WITH FAMV. Further attenuated measles vaccine (FAMV), the only available measles vaccine, is given subcutaneously. MIG is unnecessary. In situations in which any febrile reaction is unwanted, a small amount (a *total* dose of 0.2 ml.) of MIG can be given. This dose of MIG will not interfere with the immune response. FAMV is administered at 15 months of age or older.

IMMUNIZATION OF CHILDREN PREVIOUSLY IMMUNIZED WITH KMV. Since these children may experience untoward reactions to LMV and are susceptible to atypical measles on exposure to wild virus, specific discussion with parents and consent for further use of measles vaccine should be obtained.

The recommendation is to immunize such children with a single subcutaneous dose of FAMV. In 10 to 50 per cent of children, one can expect a local reaction (heat, induration, and tenderness), and in 3 to 10 per cent of children systemic symptoms (fever, malaise, and regional adenopathy) are expected. I have encountered reactions severe enough to require hospitalization.

COMBINATION OF LIVE VIRUS VACCINES. LMV has been combined with other viruses.

SPECIAL CIRCUMSTANCES. If an unimmunized child is exposed to natural measles and promptly brought to a physician's attention, LMV administration may result in prevention of measles. This protection occurs because LMV has a shorter incubation period than natural measles (7 days as opposed to 11 days).

If clinical tuberculosis is present, or the unimmunized child has a positive tuberculin test, measles prevention is desirable. Natural measles occurring in patients with tuberculosis can exacerbate the disease. If adequate chemotherapy is administered, LMV can be given. Temporary depression of tuberculin sensitivity may occur following LMV, commencing in 4 to 7 days and lasting several weeks.

Children who received LMV prior to 15 months of age pose a dilemma for practitioners. Current recommendations suggest the following approach:

1. All who received LMV prior to 12 months of age should receive another dose of LMV at whatever age they are discovered after 15 months.

2. Children who received LMV between 12 and 15 months of age. As only 15 to 20 per cent of such children will not be immunized it seems unnecessary routinely to seek all out. In fact, 80 to 85 per cent will be fully protected and would receive a second dose unnecessarily. Thus, *routine* reimmunization is not recommended. However, if a miniepidemic occurs in which patients of a given practice are in danger of exposure, reimmunization for this group is warranted.

In measles epidemics, with high risk of exposure in infants, one may wish to immunize infants between 6 and 15 months of age with LMV without simultaneous MIG. It must be appreciated that some infants will not be immunized, but will be protected by natural transplacental immunity. All infants immunized during epidemic conditions who were under 15 months of age must receive a second dose of LMV at or after 15 months of age.

For persons who cannot be given LMV due to risks associated with their underlying disease, condition, or age, one must consider use of preventive amounts of MIG on exposure.

Adverse Effects of LMV. The usual fever and rash in association with LMV have been described. LMV has resulted in disseminated disease and death in persons with depressed immune function involving absent or diminished cell-mediated immunity. Although a variety of acute CNS disorders have occurred within 30 days of LMV administration, none has definitely been attributed to LMV, and a few have been identified as caused by other viruses.

Subacute sclerosing panencephalitis, the slow measles-virus infection of the central nervous system, has been described following LMV. The exact incidence is extremely low, less than that associated with wild virus infection.

Theoretically, tuberculosis can be exacerbated by LMV administration. Several instances of tuberculous meningitis were described within 30 days of LMV administration. However, direct evidence for worsening of tuberculosis secondary to LMV is lacking. Treated tuberculosis is not a contraindication to measles vaccine.

Although a potential problem, egg-sensitive children deliberately immunized with the vaccine virus grown from chick embryo tissue culture have not reacted unusually.

Passive Immunization. Immune serum globulin (ISG) contains a variable amount of measles antibody; measles immune globulin (MIG) has been adjusted to contain 4000 measles virus-neutralizing units per milliliter. Use of the calibrated product, MIG, results in more certain dosage and effect.

MIG or ISG may be used to prevent or modify measles in an exposed, susceptible person. I believe that prevention, with subsequent LMV immunization in 8 to 12 weeks, should be the goal of MIG use. The doses are 0.25 ml. per kg. for prevention.

Protection of children suspected or known to have CMI defects may require 20 to 30 ml. ISG on exposure.

All MIG or ISG is given deep intramuscularly in a large muscle mass; no more than 5 ml. is given at one site. Care should be exercised to avoid intravenous injection.

Smallpox

Today smallpox is limited geographically to certain areas of the world. Since 1976, Ethiopia and Somalia remain the foci of smallpox. World health experts anticipate the total eradication of smallpox. With the decreasing reservoir, the risk of importation diminishes. Inasmuch as for decades there has been no endemic disease, and given the rarity of importations, all official advisory bodies recommended the abandonment of mandatory, routine smallpox vaccination in the United States. Significant numbers of children were suffering from mild to lethal complications in the absence of risk of exposure to smallpox.

All these factors have led to the current rationale for smallpox vaccination. Only persons at risk from exposure are to be vaccinated. These include (1) those contemplating travel to an endemic region, (2) military personnel, (3) health personnel who may be the first to contact an imported case, (4) travel workers on international routes and in terminals serving areas of endemicity, and (5) in event of importation or local epidemic, "ring" vaccination of persons in contact with infected patients.

Immunizing Antigens.   A variety of products are available for vaccination. All depend on the viability of vaccinia virus to be delivered to a wound in the dermis. Required is an adequate titer of virus in a form preserving infectivity. This is especially critical for areas of the world in which adverse environmental circumstances may destroy virus inadequately protected.

Rubella (German Measles)

Active Immunization.   The original vaccine candidate strain HPV-77 has been passaged in avian cell lines; a duck embryo tissue culture product is the most widely used vaccine. Canine kidney tissue culture vaccine also has been employed; reactivity with this vaccine is at an unacceptable level for many physicians; hence, its use has diminished. Other candidate strains and formulations may be on the market. The physician is urged to consult expert recommendations and the manufacturer's brochure for specific information.

Rubella vaccine is a biological that contains live virus, and all of the usual precautions in storage, maintenance, and administration should be observed.

It is likely that cell-mediated immunity is responsible for recovery from an immunity to rubella. Antibody plays a role, but infection has been noted in persons with detectable titer. Most reinfection is subclinical, evidenced only by antibody increases following exposure.

Infants with congenital rubella demonstrate persistent or chronic infection with the agent despite high levels of serum antibodies. It is suspected that persistent rubella virus infection results from direct viral infection of lymphocytes, rendering them unresponsive to rubella antigens. With recovery from lymphocyte infection, cell-mediated immunity is restored and the virus is eradicated.

The fetus is susceptible to rubella virus and initially offers no defense. With persistence of the virus, an immunologic response characterized by specific IgM antibody develops. Thus the neonate with congenital rubella has both virus and antibody present.

A syndrome analogous to subacute sclerosing panencephalitis has been ascribed to rubella. These data suggest rubella virus may become latent in brain cells, despite a persistent and brisk antibody response. Thus far, the situation resembles measles virus subacute sclerosing panencephalitis.

Schedules for Immunization.   PRIMARY IMMUNIZATION IN CHILDHOOD.   Any child, from 12 months to prepuberty, is a candidate for rubella immunization. Although rubella virus vaccine will be effective at 12 months of age, it can most conveniently be given with measles vaccine at 15 months of age. Routine immunization at or near 15 months of age is recommended. The need for identifying nonimmunized children on entry into school and at intervals thereafter and for providing rubella immunization is important also. Many states have adopted mandatory rubella immunization policies as part of their health code.

Rubella immunization is accomplished by subcutaneous injection of the single antigen or as part of a combined vaccine. More than 95 per cent of recipients can be expected to develop serum antibody.

PRIMARY IMMUNIZATION FOR FEMALES ONLY. In this strategy, only those whose potential offspring are at risk receive the vaccine. All females at the following life stages are candidates: (1) female children just prior to menarche and (2) females in the childbearing years who lack rubella antibody. For all postmenarchal females the following conditions must be met:

1. A serum antibody titer from a reliable laboratory must demonstrate absence of rubella antibody.

2. The candidate must not be pregnant.

3. Measures to prevent pregnancy must be taken for at least 3 months following immunization.

4. Full knowledge of the risks of immunization if pregnancy occurs within 3 months must be available to and understood by the recipient (and parents of minors).

5. The recipient (and parents) should be aware of the possible occurrence of arthralgia and arthritis following immunization.

The actual immunization procedure does not differ from that for children.

SPECIAL CIRCUMSTANCES. Exposure to rubella cannot be "treated" by rubella vaccination; vaccine may be given in the hope that no disease will occur and to protect against future exposure.

In certain closed or limited population groups, such as colleges, institutions, and military camps, it may be desirable to immunize exposed persons in an attempt to limit or halt an epidemic. All precautions related to postmenarchal females should be observed.

Adverse Effects of Vaccine. Rubella vaccine is a live virus preparation. It produces an infection unassociated with typical rubella symptoms. However, virus may be present transiently in the throat of 75 per cent of recipients.

Arthralgia and arthritis occur in 1 to 5 per cent of all children immunized. Many clinicians report a frequency as high as 15 per cent . The arthritis may occur several weeks after immunization and may not be associated with the vaccine. Since the symptoms resemble rheumatoid or other forms of arthritis, unnecessary costly diagnostic evaluations have been undertaken. Arthralgia and arthritis are more frequent in older female children and adults; 10 to 30 per cent of recipients may experience symptoms.

A peculiar set of syndromes occurs infrequently in recipients of rubella vaccine. Non-localized pain about the joints of the upper and lower extremities is believed to be due to a neuropathy induced by the vaccine. Two forms have been described: one involves the upper extremities, with severe recurrent pain often occurring at night, and the other involves the lower extremities, with pain producing a crouching posture (catcher's crouch syndrome). The onset is variable but may be as late as 70 days after vaccine administration. Episodes may recur at varying intervals; one patient in Arizona had recurrent symptoms in the lower extremities for almost 2 years.

Other adverse effects include infrequent instances of thrombocytopenia, rash, or lymphadenopathy.

Passive Immunization. There is no available specific rubella immune globulin. Different lots of immune serum globulin (ISG) have markedly varied rubella antibody content. Protection against infection has not been consistently demonstrated. Rash and other symptoms may be suppressed, but infection occurs. There is no convincing evidence that ISG can protect an exposed, susceptible pregnant woman from rubella or her fetus from congenital rubella. Inapparent infection may occur with virus transmission to the fetus following ISG administration.

Some clinicians utilize 20 to 30 ml. of ISG in situations when pregnant women susceptible to rubella are exposed. They should do so only if they and their patients are aware of the futility of this approach.

Mumps

Mumps is a variable disease affecting mostly preteenagers. It usually produces a mild disease. On occasion, it can be severe, and complications occur frequently enough to warrant immunization with a safe, effective vaccine. Mumps in adults poses a problem for the male, in that as many as 20 per cent of postpubertal males with mumps develop orchitis. Orchitis is a painful, incapacitating disease, although sterility, a feared consequence, is extremely rare.

Mumps is a leading cause of overt meningoencephalitis, and greater numbers of persons have subclinical infection of the meninges. Mumps has been suspected as one cause of juvenile diabetes mellitus, based on its predilection for infection of the pancreas and the concordance of incidence between waves of mumps infection and the occurrence of juvenile diabetes mellitus 2 to 4 years later.

Thus, there was ample reason to welcome a vaccine, which appeared to parallel measles virus vaccine development. Live mumps virus, isolated from Hilleman's daughter, was attenuated by passage in chick embryo tissue culture. All subsequent vaccine used in this country is derived from this strain.

Despite early concerns over mumps vaccine's efficacy, prolonged experience has indicated that it appears both safe and effective. Today it has assumed a place in routine immunization and is often given in combination with measles and rubella vaccines.

Active Immunization. Live mumps virus vaccine is grown in chick embryo tissue culture and is a derivative of the Jeryl Lynn isolate (3). It produces no significant symptoms following inoculation. More than 95 per cent of recipients develop antibody.

The vaccine is a live virus preparation, and all precautions applying to this type of biological should be observed.

Mumps is one of the few viruses for which a direct demonstration of cell-mediated immunity is possible. Mumps virus antigens injected intradermally result in a delayed-type response. The precise role of cell-mediated immunity in immunity is not known. There is some evidence that suggests that cell-mediated immunity response plays a role in disease as well as recovery. Immunity against rechallenge with mumps virus, as with other agents, is generated with the presence of antibody.

Durable immunity follows natural disease; instances of two or more episodes of "mumps" may be related to other viral agents that can produce parotitis.

Schedules for Immunization. PRIMARY IMMUNIZATION IN INFANTS. Inclusion of mumps virus vaccine in routine pediatric immunization procedures is becoming a reality. A single dose of mumps virus vaccine, attenuated, is injected intradermally. This usually is accomplished at 15 months of age in a combined measles-mumps-rubella vaccine.

PRIMARY IMMUNIZATION IN PREPUBERTAL MALES AND ADULT MALES. If desired, mumps virus vaccine can be administered to prepubertal and adult males. A history of mumps can be deceptive, as other viruses occasionally produce parotitis. Failure to recall mumps is no guarantee that one has not been infected; 30 per cent of childhood mumps are asymptomatic.

A single subcutaneous dose of live mumps virus vaccine is sufficient.

SPECIAL CIRCUMSTANCES. Persons exposed to mumps, particularly susceptible adolescent or adult males, can be immunized with live mumps virus vaccine, but there is no guarantee that mumps will be averted. However, if mumps does not occur, the person will be protected against subsequent exposures.

Adverse Effects of Vaccine. There are no significant adverse effects that have been attributed to live mumps virus vaccine.

Passive Immunization. A specific mumps immune globulin is commercially available but is of unproved efficacy and not recommended.

Combined Viral Vaccines. Considerable success has been achieved in the efforts to combine two or more viruses into single vaccines. The advantages are obvious for commonly employed agents, viz., ease of administration, economy, and sparing the patient multiple visits and injections. There are some disadvantages: loss of flexibility of individual indication for the single components, inability to distinguish adverse effects from among the components, and potential combinational accumulation of adverse effects.

Available for use are the following combinations:

1. Polioviruses 1, 2, and 3.

2. Measles-Mumps-Rubella. This combination is designed as a primary immunizing agent for infants and children. It has the virtue of simultaneous early protection against all three diseases without sacrificing the efficacy of the individual components. It has the disadvantage of removing individual vaccines from selective use.

3. Measles-Rubella. This is designed for use among children in whom mumps virus immunization is not desired, or for children who have already experienced clinical mumps but not measles or rubella.

4. Rubella-Mumps. This is designed for use among children who have already had measles vaccine or the natural disease. It can conveniently be administered to preadolescents.

Other combinations have been experimentally evaluated, but convenient, tested formulations of proved efficacy are not available. The physician is cautioned about the following practices:

1. Making his own "combinations." Little or no data exist for simultaneous administration of individual viral vaccines. One cannot be guaranteed that such combinations will not result in interference or will not be associated with cumulative adverse consequences. Certainly individual vaccines should not be admixed in a single syringe.

2. Administration of viral vaccines in a sequence that does not allow a "safe" interval. It is recommended that viral vaccines, if administered singly, be given at least 30 days apart. This recommendation is made to avoid the potential problem of the first vaccine interfering with the second. Also, the cumulative effect of expected reactions following individual vaccines can be avoided. Intervals of 2 days to 2 weeks are particularly hazardous in these respects. Whenever possible, a full month should elapse between viral vaccines.

3. Administration of viral vaccines in conjunction with or shortly after human gamma globulin or blood transfusions. Passively administered antibody can interfere with active immunity. Except in cases specifically indicated (e.g., measles vaccine and gamma globulin, rabies vaccine, and

rabies immune globulin) no viral vaccine should be administered within one month of gamma globulin administration. In designing rapid immunization schedules for overseas travel, gamma globulin should be given last, after all viral vaccines have been administered, and after at least a 2-week interval from the last vaccine.

Rabies (See also p. 54)

Active Immunization. Two types of vaccines are available for use in rabies prophylaxis in humans: duck embryo grown virus and infected rabbit brain. Both are inactivated antigens.

Duck embryo vaccine (DEV) is more commonly used; it is standardized for adequate potency. It does not result in as high a titer as traditional brain tissue vaccines, but appears associated with less risk of neuroparalytic accidents. The virus is killed by exposure to β-propiolactone.

Rabbit brain vaccine (Semple) is prepared from brain tissue of infected rabbits. Rabies virus is inactivated by phenol. Some preparations are inactivated by ultraviolet light. More potent than DEV, Semple vaccines have the disadvantage of inducing a demyelinating disease in some recipients.

Both vaccines stimulate adequate amounts of neutralizing antibody, although extra doses of DEV may be required to achieve maximal effect. Both must be given in prolonged fashion, resulting in inconvenience and extended discomfort.

Effectiveness of these vaccines in human exposure is impossible to judge. There are too many variables determining actual risk, and the baseline of exposed persons is unknown. Both vaccines have failed, i.e., rabies has occurred in persons treated. Some have been true failures; prompt therapy was initiated and an appropriate course followed. Other failures were associated with delayed or inappropriate therapy.

Schedules for Immunization. Prophylaxis against rabies can be divided into three categories: candidates for treatment, management of the animal bite, and specific procedures in immunization.

CANDIDATES FOR PROPHYLAXIS. Not all humans bitten by animals should be treated for rabies exposure. The World Health Organization (WHO) has attempted to establish worldwide guidelines, which must be modified by both individual and local epidemiologic circumstances. Firm rules governing each bite cannot be stated unequivocally. Rather, certain generalizations and principles are the best guide in evaluating a specific instance. Some of these follow:

1. All wild animals that bite, except rodents, must be considered rabid. (However, skunks, bats, coyotes, bobcats or mountain lions, foxes, and raccoons are among the species at the highest risk of infection.) All wild animal bites must be treated on notification; do *not* await laboratory confirmation. If the laboratory results are positive, treatment is already started; if negative, treatment can be discontinued.

2. Treatment of persons bitten by domestic animals is best evaluated in the light of local epidemiologic knowledge. If cats have not been rabid in a particular locale and exposure to wild animals is minimal, then rabies prophylaxis is unnecessary for a cat bite. Conversely, if cats have been shown to be rabid locally or if there is ample exposure to wild animals or both, then a bite becomes suspect for rabies.

3. A fully immunized family pet that bites because it is provoked is seldom, if ever, rabid. Unless the animal is sick or has been exposed to animals which could be rabid, it usually is unnecessary to do other than observe the animal.

4. Vigorous efforts should be made to have laboratory examination of any animal suspected of being rabid. Disposal of the animal deprives the clinician and patient of a vital bit of information.

5. Penetration is usually necessary for virus to gain entry; a notable exception is saliva that contains rabies virus contaminating an open wound or skin lesion. If no penetration has occurred and the skin is intact, rabies prophylaxis is unnecessary.

6. Confinement and observation of biting animals is an important component in the decision-making process. Healthy domestic animals should be kept under professional observation for 10 days. If the animal becomes ill it should be killed (avoiding damage to the brain). The entire head should be shipped to an expert laboratory *after* consultation with that laboratory as to correct procedure in handling and shipping. Inadequate attention to these critical details can prevent acquisition of important information and can be hazardous to health.

Wild animals should not be confined if captured. They should be immediately killed and examined in a competent laboratory. All the precautions listed here should be observed.

7. Evidence of adequate rabies immunization in a biting animal almost always precludes rabies.

8. All possible information should be gathered promptly to assist the physician in selecting candidates for treatment. Delays can interfere with the maximal efficacy of immunization.

MANAGEMENT OF THE BITE (see p. 55).

SPECIFIC PROPHYLAXIS (BOTH ACTIVE AND PASSIVE). Local epidemiologic circumstances and individual case factors will modify WHO recommendations, given in Table 2. There are several possibilities when choosing vaccines and serums.

TABLE 2. **Recommendations for Rabies Prophylaxis***

ANIMAL	RABIES STATUS (CLINICAL JUDGMENT)	TREATMENT†	
		Bite	*Other Exposure‡*
Wild	Consider all wild animals, except rodents,§ as rabid	RIG** and Vaccine	RIG and Vaccine
Domestic	Healthy	None	None
	Escaped	RIG + Vaccine	(Vaccine)¶
	Rabid	RIG + Vaccine	RIG + Vaccine

*Modified from WHO recommendations
†Individualize all rabies prophylaxis therapy
‡Includes nonbite wounds (scratches, and others) and open skin lesions contaminated with saliva from animal. May also be extended to include heavy aerosol contamination
§No human rabies has ever been reported in bites of a rodent or lagomorph in the United States
**RIG, rabies immune globulin (human)
¶Controversial—authorities recommend initiation of DEV but individual factors may modify

1. Use of DEV or Semple vaccine for exposure. From 14 to 21 daily doses of DEV should be injected subcutaneously. Since multiple sites are required, both the thigh and the abdomen are usually selected for the injections. Local reactions are common, particularly after the fourth or fifth dose; both current and past sites may flare up simultaneously.

Although rare, anaphylaxis can occur, and epinephrine should be available in a syringe in the room where the patient is inoculated. The more usual local symptoms can be partially alleviated by administration of an antihistamine. Patients and parents should be informed of the expected local reactions. Their cooperation is essential in completing the prolonged course.

If rabies immune globulin (RIG) is indicated, vaccine dosage must be extended to 21 days and two booster doses given, one on the tenth day after completion of the series and the second 10 days later. The 21 doses can be given on 21 consecutive days or as double doses on the first 7 days (total of 14 doses) and single dose for the next 7 days.

In instances of proved exposure, consultation with the Center for Disease Control can result in assay of specific antibody. Such determinations can assist in modifying the immunization schedule to ensure adequate antibody stimulation.

When there are significant allergic reactions to one vaccine, the other may be substituted. If a neurologic complication develops, *all* vaccine administration must be suspended.

2. Use of human rabies immune globulin (RIG). A major advance in rabies prophylaxis was afforded in 1975 with the availability of RIG. This product avoids all the ill effects of horse serum and provides reliable human antibody, which persists for longer periods than that from the horse.

RIG is given intramuscularly both at the bite site (up to one half the total dose) and at the usual intramuscular injection sites. The recommended dose is 20 I.U. per kg. (0.133 ml. per kg.) of body weight.

3. Use of rabies antiserum (horse). Equine rabies antiserum should be totally replaced by human RIG. However, information concerning its use is provided here in the event RIG is not available. *Equine antiserum is not recommended for rabies prophylaxis as long as RIG is available.*

The dose is 40 I.U. per kg. Up to 50 per cent of the antiserum should be infiltrated around the bite; the rest is given intramuscularly. The patient must always be tested for horse serum sensitivity prior to administration. If the patient is sensitive, horse serum can still be administered utilizing a desensitizing schedule. Serum sickness may occur in 20 per cent of persons receiving horse serum, regardless of the history or results of testing.

SPECIAL CIRCUMSTANCES. Some occupations expose persons to possible rabies contact, e.g., veterinarians, animal handlers, and zoo keepers. Pre-exposure immunization is possible with duck embryo vaccine (DEV). Two 1.0 ml. injections of DEV are recommended. They are given subcutaneously in the area of the deltoid at an interval of 1 month. A third dose of 1.0 ml. is given 6 months later. Neutralizing antibody will develop in 80 to 90 per cent of recipients; serum titers can be assayed 3 to 4 weeks after completion of the series. Booster doses can be repeated until antibody is demonstrated.

Recall injections to maintain immunity are administered every 2 to 3 years and can be guided by serum titers.

On exposure to a rabid animal, five daily doses of DEV are administered, with a booster dose 20 days after the last one. Nonbite exposures are treated with a single booster of DEV. RIG should not be used in persons who have been preexposure immunized and exposed; it inhibits antibody responsiveness.

If rapid preexposure immunization is desired, three weekly injections of 1.0 ml. DEV are administered, with a booster 4 months later.

Adverse Effects of Immunization. Both duck embryo vaccine (DEV) and Semple vaccines give rise to painful or pruritic areas of induration and erythema or both at sites of injection. This usually begins after the fourth or fifth dose; each subsequent dose reacts, as do the sites of previous antigen inoculation.

Systemic symptoms, notably fever and malaise, occasionally occur. These are more common late in therapy, usually after the first week. Serum sickness has been noted, but whether it is related to vaccine or to the simultaneously administered horse serum is uncertain. Rarely, anaphylaxis has occurred; this possibility should be anticipated by the ready availability of epinephrine drawn into a syringe.

The most serious adverse effects are those related to neuroparalytic disease. The Semple vaccines are associated with a 1:6000 risk after a 14 day course; some studies have reported a 10-fold higher incidence. DEV is far safer in this regard; only 1:106,000 develop CNS sequelae.

RIG has no significant adverse effects if administered properly.

Horse serum (rabies antiserum) has the usual hazards associated with this product, ranging from serum sickness to anaphylaxis.

VACCINES USED UNDER SPECIAL CIRCUMSTANCES

Cholera

Cholera is caused by *Vibrio cholerae*. The effects of the disease are the direct result of the elaboration of a powerful exotoxin that leads to profuse and continuing water loss with accompanying electrolyte depletion. Cholera is endemic in India, Pakistan, Bangladesh, and southeast Asia and has spread both east and west from that focus.

Active Immunization. Cholera vaccine consists of 10 billion killed vibrios per ml. It is a weakly protective vaccine with variable estimates of its effectiveness. Although experimental trials with an oral vaccine are encouraging, none is available to date.

Two doses of vaccine are administered one month apart for children under the age of 5; 0.1 ml. is initially given followed by 0.3 ml. 30 days later. Within the next 6 months, a booster dose of 0.1 ml. is given. For children between the ages of 5 and 10, the initial dose is 0.3 ml. followed by a 0.5 ml. dose to complete the primary series and 0.3 ml. for booster. For children over 10, the corresponding doses are 0.5 ml., 1 ml., and 0.5 ml. Discomfort at the site of immunization with accompanying induration and stomach symptoms of malaise, fever, and headache may occur within the first 24 to 48 hours after immunization.

Plague

Yersinia pestis causes human plague, usually as a result of contact with rodents, fleas, or, in the case of pneumonic plague, human contact. Although plague occurs throughout the world, an endemic focus in the western states, principally in Arizona, New Mexico, and Colorado, is of concern to pediatricians in this country.

Active Immunization. Plague vaccine consists of either heat or formalin inactivated organisms grown in laboratory media and preserved with phenol. Plague immunity is an enigma, but the vaccine appears to protect against the disease. It is recommended only for those at high risk, including field workers with high contact and laboratory workers dealing with the organism.

Three intramuscular doses of vaccine are given; the first two, 30 days apart and the third, 1 to 3 months later. Booster doses can be given every 6 to 12 months. Children less than 1 year of age should receive 0.1 ml. for the first two doses and then 0.4 ml. for subsequent boosters. For children between the ages of 1 and 4, 0.2 ml. with 0.08 ml. boosters are used, and for children between the ages of 5 and 10, 0.3 ml. with 0.12 ml. boosters. Children over 10 and adults should receive 0.5 ml. thirty days apart with 0.3 ml. as subsequent boosters.

Plague vaccine results in frequent local reactions and, with multiple doses, in systemic reactions. Local induration with tenderness and erythema are noted. Fever, headache, and malaise are common systemic reactions and may increase in severity with repeated doses.

Typhoid Vaccine

Salmonella typhi (Group D) is the cause of typhoid fever. In children in the United States the greatest risks of contracting this disease are in the following circumstances:

1. During exposure to the disease or to a carrier of *S. typhi*.
2. During outbreaks of typhoid fever, and during travel to primitive areas where typhoid fever is endemic.

Most experts advise immunization for persons in these circumstances. However, it is important to understand that local disasters such as floods and earthquakes do not qualify as indications for immunization, nor does travel confined wholly within the United States.

Active Immunity. Current typhoid vaccines are protective. Unfortunately, the history of typhoid immunization is such that the high reaction rate and the low effectiveness of previously formulated vaccines have led many to believe that this product is not useful. Current vaccines usually are acetone inactivated and consist of suspensions of organisms containing all the appropriate antigens.

Active Immunization. Immunity to *Salmonella typhi* is a relative phenomenon, although the vaccine appears to confer protection against relatively low-dose exposure. Persons can acquire the disease from ingestion of large numbers of organisms. Thus it appears the immunized person is protected against typhoid fever in such circumstances as moderately contaminated water ingestion but would not be expected to withstand the challenge of teeming organisms in an undercooked or badly stored poultry dish. Protection against low to moderate bacillary exposure should result in 70 to 90 per cent protection against disease.

Children should receive two doses of 0.25 ml. each, administered subcutaneously at least 4 weeks apart. *Although some recommendations include intradermal inoculation with 0.10 ml., it is important to underscore that this route cannot be used with acetone-killed vaccine.* For children older than 10 years of age, the doses increase to 0.5 ml. administered subcutaneously at least 4 weeks apart. Recall immunization is accomplished with the same dose that was used for primary immunization at approximately 3 year intervals if exposure continues. Rarely, time does not permit the 4 week interval between doses. In this case, a single dose is given at weekly intervals, and may protect the individual. A booster dose should be given 4 or more weeks later.

Typhoid vaccine produces a large number of reactions. Local induration with pain and regional adenopathy accompanied by fever are common.

Influenza Vaccine

The influenza viruses are classified according to their antigenic structure into types A, B, and C. Type C infrequently produces upper respiratory tract infections such as croup in small numbers of children in localized epidemics. Type B is present periodically in any given community in the form of epidemic influenzal infection, but never reaches the proportion that Type A does. Type B influenza has been observed to be followed in certain situations with Reye's syndrome. The major cause of disease in children is the epidemic Type A infection. Usually occurring yearly in a given location, Type A infections will vary in the extent of epidemicity from year to year. At varying intervals of a decade or more, they will undergo enough antigenic change so that a larger epidemic, involving whole countries or even the entire world (pandemic), will occur. During these periods of high epidemicity or during a pandemic, morbidity and mortality from the disease in children is excessive. It appears that persons with chronic respiratory, cardiovascular, and neurologic disease are particularly vulnerable.

Except during epidemics, the previously available vaccines were sufficiently toxic that they have never been recommended for general use in children. These vaccines were prepared from inactivated whole virus particles and their use was associated with an unacceptable local and systemic reaction rate. In 1976 a new antigenic variant of Type A appeared. This virus resulted in a restricted epidemic in Fort Dix, New Jersey, among military recruits. As this virus shared many characteristics with the virus that produced the 1918 pandemic, a full scale effort was launched by public health authorities to encourage the manufacture, testing, and deployment of swine influenza vaccine for as much of the population as could be reached. Sequential testing of two types of product, the usual whole virus vaccine and a vaccine prepared by treatment of a virus particle, which resulted in disruption and isolation of fragments of the virus (so-called split product vaccine), indicated that adults could produce antibody in response to it with a minimum of side-effects. However, children still experienced unacceptable reactivity to whole virus vaccine. This resulted in a recommendation that only the split product type vaccine be employed in children. The entire effort at immunization against swine influenza was hampered by a variety of problems ranging from the ethical and social to the biologic. The effort finally ended with the occurrence of Guillain-Barré syndrome among vaccine recipients at a rate some nine times that occurring in the unimmunized. As a result of this experience, plus the fact that swine influenza was not identified anywhere else in the world following the Fort Dix epidemic, all efforts to immunize against swine influenza for the 1977–1978 epidemic year were abandoned.

Since influenza virus undergoes subtle antigenic change over time, vaccines employed in any given year are so manufactured to include the anticipated prevalent antigens. As of this writing, it is anticipated that A-Victoria and its variants will be the Type A antigens to be included in influenza vaccines. The exact composition for any given year is predicated on then current epidemiologic information about the prevalent virus. As a result, in future years the physician can look to the United States Public Health Service and to the various recommending groups for advice concerning which vaccine should be employed in the patient population.

Active Immunization.   Given all the complex factors involved in influenza epidemiology, the current recommendation is to immunize only those children deemed at high risk from influenza infection. Almost all experts agree that children with chronic respiratory and cardiovascular disease are candidates for immunization. There is less agreement on other groups. Some experts recommend that children with asthma, neurologic disorder, and certain metabolic diseases such as diabetes also be included. In addition, children with malignancies or those receiving immunosuppressive therapy or congenitally immunodeficient are also thought by some to require protection. As there is great variability in expert recommendations, the physician is advised to consult the current recommendations of the American Academy of Pediatrics Committee on Infectious Diseases (the Redbook Committee).

The exact product to be used in any given year and its mode of administration has similarly undergone changes in recent years. Currently, the thinking is that only split product vaccines should be used for young children, and should probably be administered in split doses. The physician is advised to follow current recommendations extant at the time influenza vaccine is to be employed. Public health agencies and the American Academy of Pediatrics will announce recommendations for any given year based on the epidemiology of influenza that year and the specific products available and useful.

Pneumococcal Polysaccharide

The clinical problem in children: pneumococci are among the most frequent infectious agents producing significant clinical illness in children. Although there are more than 80 types, only a few account for more than 80 per cent of infections. For most children infection with pneumococci is an event for which there is no predictability; i.e., we do not know much about specific individual susceptibility in otherwise normal children. For a few children, a disease or condition exists that is associated with an increased risk of serious, even life-threatening, disease. Examples include functional or anatomic asplenia (such as is seen in congenital absence of the spleen, in surgical removal of the spleen in a variety of settings, in sicklemia [infarction of the spleen with so-called autosplenectomy]) in nephrotic syndromes, in B cell immune deficiency states, in anatomic connections between the meninges and the nasopharynx, and so on.

Clinical infections range from subtle dermatitis through otitis media and pneumonia to bacteremia and meningitis. Ordinarily, recognition is easy and therapy efficacious with penicillin, or an appropriate substitute in the host who is hypersensitive to penicillin. An exception is bacterial meningitis, which is among the more lethal and devastating infections, probably because of the extensive damage done prior to the diagnosis and institution of penicillin therapy.

In recent years, both penicillin resistance and decreased susceptibility of certain pneumococci have been described. Multi-drug resistant strains have been noted in adults in Africa. These findings give more emphasis to an immunologic approach to control of pneumococcal infections.

Active Immunization. Pneumococcal vaccine, polyvalent (Pneumovax) is composed of 50 micrograms of each of 14 types of pneumococcal capsular polysaccharide. It is administered as a single dose of 0.5 ml. intramuscularly or subcutaneously. The polysaccharide is suspended in isotonic saline solution and contains 0.25 per cent phenol as preservative. The types of pneumococci included are 1,2,3,4,6,8,9,12,14,19,23,25,51, and 56.

Adverse Effects of Immunization. At least 90 per cent of *adults* had a four times or greater antibody increase to each of the 14 specific polysaccharide types in the licensed vaccine. Nearly 86 per cent of adults and all children in one series experienced reactions at the site of administration consisting of erythema, tenderness, and induration in varying combinations.

Mild fever was recorded in about 40 per cent of 42 children, one of whom had a moderate reaction. There were no permanent sequelae, and reactions were usually short-lived, lasting at most for 4 to 5 days.

Part of the difficulty in assessing efficacy and side-effects lies in the many variations of vaccines tested other than the one licensed. For example, the only comprehensive study in children in reference to efficacy utilized an octovalent vaccine, not the 14-valent one licensed.

Efficacy, as judged by antibody production in children less than 2 years of age, is not present with this product. This result is similar to that observed with other polysaccharide antigens (*H. influenzae* and meningococcus A & C).

Vaccine efficacy in adults has been most satisfactory in terms of preventing pneumococcal disease. Up to 92 per cent reduction of type-specific pneumococcal infections has been observed in adults in various trials.

The only published efficacy trial in children indicated significant protection against serious pneumococcal disease in patients with sicklemia older than 2 years.

CURRENT RECOMMENDATIONS. Pending specific trials in children with the 14-valent available vaccine, it seems prudent to make the following recommendations:

1. Children under 2 years of age should not receive the vaccine.

2. Asplenic children, functional or anatomic, should be given a single 0.5 ml. dose, preferably before the asplenic state is achieved but at any time if this is not possible.

3. Consideration should be given to administration of the vaccine to children with the nephrotic syndrome.

4. All other children should not receive the vaccine until further data justify a specific recommendation.

Meningococcal Vaccines

Meningococcal disease in infants and children affects a smaller number than either the pneumococcus or *Hemophilus influenzae*. Approximately 3000 to 6000 cases a year occur in all age groups and epidemics are noted approximately every 10 years.

Seragroups B and C produce the majority of disease in the continental United States. Group B is the predominant strain and, for the most part, is sulfonamide-sensitive. In addition, instances of seragroups other than A, B, and C have occurred.

The Vaccine.   There are two polysaccharide vaccines available, for types A and C. They are specific to the type and do not provide any cross-protection.

Vaccine Efficacy.   These vaccines are highly antigenic for persons older than 2 years of age. Like the other polysaccharide vaccines they fail to stimulate significant antibody in young infants. Both A and C appear to be highly effective in reducing the corresponding meningococcal disease rate, especially in epidemic situations.

Side-effects are minimal and infrequent. Localized erythema and tenderness lasting 1 to 2 days is observed in a few vaccinees.

Long-term immunity is not yet established, as these products have been employed for too short a period to permit judgment.

CURRENT RECOMMENDATIONS.   Routine immunization is *not* recommended.

Selective uses include:

1. Travelers to epidemic areas.

2. Possible use in household contacts in conjunction with antimicrobial prophylaxis. This will work only if there is a sufficient lapse between exposure and presumed onset of disease, allowing the vaccine to stimulate antibody.

3. Population at risk in epidemic situations. Public Health authorities should notify practitioners of the existence of an epidemic, and residents in the area should be immunized. Consultation with the Center for Disease Control and Bureau of Biologics is mandatory.

The vaccine should not be given to children less than 2 years of age.

The Respiratory System

ACUTE RESPIRATORY FAILURE

method of
BARRY MAKE, M.D.,
and JEROME S. BRODY, M.D.
Boston, Massachusetts

Human tissues use oxygen as a soure of fuel and produce carbon dioxide as a byproduct of cellular metabolism. The lungs play an integral role in the regulation of oxygen and carbon dioxide by providing a gas-exchanging surface across which oxygen from the ambient environment enters the oxygen-deficient venous blood from the body's tissues and excessive carbon dioxide is eliminated.

"Respiratory failure" is the term applied to the result of a number of pathologic entities in which there is a failure of the respiratory system to maintain an adequate level of oxygen or a normal level of carbon dioxide in the arterial blood. More specifically, respiratory failure can be defined by certain arterial blood levels of oxygen and carbon dioxide, i.e., a partial pressure of oxygen in the arterial blood (Pao_2) of less than 50 mm. Hg or a partial pressure of carbon dioxide in the arterial blood ($Paco_2$) of over 50 mm. Hg. Although the choice of these values of Pao_2 and $Paco_2$ for defining respiratory failure is somewhat arbitrary, these levels of arterial blood gases indicate the presence of a severe degree of dysfunction of the respiratory system that may have profound clinical effects on other body systems. It should be noted that a Pao_2 of 50 mm. Hg is associated with an O_2 saturation of approximately 85 per cent, assuming a normal oxygen-hemoglobin dissociation curve. Below this Pao_2, the shape of the oxyhemoglobin dissociation curve is not curvilinear, but rather it demonstrates a sharp downward slope such that, with small changes of Pao_2, arterial desaturation develops and the oxygen content falls dramatically. The prefixes "acute" and "chronic" are appended to the term respiratory failure and indicate not only the time period over which the clinical process has developed but also the presence of physiologic compensation, which serves to modify the acute effects of the disease.

When respiratory failure develops over a very short period of time (minutes to days) the term "acute" is used. In acute respiratory failure there is insufficient time for compensatory mechanisms to develop, and such patients thus develop signs and symptoms attributable to their lung disease. The term "chronic" implies that the hypoxemia or hypercapnia has been present for a longer period (from months to years). In chronic respiratory failure there are fewer symptoms because the body has been given time to adjust slowly to the presence of altered levels of carbon dioxide or oxygen. Both acute and chronic respiratory failure can be present at the same time, as when a pneumonia rapidly develops in a previously well-compensated patient with chronic respiratory failure. In such a situation, the patient can not acutely compensate for the additional respiratory insult and develops acute respiratory failure associated with clinical deterioration.

A Pao_2 that acutely falls below 50 mm. Hg may fail to provide adequate oxygen for cellular metabolism, resulting in marked tissue dysfunction with the subsequent production of lactic acidosis and clinical signs of hypoxia. A Pao_2 that falls below 50 mm. Hg insidiously will lead to compensatory polycythemia, increased cardiac output, and a shift of the oxyhemoglobin dissociation curve; all of these compensatory mechanisms increase tissue oxygen delivery. Thus, a Pao_2 of 50 mm. Hg in chronic respiratory failure may not cause any symptoms. A $Paco_2$ that acutely rises above 50 mm. Hg is associated with a pH below 7.3; this subsequent acidosis may impair tissue function, with resultant signs and symptoms. Levels of $Paco_2$ above 50 mm. Hg that develop chronically lead to bicarbonate retention by the kidneys, which buffers the respiratory acidosis. Therefore, chronic hypercapnia in chronic respiratory failure is not associated with acidosis and thus manifests few, if any, clinical symptoms.

Treatment

The treatment of acute respiratory failure depends on the major cause of the respiratory derangement. Therefore, the first step in approaching such a patient is to determine the type of respiratory failure that is present. There are three distinct pathophysiologic types of respiratory failure, each associated with specific patterns of arterial blood gas abnormalities and different clinical pictures. If a pathophysiologic diagnosis of the cause of acute respiratory failure can be made, then a specific etiologic diagnosis is not always necessary in order to initiate treatment.

The three major pathophysiologic types of respiratory failure are: (1) ventilation failure with normal lungs, (2) ventilation failure with abnormal lungs, and (3) oxygenation failure. Ventilation failure with normal lungs occurs in patients who have no intrinsic pulmonary pathology but who can not maintain adequate movement of air into and out of the lungs. This hypoventilation results in an increase in $Paco_2$ and a proportional decrease in Pao_2.* Ventilation failure with abnormal lungs occurs in either patients with prior intrinsic lung disease or those who have an acute pulmonary process that also prevents adequate maintenance of gas exchange at the alveolar level. In such subjects, the $Paco_2$ is elevated and the Pao_2 is reduced out of proportion to the change in $Paco_2$. Oxygenation failure suggests the presence of pulmonary pathology that interferes predominantly with oxygen transfer, thus producing a low Pao_2 but decreased or normal levels of $Paco_2$ until late in the disease.

The signs and symptoms of respiratory failure are nonspecific and are related in part to the presence or absence of compensatory mechanisms. Thus, since clinical evaluation may be misleading, measurement of arterial blood gases is the only way to make a definitive diagnosis of acute respiratory failure. The importance of this as an aid to the diagnosis of respiratory failure can not be overemphasized. Before the results of arterial blood gases can be interpreted, the physiologic basis of a normal Pao_2 and $Paco_2$ must be understood.

The determinants of the $Paco_2$ are the amount of CO_2 produced by the tissues and the amount excreted from the body. When more CO_2 is produced by the tissues, more CO_2 enters the blood. The only clinically important route of excretion of CO_2 from the body is through the lungs and the amount of CO_2 excreted through the lungs is proportional to the alveolar ventilation (i.e., the amount of ventilation which is able to exchange gas with pulmonary capillary blood). Thus, $Paco_2$ is directly proportional to CO_2 production and indirectly proportional to alveolar ventilation. Since carbon dioxide production is reasonably constant in a person at rest, the only cause of an increased $Paco_2$ is a reduction in effective alveolar ventilation.

The level of oxygen in arterial blood is determined by several distinct physiologic factors. First, sufficient quantities of oxygen must be present in alveolar gas. When the inspired concentration of oxygen is reduced, less oxygen reaches the capillaries. Such situations are uncommon in clinical medicine and occur only at high altitudes. Second, the oxygen must reach the gas exchanging surface. If total ventilation is decreased, the amount of oxygen reaching the air-blood interface will be reduced and the Pao_2 will decrease. As noted, decreased ventilation also causes an increased $Paco_2$. Third, unoxygenated blood must reach the pulmonary gas-exchanging surface. If intra- or extrapulmonary anatomic shunts are present, some unoxygenated blood may not reach the pulmonary capillaries and that portion bypassing the lungs will remain unoxygenated. Fourth, the amount of ventilation must be closely matched to the amount of perfusion in each alveolus to achieve the most efficient oxygen exchange between the alveoli and the pulmonary capillaries. Alterations in the relative amounts of ventilation and perfusion are the most common causes of arterial hypoxemia. Because of the different shapes of the oxygen-hemoglobin (sigmoid) and carbon dioxide–hemoglobin (relatively linear) dissociation curves, uninvolved portions of lung can compensate by hyperventilation for low ventilation-perfusion areas of lung in terms of CO_2 but can not add more O_2 to their already oxygen-saturated blood. Thus, ventilation-perfusion imbalance leads to decreased Pao_2 with normal $Paco_2$. Fifth, the oxygen must be able to diffuse through the alveolar wall into the pulmonary capillaries. Reduction in the ability of the lungs to allow diffusion of oxygen does not affect carbon dioxide exchange because CO_2 is much more soluble in the interstitial fluids and more readily diffusible than oxygen.

VENTILATION FAILURE WITH NORMAL LUNGS

In order to achieve adequate gas exchange, the function of several different organs of the human body must be integrated in a coordinated fashion to act as a single unit. Thus, the *respiratory system* includes not only the lungs but also the central and peripheral nervous systems, respiratory muscles, bony chest wall, and upper respiratory tract.

The respiratory center in the *brain* must initiate an impulse to trigger inspiration and expiration. This impulse must be sent through the central nervous system to the *spinal cord* and then to the respiratory muscles by way of the cervical efferents. The *peripheral nervous system* and ganglionic connections must be intact to deliver the impulses to the *respiratory muscles* of the chest wall, diaphragm, and abdomen. The *bony chest wall* must be intact to allow the respiratory muscles to exert sufficient pull to achieve adequate inspired volume.

---

*The "alveolar-air equation" $(P_AO_2 = P_IO_2 - Paco_2/R$, where the respiratory quotient $R = CO_2$ produced/O_2 consumed is normally 0.8) implies that the Pao_2 will decrease 1.25 mm. Hg for each 1 mm. Hg increase in $Paco_2$ if there is no defect in gas exchange.

Once the signals are properly integrated and inspiration is initiated, the *upper air passages* must be patent to allow free movement of air into the *trachea* and *bronchi,* and finally to the *alveoli* where gas exchange actually occurs. A failure of any of the individual components of the respiratory system can lead to insufficient ventilation. Respiratory failure in this setting due to disease outside the lung is called ventilation failure with normal lungs.

The cause of this type of respiratory failure usually lies outside the lung parenchyma. In such patients, the lung parenchyma is normal and oxygen exchange is preserved. The decrease in total alveolar ventilation results in an elevated $Paco_2$ with a proportional decrease in Pao_2. Examples of specific causes of ventilation failure with normal lungs include:

1. Central nervous system (CNS) disorders: sedative overdose, narcotic overdose, CNS trauma and cerebrovascular disease.

2. Peripheral nervous system dysfunction: spinal cord transsection, Guillain-Barré syndrome, tetanus, and myasthenia gravis.

3. Chest wall disorders: multiple rib fractures with flail chest.

4. Muscles of respiration: polymyositis.

5. Upper respiratory tract disease: acute epiglottitis of children, anaphylactic reaction with laryngeal edema, aspiration of foreign body, and laryngeal edema secondary to prolonged intubation or surgical procedures.

In ventilation failure with normal lungs, the goal of therapy is to support ventilatory function until the specific cause of the respiratory failure can be determined and treated. Early intervention with supportive therapy helps prevent the pulmonary complications (atelectasis and pneumonia) of this form of respiratory failure.

Immediate Lifesaving Treatment

When ventilatory failure occurs suddenly, such as following trauma to the spinal cord, immediate cardiorespiratory resuscitative efforts may be required before the patient can be transported to a hospital. These measures should be performed in the following sequence:

1. Perform a rapid clinical assessment of the patient. The most important aspect of this brief initial examination is to determine whether the patient is breathing. At the same time the pulse should be palpated to ascertain the presence of a reasonable cardiac output.

2. If the patient is not breathing, the respiratory rate appears to be very slow, or the respirations appear to be shallow and inadequate to sustain life, then emergency treatment is indicated.

3. Establish an airway. In acute situations this can be done most rapidly by hyperextending the patient's neck to allow a direct passage from the oropharynx to the trachea. Airway patency should be further assured by pulling the tongue forward, searching the mouth quickly, and removing any foreign material which might obstruct the free flow of air. Use of a mechanical oropharyngeal tube may aid in keeping the tongue forward. In the case of a foreign body obstructing the upper airway, use of the Heimlich maneuver (rapid epigastric compression) may dislodge the obstructing lesion. When the upper airway can not be cleared, performance of emergency tracheostomy may be lifesaving. In ventilatory failure without upper airway lesions in a hospital where there is a physician skilled in the performance of endotracheal intubation, passage of an endotracheal tube will establish a more permanent airway. Establishment of an airway with an endotracheal tube is a reasonable goal of therapy only after other emergency procedures to reestablish breathing and circulation have begun and the patient is stabilized.

4. Assure adequate ventilation. Once an airway is established, ventilation of the lungs must be assured. Outside the hospital setting, mouth-to-mouth resuscitation can achieve satisfactory ventilation. In the hospital, manual compression of a hand resuscitator (such as an "Ambu"-type bag) can force air into the patient's lungs and achieve effective ventilation. A rate of approximately 14 breaths per minute should be satisfactory if each breath results in observable expansion of the chest wall.

5. Establish adequate cardiac function. If the pulse is absent or blood pressure is unobtainable, appropriate cardiac resuscitative measures should be instituted.

6. Consider oxygen administration. If there is no indication that the patient has chronic obstructive pulmonary disease (COPD), such as emphysema or chronic bronchitis, then it is reasonable to administer high concentrations of oxygen until the results of the initial blood gases are obtained. In patients with COPD with ventilation failure, administration of O_2 may further depress the respiratory system (discussed below), but oxygen does not cause significant respiratory depression in patients who have ventilation failure with normal lungs. However, Pao_2 over 80 mm. Hg results in nearly full saturation of hemoglobin with oxygen. Use of excessive concentrations of inspired O_2 is therefore unnecessary and may lead to oxygen toxicity.

7. Measure the effectiveness of ventilation. The most accurate and rapid method of measuring the ventilation reaching the alveoli is by determining the $Paco_2$. A $Paco_2$ below 36 mm. Hg indicates overventilation, and a $Paco_2$ over 44 mm. Hg indicates underventilation. Therefore, an arterial blood gas measurement should be performed once the acute situation has been stabilized.

8. Perform clinical assessment. If the patient appears stable or when adequate spontaneous respirations and cardiac function are established, further clinical evaluation can be performed. A physical examination should be performed to search for clues to the specific causes of ventilation failure, and such causes should be treated. For example, needle tracks over the arms should suggest a possible intravenous narcotic overdose and a narcotic antagonist should be administered.

Intubation

Patients with ventilation failure and normal lungs who are awake with a good cough and gag reflex do not usually require endotracheal intubation. However, endotracheal intubation is often useful early in the course of the disease in such patients to prevent complications and to (1) provide access to the lower respiratory tract when mechanical ventilation is required; (2) protect the lower respiratory tract from secretions from the mouth and vomitus from the stomach, particularly when patients have an altered level of consciousness with absent cough, poor gag reflex or active vomiting; (3) allow removal of excessive pulmonary secretions by suction catheters when patients are unable to cough up these secretions spontaneously; and (4) provide intermittent deep breaths via a hand resuscitator to prevent atelectasis and hypoxemia.

Specifically, endotracheal intubation is required in patients with ventilation failure and normal lungs in the presence of coma; altered level of consciousness, especially if the patient is vomiting; significant hypoventilation; hypoxia, i.e., a Pao_2 so low that symptoms result (hypotension, cardiac ischemia, cardiac irritability or arrhythmias, oliguria, altered mental status, seizures, or cool, pale extremities); hypoxemia due to atelectasis related to inability to sigh and take deep breaths (atelectasis may involve relatively small numbers of alveoli and not be associated with radiographic abnormalities but nevertheless cause significant physiologic complications related to altered ventilation/perfusion ratios); excessive airway secretions which can not be spontaneously cleared, particularly when they lead to atelectasis, hypoxemia disproportionate to the hypercapnia, or infection.

If there is a question concerning the necessity of an endotracheal tube, it is safer to insert a tube when it is unnecessary and thus assure protection of the lower respiratory tract and a patent upper airway than to not place a tube when it is really necessary and allow the patient to suffer the possible consequences of respiratory acidosis and aspiration pneumonitis. Therefore, we suggest error on the side of conservatism when considering endotracheal tube placement in order to protect the patient. It must be remembered, however, that intubation is not without hazards. Endotracheal tubes bypass the normal upper respiratory tract defense mechanisms that protect the lungs from injury and environmental exposure. Patients with endotracheal tubes can not cough and normally clear their airways of secretions.

Mechanical Ventilation

It is difficult to specify every condition that may be an indication for ventilatory support in patients with respiratory failure. The physician must rely on a combination of objective findings and subjective feelings and impressions. The art of knowing when to initiate ventilatory support requires an understanding of the pathophysiologic mechanisms and the natural history of the underlying disease process. The goal of mechanical ventilation is to prevent complications of severe ventilatory failure and to allow time to reverse the basic underlying disease that led to the respiratory failure. Not all patients who are intubated require mechanical ventilatory support. Nevetheless, the following are indications for ventilatory support in patients with ventilation failure and normal lungs:

APNEA. Patients without spontaneous respirations obviously need ventilatory support.

INADEQUATE ALVEOLAR VENTILATION. Since the $Paco_2$ is the best indicator of alveolar ventilation, the measurement of blood gases can provide the best indication of the severity of ventilatory failure. In previously healthy patients without metabolic alkalosis, a $Paco_2$ above 45 is a poor prognostic sign and an indication for mechanical ventilation.

POOR PULMONARY MECHANICS. Patients who have a respiratory rate greater than 35, small tidal volumes below 5 ml. per kg., vital capacity less than 15 ml. per kg., or who are unable to generate an inspiratory force of more than 25 cm. H_2O are prone to develop inadequate alveolar ventilation and hypercapnia. Therefore, in this group of patients respiratory support might be accomplished at an early stage before gross elevation in $Paco_2$ to prevent complications of severe respiratory failure.

LOW Pao_2. Since these patients have normal lungs, their arterial oxygen values will be decreased only in proportion to the elevation in $Paco_2$. However, in patients who develop atelectasis, infections, or retained secretions due to inadequate sigh or cough, the Pao_2 may decrease significantly. In patients with these complications mechanical ventilation may be required.

Ventilator Care. When patients with ventilation failure and normal lungs require mechanical ventilation, certain guidelines for ventilator care should be followed.

1. Provide adequate ventilation. A tidal volume in the range of 10 to 15 ml. per kg. should be prescribed at a rate of 10 to 12 breaths per minute as initial ventilator orders. In this form of respiratory failure the $Paco_2$ should be maintained at about 40 mm. Hg. If the $Paco_2$ is below 35 mm. Hg (indicating hyperventilation), then the respiratory rate or tidal volume should be lowered. If there is hypoventilation with a $Paco_2$ above 45 mm. Hg, then the respiratory rate or tidal volume should be increased. We suggest changing only one ventilator setting at a time. It should be noted that tidal volumes below 10 ml. per kg. without periodic deep breaths may lead to progressive atelectasis with impaired oxygen exchange. Therefore, larger tidal volumes are recommended to prevent these complications. The adequacy of alveolar ventilation must be assessed whenever a patient is placed on mechanical ventilation, and reassessed after each change in the ventilator parameters by measurement of arterial blood gases and clinical evaluation.

2. Maintain normal pH. Once adequate alveolar ventilation has been achieved and the $Paco_2$ is normal, the pH should be in the normal range of 7.38 to 7.43. If metabolic alkalosis or acidosis is present, maintaining a relatively normal pH should be the primary therapeutic goal, rather than achieving a normal $Paco_2$. Rapid changes in $Paco_2$ may not be acutely reflected in the cerebrospinal fluid (CSF), thus causing a discrepancy between the blood and cerebrospinal fluid pH, leading to profound complications such as seizures. Thus, if a severe metabolic derangement is present, the $Paco_2$ should be modified slowly to prevent complications due to rapid pH changes. Until the underlying metabolic problem can be adequately corrected, respiratory compensation via the mechanical ventilator may be necessary to prevent severe acidemia or alkalemia. For example, a patient with diabetic ketoacidosis who also requires mechanical ventilation for ventilation failure may have an acidotic pH once normal alveolar ventilation and $Paco_2$ are reestablished. To compensate temporarily for the metabolic acidosis until specific therapy for the diabetes is effective, it may be necessary to temporarily hyperventilate the patient to achieve a $Paco_2$ below 40 mm. Hg and partially correct the acidemia. In such patients, the goal of therapy is to compensate partially for the metabolic problem by adjusting the level of alveolar ventilation.

3. Consider supplemental oxygen administration. Supplemental oxygen may be necessary if complications such as atelectasis occur. The patient's Pao_2 should be kept within a range which is normal for that patient's age and pulmonary status. This usually means a Pao_2 between 80 and 90 mm. Hg.

Prevention of Complications. Adherence to the following guidelines can minimize complications related to endotracheal tubes.

1. Humidify the inspired air. One function of the upper respiratory tract is to humidify the ambient air before it reaches the alveoli. Nonhumidified air can dry the lower respiratory tract and impair its normal mucociliary function.

2. Warm the inspired air. The upper respiratory tract normally warms the inspired air to body temperature. Superheated inspired air may cause respiratory tract burns, while underheated air may cause a significant loss of body heat through the lungs.

3. Provide periodic deep breaths. Some ventilators are capable of providing intermittent deep breaths to replace the normal sighs of nonintubated subjects and thus prevent atelectasis. With the use of the larger tidal volumes mentioned, periodic sighs with the ventilator may not be necessary. When tidal volumes below 10 ml. per kg. are used, periodic deep breathing must be performed several times an hour with larger volumes in the range of 15 ml. per kg. Sighs can also be administered by nursing personnel when patients are taken off the ventilator and suctioned to remove secretions from the airways. Sighs delivered in this manner with a manually compressed Ambu bag are an effective means of providing deep breaths.

4. Remove secretions. Since patients with endotracheal tubes can not cough effectively, the airways must be kept free of secretions by intermittently passing a catheter into the trachea through the endotracheal tube and applying suction to remove the excess tracheobronchial secretions. Care must also be taken to change the patient's position frequently throughout the day so that one area of the lungs is not constantly in a dependent position, causing secretions to pool in dependent lung segments. If there is difficulty mobilizing secretions and the medical condition permits, the patient can be intermittently positioned with the head lower than the thorax to facilitate drainage of secretions to more central airways where they can be removed with a suction catheter. In addition, chest percussion and vibration are often helpful in mobilizing secretions. If bronchospasm is present, bronchodilator drugs may be a useful adjunct to mobilize secretions.

5. Prevent complications related to the endotracheal tube. Because of the possible complications of laryngeal and tracheal damage with sub-

sequent tracheal stenosis from endotracheal tubes (ET), proper nursing care is most important. The pressure in the balloon cuff of the ET must not be excessive; only the minimal amount of air necessary to occlude the trachea and prevent air from leaking from the lungs and secretions from leaking into the lungs should be placed in the cuff. Only endotracheal tubes with soft, "low-pressure," high-compliance balloon cuffs should be used for prolonged intubation.

Unnecessary movement of the endotracheal tube that may irritate the trachea should be avoided. To prevent excessive movement, the endotracheal tube should be securely fixed in place with tape around the patient's head or neck. Nasotracheal tubes provide somewhat more support and less movement than orotracheal tubes, but may cause nasal irritation and sinusitis and may not be as large in internal diameter. As patients with endotracheal tubes may have difficulty coughing effectively, secretions must be removed from the lower respiratory tract by suctioning. The presence of worsening hypoxemia, increased respiratory difficulty, or increasing airway pressure with mechanical ventilators suggests the need for immediate suctioning. However, suctioning should be performed prophylactically to prevent such complications, using the following technique:

1. Remove the patient from the mechanical ventilator and connect a hand resuscitator to the endotracheal tube.

2. Provide deep breaths with the hand resuscitator connected to an oxygen source with sufficient oxygen concentration to prevent hypoxemia (in most patients without chronic obstructive pulmonary disease, 100 per cent oxygen is recommended).

3. Insert the suction catheter through the endotracheal tube and apply intermittent suction while withdrawing the catheter in a circular motion. Limit tracheal suction time to less than 15 seconds to prevent prolonged apneic periods.

4. Repeat the procedure for deep breathing with a hand resuscitator.

5. Place the patient back on the mechanical ventilator.

The cuff on the endotracheal tube should be intermittently deflated to remove pooled hypopharyngeal secretions, which can cause a local irritation at the cuff site or be aspirated into the lungs. Cuffs are usually deflated at least every 3 hours as follows:

1. Place the suction catheter in the hypopharynx either through the mouth or nose and apply constant suction.

2. Remove the patient from the mechanical ventilator and connect a hand resuscitator to the endotracheal tube.

3. Slowly deflate the cuff during inspiration while the patient is being ventilated with a hand resuscitator. Once the cuff is fully deflated begin reinflating the cuff slowly with only the minimal amount of air necessary to occlude the trachea.

4. Place the patient back on the ventilator.

5. Suction the patient's mouth of any residual secretions.

6. The patient's lower respiratory tract must then be suctioned as outlined above.

Careful adherence to these guidelines will effectively remove secretions, provide deep breaths, assure adequate oxygenation during the suctioning procedure, and prevent aspiration of mouth contents and secretions from above the endotracheal tube cuff.

As this discussion implies, all patients with respiratory failure require skilled, intensive nursing care in addition to careful management by the physician. It is therefore imperative that appropriate nursing care and observation be available around the clock. An intensive care unit or respiratory care unit provides the optimal hospital setting for such patients.

Discontinuing Mechanical Ventilation. If mechanical ventilation is to be discontinued, the patient must have sufficient respiratory function to allow adequate alveolar ventilation without mechanical assistance. Patients must also be rested, have adequate nutritional status, and have improvement or reversal of the precipitating factors for the respiratory failure. Specific measurements of respiratory mechanics have been shown to correlate with ability to discontinue mechanical ventilation. Such measurements do not provide an absolute answer as to when to discontinue mechanical ventilation, but the following objective measurements may be helpful in arriving at a decision to begin weaning:

1. Nonassisted tidal volume more than 5 ml. per kg.

2. Inspiratory force greater than -20 cm. H_2O.

3. Minute ventilation less than 10 liters per minute.

4. Ability to double minute ventilation with a maximal voluntary ventilation maneuver.

5. Pao_2 on 100 per cent inspired O_2 of greater than 350 mm. Hg.

6. Vital capacity greater than 10 to 15 ml. per kg.

7. Dead space/tidal volume ratio of less than 60 per cent.

The process of discontinuing mechanical ventilation can be very stressful for the patient, both physically and psychologically. For this reason, attempts at weaning should not be initiated unless there is a reasonable chance the procedure will be successful. The patient's cooperation is mandatory. The goal of close observation by nurses and physician during weaning is to protect the patient and avoid complications should the procedure be unsuccessful. Initial weaning periods should be brief as an encouragement to the patient and to prevent medical complications.

There are two basic methods used to wean patients from mechanical ventilation. The first, more traditional method is simply to take the patient off the ventilator and connect him by means of a T-shaped adapter on the endotracheal tube to a source of humidified inspired air with an appropriate O_2 concentration to prevent hypoxemia. The following procedure may be helpful.

1. Before weaning is begun, the vital signs and respiratory mechanics should be measured.

2. Place the patient in a sitting position.

3. Inform the patient of the procedure to elicit his cooperation.

4. Once the patient is taken off the mechanical ventilator for the first time, vital signs should be taken every 5 to 10 minutes and cardiac rhythm monitored.

5. During the first weaning period, arterial blood gases should be determined after 15 minutes.

6. If the patient is doing well clinically without arrhythmias, hypertension, tachycardia, cyanosis, agitation, signs of hypoxia, inadequate ventilation, or acidosis, the weaning period can continue until the patient appears tired, the vital signs deteriorate, or the patient becomes symptomatic.

7. Initial weaning periods should be for relatively brief periods of time, and the patient should be returned to the mechanical ventilator to rest and improve gas exchange between weaning periods. The frequency with which the patient should be placed on the T-piece is determined by the results of the previous weaning procedure.

8. If the weaning procedure has gone well, the length of time can be increased slowly from 15 minutes to one half hour or an hour at a time. The factors limiting abrupt discontinuation of mechanical ventilation are usually the patient's lung mechanics.

9. Careful records should be maintained that include lung mechanics measurements, blood gases, vital signs, and clinical observations. Such records are invaluable aids in determining the success of the procedure and further therapy.

A newer method of weaning from mechanical ventilation employs a technique called intermittent mandatory ventilation (IMV). During this procedure, the patient is allowed to breathe on his own but is given periodic deep breaths by the ventilator at a rate determined by the physician. Intermittent mandatory ventilation requires a slight modification of the normal ventilator circuitry but is available as an addition to most newer mechanical ventilators. As an initial step, the patient may begin at a ventilator respiratory rate of 6 to 8 per minute, thus allowing him to provide the remainder of the necessary alveolar ventilation. Weaning by IMV is a slower process, but may possibly avoid some of the complications that tend to occur when patients are abruptly taken off mechanical ventilation and placed on a T-piece. Signs that the patient is not tolerating this procedure are similar to those mentioned previously and should be an indication to return the patient to his original ventilator settings. If the patient tolerates the procedure, then the number of IMV breaths per minute provided by the ventilator is slowly decreased. Once the patient is receiving one to two breaths per minute he can usually be taken off the mechanical ventilator completely and placed on a T-piece. Arterial blood gases should be monitored closely during the IMV weaning procedure to assure adequate alveolar ventilation and the absence of respiratory acidosis.

VENTILATORY FAILURE WITH ABNORMAL LUNGS

Patients with chronic bronchitis, emphysema or asthma may develop acute ventilatory failure. Severe obstructive airway disease with increased dead space and airway resistance produces an increased work of breathing and may chronically and insidiously lead to the development of hypercapnia and inadequate alveolar ventilation. In these patients, chronic hypercapnia and chronic respiratory failure are signs of severe lung disease and may not be associated with clinically significant acute deterioration. However, when hypercapnia develops acutely in chronic obstructive pulmonary disease (COPD) patients who have not previously had an elevated $Paco_2$, or when the level of $Paco_2$ rises acutely to higher levels, causing respiratory acidosis in association with clinical deterioration, then such patients have acute respiratory failure. This acute respiratory failure requires more specific acute therapeutic intervention. Causes of acute exacerbations in patients with chronic obstructive pulmonary disease include:

1. Acute infectious bronchitis. This may be due to either viral or bacterial organisms and is usually associated with a change in the patient's sputum. Often the patient notes a gross change in the amount, consistency, or color of his sputum. Increased or decreased amounts, increased viscosity, or purulent sputum may indicate an infection. The physician should examine the sputum grossly and microscopically. Microscopic examination of a wet preparation will show large numbers of polymorphonuclear leukocytes (PMN) in infectious diseases and high percentages of eosinophils in patients with extrinsic asthma. Sputum Gram stain should be used as a guide to initial antibiotic selection. Bacterial organisms most commonly seen in this group of patients include *Hemophilus* and pneumococci. Large numbers of polymorphonuclear cells (PMN) without bacteria suggest a viral process. Sputum culture should be sent for further bacteriologic confirmation.

2. Pneumonia. As these patients usually have impaired cough and mucociliary clearance mechanisms due to their chronic pulmonary disease, they are susceptible to more frequent bacterial pneumonias.

3. Retained secretions. Increased sputum viscosity because of dehydration, infections, and impaired cough and clearance mechanisms may impair ventilatory reserve.

4. Congestive heart failure. Patients with chronic hypoxemia develop pulmonary vasoconstriction and hypertension, resulting in right ventricular hypertrophy and eventual right ventricular failure. Signs of jugular venous distention, peripheral edema, hepatomegaly, hepatojugular reflux and cardiomegaly are signs suggestive of this complication. Left ventricular failure caused by coronary artery disease or other mechanisms may also precipitate respiratory failure.

5. Polycythemia. Patients with markedly elevated hematocrits over 60 per cent may develop cardiorespiratory complications due to increased blood viscosity.

6. Pulmonary embolus. Patients with severe pulmonary disease may have markedly decreased exercise tolerance and often become bedridden. They are then prone to develop deep vein thrombosis and pulmonary emboli related to their inactivity.

7. Pneumothorax. Rupture of a subpleural bulla or bleb resulting in air in the pleural space with lung collapse may impair pulmonary function sufficiently to cause respiratory failure.

8. Gastrointestinal bleeding. Patients with obstructive lung disease have an increased incidence of peptic ulcer disease. Gastrointestinal bleeding and anemia may cause increased dyspnea and decreased oxygen delivery to the tissues.

9. Respiratory depressant drugs. Sedatives, narcotics, or analgesics that depress the respiratory center may precipitate respiratory failure. COPD patients need maximal respiratory drive and respiratory muscle function in order to maintain their chronic compensated state and increased work of breathing.

10. Oxygen. Since patients with chronic hypercapnia have respiratory centers that are relatively insensitive to additional levels of $Paco_2$ (because of renal HCO_3^- retention and highly buffered respiratory centers), their respiratory drive is normally stimulated by hypoxemia. If the hypoxemia is corrected, the respiratory center will be depressed with resultant alveolar hypoventilation and possibly apnea.

11. Surgery. Surgical procedures, particularly those associated with upper abdominal incisions and significant postoperative pain, may impair not only deep breathing and coughing but also normal breathing in patients with severe COPD.

12. Nonspecific causes of increased airway resistance. In the absence of any of these causes for ventilatory failure in a patient with abnormal lungs, the patient's underlying lung disease may be so severe that even small changes in airway mechanics produced by environmental pollutants, changes in the weather and humidity, or other nonspecific respiratory irritants such as dust or fumes, may lead to acute respiratory failure. Progression of the underlying lung disease has been cited as another possibility for respiratory failure in these patients, but this diagnosis should be made only after more treatable causes of the condition are excluded.

It is often difficult to specify a single cause for the development of acute ventilatory failure in patients with abnormal lungs, either because multiple precipitating factors may be present or because even subtle subclinical conditions may be sufficient to lead to respiratory failure.

Treatment

The goal of treatment in this form of respiratory failure is to maintain adequate gas exchange while treating the underlying precipitating factors responsible for the ventilatory failure.

1. Administer low flow oxygen. Because of intrinsic lung disease and hypercapnia, the Pao_2 in these patients tends to be very low. However, excessive administration of oxygen and complete correction of hypoxemia in patients with chronic hypercapnia may lead to further respiratory depression and should be avoided. Normally, $Paco_2$ is the most important stimulant of ventilation. However, as previously mentioned, patients with chronic hypercapnia and compensatory bicarbonate retention become insensitive to further increments in carbon dioxide. These patients with severe COPD, therefore, continue to breathe primarily because of hypoxic respiratory drive. Hypoxemia is not a potent respiratory stimulant in healthy persons with normal Pao_2, but it does cause a significant increase in ventilation at levels below 50 mm. Hg. The goal of oxygen therapy in this form of acute respiratory failure is to increase oxygen delivery to the tissues by increasing oxygen content without increasing Pao_2 to levels that no longer stimulate hyperventilation via the oxygen receptors in the carotid bodies. Below a Pao_2 of 50 mm. Hg, the shape of the oxyhemoglobin dissociation curve is very steep and small increments in Pao_2 are sufficient to cause significant increases in arterial oxygen content and, thus, tissue oxygen delivery. For these reasons low flow oxygen sufficient to correct the hypoxemia only partially is the treatment of choice. Oxygen therapy should be initiated with a 24 or 28 per cent "Venturi" mask. Such facemasks may be uncomfortable to some patients and lead to a feeling of suffocation. In such cases, oxygen administration by nasal cannula at 1 to 2 liters per minute will provide fairly low inspired oxygen concentrations in the range of 24 to 28 per cent.

The disadvantage of the latter form of therapy is that the exact inspired oxygen concentration is unknown, as it varies depending on the patient's respiratory rate and pattern. The effects of oxygen administration should be carefully monitored by repeat analyses of arterial blood gases to assure that the hypoxemia has been relieved without causing excessive respiratory depression and respiratory acidosis. In many patients with ventilatory failure and abnormal lungs, there is a very fine line between too much oxygen administration with further respiratory depression and too little oxygen administration with severe hypoxemia.

2. Remove secretions. One commonly associated event in these patients is excessive, often inadequately cleared airway secretions. Secretion clearance may be aided by the following therapy.

a. Encourage deep breathing and coughing. The most effective means of clearing the airways of secretions is to encourage the patient to cough on his own. However, the cough may be relatively ineffective because of the severe degree of obstructive airway disease.

b. Perform chest physical therapy. Chest percussion, frequent turning of the patient from one position to another, and postural drainage, if tolerated, may all be effective in aiding the clearance of secretions from the airways.

c. Administer fluids. Fluids given intravenously or orally may decrease sputum viscosity and thus allow easier expectoration.

d. Expectorants. The role of expectorants in decreasing secretion viscosity is controversial. Adequate doses of guaifenesin (glyceryl guiacolate) may be helpful in decreasing sputum viscosity. Aerosolized mucolytics such as acetylcysteine have been reported to be helpful in some instances, but may be irritating to the bronchial mucosa and increase bronchospasm. We do not routinely recommend these measures unless other modalities of therapy are ineffective or the sputum is particularly viscous. Direct delivery of aerosolized saline solution to the respiratory tract by way of in-line neubulizers and prior humidification of the inspired air may be as effective as mucolytics.

3. Reverse bronchospasm with bronchodilators. Even though some patients in this group may have little reversible airway disease, a trial of bronchodilators in all such patients should be a routine part of therapy for acute respiratory failure. The drug of choice is intravenous aminophylline. The initial dose of aminophylline is 5.6 mg. per kg. delivered over a period of 20 to 30 minutes intravenously. In patients who have been on prior theophylline therapy, the initial loading dose should be halved. Maintenance aminophylline requirements are 0.9 mg. per kg. per minute delivered as a continuous intravenous infusion. It should be remembered that even though these doses have been calculated to achieve a blood level of 10 micrograms per ml. in most normal patients, there is a certain degree of variability in the blood levels actually achieved. Patients who have decreased theophylline metabolism include those with liver disease or congestive heart failure, and those on other medications that interfere with metabolism of theophylline such as erythromycin. The side effects of excessive doses of aminophylline include seizures, cardiac arrhythmias, and gastrointestinal symptoms such as nausea and vomiting. At the first sign of any of these complications, aminophylline should be discontinued for a period of 2 to 3 hours, after which a slightly lower maintenance dose can be resumed. It is often helpful to obtain blood levels of aminophylline as a guide to therapy; the optimal blood level to achieve significant bronchodilatation without side effects is 10 to 20 micrograms per ml. If additional bronchodilatation is desired, one of the newer beta-adrenergic stimulants such as metaproterenol or terbutaline can be added to the theophylline preparations.

Theophylline preparations and beta-adrenergic agents act by different intracellular mechanisms and their concurrent administration has been shown to achieve a synergistic effect, with a level of bronchodilatation greater than with either agent used alone. Beta-adrenergic agents have a more specific action on bronchial smooth muscles and less cardiotoxicity than theophylline preparations.

The beta-adrenergic agents currently available for oral use are metaproterenol and terbutaline. Metaproterenol is administered at a dose of 10 or 20 mg. every six hours. Terbutaline has a longer half-life and 2.5 or 5.0 mg. may be given every 8 hours. We usually begin at the lower dose and if there are no significant side effects, proceed to increase the dose. The most common side effect is muscle tremor, which may disappear or lessen with long-term use. Metaproterenol is available in a metered-dose inhaler, but most patients with respiratory failure can not cooperate sufficiently to use such devices because of respiratory distress. Terbutaline is also available for subcutaneous injection and may occasionally be helpful for rapid relief of acute bronchospasm in a dose of 0.25 mg., but may cause hypertension, tachycardia, or palpitations.

Aerosolized bronchodilators (isoproterenol or isoethrine) may be nebulized for additional effect. Even in patients who have little reversibility bronchodilators should be administered. When obstructive disease is very severe, even minor improvements in lung mechanics may be significant in terms of clinical response.

Corticosteroids are of greatest use in the treatment of patients with asthma. The presence of significant sputum eosinophilia, a definite diagnosis of extrinsic asthma as the cause of severe acute respiratory failure, or the administration of steroids within the previous 6 months are indications for steroid administration. Steroids should be given intravenously in initial doses equivalent to 100 to 200 mg. of hydrocortisone every 6 hours. Early administration of steroids is essential, since their effect is not seen for 4 to 8 hours. Aerosolized steroids are not useful acutely and should only be prescribed for stable ambulatory patients.

4. Antibiotics. The sputum should be examined to evaluate the presence of infections, and a chest roentgenogram should be obtained to look for infiltrates indicative of pneumonia. If infection is identified either clinically, by chest roentgenogram, or on the basis of sputum examination, appropriate antibiotic therapy should be initiated. If no infections and no other acute, precipitating events for the ventilatory failure can be ascertained, an empiric trial of antibiotics is warranted in this group of patients. In acute exacerbations of chronic obstructive lung disease, ampicillin is a reasonable antibiotic choice to cover most of the bacteria usually encountered.

5. Treat other precipitating factors. A careful search for and treatment of the other possible precipitating factors listed are essential. Even what would appear to be trivial insults in patients with normal lungs (such as mild sedatives or tranquilizers) may be significant factors in precipitating acute respiratory failure in patients with severe obstructive airway disease.

6. Improve cardiac function. If evidence of right heart failure is present, the administration of diuretics to reduce plasma volume and the use of oxygen to reduce pulmonary hypertension are indicated. Care must be taken in the administration of diuretics to prevent contraction metabolic alkalosis, which may lead to further CO_2 retention as a respiratory adjustment for the metabolic alkalosis. Therefore, potassium chloride should be administered routinely whenever diuretics are prescribed. Digitalis preparations are usually not very effective in treating right heart failure. However, if any evidence of left ventricular dysfunction is present, digitalis should be administered cautiously, since hypoxemia in the presence of digitalis may lead to significant arrhythmias.

7. Pneumothorax. If a pneumothorax is present, a chest tube should be inserted percutaneously to expand the underlying lungs and improve lung function.

8. Anticoagulants. If a pulmonary embolus is suspected, heparin should be administered as a continuous intravenous infusion. The diagnosis of pulmonary embolus may be difficult to prove, as these patients have abnormal perfusion scans on the basis of their chronic lung disease rather than because of acute vascular occlusion. Therefore, ventilation-perfusion scans or arteriograms may be necessary to confirm the diagnosis.

9. Phlebotomy. Phlebotomy should be performed if the hematocrit exceeds 55 per cent after the patient is well hydrated.

10. Electrolyte disturbances should be corrected. Metabolic alkalosis is poorly tolerated because of compensatory respiratory acidosis and further alveolar hypoventilation.

11. Sedation. Sedation is to be avoided in these patients in order to prevent further ventilatory failure.

Mechanical Ventilation

In contrast to ventilation failure in patients with normal lungs on whom mechanical ventilation should be employed early, before pulmonary complications occur, mechanical ventilation is usually indicated in patients with abnormal lungs only when significant respiratory acidosis or severe hypoxemia is present.

Significant respiratory acidosis that is not improved by the conservative measures outlined earlier is an indication for mechanical ventilation. Because of the increased work of breathing owing to increased airway resistance and the large tidal volumes necessitated by increased physiologic dead space, these patients may tire physically and be unable to maintain adequate alveolar ventilation for long periods. This is associated with additional ventilatory failure, hypercapnia, and respiratory acidosis, despite maximal conservative therapeutic measures. An initial pH below 7.20 or worsening respiratory acidosis despite maximal therapy should be treated with mechanical ventilation. The absolute level of Pa_{CO_2} is not helpful in determining the urgency of therapy, as patients with severe chronic obstructive pulmonary disease and chronic hypercapnia with renal compensation may have high levels of Pa_{CO_2} with pH values greater than 7.30.

When arterial hypoxemia is associated with evidence of lack of oxygen in the body tissues, mechanical ventilation is indicated. Hypoxia may be evidenced by central nervous system, cardiac, or renal complications such as cardiac arrhythmias, hypotension, myocardial ischemia, lethargy, altered mental status, disorientation, poor urine output, or metabolic acidosis. Any of these signs is an indication for mechanical ventilation, which would enable administration of adequate oxygen without fear of further respiratory depression. The following are guidelines for patients who require mechanical ventilation:

1. Assure adequate alveolar ventilation. Initially, a tidal volume in the range of 10 to 12 ml. per kg. and a respiratory rate of 10 to 12 per minute may be specified. Repeat measurements of arterial blood gases following institution of me-

chanical ventilation and whenever ventilator settings are changed are mandatory to assure adequate ventilation. Respiratory alkalosis should be avoided in these patients by maintaining the $Paco_2$ above 40 mm. Hg if the patient has chronic hypercapnia. In patients with chronic CO_2 retention whose $Paco_2$ is rapidly corrected on the ventilator, the pH will become markedly alkalotic, which might be reflected in severe complications such as seizures. Therefore, the pH should be kept in the range of 7.35. Within several days renal compensation will slowly bring the pH up toward 7.40. The goal of therapy with mechanical ventilation is to assure not only adequate alveolar ventilation but, more important, a relatively normal pH.

2. Administer oxygen. These patients usually do not require high concentrations of oxygen unless there are other major coexisting complications such as severe heart failure or pneumonia. Oxygen concentrations in the range of 30 to 40 per cent are usually adequate to achieve a reasonable Pao_2. The Pao_2 should be continually assessed by repeated blood gas analyses to assure adequate oxygenation. Since these patients have chronically adapted to low Pao_2, the Pao_2 should be kept around 60 mm. Hg, a level sufficient to achieve over 85 per cent O_2 saturation of the blood but should not cause further respiratory depression once the patient begins to breathe on his own; it is also a level that relieves hypoxia-induced pulmonary vasoconstriction.

3. Inspiratory flow rates. These should be kept relatively slow to allow more even distribution of inspired air throughout the lungs. Because these patients have airway obstruction, the expiratory time should be long enough to allow complete expiration before the next breath is initiated.

4. All the procedures mentioned in the previous section concerning proper endotracheal tube care and suctioning techniques should be followed in these patients.

Discontinuing Mechanical Ventilation. The basic guidelines, methods, and techniques for discontinuing mechanical ventilation in this form of respiratory failure are similar to those outlined in the previous section. However, several differences in approach are necessary because of the underlying severe pulmonary disease in patients with acute ventilatory failure and abnormal lungs.

1. The guidelines for discontinuing mechanical ventilation must be thought of as relative rather than absolute indications for successful weaning. In patients with severe COPD, nonpulmonary factors such as nutritional status and muscle strength may prevent successful long-term weaning. Subjective clinical impressions concerning the patient's course are often helpful in assess-

ing whether the patient can discontinue mechanical ventilation.

2. Weaning in COPD patients may be a lengthy process, requiring days or weeks to complete. Physicians must provide continual encouragement to the patient and nursing personnel during the stressful and often depressingly slow weaning period.

3. Prior to weaning, blood gas values should be adjusted to levels which the patient can maintain without mechanical assistance. For example, if a patient has chronic CO_2 retention when stable, it is reasonable to attempt to keep his $Paco_2$ high during weaning.

4. Patients with COPD should be mobilized by sitting up in a chair and getting out of bed as an aid to gas exchange, secretion clearance, and improved muscle strength.

5. Patients with COPD may require reinstitution of mechanical ventilation so they can obtain adequate rest. It is often helpful to wean these patients only during the day and to allow them to sleep on the ventilator at night without weaning attempts.

OXYGEN FAILURE

This form of acute respiratory failure is sometimes called shock lung, noncardiogenic pulmonary edema, or adult respiratory distress syndrome (ARDS). Most cases of acute depression of Pao_2 below 50 mm. Hg are related to pathologic accumulation of fluid in the interstitium and alveoli of the lung. Edema in the airways and parenchyma lead to intrapulmonary shunting of blood; i.e., blood flowing through nonventilated alveoli is not oxygenated. Patients with pulmonary edema are usually tachypneic, severely hypoxemic, and in significant respiratory distress. Pulmonary edema may be caused by cardiac or pulmonary disease. As the treatment of cardiac and pulmonary diseases differs, it is mandatory to search for the underlying cause of the pulmonary edema. Clinical signs of left ventricular failure are often absent or misleading in these patients, and right heart catheterization is helpful in ruling out a cardiac basis for pulmonary edema. Right heart pressures can be measured with the aid of the Swan-Ganz balloon-tipped flow-directed catheter. A pulmonary capillary wedge pressure greater than 10 to 12 mm. Hg indicates elevated left atrial pressure and cardiac dysfunction. Routine Swan-Ganz catheterization of patients with acute oxygenation failure is common in large medical centers and provides the additional benefit of allowing precise monitoring of intravascular volume to guide fluid and diuretic therapy. Specific noncardiac causes of oxygenation failure include: massive trauma; excess fluid or blood administration; hypotension; surgery; head trauma; overwhelming pneumonia, either viral, bacterial or secondary to aspiration; drugs, particularly narcotics; environmental and industrial exposures such as with chlorine gas; pancreatitis; excessive oxygen administration; and fat or thrombotic emboli.

Treatment

The goal of therapy in adult respiratory distress syndrome is to improve oxygenation and allow the lung to heal itself while treating the underlying precipitating factors. Oxygenation can be improved by the following measures:

1. Administer oxygen. In mild cases of adult respiratory distress syndrome, oxygen may be administered without the use of an endotracheal tube and mechanical ventilator. Because of the large shunt, high concentrations of oxygen are necessary to correct the hypoxemia. Adequate oxygenation must be assured by repeat analyses of arterial blood gases. Often, the highest oxygen concentrations possible are necessary to achieve adequate oxygenation and prevent tissue hypoxia. Oxygen may be administered by nasal prongs but this can not achieve over 70 per cent inspired oxygen concentration. Nonrebreathing masks, which have a reservoir bag of oxygen, can achieve inspired oxygen concentrations in the range of 80 to 100 per cent, depending on the patient's respiratory pattern. Patients with ARDS are markedly tachypneic with an increased minute ventilation, and even these masks may fail to provide sufficient oxygen.

2. If tissue hypoxia occurs or Pao_2 is below 50 mm. Hg on maximum oxygen administration, the patient should be intubated and mechanical ventilation initiated. The use of mechanical ventilation with intermittent positive pressure breathing assures a more even distribution of inspired air, larger tidal volumes and higher oxygen concentrations, all of which improve gas exchange.

3. Because these patients are often markedly tachypneic, their respiratory pattern may be difficult to control once mechanical ventilation is begun. In such cases, patients must be sedated with diazepam or morphine to allay anxiety and to depress the respiratory center sufficiently to allow total control of ventilation by mechanical means. If the respiratory rate is still uncontrollable and the patient is still hypoxemic, paralyzation with pancuronium bromide should be initiated. Peripheral muscle paralysis also reduces peripheral oxygen consumption by the voluntary muscles. Initial doses of 0.06 to 0.10 ml. per kg. intravenously are recommended. Dosage must be individualized, and incremental doses often need to be repeated every half to one and a half hours. Pancuronium administration may be associated with tachycardia but is not usually accompanied by hypotension.

4. With mechanical ventilation, large tidal volumes of 10 to 15 ml. per kg. at rates of approximately 12 to 14 per minute are usually required to maintain adequate alveolar ventilation because of the hypermetabolism with increased CO_2 production and intrapulmonary shunts in these patients. Because the lungs become stiff due to the interstitial and alveolar edema, high peak airway pressures are usually necessary to deliver adequate tidal volumes. The resultant elevation of intrathoracic pressure may be associated with complications of pulmonary barotrauma, such as pneumothorax, and impaired venous return to the heart with decreased cardiac output. The acute development of shortness of breath and hypotension should alert the physician to search for pneumothorax, which must be treated with chest tube insertion into the pleural space. The decreased cardiac output can usually be treated successfully by increased intravenous fluid administration.

5. Positive-end expiratory pressure (PEEP). If patients are still hypoxemic despite 100 per cent oxygen administration and large tidal volumes with a mechanical ventilator, then the use of PEEP may improve hypoxemia and allow the reduction of inspired O_2 concentrations. Positive-end expiratory pressure increases the volume remaining in the thorax at the end of a normal expiration, i.e., the functional residual capacity (FRC). The positive pressure and increased FRC result in less airway collapse during expiration with reduced shunting of blood through the lungs and improved gas exchange. Positive-end expiratory pressure should be initiated at low levels, such as 5 cm. H_2O, and its effects measured in terms of gas exchange and cardiac output. The level of PEEP should be increased in increments of approximately 5 cm. H_2O until adequate oxygenation and Pao_2 are achieved. Cardiac output should be supported with volume expansion or inotropic agents if necessary.

As oxygen delivery to the tissues is proportional to the product of cardiac output and arterial oxygen content, if the increased mean airway pressure caused by PEEP impedes cardiac function, tissue oxygenation would decrease. Even if the Pao_2 increased, a reduced cardiac output might be associated with reduced oxygen delivery to the tissues. Both Swan-Ganz catheterization with a thermodilution tip to measure cardiac output and measurement of Pao_2 are necessary to completely define the state of oxygenation of the tissues. In this regard measurement of mixed venous Po_2 (drawn through the proximal pulmonary artery port of a Swan-Ganz catheter) may be helpful in assessing tissue oxygenation. The normal value for mixed venous Po_2 is 40 mm. Hg. A level below 35 mm. Hg indicates the presence of tissue hypoxia, which may be caused by a reduced arterial oxygen content or a reduced cardiac output.

6. Other measures to improve oxygenation include correction of alkalosis, maintenance of a normal hemoglobin level, and measures to reduce oxygen consumption. Alkalosis results in a leftward shift in the oxyhemoglobin dissociation curve such that less oxygen is available to the tissues. Therefore, respiratory and metabolic alkalosis should be prevented or corrected, when present. Since arterial oxygen content* also depends on the amount of hemoglobin available to carry oxygen, anemia in patients with severe hypoxemia should be treated with red blood cell transfusions.

Another therapeutic approach in patients with severe uncorrectable hypoxemia is to reduce tissue metabolism and thus decrease tissue oxygen consumption. Peripheral neuromuscular blockade and the use of cooling blankets to reduce body temperatures below the normal range have been advocated by some.

Measures to Reduce Extravascular Lung Water. The techniques purported to reduce extravascular lung water are largely unsubstantiated at the present time, but the concepts underlying these therapies are important.

1. Dehydration. Patients with noncardiogenic pulmonary edema should not have an overexpanded vascular space. Excessive fluids should not be prescribed, as these may end up in the lungs and increase the degree of pulmonary edema. Fluids should be administered cautiously and guided by the measurement of electrolytes and pulmonary capillary wedge pressure.

2. Diuretics. Administration of diuretics may be helpful to deplete intravascular volume and thus reduce extravascular lung water.

3. Plasma proteins. By increasing plasma oncotic pressure it might be theoretically possible to draw fluids from the lung into the vascular space. Some centers routinely use large amounts of albumin and plasma as opposed to electrolyte solutions in water to support blood pressure. Certainly, a decrease in plasma proteins should be treated with protein administration, but the effectiveness of this procedure in patients with normal protein levels has not been definitively proved.

4. Cardiac function. Patients with increased pulmonary capillary wedge pressure and signs of left ventricular failure not due to increased plasma volume should receive digitalis. In the absence of congestive failure, wedge pressure can usually be controlled by diuretics and dehydration. In ARDS patients with severe hypoxemia uncorrected with O_2, mechanical ventilation, and PEEP, O_2 delivery may be improved by increasing the cardiac output with the use of inotropic agents such as intravenous infusion of dopamine or isoproterenol. The effects of cardiac drugs must be closely monitored by measurement of cardiac output and Pao_2.

5. Corticosteroids. Administration of large doses of systemic steroids has been advocated as a means of reducing the capillary endothelial damage that causes fluid to leak into the pulmonary parenchyma. We do not routinely use steroids unless indicated for other reasons.

6. Secretion clearance. In any patient on mechanical ventilation, secretions may pool in the airways and lung parenchyma. The airways should be kept clear of secretions by intermittent suctioning of the airways, changing the patient's position frequently, and performing chest physical therapy.

7. Bronchodilators. If bronchospasm is present, bronchodilators should be administered to decrease airway resistance and improve distribution of inspired gas.

Discontinuing Mechanical Ventilation. The most important of the previously listed criteria in determining the ability of patients with oxygenation failure to be weaned from mechanical ventilation is not their lung mechanics but rather the gas-exchanging function of their lungs. Once oxygenation improves such that an adequate Pao_2 can be maintained without mechanically assisted ventilation (suggested by a Pao_2 on 100 per cent oxygen without PEEP of over 300 to 350 mm. Hg and a respiratory rate under 35 per minute), weaning can begin.

Weaning can often be initiated earlier by using continuous positive airway pressure (CPAP). With CPAP, a T-shaped adapter is attached to the endotracheal tube. A source of high flow humidified oxygen for inspiration is attached to one end of the T-piece while the expiratory line is kept under positive pressure (such as below water in a large plastic jar). Continuous positive airway pressure (CPAP) increases the functional residual capacity (FRC), prevents airway closure, and improves oxygenation in a manner similar to PEEP while allowing the patient to breathe on his own with lower inspired oxygen concentrations. The level of positive airway pressure may then be decreased slowly. Once airway pressure is atmospheric, the patient can usually be extubated successfully.

---

*Oxygen content = oxygen bound to hemoglobin + oxygen dissolved in plasma = hemoglobin × 1.34 ml. O_2 per gram of HgB × O_2 saturation + Pao_2 × 0.003 ml. O_2 per mm. Hg. Most of the oxygen is carried bound to hemoglobin; the amount of oxygen dissolved in plasma is minimal.

CHRONIC BRONCHITIS AND EMPHYSEMA

method of
STEVEN G. KELSEN, M.D.,
HUGO D. MONTENEGRO, M.D.,
and NEIL S. CHERNIACK, M.D.
Cleveland, Ohio

Chronic bronchitis produces inflammation of the airways with excessive mucus production and can be diagnosed *clinically* by a history of cough and sputum production on most days for 3 consecutive months in 2 successive years. Emphysema, on the other hand, produces dilatation and destruction of air spaces distal to the terminal bronchiole and is diagnosed *pathologically*. In chronic bronchitis, the functional disturbances result from inflammatory narrowing and an increase in secretions within the airway lumen. In emphysema, they result from a disruption of the lungs' tissue elements which act to "tether" and maintain the patency of the intrapulmonary airways. Collectively, the two diseases make up the category of lung diseases described by the term chronic obstructive pulmonary disease (COPD). They are characterized functionally by (1) obstruction to airflow, (2) hyperinflation of the lungs with air trapping, (3) impaired efficiency of oxygen and carbon dioxide exchange, and (4) an increased work of breathing. The effects of emphysema and chronic bronchitis can be distinguished in the laboratory. Emphysema decreases lung elastic recoil and the $D_L CO$. This is, however, of little help clinically, because in the vast majority of subjects both processes are present simultaneously so that the therapeutic approach is the same.

Of great importance is recent evidence suggesting that the earliest lesions in COPD occur in the small (less than 2 mm. diameter) airways which produce no symptoms. Symptomatic, clinically evident disease develops only after many years when extensive involvement of the small airways has occurred. Detection of the disease in its subclinical form is now possible with readily available noninvasive techniques. These tests can be incorporated easily in the routine of the regular health check-up. Lesions detected at this stage of the disease may be completely reversible with elimination of the inciting factors such as cigarette smoke or industrial toxins.

Unfortunately, the majority of patients are first seen by the physician when the characteristic symptoms of shortness of breath and exercise limitation are already present. At this stage, normal lung function cannot be restored and the aims of medical management become (1) prevention of conditions which can accelerate pulmonary dysfunction, such as infection or exposure to bronchial irritants; (2) correction of reversible factors contributing to airflow obstruction (e.g., relief of bronchospasm and elimination of secretions); (3) treatment of secondary complications, such as congestive heart failure and acute respiratory failure; and (4) various supportive measures which improve the life style of the patient.

Overall Approaches

Minimizing the Progressive Loss of Pulmonary Function. The slow decrease in pulmonary function over time which occurs in most patients with chronic bronchitis and emphysema is greater than can be accounted for by an aging process alone. It is suspected that multiple factors contribute to the loss of lung function. One factor may be continued cigarette smoking. Although lung function deteriorates with age more rapidly in smokers than in nonsmokers, it is not clear if the rate of deterioration is affected by smoking in patients with *established* bronchitis and emphysema. It is known, however, that an acute increase in airway resistance may be produced by smoking only a single cigarette. Furthermore, most patients will report a reduction of the volume of sputum produced when cigarette smoking is discontinued, as well as a subjective improvement in the state of well-being. Therefore cessation of smoking is the first step in the therapeutic regimen for all patients.

A careful history is the key to pinpointing irritants in the work place and home environment which should be avoided. It is well known that the number of respiratory deaths increases during periods of severe atmospheric pollution. Patients living or working in areas with continuously high levels of air pollution which produce symptoms may benefit from a temporary or permanent change in their living or working location.

Inflammatory reactions introduce proteolytic enzymes which may digest lung tissue. Tissue destruction is accelerated in patients with alpha-1-antitrypsin deficiency. Younger patients (below age of 40) with chronic obstructive lung disease should be tested to see whether or not this deficiency is present.

Significant reductions in lung function may occur after acute respiratory infection. For example, a single acute bacterial pneumonia can produce respiratory failure in patients with borderline respiratory function. Furthermore, viral respiratory tract infections may account for as many as two thirds of all symptomatic episodes. Viral infections may interfere with lung clearance mechanisms and increase the susceptibility of the lung to bacterial colonization.

Given these considerations, patients with COPD should receive annual influenza vaccination against the prevalent strains. Vaccinations should be completed before the winter season. Studies have indicated that patients with chronic bronchitis given antibiotics prophylactically at the first sign of a respiratory tract infection (upper or lower) or simply when the sputum becomes purulent tend to have less morbidity in terms of hospitalizations and days lost from work. Furthermore, the duration of acute symptomatic exacerbations is reduced. This indicates that antibiotic therapy should be instituted early in all respiratory tract infections. Continuous administration of antibiotics over the winter months in some patients with repeated infections seems to be advisable.

Correction of Reversible Factors Which Contribute to Airflow Obstruction. In emphysema, airflow is reduced by airway collapse and by a decrease in the "driving" pressures (elastic recoil of the lung) which account for maximal flow. These factors cannot be reversed directly. However, the factors which produce airflow obstruction in chronic bronchitis are partly reversible and are present to some degree in all patients with COPD. Airflow obstruction in chronic bronchitis is produced by (1) increases in bronchomotor tone, (2) intraluminal mucus, and (3) mucosal edema.

Augmented parasympathetic nervous activity contributes to the heightened bronchomotor tone. A variety of α- and β-adrenergic agonists and anticholinergic blocking drugs are useful in relaxing bronchial smooth muscle.

Elimination of mucus may be achieved by physical measures which stimulate coughing and liquefaction of secretions and by the use of gravity or percussion to mechanically facilitate clearance. β-adrenergic drugs also increase the rate of mucociliary clearance.

Edema of the airways occurring in the acute stage of inflammation produced by exposure to noxious agents in the air or by antigen-antibody reactions is sometimes relieved by corticosteroids.

Treatment of Secondary Complications. RESPIRATORY FAILURE. Respiratory failure is usually considered to be present when the Po_2 is less than 50 mm. Hg or the Pco_2 is greater than 50 mm. Hg (at sea level in the absence of an accompanying metabolic alkalosis).

Subtle impairment of oxygen exchange, as indicated by increases in the alveolar-arterial oxygen tension gradient, is one of the earliest changes in COPD. However, because of the sigmoid shape of the oxyhemoglobin dissociation curve, the oxygen content of arterial blood is well maintained until the Po_2 falls below 60 mm. Hg. Hypoxemia results from poor distribution of inspired gas relative to pulmonary blood flow (ventilation-perfusion mismatch). However, reduction in the level of total ventilation (alveolar hypoventilation) may contribute to the development of hypoxemia when CO_2 retention is present. In most patients, increases in arterial CO_2 occur only when airway obstruction is severe and forced expiratory flow rates are less than 25 per cent of the predicted normal values (e.g., FEV_1 values of 1.0 to 1.5 liters or less). However, in some patients, impaired chemosensitivity with a failure of respiratory activity to increase appropriately in response to changes in blood gas tensions may also contribute to CO_2 retention.

COR PULMONALE AND CONGESTIVE HEART FAILURE. The prognosis of patients with COPD is poorer when there is pulmonary hypertension. The level of pulmonary artery pressure rises because hypoxia and hypercapnia produce vasoconstriction. Reduction in the volume of the pulmonary capillary bed caused by anatomic destruction of alveolar septa appears to be less important a cause of hypertension. In addition, severe hypoxia in patients with COPD may cause left ventricular dysfunction. Oxygen therapy and careful management of fluid and electrolyte balance are therefore important in the management of these patients.

Surgery. Resection of lung bullae rarely is of long-term benefit. Infrequently, a single bulla may expand sufficiently to produce symptoms that may be alleviated by removal of the bulla. Other surgical measures do not appear to be helpful in treating COPD. Intensive bronchodilator and antibiotic treatment to optimize lung function should precede elective surgical procedures in these patients.

Outpatient Management

Bronchodilators. In the past several years, significant advances have been made in understanding the physiology of bronchial smooth muscle constriction and in the development of improved bronchodilator drugs. These drugs can be given orally or in aerosol form and so are well suited for chronic outpatient care.

β-ADRENERGIC AGONISTS. β agonists relax bronchial smooth muscle by activating adenylcyclase and increasing the production of cyclic AMP. This bronchodilating action is mediated by a different set of β receptors (β_2) than those which produce cardiovascular (tachycardia and increased cardiac output) and central nervous system (CNS) effects (β_1). Newer preparations which have selective affinity for β_2 receptors are now available and provide potent bronchodilatation without the frequent adverse effects previously noted with isoproterenol, which has both β_1 and β_2 effects. Furthermore, the structure of the new drugs makes them less susceptible to the action of catechol-o-methyl transferases and monoamine oxidases, thereby prolonging their duration of action. Salbutamol, terbutaline, and metaproterenol are examples of these newer drugs that have been shown in clinical trials to be effective and safe in man. When given orally, these drugs have an earlier onset of action than ephedrine (a combined α- and β-adrenergic agonist) and greater degree and duration of bronchodilatation (4 to 6 hours). Because the onset of action of the oral β_2 preparations is sufficiently rapid for most outpatients, it is seldom necessary to prescribe aerosol preparations. We use terbutaline, 5 to 7.5 mg. orally every 6 hours, as the β stimulant in most outpatients. Ephedrine is rarely used because of its relatively low potency and high incidence of side effects such as palpitations, insomnia, and urinary retention if prostatic enlargement is present. A frequent but short-lived side effect of terbutaline has been the development of hand tremor (a manifestation of β_2 stimulation on skeletal muscle). To date, there is no evidence of tachyphylaxis or paradoxical bronchospasm with terbutaline—either of which can occur when isoproterenol is used. In patients who cannot tolerate oral terbutaline because of idiosyncratic reactions, we use metaproterenol by Freon propellant aerosol (two to three inhalations [0.65 mg. metered dose each breath] every 6 hours).

XANTHINES. Xanthines such as theophylline increase the intracellular concentration of cyclic AMP, but do so by inhibiting the activity of diphosphoesterase which breaks down cyclic AMP. There is in vitro evidence for a synergistic interaction between adenylcyclase activators like the β agonists and diphosphoesterase inhibitors like theophylline. However, theophylline can be effective even when the sympathomimetics are not. Theophylline and its derivatives (methylated xanthines) are available in anhydrous form or in a variety of salts and solutions. About 90 per cent of uncoated aminophylline (theophylline ethylenediamine) and the choline salt of theophylline (oxtriphylline) are absorbed in the fasting state. They have a plasma half-life of 4 to 5 hours. The rates of excretion of the drug vary somewhat between individuals but are sufficiently close to allow dosage to be based on body weight and the amount of anhydrous theophylline in each preparation. We generally use aminophylline tablets (80 per cent anhydrous theophylline by weight) in an initial dose of 3 mg. per kg. of anhydrous theophylline every 6 hours around the clock. This dose may be increased to a maximum of 6 mg. per kg. every 6 hours until the desired effect has been reached or toxicity develops. The blood level of the drug will plateau by 1 to 2 days. Thereafter, the dose of the drug can be increased every 2 to 3 days in an attempt to find an optimal level. Because rates of absorption are slower with oral administration, cardiovascular toxicity (hypotension, arrhythmias) and CNS toxicity (seizures) are rare, but anorexia, nausea, and vomiting can occur. Toxicity is usually associated with blood levels in excess of 20 micrograms per ml.

In Elixophyllin (a 20 per cent alcohol solution of anhydrous theophylline), the concentration of theophylline (80 mg. in 15 ml.) is relatively low. A substantial volume (45 to 60 ml.) must be ingested (9 to 12 ml. of alcohol) to deliver an adequate dose of theophylline.

ANTICHOLINERGICS. Recent evidence suggests that vagal reflexes contribute to the airway constriction that occurs in response to inhaled irritants or antigen-antibody reactions. The responses are diminished in animals by vagotomy and in man by blockade of efferent vagal fibers with an anticholinergic such as atropine. The role of these drugs in COPD is as yet unsettled. However, atropine, when given as an aerosol, increases the FEV_1 in patients with COPD. Concern about side effects of atropine (tachycardia and drying effects on tracheobronchial secretions) has led to the development of derivatives of atropine without these adverse actions. The most promising seems to be the methyl bromide of N-isopropyl nortropine known as Sch 1000. This is an inhaled bronchodilator with a potency equivalent to or greater than atropine and may be of particular value in patients with COPD and cardiovascular disease.

CORTICOSTEROIDS. The role of this class of drugs in COPD is controversial. Corticosteroids are available both as oral preparations and as aerosols containing derivatives with prominent pulmonary effects but little systemic effects because of poor absorption. Corticosteroids may help dilate bronchi and decrease inflammation. Their use is best limited to patients with (1) a substantial allergic component to their disease, (2) sputum or blood eosinophilia, (3) episodic bronchospasm, and (4) no evidence of pulmonary infection (e.g., inactive tuberculosis, suppurative bronchiectasis). Steroids are employed only when maximal doses of other bronchodilators have been given without sufficient improvement.

Antibiotics. In contrast to normal subjects, in whom the lower respiratory tract is sterile, the lower respiratory tracts of patients with COPD appear to be colonized with gram-positive and gram-negative organisms (most commonly *Streptococcus pneumoniae* or *Hemophilus influenzae*). Continuous antibiotic treatment is helpful in some patients. In all patients, antibiotics should be used at the first sign of a respiratory infection or when the sputum becomes discolored. Either ampicillin, 500 mg. orally four times daily, or tetracycline, 250 mg. orally four times daily, for 7 days can be used. Amoxicillin, a derivative of ampicillin, is also reported to be well absorbed and to produce high levels in blood and sputum. Chloramphenicol is effective but should be used only as a last resort because of its hematologic toxicity. Clinical trials suggest that penicillin is relatively ineffective. Gram stain and culture of the sputum are of little help in most cases but should be obtained in patients with significant febrile illnesses or clinical or radiologic evidence of pneumonia before antibiotics are changed.

Chronic Oxygen Therapy. Recent studies indicate that in severely hypoxemic subjects (Po_2 of less than 55 mm. Hg), chronic oxygen administration for at least 15 hours a day may be of value in (1) decreasing pulmonary artery pressure both at rest and during exercise, (2) minimizing polycythemia, (3) improving exercise tolerance, and (4) improving electroencephalographic (EEG) tracings and intellectual function. Furthermore, episodes of congestive heart failure seem to occur less frequently with oxygen administration. The effects of chronic oxygen therapy on long-term survival are less clear cut, however, but appear to be of benefit in patients living at high altitude.

Oxygen therapy may be particularly helpful during sleep. Arterial Po_2 may drop substantially during sleep in some patients with COPD because of an exaggeration of the normal hypoventilation of sleep and a worsening of ventilation-perfusion relationships. These changes may be most marked during rapid eye movement (REM) sleep.

Patients in whom chronic oxygen administration is considered should be hospitalized (1) to ascertain the effects of various oxygen flow rates on the Pao_2 and (2) to determine the increase in $Paco_2$ (generally slight) which results from the decrease in hypoxic chemical drive.

Several methods are now available to provide oxygen conveniently at home. A liquid oxygen system (Linde), consisting of a reservoir tank and portable (7 lb.) "walker," and a device which acts as a molecular "sieve" to concentrate oxygen by extracting nitrogen from room air are available. Regardless of the method chosen, domiciliary oxygen is expensive. Its use should be reserved for patients with (1) a Po_2 of less than 55 mm. Hg at rest, which declines still further with exercise or sleep, or (2) evidence of cor pulmonale.

Diuretics and Digitalis. Intravascular volume is increased and peripheral edema is common even in the absence of heart failure in COPD. Diuretics are useful when extravascular salt and water are increased to prevent simultaneous accumulations in the lungs which can interfere with gas exchange.

The effectiveness of digitalis in improving right ventricular function even in the presence of heart failure is controversial. Also, patients with COPD develop serious arrhythmias with even small amounts of digitalis.

Improvement in Respiratory Drive. Reduced sensitivity of the respiratory "center" to chemical stimuli may aggravate hypoxemia and hypercapnia. In some patients with inherent disturbances in the function of the respiratory "center," respiratory failure may be produced by only slight degrees of airway obstruction. In such patients agents to stimulate respiratory drive (e.g., medroxyprogesterone) may be of benefit. More common, however, are decreases in chemosensitivity "acquired" during the course of treatment.

For example, metabolic alkalosis caused by intensive diuretic therapy may substantially blunt the response to CO_2. This should be prevented by administering adequate potassium and chloride. Also, sedatives and tranquilizers can diminish the responsiveness of the respiratory "center" to changes in Pco_2 or Po_2 and should be avoided.

Physical Therapy. Patients with copious, thick secretions which are difficult to raise by coughing alone may be helped by postural drainage and chest percussion performed three to four times a day. These measures are generally more effective in mobilizing secretions than available expectorants and mucolytics. Incoordination of the breathing muscles has been implicated in some patients in causing poor gas exchange. In these patients breathing exercises are helpful, but in the majority of patients they are not. Patients with COPD are occasionally found to spontaneously employ pursed-lip breathing. This technique has been shown to be effective in some patients in relieving dyspnea and decreasing minute ventilation. The physiologic effect of pursed-lip breathing appears to be related to a reduction in expiratory flow and an increase in intra-airway pressure which minimizes airway collapse.

Left to themselves patients with obstructive pulmonary disease tend to become inactive, and deconditioning further limits exercise tolerance. A regular schedule of physical activity is beneficial in improving exercise performance. Physical training programs increase exercise tolerance and decrease oxygen consumption at any level of exertion. This improvement occurs without a measurable change in pulmonary function and appears to be the result of improved efficiency of both skeletal and cardiac muscle. Any attempt to increase the exercise tolerance of inactive patients should be attempted cautiously and only after physiologic studies of the effect of exercise on blood gas tensions and the cardiovascular system have been obtained.

Inhalation Therapy. NEBULIZATION-HUMIDIFICATION. A variety of devices have been employed to increase the water content of inspired air to help liquefy secretions and facilitate their removal. In normally hydrated patients breathing takes place through the nose and mouth, and the inspired air is 100 per cent saturated by the time it reaches the trachea. In addition, in nose- or mouth-breathing patients, very little of the water emitted by humidifiers and nebulizers reaches the lungs. Most is deposited in the upper airway or swallowed. Accordingly, we prefer to maintain hydration and sputum fluidity by having our patients drink 2 to 3 quarts of liquid daily.

IPPB. Intermittent positive pressure breathing (IPPB) per se does not improve pulmonary function and may even increase airway resistance and the work of breathing in subjects with reactive or easily collapsible airways. In patients with COPD, its use should be confined to the delivery of aerosol medication. Although IPPB is an effective means of delivering bronchodilator medication, several recent studies have shown that it is no better than hand-powered or propellant nebulizers. However, in subjects who cannot take or hold a deep breath, are weak, or lack coordination, IPPB "assist" may allow greater penetration of the drugs. Long-term use of IPPB as a means of delivering bronchodilators may produce overdistention of the lung, and it should not be used routinely in outpatient care.

Hospital Management

Acute respiratory failure, precipitated by acute infection, congestive heart failure, bronchospasm, or retention of secretions, is the most common cause of hospitalization in patients with COPD. Recognition of the precipitating factor(s) is the first step in hospital management. In general, however, the modalities used during hospitalization are the same as those used in the outpatient setting except for a greater intensity of application.

Oxygen Therapy. In most patients in acute respiratory failure, the most immediate threat to life is that of severe hypoxemia. Continuous administration of O_2 is mandatory. Small, precise increases in oxygen concentration must be given so as to improve the arterial oxygen content without an excessive rise in P_{CO_2}. This can best be accomplished by any of a number of devices using the Venturi principle to deliver large volumes of gas with small (24 and 28 per cent) increases in oxygen concentration. Use of these Venturi devices (e.g., Ventimask) also prevents changes in either the level or pattern of breathing from affecting the inspired oxygen concentration in contrast to low flow systems.

Most patients in acute respiratory failure may be adequately treated without mechanical ventilation. Rather, intubation and mechanical ventilation should be reserved for the minority of patients in whom a progressive rise in P_{CO_2} occurs to the point at which either severe respiratory acidosis (pH < 7.25) or a CO_2-induced obtundation occurs. Rarely, the failure to obtain adequate oxygenation (P_{O_2} greater than 55 to 60 mm. Hg) using a facial mask may require mechanical ventilation. Patients on O_2 therapy with or without the aid of mechanical ventilation should be followed with measurements of arterial blood gases at regular intervals even when the clinical condition is apparently stable.

Bronchodilators. In the acute stage of the disease, aerosol and intravenous bronchodilators should be given because of their rapid onset and assured delivery.

We use aminophylline as a continuous infusion. This is always begun with a loading dose of 6.0 mg. per kg. given over 20 minutes, followed by a maintenance dose of 0.9 mg. per kg. per hour. In most patients, this dose will give a blood level of 10 to 15 micrograms per ml. Use of a loading dose produces a peak effect in 15 minutes, compared to 8 hours when the loading dose is not given. When a greater effect is desired, an additional dose of 3.0 mg. per kg. may be given over 20 minutes and the continuous dose increased to 1.35 mg. per kg. per hour. This larger dose will produce a blood level of 15 to 20 micrograms per ml. Patients with congestive heart failure or severe liver disease appear to have a decreased rate of clearance of the drug, and their maintenance dose should be decreased by one third and one half, respectively. The loading dose remains unchanged, however.

AEROSOL. There are at present no readily available β_2 aerosol *solutions*. We therefore make use of aerosolized isoproterenol, 0.5 ml. of 1:200 dilution given by IPPB machine over 15 minutes and repeated no more often than every 4 hours. In patients with cardiovascular disease, we use isoetharine in equivalent dose, because it may have less β_1 effect.

All bronchodilators may produce an initial decrease in P_{O_2}, because they dilate pulmonary blood vessels and may increase the perfusion more than the ventilation of some poorly ventilated regions. Consequently, bronchodilators in acute respiratory failure should be given only in conjunction with oxygen therapy.

ATELECTASIS

method of
RICHARD M. PETERS, M.D.
San Diego, California

Atelectasis means absence of air within the lung. The nonaerated area of lung may be an anatomic segment, lobe, or entire lung, or it may be smaller portions of lung in various anatomic areas.

Atelectasis of anatomic segments of lung most often results from retained secretions that block bronchi, usually in areas where ventilation has been limited by splinting of chest cage or diaphragm. The likelihood of such atelectasis is increased in patients with increased bronchial secretions. If such patients become dehydrated or are given atropine, these secretions can become thick and tenacious. Such thick, tenacious secretions are a major cause of atelectasis.

Anatomic obstruction of major bronchi with subsequent development of atelectasis also can be due to endobronchial tumors or an aspirated foreign body. In both circumstances, patients develop dyspnea and then infection behind the obstructing tumor or foreign body. A particular form of anatomic obstruction that occurs most frequently in the middle lobe results from enlargement of lymph node, compressing the membranous portion of the bronchus. These patients also usually present with fever and dyspnea.

In children, aspiration of anything from peanuts to toy bullets takes place when they are upright. In this position, the most likely site for the foreign body to lodge in the tracheobronchial tree is in the right lower lobe; next, the left lower lobe. Aspiration occurring with seizures, unconsciousness, substance abuse or anesthetics usually occurs in the supine position and the affected segments are the superior segments of the lower lobes and the posterior segments of the upper lobes. These are the dependent segments when a patient is supine.

In the postoperative patient, atelectasis results from disruption of the chest wall function so that deep breathing and coughing are inhibited. Pain also results in immobilization of the patient, leading to increased fluid in the dependent lung. This makes the lung less compliant and more subject to collapse. Atelectasis can also be due to lung compression from pneumothorax or pleural fluid or blood.

Prevention and treatment of atelectasis require the following:

1. *Prevention of aspiration.* Unconscious patients should be nursed whenever possible, lying on their side with mouth dependent. Small children should not be given objects that can be aspirated.

2. *Maintenance of adequate hydration of the patient.* Adequate fluid therapy is essential. Intravenous fluids should be continued in postoperative or seriously ill patients until it is clear that the patient's oral intake will be adequate.

3. *Avoidance of atropine-like compounds.* These drugs thicken secretions and prevent the patient from coughing them up.

4. *Control of chest wall and abdominal pain.* Coughing and deep breathing are essential in postoperative patients to prevent retention of secretions and atelectasis.

Too often patients are manipulated and placed in great pain; then large amounts of analgesics are needed to control the pain. Instead, the analgesic should be given in anticipation of the activity. The best method of controlling pain is local nerve blockade with intercostal block or thoracic epidural anesthesia. If nerve block is not practical, morphine analgesia 0.1 to 0.15 mg. per kg. should be given every 2 to 4 hours. Morphine analgesia should be adjusted for age and general health. Young, heavy muscled patients will require high doses of narcotics; debilitated and elderly patients, low doses. Morphine should be avoided and local blocks used in patients with chronic obstructive pulmonary disease (COPD). Deep breathing, coughing, bed making, or ambulation should be scheduled so that they are attempted when analgesia is at its maximum, 5 minutes after intravenous morphine or 30 minutes after subcutaneous morphine.

5. *Mobilization and, if feasible, ambulation.* Patients who remain immobile fail to expand their lungs and do not cough well. The supine posture causes elevated diaphragm and low lung volume. If the patient cannot sit up, he should be rolled to full lateral decubitus position at least 50 per cent of the time. This position hyperexpands the superior lung by the gravitational pull of the diaphragm and mediastinum. If a lobe is atelectatic, the patient should be positioned with that side up and encouraged to cough and take deep breaths while chest physiotherapy is administered.

6. *Blow bottles and incentive spirometers.* Blow bottles and incentive spirometers motivate the patient to take deep breaths and prevent low lung volumes leading to atelectasis. Patients must be instructed in their use. Too often they are just given the devices without effective instructions.

7. *Bronchodilators.* In patients with bronchoconstriction due to asthma or chronic obstructive airway disease, bronchodilators are important. These patients can be recognized by the presence of wheezes and ronchi. If not contraindicated because of cardiac status, nebulized isoproterenol 1:200 can be used, and if not effective, 1:100 solution may be tried. Aminophylline by intravenous drip should be given if not contraindicated by cardiac disease.

8. *Endotracheal suction.* Suction induces cough and helps raise secretions. Remember to give analgesics prior to suctioning in patients with chest wall pain.

9. *Bronchoscopy.* The ease of fiberoptic bronchoscopy and its effectiveness demand that it be used early in case of lobar or segmental atelectasis. Rarely will one see a mucus plug in a large bronchus. However, lavage almost always brings up multiple small plugs, which, when removed, increase the ability to aerate the lung. Bronchoscopy is effective only if steps 1 to 8 precede and follow its use. In some patients, multiple bronchoscopies are required. Bronchoscopy is also essential to evaluate whether a foreign body or endobronchial lesion is the basis for the atelectasis.

10. *Pneumothorax or pleural effusion.* If present, they should be aspirated or drained using closed chest bottle drainage to relieve compression of the lung. If complete atelectasis due to compression has been present for more than 12 hours,

closed drainage alone may not result in re-expansion. Such patients require steps 1 to 8 as well as aspiration of pleural air or fluid. If these conservative measures do not promptly relieve atelectasis, bronchoscopy is essential.

11. *Chest x-rays.* The assessment of the presence of atelectasis and success in treatment requires frequent chest x-rays to ascertain that lung collapse has been corrected.

Foreign Bodies and Endobronchial Tumors

If atelectasis is due to a foreign body, prompt removal is imperative. This should be done by a bronchoscopist skilled in foreign body removal. In children, life can be endangered if the grasp of the foreign body is lost during extraction and it falls into the opposite bronchus. It is always safest to remove foreign bodies under local anesthesia, when the patient's cough can be used as an adjunct. If atelectasis is due to bronchial stenosis, tumor, or a foreign body that cannot be extracted transbronchially, then surgical correction is indicated. Inoperable obstructive bronchial tumors should be treated by radiation therapy.

Diffuse Miliary Atelectasis—Adult Respiratory Distress Syndrome

Another form of atelectasis is diffuse atelectasis of small groups of alveoli. This type of atelectasis has been labeled adult respiratory distress syndrome (ARDS). It has a number of causes. It is most frequently seen after massive trauma or severe sepsis. ARDS is characterized by increase in lung water and fall in lung compliance (stiff lungs). In this syndrome, the capillaries and alveolar epithelium are injured and they allow both fluid and protein to leak into the interstitium and the alveolar lumen. The increased fluid makes the lungs stiff and thus lowers functional residual capacity (the volume of air left in the lungs at the end of expiration). The partially fluid-filled alveoli are unstable and, as expiratory lung volume falls, the unstable alveoli collapse.

As with lobar atelectasis an intrapulmonary shunt results; that is, blood perfuses unventilated alveoli, causing unoxygenated blood to reach the left ventricle. Calculation of the portion of total flow going to unaerated alveoli, shunt fraction, is a good index of the severity of ARDS. A shunt fraction over 20 per cent represents moderately severe ARDS; over 30 per cent, severe ARDS. Blood gas determinations in these patients show a low Pao_2 and $Paco_2$, the latter evidence of hyperventilation in an attempt to correct the depressed O_2. Administration of a high concentration of oxygen to these patients is futile because the low Pao_2 is due to blood perfusing unventilated alveoli. Treatment that has proved successful is to keep the airway pressure above atmospheric at the end of expiration—positive end expiratory pressure (PEEP). The elevated end expiratory pressure raises the functional residual capacity of the lungs. By increasing the lung volume in this manner, alveoli are reopened and the shunt fraction decreased. In severe ARDS, the PEEP level may have to be raised to high levels. High levels of PEEP can result in alveolar rupture and pneumothorax. It also can depress venous return to the heart, thus lowering cardiac output.

Patients with ARDS require ventilator assistance because of the hypoxemia and increased work required to ventilate their stiff lungs. I feel the best method of treating these patients is with continuous positive airway pressure (CPAP) and intermittent mandatory ventilation (IMV). The IMV rate and volume are set to maintain $Paco_2$ at about 35 mm. Hg. The CPAP level is increased to try to bring the Pao_2 above 70 or shunt fraction to less than 0.15. Often this may not be possible in very sick patients. These patients require skilled care, with monitoring of cardiac output, lung compliance, and frequent blood gas determinations as CPAP is increased to optimum level. In patients who show progressive fall in Pao_2, early transfer to a facility where these skills are available is lifesaving. Delay can allow fibrosis of the lung to occur and result in irreversible changes.

High concentrations of oxygen, above Fio_2 of 0.5, should be avoided as they aggravate the lung injury, leading to collapse of poorly ventilated alveoli and injury to alveolocapillary membrane of aerated alveoli.

Antibiotics

Since segmental atelectasis and ARDS are both frequently associated with infection, cultures should be obtained and appropriate antibiotics administered.

CHRONIC BRONCHITIS AND BRONCHIECTASIS
method of
ROBERT A. BARBEE, M.D.
Tucson, Arizona

Terminology

The common denominator in the pathogenesis and subsequent clinical picture of chronic bronchitis is longstanding exposure to one or more of a variety of bronchial irritants. Cigarette smoke and toxic air pollutants are the most common. Without such an exposure history, in fact, the diagnosis may be in question. As a result of these chronic inflammatory stimulants, three specific pathologic features develop: (1) an absolute increase in the number of mucus secreting glands in the bronchial walls, (2) a decrease in the ciliary clearance activity of the bronchi, and (3) a decrease in resistance to infection, probably secondary to lessened alveolar macrophage activity. A majority of subjects with this pathologic triad remain subclinical, provide a history of "morning cigarette cough," and have little or no evidence of significant airway obstruction between acute infectious exacerbations. To this group the term chronic simple bronchitis is applied.

A susceptible subgroup of those with this picture, usually without a significantly different exposure history, develops obstructive airways disease, most commonly in the smaller bronchi, less than 2 mm. in diameter. The term chronic obstructive bronchitis is given to this clinical entity, which in the British literature makes up a major portion of those with chronic obstructive pulmonary disease (COPD). Mucopurulent bronchitis has been used to describe the presence of chronically purulent sputum but has little current value.

Bronchiectasis defines an entity in which local or more generalized destruction of the bronchial wall, usually secondary to infection, produces a dilated saccular change: such a change may be diagnosed by a bronchogram, but this is usually not necessary, as the principles of management are similar to those for chronic bronchitis.

Clinical Presentation

In terms of their dominant symptoms of cough and sputum, chronic bronchitis, simple and obstructive, and bronchiectasis represent a spectrum of disease states, both in severity and the frequency with which therapeutic intervention is required. In addition to the sputum production that characterizes all three conditions, hemoptysis and a variable amount of bronchospasm and resultant wheezing may be prominent during acute exacerbations. In bronchitis, hemoptysis is usually scanty, associated with particularly strenuous coughing episodes, and often accompanied by burning substernal chest pain. Patients with bronchiectasis are subject to greater quantities of hemoptysis, which intermittently is quite heavy.

Although wheezing is not a constant feature, bronchial edema and spasm caused by severe coughing paroxysms may produce a clinical picture that simulates the more readily reversible physiologic features of the patient with chronic asthma.

General Principles of Management

The history of patients with chronic bronchitis and bronchiectasis virtually always includes exposure to the chronic irritation of cigarettes or other airborne pollutants or both. In children and young adults, chronic cough and wheezing in the absence of respiratory infection is more typical of allergic disease than of chronic bronchitis. Recurrent episodes of acute bronchitis or upper respiratory infections that "settle in the chest" and persist longer than a few days are characteristic

histories provided by patients with mild disease and in the early years in those with airways obstruction. Rarely, the family history will disclose an increased incidence of obstructive disease and lead one to suspect an Alpha$_1$-antitrypsin deficiency. Similarly, young adults with a mild form of cystic fibrosis may present with symptoms of chronic cough and sputum in the absence of the more classic pulmonary and systemic findings usually associated with this disease. Childhood asthma, which has become subclinical during the teen years, may surface after years of smoking as a chronic bronchitis with a significant allergic component. Some authors, because of the cough and sputum that continue between acute asthma attacks, prefer the term chronic bronchitis with bronchospasm to describe this picture, which combines the features of both diseases. For the bronchitis component the principles of therapy, described as relief of infection and facilitation of good bronchial hygiene, are the same with or without bronchospasm. Avoidance of cigarettes and pollutant-filled environments is the first step in successful management of all forms of bronchitis and bronchiectasis.

Radiologic examination of the chest is usually normal in simple bronchitis and often also when physiologic evidence of obstruction is present. A "heavy" appearance of the bronchial markings, especially at the lung bases, may be present, or perihilar bronchi, when seen on end, may show an increase in the thickness of the wall. Localized fibrosis and cystic changes, associated with a decrease in surrounding lung volume, are characteristic of segmental or lobular bronchiectasis.

Because one may expect to manage patients with bronchitis and bronchiectasis over a period of many years, simple office spirometric studies serve as a valuable adjunct, both for diagnosis of airway obstruction and as an objective guide to the effectiveness of therapy. The forced vital capacity (FVC) and forced expiratory volume in the first second (FEV$_1$) require minimal equipment, can be performed on each visit, and provide both physician and patient with an objective guide by which to assess progress. Similarly, examination of the blood and sputum for the presence of eosinophils is helpful in determining the extent to which allergy may be playing a role in the individual patient. Greater than 300 eosinophils per cu. mm. of blood, or a predominance of eosinophils in the sputum (Hansel's stain) may indicate not only that allergy is present, but also that considerable reversibility of obstruction is possible with the use of bronchodilators.

Finally, all patients must be thoroughly educated concerning the pathology of their disease, the results of that pathology, and the rationale for the proposed treatment. Patient compliance with the specific aspects of management occurs in direct proportion to understanding of the patient concerning the purpose of the total management program. For example: the physician who demands that the patient stop smoking usually achieves less than one who takes the time to advise his patient about the specific effects of cigarette smoke on the bronchial tree. Successful management of chronic bronchial diseases can occur only when the educated patient is "actively" involved in therapy. Because tremendous variation exists from patient to patient and from time to time in the same patient, the specific recommendations listed here must be individualized. Sputum production or bronchospasm or both may dominate the picture in some patients, requiring more vigorous attention than in others. However, each major area—antibiotics, respiratory therapy, and bronchodilators—address the primary pathologic and clinical features of these diseases.

Treatment

Antibiotics. The use of antibiotics is determined by the nature of the sputum, its color, character, and quantity, rather than the identification of a specific causative organism. Most episodes of acute bronchitis that are superimposed on chronic bronchitis or bronchiectasis are viral in nature, and in the absence of radiographic evidence of pneumonia are not associated with a dominant organism or change in the usual flora of the sputum between episodes. Thus, sputum culture commonly produces growth of *Hemophilus influenzae* and *Streptococcus pneumoniae* in addition to the normal nasopharyngeal flora. Less often, in the presence of a parenchymal infiltrate the pneumococci predominate. Treatment, therefore, is based upon an increase in quantity and purulence of the sputum, associated commonly with decreased respiratory status, even in the absence of a specific causative organism. Hemoptysis, mild in bronchitis, and possibly more severe in bronchiectasis, frequently accompanies the other sputum changes and of itself warrants antibiotic therapy.

Ampicillin and tetracycline are the antibiotics of choice, both because of their broad spectrum of coverage and relatively minor (usually gastrointestinal) side effects. Doses of 250 or 500 mg. every six hours for 10 to 14 days are usually sufficient to bring the sputum to its preexacerbation status. When pneumococci dominate the sputum, penicillin may be used but should not be considered a first line drug for most exacerbations. Erythromycin may be used in place of ampicillin in patients who are allergic to penicillin.

Patients who have been educated concerning the nature of their disease and the specific bronch-

ial pathology are perfectly capable of determining their need to begin a course of antibiotic therapy. It is better to provide them with a prescription for either tetracycline or ampicillin, to be filled and started at the onset of an exacerbation, than for them to maintain a supply of either antibiotic at home. Tetracycline, especially, deteriorates after 6 months. Intermittent treatment courses based upon objective clinical evidence of sputum change coupled with a regular program of bronchial hygiene are recommended, rather than chronic long-term low-dose antibiotic therapy. Sterilization of the lower respiratory area is not possible by chronic antibiotic administration, which only encourages the growth of fungal and Pseudomonas infections. For the patient who is not capable of assessing exacerbations, a regularly scheduled antibiotic program may be used. Ampicillin or tetracycline is prescribed 1 week out of 4 or 6 as indicated. Newer sulfa preparations containing trimethoprim and sulfamethoxazole are well tolerated and may have a role in acute bronchial infections (see manufacturer's official directive before using). Four tablets per day are usually prescribed initially, followed by 1 or 2 tablets twice daily for the remainder of the 10 to 14 day treatment course.

Following a course of antibiotics, it is often possible to culture Pseudomonas from the sputum as the predominant organism. Rarely is it necessary to treat such a culture. Within days, the *H. influenzae* return and the usual bacterial flora in these patients is restored. Attempting to eradicate the Pseudomonas runs the risk of producing significant Candida infection or unnecessary drug side effects or both from the colistimethate or gentamicin (Garamycin), which are necessary to treat clinical Pseudomonas infections effectively. Aerosolization of antibiotics into the tracheobronchial tree is of little or no value, and should be avoided. Patients with serious infectious exacerbations that are accompanied by high fever, radiographic evidence of pneumonia, or significant arterial blood gas abnormalities should be hospitalized and treated with intravenous antibiotics, ampicillin, or one of the cephalothin group, in addition to supplemental oxygen and respiratory support, as necessary.

Respiratory Therapy. No patient with significant bronchitis or bronchiectasis can be successfully treated with antibiotics alone. A long-range program to facilitate the prompt and continuous removal of bronchial secretion must also be included. To be effective, such a program should be based upon education of the patient (and frequently his family also) by the physician, nurse, or respiratory therapist concerning the need to maintain good bronchial hygiene. Daily sputum production often requires daily postural drainage, especially before retiring and after arising. For many, postural drainage alone, 15 minutes twice each day, may be sufficient. Illustrated booklets are available to assist patient understanding of the principle of this procedure. Because the results of such drainage will vary from day to day and week to week, frequent reinforcement is usually necessary to ensure continued patient compliance. Those who understand the pathology of their disease and the rationale for a therapeutic approach that is both tedious and time consuming are more likely to be successful. When percussion is added to postural drainage additional benefit is achieved. Training of the patient's spouse or other family member requires little time, and has the additional advantage of involving a person close to the patient in the therapy of this chronic debilitating disease.

For patients with more severe obstructive disease who produce large quantities of sputum, the addition of daily mist inhalation, usually twice daily, further enhances the effectiveness of respiratory therapy. Small mist generators are available for a fraction of the cost of intermittent positive pressure breathing (IPPB) machines and are equally (or more) effective. No advantage has thus far been demonstrated for the addition of positive pressure, and its use is not recommended. The primary objective of mist treatment is to liquefy and facilitate sputum removal through subsequent percussion and drainage. Distilled water (15 ml. per treatment) is often sufficient when used alone. Because the coughing, which necessarily is a part of respiratory therapy, often increases airway resistance and bronchospasm, bronchodilators are often added to the mist solution. Five to 10 drops of isoproterenol (Isuprel), isoetherine, or terbutaline (0.25 mg.) has proved effective when used in this way. Alternatively, an inhalation of a measured dose bronchodilator before and after a mist and drainage treatment may accomplish sputum removal without producing persistent bronchospasm. The best argument for the importance of these measures in the overall treatment program is the improvement of the patient's symptoms, and those that make believers of skeptical patients are the increased sense of well-being, improvement in arterial oxygen tension, and reduced requirement for antibiotics to treat acute infectious exacerbations that occurs as a result of maintaining good bronchial hygiene.

Bronchodilators. Most patients with obstructive bronchitis and bronchiectasis and those with simple bronchitis during exacerbations have a degree of reversible spasm that accompanies their chronically infected bronchi. Thus, a clinical trial of both oral theophylline preparations and inhaled sympathomimetics is indicated. Aminophylline or one of its many variations is given 4 times daily, usually before meals and at bedtime, to a usual daily dose of 800 mg. Single drug therapy is preferred to drugs which contain ephedrine and a sedative in addition. Gastrointestinal side effects can usually be minimized by either decreasing dosage or varying the form of theophylline used. Toxic blood levels are seldom reached with 800 mg. per day. Longer acting sympathomimetics such as metaproterenol allow their usage on a regular schedule rather than the as-necessary basis which in the past had led to frequent inhaler abuse. When coupled with theophylline, and given as two inhalations four times daily, they contribute greatly to the relief of bronchospasm and removal of sputum. Rarely, especially during acute exacerbations, when bronchospasm may be prominent, short courses of steroids, usually not longer than 7 to 10 days may be beneficial. Usually, however, their use on a more chronic basis can and should be avoided.

Ancillary Measures. Because cigarette smoking is so intrinsically related to chronic cough and sputum, cessation should be strongly recommended. A sympathetic approach based upon patient understanding of the effects of smoking on the pathologic process is probably more effective than self-righteous indignation.

Maintenance of adequate hydration, especially during periods of warm dry weather seems obvious but warrants mention. Sputum consistency mirrors the status of body hydration in general and may be raised more effectively when positive fluid balance is maintained. During acute exacerbations patients are frequently dry and require reminders concerning the need for increased fluid intake. On a short-term basis the old standby, saturated solution of potassium iodide (SSKI), may be of some help in thinning secretions, but has little or no role in chronic administration. Uncomfortable iodine side effects are common. Cough preparations containing glycerol guaiacolate are generally of little help, and cough suppressants should be avoided. Mucolytic agents, enzymes, and detergents are of no value in chronic management and often induce bronchospasm.

Both influenza and the newly available pneumococcus vaccine are recommended for this patient group, in which both viral and bacterial infections are frequent and potentially life-threatening.

Surgical management of bronchomucosis is rarely indicated at the present time and is employed only for documented localized disease when medical management has been unsuccessful. In no case should excision be carried out without prior documentation through bronchography that disease does not exist in areas other than the special area in question.

PRIMARY LUNG CANCER

method of
DONALD L. PAULSON, M.D.
Dallas, Texas

Cancers of the lung and bronchus account for 10 per cent of all malignant neoplasms and about 80 per cent of all respiratory tract cancers. In men, bronchogenic carcinoma is the most common visceral cancer, accounting for 17 per cent of all malignancies; in women, it is the third most common cancer, only 3 per cent. The male-female ratio, which was 6.3:1 in 1950 to 1959, has steadily decreased to 5.3 in 1960 to 1964 and 4.2 in 1965 to 1969. Age-adjusted incidence rates show an increase in men from 15 per 100,000 in the 1940s to 63 per 100,000 in the 1960s, and in women from 3 per 100,000 to 10 per 100,000 in the 1960s. In the last 20 years, there has been a 2-fold increase in men and a 3-fold increase in women.

For all stages of the disease combined, the 3-year relative survival rate for males increased from 5 per cent in 1940 to 1949 to 10 per cent in 1965 to 1969; the corresponding rate for females increased from 10 per cent in 1940 to 1949 to 16 per cent in 1965 to 1969. The 5-, 10- and 15-year survival rates show a similar trend. The same trend is found in the localized and regionally involved cases.

One third of cancers of the lung and bronchus in women are diagnosed in those under 55 years of age; only one fifth of male patients are in this younger group. Women also have a better survival experience than men in all age categories for all stages combined, but the difference is small for patients over 65 years of age. The survival advantage for women is most apparent among patients with localized disease; there is little sex difference in survival rates among patients with regional spread of the disease or distant metastases.

Among both males and females, the natural history of carcinoma of the lung is such that diagnosis in a localized stage is possible in less than 20 per cent of all patients. Another 25 per cent have evidence of regional spread, and the remainder, or 55 per cent, have demonstrable remote metastases at the time of diagnosis.

Management

Resection, when applicable, is the generally accepted treatment of choice for bronchogenic carcinoma. There is evidence that resections done in the early localized stages of cancer of the lung do actually prolong life and improve physical and mental comfort, at least improving the quality of survival. In later stages, there is less opportunity for good results, simply due to greater extent of the disease. It must be admitted, however, that not all resections are beneficial and that prolonged survival depends mainly on the natural history of the lesion, its extent, and stage of involvement at the time of diagnosis. Efforts to increase the usefulness of surgery through extended operations on an unselective basis for the advanced stages of the disease have, in general, resulted in higher morbidity and mortality rates without benefit to survival time.

Since resection is possible in less than one third of patients with bronchogenic carcinoma, other modes of treatment, such as irradiation and chemotherapy, are applicable to many of the remaining patients. Judicious application of these techniques, singly or in combination, may induce quiescence in growth, relief of distressing symptoms, and, in some patients, prolongation of life. Preoperative irradiation employed on a selective basis is apparently of adjunctive value to attain better localization and improved results of resection. Some patients with limited regional spread may thereby become suitable candidates for definitive procedures.

The efficacy of treatment is usually gauged by survival time measured from the date of diagnosis. Prolonged survival is frequently attributed solely to the mode of therapy, although it may be improved simply by making the diagnosis at an earlier stage. It does not necessarily follow that treatment instituted after earlier diagnosis exerts a significant influence on the natural course of the disease. Although earlier diagnosis results in increased survival time, earlier treatment may have no effect on the eventual prognosis for cure.

Selection of Patients for Treatment

Optimal results of treatment can best be achieved at the present time through better selection of patients for specific modes of therapy, improved therapeutic techniques, and the use of adjunctive measures such as irradiation in combination with resection or chemotherapy with irradiation therapy.

Resectability is not synonymous with operability. A particular lesion may be locally resectable but be inoperable due to location, extent or stage of the disease, cell type, or evidence of distant metastases. Similarly, a given neoplasm may be assessed as operable but found anatomically nonresectable by exploratory thoracotomy. The presence of a cancer and the presumed ability to resect it must be balanced against the benefits to be reasonably expected, based on (1) knowledge of the natural history of the disease; (2) the stage, extent, and cell type of the lesion, its rate of growth, and duration of symptoms; (3) the presence or absence of metastases; and (4) the patient's age and cardiac and pulmonary functional status. Some lesions, such as small cell undifferentiated carcinoma or most lesions with mediastinal nodal involvement, are best treated by irradiation alone or in combination with chemotherapy.

Staging

Complete pretreatment evaluation of the patient permits classification of the lesion according to its extent and stage of lymph node involvement. Classification of the stage of bronchogenic carcinoma at the time of diagnosis facilitates the choice of treatment, provides important correlative information for survival and clarifies the results of treatment on an objective basis.

Although it is generally agreed that tumor invasion of regional lymph nodes is evidence of a more advanced stage of disease, much confusion remains both as to the significance of precise localization and the extent of tumor invasion. There are reports of relatively high 5-year survival rates with invaded intrathoracic nodes, but precise localization and extent of nodal involvement is often difficult to ascertain from these reports. In other series, with documented evidence of localization and extent of invasion of mediastinal nodes, the 5-year survival rate is without exception less than 10 per cent.

Regional lymph node involvement may be broadly classified as *hilar* or *mediastinal* in location. The hilar nodes may be divided into intersegmental and interlobar groups, including the lymphatic "sump" nodes. The mediastinal nodes can be divided into the anterior and posterior mediastinal groups, the tracheobronchial nodes, and the paratracheal nodes. The anterior nodes lie parallel to and anterior to the phrenic nerve and on the left side in close proximity to the origin of pulmonary artery and innominate veins. The posterior nodes are largely paraesophageal and are found in the inferior mediastinum in the pulmonary ligament. The tracheobronchial nodes constitute the most important group, since the lymphatic drainage of the lung is mainly proximal and since they are accessible for biopsy by mediastinoscopy. They are divided into inferior and superior groups. The inferior tracheobronchial nodes are situated in the angle of the bifurcation of the trachea and are also known as subcarinal nodes. The superior tracheobronchial nodes, right and left, are located in the lateral angle between the trachea and corresponding main bronchus. The paratracheal nodes are situated higher up in the superior mediastinum, anterolaterally to the trachea.

The surgical classification for carcinoma of the lung originally proposed by Salzer and modified by Nohl records (1) the extent of growth in the lung, (2) the stage of lymph node involvement, and (3) the presence or absence of pulmonary vein invasion (see Table 1). The factors of involvement of the visceral pleura and infiltration of neighboring structures as in "B" and "C" cases are frequently established by operation only, as is the case with vascular involvement. A high correlation, however, exists between survival after resection and the stage of lymph node involvement and the extent of tumor in the lung as well as venous

TABLE 1. Salzer's Classification (Modified)

EXTENT OF GROWTH

A = Growth confined to lung
B = Involvement of visceral pleura, including interlobar fissure
C = Infiltration of neighboring structures; for example, parietal pleura, chest wall, esophagus, pericardium, myocardium

LYMPH NODE INVOLVEMENT

0 = None
1 = Intersegmental nodes
2 = Interlobar or hilar nodes
3 = Mediastinal nodes
4 = Distal metastases; for example, supraclavicular nodes, liver metastases

VASCULAR INVOLVEMENT

V = Demonstrable invasion of intima of pulmonary veins

---

invasion. Salzer's classification is useful surgically but does not lend itself to precise staging in the usual sense preoperatively.

A similar classification known as the TNM system has been developed and is used internationally for clinical staging of cancer primary at any site in the body. Based on TNM principles, the Lung Task Force of the American Joint Committee for Cancer Staging and End Results Reporting has developed a classification for the clinical and surgical staging of lung cancer (see Tables 2 and 3). Various additions and modifications of this system have been proposed in the interest of greater precision in staging, based on location (central or peripheral), extent and size of the primary tumor, and location and type of nodal involvement.

Within the T category, tumors located centrally have been defined according to proximal spread in the bronchial tree, and categories of carcinoma of the peripheral type based on size have been added. Mediastinal nodal involvement has been divided according to location (tracheobronchial, paratracheal, ipsilateral, or contralateral) and character (intranodal or paranodal).

Clinical pretreatment staging of bronchogenic carcinoma can be attained with a high degree of accuracy by means of x-rays (tomograms and pulmonary angiography), bronchoscopy, mediastinoscopy, and scanning techniques. Clinical staging is confirmed and added to by careful, precise surgical staging. In various series, preoperative classification of the anatomic extent of the disease has been confirmed in more than 80 per cent of resected cases. Surgical staging is more accurate than clinical staging, but clinical staging, completely performed before treatment, will suffice for clarifying and comparing the results of radiotherapy on an objective basis.

TABLE 2.   **The Definitions of T, N, and M Categories for Carcinoma of the Lung**

T PRIMARY TUMORS

T0	No evidence of primary tumor
TX	Tumor proven by the presence of malignant cells in bronchopulmonary secretions but not visualized roentgenographically or bronchoscopically
TIS	Carcinoma in situ
T1	A tumor that is 3.0 cm. or less in greatest diameter, surrounded by lung or visceral pleura and without evidence of invasion proximal to a lobar bronchus at bronchoscopy
T2	A tumor more than 3.0 cm. in greatest diameter, or a tumor of any size which invades the visceral pleura or with its associated atelectasis or obstructive pneumonitis, extends to the hilar region. At bronchoscopy the proximal extent of demonstrable tumor must be within a lobar bronchus or at least 2.0 cm. distal to the carina. Any associated atelectasis or obstructive pneumonitis must involve less than an entire lung, and there must be no pleural effusion
T3	A tumor of any size with direct extension into an adjacent structure such as the chest wall, the diaphragm, or the mediastinum and its contents; or bronchoscopically demonstrated to involve a main bronchus less than 2.0 cm. distal to the carina; any tumor associated with atelectasis or obstructive pneumonitis of an entire lung or pleural effusion

N REGIONAL LYMPH NODES

N0	No demonstrable metastasis to regional lymph nodes
N1	Metastasis to lymph nodes in the peribronchial and/or the ipsilateral hilar region (including direct extension)
N2	Metastasis to lymph nodes in the mediastinum

M DISTANT METASTASIS

M0	No distant metastasis
M1	Distant metastasis such as in scalene, cervical, or contralateral hilar lymph nodes, contralateral lung, brain, bones, liver

Each case must be assigned the highest category of T, N, and M which describes the full extent of disease in that case.

Results of Clinical and Surgical Staging

Five-year survival for patients after resection with surgical stage I disease is in the range of 40 to 50 per cent; Stage II, 25 to 30 per cent; and Stage III, 10 to 15 per cent. For patients with limited extent of tumor and less than 3 cm. in diameter and no lymph node involvement (T1 N0 M0), survival at 5 years is in the range of 40 to 60 per cent. Five-year survival in resected Stage III cases with positive mediastinal nodes is less than 10 per cent, with negative mediastinal nodes 25 per cent.

Dominant factors in survival are the extent of the disease and the stage of nodal involvement. The greater the extent of the lesion, the higher is the incidence of positive mediastinal nodes. No patients with direct extension to the adjoining structures, such as chest wall, pericardium, or myocardium, and mediastinal nodal involvement (T3 N2) have survived much more than 1 year. Extended resections for T3 cases may be justified in patients with no nodal involvement.

Mediastinoscopy

In the case of bronchogenic carcinoma, a unique situation is afforded for the clinical classification of the stage of regional nodal involvement by the routine use of mediastinoscopy. The most important mediastinal lymph node groups are accessible, and the presence of metastases can be confirmed by biopsy. In addition, careful

TABLE 3.   **Stage Grouping in Carcinoma of the Lung**

Occult Carcinoma	
TX N0 M0	An occult carcinoma with bronchopulmonary secretions containing malignant cells but without other evidence of the primary tumor or evidence of metastasis to the regional lymph nodes or distant metastasis.
Stage 1	
TIS N0 M0	Carcinoma in situ
T1 N0 M0	A tumor that can be classified T1 without any metastasis or with metastasis to the lymph nodes in the
T1 N1 M0	ipsilateral hilar region only, or a tumor that can be classified T2 without any metastasis to nodes or dis-
T2 N0 M0	tant metastasis.
	Note: TX, N1, M0 and T0 N1 M0 are also theoretically possible, but such a clinical diagnosis would be difficult if not impossible to make. If such a diagnosis is made, it should be included in Stage 1.
Stage II	
T2 N1 M0	A tumor classified as T2 with metastasis to the lymph nodes in the ipsilateral hilar region only
Stage III	
T3 with any N or M	Any tumor more extensive than T2, or any tumor with metastasis to the lymph nodes in the medi-
N2 with T or M	astinum, or with distant metastasis
M1 with any T or N	

mediastinal exploration will determine the location, extent of involvement, and histologic type of tumor tissue with a high degree of accuracy.

Mediastinoscopy is therefore mandatory for clinical staging and pretreatment evaluation of the anatomic extent of the disease in bronchogenic carcinoma. It may be performed either through a cervical incision for the evaluation of superior mediastinal nodes or by an anterior mediastinotomy through an extrapleural approach in the second interspace for subaortic lymph nodes.

Information regarding regional nodal involvement provides important correlative information for survival and emphasizes the concept of careful selection of patients for treatment. For patients with no nodal involvement observed, survival at 5 years after resection is in the range of 45 per cent; for those with hilar nodes involved, 30 per cent; but less than 10 per cent for those with mediastinal nodes involved.

Accurate localization and the extent of nodal involvement are of significance to prognosis. Ipsilateral or contralateral spread and tracheobronchial or paratracheal nodal involvement must be distinguished. The extent of nodal involvement is defined as being intranodal or perinodal. High paratracheal or contralateral nodal metastases portend a poor prognosis, as does perinodal involvement. Perinodal involvement predominates in all histologic types, and survival after resection is limited to 2 years. Operative mortality is four times that of patients with intranodal spread. Unfortunately, intranodal involvement has been found in only 15 per cent of patients with mediastinal nodal involvement.

In patients with ipsilateral intranodal involvement, 3-year survival rates as high as 40 per cent may be obtained by resection. If patients with contralateral spread or perinodal growth be excluded from operation, there remains only 12 per cent located ipsilaterally and having only intranodal growth. Selection of these patients for resection is justifiable and constitutes the only instances of long-term survival in patients with mediastinal nodal involvement.

There is also a highly significant association between histologic type and mediastinal node metastases. In both small cell undifferentiated carcinomas and adenocarcinomas, a much higher percentage of mediastinal nodal involvement is found than in epidermoid carcinoma, providing important information regarding both diagnosis of histologic type and operability. No significant differences have been found in survival at 5 years between squamous cell carcinoma, adenocarcinomas, or other undifferentiated carcinomas (exclusive of small cell undifferentiated types) in patients with negative lymph nodes. However, mediastinal nodal involvement in a patient with squamous cell carcinoma does not carry as serious a prognosis as it does in a patient with undifferentiated carcinoma or adenocarcinoma. Resection may be done in patients who have squamous cell carcinoma and ipsilateral, intranodal involvement. In the case of undifferentiated carcinoma or adenocarcinoma, mediastinal nodal involvement is significant of distant dissemination.

By means of mediastinoscopy, histologic proof is obtained in 45 per cent of all patients and in at least 75 per cent of those with small cell undifferentiated carcinomas. Positive nodes are found in a significant number of patients in spite of negative x-ray studies and in 1 of 3 patients with lesions otherwise considered operable. A 90 per cent correlation between a negative exploration and resectability has been found in most reported series, and the resectability rate of patients operated on raised from an average of 65 per cent to better than 90 per cent. The morbidity of mediastinoscopy is less than 3 per cent and the mortality less than 1 per cent, in contrast to a mortality of 4 to 12 per cent for indiscriminate, unwarranted, and harmful standard exploratory thoracotomies for nonresectable lesions, performed in 35 per cent of patients otherwise presumed to have an operable lesion.

Operation

The concept of selectivity for operation, based on complete pretreatment evaluation of the patient, has resulted in improved resection rates and survival figures, with a low surgical mortality and increased surgical salvage in the long run. Resection rates improved from 65 to 90 per cent and the percentage of lobectomies rose as high as 74 per cent. Increased resection rates, with increased proportions of lobectomies, lessen the overall mortality risks of operation and improve the quality of survival with greater physical and mental comfort to the patient.

Lobectomy with complete clearance of the areas of lymphatic drainage has become the operation of choice for peripheral or localized hilar lesions with or without minimal involvement of the hilar nodes. There is no significant difference in long-term survival rates for patients with central or peripheral lesions either with no nodes involved or for those with nodal involvement as well. Differences in mortality, morbidity, and quality of survival favor the lesser resection and make lobectomy attractive where it is applicable, Cell type, location, extent, and stage of involvement, together with the patient's age and cardiac and pulmonary function, are the determining factors in the choice between lobectomy and pneumonectomy. Better survival rates for lobectomy in large part reflect better localization of the lesions resected in many cases, and in this sense are not comparable to the results obtained following pneumonectomy for the more extensive carcinomas. However, comparison of different series in which varying proportions of lobectomies were done indicates at least as good or better survival associated with a high proportion of lobectomies in contrast to a series composed largely of pneumonectomies.

Lobectomy is justifiable selectively for hilar or centrally located lesions, provided the lymphatic "sump" in the hilum is excised. One third of squamous cell carcinomas reveal either no lymphatic involvement or only infiltration of the intrapulmonary nodes. Bronchial involvement far beyond the point of palpable tumor is unlikely, and submucosal spread, when it occurs, is usually associated with lymphatic nodal involvement. A margin of 1.5 to 2 cm. beyond visible carcinoma constitutes adequate clearance for bronchial wall extension as well as most instances of epithelial metaplasia.

Lobectomy in combination with a bronchoplasty, such as sleeve resection of the main bronchus to permit wider excision of the major bronchi, may be done deliberately as an adequate procedure in selected cases with or without preoperative irradiation. Survival rates for localized stage I cases are 55 per cent at 5 years.

Pneumonectomy is indicated to achieve complete clearance for patients in whom the interlobar or hilar nodes are involved. Lobectomy under these circumstances yields poorer survival than pneumonectomy. The deciding factors of poor pulmonary or cardiac reserve and age of the patient, however, may dictate the lesser resection in spite of the stage of lymph node involvement. Under these circumstances, preoperative irradiation combined with sleeve resection of the main bronchus and radical lobectomy in selected cases is the procedure of choice as a compromise with pneumonectomy. Five-year survival of 18 per cent has been reported in such patients.

In general, pneumonectomy in patients over the age of 70 is to be avoided, since long-term survival is poor. Pulmonary arteriography is useful in centrally located lesions, particularly for those involving the upper lobes to determine operability and the extent of resection necessary for complete removal. This information may be crucial for patients who can not tolerate a pneumonectomy and in those over the age of 70. Under these circumstances, irradiation therapy may yield at least as good survival time without the morbidity and mortality of operation.

Extended resections on a selective basis are justified, particularly with the use of preoperative irradiation. Resections of extensions to the chest wall, pericardium, blood vessels, or heart may be done in individual patients in the hope of prolonged survival. The best results of extended resections are obtained in those patients without mediastinal nodal involvement. In those with nodal involvement, survival over 1 year is rare. Indiscriminate extended surgery, often in the presence of mediastinal nodal involvement, results only in high morbidity and mortality without benefit to survival time.

Radiation Therapy

Irradiation in the treatment of bronchogenic carcinoma may be used for (1) inoperable and poor risk patients, (2) operable lesions in patients who refuse surgery, (3) palliative therapy for metastases (brain or bone), and (4) an adjunct to surgery either postoperatively (immediate for residual carcinoma, late for recurrence) or preoperatively to attain better localization and sterilization of the lymphatics.

Radiotherapy is subject to limitations of extent and stage of disease similar to surgery, but better survival time with lower mortality is probably obtained in patients with comparably extensive disease. Irradiation results in approximately 5 per cent survival at 5 years for the inoperable and 10 per cent for nonresectable lesions found by exploratory thoracotomy. Indiscriminate extended resections for Stage III cases, on the other hand, result in a high surgical mortality (over 20 per cent), only about 15 per cent survival at 1 year, and few long-term survivors, a negative surgical salvage.

Postoperative radiotherapy for carcinoma of the lung has been used with the aim of improving survival by sterilization of regionally involved areas inaccessible or invisible to the surgeon. Generally, it has been reserved for known residual or recurrent carcinoma. Although its value has not been proved, it appears to be of palliative advantage for individual patients in apparent prolongation of life and prevention or control of distressing symptoms of pain, cough, hemoptysis, or venous obstruction. Since the prognosis in advanced stages of involvement is poor due to associated occult distal metastases, any increment to survival would be small, whatever the mode of local treatment.

Recently, postresection radiotherapy has been used for all stages of the disease, particularly for those with mediastinal nodal involvement. The apparent improved survival time may be due to selection of favorable cases. It is not of proved value.

Preoperative irradiation is defined as a means of preparation of the patient with a resectable lesion for surgery by modification of the extent of disease through moderate dosage therapy to facilitate complete resection without increase in morbidity or mortality. Aims of presurgical therapy are (1) to limit extent of the tumor by destruction of cancer cells at the periphery, (2) to produce sclerosis of the vascular bed and sterilize the lymphatics, and (3) to damage the viability of the remaining malignant cells to decrease their ability to implant and proliferate if disseminated or left behind at operation.

The theoretical advantages of preoperative over postoperative irradiation depend on the treatment being administered prior to surgical interference with its attendant risks of dissemination, implantation, or inflammation, together with violation of the vascular bed of the tumor and its lymphatics, resulting in reduced oxygen tension and decreased radiosensitivity.

Carcinoma spreads by direct extension, lymphatic involvement, vascular invasion, dissemination, and implantation. Disappointments in operative treatment, although most commonly attributed to unappreciated occult distal metastases occurring prior to diagnosis, may result from dissemination, implantation or incomplete resection of all carcinoma at operation.

The combination of surgery with radiation probably compounds the inherent risks of these modes of therapy individually. Although optimal dosimetry and method of delivery are not established for bronchogenic carcinoma, in practice the dose administered will be that which presumably results in maximal increase in patient survival with minimal morbidity and mortality.

Bronchogenic carcinomas in the superior pulmonary sulcus produce a characteristic clinical syndrome described by Pancoast. Although locally invasive of adjacent nerve roots, the sympathetic chain, ribs, and vertebrae, they are frequently low-grade epidermoid or large cell undifferentiated carcinomas that do not metastasize distally until late. In the past, lesions in this location have been generally considered inaccessible to complete resection and resistant to irradiation therapy. Previous experience of treatment was poor, whether the patient received no treatment, irradiation alone, or surgery followed by irradiation.

Preoperative irradiation in moderate dosage (3000 rads in 10 fractions over 12 elapsed days) combined with extended resections for bronchogenic carcinoma in the superior pulmonary sulcus (at a 3- to 4-week interval) has been used for 21 years, with low morbidity and an operative mortality of 3 per cent in 65 cases. Eighteen of 54 patients (33 per cent) survived more than 5 years and 10 of 35 (29 per cent) more than 10 years after completion of the combined treatment. None of 15 patients with hilar or mediastinal nodal in-

volvement (Stage III T3 N2) survived much more than 1 year, whereas 21 of 44 patients with no nodal involvement (Stage III N0) survived more than 3 years. Stage of nodal involvement and the pathologic effects of irradiation at the level of the chest wall were the dominant factors in survival.

The results of combined preoperative irradiation and resection compared to primary resection in patients with central lesions similar in cell type, extent, and stage of disease reveal improved survival for the preoperative radiotherapy group in the relatively localized lesions but no significant differences for the more extensive lesions. Complications are more frequent in the prior radiotherapy group. In general, morbidity and mortality are proportionate to the stage of disease and the extent of resection necessary.

Improved survival is obtained with preoperative irradiation for the relatively localized epidermoid carcinomas of the type for which sleeve resection of the bronchus in combination with lobectomy can be done. Moderate dosage of 3000 rads in 3 weeks or 4000 rads in 4 weeks, with a 3- to 4-week interval between completion of irradiation and surgery, has increased survival to 76 per cent at 5 years, compared to 44 per cent for those treated by resection only. There was no increase in morbidity or mortality, and the radiation therapy appeared to be effective in the prevention of recurrence of the carcinoma locally.

The results of published individual and collaborative studies concerned with preoperative irradiation of carcinoma of the lung on an unselective basis confirm the poor prognosis in advanced stages of involvement and reveal no significant differences in survival or better survival in the nonirradiated group. Morbidity and mortality were higher with preoperative irradiation in the dosage used (over 4000 rads). Similar limitations of extent and stage of disease apply equally to radiation therapy and surgery.

At present, preoperative irradiation in preparation for radical or extended resection appears to be of value in moderate dosage on a selective basis for (1) extreme peripheral lesions with chest wall involvement, including carcinomas in the superior pulmonary sulcus; (2) localized lesions, particularly to facilitate a lesser resection in combination with bronchoplasty; (3) those lesions with regional hilar node involvement otherwise considered resectable; and (4) any case in which an extended resection is contemplated, provided there is no mediastinal nodal involvement.

Chemotherapy

At present, chemotherapy is of palliative value for patients with disseminated disease. Patients with disseminated disease have benefited by treatment with alkylating agents, and median survival time improved to 36 weeks in those with limited disease of various histologic types.

In patients with superior vena caval obstruction, the combination of chemotherapy (alkylating agents) and radiotherapy is of proven palliative value.

Encouraging results of chemotherapy for small cell undifferentiated carcinoma have been reported using various combinations of chemotherapeutic agents. The response rate of cyclophosphamide-vincristine combined with radiation therapy was 71 per cent (36 per cent complete responses). Eighteen per cent of patients with limited disease survived 3 years with no recurrence of disease. Studies of various combinations of chemotherapy and radiotherapy are continuing for other histologic types as well as small cell carcinomas.

Steroids are of value in terminal cases, producing subjective improvement. The combination of steroids and chemotherapy is of palliative value in patients with diffuse bronchio-alveolar carcinoma and those cases of diffuse lymphatic spread.

The combination of chemotherapy and surgery has been studied and reported to be of no benefit, with increased morbidity and adverse effects on survival.

COCCIDIOIDOMYCOSIS

method of
JOHN F. BROWN, JR., M.D.
Los Angeles, California

Introduction

Coccidioidomycosis is best known as an endemic fungal disease of southwestern United States and northern Mexico. On return to their homes, some of the many nonimmune tourists may develop coccidioidal disease. With the increased use of immunosuppressive measures and of organ transplantation, old coccidioidal infections may be reactivated long after and far removed from the patient's stay in the endemic area. Only one third of all infected patients are ill enough to see a physician. Less than 1.0 per cent of infected persons develop disseminated disease. Severe infection or disseminated infection is more

likely to occur in the very young and in the elderly debilitated individual, among nonwhites, among males, and among pregnant females.

General Therapy

Usually the primary coccidioidal infection is pulmonary. Often the healing is rapid and complete. Residual cavities or granulomas may require excision. Unless the surrounding lung is contaminated by the operative procedure amphotericin B is rarely required.

1. Patients do not require isolation procedures.

2. Bed rest is needed only during symptomatic illness.

3. Symptomatic relief should be given for aches, pains, and cough.

4. Corticosteroids rarely are required for the allergic manifestations.

Specific Therapy

Amphotericin B is the drug of choice. It is required for the following conditions.

Primary Pulmonary Coccidioidal Disease. 1. Infants and debilitated elderly patients.

2. Severe pneumonias with high complement fixation titers especially in nonwhites, pregnant women, diabetics, and patients with immunosuppressive diseases or receiving immunosuppressive therapy.

3. Persistent hilar or mediastinal adenopathy after pneumonia clears.

4. Amphotericin B coverage prior to and after thoracic surgery; during an acute pulmonary infection, extensive pulmonary involvement, postoperative complications, and repeat surgery.

Disseminated Disease. Intravenous amphotericin B therapy is necessary irrespective of low antibody titers or absence of pulmonary lesion.

1. *Skin and lymph nodes:* if draining lesions present add local therapy with use of 10 per cent amphotericin B solution.

2. *Bones and joints:* currettage, sequestrectomy, and synovectomy plus local irrigation with 10 per cent amphotericin B solution.*

3. *Viscera and genitourinary tract:* only intravenous therapy unless abscesses present requiring drainage.

4. *Meninges:* Local therapy required, usually given intracisternally.* Less often given intraventricularly via Ommaya reservoir or hyperbaric glucose administration via lumbar puncture.

---

*This use of amphotericin B is not listed in the manufacturer's official directive.

Methyl prednisolone may be added to the solution to minimize amphotericin-induced arachnoiditis.

Administration of Amphotericin B

Preparation. Add 10 ml. of distilled water (no preservatives) to 50 mg. vial. Add the diluted amphotericin B to 5 per cent dextrose in water (incompatible in saline) to make a final concentration of 0.1 mg. per ml. Mixture does not need protection from light during administration.

Premedication is usually required to prevent the acute adverse effects (fever, chills, nausea, vomiting, headaches, anxiety) of amphotericin B. Diphenhydramine (50 mg.) and prochlorperazine (10 mg.) are given orally or intramuscularly as well as oral aspirin 30 minutes prior to infusion. If the preceding is not effective, oral or intramuscular corticosteroids may be added to the premedication. One of the most important aspects of therapy is to keep the patient fully informed as to the state of his disease, changes in therapy, and current results of the therapy.

Dosage. Initial dose is 10 mg. and increased 10 mg. each day until the usual maximum dose of 50 mg. is reached. Some patients may tolerate an individual dose of 1 mg. per kg. After the maximum individual dose is reached, it is given every other day. Most patients tolerate the amphotericin B better if the dose is given within a 1 hour rather than over a 4-hour period (see manufacturer's official directive).

Total dose is determined by the clinical condition of the patient. Usually 2 grams are sufficient. In some patients 1 gram may be adequate.

Monitor the treatment with complete blood count (CBC) urinalysis, serum electrolytes particularly potassium, creatinine clearance, blood urea nitrogen (BUN), serum proteins, and Coombs' test. Most patients develop decreased renal function and a normochromic, normocytic anemia. Reduction of the daily dose or the frequency of treatment or both usually minimizes the toxic effects of amphotericin. During the treatment period oral potassium supplement usually prevents hypokalemia. Blood transfusions are given only for occasional severe anemia.

Prognosis. When the treatment has been individualized as to careful supportive therapy as well as closely supervised amphotericin B therapy, the mortality of nonmeningeal disseminated coccidioidal disease has dropped to 10 per cent. The mortality of coccidioidal meningitis is 40 per cent.

New Therapies. Miconazole is the most extensively studied new antifungal drug. Results of transfer factor immunotherapy make it desirous that these investigational studies be continued.

HISTOPLASMOSIS
method of
HAROLD G. MUCHMORE, M.D.
Oklahoma City, Oklahoma

Histoplasmosis is a common fungal infection that has worldwide distribution. Human and animal infections follow inhalation of small spores (microconidia) produced by the soil phase of a dimorphic fungus that has long been called *Histoplasma capsulatum*. The characteristic tuberculate chlamydospore (macroconidium) that aids in identifying this fungus is not the infectious particle. Recently, the perfect (sexual) form of this fungus has been described, and it has been identified as a heterothallic ascomycete. However, it is not likely that its new name (*Emmonsiella capsulata*) will achieve rapid clinical popularity.

The fungus grows in soil whose nitrogen content is enriched with animal droppings, especially of birds and bats. Many simultaneous group infection episodes have been described that resulted from disturbing soil under bird roosting sites and in bat caves. In the United States, human infections, as measured by skin test reactivity, are most frequent in the vast Mississippi River drainage area, particularly along the Ohio-Mississippi area where more than 90 per cent of young adults may be skin reactors. Histoplasmosis is a "place" disease, showing wide variation in its occurrence even in apparently suitable sites.

Following inhalation into the lung and phagocytosis by macrophages, the fungal spores transform into small (2 to 5 microns) yeast cells whose single buds exhibit a narrow neck (bud base). Dissemination throughout the body occurs early and foci of infection may be established in almost any organ, especially lymph nodes, liver, spleen, and adrenals. The characteristic tissue response to this infection is granuloma formation, complete with giant cells. Because of the toxicity of amphotericin B, a firm diagnosis should be established, if possible, before therapy is instituted. Preferably the fungus should be recovered on culture and identified in the laboratory prior to therapy. In tissue the yeast cells may be difficult to see, requiring staining of the polysaccharides in the cell wall with silver (Gomori method) or the Schiff reagent (PAS). Immunofluorescence on tissue sections may be used to identify the yeast in tissue if it fails to grow in culture.

Clinical Forms of the Disease

Asymptomatic Primary Histoplasmosis. This is the usual presenting form of this infection, and the patient will show only a reactive skin test and perhaps single or multiple calcifications on the chest x-ray film. No treatment is needed.

Symptomatic Primary Histoplasmosis. The incubation period following inhalation of *Histoplasma* spores is short (1 to 2 weeks), and the severity of the illness will vary in proportion to how heavy the exposure. Onset is typically rapid, and the illness is characterized by dry cough, dyspnea, and pleuritic chest pains. There may be cyanosis, fever, headache, malaise, night sweats, and weight loss. Chest x-rays may show a variety of lung infiltrates and hilar lymph node enlargement. The fungus may be recovered from sputum during the acute illness. The duration of symptoms is usually short (1 to 2 weeks), but convalescence may be slow with recurrent fever and fatigability. Almost all patients with this form of histoplasmosis recover spontaneously, and only rarely will any of this group require amphotericin B.

Acute Reinfection Pulmonary Histoplasmosis. Otherwise healthy persons previously infected with *Histoplasma* may exhibit an acute febrile illness after inhaling the microconidia subsequent to their primary infection. This acute illness of widely varying severity begins abruptly 7 to 10 days after exposure and is a hypersensitivity pneumonitis. In severe cases a short course of steroids, given simultaneously with amphotericin B, will quickly reduce symptoms and speed recovery. It is emphasized that patients of this group who require such treatment are rare.

Chronic Pulmonary Histoplasmosis. This is the most frequent clinical form of histoplasmosis and, as it presents, is indistinguishable from pulmonary tuberculosis and indeed, the two may occur together. The variable symptomatology is that of chronic pulmonary infection, and the patient may have dyspnea, weight loss, fever, and hemoptysis. The chest roentgenogram may show fibronodular or cavitary lung disease.

The published results of the Veterans Administration Armed Forces Fungus Study Group show clearly that chronic pulmonary histoplasmosis should be treated and that progression of the disease is usually stopped by amphotericin B. The total dose of amphotericin B required in these patients ranges from 500 to 2500 mg. The role of lung resection in chronic cavitary pulmonary histoplasmosis is not so clear. If resection is to be performed, then amphotericin B administered afterward will reduce the frequency of relapses.

Surgery may also be required to differentiate a histoplasmoma from a lung neoplasm. Histoplasmomas present as solid pulmonary nodules, often solitary and of varying size. Patients with such nodules usually have negative sputum cultures, and may have negative serologic tests. The resected lesion should be cultured, but this too may be negative. Tissue sections, with the stains noted above, may show only the empty cell walls of the apparently defunct yeast. Identification by immunofluorescence is possible in such cases.

Disseminated Histoplasmosis. Early dissemination presumably occurs subclinically in most if not all patients at the time of initial infection. This is usually a benign process that is recognized incidental to discovery of a calcified extrapulmonary focus, and treatment is seldom required.

Clinically recognizable disseminated histoplasmosis is a serious process, requiring therapy. In children this form may exhibit lymphadenopathy, hepatosplenomegaly, and bone marrow involvement. The disease has been confused with leukemia and lymphoma, and vice versa.

Adults with disseminated histoplasmosis usually have hepatosplenomegaly, anemia, and weight loss. Mucocutaneous lesions are frequent and when present are helpful in establishing the diagnosis, since these ulcerations are usually teeming with the yeast cells that can be readily demonstrated microscopically in touch preparations, scrapings, or biopsy, as well as be recovered in cultures. The mucosa of the small bowel may have similar lesions. The adrenals are frequently involved, and the patient may present with adrenal insufficiency. Adrenal function tests should be obtained in all patients and repeated as indicated. Adrenal histoplasmosis may respond poorly to treatment. Histoplasmal meningitis occurs and may require some form of localized amphotericin B therapy such as intrathecal instillation, or the use of the Ommaya reservoir (the use of amphotericin B intrathecally is not listed in the manufacturer's official directive).

Treatment

Amphotericin B is the drug of choice in the treatment of histoplasmosis. This drug is very poorly soluble and for practical purposes is not absorbed from the gut. It is supplied as a mixture with sodium desoxycholate, which serves to disperse the amphotericin B as a crystalloid suspension when added to 5 per cent glucose in water. Mixing with saline or acidic solutions may produce a cloudy dispersion or a precipitate, and these are unsatisfactory for patient administration. In 5 per cent glucose in water the drug is stable at room temperature and need not be protected from light. Ordinarily, the drug is administered the same day it is added to the glucose solution. Once mixed, the final infusion mixture should be used, and any residual amount should be discarded.

The drug is supplied in vials containing 50 mg. of amphotericin B as a dry powder. Add 10 ml. of sterile water (preservative-free) or 5 per cent glucose in water and shake until the liquid is clear. This liquid, which contains 5 mg. per ml., is added to 5 per cent glucose in water, to achieve a final concentration for infusion of 0.1 mg. per ml. In other words the entire 50 mg. content of the original vial would be added to 500 ml. of 5 per cent glucose in water. However, when lesser amounts are to be administered, such as at the beginning of therapy, smaller volumes of the infusion concentration can be mixed.

Ordinarily, I begin with a 10 mg. dose on the first day of therapy, and increase the dose each day, so that 10, 20, 30, 40, and 50 mg. are given on successive days. When the 50 mg. dosage is reached, it is continued on Monday, Wednesday, and Friday. The 50 mg. dosage given 3 times each week is adequate for treating most adult patients, but some, particularly those weighing over 70 kg., may require larger doses. The usual upper dosage limit is 1 mg. per kg. for any one dose, but larger amounts have been given. Some patients may not tolerate the 50 mg. dosage, or the 1 mg. per kg. dosage. Children usually do tolerate the 1 mg. per kg. dosage.

Amphotericin B is given intravenously through a carefully placed scalp vein needle. Vein rotation and alternating arms will help reduce the incidence of local reactions. Care must be taken to avoid interfering with local blood flow, resulting in drug stasis and increased incidence of phlebitis. Constrictive bandages, tight clothing, and venous obstruction by arm or body position should be avoided. Satisfactory needle placement is determined with a glucose-in-water infusion before switching to the amphotericin B. Flow rates will vary, but usually the infusion of 50 mg. in 500 ml. can be completed in less than 2 hours. Cardiac patients may require slower infusion rates. These infusions may be given on an out-patient basis, particularly after the patient's tolerance to the drug has been established. Consistent with the patient's other health problems, I prefer to administer the drug on an out-patient basis if at all possible. My routine then is to give the drug on Monday, Wednesday, and Friday after first obtaining any necessary laboratory work, and allow the patient to go home on completion of the infusion. Obviously, seriously ill patients are treated in the hospital and their dosage schedules adjusted individually.

Amphotericin B is a toxic drug and often causes nausea and vomiting, fever, shaking chills, and sometimes deep, aching bone pain. These manifestations vary widely among patients. Fortunately, as treatment continues these reactions usually decrease in frequency but may recur unexpectedly with any individual dose. The reactions may be reduced or eliminated by slower infusion or by premedication. A variety of premedication drugs have been recommended, including sedatives, tranquilizers, antihistamines, and steroids, as well as aspirin. In my experience aspirin one half hour before the infusion is generally the most useful and does not interfere with administration

of the infusion on an out-patient basis. Amphotericin B depresses renal function, both glomerular and tubular, and results in azotemia with elevated serum creatinine and urea concentrations. Renal function improves after amphotericin B is discontinued but does not return completely to pretherapy values. Patients who already have reduced renal function will require downward adjustment of amphotericin B schedules. Anemia is also a usual result of amphotericin B therapy. Bone marrow activity is depressed, and there is interference with reincorporation of red cell iron into hemoglobin. Transfusion is only seldom required. Depression of white cell production is rare but may occur. Liver toxicity is not frequent but also occurs with transaminase and other enzyme elevations. Kaliuresis occurs in all patients, and prophylactic oral potassium is indicated in virtually every patient. The serum potassium values may not reflect this potassium loss.

The degree and variety of amphotericin B toxicity requires monitoring, and this is accomplished by blood chemistries (profile 18), a complete blood count (with differential), and a urinalysis, looking particularly for white cells and protein. These are repeated at least once each week. Usually, the derangements observed will stabilize on some constant dosage of amphotericin B, and treatment can continue at that rate. However, steadily rising (or falling) values for the creatinine, blood urea nitrogen (BUN), hemoglobin, or serum enzymes is an indication that therapy may have to be reduced or interrupted. Despite this impressive list of toxicities, most patients improve during the course of amphotericin B therapy, and the appearance of a toxic manifestation itself is not necessarily an indication to interrupt therapy. The extensive and impressive toxicity emphasizes the need for a well-established diagnosis before therapy is begun, as the physician is then less likely to interrupt therapy as the toxicity appears.

Most patients with histoplasmosis will respond to amphotericin B, and a total dose in the vicinity of 2.0 grams is usually adequate. The total amount each patient receives is often governed by the extent of clinical improvement and the degree of toxicity encountered. Studies on other drugs have not progressed far enough to allow any clear recommendations. Included in this group are the methylester of amphotericin B, rifampin, and miconazole and its congeners and transfer factor. A more satisfactory drug would be desirable, but despite its toxicity, amphotericin B has remained the drug of choice for histoplasmosis and other deep mycoses throughout the past 20 years.

NORTH AMERICAN BLASTOMYCOSIS

method of
JOHN F. BUSEY, M.D.
Jackson, Mississippi

Despite the geographical connotation of its name, North American blastomycosis is not confined to the North American continent but has occasionally been found in Africa and Central America. Most cases recognized are from the Mississippi-Ohio River Valley and mid-Atlantic states in the United States and from several Canadian provinces. Migration from any of these endemic areas accounts for many of the cases found elsewhere. Following migration, the manifestations of the disease may be delayed for several years in some instances.

The disease is acquired through the inhalation of the infective spores, a product of the filamentous phase of the organism *Blastomyces dermatitidis*. The tissue response in the lung may be quite variable from patient to patient. Pneumonic, infiltrative, nodular, and miliary patterns are seen. Cavitation is not uncommon. Symptomatology depends on the type and extent of the lung reaction. Fever, chest pains, cough, and sputum production are common symptoms and hemoptysis may occur.

The course of the disease may range from its most usual one of a chronic slowly progressing disorder to an acute and fulminating process. Dissemination may occur at any time and with any of the lung patterns. In some instances widespread dissemination develops with only minimal pulmonary involvement or, in other instances, when the lung lesion is no longer apparent. In some patients extensive pulmonary disease may be present but with no dissemination. The skin, subcutaneous tissue, genitourinary tract, bones, and central nervous system are the most common sites for dissemination.

Management

Until very recently it has been generally believed that all human patients with North American blastomycosis require treatment. Recently, several acute cases of this disease were reported that had self-limited courses and required no specific therapy. These patients are being closely followed by a group of investigators. Until it has been clearly established that the disease in these patients does not recur, despite these reports and because of the serious prognosis associated with dissemination it continues to appear rational to treat all patients in whom the diagnosis is established. This decision to treat should include instances in which the correct diagnosis of blastomycosis was made subsequent to what appeared to have been the complete excision of a pulmonary lesion.

Treatment

Amphotericin B. Amphotericin B (Fungizone) is the most effective agent for the treatment of blastomycosis. Unfortunately, it has toxic and undesirable side effects that often create major problems in its administration. Immediate reactions include nausea, vomiting, chills, fever, headaches, and malaise. These immediate reactions may be so severe as to cause the patient to abandon treatment, but they tend to become less severe or disappear after several days of treatment. An occasional patient will experience no side effects. Phlebitis may develop in the vein receiving the infusion. Toxic side effects occurring throughout the course of therapy are usually more significant than are the immediately annoying ones. Amphotericin B has a nephrotoxic property and rising blood urea nitrogen levels can be expected. Moderate degrees of anemia may occur but seldom cause any curtailment in therapy. Hypopotassemia may also occur but is easily corrected.

Amphotericin B therapy is begun with 10 mg. in 100 ml. of 5 per cent dextrose in water. A saline solution is not used, as it will cause precipitation. The medication is usually given on an alternate day basis except in instances in which daily administration is advised for a few days in acutely ill patients. Thereafter, the every-other-day schedule is maintained. The dosage should be increased with each infusion by 5 mg. of the drug and 50 ml. of 5 per cent dextrose in water until the patient is receiving 50 mg. of the drug in 500 ml. of solution. It is only an exceptional patient who can be uninterruptedly brought to this 50 mg. dosage, for most patients develop rising blood urea nitrogen levels. With mild rises in the blood urea nitrogen, the dosage may be slowly increased, but when blood levels reach 50 mg. per dl. (100 ml.), the increases in dosages should be stopped and a decrease of 5 mg. made. After a few days at reduced dosage, it may be possible to increase the drug dosages again.

Not infrequently it is impossible to give more than 25 or 30 mg. three times a week because of the renal toxicity. This situation lengthens the duration of the therapy but does not necessarily decrease its effectiveness. The total dosage of 1.5 to 2 grams of amphotericin B is adequate in most instances and is the recommended dosage. Some patients who have received only 1 gram have been cured. Relapses have also occurred following the administration of 2 grams. Should a relapse occur, retreatment using the same drug and same regimen is usually successful.

The drug manufacturer's package insert ma-

TABLE 1. **Guidelines for Amphotericin B Therapy**

1. Prior to starting therapy obtain the following:
   Blood urea nitrogen (BUN)
   Serum creatinine
   Serum potassium (K)
   Hemoglobin (Hgb)
2. Oral administration of 50 mg. diphenhydramine hydrochloride (Benadryl) one hour prior to each infusion
3. Incorporate 2500 units of heparin into each infusion
4. Give each infusion intravenously in 45 to 75 minutes
5. Infusions are given three times a week. If severely ill, daily administration for the first 4 to 7 days is advised and the starting dose may be higher
6. 1st Infusion: 10 mg. amphotericin B in 100 ml. 5 per cent dextrose in water (5D/W)
7. 2nd Infusion: 15 mg. amphotericin B in 150 ml. 5D/W
8. 3rd Infusion: 20 mg. amphotericin B in 200 ml. 5D/W
9. 4th Infusion: 25 mg. amphotericin B in 250 ml. 5D/W
10. Increase each subsequent infusion by 5 mg. of amphotericin B and 50 ml. 5D/W until 50 mg. amphotericin B is being given in 500 ml. 5D/W
11. Should BUN reach 50 mg. per dl. temporarily halt increases in drug dosage. Decrease in dosage may be necessary
12. In some instances it may not be possible to attain more than 25 to 30 mg. dosages
13. BUN, K, and Hgb determinations after the 3rd infusion and at least weekly thereafter. When the BUN begins to rise, and it usually does, that determination may be desirable on alternate days
14. Give an oral potassium supplement if hypokalemia develops
15. Total amphotericin B dosage is 1.5 to 2 grams
16. After the patient feels better, the dosage and schedule established, the patient may be discharged from the hospital and receive the treatment on an out-patient basis

terial indicates a daily dosage to range up to 1.0 mg. per kg. of body weight and a dosage of 1.5 mg. per kg. of body weight when the drug is used on an alternate day schedule. In our experience, those high dosages are only rarely attainable due to the nephrotoxicity produced. We have found that lower dosages, such as 50 mg. three times a week, have usually been equally effective.

The administration of the amphotericin B infusion in approximately 1 hour (range 45 to 75 minutes) results in fewer and less severe immediate reactions of chill, fever, and nausea. The package insert brochure supplied by the drug manufacturer recommends *slow* intravenous administration over a period of 6 hours. In this community, where there has been extensive use of the drug for the treatment of blastomycosis and occasional usage in other fungal infections, the rapid administration method has been employed for the past 16 years. We know of no untoward results attributable to this rapid administration. The method is better accepted by the patient and the end therapeutic results are identical with the prolonged administration.

The drug manufacturer's brochure advises the solution be protected from light during its administration. Existing evidence suggests the light protection is unnecessary. The brochure also cautions against the use of dextrose solutions with pH below 4.2 in the preparation of the infusion solution. It advises ascertaining the pH of each container of dextrose injection and recommends a buffer to be used to bring it above 4.2. This is not necessary because there is available 5 per cent dextrose in water solutions with a pH of 5.

2-Hydroxystilbamidine Isethionate. 2-Hydroxystilbamidine isethionate is an antifungal agent that may be used in selected cases of blastomycosis. It is less toxic than amphotericin B but it is also less effective. In patients who have limited pulmonary involvement, no evidence of cavitation, and no dissemination to any area other than the skin, the drug has been used effectively. It should also be considered for management of amphotericin B treatment failures. Toxic reactions are only occasionally experienced but sometimes are quite severe. The principal damage from the use of 2-hydroxystilbamidine is to the liver; jaundice may develop and death has been reported. Serum glutamic oxaloacetic transaminase elevations of low or moderate levels have been frequently observed but without other evidence of toxicity.

The daily administration of 225 mg. of the drug in 200 to 250 ml. of 5 per cent dextrose or sodium chloride U.S.P. should be accomplished in 30 minutes or longer. The total dosage is 8 to 16 grams. The most extensive experience has been with the administration of 16 grams, but it is known that 8 grams have effected cures in some instances. Twelve grams should be the goal in most cases, with the extent of involvement and the nature of the therapeutic response dictating the total dosage.

EMPYEMA THORACIS

method of
R. RANDOLPH BRADHAM, M.D.
Charleston, South Carolina

Causes

The more common causes of empyema are infection by pneumococci and staphylococci and mixed infections. Coliform empyema usually originates below the diaphragm. Empyema resulting from infection distal to an obstructing bronchogenic carcinoma is becoming more common. A post-traumatic hemothorax occasionally becomes infected, especially after repeated thoracenteses. Fungal amebic empyemas are not very common except in endemic areas. These infections, tuberculous empyema, and space problem infections are complicated and require specific considerations beyond the scope of this paper.

Aims of Treatment

1. Control of infection.
2. Expansion of the lung and obliteration of the pleural space.
3. Restoration of pulmonary function.

Thoracentesis. Initially it is important to remove as much of the pleural fluid as possible and to establish the diagnosis with bacteriologic studies. Thoracentesis is the first method of drainage employed and is performed as follows:

1. Select the site carefully by examination of the x-rays, by physical examination, and by fluoroscopy when necessary.
2. Use 1 per cent lidocaine (Xylocaine) locally. Explore site first with 21 gauge needle to verify site.
3. After puncturing skin with a No. 11 scalpel blade, insert large-bore, short-beveled needle to remove fluid. Position needle just inside pleura. Insert at superior border of bottom rib in the interspace used.
4. Obtain cultures and sensitivity studies for acid-fast bacilli (AFB), fungi, and pyogens. Have immediate Gram stain done.
5. Repeat thoracentesis if fluid reaccumulates, provided removal of fluid by thoracentesis is effective.
6. Give systemic antibiotics as indicated by Gram-stained smear and sensitivity studies.

Tube Thoracostomy. If the fluid reaccumulates rapidly or if it becomes too thick to withdraw with a needle, tube drainage will be necessary. Development of a bronchopleural fistula, usually heralded by an air-fluid level, requires immediate tube drainage as follows:

1. Select site near base of cavity.
2. Infiltrate with 1 per cent lidocaine (Xylocaine). Test location with aspirating needle. Make a ½-inch incision.
3. Introduce a tube, No. 28 to 32 French, with trocar or with hemostat after separating the tissues. Secure tube to chest wall with suture.
4. Connect tube to underwater sealed drainage.
5. Suction of 10 to 20 cm. water pressure sometimes aids in evacuating the cavity.
6. Maintain patency of tube by stripping or flushing.
7. Tube can usually be cut off and left for open drainage after 8 to 14 days if pleural space is obliterated.
8. Remove tube slowly, allowing tube tract to close.

Rib Resection and Drainage. Rib resection and drainage is necessary when an empyema cavity becomes chronic, loculations occur, fibrinous deposits form, and the pus becomes thicker and more difficult to remove.

1. Local or general anesthesia is selected depending upon the status of the patient.
2. Check site of cavity with an aspirating needle.
3. An 8- to 10-cm. incision is made conforming to a rib near the base of the cavity in the lateral position, provided that the cavity extends laterally.
4. The rib is exposed and a 5- to 8-cm. segment is resected.
5. The cavity should be evacuated by suction as soon as it is opened to avoid aspiration into the tracheobronchial tree, should a communication exist.
6. Explore cavity with finger to break up loculations and to ascertain the base of the cavity.
7. Remove clumps of fibrin with sponge forceps.
8. Biopsy pleura and repeat culture and sensitivity studies.
9. Insert large-bore tube and connect to underwater sealed drainage.
10. Close tissue securely around tube.
11. Tube can be cut off and incorporated into bandage after 6 to 10 days. It might have to be kept in place for weeks or months.
12. Make sure that space is obliterated before tube is removed. This can be done by placing contrast material into the cavity through the tube.
13. The patient should be given breathing exercises to mobilize the affected chest.

Decortication. In long-standing, chronic empyema with a fixed wall cavity and restricted lung expansion, decortication may be necessary to free the trapped lung to restore maximal pulmonary function and obliterate the pleural space. The "peel" should be removed from the diaphragm as well as from the lung surface. Such procedures as closure of a bronchopleural fistula and thoracoplasty must sometimes be employed to deal with the more severe cases.

PRIMARY LUNG ABSCESS

method of
CHARLES F. TATE, JR., M.D.
Miami, Florida

Primary lung abscess usually presents in the upper lobes or superior segment of the lower lobes as a single lesion with an air fluid level on x-ray. There is a productive cough with purulent and, in the classic case, a very foul-smelling sputum, denoting the anaerobic abscess. Usually the abscess is secondary to aspiration of mouth secretions from around carious teeth and pyorrhea and is an unusual problem is the edentulous patient. The mouth flora usually consists of anaerobic streptococcus, diphtheroids, fusiform bacilli, spirochetes, and others that grow only with proper anaerobic culture techniques. Anaerobic culture material should be transported to the laboratory in an airtight syringe, no air bubbles, and specific instructions given to culture anaerobically. These organisms act synergistically with one another, it seems, and are rapidly destructive to lung tissue if the area is plugged off. Aspiration into a dependent segmental bronchus may occur following almost anything that paralyzes or depresses the gag reflex, such as a drunken stupor, convulsion, postictal state, tonsillectomy, dental extraction, head injuries, stroke, or general anesthesia.

Routine aerobic and anaerobic cultures are indicated, plus Gram stain. In addition, acid-fast bacilli, and fungal smears and cultures are done. Actinomycosis is an anaerobic organism and has to be specifically asked for on smear and culture. This is the reason this diagnosis is almost always made at thoracotomy. Other causes of lung abscesses may be septic emboli, Friedlander's pneumonia, staphylococcal pneumonia, and septicemia. The particular clinical picture must be carefully evaluated. Sputa cytology for malignancy should always be done, especially in the smoker.

Therapy

Therapy is initiated immediately for the specific or suspected problem. Penicillin G, 2 to 6 million units per 24 hours, is adequate for the anaerobic abscesses and the nonspecific abscesses, and is given either intramuscularly or intravenously for 8 to 12 days; then administration may be switched to oral tablets of 250 mg. potassium salt of phenoxymethyl penicillin or the equivalent 4 times daily until all evidence of purulent sputa has cleared.

Careful reevaluation of the drug program after return of the cultures, in light of the clinical progress, should be carried out. If *Bacillus fragilis* is cultured and the patient is not responding to medication, clindamycin is the drug of choice, 8 to 12 mg. per kg. per day by intravenous fluids.

If gram-negative organisms predominate, gentamicin, 1.5 to 2.0 mg. per kg. per day, or kanamycin, 15 mg. per kg. per day, should be considered.

If staphylococcal organisms predominate, oxacillin sodium or nafcillin sodium, 50 to 100 mg. per kg. intravenously daily, divided into four doses, should be used, until the penicillinase status is known. Antibiotic therapy should be continued until all purulent sputa have cleared.

If the intermediate strength purified protein derivative (PPD) is positive and the x-ray suggestive, cover with 300 mg. isoniazid (INH), 50 mg. of pyridoxine, and 1.0 gram intramuscularly of streptomycin (0.5 gram if over age 45) if not already on an aminoglycoside. Watch creatinine and serum glutamic oxaloacetic transaminase values (SGOT) frequently. When discharge occurs, substitute ethambutal, 15 mg. per kg. daily, for the aminoglycoside until the acid-fast bacilli cultures are reported. If negative, the ethambutal should then be stopped. Advise bed rest until toxicity subsides, and a high caloric diet and vitamins are routinely given.

Bronchoscopy to establish bronchial drainage should be done as an emergency if a necrotizing lesion is closely adjacent to the visceral pleura, the patient is toxic, and no sputum is being raised, with the idea of preventing development of a bronchopleural fistula and pyopneumothorax with very serious consequences. Otherwise, bronchoscopy should be done after the purulent sputum has cleared, to prevent aspiration. It is important to rule out definitely carcinoma with partial obstruction or the presence of a nonopaque foreign body. Fiberoptic bronchoscopy under fluoroscopic control, with suction and brushing, may be done multiple times if necessary to facilitate drainage.

Postural drainage is extremely important, 3 to 6 times a day, and should be carried out as long as the patient is raising significant sputum. The patient should be positioned for sleep to encourage drainage during the night.

Good dental care is essential for prevention of future aspiration.

The lesion may remain in the form of a localized area of bronchiectasis or a thin-walled cavity. If the area drains readily, no further treatment may be necessary. If, however, the lesion is in a dependent area, e.g., a basilar segment of the lower lobe, drainage is usually not adequate, and recurrence of symptoms is common, with hemoptysis and purulent sputum. In these patients, after maximal improvement, a bronchogram to localize the involved segment and the extent of the lesion may be done. Resection may then be considered if the opposite side is clear on a bronchogram.

Some 90 to 95 per cent of primary lung abscesses clear without significant residual following adequate antibiotic treatment and good drainage.

Weekly or more frequent x-rays, daily sputum collection and observation, temperature checks, and laboratory studies as indicated should be done to expedite the patient's care while in the hospital. Often, the patient can be discharged after 2 weeks, if reliable, but will definitely need to be followed carefully on antibiotics until the sputum is clear of pus and by serial x-rays until the lesion has stabilized.

ACUTE OTITIS MEDIA

method of
PAUL E. HAMMERSCHLAG, M.D.,
and JAMES A. DONALDSON, M.D.
Seattle, Washington

Acute otitis media is commonly seen in one of two forms: acute suppurative otitis media and seromucinous otitis media.

Acute Suppurative Otitis Media

Bacterial upper respiratory infections, particularly in pediatric patients, may lead to acute suppurative otitis media. The causative organism may be a pneumococcus, streptococcus, or *Hemophilus influenzae*. Although the *H. influenzae* organism is more commonly found in patients under 5 years of age, it has been identified as a causative organism in all age groups. Other organisms isolated include *Neisseria catarrhalis* (5 to 10 per cent) and Group A *β*-hemolytic streptococcus (5 per cent). A significant percentage (25 per cent) of the fluid isolated from acute otitis media is bacteriologically sterile. In neonates, *Escherichia coli* must be considered. Limited studies have reported the isolation of viruses in acute otitis media.

In addition to the symptoms associated with the underlying upper respiratory infection, the patient complains of severe otalgia, aural pressure, and decreased hearing. The diagnosis is readily made upon visualizing an erythematous bulging tympanic membrane, or distention of the membrane by purulent material, but without marked erythema. In a cooperative patient, tuning fork tests indicate a conductive loss, with a negative Rinne (BC > AC), and a Weber lateralizing to the affected ear. The causative organism is identified most dependably in material obtained by paracentesis or by performing a myringotomy and streaking the tip of the myringotomy knife directly on culture medium. Prior to this procedure, the external auditory canal should be sterilized by isopropyl alcohol irrigation to prevent contamination of the bacteriologic specimen. Criteria for tympanocentesis are limited, but include patients with compromised immunologic defense mechanisms, infections not responding to a previously instituted antibiotic regimen, and severe otalgia refractory to analgesics.

Treatment

Treatment consists of the following measures:

1. Antibiotics effective against pneumococci and *Hemophilus influenzae:* (a) Amoxicillin, 25 to 40 mg. per kg. per 24 hours divided into three doses, or ampicillin, 50 to 100 mg. per kg. per 24 hours orally in four divided doses; (b) penicillin V or G, 25,000 to 50,000 units per kg. per 24 hours, and triple sulfonamides or sulfisoxazole, 125 mg. per kg. per 24 hours orally in four divided doses. For the penicillin-allergic patient and the ampicillin-resistant *Hemophilus* infection, erythromycin, 40 to 50 mg. per kg. per 24 hours, concomitant with the above sulfa antibiotics, is recommended. Adult dosages are: amoxicillin, 250 mg. orally three times daily; ampicillin, 250 mg. orally four times daily; penicillin VK, 250 mg. orally four times daily; sulfisoxazole, 500 mg. orally four times daily; and erythromycin, 250 mg. orally four times daily. The therapeutic course should be for 10 days.

2. Decongestants electively combined with an antihistamine, e.g., triprolidine hydrochloride and pseudoephedrine (Actifed), may be effective.

3. Analgesics: Acetaminophen or codeine or both.

4. For acute otitis media with a purulent otorrhea from a tympanic membrane rupture: Clean the external auditory canal of purulence and then, in addition to the systemic antibiotics, start the patient on topical antibiotic solution, e.g., polymyxin B, neomycin, and hydrocortisone (Cortisporin otic).

5. Myringotomy is performed if the pain is severe or rapidly increasing or if the tympanic membrane is bulging to the bursting point. It can be performed in infants without anesthesia, in cooperative children following the application of a 2-mm. pledget of cotton moistened with Bonain's solution (equal parts cocaine, menthol, and phenol crystals), or in the uncooperative child under 75 pounds, following the intramuscular injection of 1 mg. of meperidine hydrochloride (Demerol) per lb. (0.45 kg.) and 2 mg. of pentobarbital sodium (Nembutal) per lb. (0.45 kg.). In some patients, a general anesthetic is necessary. A generous curvilinear incision is made in the posteroinferior quadrant, halfway between the umbo and the canal wall.

6. A careful follow-up examination includes evaluation of the appearance of the tympanic membrane, together with its motion and the patient's hearing. At the time of follow-up, incomplete resolution of seromucinous otitis media must be sought and appropriately treated, if present.

Infants with recurrent acute suppurative otitis media should not receive a bottle while supine. Recurrent otitis media may be treated with myringotomy and insertion of pressure equalizing ventilation tubes. Prophylaxis with ampicillin or sulfisoxazole, 125 mg. to 250 mg. every day for 3 months or longer, has been successful in limited clinical trials.

Potential complications of acute otitis media, which are rare, include acute mastoiditis, facial nerve paralysis, labyrinthitis, otogenic meningitis, brain abscess, and lateral sinus thrombosis.

Seromucinous Otitis Media

Seromucinous otitis media is a collection of fluid in the middle ear cleft. The fluid is of variable viscosity, ranging from a clear, thin, serous effusion (serous otitis media) to a thick, tenacious, mucoid exudate ("glue ear"). The pathogenesis of the thin fluid appears to be related to an inadequate aeration of the tympanum, in which a vacuum forms after absorption of oxygen, thus causing transudation from the middle ear mucosa. The thick mucoid exudate may be the residual of treated acute suppurative otitis media or secretions from the middle ear mucous glands for incompletely understood reasons. Multiple causes for the underlying eustachian tube obstruction include lymphoid (adenoid) hyperplasia, tumor in the nasopharynx, mucosal swelling from allergies, granulomatous disorders, or preliminary nasopharyngeal irradiation. Eustachian tube dysfunction secondary to developmental anomalies, such as cleft palate, Down's syndrome, and craniofacial anomalies, e.g., Apert's syndrome, is common in this group of patients. Incomplete resolution of acute otitis media or barometric trauma following an upper respiratory infection may exceed the functional capacity of the eustachian tube, thus producing serous middle ear effusion. Seromucinous otitis media is most common in young children and decreases with maturity as the peritubal lymphoid tissue regresses and the eustachian tube anatomy assumes a more efficacious contour.

The patient may complain of aural fullness or pressure and a variable hearing loss, or blockage. The tympanic membrane may be straw colored, dull, opaque, edematous, blue, or translucent, with a distinct air fluid level. A tympanic membrane retraction is usually present, with reduced motility on pneumatic otoscopy and decreased compliance on tympanometry. A conductive hearing loss may be verified with the tuning fork.

Treatment is directed towards correcting the underlying cause of the eustachian tube dysfunction, when possible, e.g., desensitization for allergic control, adenoidectomy for obstructing adenoid hypertrophy, and continuation of antibiotics for incompletely treated otitis media. Many times resolution can be achieved by the use of self-inflation (Valsalva's maneuver), inflating balloons while occluding the nose, or by using the Mathes inflator or the Politzer bag. The use of decongestants has produced variable results.

A pressure-equalizing ventilating tube may be used in patients with chronic seromucinous otitis media with a significant hearing loss. These tubes usually stay in place 3 to 12 months, giving the middle ear mucosa and the eustachian tube time to resume their normal status. In the pediatric patient, this temporizing measure may suffice until the patient matures, with resultant adenoid tissue atrophy and eustachian tube anatomic changes. Those with craniofacial anomalies or permanent eustachian tube dysfunction may benefit from a permanent pressure-equalizing ventilating tube or hearing aid to manage the problems of hearing deficits.

Acute Mastoiditis

Acute mastoiditis is a complication of acute suppurative otitis media. Since the introduction of antibiotic therapy, this has become a very unusual entity. It should be suspected following untreated, or inadequately treated, acute otitis media, with the development of a low-grade nocturnal otalgia, continued or recurrent otorrhea, a slight fever, postauricular swelling and tenderness, and a sagging of the medial aspect of the external auditory posterosuperiorly. At times, dissolution of bone can be detected on x-ray examination. Intensive therapy is begun with systemic penicillin or amoxicillin, and the patient is carefully observed. If the course during the next 24 to 36 hours becomes one of gradual improvement, therapy may be continued for 2 weeks. If, by the end of 36 hours, improvement is not noted, or earlier if the symptoms are worsening, a complete mastoidectomy should be performed.

BACTERIAL PNEUMONIA
method of
JAMES R. BONNER, M.D.
Mobile, Alabama

Effective treatment of patients with bacterial pneumonia requires both general supportive measures and specific antimicrobial agents directed against the causative microorganisms.

General Measures

Most patients need hospitalization, at least initially, in order to assure adequate rest, good diet, and prompt treatment of any complications which may arise. Dehydration is a frequent concomitant of pneumonia, and proper fluid balance should be assured either orally or by the administration of appropriate intravenous fluids. Mobilization of purulent material should be promoted, if necessary, by humidified air, vibropercussion, and postural drainage. Airway obstruction can result from inflammatory edema, secretions, or bronchospasm. When wheezing is heard, bronchodilators such as aminophylline, 100 or 200 mg. every 6 hours (adult dose), may be helpful. Therapeutic bronchoscopy is sometimes indicated to remove inspissated secretions. Supplemental oxygen may be required for hypoxia, and arterial blood gases should be measured in all patients with cyanosis or respiratory distress. Patients with chronic obstructive lung disease may need a hypoxic stimulus for respiration, and oxygen therapy may result in respiratory depression and carbon dioxide retention. Limited amounts of oxygen with careful monitoring of arterial blood gases is necessary in these patients. Ventilatory support may be needed in seriously ill patients and is discussed in the article on Acute Respiratory Failure. The use of aspirin or other antipyretics is of doubtful value, as it may negate the usefulness of the temperature response in following the patient's course and sometimes causes wide swings in temperature, resulting in uncomfortable chills and sweats. Fever should be treated in patients with heart disease, in whom the accompanying tachycardia could be dangerous, and in patients with temperatures above 105°F. (40.5°C.). Pleuritic pain leads to shallow respirations and should be relieved by analgesics such as indomethacin, 25 mg. three times daily (with meals) (this use of indomethacin is not listed in the manufacturer's official directive), or codeine, 15 to 30 mg. intramuscularly or 30 to 60 mg. orally every 4 hours. Codeine is a cough suppressant but has the advantage of not affecting temperature

Identification of Pathogen

Attempts to identify the specific pathogen should precede initiation of antimicrobial therapy. Careful examination of a Gram stain of a good sputum specimen remains the best test in determining initial therapy. The presence of numerous polymorphonuclear leukocytes is evidence that an adequate specimen has been obtained. Transtracheal aspiration is recommended by some in order to avoid contamination of sputum by upper respiratory bacteria. This procedure is particularly useful if precise anaerobic cultures are desired but carries some risk and should not be performed routinely. Specimens obtained by bronchoscopy offer little advantage over expectorated sputum except in patients who are unable to produce a proper specimen. Sputum can sometimes be obtained by nasotracheal or oro-

tracheal suctioning. Before initiating treatment, sputum and blood cultures should be obtained.

The drugs of choice for specific bacterial infections, along with alternative drugs, and the usual doses are listed in Table 1.

Specific Treatment

Pneumococcal Pneumonia. *Streptococcus pneumoniae* is still the most common cause of bacterial pneumonia, especially in previously healthy young adults. It characteristically produces an acute illness with fever, a single chill, pleuritic chest pain, and expectoration of rusty brown sputum. Patients sometimes develop a sterile pleural effusion, but empyema and abscess formation are unusual. Demonstrable bacteremia occurs in about 30 per cent of patients with pneumococcal pneumonia, and these patients have a poorer prognosis than patients whose blood cultures are negative. Arthritis, endocarditis, and meningitis are infrequent complications of pneumococcal bacteremia. Confusion and lethargy should not be attributed to "toxicity" or hypoxia without first examining the cerebrospinal fluid.

The drug of choice for pneumococcal pneumonia is penicillin G. For patients allergic to penicillin, erythromycin may be substituted. Antibiotics should be continued for 1 week or until the patient has been afebrile for 2 to 3 days, whichever is longer. Patients usually show marked clinical improvement with defervescence within 24 to 48 hours, but occasionally 3 to 4 days elapse before improvement is noted. It is important to remember that radiographic clearance often does not accompany clinical improvement. Signs of consolidation may persist for up to 10 weeks, and volume loss and streaking may persist for over 4 months. Clinical improvement and radiographic clearance are most often delayed in patients with chronic obstructive lung disease, elderly patients, and those with extensive disease. Patients with persistent radiographic changes should have chest x-rays repeated every 4 to 6 weeks to rule out other pulmonary disorders.

Staphylococcal Pneumonia. *Staphylococcus aureus* is responsible for 1 to 2 per cent of adult bacterial pneumonia. The pneumonia may be "primary" or may result from hematogenous spread from staphylococcal disease elsewhere. Primary staphylococcal pneumonia occurs most commonly in patients with chronic debilitating disease, as a nosocomial infection, or following an episode of influenza. Hematogenous staphylococcal pneumonia can complicate staphylococcal bacteremia from any cause such as skin infection, drug addiction, acute bacterial endocarditis, or

TABLE 1. **Antibiotic Treatment for Adult Bacterial Pneumonia**

MICROORGANISM	DRUG OF CHOICE*	ALTERNATIVE DRUGS‡
Streptococcus pneumoniae	Procaine penicillin G, 600,000 U. I.M. q. 12 h.	Erythromycin, 500 mg. P.O. q. 6 h. Cephalothin, 1–2 grams I.V. q. 4 h.
Staphylococcus aureus	Nafcillin, 1–2 grams I.V. q. 4 h. *or* Aqueous penicillin G, 20 million U. I.V.q.d. in divided doses (when bacteria susceptible)	Cephalothin, 1–2 grams I.V. q. 4 h. Vancomycin, 1 gram I.V. over 30–40 min. q. 12 h.
Hemophilus influenzae	Ampicillin, 1–2 grams I.V. q. 6 h. *or* Amoxicillin, 500 mg. P.O. q. 8 h.	Chloramphenicol, 0.5–1 gram I.V. q. 6 h.
Streptococcus pyogenes	Penicillin, 10–20 million U. I.V. q.d. (in divided doses)	Cephalothin, 1–2 grams q. 4 h.
Klebsiella	Gentamicin, 1–1.5 mg./kg. I.V. or I.M. q. 8 h. *plus* Cephalothin, 1–2 grams/kg. I.V. q. 4 h.	Chloramphenicol, 0.5 gram I.V. q. 6 h.
Enterobacter	Gentamicin, 1–1.5 mg./kg.I.V. or I.M.q.8h. *plus* Carbenicillin, 5 grams I.V. q. 4 h.	Chloramphenicol, 0.5–1 gram I.V. q. 6 h.
Escherichia coli	Ampicillin, 1–2 grams q. 6 h. I.V. (when bacteria susceptible) *or* Gentamicin, 1–1.5 mg./kg. I.V. or I.M. q. 8 h.	Cephalothin, 1–2 grams I.V. q. 4 h. Chloramphenicol, 0.5–1 gram I.V. q. 6 h.
Proteus mirabilis	Ampicillin, 1–2 grams q. 6 h. I.V. (when bacteria susceptible) *or* Gentamicin, 1–1.5 mg./kg. I.V. or I.M. q. 8 h.	Cephalothin, 1–2 grams I.V. q. 4 h. Chloramphenicol, 0.5–1 gram I.V. q. 6 h.
Other Proteus species	Gentamicin, 1–1.5 mg./kg. I.V. or I.M. q. 8 h. *plus* Carbenicillin, 5 grams I.V. q. 4 h.	Chloramphenicol, 0.5–1 gram I.V. q. 6 h.
Serratia marcescens	Gentamicin, 1–1.5 mg./kg. I.V. or I.M. q. 8 h. *plus* Carbenicillin, 5 grams I.V. q. 4 h.	Chloramphenicol, 0.5–1 gram I.V. q. 8 h.
Pseudomonas aeruginosa	Tobramycin, 1–1.5 mg./kg. I.V. or I.M. q. 6 h. *plus* Carbenicillin, 5 grams I.V. q. 4 h.	
Aspiration pneumonia	Penicillin, 20 million U.I.V. q.d.† (in divided doses)	Clindamycin, 300 mg. I.V. q. 6 h. Chloramphenicol, 0.5–1 gram I.V. q. 6 h.

*Dosages are for adult patients with normal renal function. Except for *Streptococcus pyogenes* and pneumococcal pneumonia, the final choice for antibiotics is dependent upon laboratory sensitivity studies.

†For aspiration pneumonia, high dose penicillin is recommended when the patient is first seen and is severely ill. Once there is clinical improvement with defervescence, low dose penicillin such as that used for pneumococcal pneumonias can be given.

‡Cephalosporins should not be used in patients with penicillin allergy if the allergy is of the anaphylactic type.

contaminated intravenous sites. Staphylococcal pneumonia is characterized by early empyema, pneumatocele, and pyopneumothorax.

Except in those rare instances in which the organism is susceptible to penicillin G, a penicillinase-resistant semisynthetic penicillin such as nafcillin is the drug of choice. Alternative drugs are vancomycin and the cephalosporins.. Cephalosporins should probably be avoided in patients with a history of immediate anaphylactic reactions to penicillin.

Drainage of empyema is an important part of therapy; this usually requires surgical placement of a chest tube. Recovery is characterized by gradual clinical improvement, with complete defervescence only after a 1 to 2 week period. Treatment should be continued for a total of 3 to 4 weeks in patients with primary pneumonia and for 4 to 6 weeks in pneumonia of hematogenous ori-

gin. In either case antibiotics should be continued until the patient is clinically better and the x-ray changes have cleared or become stable (this is a necrotizing pneumonia, and residual scarring is not uncommon).

Hemophilus Pneumonia. *Hemophilus influenzae* is being increasingly recognized as an important cause of pneumonia in adults. This entity is usually seen in older adults, and especially persons with chronic obstructive pulmonary disease. Both bronchopneumonia and lobar pneumonia are seen, and the infiltrates most often involve the lower lobes. Sterile pleural effusion is common, but empyema and abscess formation are rare. Bacteremia is detected in one third of cases, and as for pneumococcal pneumonia, these patients have a poorer prognosis than patients whose blood cultures are negative. Diagnosis depends on finding a predominance of small, gram-negative rods on Gram stain of sputum or culturing the organisms from blood, pleural fluid, or transtracheal aspirates. Sputum cultures are difficult to interpret because *Hemophilus influenzae* is sometimes part of the upper respiratory flora of healthy adults, and many laboratories do not use media suitable for the identification of hemophilus in sputum.

Ampicillin is the drug of choice. *Hemophilus influenzae* is occasionally resistant to ampicillin, and in these instances as well as in patients allergic to penicillin, chloramphenicol should be used. This is not a necrotizing pneumonia, and clinical improvement is usually rapid.

Streptococcal Pneumonia. *Streptococcus pyogenes* (group A beta-hemolytic Streptococcus) is presently a rare cause of pneumonia. The disease is associated with streptococcal outbreaks in the community and sometimes follows influenza or measles. Characteristically there is abrupt onset of chills, fever, and cough productive of thin pink sputum. In contrast to pneumococcal pneumonia, bacteremia is infrequent, and early empyema formation is common. The antibiotic of choice is parenteral penicillin, and empyema formation requires prompt drainage. The fever is often prolonged, and this should not lead to a change in antibiotics. Treatment for 2 to 4 weeks is usually necessary.

Aerobic Gram-Negative Rod Pneumonia. Klebsiella is a cause of acute lobar pneumonia in debilitated patients, especially alcoholics. It may have a predilection for the right upper lobe and is characterized by acute illness with fever, chills, and production of tenacious brown sputum. Klebsiella and other gram-negative bacilli also cause nosocomial infections, often in severely ill patients who are already receiving antibiotics and those requiring respiratory support. Microorganisms involved include *Escherichia coli*, Proteus species, *Serratia marcescens*, Enterobacter, and *Pseudomonas aeruginosa*. These bacteria produce necrotizing pneumonias sometimes complicated by abscess or empyema. Antibiotic sensitivities may vary in these species, and therapy must be based on susceptibility data. Pending sensitivity data a cephalosporin and an aminoglycoside such as gentamicin or tobramycin should be started (tobramycin is recommended as the initial drug in suspected or proved Pseudomonas pneumonia, and in this situation carbenicillin is included, as it may be synergistic with the aminoglycosides against Pseudomonas). Treatment should be continued for 2 to 3 weeks or until there is clinical improvement and x-rays show complete clearing or stabilization of the infiltrates (gram-negative pneumonia often leaves residua of scar tissue apparent roentgenographically).

Aspiration Pneumonia. Aspiration of oropharyngeal or gastric contents can cause severe necrotizing pneumonia and lead to formation of chronic lung abscess. Aspiration can occur secondary to swallowing disorders or unconsciousness (e.g., alcoholism, seizures, general anesthesia). Antibiotic coverage is directed against upper respiratory flora, e.g., alpha-hemolytic streptococci and anaerobic bacteria such as Fusobacterium and Bacteroides species. Most of these microorganisms are susceptible to penicillin, and this drug has been proved effective even when resistant anaerobes such as *Bacteroides fragilis* are involved. If the patient does not respond to penicillin or has a history of penicillin allergy, chloramphenicol or clindamycin should be substituted. If the patient was seriously ill before the aspiration event or was receiving antibiotics, prior colonization of the upper respiratory tract by penicillin-resistant organisms may be assumed. In such situations staphylococci or enteric gram-negative bacilli may predominate, and treatment should be based on the results of Gram stain and culture. Many of the complications of pulmonary aspiration are due to a chemical pneumonitis or obstructive pneumonitis, and the treatment of these aspects of aspiration is discussed in the article on Nonbacterial Pneumonia.

Patients severely ill with bacterial pneumonia of any cause in whom the specific pathogen is uncertain should initially receive therapy for *Staphylococcus aureus* and gram-negative enteric bacilli. The combination of tobramycin and cephalothin is recommended in these situations. When results of sputum and blood cultures are available, therapy may be modified.

VIRAL AND MYCOPLASMAL PNEUMONIAS
method of
JOHN P. GRIFFIN, M.D.
Memphis, Tennessee

Introduction

Viral and mycoplasmal agents can produce a lower respiratory infection with pneumonitic reaction, clinically and radiographically, as the most severe manifestation. This illness has been termed "atypical pneumonia," because it usually is characterized by an absence of rigors and high fever, of purulent and rusty sputum and of true pleuritic pain, so typical of pneumococcal pneumonia, the prototype of bacterial pneumonias. Additionally, viral and mycoplasmal pneumonias most often do not evidence physical findings and roentgenographic features of the lobar consolidation of classical pneumococcal pneumonia. The clinical manifestations of these "atypical pneumonias" tend to be similar, irrespective of their specific causative agent. *Mycoplasma pneumoniae* is the only mycoplasmal species recognized as capable of producing pneumonia in man; however, almost the entire spectrum of respiroviruses, from influenza to rhinovirus, can cause this syndrome. Since cultures of respiratory secretions for viruses and mycoplasmas are not performed in the clinical laboratory, etiologic diagnosis in this group of pneumonias must be serologic. Demonstration of four-fold or greater increases in serum antibody requires several weeks, and thereby is retrospective and of no practical value to the physician responsible for treatment. The exception to this is the demonstration of cold agglutinins by a positive screening test or by serum titration of greater than 1:40, both of which are presumptive evidence of pneumonia due to *Mycoplasma pneumoniae* and suggest appropriate antibiotic treatment.

Viral Pneumonias

Treatment. No specific antimicrobial treatment is currently available for any of the true viral pneumonias. Hypoxemia often exists in these disorders, by a mechanism of ventilation-perfusion inequality, so that supplementary oxygen should be administered with interval determination of arterial blood gas values. Alveolar hypoventilation may exist because of underlying chronic obstructive pulmonary disease, owing to the use of respiratory-depressant medications of the sedative, narcotic, or tranquilizer type, or from fatigability with a severe and prolonged illness; the possible need for assisted ventilation by a volume respirator must also be assessed by monitoring blood gases. Although viscid purulent sputum is not characteristic, aerosol therapy is often of help in improving pulmonary clearance; cilioplegia (paralysis of the ciliary apparatus of the respiratory mucous membrane) may result in patchy atelectasis and areas of apparent consolidation; denuding of the respiratory mucosa is occasionally seen with severe influenzal pneumonia and can result in not only associated clearance problems but additionally significant hemoptysis. A heated fine particle mist of water, as available by ultrasonic nebulization, is often helpful in management of these pneumonias. If wheeze or other evidence of bronchospasm is present, I additionally nebulize sympathomimetic amines 4 to 6 times daily, preferably prior to superwetting of the respiratory tract by heated water mist. Expectorant drugs have been of little value in this setting, but maximal bronchorrhea is encouraged by high fluid intake orally or intravenously in seriously ill patients. Physiotherapy in the form of postural drainage or chest percussion has been discouraging in the treatment of viral pneumonia.

Hacking nonproductive cough can be fatiguing to the patient, and cautious use of cough suppressants, preferably parenteral codeine in hospitalized patients, is indicated. Additional symptomatic and supportive care is important, including antipyretics for high fever, maintenance of adequate fluid and electrolyte balance, and analgesics occasionally, since pleuritic pain and splinting are rarely observed in uncomplicated viral pneumonia.

Complications. The most common complication of viral pneumonia is secondary bacterial infection, as exemplified by influenza. Most morbidity and mortality from pneumonia complicating influenza is due to secondary infection, usually with the Pneumococcus, but also in this setting with Staphylococcus, Streptococcus, and Hemophilus. Therefore, seriously ill patients with viral pneumonia should be carefully observed for clinical signs of bacterial complications; their sputum should be monitored by Gram-stained smear and culture for pyogens. Myopericarditis is occasionally seen in association with viral pneumonia due to influenza or some enteroviruses, and cardiac decompensation might result from either congestive failure or cardiac tamponade. Rarely, viral pneumonia may be accompanied by meningoencephalitis or in overwhelming infection by a viral-induced endotoxin-like shock syndrome.

Prevention. One drug, amantadine hydrochloride, has proven efficacy in the prevention of viral respiratory infection and is used to inhibit cellular penetration of influenza A viruses. The recommended dose is 100 mg. twice daily for persons over the age of 9 years. Children aged 3 to 9 years should receive 2 to 4 mg. per pound of body weight, not to exceed a total daily dose of 150 mg. Gastrointestinal and central nervous system symptoms occur in 1 to 2 per cent of cases if the recommended dose is followed, but side effects are greatly increased if it is exceeded. It is contraindicated for patients with a history of central nervous system disease or for patients taking depressant, stimulant, or tranquilizer drugs. The principal use of amantadine is for patients at high risk of mortality from influenza during an epidemic in which such persons have not received appropriate vaccine prophylaxis within weeks of expected infectious exposure. In practice, because of the short incubation period and rapid spread of epidemic influenza, this requires prevention with amantadine as soon as influenza infection is confirmed in the community. The major disadvantage of this drug is that it must be administered daily throughout the entire season of possible influenza infection.

The most important tool in the management of serious respirovirus infection is the timely use of effective vaccines for immunoprophylaxis. The prototype of such biologicals is the influenza A vaccine. Because of the changing antigenicity of these viruses, with respect to both hemagglutinin and neuraminidase antigens, viral surveillance by all available methods must be continuously utilized to permit new vaccine production and administration to those at high risk prior to likely exposure in order to prevent the devastating morbidity and mortality of these most pathogenic of the respiroviruses. The American population, as well as the medical community, is attempting to recover its confidence in immunization for influenza prevention, after the unfortunate fiasco of the "swine-flu" universal vaccination program, and the identification of a rare but apparently true association between receiving this vaccine and the development of the serious Guillain-Barré syndrome of paralysis. It is suggested that the annual recommendations of the United States Public Health Service Advisory Committe on Immunization Practices be carefully followed for yearly influenza vaccination only for patients at high risk.

Vaccines against other specific respiratory viruses have been prepared and to some extent clinically tested. They have certain areas of usefulness—for example, the favorable effect of adenovirus vaccine immunization in closed groups such as those in military training centers. Effective immunization to the parainfluenza viruses and respiratory syncytial virus, the chief causes (in children) of croup and bronchiolitis, respectively, and also important causes of pneumonia, would be gratefully welcomed. However, results to date in these areas have not been satisfactory, and therefore it can be stated that they have no present usefulness in clinical practice. Neither have rhinovirus or respiratory enterovirus vaccines been satisfactory.

Mycoplasmal Pneumonia

Treatment.   Antibiotics of both the erythromycin and tetracycline classes have been demonstrated in controlled studies to shorten the period of fever, decrease morbidity, and hasten resolution of pulmonary infiltration. The response to these drugs is not striking in comparison to the dramatic resolution of infectious signs in patients with pneumococcal pneumonia treated with penicillin. It is considered unnecessary to treat all patients with atypical pneumonia with antibiotics, on the supposition that *Mycoplasma pneumoniae* might be the causative agent. It is my practice to test immediately for the presence of significant titer of cold agglutinins either by the rapid screening tube test or by an overnight incubation and to reserve antibiotic treatment for those who demonstrate positive results. Since in some patients with *M. pneumoniae* infection cold agglutinins fail to rise during the illness, or, as is more usual, they have not developed to significant levels at the time of

first examination, antibiotic treatment should be prescribed in patients who are seriously ill regardless of an initial negative cold agglutinin test. Clinical trials have demonstrated only marginal superiority of erythromycin, but the exquisite sensitivity of representative isolates of *M. pneumoniae* to 0.1 microgram per ml. of erythromycin as opposed to a lesser degree of sensitivity to tetracycline has favored erythromycin as the drug of choice. It should be given at 2 grams per day in four divided doses by mouth for a 7 to 10 day period. Penicillin has no effect in the treatment of this infection because of the lack of a cell wall in these microorganisms; in fact, the laboratory incorporates large amounts of penicillin into the medium for growth of mycoplasma to prevent the growth of bacteria contained in the respiratory tract flora. Occasionally, it is difficult to differentiate pneumococcal pneumonia from atypical pneumonia caused by *Mycoplasma pneumoniae*. In this instance, erythromycin is preferred because of its expected optimal effect in both of these types of bronchopneumonia.

Complications.   Complications of this disease are rare and are seldom of consequence. A small percentage of patients with mycoplasmal pneumonia will develop hypersensitivity dermal eruptions of the erythema multiforme type, with an occasional patient afflicted by the more severe Stevens-Johnson syndrome. These patients require specific antimicrobial treatment plus the use of corticosteroids to suppress inflammation. Less frequently, bullous myringitis, meningoencephalitis, or pleuritis with minimal effusion will be noted. Bacterial superinfection of mycoplasmal pneumonia is unusual, despite the observation that colonization with various bacterial species and a neutrophilic leukocytosis are seen during convalescence. Such laboratory data should be cautiously interpreted to resist the impulse to rotate antibiotics. Some patients experience a prolonged period of dry cough, a problem that can be expected to resolve with only symptomatic treatment. There is no evidence supporting a role of mycoplasmal pneumonia in the development of bronchiectasis or in the initiation of chronic bronchitis.

Prevention.   Mycoplasmal pneumonia is usually an endemic disease, with unpredictable epidemic behavior. In closed populations, such as military camps, university complexes, and institutions, particularly where the personnel are of a younger age group, higher prevalence of this infection is observed and effective prophylaxis would be indicated. Parenteral vaccines composed of inactivated organisms have been found to be partially immunogenic and somewhat helpful in reducing morbidity. In the Syrian hamster model of mycoplasmal pneumonia, evoking local immunity in the respiratory tract provides optimal prophylaxis. Living attenuated *Mycoplasma pneumoniae* vaccines have been produced for administration intranasally. The most promising of these new biologicals is produced by mutagen exposure of conditional-lethal temperature-sensitive variants of this organism. These mutants grow well at 32°C., the temperature of the upper respiratory tract, but poorly at 38°C., the temperature of the lower tract. This permits development of local immunity on intranasal growth, but prevents spread to the bronchi, allowing vaccine-induced pneumonia. Further field trials of novel live vaccines are under way, but no *Mycoplasma* immunoprophylactic agent has yet been approved for use in civilian medical practice.

PULMONARY EMBOLISM

method of
HAROLD L. ISRAEL, M.D.,
and G. WILLIAM ATKINSON, M.D.
Philadelphia, Pennsylvania

There is consensus that heparin is the most effective agent for treatment of pulmonary embolism, with lesser roles for oral anticoagulants, fibrinolytic agents, and surgery. There is growing agreement regarding the details of administration and on the duration of anticoagulant therapy. What remains divergent is opinion regarding the accuracy of diagnosis of pulmonary embolism and the evidence necessary to justify institution of anticoagulant therapy. Although the efficacy of treatment is established beyond any possible doubt, opinions vary concerning the hazards of the available therapeutic measures and the degree of certainty necessary to justify their use. In the past pulmonary embolism was often unrecognized prior to fatal episodes. Despite the proliferation of diagnostic techniques in the past 2 decades, there has not been a corresponding increase in accuracy of detection of thromboembolism.

Treatment on suspicion of thromboembolism has been advocated by most authorities as the wisest response to the recognized uncertainty of diagnosis. Recently, it has been argued that the pendulum has swung too far, that many patients are being treated for pulmonary embolism on flimsy evidence, and the hazards of overtreatment exceed those of undertreatment. Fatal bleeding occurs in 1 of each 1000 patients treated with heparin, so that treatment for pulmonary embolism has a small but inescapable risk. The hazards of undertreatment are more difficult to measure. In a study carried out at one medical center with special expertise in angiography, pulmonary arteriograms were performed in 157 patients because of strong suspicion of embolism based on clinical and isotopic study. Angiographic evidence of embolism was found in only 27 per cent. If a positive arteriogram is regarded as a sine qua non for diagnosis of pulmonary embolism, then this experience is interpreted as demonstrating that all other available methods of diagnosis are inaccurate and that overdiagnosis is the rule in hospitals that do not employ pulmonary angiography as a routine. It may be argued to the contrary, however, that when clinical, roentgenographic and scan evidence arouses suspicion of pulmonary embolism, failure to secure angiographic confirmation in three quarters of such patients indicates that arteriographic visualization of thrombosis is no more reliable than other methods.

The difficulties in obtaining objective evidence of pulmonary embolism has led some physicians to recommend that antiembolic therapy be instituted, not on the basis of cardiopulmonary changes but on objective evidence of disease in the veins of the lower extremities, where most pulmonary emboli originate. The three principal methods that have been developed are ^{125}I fibrinogen thigh and leg scanning, impedance phlebography, and Doppler ultrasound. These methods have contributed greatly to our knowledge of the epidemiology and pathogenesis of pulmonary embolism. There is evidence that deep vein thrombosis in the legs is much less important than thigh thrombosis as a source of embolism. Again, however, the practical value of these studies in clinical diagnosis is limited by the difficulty in accomplishing these studies before heparin therapy is started. Fibrinogen scanning takes 48 hours to complete and there is often equal delay in scheduling the specialized radiologic and ultrasound studies. In most instances in which pulmonary embolism is considered delays of this length cannot be justified. Moreover, one recent study has demonstrated that our methods for recognition of venous thrombosis are no more reliable than our techniques for detection of embolism to the lungs. Impedance phlebography in 136 patients with strong evidence of pulmonary embolism revealed thigh involvement in 26 per cent, calf involvement in an equal number, and no deep vein thrombosis in 48 per cent.

Indications for Treatment

The sudden onset of pleuritic pain or dyspnea in patients with chronic venous disease, patients with recent injuries to the lower extremities, patients who have undergone surgical procedures, or those who have been immobilized by congestive heart failure, strokes, or other incapacitating illness should be regarded as indicative of pulmonary embolism until some other cause is established. A history of prior pulmonary embolism supports the diagnosis, although the possibility of perpetuating error by this criterion must be recognized.

The demonstration of tachycardia, a localized pleural rub or rales, signs of edema or tenderness in the lower extremities, a normal chest roentgenogram or one showing unilateral or bilateral areas of segmental basal atelectasis with or without effusion, acute or transient electrocardiographic evidence of pulmonary hypertension, and diminished left ventricular output all support the diagnosis, which should be regarded as highly probable unless a normal perfusion lung scan is obtained. If a satisfactory lung scan is entirely negative, pulmonary embolism is virtually excluded. The converse, of course, is not true. Abnormal lung scans may be due to asthma, pneumonia, neoplasm, or emphysema, and only if these diseases are excluded may perfusion abnormalities be regarded as diagnostic of pulmonary embolism. Measurement of arterial oxygen tensions is an even less reliable indication of pulmonary embolism. Tensions below 80 mm. Hg may be due to any of the diseases enumerated above as well as others. Demonstration of normal oxygen tension, above 80 mm. Hg, makes large emboli improbable but does not absolutely exclude the diagnosis.

The role of pulmonary angiography in clinical diagnosis of pulmonary embolism remains debatable. Use of this method of diagnosis has declined in recent years except in centers with special interests in this procedure. As with perfusion scanning, a completely normal arteriogram taken prior to institution of anticoagulant treatment virtually excludes embolism, but abnormal vascular shadows are not invariably the result of clots. In most cases the decision as to whether therapy for embolism is to be instituted should not be postponed until an arteriogram can be secured.

Therapy of pulmonary embolism is based on the fact that in most patients an intrinsic and highly efficient thrombolytic system exists that will clear most veins of clot within a 5 to 7 day period. Treatment is directed at the relief of symptoms, correction of hypoxemia, acute pulmonary hypertension, consequent heart failure, and the prevention of further clot formation. Although urokinase and streptokinase have been shown to promote clot lysis in the first 24 hours and favorably influence mortality and morbidity from massive pulmonary embolism in the first day of treatment, the basic treatment for this disease remains heparin.

Heparin

Heparin should be given to every patient with a presumptive diagnosis of pulmonary embolism unless it is absolutely contraindicated. Use of a continuous infusion of 1000 units of heparin per hour, or intermittent intravenous administration of 5000 units of heparin every 4 to 6 hours are the preferred methods of treatment, but subcutaneous administration of 10,000 units of heparin every 8 hours is acceptable. Therapeutic range of

effectiveness is approximately 1.5 to 2.5 times control value for the partial thromboplastin time (PTT) in the constant infusion method and 1.5 times the PTT control value in a blood specimen taken just before the next heparin dose in the intermittent schedule. Most patients kept within this range have little risk of hemorrhagic complications and are in an area that is effective therapeutically. Oxygen is ordinarily given to correct hypoxemia, and cardiac failure is treated with digitalis and diuretics. Codeine is useful for palliation of pleuritic pain. Application of elastic stockings to accelerate deep vein flow is of dubious prophylactic value and is superfluous once heparin has been started. Antibiotic therapy should be given if there is uncertainty as to whether the pulmonary disease is of thrombotic or infectious cause. Stool examinations are done routinely for occult blood to monitor the possibility of gastrointestinal bleeding as a complication of heparin use. When symptoms subside, bed rest is no longer required.

The recurrence rate after 8 to 10 days of heparin administration is low in patients who have recovered from their underlying illness and are fully ambulatory. Patients who are bedfast or who have chronic venous disease are candidates for long-term anticoagulant therapy or surgical measures.

Methods of Heparin Administration.   Heparin is effective when given intravenously by continuous infusion or by bolus injections at 6 hour intervals. The former method requires more constant laboratory surveillance but is not demonstrably more effective than interrupted intravenous administration. Despite its disadvantages, its use has been .advocated on the grounds that bleeding complications were fewer with this technique. Recent studies have failed to support this view, and we prefer use of bolus administration of heparin. Heparin therapy is somewhat less effective when given subcutaneously in doses of 10,000 units every 12 hours, but this treatment may be regarded as equal in efficacy to oral anticoagulants.

Although control of heparin dosage by measurement of partial thromboplastin times is commonly recommended, in practice there is little use to such determination in patients receiving interrupted venous or subcutaneous injections. Many physicians omit PTT measurements unless bleeding occurs or recurrent embolism is suspected. In the latter case it is urgent to determine whether heparin in usual doses is being effective. In rare instances massive doses of heparin are needed to inhibit coagulation, and close monitoring of dosage by coagulation tests is required. Heparin is not often indicated during pregnancy or in patients with liver disease but can be safely used in these circumstances.

Oral Anticoagulants

Prolonged anticoagulant therapy requires cooperative patients and close and careful outpatient surveillance. If a patient is uncooperative, unmotivated, or misses clinic visits, anticoagulants should not be given. Although "minidose" subcutaneous injection of 5000 units of heparin every 12 hours is a most effective preventative, it is expensive and requires daily self-administered injections. The partial thromboplastin time does not have to be monitored with this regimen, as the risk of hemorrhage is nil. An alternative, however, is warfarin, which can be given orally and is more acceptable to patients. Usually doses are employed that maintain prothrombin times from 1.5 to 2.5 times control values. The risk of hemorrhagic complications is higher with warfarin than heparin but it remains the only alternative.

Warfarin is the only oral anticoagulant widely used in the United States. In contrast to heparin, rather close limits between efficacy and safety exist. The prothrombin time should be kept at twice the duration of controls, with permissible limits between 1.5 and 2.5 times control values. Many cooperative patients having access to superior laboratory facilities can often achieve satisfactory therapeutic effects for prolonged periods with safety. When these conditions are not fully met, bleeding not infrequently becomes a serious problem, necessitating an end to oral anticoagulant treatment.

It should be noted that warfarin cannot be used in pregnancy because it crosses the placenta, or in patients with liver disease sufficiently severe to affect the prothrombin time, where it is impractical to monitor the dosage of warfarin.

The daily dose of warfarin in most patients ranges from 2.5 to 10 mg. It should be emphasized that warfarin does not become fully effective for 96 hours after initiation of treatment; heparin should not be discontinued earlier.

Surgical Prevention of Pulmonary Embolism

The management is quite different when pulmonary embolism occurs in a patient who is bleeding or who has just had neurosurgery or prostatic resection. Fibrinolytic and anticoagulant therapy is contraindicated in these circumstances, and there is no other way to prevent further thromboembolism. However protection against massive and possibly fatal embolism can be provided by reducing the caliber of the abdominal vena cava, either by suture, clipping, or insertion of an "umbrella" device. These are temporary expedients, since thrombosis is likely to recur proximal to the clip or ligature and collaterals quickly develop through which small clots from the legs can pass. The indication for surgical interruption of the abdominal cava is fortunately rare, but it cannot be avoided if a patient has definite pulmonary embolism, and anticoagulants for whatever reason cannot be used.

A more common pretext for surgical interruption is failure of anticoagulant therapy; that is, the recurrence of pulmonary embolism in a patient being treated with anticoagulants. Greater experience with heparin therapy has made it clear that such failures are extremely uncommon and are usually the result of some lapse in dosage or administration. Better controlled or more vigorous use of heparin almost invariably corrects the problem, and surgical interruption is rarely required in these circumstances. Interruption of the inferior vena cava may be accomplished by ligation, plication, and the passage of an umbrella sieve percutaneously that subsequently opens and is seated in the proximal inferior vena cava. These techniques should be reserved for patients who have repeated embolism despite seemingly adequate heparin therapy, as well as patients to whom heparin cannot be given because of absolute contraindications such as gastrointestinal bleeding. The results of vena cava interruption are usually short-lived, in that venous bypasses of the caval interruption develop in the ovarian and renal system, and postsurgical emboli not infrequently travel through these bypass vessels, as well as from thrombosis developing at the proximal side of the vena caval obstruction.

Treatment of Massive Pulmonary Embolism

The patient in shock represents a special problem. In these circumstances, fatal impairment of left ventricular output must be averted by emergency medical or surgical means. Vigorous intravenous heparin therapy should prevent additional embolic insults, but the patient's own fibrinolytic system may fail to lyse the clot in time to restore circulation. Fibrinolysin has recently been released for clinical use with the recommendation that its use be restricted to medical centers with "facilities for pulmonary angiography and laboratory monitoring of coagulaton disturbances." If a pulmonary arteriogram can be scheduled without delay, it is desirable to confirm the diagnosis of massive embolism by this method before employing fibrinolysin, but if the procedure cannot be carried out within a few hours, and if other evidence for massive embolism is strong, fibrinolytic therapy should be utilized. If these agents are not available, isoproterenol may be used in an effort to reduce pulmonary hypertension. A 2 mg. dose of isoproterenol in 500 ml. of water is infused at a rate of 1 microgram per minute. The use of surgical embolectomy has declined because of the low yield of successes, and maintenance of circulation by cardiopulmonary bypass is available only in a few centers.

Fibrinolytic Therapy

Streptokinase and urokinase have recently been licensed for treatment of acute massive pulmonary embolism, and the former is now commercially available. It is recommended that it be used only by physicians with wide experience in management of thromboembolic disease. Bleeding during fibrinolytic therapy is more severe and difficult to control than bleeding induced by anticoagulants. The list of contraindications is long: surgery within the preceding 10 days, liver or kidney biopsies, parturition, recent gastrointestinal bleeding, intra-arterial diagnostic procedures, trauma, visceral neoplasms, hypertension, liver or kidney disease, thrombocytopenia or other coagulation defects, or subacute bacterial endocarditis.

The usefulness of fibrinolytic therapy is sharply limited to acute massive pulmonary embolism resulting in profound drop in left ventricular output and shock. In these circumstances, when an obstruction of a major pulmonary arterial trunk is confirmed by arteriography, a trial of fibrinolytic therapy should precede attempts at surgical embolectomy.

A loading dose of 250,000 units of streptokinase is administered over a 30 minute interval. A maintenance infusion is continued at a rate of 100,000 units per hour for 72 hours. The thrombin clotting time should be checked at 2 to 3 hour intervals, and kept at 2 to 5 times normal. At the end of 72 hours, streptokinase therapy is replaced by heparin infusion, with the institution of oral anticoagulant treatment if this is thought to be necessary.

Prevention of Thromboembolism

The problems in recognition, both of venous thrombosis and of pulmonary embolism, could best be averted by effective methods of preventing thromboembolism. The safety and value of "mini-dose" heparin prophylaxis have been firmly documented in recent years. Although heparin in dosage of 5000 units subcutaneously 2 or 3 times daily has no effect on the partial thromboplastin time or other coagulation factors, it significantly reduces the incidence of thromboembolism both in surgical and medical patients. The frequency of fatal postoperative embolism has been reduced from 7 per 1000 to zero, with little increase in bleeding complications. Cessation of heparin prophylaxis because of bleeding has been necessary in less than 3 per cent of patients treated. There has been no significant difference between treated and control subjects in frequency of wound hematomas or transfusion requirements.

Significant reduction in thromboembolic complications has also been demonstrated in medical patients with stroke and myocardial infarction. Heparin prophylaxis is recommended for other medical patients confined to bed longer than 6 days, especially those with increased risk factors such as cancer, congestive heart failure, obesity and prior thromboembolic manifestations. Mini-dose heparin prophylaxis (5000 units 2 hours prior to operation and every 12 hours thereafter) is recommended for all surgical patients over the age of 40 undergoing cardiothoracic, gynecologic, and other abdominal surgery. It is insufficient to avert thromboembolism in patients with hip fractures but is contraindicated in patients having neurosurgery or ocular and prostatic surgery. The frequency of pulmonary embolism in patients with hip fractures is high, and vigorous therapy with heparin or oral coagulants is indicated in this group, although there are recent reports that aspirin prophylaxis is effective in such patients.

Despite the numerous reports attesting to the efficacy and safety of low-dose heparin therapy, it has not been as widely or as rapidly adopted as one might expect. A recent survey of 84 surgical patients of Thomas Jefferson University Hospital for whom low-dose heparin prophylaxis appeared indicated showed that only 14 received this medication, 32 patients had elastic stockings applied, 6 received prophylactic aspirin, and 32 received no treatment. It appears that many surgeons are not yet convinced of the safety and practicality of low-dose heparin prophylaxis.

Septic Embolism

Protracted fever after parturition, abortion, or gynecologic surgery is frequently the result of infectious pelvic thrombophlebitis, often resulting in septic pulmonary embolism. Blood cultures may reveal various gram-positive or gram-negative organisms, sometimes anaerobes, but in a majority of instances blood cultures are sterile. The fever is unresponsive to antibiotics but a characteristic feature of this illness is a prompt lysis of fever when heparin therapy is added: the uniformity of this response is such that it represents a diagnostic test. Heparin therapy is usually continued for 7 to 8 days; oral anticoagulants are unnecessary.

Septic pulmonary emboli occasionally result from septic phlebitis elsewhere: osteomyelitis in children, abscesses of head and neck, and right-sided endocarditis.

In recent years intravenous drug abuse has become a major cause of septic embolization, but an even greater source is iatrogenic, due to prolonged use of intravenous catheters for purposes of nutrition or medication.

SARCOIDOSIS

method of
OM P. SHARMA, M.D.,
and NORMAN E. LEVAN, M.D.
Los Angeles, California

Definition

Sarcoidosis is a multisystem granulomatous disorder of unknown cause most commonly affecting young adults and presenting with bilateral hilar lymphadenopathy, pulmonary infiltration or fibrosis, skin lesions, eye involvement, or peripheral lymphadenopathy. Indeed, no tissue system is immune from the disease. The diagnosis is established when clinical or radiographic findings are supported by histiologic evidence of epithelioid cell granulomas in the affected tissue. These granulomas lack caseation, show no evidence of bacterial or fungal organisms, and they may either resolve or convert into an acellular hyaline fibrous tissue.

Management

Once the diagnosis of sarcoidosis is established, treatment decisions and evaluation of its effectiveness must take into consideration the natural history of sarcoidosis and extent of organ involvement.

Acute sarcoidosis is a benign, self-limiting disease with abrupt onset. As patients are usually asymptomatic, the condition is frequently diagnosed on routine chest roentgenograms, which usually show bilateral hilar lymphadenopathy, and, occasionally, diffuse pulmonary infiltration. Erythema nodosum may be present at the onset. The chest roentgenographic abnormalities clear within a year in more than 65 per cent of patients, particularly in white patients with erythema nodosum.

Chronic sarcoidosis has an insidious onset and a course that is slow, progressive, and highly variable. In more than 90 per cent of patients the chest roentgenograms are abnormal, usually showing pulmonary infiltration with or without advanced fibrosis. Other frequent findings are chronic skin lesions, including lupus pernio and firm small plaques, and small multiple papules; chronic uveitis, glaucoma, and cataract; nose and upper respiratory tract lesions; persistent parotitis; hypercalcemia and hypercalciuria; hypersplenism; and bone marrow granulomas.

Indications for Treatment

The goal of treatment is to prevent fatal or crippling sequelae such as extensive pulmonary fibrosis, cor pulmonale, blindness, and renal failure.

Lungs. The use of corticosteroids, or indeed any therapy now available for pulmonary sarcoidosis, is somewhat controversial, in that it is uncertain whether treatment confers any long-term benefits or alters favorably the natural course of the disease. We administer corticosteroids if an abnormal chest roentgenogram fails to show improvement in 6 months. Other indications for systemic corticosteroids are diminished lung volumes, evidence of airway obstruction, impaired diffusing capacity, and hypoxemia sufficiently severe to produce symptoms. Conversely, bilateral hilar adenopathy, particularly if associated with erythema nodosum, generally subsides without treatment.

Eye. All patients with sarcoidosis should have an adequate ophthalmologic evaluation, including slit-lamp examination. Fortunately, ocular sarcoidosis tends to respond well to treatment, often to local therapy alone. Topical corticosteroids, as in eye drops or ointment form, are usually adequate for control of anterior uveitis. Failure to improve in a week or two, or the presence of posterior uveitis as revealed by slit-lamp examination, indicates concurrent use of systemic corticosteroids.

Upper Respiratory Tract. Involvement of this area by sarcoidosis is less frequent but most disabling. Nose, nasopharyngeal mucosa, and larynx may all be affected. We regard upper respiratory tract sarcoidosis as an indicator of chronic fibrotic sarcoidosis and an indication for mandatory treatment.

Abnormal Calcium Metabolism. Estimation of the 24-hour urinary calcium excretion is essential to uncover abnormal calcium metabolism, inasmuch as hypercalciuria is three times as common as hypercalcemia. Corticosteroids are believed to prevent urinary excretion of calcium and resultant nephrocalcinosis indirectly by blocking calcium absorption from the gut and diverting it to harmless fecal excretion.

Heart. Myocardial involvement may be indicated by heart block or cardiac arrhythmia and is an indication for corticosteroid therapy.

Central Nervous System. Diabetes insipidus, epilepsy, and papilledema caused by sarcoidosis respond well, generally, to corticosteroids.

Miscellaneous. Other situations occasionally requiring treatment are hypersplenism, enlarged parotid or lacrimal glands, disfiguring skin lesions, symptomatic bone or lymph node involvement, and systemic symptoms of persistent fever, chills, and weight loss.

Methods of Treatment

Corticosteroids. At present, corticosteroids are the most effective agents for influencing the clinical, biochemical, and radiologic abnormalities of sarcoidosis. When there are contraindications or inadequate response to corticosteroids, other anti-inflammatory agents may be tried. We generally administer initially 30 to 40 mg. of prednisone daily, in divided oral doses, gradually reducing this dosage to maintenance levels, about 5 to 10 mg. for most of the medications given. In many patients, after the initial 4 to 6 week period with 30 to 40 mg. of prednisone daily, we have used 30 to 40 mg. every other day. The alternate day use of prednisone seems to be at least as effective as the daily administration.

Acute uveitis requires somewhat higher dosages, 60 to 80 mg., of prednisone. Local corticosteroids alone, as mentioned, are often effective for controlling anterior uveitis, and may be administered in the form of eye drops alone or reinforced by one subconjunctival injection.

An attempt should be made to treat cutaneous lesions by local corticosteroids alone. Triamcinolone acetonide diluted with 1 per cent procaine to a final concentration of 2 to 5 mg. per ml. may be injected intralesionally and the injections repeated at 1 to 2 week intervals. On occasion, high potency corticosteroid creams or lotions, massaged in well three or four times daily, are helpful.

Other Anti-inflammatory Agents. Chloroquine is useful, particularly in the management of chronic skin lesions and pulmonary fibrosis, starting with 250 mg. twice daily for 6 months (this use of chloroquine is not listed in the manufacturer's official directive). It may also be used concurrently with corticosteroids to reduce their dosage. Chloroquine administration poses hazards to the eye and may lead to irreversible retinopathy and blindness, so that frequent and careful ophthalmic examinations are a strict requirement. Oxyphenbutazone, in a controlled study, was found to be quite similar to the corticosteroids in its effect on the radiologic pulmonary findings and in the prevention of the evolution of the Kveim test. It is given in a dose of 100 mg. four times daily for 3 to 6 months (investigational use). Allopurinol, 100 mg. four times a day (this use of allopurinol is not listed in the manufacturer's official directive), and colchicine, 0.5 mg. twice daily, have been found helpful in the management of arthritis caused by sarcoidosis.

Immunosuppressive drugs such as methotrexate, chlorambucil, or azathioprine (investigational) have been used when there has been inadequate response to corticosteroid therapy, with good results in some patients.

Antituberculosis therapy is not administered routinely to our patients. The patients with positive tuberculin skin test receiving corticosteroids are given prophylactic isoniazid.

SILICOSIS

method of
HOWARD A. BUECHNER, M.D.
New Orleans, Louisiana

Silicosis, the oldest of the pneumoconioses, is caused by inhalation of small particles of silicon dioxide (SiO_2) which are capable of reaching the alveoli of the lungs. Particles in the range of 0.1 to 5 microns are most likely to cause disease, and the smaller the particle size, the greater the hazard to the individual.

Silicosis has been known by a variety of terms in the past, such as "miner's consumption," "grinder's rot," "stone mason's phthisis," "potter's asthma," and "stonecutter's disease." As these names imply, the disorder is almost exclusively related to occupational exposure to silica and is a potential hazard in hard rock miners of coal, gold, lead, copper, iron, zinc, and silver, tunnel drillers, jack hammer operators, handlers of abrasive materials containing silica, talc workers, sand pulverizers, and sandblasters.

There are three main types of silicosis:

1. The simple form, characterized by small nodular densities throughout the lung and rarely associated with symptoms or pulmonary disability.

2. Conglomerate silicosis, characterized by the formation of large masslike fibrotic lesions in the lungs and frequently associated with bronchitis, emphysema, various infections, cor pulmonale, and progressive respiratory disability.

3. Accelerated, acute, or fulminating silicosis, which results from relatively short periods of exposure to high concentrations of very small silica particles. Pulmonary lesions are massive, diffuse, and relentlessly progressive. Early death is inevitable. Histologically, the picture is a mixture of diffuse interstitial pneumonitis and fibrosis, desquamative interstitial pneumonia (DIP), and alveolar proteinosis. This form of silicosis is most frequently seen in sandblasters who have worked in closed spaces without adequate protection.

Pathogenesis. The exact mechanism by which silica produces pulmonary damage is still poorly understood but recent studies have indicated that various immunologic reactions are probably involved. In addition, silica is lethal to the macrophages of the lung. When tiny sand particles are inhaled they are engulfed by the defending macrophages, and these cells attempt destruction and removal of the foreign material. Instead, the macrophages themselves are destroyed and release various enzymes, which produce tissue necrosis and eventual fibrosis. Macrophage destruction also plays a primary role in rendering the host more susceptible to infection.

Prevention

There is no specific treatment for silicosis, but in the light of present knowledge of the disease, there is no reason why it should exist at all. If proper preventive measures were utilized in all industries involving exposure to silica dust, the disease would disappear or greatly decrease in prevalence. Preventive measures include the total elimination of silica from the industrial process whenever possible, stringent dust control, and the use of effective, high quality protective equipment such as airtight hoods with an external air supply. Sandblasting should be "outlawed," as it has been in Great Britain for many years. In the United States, many, but not all, companies have substituted nonsilica-containing materials for sand in the blasting process and this is a major, but still incomplete, step in the right direction.

Treatment

When preventive measures fail, usually because they have not been properly designed or enforced, and the patient does develop detectable silicosis he should be removed forever from further contact with silica dust. Even so, the disease may continue to progress.

Acute or Accelerated Silicosis. This form of the disease is likely to be fatal. However, the toxic effects of the illness, such as high fever, can be suppressed and other symptomatic improvement attained by the administration of corticosteroids. Whether or not this form of therapy actually delays the progression of the pathologic process and prolongs life is uncertain. Prednisone appears to be the drug of choice. Treatment is started with daily doses of 60 to 100 mg. After 4 to 6 weeks of therapy, the dosage is gradually reduced to that level at which symptoms are adequately controlled, but relatively high doses will probably be required for the duration of the patient's life. Since acute silicosis usually resembles alveolar proteinosis, with accumulation of a proteinaceous fluid in the alveolar spaces, pulmonary lavage might be of some benefit in the relief of dyspnea, which cannot be controlled by oxygen administration. If the patient has a positive tuberculin skin test or a clinical mycobacterial infection he should be treated as discussed below.

Simple Silicosis. No treatment of any kind is usually required for this type of silicosis, other than removal of the patient from further contact with silica dust. Tuberculin skin testing should follow, with appropriate management as described in the section on Infections below.

Conglomerate Silicosis. Although there is no specific treatment for the silicotic process, the management of its many complications may be very helpful. Bronchitis, emphysema, cor pulmonale, and respiratory failure should be treated as described elsewhere in this volume.

Infections

As previously indicated, silica is lethal to pulmonary macrophages and thus robs the lungs of an important defense mechanism, rendering the patient with silicosis more susceptible to various infections. The organisms that most frequently cause infection are *Hemophilus influenzae*, the *pneumococcus, Mycobacterium tuberculosis, M. kansasii, M. intracellulare, Cryptococcus neoformans, Sporotrichum schenckii,* and *Nocardia*. In a study of 83 sandblasters with silicosis in the New Orleans area, approximately 25 per cent had clinical mycobacterial infections, almost equally divided between *M. tuberculosis* and other ("atypical") mycobacteria. The risk of a patient with silicosis developing clinical tuberculosis has been estimated as 758 times greater than the risk to a normal person and the silicotic is at approximately 6000 to 7000 times greater risk of developing an atypical mycobacterial illness. About 5 per cent of silicotics develop systemic fungus infections.

In view of the high risk of tuberculosis, every patient with silicosis should be skin tested with tuberculin, purified protein derivative (PPD) by the Mantoux technique, and managed as follows:

1. If the intermediate strength (5 T U) tuberculin skin test is positive (induration of 5 mm. or more), the patient is considered to have a tuberculous or other mycobacterial infection and treatment is indicated. If there is no evidence of clinical disease as indicated by symptoms, radiographic findings, or bacteriologic studies of the sputum, the patient should be treated with isoniazid (INH), 300 mg. in one dose each day for at least 1 year. Although there is no evidence to support the benefit of giving INH for longer periods, I prefer to administer the drug for 2 years or more, and some physicians prescribe INH for life. I recently encountered a patient who had been taking the drug for 19 years. Pyridoxine, 50 mg. daily, should be given during the course of INH therapy to prevent peripheral neuritis.

2. If the tuberculin skin test is negative, it should be repeated every 6 to 12 months for the rest of the patient's life. If conversion to a positive reaction occurs in the absence of clinical disease, the patient should be treated with INH and pyridoxine as described above.

3. If active tuberculosis is detected (silicotuberculosis) by demonstrating tubercle bacilli in the sputum or gastric contents, or even if the diagnosis is only suspected because of radiographic or other clinical findings, the patient should receive "double" or "triple chemotherapy," depending on the severity of the disease. For minimal tuberculosis, INH, 300 mg., and ethambutol, 15 mg. per kg. (not to exceed 1 gram) in one dose daily, is adequate. For more than minimal tuberculosis, rifampin, 600 mg. in one daily dose, is added to the above two drugs. In all cases, treatment is continued for 24 months or longer if the response is slow and significant residual lesions persist.

4. Atypical mycobacterial infections (Mycobacteriosis) are treated with "triple chemotherapy" as described, and treatment is altered by addition of other antimycobacterial drugs as indicated by bacterial sensitivity studies.

5. Infections with other bacteria or fungi are treated by the methods described elsewhere in this volume.

Recently it has been noted that various autoimmune diseases such as rheumatoid arthritis, scleroderma, or lupus erythematosus may occur in association with silicosis. In these situations appropriate treatment of the coexisting disorder must be carried out. However, it must be remembered that agents used in the treatment of these diseases are usually immunosuppressive and the risk of infection with fungi, mycobacteria, and other organisms increases accordingly. The physician must be extremely alert to this danger.

Various agents have been tried in an attempt to block the fibrogenic effects of inhaled silica, including aluminum powder, D-penicillamine, polyvinylpyridine-N-oxide and poly-betaine, but they are either ineffectual, too toxic, or of uncertain benefit. Other agents are now under investigation.

BAGASSOSIS, FARMER'S LUNG, AND OTHER FORMS OF HYPERSENSITIVITY PNEUMONITIS

method of
HOWARD A. BUECHNER, M.D.
New Orleans, Louisiana

Hypersensitivity pneumonitis, referred to in the British literature as "extrinsic allergic alveolitis," may be caused by a variety of inhaled antigens contained in organic dusts. The list of these disorders has grown rapidly in recent years and includes bagassosis, farmer's lung, mushroom grower's disease, and humidifier or air conditioning-heating system disease all caused by thermophilic *Actinomycetes* contained in organic dusts of various origins.

Various fungi such as *Aspergillus, Penicillium, Mucor, Altenaria, Graphium, Pullularia,* and *Coniosporium corticale* cause similar illnesses designated as maltworker's lung, suberosis, cheese washer's lung, paprika slicer's disease, sequoiosis, pulp wood handler's disease, maple bark stripper's disease, and others.

Animal protein from birds, cows, and pigs may produce hypersensitivity pneumonitis in pigeon breeders, parakeet fanciers, chicken and turkey handlers, and users of pituitary snuff.

This list is by no means complete and new entries seem to occur on an almost yearly basis.

Bagassosis is a typical example of this type of disorder. The thermophilic *Actinomycete, Thermoactinomyces saccharii,* flourishes in old stored sugar cane fiber (bagasse). When this material is disturbed, the worker inhales these agents and shortly thereafter suffers an acute pneumonia-like illness. Repeated exposures may lead to chronic interstitial fibrosis.

Treatment of bagassosis or other forms of hypersensitivity pneumonitis is relatively simple and consists primarily of recognition of the disorder and separating the patient from further contact with the offending antigen. Ordinarily, this will result in gradual improvement over a period of days, weeks, or even months. Relapses almost always occur following reexposure, and the danger of permanent lung damage and disability increases proportionately.

Acute episodes of hypersensitivity pneumonitis frequently require bed rest and supportive care, including oxygen, cough suppression, relief of pain, hydration, and antipyretics. Severe symptoms can be modified and the duration of the illness shortened by the use of corticosteroids. Prednisone is usually administered in doses of 60 mg. daily, with gradual reduction of dosage and termination of therapy after a period of 2 to 6 weeks. No benefit can be expected from antibiotics.

Prevention of bagassosis and other forms of hypersensitivity pneumonitis can be accomplished by eliminating the offending antigen from the worker's environment or, when this is impossible, by providing and enforcing the use of good quality respirators.

SINUSITIS

method of
C. THOMAS YARINGTON, JR., M.D.
Seattle, Washington

Incidence and Etiology

Sinusitis is probably one of the most frequently misdiagnosed conditions affecting Americans and is also most often managed by self-treatment. Fortunately, the vast majority of patients who have diagnosed or have been diagnosed as having sinusitis actually suffer from some other minor abnormality of the upper respiratory tract. Conditions that are frequently erroneously considered to be sinusitis are postnasal discharge, allergic rhinitis, nasopharyngitis, vasomotor rhinitis, headaches from a variety of sources, and mechanical nasal obstruction.

The supposed incidence of sinusitis, therefore, greatly exceeds the actual incidence of the disease. A vast array of medications is available to the consumer for the treatment of this disease and the majority are combination drugs designed to relieve minor headache, to relieve minor allergic symptoms, and to provide some nasal decongestion through vasoconstriction. In the face of significant public misconception pertaining to sinusitis, a strong trend toward self-diagnosis and treatment with proprietary medications, and failure in recognizing the possibility of complications, the physician treating sinusitis should give particular attention to accurate diagnosis and appropriate follow-up.

Treatment

The goals in the treatment of sinusitis are primarily the establishment of drainage and the management of bacterial infection. Since physical examination of the paranasal sinuses is limited and transillumination is of little value without considerable experience and known normal evaluations in the same patient, x-rays of the paranasal sinus remain the only mechanism available for clear-cut diagnosis and meaningful follow-up.

The first step in the disease process should be directed toward establishing drainage, which can be accomplished with the use of local or systemic decongestants. The use of local decongestants in the form of nose sprays or drops, such as 2 per cent ephedrine or other similar preparations, has distinct disadvantages. These are the rebound phenomenon (which frequently occurs), the apparent addiction of the patient to the use of the medications, and the resulting rhinitis medicamentosa, which can be a long-term complication. For this reason, we do not prescribe nasal topical decongestants and limit their use to the patient in the hospital or in the office. We recommend the use of systemic decongestant and employ one of a number of combination drugs utilizing ephedrine or pseudoephedrine with an antihistamine, usually chlorpheniramine or others of the propylamine class. Although there is some controversy over the use of combination decongestants and antihistamines, the rationale is that benefit is achieved from the decongestant and vasoconstriction activity, as well as the antihistamine activity in the patient with mild or severe allergic rhinitis. We select a combination drug with a sustained relief mechanism such that the prescribed medication need only be taken every 12 hours. In some patients the mild sedative effect of the antihistamine also proves advantageous.

The normal contraindications should be considered in patients with hypertension, diabetes, glaucoma, or those who may be taking a monoamine oxidase inhibitor or tricyclic antidepressant. Also, the patient should be advised of the possible mild sedative effect of the medication. We provide the patient with sufficient medication for symptomatic relief for at least a week following relief of the acute symptoms.

A second important adjunct to therapy is the local use of heat and humidity. Steam inhalation and the use of hot, moist compresses to the nose and face have demonstrated considerable effect toward relieving the symptoms of sinusitis.

The management of the bacterial infection accompanying or causing acute sinusitis is usually achieved through the use of penicillin, utilizing oral phenoxymethyl penicillin (V-Cillin) in doses of 250 to 500 mg. four times a day for adults, with equivalent doses for children. In the patient who is allergic to penicillin, doxycycline hyclate (Vibramycin), with 100 mg. twice a day the first day followed by 100 mg. daily, is a reasonable alternative. Either medication should be maintained for a minimum of 10 days.

Cultures of nasal drainage are notoriously lacking in correlation with organisms within the sinus. Therefore, routine culture, other than at surgery, may be impractical.

It should be remembered that in young children the frontal sinuses have not yet developed and the maxillary sinuses have not usually developed to a point of clinical significance. In youngsters, ethmoiditis, with the frequent complication of orbital cellulitis, is the most common manifestation of sinusitis. Here consideration should be given to the use of ampicillin in appropriate dosage, due to the high incidence of *Hemophilus influenzae* and *Bacillus pneumoniae* as the primary cause of bacterial disease.

Local relief of pain can usually be provided with nonnarcotic analgesics of the physician's choice. The use of narcotics should usually be limited, inasmuch as progressive or severe pain resulting from sinusitis frequently is a manifestation of an impending complication such as osteitis or osteomyelitis. In the patient with progressive disease, in the face of adequate treatment, consideration should be given toward hospitalization and surgical drainage of the involved sinuses.

The place of antral lavage or puncture is a subject of some controversy today. It is thought by some that these procedures should not be carried out unless the patient has been on a course of antibiotics and decongestants for a sufficient period to achieve adequate blood levels to prevent complications of the procedure. Others feel that if this has been achieved, then the indications for drainage by lavage are no longer necessary and that more extensive procedures should be undertaken if response to medication alone is not adequate. In our practice, lavage and drainage are limited to patients in whom acute relief of severe symptoms due to obstruction is indicated. In those patients who do not respond adequately to therapy or in whom the symptoms worsen while on adequate treatment, it is our practice to consider surgical drainage of the sinus involved. Particularly in unilateral maxillary disease, we prefer the Caldwell-Luc approach rather than antral windows, so that we may explore visually the involved sinus and rule out the possibility of neoplasm, as well as to be able to create a larger antral window for future drainage and remove nonviable mucous membrane or disease.

The Frontal Sinus. A word about the peculiar problems of the frontal sinus is in order. Because of the intimate relationship between the frontal sinus and the cranial cavity and the connection afforded by the veins of Breschet to the epidural space, frontal sinusitis should be regarded as presenting an ominous threat. A patient with frontal sinusitis in which a fluid level can be seen on x-ray or in whom the sinusitis does not respond rapidly and adequately to medical therapy should be hospitalized. Drainage should be achieved surgically if medical efforts do not afford prompt regression of symptoms and adequate drainage. Office procedures, such as infracture of the middle turbinate, local decongestion and suction, and Proetz irrigation, may be utilized prior to surgical drainage.

Chronic Sinusitis. Patients who have responded to medical therapy but retain x-ray evidence of disease should be evaluated further to differentiate between chronic sinusitis, allergic polyposis, or neoplasm. The patient with recurrent symptomatic disease or chronic x-ray evidence of disease, particularly of a single, unilateral sinus, should be seriously considered for surgical exploration for purposes of differential diagnosis as well as for prevention of further problems. Patients falling in this category should be referred to an appropriate otolaryngologic surgeon for consultation.

STREPTOCOCCAL PHARYNGITIS

method of
MARTIN F. RANDOLPH, M.D.
Danbury, Connecticut

With rare exceptions, in the child presenting with sore throat, if one excludes the beta-hemolytic streptococcus as the causative agent, one excludes the need for antibiotic therapy. Because of the lack of association of specific signs and symptoms with streptococcal infections of the pharynx, the definitive diagnosis of streptococcal pharyngitis is dependent upon the isolation of *Streptococcus pyogenes* by throat culture. A throat culture properly taken and processed in the office laboratory will detect throat infections caused by beta-hemolytic streptococci with an accuracy of 95 to 97 per cent. Only through prompt recognition and treatment of beta-hemolytic streptococcal infection can the suppurative and nonsuppurative sequelae of these infections be prevented.

The objectives of therapy are (1) to eliminate the organism from the throat, (2) to gain prompt relief of symptoms, (3) to reduce the threat of infection within the family and classroom, and (4) in the process to educate parents and patient to the value of the throat culture in the early diagnosis of streptococcal pharyngitis.

In practice the first three objectives are met in the first 24 to 36 hours of effective antibiotic therapy; the child gains rapid cure of his clinical illness and returns to the classroom in 2 to 3 days. His throat culture is rendered negative for beta-hemolytic streptococci after 24 hours of specific therapy and he is no longer contagious to those around him. Prevention of rheumatic fever is accomplished by early eradication of the organism, but it is less clear if early treatment can prevent nephritis.

In the treatment plan for streptococcal sore throat both parents and patient must be educated to the early signs and symptoms of Group A streptococcal pharyngitis. We instruct our patients in the positive and negative criteria for "strep sore throat"; the positive criteria are fever, sore throat, nasal speech, tender anterior cervical glands, and characteristic breath odor; the negative criteria are rhinorrhea, cough, hoarseness, and sneezing. Parents are advised that a throat culture is warranted with any two positive criteria, but the simultaneous presence of two negative criteria makes strep sore throat unlikely. We find parent education promotes greater responsibility for obtaining throat cultures when indicated. Additionally, the educated parent is more likely to comply fully with oral antibiotic regimens.

Antibiotic Therapy

Penicillin remains the drug of choice in the treatment of streptococcal pharyngitis and has been the antibiotic most completely evaluated in terms of its efficacy in the prevention of rheumatic fever. It has been established that therapy should be maintained for 10 days to eradicate the infecting organism and to prevent acute rheumatic fever. This is most reliably accomplished by a single intramuscular injection of benzathine penicillin G. The recommended dose of benzathine penicillin is 600,000 units in young children, 900,000 units in older children (10 years or more) and adolescents, and 1.2 million units in adults. A single intramuscular injection ensures patient compliance, is convenient, and is quite inexpensive. The risk of severe drug reaction is very uncommon in children and adolescents.

Oral administration of penicillin is less reliable in eradicating the streptococcus, in part because of the difficulty in completing a full course of therapy once symptoms have improved, usually within 2 days. Nevertheless, oral penicillin is effective and widely accepted therapy. Both phenoxymethyl penicillin (penicillin V [Pen-Vee-K]) and penicillin G are acceptable. Phenoxymethyl penicillin provides more uniform absorption and is no longer more expensive than penicillin G. The dose schedule is 125 mg. four times a day for the child under 60 pounds and 250 mg. three or four times a day for those over 60 pounds. The same total dose given twice daily may be as effective as the four-times-a-day schedule. Although there may be some advantages in having the child take medication twice a day there is also the risk that if one dose is missed the streptococci will not be eradicated because it has been established that one dose of penicillin a day is ineffective. Treatment failure rates associated with 10 days of any of the forms of oral penicillin range from 10 to 20 per cent and are considerably higher in most studies than the treatment failure associated with a single injection of benzathine penicillin.

Although the broad-spectrum penicillins (e.g., ampicillin) and penicillinase-resistant penicillins (e.g., oxacillin, sodium [Prostaphlin]) are effective antistreptococcal drugs, they have no place in routine therapy.

In the patient with a history of allergy, either documented or suspected, other antibiotics should be considered. Of these, erythromycin is the drug of choice administered for 10 days in a daily dosage of 30 to 40 mg. per kg. divided into 2 or 4 doses. Resistance of Group A streptococci to erythromycin has been reported but is rare. There are a number of other antibiotics capable of eradicating streptococci from the upper respiratory tract when administered orally for 10 days, including the cephalosporins and clindamycin. These antibiotics are more expensive and are reserved for patients in whom there have been adverse reactions to penicillin or erythromycin.

Follow-up. Despite apparently adequate therapy, 10 to 20 per cent of children experience a second attack of streptococcal sore throat or a bacteriologic recurrence within one month of initial treatment. This high recurrence or reinfection rate dictates the need for routine follow-up throat cultures 7 to 10 days after the completion of a full course of penicillin therapy, or 3 weeks after an injection of benzathine penicillin G. Follow-up throat cultures are especially indicated in patients treated with oral antibiotics and in patients who are members of high risk families, including individuals with a history of acute rheumatic fever. Children still harboring group A streptococci should receive a second course of treatment. Intramuscular benzathine penicillin is a good choice and usually eradicates the organism from the throat.

Rheumatic Fever Prophylaxis. Prophylaxis against beta-hemolytic streptococcal infection is recommended for all patients who have had acute rheumatic fever. Any one of the following regimens may be used: (1) Benzathine penicillin G, 1,200,000 units intramuscularly once a month; (2) oral phenoxymethyl penicillin, 125 mg. twice a day to children under 23 kg. (50 lb.) and 250 mg. twice daily to children over 23 kg. and to adults; or (3) sulfadiazine, 0.5 gram daily to children weighing less than 23 kg. and 1.0 gram daily to those patients weighing more than 23 kg.

TUBERCULOSIS AND OTHER MYCOBACTERIAL DISEASE

method of
J. E. KASIK, M.D.
Iowa City, Iowa

There has been a century long, progressive decline in the incidence of tuberculosis. At present, the overall prevalence of skin test reactivity to purified protein derivative (PPD) of the population of the United States is below 25 per cent.

Nevertheless, more than 30,000 new cases of active tuberculosis were reported in the United States in 1977, and a physician's chance of encountering a new case is still significant. Population groups particularly at risk are the aged, recent immigrants, or those who live in certain areas, such as the inner city. Some social groups such as alcoholics or custodial patients also have a significantly increased risk of active disease when compared to the general population.

Unfortunately, the overall decline in the incidence of active tuberculosis has not been as rapid as the decline in the index of suspicion of the disease among physicians who are likely to encounter it. Anyone who appears in a physician's office with cough, sputa, hemoptysis, malaise, fever, and weight loss is very likely to be treated for pneumonia or evaluated for a tumor, often repeatedly, before the possibility of mycobacterial infection is considered.

General Principles of Therapy

The therapy of most forms of tuberculosis is neither difficult for the physician nor dangerous for the patient. The basic principle of therapy is the use of multiple drugs that are given for a sufficient period of time to establish control of the infection and prevent relapse. The number of drugs used depends on the extent of disease. In instances in which the number of organisms is relatively small, such as a tuberculous pleural effusion, two drugs are sufficient. In patients with widespread disease and a large bacterial population, such as in pulmonary tuberculosis with multiple cavities, three or more drugs are often needed to eliminate the bacteria and prevent relapse. In most instances therapy should be continued 18 months or longer. If a patient is started on two or more drugs and therapy is continued for a sufficient period of time, the prognosis is usually excellent.

The cardinal sins in the therapy of tuberculosis are the failure to use multiple drugs and to maintain therapy for a sufficient period of time.

When to Institute Therapy

Therapy for tuberculosis can be initiated on clinical indications alone, without bacteriologic confirmation, if the situation warrants. The usual criteria for instituting therapy are a suspicious history, a compatible x-ray, and a positive skin test. The circumstances compelling presumptive therapy include a serious illness, the danger of infecting others, or a complicating illness that increases the risk of the infection to the patient. It is important to stress that bacteriologic confirmation of active disease may take several weeks and, in some instances, such as in tuberculous meningitis, may never be obtained. As a result, therapy can and should be initiated solely on clinical grounds, if in the judgment of the physician delay in therapy may be hazardous.

A positive skin reaction to intradermal purified protein derivative (PPD) is usually, but not always, found in patients with active disease. It is reasonably safe to begin testing with 5 TU of PPD injected intradermally. A positive skin test is indicated by induration of the skin greater than 10 mm. in diameter, but any reaction larger than 5 mm. is worthy of note. If the reaction to 5 TU is negative, a repeat test with 250 TU should be made. It is accepted that 250 units has a higher incidence of false positive rections than 5 TU, caused by either prior exposure to atypical mycobacteria or to nonspecific reactions. If the test with 250 TU is negative, this is important enough to make the physician reassess the situation, since patients with active tuberculosis who fail to react to this higher concentration are not common. Patients with active disease who are nonreactors to PPD can be encountered among persons who are immunosuppressed, severely ill, malnourished, or aged, and this usually occurs as the result of several simultaneous events. A positive skin test is expected in patients with active disease, but it is not a universal occurrence. Although the test is very helpful in the presumptive diagnosis of tuberculosis, it must be used in the context of the whole clinical picture.

Sputa smears for acid-fast bacilli are often positive in patients with active pulmonary disease, particularly if cavities are present. Smears should be obtained promptly, by induction if necessary, if the disease is suspected. Concentration of the mycobacteria in the sputa specimen significantly increases the yield on smears. Cultures should be obtained, as they are more productive than smears and provide definitive data about the species of mycobacteria causing the infection and its drug sensitivity. If sputa is obtained for culture by induction, the saline solution used must be free of preservatives and the use of propylene glycol in conjunction with the generation of a saline aerosol must be omitted, as both interfere with the growth of the organisms. Simultaneous drug therapy will not interfere with diagnostic bacteriology in primary tuberculosis and should not be withheld on these grounds.

Therapy of genitourinary tuberculosis should be withheld until cultures have been submitted. Forty eight hours of therapy with drugs may sterilize the urine, at least to the extent that cultures will not grow. Genitourinary tuberculosis is diagnosed by a compatible intravenous pyelogram, a positive skin test, and identification of mycobacteria in the urine. A fresh morning specimen is used for cultures.

Therapy of Tuberculosis

Pulmonary Tuberculosis. For minimal to moderate disease, including tuberculous effusion (in adults), use isoniazid, 300 mg. per day, ethambutol, 15 mg. per kg. per day, and pyridoxine, 25 to 50 mg. per day. An optional alternate program uses INH + rifampin (600 mg. per day) + B_6. The concomitant use of pyridoxine (vitamin B_6) is probably not needed in most patients, but it is inexpensive, safe, and precludes INH-induced B_6 deficiency. Drugs are given as a single daily dose for 18 months to 2 years.

For moderate to extensive disease (in adults), use the same combination for minimal disease plus rifampin (600 mg. per day for 1 year).

Optional alternate program: Streptomycin, 1 gram per day for 30 days, then 1 gram three times

TABLE 1. **Drugs Commonly Used to Treat Tuberculosis and Their Side Effects**

DRUG	DOSAGE (ADULT/DAILY)	SIDE EFFECTS	DETECTION	REMARKS
Isoniazid (INH)	5–10 mg./kg.: 300 mg.	Peripheral neuritis, hepatitis, hypersensitivity, convulsions	SGOT/SGPT	For neuritis, B_6 25–50 mg. as prophylaxis; hepatitis rare in young (less than 35)
Ethambutol (EMB)	15 mg./kg.	Optic neuritis (reversible with d/c of drug) very rare at 15 mg./kg., skin rash	Visual acuity, red-green color discrimination (Snellen chart)	Ocular history and funduscopic exam before use; contraindicated with optic neuritis
Streptomycin (SM)	0.75 gram–1.0 gram	Otic and vestibular toxicity, decreased hearing, vertigo, tinnitus	Gross hearing; audiograms; avoid BUN and creatinine	More common in older patients (more than 60); decrease dose or avoid drug if renal insufficiency
Rifampicin (Rif)	600 mg.	GI disturbance, liver dysfunction, thrombocytopenia may interfere with oral contraceptives, and anticoagulation; rare renal damage	SGOT/SGPT Bilirubin BUN & creatinine	Adverse reactions are more common and severe with intermittent therapy. Patients should be warned about intermittent therapy

a week for 12 to 20 weeks, in place of rifampin. Some therapists prefer to save rifampin for possible later reactivation of the disease. The cost and inconvenience of administration and possible ototoxicity of streptomycin are factors to consider. The association of ototoxicity in older patients or patients who have impaired renal function often precludes the use of this antituberculosis medication in those patients.

Miliary Tuberculosis and Other Extrapulmonary Infections (lymph node, osseous, renal, gastrointestinal) (in adults). Use same therapy as for moderate to extensive pulmonary tuberculosis. Some therapists advise an additional year of treatment with INH with B_6 for renal, osseous, or lymph node infection (total INH therapy: 3 years).

Tuberculous Meningitis (in adults). Use same initial therapy as for moderate to extensive pulmonary tuberculosis.

There is evidence that therapy of meningitis with INH-ethambutol alone yields the same results as triple drug regimens, but concomitant miliary disease is possible and sometimes difficult to eliminate as a possibility.

It should be pointed out that there have been reports of tuberculous meningitis produced by organisms resistant to one or more drugs commonly used in the therapy of tuberculosis. These infections usually occur in children from households where another patient resides who had been unsuccessfully treated for pulmonary tuberculosis. The prudent physician who encounters a case of tuberculous meningitis will inquire about this possibility and modify chemotherapy to include two drugs different from those used in the treatment of the contact.

Another problem in tuberculous meningitis occurs in obtunded patients who cannot take oral medication. INH is available for intramuscular injection and should be used with streptomycin.

Childhood Tuberculosis. Primary tuberculosis is treated with INH and ethambutol (see minimal pulmonary tuberculosis). Usual dose of INH in children is 10 mg. per kg. per day (up to 300 mg.) with ethambutol 15 mg. per kg. per day. Duration of therapy is usually 18 months.

Where indicated, rifampin can be added. The usual dose is 10 to 20 mg. per kg. per day, up to 600 mg. per day.

It is important to remember that childhood tuberculosis, particularly primary disease, is seldom infectious.

Triple drug therapy, if possible, should be employed in tuberculous meningitis in children.

Ethambutol has not been approved by the Food and Drug Administration for use in children, but it has been widely employed for this purpose. Its use avoids the use of other drugs with significant toxicity.

Steroids in Tuberculous Infections

Steroids have a mixed effect on tuberculosis. Although they inhibit delayed-type hypersensitivity and thus may activate a latent infection, they also ameliorate the symptoms of the disease. If used in combination with adequate chemotherapy, they have demonstrated value in patients with widespread disease with severe accompanying symptoms such as fever, malaise, anorexia, and debility. As a result, steroids are helpful while awaiting the control of infection by chemotherapy in the patient with widespread tuberculosis who is critically ill.

Steroids are also used in meningeal tuberculosis in patients with impending or overt cerebrospinal fluid block and possible internal hydrocephalus. Because of the serious nature of this complication, some clinicians advocate the use of steroids in all patients with tuberculous meningitis.

Usual dose is prednisone (or equivalent drug), 20 to 30 mg. twice daily or 2 mg. per kg. per day in infants and children up to 60 mg. per day in divided doses.

After one week, the dose can be gradually reduced to one that maintains the patient reasonably free of symptoms. Usually steroids can be discontinued in 4 to 6 weeks.

In meningitis, therapy with steroids should be continued until signs of infection have cleared from the cerebrospinal fluid.

Problem of Dissemination

The close contacts of a patient with active pulmonary tuberculosis must be skin tested. Close contacts are members of his household, coworkers in his immediate vicinity, and those who might also be confined with the source case in the same room for significant periods of time. The incidence of skin test conversion among those in contact with a known case of tuberculosis is a reliable index of the infectiousness of that case.

In childhood tuberculosis or in persons with a recent skin test conversion with a normal chest x-ray, infection of others is seldom a problem. It does indicate, however, recent contact with a patient with active disease. The source case must be identified.

The physician treating tuberculosis must avail himself of the visiting nurse and social service agencies to assure continuing adequate therapy of the patient at home and suitable evaluation of the public health aspects of the patient's illness.

Hospitalization and Isolation

Hospitalization for tuberculosis should be based on the relative needs of the patient, how ill he is, the need for therapy of other problems, and whether diagnostic evaluation is required. As soon as the patient is able to be cared for at home, he may be discharged.

It is important to stress, however, that discharge is not simply giving the patient a supply of medicine and a return appointment. The patient must be educated as to the seriousness of his illness, the excellent prognosis that follows strict adherence to the plan of therapy, and the need for communication with the physician if difficulties are encountered. The patient must be monitored in these regards and reevaluated if compliance is in doubt. The patient must be informed of the potential infectiousness of his illness, the necessity to take his medications, and to be aware of his responsibilities to others.

Tuberculosis is spread by inhalation of droplets containing viable mycobacteria. This is the only significant mode of dissemination. Therefore, the single most important factor in controlling the infection is isolation of the patient in a room with exhaust ventilation. Generation of an infected aerosol can be interrupted by having the patient cough into a disposable tissue and wear a mask, and by prompt, appropriate chemotherapy.

It is obvious that many well-established procedures such as gowns, caps, room sterilization, special eating utensils, and the masking of hospital personnel and visitors have little or no value. The masks commonly employed as a part of isolation for tuberculosis do not significantly limit inhalation of infected droplets generated by infectious patients (0.5 to 5 micron in diameter) and simply give a false sense of security.

The keys to limitation of the spread of tuberculosis at home, in custodial institutions, or in the hospital are a high index of suspicion by the physician followed by prompt diagnosis and institution of adequate chemotherapy. The infectiousness of patients with disease rapidly diminishes on multidrug therapy, and the cessation of the patient's cough limits the dissemination of mycobacteria.

Atypical mycobacterial infections are not transmissible.

Prophylaxis of Tuberculosis

It has been demonstrated that isoniazid (INH), 300 mg. per day (in adults) for 9 to 12 months, can substantially reduce the incidence of active tuberculosis in certain groups of patients. Not only does this prophylactic effect occur during the administration of the drug but the protective effect persists for several years after cessation of therapy. The groups that have been identified in which a program of INH prophylaxis is useful are listed, in order of priority, as follows:

1. Household contacts of patients with active tuberculosis (skin test positive or negative).

2. Recent skin test converters.

3. Previously diagnosed patients with active tuberculosis who are currently inactive but have had no or inadequate chemotherapy.

4. Patients with a positive skin test who have certain other illness such as Hodgkin's disease, lymphoma, carcinoma, silicosis, and who are on

immunosuppressants or antineoplastic therapy, or have had a gastric resection.

5. Patients with a positive skin test who have an abnormal chest x-ray, which suggests inactive granulomatous disease.

6. All tuberculin-positive children and adolescents (in immigrants to the United States the physician should ascertain if the child has been immunized with Bacillus of Calmette and Guérin [BCG], as the vaccine converts the skin test).

7. Tuberculin-positive adults with a normal chest x-ray.

Because the risk of INH hepatitis significantly increases with age and the incidence of tuberculosis is much lower in category 7 than in others, INH prophylaxis in this group is usually limited to persons less than 35 years of age. This limit is not fixed, however, and should be used as a guide only, recognizing that the incidence of INH hepatitis is still relatively low, even in those above this age.

INH Toxicity

Hepatitis produced by INH has been demonstrated to be a common problem in patients treated with the drug. Fortunately, in most patients the problem is only an asymptomatic, minor, and transient elevation of hepatic enzymes.

Only in a few patients, usually in those over the age of 35, does this progress to frank jaundice or on rare occasions death from liver failure. In general, serious liver problems have occurred in those patients who continued to take the drug in spite of signs of toxicity such as anorexia, malaise, and jaundice.

INH toxicity appears to be nonallergic, and the result of direct hepatocellular damage. It is reversible and may not be a problem if the patient is cautiously restarted on the drug with careful monitoring of hepatic function. Current practice is to administer INH to most patients without monitoring hepatic function, warning the patient to discontinue the drug and see the physician if he develops signs of toxicity. There has been a report which has indicated that clinical symptoms of a relatively minor nature may not be a reliable indication of early, reversible hepatic damage. Although this is disquieting, the practice of using INH without monitoring hepatic enzymes is widespread. In certain patients, particularly those who are older or who have preexisting hepatic disease, periodic monitoring of hepatic enzymes during therapy seems advisable, at least during the first months of therapy.

Infections with Atypical Mycobacteria

The atypical mycobacteria are a special problem because of their almost universal resistance to the available antituberculosis drugs.

Rather surprisingly, infections produced by *Mycobacteria kansasii,* the photochromogens, and Runyon Group I organisms respond to therapy almost as well as infections produced by sensitive strains of *Mycobacteria tuberculosis.* These infections are usually treated with a minimum of three drugs: isoniazid, ethambutol, and rifampin, with some clinicians advocating adding therapy with streptomycin 1 gram per day for 30 days, followed by 1 gram 3 times a week for an additional 12 to 14 weeks. Results with this regimen have been good.

The therapy of Runyon Group III mycobacteria such as *Mycobacterium avium* has a much poorer outcome, irrespective of drugs used. Commonly, five or more drugs are used, but the advantages of this approach over less massive and less toxic programs have not been clearly established. Surgery, which is rarely used in the therapy of *M. tuberculosis* infections, is still useful in infections of Group III species if the disease is limited to a resectable area of the lung.

A physician encountering an infection due to the *M. avium-intracellulare* group who has not had experience with these organisms would be wise to seek consultation.

A similar statement should be made of other atypical mycobacterial infections such as the Group IV species and the scotochromogens. These infections are difficult to treat and have a guarded prognosis.

The Problem of Tuberculosis in the Nursing Home

Active tuberculosis is a relatively common problem in nursing homes. The coincidence of debility and a relatively high rate of skin test reactivity to PPD leads to a high risk of reactivation of latent infection. Cases that develop in nursing homes are often overlooked among the many medical problems of the patients who reside in these facilities. As a result, physicians who care for patients in these facilities must be alert for the possibility of active tuberculosis and the facility must have a program of control.

The problem of tuberculosis in a nursing home is simple to deal with if a preventive program is implemented. All patients must have skin tests on admission, and those with positive reactions should have a chest film taken. Those with positive skin tests must be identified as special risks and have biannual chest x-rays. Those with abnormal films, either on admission or later, need to be evaluated with appropriate diagnostic studies. Isoniazid prophylaxis is not recommended for elderly patients with normal chest films. In view of the relative risks, isoniazid should be used only if active disease is suspected.

Nursing home personnel should have skin tests when first employed, and those with negative reactions should be retested every six months. If an employee's test undergoes a conversion, prophylaxis with isoniazid is often indicated. The physician should reevaluate the employee's patient contacts to ascertain how the infection occurred. Evaluation of the rate of skin test conversions in health personnel is an index of the effectiveness of an antituberculosis program in a chronic care facility.

Short Course Chemotherapy

Recent data have indicated that therapy with INH, ethambutol, and rifampin, usually with an initial period of treatment with streptomycin, can control pulmonary tuberculosis and has a low rate of relapse, even if administered for only 9 months. This program of therapy has the major advantage that supervision of the patient is brief, drug toxicity is reduced, and overall costs are minimized. It seems probable that this major advance in the chemotherapy of tuberculosis will have a significant influence on future therapy programs. At present, however, the physician should be reminded that older, standard therapy programs are well established, have a low incidence of toxicity, and, if completed properly, a very low incidence of relapse. In the compliant patient on a well-established drug program, conventional therapy would seem to be the most conservative approach.

Intermittent Therapy

Intermittent therapy is reserved for patients who, for various reasons, require close supervision of their treatment. This is almost always limited to alcoholics or others with significant social or mental problems. It is not a substitute for routine therapy in the average patient. It can be used only in patients with disease that has not been previously treated or whose organisms have been shown to be sensitive to INH, ethambutol, and streptomycin.

Therapy consists of an initial period of in-hospital care with multiple drug therapy, usually 4 to 8 weeks, and then discharge to twice-weekly treatment. Usual doses of drugs are INH, 15 mg. per kg.; ethambutol, 40 mg. per kg.; and streptomycin, 20 mg. per kg. given 2 times a week. The drugs must be given under direct supervision by a visiting nurse who ascertains ingestion. No compromise on the latter point is allowed. Duration of therapy is 2 years.

Other Drugs Used to Treat Tuberculosis

There is a substantial list of drugs such as para-aminosalicylic acid, cycloserine, viomycin, pyrazinamide, kanamycin, and ethionamide that are available for therapy. Their use is limited to retreatment of drug-resistant organisms, therapy of Group III mycobacteria, or where various allergies to one of the conventional drugs exists. Their use should be limited to experienced physicians, as their toxicity can be substantial, and the situations in which they are indicated are complex and often difficult to manage.

Follow-up Procedures

During therapy, the physician should expect improvement in all the findings associated with the infection. Clinical symptoms usually decrease within the first month except in those with very extensive disease. The chest x-ray usually has clear signs of improvement by the tenth to twelfth week of treatment. Sputa may continue to be positive for several months but this is not a sign of infectiousness. Failure to achieve these goals or the late reappearance of mycobacteria in the sputa may indicate a failure of therapy and always demands reevaluation of the patient with particular reference to drug sensitivity studies. In those instances in which this has occurred or is suspected, additional drugs must not be prescribed singly. In a failing program, two or more drugs must be added to or substituted for those in use.

Upon completion of therapy, most patients need periodic follow-up for 2 years, with chest x-ray and sputa cultures. If progress is satisfactory, most can be discharged from care. Those who need longer follow-up are patients who are suspected to have been noncompliant or have other serious illnesses that inhibit cell-mediated immunity.

VIRAL RESPIRATORY INFECTIONS
method of
ROBERT B. BELSHE, M.D.
Huntington, West Virginia

Introduction

Adults living within the United States suffer an acute viral respiratory illness on an average of twice a year, and children become ill with viral respiratory disease with even greater frequency. Collectively, more time is lost from work and school due to viral respiratory disease than to any other illness. This high frequency of morbidity is due to the more than 200 antigenically different viruses that can produce acute respiratory disease. These viruses are a heterogenous lot, including rhinoviruses, myxoviruses, paramyxoviruses, adenoviruses, and coronaviruses. Although each of these groups is classically associated with a specific illness (rhinoviruses and coronaviruses with the common cold, myxoviruses with influenza, paramyxoviruses with croup and bronchiolitis, and adenoviruses with pharyngitis), each of these agents can cause a spectrum of respiratory tract illnesses, ranging from mild rhinorrhea to severe febrile, life-threatening, lower respiratory disease. Thus, a causative association of a specific respiratory illness with a given virus cannot be made on clinical criteria alone.

Establishing a specific etiologic diagnosis requires recovery of virus from secretions of the respiratory tract, the detection of viral antigens in smears of nasal secretions by immunofluorescence, or the detection of a diagnostic four-fold rise in antibodies between serum collected at the onset of illness and that collected during convalescence. These tests are available on a limited basis and usually only in a specialized laboratory. Furthermore, the results from tests other than immunofluorescence usually cannot be obtained for 2 or 3 weeks. Therefore, treatment must be instituted without access to the definitive diagnostic laboratory examination.

Management

Among adults, most viral disease is limited to the upper respiratory tract. Except for influenza A virus infections the illnesses are generally brief, less than 1 week in duration, and fever is usually absent or mild. Treatment, therefore, is limited to the relief of uncomfortable symptoms in adults, with close observation for complicating bacterial infection. In contrast, infants and young children may become very ill, with high fever, airway obstruction, and pneumonia, during infections with one of several viruses. Treatment of infants and children may be lifesaving, particularly if airway obstruction (bronchiolitis) is present. Unfortunately, treatment is limited to supportive care during the acute illness, since (with the exception of amantadine for influenza A virus infection) no specific antiviral chemotherapy exists.

Symptomatic Treatment of Upper Respiratory Viral Infections

Fever, Malaise, Fatigue, and Myalgia. The extent of activity should be curtailed in keeping with the severity of symptoms. Bed rest and aspirin are advised for febrile patients. The dosage of aspirin is 650 mg. (two 325 mg. tablets) orally, every 3 to 4 hours for adults and 60 mg. (one chewable baby aspirin) for every year of age under 10, given every 4 to 6 hours for children. Acetaminophen may be substituted in persons sensitive to aspirin or if aspirin is otherwise contraindicated (patients with peptic ulcer disease, bleeding tendency, or those taking oral anticoagulants). The dosage of acetaminophen is 600 mg. (two 300 mg. tablets) orally every 3 to 4 hours in adults. Acetaminophen may be substituted, alternated, or added to aspirin for children who cannot take or fail to respond to aspirin therapy. A liquid preparation of acetaminophen is easiest to administer to children; the dosage is 16 to 32 mg. every 4 to 6 hours for infants less than 1 year old, 60 to 120 mg. for children 1 to 3 years old, 120 mg. for those aged 3 to 6 and 240 mg. for those aged 6 to 12 years. High fever also may require sponging with tepid water or alcohol to avoid febrile seizures in susceptible children.

Nasal Obstruction and Rhinorrhea. Relief of nasal obstruction is best accomplished with topical applications of long-acting nasal decongestant sprays or drops. For adults, I prefer oxymetazoline 0.05 per cent (Afrin 0.05 per cent) nasal spray, applied with 2 sprays in each nostril every 12 hours. More frequent use or use for more than 3 or 4 days uniformly results in the development of rebound nasal congestion, which may cause a patient to chronically administer such sprays. Xylometazoline 0.1 per cent (Otrivin 0.1 per cent) nasal spray used every 4 to 6 hours or phenylephrine 0.5 per cent (Neo-Synephrine 0.5 per cent) nasal spray used every 3 to 4 hours is equally efficacious but requires more frequent application and also may cause rebound nasal congestion. For children over 1 year of age, I recommend oxymetazoline 0.025 per cent (Afrin 0.025 per cent) every 12 hours and for children less than 1 year, 0.125 per cent phenylephrine drops (Neo-Synephrine 0.125 per cent) every 6 hours. Frequent removal of nasal mucus using a plastic dropper syringe for aspiration and isotonic saline solution to loosen secretions also is beneficial in infants. Neither oxymetazoline nor xylometazoline should be used by patients taking monoamine oxidase (MAO) inhibitors.

Oral medications for nasal obstruction may be used also. There are many over-the-counter and prescription drugs marketed for relief of the symptoms of upper viral infection, and most of these drugs are combinations of decongestant, to relieve nasal obstruction, and an antihistamine, to relieve rhinorrhea. Before prescribing an oral decongestant or antihistamine the physician should inquire as to what medication the patient has self-administered in order to avoid overdosage of decongestants and antihistamines. I recommend pseudoephedrine (Sudafed) for relief of nasal obstruction alone. The dosage is 15 mg. orally every 8 hours for infants less than 4 months old, 30 mg. every 6 to 8 hours for patients aged 4 months to 6 years, and 60 mg. every 6 hours for patients 6 years and older. I recommend chlorpheniramine (Chlor-Trimeton) for relief of rhinorrhea alone. The dosage should be titrated for each patient. The maximum recommended dose is 1 mg. for infants every 8 hours, 2 mg. for children less than 12 years old every 6 to 8 hours, and 4 mg. every 6 hours for adults. Fixed combinations of these 2 drugs or their analogs may also be given (Chlor-Trimeton decongestant, Dimetapp, Drixoral, etc.). Fixed combinations do not allow for titration against individual symptoms, but this is not a major drawback in most patients. Drowsiness is a common side effect in patients who take antihistamines alone or in combination for relief of rhinorrhea.

Nonspecific measures, such as humidification of air, also are beneficial for nasal obstruction for patients in whom this maneuver is practical.

Cough, Sore Throat, and Hoarseness. Persistent cough or cough productive of purulent sputum should always raise the question of lower respiratory infection—of either viral or bacterial cause—and be treated appropriately (see below). Minor cough should be treated with the expectorant guaifenesin (glyceryl guaiacolate [Robitussin]), and if this fails, the cough suppressant dextromethorphan or codeine can be added to the medication. Only plain guaifenesin, ½ teaspoon orally every 4 to 6 hours, should be given to infants. The dosage of guaifenesin-dextromethorphan (Robitussin-DM) is ¼ to ½ teaspoon every 4 hours for children 2 to 6 years old, ½ to 1 teaspoon every 4 hours for children aged 6 to 12, and 1 to 2 teaspoons every 3 to 4 hours for adults. Reduction of rhinorrhea with antihistamines as recommended above also will alleviate cough induced by postnasal drip.

Sore throat is best treated with aspirin in doses listed earlier and frequent warm saline gargle (1 tablespoon of salt dissolved in ½ cup of warm water). Prevention of aggravating factors, cough, and inhalation of irritants such as tobacco smoke also will improve throat irritation.

Hoarseness may be improved by relief of cough with expectorants as recommended above; these loosen mucous secretions trapped in the larynx. Other measures, such as inhalation of humidified air, hydration, and minimizing speaking will help in some patients.

Treatment of Complications of Upper Viral Respiratory Infections. In most patients with viral respiratory disease, the illness resolves without sequelae. In occasional patients serous otitis media, otitis media, or acute sinusitis develops. Serous otitis media is best treated with oral decongestants in addition to liberal use of nasal decongestant drops, which trickle down the nasopharynx and may relieve eustachian tube blockage; use dosages as suggested above. Acute sinusitis also frequently responds to this regimen; however, the addition of an antibiotic, such as ampicillin, is also of benefit in patients with acute sinusitis due to bacterial infection. Acute otitis media should be treated with antibiotics in addition to decongestants.

Viral Infections of the Lower Airways and Lungs

Influenza. Influenza A is the most common cause of serious viral respiratory disease in adults. Influenza A virus infection is generally limited to the upper airway but infection of the lower airways and lungs is not uncommon. When lower respiratory involvement does occur, this infection and its sequelae are life-threatening in certain groups of "high-risk" patients. These "high-risk" persons include those with diabetes mellitus, heart disease, pulmonary disease, other chronic debilitating conditions, and those over 65 years of age. Prevention of influenza A virus infection is best accomplished through immunoprophylaxis. I recommend yearly vaccination with the killed virus vaccine, either the split product or whole virus vaccine, for "high-risk" patients and for persons who provide essential services to the community. The vaccine is efficacious only for the antigenic types of influenza viruses from which it is prepared. Therefore, the vaccine should contain viral antigens of similar serotype to those viruses circulating in the community. Most vaccine contains antigens of one or more influenza A strain and one influenza B strain. The production of vaccine lags one year behind the emergence of new antigenic types of influenza A virus. In 1977–1978, three antigenic types of influenza A virus circulated (A/Victoria/3/75, A/Texas/1/77, and A/USSR/90/77), but influenza vaccine was available only against one of these serotypes which provided protection against A/Victoria/3/75 and partial protection against A/Texas/1/77. Vaccine against the A/USSR/90/77 strain was not available until the 1978–1979 epidemic season.

Fortunately, amantadine can be used for influenza chemoprophylaxis and treatment. This drug is effective in preventing all types of influenza A virus infections but not influenza B or other viral infections. The drug should be given daily to "high-risk" persons when influenza A is known to be circulating in the community. It can also be given at the time of immunization and continued until such time as sufficient antibodies produced by the vaccine have developed (3 weeks). Alternatively, the drug can be given for the duration of the community's epidemic if no vaccine is available. For patients with recent known exposure to influenza A virus, I recommend 10 days of amantadine administration if no repeat exposure is anticipated. The dosage is 100 mg. of amantadine (Symmetrel) orally twice a day for adults. Children, aged 1 to 9 years, can be given 2 to 4 mg. per pound (4.4 to 8.8 mg. per kg.) of body weight in two divided doses and should not exceed 150 mg. daily. The more common side effects include confusion, dizziness, nervousness, anxiety, anorexia, and occasionally depression. I avoid using amantadine in pregnant women.

The efficacy of amantadine in treatment of acute influenza A virus infections is difficult to establish, since in most patients this disease is brief.

However, patients severely ill with influenza A virus infections may be benefited by amantadine treatment. The dosage is the same as given earlier for chemoprophylaxis.

Bacterial pneumonia not infrequently follows influenza virus infections in "high-risk" patients. The reason for this phenomenon is not known but has been ascribed to impaired ciliary action leading to reduced ability to clear foreign substances, depressed pulmonary macrophage function, or other factors. In patients convalescing from influenza, occurrence of fever, increased shortness of breath, chest pains, increased sputum production, or sudden deterioration in general clinical status should alert the physician to the development of bacterial pneumonia. Sputum and blood cultures should be obtained and the initial antibiotic therapy guided by the Gram stain of a sputum sample that the physician is confident has come from the lungs and not the nasopharynx. It should be noted that staphylococcal pneumonia is distressingly common in patients convalescing from influenza infection.

Croup, Bronchiolitis, and Viral Pneumonia in Children. Treatment of infants and children with viral croup, bronchiolitis, or pneumonia is directed at supporting the patient until the viral infection is cleared by the child's immune response. Appropriate laboratory studies should be done to ensure that the patient does not have a bacterial cause for the illness. Infants with evidence of airway obstruction require hospitalization and treatment with humidified oxygen in concentrations to maintain the arterial Po_2 between 70 and 90 mm. Hg. Intravenous fluid therapy should replace fluid losses but not overhydrate the patient, as inappropriate secretion of antidiuretic hormones may occur in patients with bronchiolitis and lead to water intoxication. Furthermore, edema fluid in the bronchioles may aggravate the airway obstruction. Antibiotic therapy is difficult to withhold in severely ill infants, especially when the viral cause of the individual patient's disease is unproven. Patients with lower respiratory infection of suspected, but not yet proved, viral cause can be treated with a broad-spectrum antibiotic such as ampicillin (25 mg. per kg. of body weight per day in equal divided doses intravenously every 6 hours), pending laboratory confirmation of a viral infection or for the duration of the illness if no viral diagnostic services are available. If *Hemophilus influenzae* type B infection is suspected, a chloramphenicol-ampicillin combination is the treatment of choice and if staphylococcal infection is suspected, methicillin (or other penicillinase-resistant antibiotic) is the treatment of choice, pending cultures to confirm or refute these suspicions.

In addition to the above measures, which are efficacious in both croup and bronchiolitis, bronchodilators may be effective in some patients with bronchiolitis. I recommend isoproterenol (Isuprel 1:200) administered by aerosol mist up to 5 times a day as a therapeutic trial. The dosage for infants is 0.25 ml. maximum of Isuprel 1:200 diluted in 2 ml. of saline solution and delivered by inhaled nebulized mist over 15 minutes. In addition, a therapeutic trial of aminophylline (5 mg. per kg. of body weight per dose) can be given administered by slow intravenous drip over 15 minutes. If bronchodilators have no effect, they should be discontinued. Corticosteroids have been shown to have no therapeutic effect on infants with bronchiolitis.

The Cardiovascular System

ACQUIRED DISEASES OF THE AORTA

method of
MICHAEL E. DEBAKEY, M.D.
Houston, Texas

Aneurysms and occlusive disease comprise the two major categories of acquired diseases of the aorta. In most patients, arteriosclerosis is the underlying pathologic condition causing both forms. Although the progress in both diseases may range from extremely slow to extremely rapid, both ultimately produce disabling and even lethal complications. In aneurysms, for example, the average duration of life after diagnosis is from one to several years, with death from rupture in most patients. In occlusive disease, life expectancy is somewhat better, but progressive arterial insufficiency ultimately produces disabling manifestations with terminal ischemic and even fatal complications.

Surgical treatment for acquired aortic disease is now fairly well standardized, with a relatively low operative risk and excellent results. Depending on the nature and extent of the disease, the following methods of surgical treatment may be indicated: (1) resection with graft replacement used primarily in aneurysmal disease, (2) thromboendarterectomy with or without patch graft angioplasty, and (3) the bypass graft.

The most satisfactory material for vascular replacement in aortic disease is the Dacron graft, which is available in various sizes and in two types of fabric construction, knitted and woven. The knitted type, which is now available as a Dacron velour graft and is considered preferable, is used under normal conditions of blood coagulation. The relatively nonporous woven graft is used in special circumstances, particularly when systemic heparinization is necessary.

Aneurysmal Disease

Aneurysms of the aorta tend to assume specific patterns depending on their location. They may be classified, in order of frequency, into: (1) aneurysms of the abdominal aorta, (2) aneurysms of the descending thoracic aorta, (3) aneurysms of the ascending aorta, (4) thoracoabdominal aneurysms, and (5) aneurysms of the aortic arch. Morphologically, they may be classified into three types: (1) fusiform or spindle-shaped, involving the entire circumference of the aorta; (2) sacciform, characterized by a pouch-like protrusion from a narrow opening in the aortic wall; and (3) dissecting, characterized by an intramural separation, usually within the medial layer.

Arteriosclerosis is by far the most common cause of aneurysms. Other less common causes are infection (including that due to syphilis); trauma; associated congenital abnormalities, such as coarctation or patent ductus arteriosus; and previous vascular operations producing false aneurysms.

Aneurysms of the Abdominal Aorta. Aneurysms of the abdominal aorta are characteristically fusiform. They arise just distal to the origin of the renal arteries, extend down to the bifurcation, and sometimes involve the common iliac arteries. They may be asymptomatic, or they may cause pain in the back extending downward toward the thigh or testicle. Pain and tenderness should be considered ominous, since they indicate progression or even imminent rupture. The most common physical sign is a pulsatile mass in the midabdomen extending toward the left side. In addition to this finding, the diagnosis may be made by plain roentgenography; in the film the aneurysm is often outlined by flecks of calcium in the outer wall. The aneurysm may also be visualized in ultrasonograms. Aortography may be necessary in occasional patients.

Treatment is essentially surgical, consisting in resection and replacement with a straight Dacron graft if the common iliac arteries are not involved, or a bifurcation graft if they are involved. The operative fatality rate for nonruptured aneurysms is about 3 per cent, as contrasted with about 33 per cent for ruptured aneurysms. Contraindications for elective operation include severe cardiac pulmonary disease or other disabling conditions. Age, in itself, is not a contraindication, provided the patient's general condition is satisfactory.

Aneurysms of the Descending Thoracic Aorta. Aneurysms of the descending thoracic aorta are primarily fusiform and of arteriosclerotic origin; they arise just distal to the origin of the left subclavian artery and extend downward for varying distances. They occur most commonly in men in the sixth to eighth decades of life. They may be asymptomatic, being discovered incidentally on routine roentgenography of the chest, or they may cause pain owing to distortion, compression, or erosion of surrounding structures. Aortography is essential in order to make a correct diagnosis and provide information regarding the precise location and extent of the disease.

Treatment is surgical excision of the diseased segment of the aorta between occluding clamps and replacement with a suitable Dacron graft. Surgical contraindications are similar to those indicated for aneurysms of the abdominal aorta. Paresis or paraplegia secondary to spinal cord ischemia is the major complication of resection of aneurysms of the descending thoracic aorta. This complication occurs in about 3 per cent of patients whether or not various prophylactic methods are used, including hypothermia, left atrial-to-femoral bypass, and femoral-to-femoral bypass. In recent years we have abandoned these procedures with no change in the incidence of this complication. The surgical risk now ranges between 5 and 8 per cent, and results up to 20 years after operation are excellent.

Traumatic lacerations of the aorta, which are often associated with false aneurysms, usually involve the descending thoracic aorta just distal to the left subclavian artery. Such injuries occur primarily after sudden deceleration in automobile accidents or a fall from a great height. If the patient survives long enough to reach the hospital, the diagnosis should be suspected from the history and evidence of widening of the upper mediastinum on plain roentgenography of the chest. Emergency aortography should establish the diagnosis, and immediate operation is then indicated, consisting in repair of the lacerated aorta or resection and graft replacement. In some patients in whom the diagnosis is not made at the time of the injury and who recover, a chronic false aneurysm develops; it can be treated in the same manner as described for fusiform aneurysms of the descending thoracic aorta.

Aneurysms of the Ascending Aorta. Aneurysms of the ascending aorta may be congenital or acquired; usually the acquired type is due to arteriosclerosis. These aneurysms are commonly fusiform and extend from the aortic annulus or just above it to just proximal to the origin of the innominate artery. Some patients have associated valvular disease with predominant aortic insufficiency. The diagnosis is established by aortography.

Treatment is surgical, consisting in resection of the aneurysm and replacement with a woven Dacron graft; cardiopulmonary bypass and coronary artery perfusion with the heart-lung machine are used. If aortic valvular disease is present, the aortic valve is replaced at the same time. The risk of operation is relatively low (about 5 to 8 per cent), and long-term results are excellent.

Aneurysms of the Transverse Arch. These aneurysms are usually fusiform and of arteriosclerotic origin; they involve part or all of the ascending aorta and the transverse arch. They occur most commonly in men in the sixth to eighth decades of life. They tend to produce symptoms from compression of the upper mediastinal structures and have a grave prognosis.

Treatment is surgical, consisting in resection of the ascending aorta and transverse arch and replacement with a woven Dacron graft; cardiopulmonary bypass with coronary and bilateral coronary artery perfusion is used. The surgical risk is about 12 to 15 per cent, and long-term results are excellent.

Thoracoabdominal Aneurysms. These aneurysms are usually fusiform and of arteriosclerotic origin. They extend from the lower descending thoracic aorta to the upper abdominal aorta, and downward for varying distances to the bifurcation of the common iliac arteries. They are usually manifested by a pulsatile mass high in the epigastrium, which is often associated with pain in the abdomen or back and, in some instances, with symptoms of chronic mesenteric insufficiency or hypertension related to renal vascular ischemia. They occur predominantly in men in the sixth to eighth decades of life. Diagnosis is established by aortography.

Treatment is surgical, consisting essentially in resection with Dacron graft replacement and revascularization of the celiac axis, superior mesenteric, and renal arteries. The surgical risk is about 12 to 15 per cent, and long-term results are excellent.

Dissecting Aneurysms of the Aorta

Dissecting aneurysm of the aorta is characterized by hemorrhagic intramural separation of the medial layer of the aortic wall, usually communicating with the normal lumen by an intimal tear. Although the cause is unknown, the predominant underlying pathologic condition is degeneration of the media in the form of cystic medionecrosis. Dissecting aortic aneurysm is often associated with Marfan's syndrome, hypertension, pregnancy, coarctation, and idiopathic kyphoscoliosis. It occurs in men about twice as often as women, most patients being in the fourth to seventh decades of life. The natural course of the disease has an extremely grave prognosis, with death in about half the patients within the first few days to weeks after onset; only a small percentage survive a few years.

There are three basic types. In Type I the dissecting process arises in the ascending aorta and extends distally throughout the remaining aorta, sometimes beyond the aortic bifurcation. In Type II the dissecting process is limited to the ascending aorta, and in Type III it arises in the descending thoracic aorta at or just distal to the origin of the left subclavian artery and extends distally for a varying distance.

Treatment is medical and surgical. Medical treatment is usually indicated during the early period in patients with acute dissecting aneurysms and is directed toward control of hypertension and reduction of cardiac contractility. Such treatment helps to stabilize the patient's condition so that subsequent elective surgical treatment may be performed. Emergency operation may be required if there is evidence of imminent rupture or if medical treatment fails to control the patient's condition. It is also indicated in the presence of continued pain, occlusion of a major branch of the aorta, severe aortic incompetence, or cardiac tamponade.

In Type I, surgical treatment consists in transection of the ascending aorta, with use of cardiopulmonary bypass, obliteration of the false lumen by approximation of the inner and outer walls of the dissecting process, and end-to-end anastomosis of the transected aorta. In some patients it may be necessary to resect the proximal segment and replace it with a woven Dacron graft. Other patients may require aortic valve replacement.

In Type II, surgical treatment consists in resection of the dissected segment of the ascending aorta, with use of cardiopulmonary bypass, and replacement with a woven Dacron graft. Most of these patients also require aortic valve replacement.

In Type III, surgical treatment consists in resection of the dissecting process in the descending thoracic aorta from just above the origin of the dissection and just distal to the left subclavian artery to a level below the end of the dissecting process or where it is relatively small, usually above the diaphragmatic hiatus, and replacement with a woven Dacron graft. If a distal false lumen remains below, it is obliterated by suture closure of the inner and outer layers before distal anastomosis of the graft.

The fatality rate after surgical treatment has been steadily reduced during the past two decades, now ranging between 10 and 12 per cent. Long-term results have been most gratifying.

Thrombo-obliterative Disease of the Aorta

This form of chronic occlusive disease, also termed Leriche's syndrome, develops because of atherosclerotic changes that sometimes arise first in the terminal abdominal aorta but most often begin in the common iliac arteries. Progressive enlargement and ulceration of the atheromatous process cause increasing constriction of the lumen until complete obstruction occurs. Depending on the rate of development of these pathologic changes, there may be incomplete obstruction of one or both iliac arteries. When both common iliac arteries become completely obstructed, the superimposed thrombus propagates proximally to produce complete obstruction of the distal aorta up to the origin of the renal arteries. In most patients the occlusive process is well localized to the aortoiliac segment, but about one third of the patients have associated segmental occlusion of the superficial femoral arteries.

The disease affects 10 men to 1 woman; most patients are in the fifth to seventh decades of life. Although the clinical manifestations vary according to the extent and duration of the disease, the most common and predominant manifestation is intermittent claudication involving the lower legs, thigh, and buttock. Sexual impotency is sometimes a prominent complaint. As the disease progresses, the pain on walking increases after shorter distances, and eventually the patient has pain at rest. Atrophy of the subcutaneous tissue and muscles of the legs, loss of hair, and even gangrenous changes may eventually occur. Important physical signs include the presence of a systolic murmur over the lower part of the abdomen and inguinal areas and absence or extremely reduced femoral, popliteal, and pedal pulses. The diagnosis may be readily made from these clinical manifestations, but arteriography is essential to determine the precise location and extent of the occlusive process in the aortoiliac region, as well as the possible associated involvement of the femoral and popliteal arteries. This information is essential in planning the operation.

Treatment is surgical unless the patient has contraindications, such as severe cardiac, pulmonary, or other disabling disease that would make the risk of operation prohibitive. The fact that in most patients this form of occlusive disease is well localized to the aortoiliac segment with a patent distal arterial bed permits performance of highly effective surgical treatment in restoring normal circulation. This is also true even in patients with associated localized occlusive segments of the superficial femoral arteries.

The method of surgical treatment depends on the location and extent of the disease. In a small percentage of patients, thromboendarterectomy may be performed, particularly if the atheroma is extremely well localized to the distal abdominal aorta or common iliac arteries. In most patients, however, the bypass graft procedure is preferable. Using a DeBakey Dacron velour bifurcation graft, the surgeon attaches the main limb to the abdominal aorta just below the origin of the renal arteries by end-to-end or end-to-side anastomosis, and he attaches the remaining two limbs below to the external iliac or common femoral arteries by end-to-side anastomosis. If the patient has associated segmental occlusions of the superficial femoral arteries, it may be necessary to perform femoropopliteal bypass grafts, depending on the age and general condition of the patient. Occasional patients may have associated stenotic occlusive lesions of the renal arteries, which may be treated at the same time by means of a bypass graft.

The operative risk is only about 1 per cent. The results of operation have been highly successful, with relief of symptoms and restoration of effective circulation in about 98 per cent of the patients. Long-term results extending from 10 to 20 years have also been highly gratifying.

ANGINA PECTORIS

method of
GILBERT H. MUDGE, M.D.
Boston, Massachusetts

Angina pectoris is a clinical syndrome and not a specific disease. Accordingly, the treatment of angina pectoris will depend on its pathogenic mechanism and not on the symptom complex. While such a principle might be intuitively obvious, it underscores the importance of the clinical presentation and necessitates a careful correlation of such presentation and laboratory data. It will be the purpose of this review to provide a rational basis for the treatment of angina pectoris due to atherosclerotic coronary artery disease. These therapeutic principles will be of potential harm if the clinical presentation of angina pectoris is not due to coronary artery disease.

Pathophysiology of Angina Pectoris

Angina pectoris is a problem of supply and demand. Angina occurs when metabolic oxygen demands of the myocardium exceeds the oxygen supply. Its clinical presentation will be identical, whether a greatly enhanced myocardial oxygen demand exceeds a normal oxygen supply or a severely limited oxygen supply cannot meet minimally enhanced metabolic needs.

The pathophysiologic mechanisms underlying changes in oxygen supply will be one of two alternatives; there must be either obstructive coronary artery disease or there will be vasospastic alterations in the caliber of the coronary arteries. Efforts to modify the former established obstructions have heretofore been unsucessful, and therapy of the latter vasospastic changes in oxygen supply has proved to be a frustrating clinical problem.

Enhanced myocardial metabolic oxygen demand will depend upon a change in the determinants of myocardial oxygen consumption. The major determinants of myocardial oxygen consumption are systolic intraventricular pressure, ventricular volume (pressure × volume is a close approximation of intramyocardial tension or stress), heart rate, contractility, and myocardial muscle mass. The minor determinants of myocardial oxygen consumption, basal oxygen requirements and energy required for myocardial activation, are of little clinical significance and will not be discussed further. In patients with angina pectoris, modifications in the major myocardial oxygen determinants will have profound beneficial clinical effects.

If proper attention is focused on two of the major determinants of myocardial oxygen consumption, the appropriate therapy for patients with angina becomes obvious. Left ventricular muscle mass and state of contractility are impossible to access at the bedside. Ventricular volume will be reflected by cardiac size, as judged by physical examination and roentgenogram. Systolic intraventricular pressure will be proportional to peripheral arterial pressure in the absence of aortic valve disease, and heart rate is routinely available. Thus, the latter two determinants, arterial pressure and heart rate, are readily measurable indices of myocardial oxygen consumption. The heart rate times blood pressure product is a reasonable approximation of myocardial oxygen needs. Angina pectoris in patients with coronary artery disease is usually provoked with an increase in either variable, and therapy is most effective when that increase is returned to basal condition.

Diagnosis of Angina Pectoris

It is most important in the therapeutic approach to angina in patients with coronary artery disease to exclude other causes of transient myocardial ischemia.

Aortic stenosis and insufficiency, idiopathic hypertrophic subaortic stenosis, and pulmonary hypertension should be suspect by cardiac auscultation. Severe hypertension is a common primary causative factor, as may be thyrotoxicosis, anemia, and paroxysmal tachyarrhythmias. Methemoglobinemia and carboxyhemoglobin may rarely induce angina. The diagnosis of angina pectoris due to coronary artery disease should be made by correlation of symptoms, physical examination, and electrocardiogram. Stress electrocardiography may be indicated, and coronary arteriography should be considered if the diagnosis is not secure.

Initial Therapeutic Efforts

The direction of initial therapeutic efforts will be obvious by the clinical presentation. Sudden onset or increase in frequency of anginal discomfort will usually necessitate hospitalization, rest, and close observation. A chronic, stable anginal pattern will require a very careful history, for minor changes in life style may be often met with marked improvement.

The most successful therapy for angina will be achieved in those patients who have an understanding of the condition, its cause, and its precipitating factors. Inciting instances may be avoided if the patient has a rudimentary pathophysiologic understanding for angina. If this can be achieved, modifications in life style and drug regimens will have wider patient compliance.

Initial therapeutic efforts should be directed at the body habitus and habits. Obesity should be vigorously attacked, for it is associated with hypertension and hyperglycemia. A dietary plan low in cholesterol should be formulated. Alcohol, in moderation, may be of help in select patients as a mild sedative, but excess alcohol is to be avoided; it has a profound myocardial depressant effect and considerable caloric value. Most importantly, smoking should be discontinued. Angina pectoris may be provoked by cigarette abuse, perhaps mediated through nicotine-induced catecholamine release. Unfortunately, this last consideration is often the most difficult to change, and dependence on smoking may be so great that any modification produces untoward psychologic stresses. In such instances, common clinical sense must prevail.

The patient's medical regimen should be vigorously explored. Amphetamines and thyroid supplement weight reduction programs must be discontinued immediately. Excessive caffeine use should be discouraged, and use of bronchodilators, nasal decongestants, many antidepressants, and L-dopa continuously monitored.

The psychologic status of each new patient with angina pectoris has to be evaluated. Emotional as well as physical stress may increase myocardial metabolic oxyen demands and should thus be avoided or at least be prepared for with vasodilator therapy. The necessary curtailment in physical activity may be associated with an understandable depression, and a compassionate approach is mandatory. Patients must be aware that angina pectoris is a chronic illness that may often be significantly modified with minimal personal limitations and drug therapy.

Precipitating factors for angina will quickly be recognized by patients. Angina with large meals is often improved with smaller proportions. Cold air–induced angina may be minimized with proper clothing. The effects of necessary strenuous physical exertion, such as sexual intercourse and travel, will be abated with prophylactic drug therapy.

Hypertension is the most commonly overlooked causative factor in the initial approach to a patient with angina pectoris. As mentioned, arterial pressure is a major determinant of myocardial oxygen consumption, and thus any efforts at reducing high arterial pressures towards normal will be directly reflected as a reduction in myocardial oxygen consumption. Patients with underlying obstructive coronary artery disease require an aggressive antihypertensive regimen; borderline normal systolic and diastolic pressures may be unacceptable. In hypertensive patients with severe angina pectoris, hydralazine (Apresoline) should be avoided because of the secondary reflex tachycardia.

Pharmacologic Therapy

Nitroglycerin.   The nitrates are the oldest and most powerful pharmacologic agents used in the treatment of angina pectoris. Amyl nitrate was first introduced, but trinitroglycerin, with less transient effects, has largely replaced it.

Although nitrates have multiple pharmacologic effects, the vasodilatory properties are most important in increasing blood supply and in lowering determinants of myocardial oxygen consumption. Dilation of both the large epicardial coronary arteries and smaller arterioles has been shown, but the enhanced total coronary blood flow seen in patients with coronary artery disease is not nearly as great as the augmentation seen in patients with normal coronary arteries. Rather, the major direct coronary effect of the nitrates on coronary blood flow is to redistribute flow from myocardium with normal perfusion to areas of transient ischemia. The extracoronary actions reduce determinants of myocardial oxygen consumption. General arteriolar vasodilation reduces systemic arterial pressure, and venous dilation leads to peripheral pooling of blood with a reduction in both end-diastolic volume and pressure. This latter effect, one of the most powerful nitrate actions, will rapidly reduce intramyocardial tension, and hence myocardial oxygen consumption. The net response to nitroglycerin administration is reduction in systemic arterial pressure and cardiac output, which will be clinically manifested by reduction in the heart rate times blood pressure product.

Angina pectoris and nitrate therapy is one instance in clinical medicine when detailed instructions in the use of nitroglycerine are just as important as its actual administration. Nitroglycerin tablets are available in multiple strength, from 0.15 to 0.6 mg., but the lowest effective dose should be prescribed. Tablets of 0.3 mg. might be tried initially. With the onset of angina, patients should be instructed to place a tablet under the tongue; a local burning sensation is a reliable marker of the tablet potency. The first trial should be done in the presence of a physician, for headache and hypotension may be untoward effects. Proper placement of the nitroglycerin tablet should be confirmed. The dosage of nitroglycerin may be reduced should vasodilatory headaches present a major problem, and patients should be instructed to assume a knee-chest position for orthostatic hypotension.

Nitroglycerin should be taken with the onset of any anginal discomfort. Should complete relief not be achieved in 5 minutes, the same dose should be repeated; a maximum of 4 fresh nitroglycerin tablets, each taken 5 minutes apart, should be adequate therapy for a single episode of angina. Prolonged pain refractory to nitrates may be an indication of infarction rather than transient ischemia, and thus patients must be advised to report to an emergency room when relief is not achieved. Nitroglycerin should be carried at all times, and the patient preferably should have different supplies, at home and at work. Nitrates must be carried in dark, opaque glass vials and replenished every 6 months because of slow loss of potency.

A major pitfall in the therapy of angina with nitrates is the patients' undue caution with its use. Patients and their families must understand that nitroglycerin is not habit forming or an analgesic. It must be emphasized that the effects of nitroglycerin permit an improvement in cardiac function, the drug being beneficial to limited myocardial oxygen supply. To this end, patients should be asked to use nitrates prophylactically when they anticipate activity that would induce angina. Sexual intercourse, meals, stair climbing, and cold exposure are prime examples, and nitroglycerin taken 5 to 10 minutes before such activity may entirely abort the ischemic response.

It is also important to ask patients to keep estimates of their daily nitroglycerin requirements. An exact record should be discouraged, for it may accentuate fixation with and reluctance to take the medication. Rather, patients might be asked to note how often they must buy a new supply. Such an approximation is an excellent index of myocar-

dial oxygen supply. Any increase in nitrate use may signal impending infarction rather than chronic ischemia.

Long Acting Nitrates. Use of oral nitrates for angina pectoris remains controversial. Animal studies indicate that hepatic degradation of nitrates is so effective that the vasodilatory properties of the medication are rapidly lost. Clinical investigations defining its efficacy with angina pectoris have been inconclusive, but studies with high dose oral nitrates for congestive heart failure are more convincing. There is no question, however, that the long-acting oral nitrates will provide prolonged subjective relief in some patients, although objective indices of myocardial oxygen consumption are little changed. Nocturnal angina is often effectively relieved with such preparations, and their use in anginal prophylaxis is occasionally successful. Isosorbide dinitrate, 5 to 10 mg. four times per day, is most commonly used and deserves consideration in patients refractory to other measures.

The most effective long-acting nitrate preparation is nitroglycerin ointment. A 2 per cent ointment applied to the skin and protected with adhesive paper covering will be slowly absorbed over 4 to 6 hours, providing sustained hemodynamic effect and subjective relief. It is applied in one half to 3 inch strips 4 to 6 times per day. Refractory, unstable, and nocturnal angina is particularly responsive to this preparation.

Beta-Adrenergic Blocking Agents. The recent introduction of the beta-adrenergic blocking agents was a breakthrough in the therapy of ischemic heart disease. While nitrates permitted reduction in arterial pressure and ventricular volume, two other major determinants of myocardial oxygen consumption, heart rate and contractility, were unaltered. Administration of beta-adrenergic blockage now provides such a means.

Beta-adrenergic receptors may be subclassified into two group, β_1 and β_2 receptors. The β_1 receptors are myocardial adrenergic receptors, and successful blockade will produce both a decrease in automaticity of pacemaker sites and a decreased contractile state. The latter type, β_2 receptors, are found in the smooth muscle of the bronchial tree, gut and arterial wall, and successful blockade may induce bronchial constriction, gastrointestinal hypermotility, and peripheral vasoconstriction.

Propranolol is the only approved beta-adrenergic blocking drug in the United States at the present time. Its most important pharmacologic effect in the treatment of angina is substantial reduction in heart rate with minimal effect on arterial pressure and cardiac output. By so doing, the double product (heart $\times$ arterial pressure) is substantially reduced. The contractile state will also be significantly depressed, with further reduction in myocardial oxygen consumption. In the exercise state, when myocardial oxygen demand is augmented, sympathetic nervous system excitation plays a primary role in increasing heart rate, blood pressure, and contractility. This response will be profoundly modified by beta adrenergic blockade. As a result, heart rate, blood pressure, cardiac output, and contractile state will increase less for a given level of exercise, and angina may be prevented.

Clinical trials have confirmed these simple pharmacologic principles. Exercise tolerance increases and nitrate consumption decreases with beta-adrenergic blockade. As this blocking agent is competitive at the receptor site with sympathetic stimulators, it stands to reason that clinical studies have also confirmed that both the degree of beta blockade and clinical response are dose-related; higher blocking doses are more effective than lower dosage. However, due to variations in hepatic metabolism, there is a wide range of effective therapy (80 to 480 mg. daily) and thus a specific protocol must be designed for each patient.

Propranolol may be started at 20 mg. four times per day. The schedule should be increased on a weekly basis until adequate relief is achieved; an increment in each dose of 10 mg. per week seems to be the most reasonable approach. If improvement is not achieved with 480 mg. per day, higher dosage will probably be ineffective. (This dose may be higher than that stated in the manufacturer's official directive.) The adequacy of beta-adrenergic blockade must be determined with each patient encounter. A resting bradycardia of 60 beats per minute or less is often an insensitive index. The response of heart rate to exercise (10 sit-ups, for example) can be readily followed as propranolol is increased, and is a far better measure of effective adrenergic blockade during enhanced metabolic stress. Heart rates of 65 to 70 with such exercise are a reasonable goal.

The side effects of propranolol are directly related to its nonselective blockade of β_1 and β_2 receptors. By depressing the contractile state, it may precipitate frank congestive heart failure in patients with significant left ventricular dysfunction. Propranolol must be avoided in acute congestive heart failure, and given at low dosage (5 to 10 mg. four times per day) in patients suspect of borderline ventricular function. In fact, hospitalization of such patients for propranolol administration is often justified. As propranolol may also provoke bronchial constriction, extreme caution is required in patients with asthma or chronic obstructive pulmonary disease. Small doses (5 to 10 mg. four times per day) should be initially administered and patients followed closely for bronchoconstriction. Pulmonary function studies can be easily followed as propranolol is increased to therapeutic range. Propranolol may also blunt recovery from hypoglycemia in insulin-dependent diabetics, and caution is encouraged with such patients. Propranolol depresses atrioventricular node conduction and should not be used in patients with second or third degree heart block. Fatigue and depression, in the absence of congestive heart failure or low cardiac output, may be particularly bothersome and may preclude the use of propranolol in some patients. Use of selective β_1 blocking agents, not currently available in the United States, may ameliorate some of these side effects.

Much attention has focused in recent years on myocardial infarction following withdrawal of propranolol therapy. Intense exacerbation of angina or frank infarction has been well documented following its abrupt cessation. The exact pathophysiologic mechanism has not yet been defined, but it may be that an enhanced exercise tolerance will suddenly provoke ischemia when the drug is removed. It is therefore imperative that patients be warned not to stop the medication precipitously. Rather, slow tapering of the drug with concomitant restricted physical activity is recommended.

It should stand to reason that the modes of action of the nitrates and beta-adrenergic blocking agent are complementary. The former decreases arterial pressure and ventricular volume, while the latter reduces heart rate and indices of contractility. Accordingly, the concomitant use of nitrates (sublingual isosorbide dinitrate) and propranolol may be significantly more effective than either agent alone.

Other Pharmacologic Considerations. The importance of controlling hypertension in patients with angina has been mentioned. Adequate blood pressure control may relieve all symptoms. Propranolol does have an antihypertensive effect, and thus should be considered in conjunction with other antihypertensives.

Cardiomegaly with congestive heart failure may worsen angina pectoris, for enlarged ventricular volume will enhance myocardial oxygen demand. Diminished perfusion pressure between the aorta and left ventricle will further limit coronary blood supply. Digitalization and diuretic therapy often significantly improves or even eliminates angina. In fact, nocturnal angina may be a manifestation of early cardiac decompensation, improved with simple medical intervention.

The patient's recognition of angina and the potential capability of myocardial infarction may initiate considerable anxiety, which should be treated with mild sedatives or tranquilizers. This is especially important if emotional stress provokes ischemic discomfort. Anticoagulation has little role to play in the management of angina pectoris, and recent evidence suggests that the antiplatelet agents (aspirin, Persantine, sulfinpyrazone) have more effect in reducing sudden infarction than in helping angina discomfort.

Exercise. Appropriate exercise programs are an integral component in the management of angina pectoris. With physical conditioning, patients may be able to perform at a higher level of activity prior to the manifestation of ischemia. Regular exercise programs can be prescribed after a multistaged treadmill exercise test. This will better define exercise capacity and correlate symptoms with electrocardiographic evidence of ischemia. Exercise can then be prescribed to a point just below that level which produces symptoms or electrocardiographic abnormalities. Repeat stress tests should be performed to document progress and direct future efforts.

Walking is probably the best initial exercise. A slow pace can be gradually increased and distance gradually lengthened. Nitroglycerin should always be carried in case angina is precipitated. When a patient can cover 3 to 4 miles in one hour, bicycling, swimming, or jogging might be considered. All exercise should be of gradual onset, with appropriate warm-up and cool-down periods. Isometric physical exertion should be avoided.

Coronary Artery Bypass Surgery. Coronary artery bypass surgery should be considered in many patients with documented coronary artery disease. Coronary and left ventricular arteriography must obviously be performed prior to such consideration for the location of obstructive lesions and patency of the distal coronary blood vessels is as important as defining left ventricular function by left ventricular angiogram. Low operative mortality and long-term success is largely a function of patent distal arteries and preserved left ventricular function.

Approximately 85 per cent of all patients who survive surgery have considerable improvement in exercise tolerance and symptoms. Many centers have shown that patients who were previously on complicated medical regimens with restricted physical activity often return to near normal life style without medication. Change from Class III to Class I cardiac symptomatology can often be anticipated. Those with obstruction to the left main coronary artery or with severe three vessel coronary artery disease may also increase their life expectancy with bypass surgery, but the latter point continues to be controversial.

Multiple factors should enter into surgical consideration. The patient's age and life expecta-

tions are important; a simple medical regimen with moderate restriction of physical exercise may be unacceptable to a young active patient. Complicated medical regimens may have poor patient compliance and might be completely avoided with coronary artery bypass surgery. Age should be no barrier; a young sedentary patient may readily accept activity restrictions distasteful to others many years more senior.

Four criteria should be fulfilled by medical centers that consider patients for coronary bypass surgery: (1) Coronary and left ventricular angiography must have a mortality of less than 0.2 per cent. (2) The operative mortality for patients with good left ventricular function and patent distal coronary vessels must be less than 2 per cent. (3) The perioperative myocardial infarction rate should be 7 per cent or less. (4) Graft patency at 1 year following surgery should be 85 per cent.

If these four criteria are met, many patients with angina pectoris and significant limitation to life style will be well served by the recommendation for coronary artery bypass procedures.

Variations of Angina

Unstable Angina. Any patient with the recent onset of severe angina or a sudden increase in anginal frequency should be considered to have unstable angina. Present evidence indicates that such patients are not at high risk for myocardial infarction or death if properly managed. Hospitalization, bed rest, sedation and close observation are usually mandatory. Propranolol and nitrates should be administered. Coronary arteriography and surgery may have to be considered if symptoms do not abate with intensive medical efforts.

Prinzmetal's Variant Angina. Coronary artery vasospasm has been shown to be the causative factor in provoking variant angina. Episodic, nonexertional, transmural ischemia and ventricular arrhythmias are the cardinal features of the syndrome, often with devastating consequences. The syndrome may be associated with obstructive coronary artery disease or with normal coronary anatomy. Therapy for variant angina is poor. Propranolol may be of little help, for enhanced myocardial oxygen consumption is not the inciting vasospastic factor. Nitrate therapy is often effective, but high dosage and constant administration is usually required. Bypass surgery has not met with overwhelming success. There are experimental direct coronary vasodilators (nifedipine) available to the European market which hold some promise in the treatment of this potentially devastating syndrome.

Specific Approach to a Patient with Angina Pectoris Due to Coronary Artery Disease

1. Careful history and physical examination, excluding nonatherogenic causes for angina. Signs and symptoms of congestive heart failure should be specifically excluded.

2. Resting electrocardiogram—is there evidence of previous infarctions?

3. Stress electrocardiography—what is patient's exercise capacity? What are the magnitudes of the S-T segment changes? Is there evidence for left main coronary artery obstruction, with 5 mm. ST depression? Which coronary arteries are involved?

4. Chest x-ray—is there evidence for heart failure?

5. Detailed discussion with patient regarding risk factors, pathogenesis, and precipitation of angina. Risk factors should be altered.

6. Detailed discussion of the therapy of angina pectoris. Mode of action of nitrates and propranolol should be explained. Coronary bypass surgery should be mentioned as a possible alternative at this point, for the general population is very knowledgeable regarding this alternative.

7. Initiation of nitrate (nitroglycerin) therapy. Patient should take first tablet in presence of physician and be warned of side effects. Prescribe exercise level.

8. Initiation of propranolol if history suggests that angina will not be controlled with 1 to 2 nitroglycerin tablets per day.

9. Increase propranolol on weekly basis, using symptoms and exercise-induced changes in heart rate as index of beta-adrenergic blockade.

10. Consider adding sublingual isosorbide dinitrate to propranolol; consider long-acting oral agents for nocturnal angina.

11. Reconsider surgical intervention at any point if symptoms do not abate or satisfactory improvement is not achieved.

CARDIAC ARREST

method of
ARTHUR A. BERENBAUM, M.D.,
AHMED C. KUTTY, M.D.,
and ROBERT BIGGANS, M.D.
Philadelphia, Pennsylvania

Definition

Cardiac arrest is defined as the sudden and unexpected cessation of effective cardiac output that maintains the metabolic requirements of the vital body organs. This catastrophic event, regardless of the cause, inevitably leads to irreversible brain damage unless immediate effective resuscitation is instituted within 2 to 3 minutes following collapse.

A rapid diagnosis is essential and is generally based on the following signs: sudden loss of consciousness, absence of heart sounds, absence of carotid and femoral pulsations, no discernible effective respiration, and other signs of circulatory collapse.

Cardiorespiratory arrest should be presumed to have occurred in a person who suddenly loses consciousness accompanied by absent pulses or ineffective respirations or both.

Etiology of Cardiopulmonary Arrest

Conditions commonly associated with cardiac arrest include: (1) acute myocardial infarction, (2) various degrees of atrioventricular block, (3) acute pulmonary embolism, (4) valvular heart disease (aortic stenosis), (5) a complication of diagnostic procedures and use of certain drugs and anesthetic agents and (6) electrolyte and metabolic abnormalities.

The most common mechanisms are: (1) ventricular fibrillation, (2) cardiac standstill (asystole), and (3) a type of electromechanical dissociation resulting in profound cardiovascular collapse. Ventricular fibrillation is frequently observed in coronary heart disease, whereas asystole is most commonly associated with anesthesia.

General Considerations

Sudden cardiac deaths, according to the American Heart Association, exceed 300,000 annually—two thirds of the patients die before reaching a hospital. The majority occur in the presence of friends, family, and bystanders. Immediate initiation of basic life support measures by bystanders might increase considerably the victim's chance of recovery. Since the cardiac arrest phenomenon is frequently encountered by nonprofessionals, it seems imperative that more people become thoroughly familiar with the immediate recognition of cardiac arrest and application of successful cardiopulmonary resuscitation (CPR) in, as well as out of, hospital surroundings.

In prehospital cardiopulmonary collapse, bystander initiated life support was associated with a more favorable outcome and decreased mortality and morbidity than when CPR is delayed, pending arrival of a trained rescue team. Lay CPR is suggested as an important means of salvaging lives in the prehospital phase of cardiopulmonary collapse.

Management of Cardiac Arrest

The fundamental techniques of CPR are:

Airway. The single most important factor contributing to successful CPR is reestablishing an open airway.

1. Should a person be suspected of having acute airway obstruction due to the inhalation of a

foreign body (e.g., food), a forceful back-slap should be attempted initially. If this fails, then the recently described Heimlich maneuver should be attempted promptly. This technique consists of a forceful "bear-hug" applied to the upper abdominal area.

2. Place patient in the supine position. When unconscious, the tongue falls backward and blocks the airway. Lift neck and tilt head backward. Place one hand behind patient's neck and the other hand on the forehead relieving mechanical blockage of airway. In addition, remove with your fingers any foreign matter in the mouth and throat. If spontaneous breathing is not resumed, begin immediate artificial ventilation by either mouth to mouth or mouth to nose breathing.

3. Mouth to mouth technique: Patient's nose is sealed with thumb and forefinger. Produce a tight seal between resuscitator's and patient's mouth. Initial ventilatory maneuver consists of four full breaths. After initial maneuver repeat respiratory cycle every 5 seconds.

Circulation. If no heartbeat is present, deliver a sharp blow to the sternum with the ulnar surface of the folded fist—the so-called "thump version." This may occasionally restore the heartbeat and terminate ventricular fibrillation. If unresponsive to the single sharp blow, start promptly external cardiac compression (ECC) and continue resuscitation until a spontaneous pulse returns. Once an oral airway is established, begin ECC and coordinate with artificial ventilation as follows:

1. If one operator is performing resuscitation, proceed initially with 4 deep breaths followed by 30 seconds of ECC. This should be followed by 2 quick lung inflations and then 30 seconds of ECC.

2. Manual technique of external cardiac compressions: Patient is supine with resuscitator's shoulder directly above the sternum. The heel of one hand is placed over the lower third of the sternum superior to the xiphoid process. The heel of the second hand is placed over the dorsum of the lower hand. Only the heel of the lower hand should be in direct contact with the patient's chest. Exert pressure vertically downward so that the sternum moves 1.5 to 2 inches.

Advanced Life Support. If "thump version" and external cardiac compression do not effectively restore cardiac output, further treatment with DC defibrillation and drug therapy should be initiated. Basic life support can be enhanced by more specialized techniques. However, more advanced life support methods only supplement, not replace, the basic life support techniques.

AIRWAY AND VENTILATION SUPPORT. In order to prevent pharyngeal obstruction by the tongue, an oropharyngeal or nasopharyngeal airway should be inserted. A well-fitting mask with a bag for manual ventilation can be used very effectively to sustain respirations. Oxygen should be administered.

Endotracheal intubation can be performed by experienced personnel if ventilation is not adequately maintained or prolonged support seems necessary. Should the intubation attempt become prolonged, further hypoxia should be minimized by continuing adequate ventilatory support by the bag-mask method. Once endotracheal intubation has been established, mechanical ventilation can be initiated.

CIRCULATORY SUPPORT. Electrocardiographic monitoring should be established immediately to determine the present rhythm and any occurrence of dysrhythmias. Arterial blood gases should be obtained and monitored at frequent intervals for detecting hypoxemia and acidosis.

VENTRICULAR FIBRILLATION. DC countershock should be applied immediately to the precordium with 400 watts per seconds. If the initial attempt is unsuccessful repeated countershocks should be delivered. If still unsuccessful, intracardiac epinephrine 1:1000, 0.5 to 1.00 ml. will on occasion enhance the ventricular response to countershock. Recent evidence suggests the effectiveness of bretylium tosylate (investigational) in primary ventricular fibrillation.

Technique of defibrillation. In an adult 400 watt-seconds (joules) should be delivered to the precordial area. One paddle is placed to the right of the sternum at the third interspace and the other near the midaxillary line in the fifth interspace. An adequate amount of electrode gel should be applied to both paddles. Children require less energy (approximately 2 watt-seconds per kg. of body weight).

VENTRICULAR TACHYCARDIA. This arrhythmia usually responds to an intravenous bolus of lidocaine 2 per cent (75 to 100 mg.). If circulatory collapse exists then direct cardioversion is the treatment of choice. Synchronized DC countershock should be used when pharmacologic intervention fails. In instances of recurrent ventricular tachycardia, propranolol (1 to 2 mg.) intravenously could be tried with repeated administration of bolus lidocaine. Procainamide can be used also effectively. One hundred mg. bolus at 5 minute intervals not to exceed 500 mg. total dose and an infusion of 2 to 4 mg. per minute may also be used to maintain therapeutic blood level.

ASYSTOLE. If there is no response to the precordial thump or intracardiac epinephrine, calcium chloride 10 ml. of a 10 per cent solution, or an infusion of isoproterenol (Isuprel) 1 to 2 mg. in

500 ml. of 5 per cent dextrose in water at a rate of 1 ml. per minute may be tried. However, these latter two pharmacologic agents are seldom effective in restoring cardiac activity in cardiac asystole. Transthoracic or transvenous pacing should be attempted promptly should these agents fail.

ELECTROMECHANICAL DISSOCIATION. This condition is diagnosed when electrical activity is maintained without effective pump or hemodynamic function of the ventricle. In addition to myocardial failure, pericardial tamponade should be considered. Emergency pericardiocentesis can be lifesaving. Calcium chloride, 0.5 to 1 gram, can enhance cardiac contractility. Large dose corticosteroids have been reported to be possibly effective (methylprednisolone, 1 to 2 grams intravenously).

Maintenance of Life Support. Close monitoring of the fluid balance and the metabolic state of the patient is critical. Blood gases should be monitored frequently and the correction of acidosis made by the administration of sodium bicarbonate, 1 mEq. per kg. Calcium chloride, 0.5 to 1.0 gram intravenously, can be used to enhance myocardial contractility if epinephrine, 0.5 ml. of 1:1000 solution given intravenously, is unable to maintain cardiac activity.

Atropine, 0.5 to 1.0 mg. intravenously, can be used if a sinus bradycardia exists, but atrial activity should be evident. Should the bradycardia be unresponsive to atropine then isoproterenol, 2.0 mg. in 500 ml. of 5 per cent dextrose in water at an infusion rate of 1 ml. per minute, can be administered. Temporary pacing can be employed if the bradycardia is resistant to pharmacologic therapy or if there is evidence of a high degree of atrioventricular block. Hypotension due to cardiac failure can be treated by an infusion of dopamine, 400 micrograms in 250 ml. of 5 per cent dextrose in water at an initial rate of 5 micrograms per kg. per minute, titrating the infusion up to 25 to 50 micrograms per kg. per minute if needed. Levarterenol, 4 mg. in 500 ml. of 5 per cent dextrose in water at a rate of 4 to 8 micrograms per minute, may be used if dopamine cannot maintain the blood pressure at a systolic level of 90 mm. Hg. The infusion of either agent must be done with care through an indwelling venous catheter which is patent and infiltration into the subcutaneous tissues has not occurred. The insertion of a central venous pressure catheter is preferable. Diuresis may be facilitated by the administration of furosemide, 40 to 80 mg. intravenously. Diuretics, coricosteroids, and total body hypothermia can be employed if the resuscitated person does not regain consciousness immediately in order to prevent further brain damage.

TERMINATION OF RESUSCITATION. Absence of effective cardiac activity persisting for more than 10 minutes despite adequate efforts to support cardiopulmonary function would indicate cardiac death. Brain death cannot be determined immediately in many instances. Should satisfactory cardiac activity be restored, further neurologic evaluation is required.

COMPLICATIONS. Numerous complications can occur following successful resuscitation. These include rib fracture, pneumothorax laceration of abdominal viscera, and aspiration pneumonitis. These conditions require immediate attention. Late complications include anoxic encephalopathy, renal failure, and sepsis.

ATRIAL FIBRILLATION

method of
ROSS D. FLETCHER, M.D.,
and ALBERT A. DELNEGRO, M.D.
Washington, District of Columbia

A thorough evaluation of the clinical setting is central to the successful management of atrial fibrillation. In the asymptomatic patient with no underlying treatable disease, chronic atrial fibrillation of longer than one year's duration and no inappropriate acceleration of ventricular response to exercise warrants no specific therapy. The majority of patients with atrial fibrillation will require therapy. In the therapy of atrial fibrillation causes such as severe mitral stenosis, thyrotoxicosis, infection, pulmonary emboli and pericardial disease, must be addressed for successful management. Other diseases in which atrial fibrillation is commonly seen such as primary myocardial disease, atherosclerotic heart disease, and mitral valve prolapse are less amenable to correction, since the underlying causes cannot be relieved but they frequently involve medication for control of the arrhythmia.

Initial Therapy

The mode of presentation of the patient determines the type of initial therapeutic intervention. The patient with hemodynamic compromise, e.g., hypotension, intractable angina, or pulmonary edema, constitutes an emergency. The patient whose hemodynamic state is well compensated may be addressed in a more leisurely fashion.

Emergency intervention in atrial fibrillation is likely to be needed in patients with mitral stenosis in which the rapid ventricular response may so shorten the diastolic filling period that incomplete atrial emptying raises the atrial pressures to the pulmonary edema range. The loss of atrial kick in patients with ischemic heart disease and compromised left ventricular compliance may drop cardiac output to hypotensive levels. This decrease in oxygen supply coupled with increased oxygen demand associated with a rapid ventricular heart rate may provoke ischemic chest pain and myocardial necrosis. Similarly, the patient with asymmetric septal hypertrophy may become hypotensive when this arrhythmia supervenes. In such patients immediate reversion of the arrhythmia to normal sinus rhythm may be life-saving. The procedure of choice in such patients is synchronized DC electrical cardioversion. Recent administration of digitalis preparations to the patient, so often done as an initial therapeutic measure, may be countered by precardioversion treatment with lidocaine, 100 mg. intravenously as a bolus, and an intravenous infusion of lidocaine, 2 to 3 mg. per minute, just prior to cardioversion.

In the patient with new onset atrial fibrillation but without hypotension, chest pain, or pulmonary edema, initial pharmacologic control is indicated. Therapy is aimed chiefly at the control of ventricular response. This is achieved by the use of intravenous short-acting digitalis preparations. The authors favor the use of digoxin, 0.5 mg. intravenously followed by 0.125 to 0.25 mg. intravenously at 2-hourly intervals until sufficient atrioventricular (AV) nodal vagal effect limits the ventricular response to 80 to 100 beats per minute.

Intravenous propranolol has also been used as a means for acute control of the rapid ventricular response to atrial fibrillation and is especially useful in mitral stenosis with good left ventricular function. Pulmonary congestion in such patients is caused by a rapid heart rate with mitral valve obstruction and resultant high left atrial pressure rather than by poor left ventricular performance. Propranolol is the initial therapy for atrial fibrillation in the setting of thyrotoxicosis and asymmetric septal hypertrophy (ASH). Indeed, the symptomatic ASH patient may become more profoundly symptomatic if an inotropic agent such as digitalis is administered. Initially, 1 mg. of propranolol HCl may be given intravenously every 3 to 5 minutes to a total of 7 mg. This should be followed up by an oral administration of propranolol titrated in dosage to achieve a ventricular response in the 80 to 100 beat per minute range.

The patient with the Wolff-Parkinson-White (WPW) syndrome and atrial fibrillation presents a special problem. An extremely rapid and irregular ventricular response with anomalous QRS forms mimicking irregular ventricular tachycardia may be the only clue to the diagnosis. The use of digitalis preparations in these patients is contraindicated, especially if the fastest ventricular response is equivalent to 290 beats per minute. Digitalis will shorten the refractory period of the accessory pathway (Kent bundle) and instances of shortening the R-R interval to less than 0.20 second with resultant ventricular fibrillation have been noted by the authors and reported by others. Propranolol in such patients increases AV nodal blockade, but accessory pathway conduction is unaffected by beta-blockade. In the WPW syndrome with atrial fibrillation, intravenous lidocaine, 50 to 100 mg. as an intravenous bolus followed by an intravenous infusion at 2 to 3 mg. per minute, or procaine amide, 250 mg. as an intravenous bolus followed by an intravenous infusion at 4 to 6 mg. per minute, will usually slow the ventricular response. Quinidine and disopyramide will lengthen bypass refractory periods. Emergent cardioversion of the atrial fibrillation may be the best way to prevent ventricular fibrillation in this unusual setting.

Electrical Cardioversion

The preferred mode of reversion to normal sinus rhythm is by synchronized DC electrical cardioversion. The patient is prepared by withholding all oral intake for at least 8 hours. Digitalis preparations are held for one half-life, (about 36 hours for digoxin, 5 days for digitoxin), and digitalis-induced arrhythmias during electrical cardioversion are decreased by pretreatment using lidocaine as outlined above immediately prior to cardioversion. A single oral dose of quinidine sulfate, 300 to 400 mg., is given about 2 hours prior to cardioversion; 5 to 10 per cent of patients revert to sinus rhythm on this alone. The cardioversion is performed in an intensive care setting, often assisted by an anesthesiologist. Proper precautions are taken to assure access to airway if needed. Oxygen and suction should be available. Diazepam, 5 to 20 mg. titrated to deep sleep or a short-acting barbiturate given by an anesthesiologist will ensure patient comfort and amnesic experience. The defibrillator's ability to synchronize its discharge with the midforces of the QRS is verified. Care must be taken to avoid synchronization on a prominent T wave. Defibrillator paddles are placed over the manubrium and the fifth intercostal space at the anterior axillary line. One paddle may also be placed anteriorly and the other one posteriorly to the right of the spine, so that the electrical energy traverses the atria more efficiently than any other part of the heart. The paddle areas are lubricated with conductive gel. If saline sponges are used, care must be taken to avoid an invisible salt bridge between the paddles that can shunt energy away from the heart. Ten pounds (4.5 kg.) of pressure is placed on the paddles and the stored energy is discharged to the patient. The majority of patients will convert with an initial dose of 75 watt-seconds. If this is unsuccessful, 150 watt-seconds and finally 400 watt-seconds are used. One must distinguish between failure to revert atrial fibrillation and successful reversion followed by premature atrial beats and resumption of atrial fibrillation. The former is treated by higher energy application to the patient. The latter is treated with the use of intravenous antiarrhythmic agents such as procaine amide, or propranolol before repeat reversion at the same energy level. Higher levels of oral quinidine prior to a repeat attempt at reversion may also be successful.

After successful reversion to normal rhythm, the patient is allowed to awaken, and quinidine, 300 mg. orally every 6 hours, is started. The quinidine dose is titrated against effect as well as against serum level one half hour prior to the next scheduled dose of 300 mg. The patient is observed for 4 to 18 hours and is thereafter discharged.

Quinidine therapy for maintenance of normal rhythm if unsuccessful may be augmented with oral propranolol or oral procaine amide. If a remediable cause of atrial fibrillation is corrected, e.g., thyrotoxicosis or mitral stenosis, antiarrhythmic therapy may eventually be discontinued.

Pharmacologic Conversion

Despite the usefulness and widespread availability of electrical therapy, pharmacologic reversion frequently occurs with general support and relatively low doses of quinidine. The ventricular response to atrial fibrillation must first be slowed by the use of digitalis preparations or beta-blockers, since quinidine's vagolytic effect increases ventricular response. Quinidine is given in increasingly higher doses, starting at 200 mg. orally every 6 hours and progressing to 400 mg. orally every 6 hours. Gradually, the fibrillation becomes less disordered, slower, and finally the arrhythmia is terminated.

Aggressive pharmacologic conversion of atrial fibrillation is fraught with the hazards of drug toxicity, both cardiac and systemic. The doses required for reversion may induce postural hypotension and vascular collapse. Tinnitus and diarrhea are commonly seen as toxic side effects. Finally, termination of the arrhythmia may result in extreme bradycardia secondary to quinidine suppression of pacemaker activity. We have observed quinidine reversion of atrial fibrillation result in profound sinus bradycardia with AV dissociation and hypotension. A more aggressive dosage schedule is 200 mg. every 2 hours for five doses followed on the next day with 300 mg., then 400 mg. every 2 hours on the third day. Increasing quinidine to high levels for purposes of reversion is more hazardous than the preferred electrical reversion.

The electrical or pharmacologic reversion of atrial fibrillation to sinus rhythm is attended by a low but real incidence of systemic embolization. The frequency of embolization peaks at about 2 to 3 days and correlates with the resumption of muscular activity of the previously fibrillating atria, which takes on the order of 1 to 4 days to recur postcardioversion for patients with fairly long-standing atrial fibrillation.

The incidence of systemic embolization is higher in patients with mitral stenosis, prosthetic mitral valves, primary myocardial disease, and patients with a previous history of emboli. Most agree that full anticoagulation with warfarin (Coumadin) to a prothrombin time of 2 to 2.5 times normal for a period of 2 weeks prior to cardioversion is indicated in the high risk patients. Not all agree on who is at risk. We recommend anticoagulation therapy for all patients with left ventricular dysfunction, mitral valve obstruction, or a history of emboli.

The object of anticoagulation is to prevent new thrombi from being present during reversion. Full anticoagulation should be present for 2 weeks to allow organization of old thrombi and prevent any new thrombi from being laid down. Similarly, since full muscular contraction of the atria in sinus rhythm may not be present for 2 to 3 days, anticoagulation therapy is continued for 1 week after reversion.

Maintenance of Sinus Rhythm after Reversion

The atrial muscle thins because of disease and becomes fibrotic after being in atrial fibrillation for more than 1 year. Sinus rhythm is difficult to maintain after two years of atrial fibrillation. It is for this reason that most patients with recent onset atrial fibrillation are given a trial after reversion to sinus rhythm on maintenance quinidine sulfate, 300 to 400 mg. every 6 hours. If diarrhea becomes a side effect, quinidine gluconate is tried at 330 mg. every 12 or every 8 hours. On occasion, the combination of propranolol and quinidine will be more effective in maintaining sinus rhythm than quinidine alone. Procaine amide is used but is less effective for maintaining sinus rhythm and more likely to create side effects. Disopyramide, 100 to 150 mg. three times daily, may control atrial fibrillation and has constipation rather than diarrhea as a side effect. Urinary retention and blurred vision are side effects and occur as its vagolytic properties are more potent than those of quinidine. This could be detrimental if the patient begins atrial fibrillation with a rapid ventricular response.

If atrial fibrillation recurs, the efficacy of the maintenance program and the need for sinus rhythm govern the decision to attempt cardioversion again. Failure to take medication or failure to achieve proper quinidine levels, would make an additional trial of sinus rhythm indicated. If the ventricular rate is controlled, an atrial kick is not needed or sinus rhythm is difficult to maintain, we permit the patient to remain in chronic atrial fibrillation.

Therapy of Chronic Atrial Fibrillation

In patients with long-term chronic atrial fibrillation who are otherwise well compensated, chronic therapy is directed at the control of the ventricular response. This is best judged by counting the apical heart rate at rest and after climbing a flight of stairs. A rate faster than 120 beats per minute to mild exercise indicates poor control of ventricular response and suggests the need for additional AV nodal blockade. The agent chiefly used is a digitalis preparation. Digoxin is the drug preparation we prefer. Much higher doses may be necessary for control of atrial fibrillation than are conventionally used for control of congestive heart failure. High serum digoxin levels have been recorded in patients treated for atrial fibrillation. Nonetheless, such patients appear to have a low incidence of digitalis-induced ventricular ectopy. The dose of digoxin should be titrated against the ventricular response. If control cannot be maintained with digoxin, occasionally, it may be achieved by changing to the longer half-life digitoxin. Again, the dose should be titrated against ventricular response. If there is concern about digitalis-induced ventricular ectopy at very high doses, augmentation of AV nodal blockade may be achieved by concomitant use of propranolol if there is no history of left ventricular decompensation.

PREMATURE BEATS

method of
ARTHUR J. MOSS, M.D.
Rochester, New York

Introduction

Premature beats may originate in the atrium, the atrioventricular junctional tissue, or in the ventricle, and from a functional point of view junctional premature beats are classified as originating in the atrium. Premature beats are omnipresent, occurring in healthy persons as well as those with organic heart disease. The spectrum of premature beats ranges from those that are isolated or infrequent to the frequent and complex patterns (bigeminy, pairing, multiform configuration, repetitive or sustained rhythms). Premature beats may occur in normal persons without specific provocation, with stress, in the setting of acute or chronic organic heart disease, during the perioperative period, with metabolic disorders, and from a variety of drugs and medications. The mechanisms underlying the production of premature beats are still controversial, but current evidence suggests reentry rather than enhanced automaticity as the predominant electrophysiologic disorder. Premature beats may be subjectively appreciated by the patient as palpitations or detected as an irregular rhythm by the physician during the physical examination. The increased probability of detecting premature beats during prolonged recordings, with oscilloscopic monitoring, telemetry, or Holter-type electrocardiographic tape recordings has enhanced the clinical recognition of premature beats. Premature beats are usually benign without major prognostic implications when they occur in the absence of organic heart disease. On occasion, premature beats may indicate the presence of previously unsuspected heart disease. Premature beats may be precursors of tachycardia and fibrillation, but, in general, the clinical significance of premature beats is determined by the severity of the underlying heart disease process and the associated comorbidity.

A variety of drugs are useful in the treatment of premature beats, and they may be classified into the following categories: (1) anxiolytics such as benzodiazepam and related compounds; (2) primary antiarrhythmic agents such as quinidine, procainamide, lidocaine, and disopyramide, the so-called membrane active agents; (3) beta blockers, an expanding group of antiadrenergic agents of which propranolol is the prototype agent; (4) digitalis preparations, with digoxin the most commonly prescribed drug; and (5) phenytoin, a primary antiepileptic agent that has therapeutic usefulness in digitialis toxic rhythms. The therapeutic decisions to initiate and terminate antiarrhythmic therapy for premature beats requires clinical judgment. As premature beats may be innocent or have ominous implications depending upon the clinical situation, and as each of the drugs utilized in the treatment of premature beats has potentially adverse effects, risk-benefit considerations must be understood. Once a decision is made to treat patients with a particular premature beat, the duration of therapy should be finite and drug therapy terminated when the risk posed by the premature beat is no longer present.

Atrial Premature Beats

Atrial premature beats (APBs) increase in frequency of occurrence with advancing age. Although they may occur as isolated phenomena in the absence of coexisting disease, and thus not require specific therapy, APBs may also be the precursor to atrial tachycardia, flutter, and fibrillation rhythms. Specific antiarrhythmic therapy is indicated when APBs are associated with troublesome subjective palpitations or when they occur in vulnerable patients with a propensity to atrial tachyarrhythmias, i.e., rheumatic mitral valve disease, preexcitation syndromes (Lown-Ganong-Levine and Wolf-Parkinson-White) with accessory pathways, hyperthyroidism, coronary heart disease, and the atrial brady-tachy syndrome. Generally, the spectrum of conditions seen in patients with APBs is quite different in ambulatory as opposed to hospitalized patients, and the therapeutic approach varies accordingly.

Ambulatory Patient. 1. APBs in individuals without evident heart disease but with troublesome palpitations: (a) Withdraw stimulants such as coffee, tea, coke, alcohol, and excitatory sympathomimetic agents that frequently trigger APBs and more complex rhythms; (b) reduce anxiety with appropriate reassurance or anxiolytic agents or both such as diazepam, 5 mg. orally three times daily; (c) antiarrhythmic therapy using quinidine sulfate, 200 to 400 mg. orally three or four times daily or the long-acting preparation quinidine gluconate 324 mg. orally every 12 hours is usually effective in eliminating most benign APBs, but these drugs may have significant adverse side effects in 20 per cent of the treated patients. Alternate drugs which may be administered singly in therapeutic trials include digoxin, 0.25 mg. orally once or twice daily, disopyramide, 150 mg. orally three or four times daily, or propranolol 20 to 40 mg. orally three or four times daily; (d) combination therapy: drug combinations are required only in the exceptional patient with frequent and subjectively troublesome APBs unresponsive to the aforementioned antiarrhythmic therapy. The most effective drug combination for suppressing APBs is quinidine and propranolol; quinidine and digoxin are an alternative combination that is also useful.

2. APBs in patients with preexcitation syndromes (short PR interval and episodic atrial tachycardias): (a) Discontinue all alcohol consumption, since ethanol appears to enhance the production of reentrant APBs and tachycardias involving the accessory pathway; (b) nonspecific therapy with the anxiolytic agent diazepam, 5 mg. orally three times daily, may be helpful in suppressing APBs and preventing emergence of tachycardias; (c) procainamide, 500 mg. orally four times daily, is the preferred agent in patients with preexcitation syndrome, although quinidine, 400 mg. orally four times daily, propranolol, 40 mg. orally four times daily, or disopyramide, 150 mg. orally four times daily, are alternate drugs with proven efficacy in this syndrome; (d) combination therapy: procainamide plus propranolol appear to act synergistically in eliminating APBs and inhibiting the occurrence of tachycardias. Propranolol plus quinidine or disopyramide are alternative combinations in patients intolerant of procainamide or in the absence of efficacy with procainamide. (e) Digoxin may enhance reentrant beats and rhythms in patients with accessory pathways around the atrioventricular node, and this drug is usually not administered as initial therapy. However, a small percentage of preexcitation patients are helped with digoxin, and this agent may be tried when more traditional therapy fails.

3. APBs in patients with chronic organic heart disease (coronary hypertensive, rheumatic heart disease): (a) Treat the underlying heart disorder to improve cardiac function and reduce myocardial ischemia. Thus, the appropriate use of cardiac glycosides, diuretics, potassium supplementation, and afterload reducing agents in congestive heart failure, antihypertensive drugs in patients with hypertension, and antianginal therapy in patients with myocardial ischemia is often effective in eliminating or markedly reducing APBs in patients with these disorders. (b) Digoxin, 0.25 mg. once or twice daily, if it has not already been administered for treatment of overt mechanical dysfunction, is the antiarrhythmic drug of first choice. There is a high probability that it will suppress APBs, and it should be effective in controlling the ventricular response rate to atrial fibrillation should the latter develop. (c) Quinidine sulfate, 200 to 400 mg. orally three or four times daily, or disopyramide, 150 mg. orally three or four times daily, may be used in conjunction with or in place of digoxin in the control of frequent and complex APBs. (d) Low dose propranolol, 10 to 20 mg. orally three or four times daily, is a very effective synergistic agent for controlling APBs when used in combination with digoxin, quinidine, or disopyramide.

Hospitalized Patient. 1. APBs complicating acute myocardial infarction: (a) Optimize circulatory and metabolic states with oxygenation, decongestion, and blood pressure stabilization as indicated by the clinical state; (b) quinidine sulfate, 200 to 400 mg. orally every six hours, should be tried initially, although procainamide, 375 to 500 mg. orally every four hours, or disopyramide, 150 mg. orally every six hours, may be used alternatively with good efficacy; (c) propranolol in doses ranging from 10 to 40 mg. orally every six hours may be used as a primary or complementary agent if the hemodynamic state permits; (d) although digoxin is relatively effective in controlling APBs and preventing complicating atrial tachyarrhythmias, this inotropic and ventricular arrhythmogenic agent should generally be avoided in patients with acute infarction. Recent evidence suggests that digoxin may extend the zone of myocardial infarction or enhance the generation of ventricular arrhythmias in this clinical setting, and thus, digoxin is relatively contraindicated.

2. APBs in association with decompensated rheumatic mitral valve disease: (a) Digoxin, 0.75 to 1.0 mg. oral loading dose in a divided schedule followed by a maintenance regimen of 0.25 mg. orally once or twice daily, is the agent of choice if this drug has not already been administered for hemodynamic stabilization; (b) quinidine sulfate, 200 to 400 mg. orally every six hours, should be administered in conjunction with the digoxin in hopes of preventing the emergence of atrial fibrillation. Procainamide, 375 to 500 mg. orally every four hours, or disopyramide, 150 mg. orally every six hours, may be substituted for quinidine in those patients intolerant of the latter drug. (c) More vigorous or involved treatment with propranolol is generally not indicated or required.

3. Multifocal APBs complicating chronic obstructive lung disease: (a) Optimize internal homeostasis—hypoxia, hypercarbia, hypokalemic alkalosis, respiratory acidosis, and congestive heart failure are metabolic and circulatory disorders frequently seen in acute exacerbation of chronic lung disease. These disorders enhance the development of multifocal APBs in the setting of cor pulmonale, and correction of the metabolic and circulatory problems will contribute to rhythm stabilization. (b) Therapy by subtraction: toxic levels of sympathomimetic amines, aminophylline and related compounds, and digitalis may develop inadvertently, and reduction of dosage or discontinuance of medication is usually effective in diminishing the frequency and complexity of APBs. (c) Antiarrhythmic therapy: when the above measures fail, a trial with quinidine sulfate, 200 to 400 mg. orally every six hours, is warranted. In the absence of prior digitalis therapy, low dose digoxin, 0.125 mg. orally once or twice daily, should be administered. Aggressive therapy is not indicated in an attempt to eliminate all APBs.

Ventricular Premature Beats

With the appreciation of the significance of ventricular premature beats (VPBs) in the early phase of acute myocardial infarction, clinicians have become increasingly concerned about the prognostic meaning of VPBs in patients with and without evident heart disease. VPBs have ominous implications in the presence of a recent coronary event, and they add additional risk to patients with cardiomyopathy. The prognostic meaning of VPBs in the presence of mitral valve prolapse is probably overestimated. In contrast, VPBs occurring in the setting of the long QT syndrome are harbingers of sudden death, yet standard antiarrhythmic therapy is contraindicated. Drug-induced VPBs, which occur with digitalis toxicity or tricyclic antidepressants, are always potentially dangerous. When VPBs exist in the absence of identifiable organic heart disease, it is reasonable not to treat the asymptomatic patient.

Ambulatory Patient. 1. VPBs in persons without evident heart disease but with troublesome palpitations or in patients with mitral valve prolapse (click-murmur syndrome, i.e., Barlow's syndrome): (a) Withdraw stimulants such as coffee, tea, coke, alcohol and excitatory sympathomimetic agents which may lower the threshold for the genesis of VPBs. Eliminate all unnecessary medication, especially tricyclic antidepressant drugs and hormonal agents. (b) Reduce anxiety with appropriate reassurance or anxiolytic agents such as diazepam, 5 mg. orally three times daily. (c) Antiarrhythmic therapy using propranolol, 20 to 80 mg. orally three or four times daily, is almost universally efficacious and is unequivocally the drug of first choice in this population. Alternate therapy with quinidine sulfate, 200 to 400 mg. orally three or four times daily, procainamide, 500 mg. orally four times daily, or disopyramide, 150 mg. orally four times daily, may be used in place of propranolol, but generally with less effective results. (d) Drug combinations that should be tried in patients with troublesome VPBs refractory to the single administration of the above agents are propranolol plus quinidine.

2. VPBs in high risk patients such as postinfarction patients or those previously resuscitated from ventricular fibrillation or both: (a) Frequently these patients have major mechanical dysfunction of the heart with congestive heart failure, low cardiac output, and limited cardiac reserve; hemodynamic stabilization with diuretics, potassium supplementation, afterload reduction, and conservative digitalis therapy (checked with blood levels) should be administered as indicated by the clinical state; (b) avoid complicating electrolyte imbalance with frequent evaluation of serum electrolytes and appropriate therapy with potassium chloride administration; (c) antiarrhythmic therapy using quinidine sulfate, 200 to 400 mg. orally every 6 hours, or procainamide, 500 mg. orally every four hours, are the mainstays of management in this high risk group. These drugs should be administered in full dosage with ade-

quacy of therapy determined by follow-up Holter-type ECG tape monitoring and by the achievement of therapeutic blood levels (4 to 8 micrograms per ml. for quinidine or procainamide). Disopyramide, 150 to 200 mg. orally every 6 hours, is an alternate agent in those patients intolerant of quinidine and procainamide. (d) Propranolol, if the hemodynamic state permits, 20 to 80 mg. orally every six hours, should be administered as a complementary agent in those patients with refractory ventricular irritability. In less hemodynamically compensated patients, small doses of propranolol, 10 to 20 mg. orally every six hours, are often beneficial in improving the efficacy of quinidine, procainamide, or disopyramide. (e) Drug combinations are generally the rule in this select group, and patient compliance in maintaining an optimal dosage interval (every six hours or every four hours as specified for the individual agents) is important for obtaining reasonably stable blood levels. (f) Persistence of frequent and complex VPBs in this vulnerable group, despite the above measures, is an indication for hospitalization, continuous monitoring, and more vigorous therapy with parenteral agents to determine the potential for suppressability.

Hospitalized Patient. 1. VPBs in association with acute myocardial infarction: (a) Oxygenation; (b) initial parenteral therapy with lidocaine, 100 mg. intravenously, followed by maintenance infusion of 3 to 4 mg. per minute intravenously (40 micrograms per kg. per minute) for 24 to 72 hours is the antiarrhythmic agent of first choice with the highest degree of efficacy. Procainamide, 100 mg. per three minutes intravenously up to a maximum of 800 mg. followed by maintenance infusion 2 to 3 mg. per minute intravenously (30 micrograms per kg. per minute) for 24 to 72 hours, may be used as an alternative agent to lidocaine with nearly equal efficacy. On occasion, procainamide will suppress and control VPBs in situations refractory to lidocaine. Quinidine can not be given intravenously, but quinidine gluconate, 300 mg. intramuscularly every six hours, is a useful agent. The onset of action of intramuscular quinidine is considerably less rapid than intravenous lidocaine or procainamide. (c) Complementary therapy with propranolol, 1 to 2 mg. intravenously or 20 to 80 mg. orally every six hours, may be used in conjunction with lidocaine, procainamide, or quinidine, especially when ventricular irritability persists after initial parenteral therapy with these agents. (d) Oral maintenance therapy with procainamide, 375 to 625 mg. orally every four hours, quinidine sulfate, 200 to 400 mg. orally every six hours, or disopyramide, 150 to 200 mg. orally every six hours, should be administered for a minimum of 1 week after discontinuance of

parenteral therapy in patients who continue to manifest ventricular irritability. Propranolol is also useful during this stage, especially when active myocardial ischemia or sympathetic hyperactivity or both are contributing factors in the genesis of the VPBs. (e) Hypokalemia, if present, should be treated with potassium chloride supplementation, 15 mEq. diluted in 100 ml. of 5 per cent dextrose in water and administered intravenously over 1 hour in urgent situations, or orally in doses of 25 mEq. when the situation is less demanding. Repeat doses may be given in 1 to 2 hours as indicated by the degree of hypokalemia. (f) Drugs such as digitalis, phenothiazines, and tricyclic antidepressants which may exacerbate ventricular irritability should be withheld. (g) Hemodynamic stabilization with control of angina, hypertension, and congestive heart failure may eliminate refractory VPBs. (h) In the setting of significant bradycardia ($<$50 per minute) unresponsive to atropine, 1.0 mg. intravenously, transvenous pacemakers should be considered for rate control.

2. VPBs in association with digitalis toxicity: (a) Stop digitalis medication for several days and obtain digitalis (digoxin or digitoxin) blood level; (b) discontinue diuretics, which may contribute to potassium loss; (c) potassium chloride should be administered if the serum K^+ level is less than 5 mEq. per liter and if digitalis-induced atrioventricular block is not present. Renal function should be evaluated (urine output, blood urea nitrogen, serum creatinine) and potassium chloride administered, 15 mEq. orally. Additional doses should be administered at dosing intervals as indicated by the persistence of the VPBs, the status of the renal function, and the serum potassium level as determined by serial electrolyte determinations. The ECG should be monitored during potassium therapy. (d) Phenytoin, 100 mg. every three minutes intravenously up to a total of 800 mg. (10 mg. per kg.), should be administered to patients with frequent and multifocal VPBs (this use of phenytoin is not listed in the manufacturer's official directive). (e) Lidocaine, 100 mg. intravenous bolus followed by a maintenance infusion of 3 to 4 mg. per minute, or procainamide, 500 to 750 mg. orally followed by 250 to 500 mg. orally every four hours, may be used interchangeably to complement phenytoin therapy or as the preferred drugs in place of this latter agent. (f) Propranolol, 1 to 2 mg. intravenously or 20 to 80 mg. orally every six hours, is useful either as a primary or as an adjunctive agent, but it should not be administered in the presence of significant sinus bradycardia or atrioventricular block. (g) In the presence of complicating high grade atrioventricular block, a temporary transvenous right ventricular pacemaker is useful in preventing excessive bradycardia and

permitting safe suppressive therapy with phenytoin, lidocaine, procainamide, or propranolol.

3. VPBs in association with quinidine or procainamide toxicity: (a) Stop the offending medication; (b) digoxin, lidocaine, and potassium chloride are contraindicated; (c) sodium bicarbonate, 40 to 50 mEq. intravenously, is useful as an immediate temporizing measure for stabilization of complex VPB patterns; (d) dopamine, 5 micrograms per kg. per minute intravenously, should be administered for correction of hypotension and low output syndrome which frequently complicates toxicity with these agents; (e) hemodialysis may be considered when primary or secondary renal insufficiency is present.

Antiarrhythmic Drug Considerations

Utilization of antiarrhythmic agents requires an understanding of basic pharmacokinetic (absorption, distribution, metabolism, and excretion) and pharmacodynamic (dose-response relationship, efficacy, selectivity, and adverse reactions) principles. For orally administered agents, the dosing interval for maintaining less than a 50 per cent fluctuation in the blood level of the drug is roughly equivalent to the half-life (procainamide, 4 hours; quinidine, 6 hours; propranolol, 4 hours; phenytoin, 20 hours; digoxin, 30 hours). Furthermore, efficacy guidelines using blood level measurements have been established for most of the antiarrhythmic agents, and blood level measurements should be used to monitor proper dosage (procainamide and quinidine, 4 to 8 micrograms per ml.; propranolol, 75 to 100 nanograms per ml.; phenytoin, 10 to 18 micrograms per ml.; digoxin, 1 to 2 nanograms per ml.; and lidocaine, 2 to 5 micrograms per ml.). Dose adjustment is often required to obtain adequate blood levels. After initiating antiarrhythmic drug therapy, the ECG should be monitored for antiarrhythmic efficacy. In ambulatory patients, follow-up Holter-type monitoring or attempts at premature beat provocation with exercise stress testing or both are useful measures that should be routinely employed for critical evaluation of the patient's response to treatment. Antiarrhythmic therapy should be discontinued when the risk posed by the arrhythmia and the associated cardiac condition is no longer present. Frequently, this decision is a difficult one, and observation of the patient's rhythm (Holter monitoring, exercise stress testing) after discontinuance of the antiarrhythmic medication will clarify whether or not continued maintenance therapy is required.

HEART BLOCK

method of
JOHN F. MORAN, M.D.,
and ROLF M. GUNNAR, M.D.
Maywood, Illinois

Heart block has many forms and composes a major portion of cardiac arrhythmias. Knowing the cause of heart block is often critical to proper patient management. The common causes of heart block are: (1) coronary artery disease, (2) idiopathic fibrosis of the bundle branches, (3) cardiomyopathies, and (4) calcific aortic valve disease. Other less common causes include congenital heart block, surgically induced block, connective tissue disorders, amyloidosis, diphtheria, syphillis, and myocarditis. Heart block may occur in the sinoatrial node by generator failure, in the perinodal area of the sinus node, the atria, the atrioventricular node, the His bundle, or the bundle branches. Symptomatic bradycardia from block in any of these areas requires treatment. The cornerstones of treatment for the various forms of heart block are atropine, isoproterenol, and electrical pacing.

Drug Therapy

Results of drug therapy for heart block are unpredictable and, therefore, are useful only in emergency or unusual circumstances. In all forms of heart block, the ventricular rate may be increased temporarily by the use of atropine intravenously. Atropine sulfate should be given intravenously at first in a dose of 0.5 mg. then repeated if there is no effect in 2 or 3 minutes. Smaller doses of atropine, or subcutaneous administration, have occasionally caused a paradoxical slowing of the sinus rate and, therefore, should be avoided. If there is still no response in the heart rate, another 1 mg. of atropine can be given in 10 to 15 minutes for a total of 2 mg. in a 10 to 15 minute space of time. Atropine can be repeated in 1 to 2 mg. doses every 4 to 6 hours if it creates the desired therapeutic result. If 2 mg. of atropine fails to induce an increased heart rate, more atropine will not likely be effective. Atropine still must be considered a temporary measure because of its side effects such as urinary retention, increased intraocular pressure, gastric retention, and psychosis, particularly in the elderly. It would be expected to obtain its greatest effect on lysis of vagal tone to the sinus and atrioventricular nodes.

Isoproterenol (Isuprel) is a potent stimulator of beta-adrenergic receptors. It has strong chronotropic effects as well as strong inotropic effects. The subsequent increase in cardiac output is due to increased left ventricular contractility as well as increased rate. A solution of 1 mg. of isoproterenol in 500 ml. of 5 per cent dextrose in water would allow an infusion rate of 1 to 6 micrograms per minute or a concentration of 2 micrograms per ml. Unfortunately, an increase in heart rate and contractility means an increase in myocardial oxygen consumption. Additionally, systemic peripheral resistance is reduced and this could mean a fall in blood pressure and a decrease in coronary blood flow if coronary flow is pressure dependent. Furthermore, ventricular irritability can be increased and ventricular ectopy can result. These factors make isoproterenol a poor choice in patients with acute myocardial infarction. However, the drug still has temporary use in patients whose heart block is on the basis of fibrosis of the conduction system as their myocardium may otherwise be normal. The heart rate and blood pressure requires careful monitoring as excess isoproterenol would decrease the cardiac output by causing excessive increases in heart rates. Heart rates should be kept below 65 beats per minute in order to avoid induction of ventricular tachycardia.

Levarterenol (L-norepinephrine) is a naturally occurring sympathomimetic drug that can increase heart rate, contractility and cardiac output. It is both an alpha and a beta receptor stimulator. It would be the drug of choice in a patient with heart block, severe hypotension or cardiogenic shock. As blood pressure increases to near normal, the reflex vagotonic effect will slow the rate and atropine or another sympathomimetic drug should be used. The dosage of levarterenol is variable. Lower doses increase the cardiac output by increasing heart rate and stroke volume. Higher doses cause peripheral vasoconstriction. The drug is supplied as levarterenol bitartrate injection (Levophed) in 4 ml. ampules containing 4 mg. One ampule in 1000 ml. of 5 per cent dextrose in water would allow an infusion of 4 micrograms per ml. This could then be titrated for the desired effect. Frequently, this requires 4 to 16 micrograms per minute. Both isoproterenol and levarterenol can be used in an emergency situation to bring the heart rate into the range of 45 to 50 beats per minutes or to stabilize the systolic blood pressure at approximately 100 mm. Hg.

Dopamine (Intropin) is a naturally occurring biochemical catecholamine precursor of norephinephrine that has been useful in the treatment of shock and refractory congestive heart failure. It has inotropic and chronotropic effects, causes dilatation of renal and mesenteric vascular beds, reduces coronary vascular resistance and causes vasoconstriction of peripheral capacitance and resistance vessels. Dopamine has been very useful in patients with left ventricular dysfunction following open heart surgery. The effect on heart rate depends on the clinical setting. In dog studies, dopamine and levarterenol produce similar dose-dependent increases in heart rate. However, dopamine was approximately one-tenth as potent as levarterenol or isoproterenol. In human patients, dopamine also has less tendency than other amines to increase the heart rate. However, clinical studies of cardiogenic shock have reported significant increases and significant decreases in heart rate. The primary indication for dopamine is cardiogenic shock or left ventricular pump failure when hypotension is present but moderate. Isoproterenol would be a better selection if bradycardia is the prime problem although if there is profound hypotension, levarterenol would be the choice. Dopamine (Intropin) is supplied in 5 ml. ampules containing 200 mg. of dopamine. It must be diluted in 250 or 500 ml. of 5 per cent dextrose in water to create a concentration of 800 micrograms or 400 micrograms per ml. respectively. This can then be titrated by intravenous infusion to bring the systolic blood pressure to 100 mm. Hg. An infusion rate of 2 to 5 micrograms per kg. per minute is a suggested starting point. Most patients will respond in the range of 8 to 15 micrograms per kg. per minute although doses up to 30 micrograms per kg. per minute have been used. Doses greater than 0.5 mg. per minute in the adult, will obliterate the renal and mesenteric vasodilator effect as the alpha vasoconstrictive effect increases.

Other drugs have also been used in the past. Isoproterenol sublingually, 10 to 20 mg. every 3 to 4 hours, sustained action isoproterenol (Proternol) 30 mg. every 4 to 6 hours, ephedrine, 15 to 30 mg. orally every 3 to 4 hours, and hydroxyamphetamine (Paredrine), 40 to 60 mg. orally every 2 to 4 hours, are all examples of drugs that have been used in the past and found to be basically undependable. Depletion of serum potassium with thiazide diuretics has also been recommended but difficulties caused by hypokalemia are more detrimental than any relief of atrioventricular block that results. This may especially be true in the presence of digitalis. This experience, however, does emphasize the deleterious effects of sudden infusion of potassium in a patient with impending heart block.

In summary, drug therapy for heart block may be useful as a temporary or an emergency measure. This will allow time for the implantation of a pacemaker. Temporary pacemaker insertion can be done easily with the floating or balloon pacing catheters. Fluoroscopy can help in catheter positioning. A direct current cardioverter should always be available during pacemaker insertion as there is a risk of ventricular fibrillation. This should be a small risk in the hands of a skilled physician.

Sinoatrial Disease, "Sick Sinus Syndrome"

Failure of the sinus node impulses can result from generator failure or block of the sinus impulse in the perinodal tissue. These cannot be differentiated easily electrocardiographically but sinoatrial block usually produces dropped P waves without disturbing the basic cycle length and if the block has a Wenckebach configuration, there will be a slight shortening of the P-P interval before the dropped beat. Often these patients do not have functioning intrinsic escape pacemakers and the ventricular impulse is also dropped. This syndrome also encompasses patients with paroxysmal supraventricular tachycardias who suffer marked sinus bradycardia when they undergo spontaneous conversion to sinus rhythm. Atropine in doses of 1 to 2 mg. intravenously can cause an increase in the sinus node rate but usually this is small. The use of atropine is impractical for long-term therapy and furthermore may only increase the rate of a subsidiary pacemaker. It also can decrease the atrial effective refractory period in these patients.

Often these patients will have disease in other areas of the conduction system, therefore, ventricular pacemakers are often recommended. If facilities are available for electrophysiologic studies that then demonstrate isolated sinus node disease, coronary sinus-atrial pacemakers are useful. More evidence is accumulating that coronary sinus pacing is safe and efficacious. However, the usual treatment for patients with symptomatic sinus bradycardia is ventricular demand pacing. Holter monitor recordings are frequently best for establishing the diagnosis.

Atrioventricular Nodal Block

Atrioventricular (AV) nodal block can be described as: (1) first degree AV block or PR prolongation, (2) second degree AV block or dropped sinus beats, and (3) third degree or complete AV block. Most chronic AV block does not involve the AV node specifically. Coronary artery disease or drug effects are the most common causes of AV block.

Prolongation of the PR interval caused by digitalis is not an indication for stopping digitalis in the absence of other symptoms. However, second degree AV block of the Wenckebach type is an indication to stop digitalis. In the setting of an acute myocardial infarction, first degree AV block requires only observation. More advanced degrees of AV block can follow, especially in the presence of anterior wall myocardial infarction.

Second degree AV block, in the setting of coronary artery disease, is often seen with acute inferior or diaphragmatic myocardial infarctions. The reason is that in 90 per cent of patients, the right coronary artery supplies blood to the artery of the AV node. Most often, second degree AV block of the Wenckebach type occurs, and an intrinsic well-functioning junctional escape pacemaker maintains the heart rate above 50 beats per minute. The patient experiences no symptoms and the arrhythmia clears spontaneously. Only observation is required in the coronary care unit. However, if symptoms of hypotension, angina, or congestive heart failure occur when the heart rate is slow, a temporary pacemaker is indicated. With the standby pacemaker in place, drugs such as digitalis can be given with more confidence. Most of these patients will not require a permanent pacemaker. If the second degree AV block is caused by quinidine, procainamide, morphine, or potassium, these drugs must be discontinued, as this is a sign of toxicity.

Congenital AV block almost always involves the AV node. Few of these patients receive pacemakers as children for a variety of reasons: (1) they are asymptomatic if they survive infancy, (2) associated inoperable congenital cardiac malformations preclude survival, (3) use of pacemakers in children is technically difficult, and (4) sudden death may be the first manifestation of complete AV block. A permanent pacemaker should be inserted in these young patients for symptoms of syncope or heart failure or slow heart rates, especially if the QRS is abnormally widened or the rate does not increase with exercise. Permanent pacing is also required in postoperative complete heart block or trifasicular disease.

Whereas second degree AV block of Wenckebach type (Type I) usually involves the AV node, second degree AV block of Mobitz (Type II) usually involves the His-Purkinje intraventricular conduction system. Most cases of chronic AV block involve fibrosis of these tissues. If type II second degree AV block is associated with a normal QRS complex, it represents a lesion in the main bundle of His. Type II AV block is either associated with disease in the bundle of His (20 per cent) or the bundle branches (80 per cent). Documentation of intermittent complete heart block can best be obtained with Holter monitor recordings if no facilities for more complete electrophysiologic studies are available.

Intraventricular Conduction Defects: Trifasicular Disease and Bilateral Bundle Branch Disease

The concept of three fasicles, the right bundle branch, the posterior division of the left bundle branch, and the anterior division of the left bundle branch, supplying conduction to the ventricles has served well to improve understanding of block below the AV node. A combination of complete right bundle branch block and left axis deviation or left anterior hemiblock is frequently found in patients' electrocardiograms preceding the onset of complete AV block. A frequency to develop complete AV block of approximately 10 per cent per year was found for patients with complete right bundle branch block and left axis deviation. The cause of trifasicular disease is critical here. If the disease is caused by an acute anterior wall myocardial infarction, the prognosis may be much worse than if the cause is idiopathic fibrosis of the bundle branches.

Recent studies suggest that trifasicular or bifasicular disease in the presence of acute myocardial infarction has a mortality of approximately 50 per cent. This is due to severe coronary artery disease and death occurs most often as a result of cardiogenic shock or left ventricular failure. Of those patients who survived the acute episode, a large number will die in the subsequent two years. Onset of the bifasicular disease in the setting of an acute myocardial infarction without documented second degree AV block, is associated with a 21 to 38 per cent incidence of progression to complete AV block. Much of the controversy surrounding permanent prophylactic pacemaking following acute myocardial infarction is clouded by a lack of any randomized series to study this problem. The number of patients is small and their coronary artery disease is usually severe. Therefore, in the absence of electrophysiologic studies to demonstrate a normal HV interval, we would permanently pace this group. We would feel more secure in this recommendation had we demonstrated a prolonged HV interval. More data may place this indication of prophylactic pacemaking in perspective, separating it from the left ventricular dysfunction and ventricular tachycardia-fibrillation causes of sudden death. These patients are probably at greater risk because they have severe coronary artery disease and severe left ventricular disease, in addition to advanced conduction system disease.

In summary, we would recommend a pacemaker in the following: (1) symptomatic bradycardia of any mechanism, (2) the bradycardia-tachycardia syndrome, a type of the sick sinus syndrome, if drug treatment fails to control the tachycardia without producing marked or symptomatic bradycardia, (3) bilateral bundle branch block, complete right bundle branch block or complete left bundle branch block, developing during an acute myocardial infarction, especially anterior wall myocardial infarction, and (4) Mobitz Type II AV block or complete AV block in the adult even if it is asymptomatic.

TACHYCARDIA

method of
DJAVAD T. ARANI, M.D.,
and DAVID G. GREENE, M.D.
Buffalo, New York

In the treatment of tachycardias the most important point to remember is that one is treating a patient with tachycardia, not treating the tachycardia. The distinction is important because appropriate treatment for one patient may miss the target completely in another patient with the same tachycardia. For example, sudden atrial fibrillation producing heart failure in one patient may demand prompt direct current (DC) cardioversion, while the same event in another patient may call for nothing but a little digoxin. The rhythm disturbance is the same; the patients and the treatments are distinct.

The heart of a healthy adult at rest usually beats 60 to 100 times per minute. When the heart rate or the rate of a cardiac chamber exceeds 100 per minute, tachycardia is present. Sinus tachycardia is caused simply by an increased rate of the sinus node. An ectopic or subsidiary pacemaker also may discharge at a rapid rate, causing tachycardia. More frequently, however, an ectopic impulse may produce sustained tachycardia by reentry or circus movement. A subsidiary pacemaker, e.g., an atrioventricular (AV) junctional pacemaker, can discharge at a rate higher than its intrinsic rate, producing tachycardia with a rate lower than 100 per minute. When the rate of an atrioventricular junctional or idioventricular rhythm is increased, but is less than 100 per minute, the term "accelerated" atrioventricular junctional or idioventricular rhythm is preferred by some authors. We have included such mechanisms under "tachycardia." Correct diagnosis, as well as an understanding of the mechanism of production of tachycardias, is important in order to provide the proper treatment. Careful analysis of the electrocardiogram (ECG) is often sufficient for diagnosis. In complex and refractory tachyarrhythmias intracardiac electrophysiologic studies may help but are infrequently essential. While the multiple antiarrhythmic agents currently available have improved the treatment of tachycardias considerably, one should not underestimate the possibility of misuse and drug toxicity with resultant serious arrhythmic complications. Plasma levels of antiarrhythmic drugs should be measured when possible in order to provide adequate therapy and avoid drug toxicity. The treatment should begin with a single pharmacologic agent. If adequate doses of the drug with therapeutic plasma levels do not control the arrhythmia, a change in drug or an additional drug should be tried.

Sinus Tachycardia

In sinus tachycardia the heart rate often ranges from 100 to 160 per minute and occasionally as high as 200 per minute. Sinus tachycardia occurs commonly and in various physiologic as well as pathologic states. Exercise, emotional stress, and anxiety usually produce physiologic sinus tachycardia. Physiologic sinus tachycardia occurs also during infancy and early childhood. Pathologic sinus tachycardia occurs in various conditions such as congestive heart failure, myocarditis, shock, hemorrhage, anemia, infections, and thyrotoxicosis. Administration of sympathomimetic agents, e.g., epinephrine, ephedrine, and isoproterenol, or vagolytic agents such as atropine, causes sinus tachycardia. Alcohol, caffeine, and nicotine may also cause sinus tachycardia. In pathologic sinus tachycardia the treatment of the underlying condition will result in a normal heart rate. In thyrotoxicosis and in conditions associated with an increased sympathetic activity propranolol (Inderal), 10 to 40 mg. four times a day, is quite effective. When anxiety plays a major role, tranquilizers such as diazepam (Valium), 2 to 5 mg. three times a day, may relieve the tachycardia.

Atrial Tachycardia

Atrial tachycardia occurs commonly both in patients without organic heart disease and in patients with various cardiac disorders. The atrial rate is usually 140 to 220 per minute but can vary between 110 and 250 per minute. The following factors influence the choice of treatment in atrial tachycardia: associated heart disease and the effect of the arrhythmia on cardiac performance, cause and precipitating factors, frequency of attacks, and the mechanisms of production.

The atrial tachycardias can be divided into two groups:

1. Atrial tachycardia due to the reentry phenomenon. Reentry often occurs in the atrioventricular node and occasionally in the sinus node.

2. Atrial tachycardia due to enhanced automaticity of the specialized atrial fibers or possibly the atrial myocardium. The term automatic or ectopic atrial tachycardia can be used for this category.

Paroxysmal Atrial Tachycardia Due to Atrioventricular Nodal Reentry. Most paroxysmal atrial tachycardias are caused by reentry within the AV node. The arrhythmia usually begins with a premature atrial beat having a prolonged PR interval. Two pathways with different refractory periods in the atrioventricular node make the reentry possible. The impulse is conducted through one pathway to the ventricle and reenters the atrium through the other pathway, causing a sustained atrial tachycardia. The initial atrial premature beat has a different morphology than the P waves caused by atrioventricular nodal reentry. Although atrial tachycardia due to reentry commonly occurs in patients without heart disease, it can occur in various organic heart diseases. If the arrhythmia is associated with severe impairment of the cardiac function such as pulmonary edema, angina pectoris, or hypotension, direct current (DC) cardioversion is the treatment of choice. When urgent treatment is not required it is useful to have a priority order of therapy starting with simple measures and gradually advancing to a more complex form of therapy. We suggest the following sequence of therapeutic measures:

1. Rest and sedation are the first measures used for the treatment of supraventricular tachycardias. Sedatives such as secobarbital, 100 mg. orally, are useful. We also use diazepam (Valium), 5 to 10 mg. intramuscularly, and continue orally three times a day if necessary.

2. Vagal stimulation is often effective in terminating reentrant atrial tachycardias. Carotid sinus pressure causes an increased vagal tone with resultant slowing of conduction and prolongation of refractoriness within the atrioventricular node and interruption of the reentrant circuit. Carotid sinus pressure should be applied to one side only and should not last more than 5 seconds. The cardiac rhythm should be monitored during this procedure. If ECG monitoring is not possible, simultaneous auscultation of the heart is an alternative. Carotid sinus pressure should not be used in patients with previous cerebrovascular accidents, and both carotids should be examined by palpation and auscultation before this procedure. The procedure should also be avoided in patients who have digitalis intoxication. Other vagotonic stimuli such as the Valsalva maneuver can convert the atrial tachycardia to sinus rhythm, and some patients are able to terminate their attacks by this maneuver. We do not recommend eyeball pressure for vagal stimulation, as this procedure can cause retinal detachment.

3. If vagotonic maneuvers and sedatives have not been effective in terminating the arrhythmia, one can use pharmacologic agents for vagal stimulation. We prefer to use edrophonium bromide (Tensilon), 10 mg. intravenously, for this purpose (this use of edrophonium bromide is not listed in the manufacturer's official directive); if there is no

response, carotid massage is applied again, since the vagotonic effect of edrophonium can be potentiated by this procedure. If edrophonium fails to terminate the arrhythmia, raising the blood pressure with pressor amines such as phenylephrine (Neo-Synephrine) and methoxamine (Vasoxyl) can initiate the carotid sinus reflex with resultant vagal stimulation. Phenylephrine is given intravenously as a bolus of 0.5 mg., or 5 mg. can be dissolved in 100 ml. of 5 per cent dextrose in water and infused intravenously until the systolic blood pressure is raised to 160 to 180 mm. Hg. Ten mg. of methoxamine may be dissolved in 20 ml. of isotonic saline solution and given intravenously while the blood pressure is monitored. We use this treatment only in patients with atrial tachycardia who otherwise have a normal heart. When the arrhythmia is associated with organic heart disease or hypertension one should avoid this form of therapy.

4. Digitalis glycosides are often effective in terminating atrial tachycardias that have not responded to the above treatment. The choice of a digitalis preparation varies among physicians. If the patient's renal function is normal, we use digoxin 0.5 mg. intravenously, and give three additional doses of 0.25 mg. every four hours and begin a maintenance daily dose of 0.25 to 0.5 mg. orally. A digitalis preparation also prolongs conduction in the atrioventricular node and interrupts the reentry circuit in most cases. If rapid digitalization is not required, 1 mg. digoxin is given orally followed by 0.25 mg. every 4 to 6 hours for four doses, followed by the maintenance dose.

5. Beta-blocking agents such as propranolol, which prolongs atrioventricular nodal conduction and refractoriness, can convert the atrial tachycardia to sinus rhythm. The recommended intravenous dose is a bolus of 0.5 to 1 mg. every 3 to 5 minutes until the arrhythmia is terminated or a total of 3 mg. is administered. Propranolol (Inderal) may be used orally, 10 to 40 mg. four times a day. We prefer to use propranolol orally and after digitalization, as some degree of heart failure may occur in patients with prolonged tachycardia. Propranolol should not be used if there is evidence of congestive heart failure or hypotension, and it is contraindicated in patients with a history of asthma or marked bradycardia.

6. Quinidine and procainamide are usually less effective than digitalis in terminating attacks of atrial tachycardia. Quinidine sulfate, 200 to 400 mg. four times a day orally, may be used after the patient is digitalized. Since DC cardioversion is an effective and relatively safe method for cardioversion of the atrial tachycardia to sinus rhythm, higher doses of quinidine should not be given before considering DC cardioversion.

7. Direct current (DC) cardioversion can terminate the arrhythmia in about 75 per cent of patients. In the absence of digitalis intoxication it is a relatively safe procedure. It is essential to omit digitalis preparations for 24 hours before the procedure. Electrical conversion should not be used in patients with digitalis intoxication, since serious ventricular arrhythmia can occur following this procedure. Small doses of diazepam (Valium) can be used intravenously in order to induce amnesia. A low-energy (50 to 100 joules) DC shock is applied.

8. Transient pervenous pacing of the right atrium is an alternative choice when an arrhythmia is refractory to the usual pharmacologic measures. A single stimulus or coupled properly timed stimuli can be used to interrupt the reentry circuit. Atrial pacing for a few seconds, with fixed rates either slower or slightly faster than the tachycardia, also is effective in conversion of the arrhythmia by interruption of the reentry pathway. This method is safe, does not require anesthesia, and is of special value in overdigitalized patients where DC countershock seems hazardous. In patients with recurrent symptomatic atrial tachycardia refractory to drug therapy a patient-controlled rapid atrial pacing can be used for conversion of the arrhythmia. This permanent pacing system has an implanted receiver-lead system and an external transmitter activated by the patient during tachycardia and gives a short burst of rapid atrial pacing, which terminates the arrhythmia. The effectiveness of this method and the appropriate pacing rate is determined by temporary atrial pacing before considering this type of pacemaker.

Digitalis is the first drug to be used for prevention of recurrent attacks of paroxysmal atrial tachycardia. Digoxin, 0.25 mg. per day, is often adequate. If digitalis does not suppress the attacks, propranolol (Inderal), 10 to 40 mg. four times a day, may be added to the regimen. Quinidine sulfate, 200 to 400 mg. four times a day, or quinidine gluconate (Quinaglute), 324 mg. three times a day, can also be used as an adjunct.

Ectopic Atrial Tachycardia. The ectopic or automatic atrial tachycardia is produced by discharge of an ectopic pacemaker with enhanced automaticity. If P waves are discernible, the initial P wave and subsequent P waves are similar to each other but different from the sinus P wave. The rate of this tachycardia is usually between 70 to 130 beats per minute. Digitalis intoxication is a common cause of this arrhythmia. Organic heart disease such as cardiomyopathy, myocarditis, myocardial infarction, and chronic obstructive pulmonary disease can be associated with this arrhythmia.

Vagal stimulation and vagotonic drugs are usually ineffective in the treatment of ectopic atrial tachycardia. Drugs affecting atrial automaticity, such as quinidine or procainamide, are useful. Quinidine sulfate, 200 to 400 mg. four times a day, or quinidine gluconate (Quinaglute), 324 mg. three to four times a day, are given orally. The incidence of gastrointestinal intolerance is lower with quinidine gluconate than with quinidine sulfate. If the patient has not been on digitalis, administration of this drug may be useful. Digitalis, through its vagal effect, decreases automaticity of the ectopic pacemaker and decreases the ventricular response by slowing the conduction in the atrioventricular node and producing atrioventricular block. If this drug is not effective in suppressing the arrhythmia, a combination of digoxin, 0.25 mg. daily, and propranolol, 5 to 20 mg. four times a day, may decrease the ventricular rate by producing atrioventricular block. DC cardioversion may be tried, although the chances of success are usually slim. In atrial tachycardia due to digitalis toxicity, digitalis is withheld and potassium is given if the patient's serum potassium is less than 4.0 mEq. per liter. In mild hypokalemia potassium chloride, 40 to 160 mEq., is administered orally in 24 hours. In more severe potassium depletion 60 to 160 mEq. should be infused intravenously over 24 hours. Propranolol is useful in digitalis-induced atrial tachycardia. The intravenous dose is 0.5 mg. every 3 to 5 minutes until the arrhythmia is terminated or a total of 3 mg. is given. If urgent treatment is not required, oral administration of this drug, 10 to 40 mg. four times a day, is preferred. Phenytoin (diphenylhydantoin, Dilantin) may be used intravenously, not more than 50 mg. per minute and not more than a total of 100 mg. every 5 minutes until the tachycardia is converted to sinus rhythm, or a total of 1 gram is administered (this use of phenytoin is not listed in the manufacturer's official directive). If digitalis-induced atrial tachycardia fails to respond to these measures or if urgent suppression of the ectopic focus is necessary, rapid atrial pacing at a rate slightly higher than the tachycardia for a few seconds is a safe and useful procedure. Conversion to sinus rhythm frequently occurs following the cessation of pacing. DC shock should be avoided in this situation.

Atrioventricular (AV) Junctional Tachycardia

Atrioventricular (AV) junctional tachycardia can be paroxysmal or nonparoxysmal. In paroxysmal junctional tachycardia the QRS complexes are usually narrow and similar to the QRS of sinus rhythm. If a previous conduction defect or aberrant conduction is present, the QRS may be wide. The P Waves, if seen, are usually retrograde, occurring just before or after the QRS complex. The rate is usually similar to paroxysmal atrial tachycardia. It is usually due to a reentrant mechanism but occasionally is caused by a rapidly discharging ectopic focus. Paroxysmal junctional tachycardia usually occurs in a healthy heart and is often self-limited and well tolerated.

The treatment of atrioventricular junctional tachycardia is usually similar to the treatment of paroxysmal atrial tachycardia. Vagal maneuvers, such as carotid massage, either convert the arrhythmia to sinus rhythm or do not change the rate at all. In nonparoxysmal junctional tachycardia the rate is usually between 70 to 130 beats per minute. This arrhythmia is seen in digitalis intoxication or organic heart disease such as acute myocardial infarction or acute rheumatic fever. Nonparoxysmal junctional tachycardia can be seen in patients with atrial fibrillation, flutter, or atrial tachycardia. The demonstration of a gradual acceleration of the junctional pacemaker and the finding of retrograde P waves are helpful in the diagnosis of nonparoxysmal junctional tachycardia. The treatment of nonparoxysmal junctional tachycardia is also similar to the treatment of nonparoxysmal atrial tachycardia. In the case of digitalis intoxication, digitalis should be discontinued and potassium should be given if the patient is hypokalemic. In acute myocardial infarction, the arrhythmia is usually transient and does not require therapy. If the rate is not too rapid and the loss of atrial contraction has deleterious effects, administration of atropine may increase the sinus rate and facilitate atrioventricular conduction. However, atropine can also have an adverse effect by increasing the rate of nonparoxysmal junctional tachycardia.

Multifocal Atrial Tachycardia

Multifocal atrial tachycardia is produced by multiple foci in the atrium discharging at different rates. The electrocardiographic manifestations of this arrhythmia consist of P waves of different configurations with different PP intervals with resultant irregular PR and RR intervals. The atrial rate may range from 100 to 250 beats per minute. The ventricular rate is slower, but is usually above 100 beats per minute. In multifocal atrial tachycardia the pulse is irregularly irregular, as in atrial fibrillation, and may simulate atrial fibrillation on the electrocardiogram if the P waves are not clearly seen. Most patients with multifocal atrial tachycardia are seriously ill. Chronic pulmonary disease is the most frequent underlying condition (85 to 90 per cent). Organic heart diseases such as rheumatic valvular disease, coronary artery disease, and malignancy are seen in a small number of patients. Digitalis intoxication is unlikely to produce this arrhythmia. However, this drug is usually not effective in slowing the ventricular rate in multifocal tachycardia and should be used with caution. Other antiarrhythmic agents such as quinidine, procainamide, phenytoin (Dilantin), and lidocaine are not usually effective. Propranolol is effective in slowing the atrial rate, but the frequent association of chronic pulmonary disease with acute respiratory distress limits the value of this agent. The most effective therapy is the treatment of underlying conditions. The hospital mortality of these patients is high, mainly due to the seriousness of the underlying diseases rather than the arrhythmia.

Atrial Flutter

On the electrocardiogram atrial flutter is recognized by regular sawtooth waves of atrial activity at about 250 to 350 per minute. In untreated atrial flutter and in the absence of an atrioventricular nodal conduction abnormality, a 2:1 atrioventricular conduction is often present, and the ventricular rate may be around 150 per minute. In patients who have received digitalis, or in those with atrioventricular node disease, atrial flutter with higher degrees of atrioventricular block may occur. The QRS complex is usually normal, but wide QRS complexes due to aberrant conduction may be present. Atrial flutter is very uncommon in the absence of heart disease. Coronary artery disease, hypertensive heart disease, and occasionally rheumatic heart disease are associated with this arrhythmia. Attacks of atrial flutter may occur in cor pulmonale and pulmonary emboli. It is not uncommon after open heart surgery. Paroxysmal atrial flutter may occur in the Wolff-Parkinson-White syndrome. If the arrhythmia is compromising the cardiac function and urgent termination is needed, DC cardioversion is the treatment of choice. Countershock is effective in more than 90 per cent of patients. A small energy shock, usually 25 to 100 joules, is usually sufficient. The procedure requires light anesthesia. In less urgent situations the drug of choice is digitalis. Digitalis, by increasing the atrioventricular block, decreases the ventricular rate. It can convert the arrhythmia to sinus rhythm. The change of the rhythm to atrial fibrillation is relatively common during digitalis therapy. Digitalis can be given orally or intravenously, depending upon the urgency of the situation. If a rapid effect is necessary, 0.5 mg. digoxin is administered intravenously followed by 0.25 mg. every 4 to 6 hours in order to produce an adequate atrioventricular block. Since large doses of digitalis are often needed for this purpose, one should consider other therapeutic regimens in order to avoid digitalis toxicity. If the usual dose of digitalis fails to decrease the ventricular rate, we use DC cardioversion with a low energy setting (25 to 50 joules) to convert the arrhythmia to normal rhythm. It is not unusual to see atrial flutter change to atrial fibrillation following this procedure. In this situation, with continuation of digitalis the ventricular rate is controlled rather easily and eventual reversion to sinus rhythm is likely. Propranolol (Inderal) is a good adjunct for increasing the degree of atrioventricular block if digitalis alone is not effective. In the absence of congestive heart failure, 10 to 30 mg. four times a day is usually sufficient. In urgent situations intravenous administration of propranolol, 0.5 to 1 mg. every 5 to 10 minutes is used. The total dose should not exceed 3 mg. Quinidine may be used to convert the atrial flutter to sinus rhythm. Quinidine sulfate, 200 to 400 mg. four times a day, or quinidine gluconate (Quinaglute), 324 mg. three to four times a day, is used for this purpose. Quinidine should not be used without digitalis as quinidine may facilitate atrioventricular conduction and increase the ventricular rate to a dangerously rapid rate. If combinations of digitalis and quinidine or digitalis and propranolol fail to convert the rhythm to sinus, DC cardioversion should be tried. Digitalis should be discontinued 24 hours before this procedure, in order to avoid digitalis-induced postcardioversion arrhythmias. Rapid right atrial pacing (400 to 800 per minute) is also used for conversion of the atrial flutter. This procedure often changes the atrial flutter to sinus rhythm or atrial fibrillation. Rapid right atrial pacing is particularly indicated in patients who are overdigitalized or after open heart surgery. For prevention of the atrial flutter digoxin, 0.25 mg. daily, with quinidine (quinidine sulfate 200 to 400 mg. four times a day or quinidine gluconate, 324 mg. three times a day) is used. Propranolol, 10 to 30 mg. four times a day, can be added to this regimen if necessary.

Atrial Fibrillation

Atrial fibrillation is more frequent than other atrial tachyarrhythmias and in the majority of patients is associated with significant organic heart disease. In these circumstances atrial fibrillation is usually a chronic and established form. Rheumatic mitral valve disease is a common underlying disorder. Atrial fibrillation is seen in coronary artery disease, thyrotoxicosis, some cardiomyopathies, hypertensive heart disease, the sick sinus node syndrome, the Wolff-Parkinson-White syndrome, and in atrial septal defects. Chronic atrial fibrillation is uncommon in chronic pulmonary disease. Attacks of atrial fibrillation, however, can occur with pulmonary emboli or pneumonia. Occasionally, atrial fibrillation is paroxysmal, occurring after consumption of alcohol or sometimes without an obvious cause. The electrocardiographic features consist of fibrillatory atrial activity of 400 to 650 per minute with an irregularly irregular ventricular response. The QRS complex is usually normal, but can be broad because of aberrant conduction. The atrial fibrillatory waves are best seen in lead VI. An untreated atrial fibrillation of recent onset usually has a rapid ventricular response of 100 to 200 per minute.

In patients who are in atrial fibrillation with rapid ventricular response requiring urgent treatment, e.g., those with pulmonary edema, cardiogenic shock, or angina pectoris, DC cardioversion is the treatment of choice. In the usual case when atrial fibrillation is not compromising cardiac function, the drug of choice is digitalis. This drug will result in slowing of the ventricular rate or conversion to sinus rhythm. One mg. of digoxin is given orally, followed by 0.25 mg. every 6 hours for four doses or, carefully, until the ventricular rate decreases to 70 to 80 per minute. In febrile patients the ventricular response should be reduced to 100 to 110 per minute. If large doses of digitalis are required, one may follow the plasma digoxin level in order to avoid toxicity. If rapid response is required, 0.5 mg. digoxin is given intravenously followed by 0.25 mg. every 4 to 6 hours for three to four doses. The maintenance dose of digoxin is usually 0.25 to 0.5 mg. daily. If the ventricular response cannot be controlled by an adequate dose of digitalis, propranolol can be helpful as an adjunct in the treatment of atrial fibrillation. The dose is significantly less than the antianginal dose, and 10 to 20 mg. four times a day is usually sufficient. In congestive heart failure, propranolol should not be used unless tachycardia plays a major role in the development of heart failure, in which case it can be used with great caution. Propranolol decreases the ventricular rate by increasing the degree of atrioventricular block. If rapid control of the ventricular rate is necessary, intravenous propranolol in small doses (0.5 to 1 mg.) can be used at 5 minute intervals up to a total dose of 3 mg. In some patients digitalis will convert the rhythm to sinus. In those who remain in atrial fibrillation, with optimal ventricular rate after administration of digitalis with or without propranolol, an attempt should be made to convert the rhythm by using other antiarrhythmic agents. Quinidine sulfate, 200 to 400 mg. four times a day, or quinidine gluconate (Quinaglute), 324 mg. three times a day, can be added to the regimen. Combinations of quinidine and propranolol may prove more effective than quinidine alone in converting the arrhythmia. In most patients who develop atrial fibrillation and do not respond to the above regimen, at least one attempt should be made to convert the arrhythmia electrically. Direct current (DC) cardioversion is administered under light anesthesia with 100 to 300 joules. Cardioversion is effective in the majority of patients, but in 70 to 80 per cent atrial fibrillation recurs by the end of 1 year. An adequate maintenance dose of quinidine confirmed by a therapeutic plasma level should be continued after sinus rhythm is obtained by DC cardioversion. In patients with rheumatic mitral valve disease cardioversion should be considered 2 to 3 months after surgery. The incidence of emboli following conversion of chronic atrial fibrillation to sinus rhythm is about 2 per cent. Although anticoagulants are used by some physicians before attempting to convert the rhythm to sinus, the value of this preventive measure is not firmly established. Cardioversion is usually not considered in the following: elderly patients, patients with atrial fibrillation of several years' duration, patients with significant cardiac enlargement, patients having a slow ventricular rate without digitalis, and patients sensitive to quinidine.

Tachycardias in the Wolff-Parkinson-White (WPW) Syndrome

In the Wolff-Parkinson-White syndrome premature activation of a segment of the ventricle occurs by an accessory atrioventricular bypass tract. The activation of the remaining portion of the ventricle is achieved through the normal atrioventricular conduction system as well as through the accessory pathway. The electrocardiogram in patients with the WPW syndrome shows a short PR interval and a delta wave at the beginning of the QRS complex. The incidence of tachyarrhythmias in the WPW syndrome is about 80 per cent. Atrial tachycardia is the most common tachycardia in the WPW syndrome (75 to 80 per cent of tachyarrhythmias) and is usually due to reentry. It is usually initiated by an atrial premature beat conducted antegrade through the atrioventricular node and retrograde through the accessory pathway, setting up a reciprocating tachycardia. The rate of this tachycardia is usually 140 to 250 per minute, and the QRS usually is normal. Broad QRS complexes due to anomalous conduction are uncommon during the attack of atrial tachycardia.

An atrial tachycardia of short duration does not require any treatment. Although the tachycardia often responds to vagal maneuvers such as carotid massage or the Valsalva maneuver, many patients require antiarrhythmic agents for control and prevention of the atrial tachycardia. Propranolol is the drug of choice in the treatment of reentrant atrial tachycardia with narrow QRS complexes. Propranolol slows conduction and prolongs refractoriness of the atrioventricular node while having no significant effect on the accessory pathways. Digitalis has a similar effect on the atrioventricular node, but usually shortens the refractory period of the accessory pathway with resultant increased conduction. In patients with the WPW syndrome who develop atrial fibrillation or flutter antegrade conduction through the accessory pathway is common. In such patients digitalis may cause extremely rapid ventricular response, which may result in ventricular fibrillation. Digitalis can be useful in patients with the WPW syndrome who develop reciprocating atrial tachycardia with a narrow QRS complex, since antegrade conduction is usually in the atrioventricular node. Digitalis is contraindicated in patients who develop atrial fibrillation with antegrade conduction over the accessory pathway. Intravenous lidocaine (Xylocaine) is an excellent choice for the treatment of the atrial flutter and fibrillation in which the antegrade conduction over the accessory pathway occurs. This drug prolongs the effective refractory period of the accessory pathway and has no effect on the refractory period of the atrioventricular node. Lidocaine is given intravenously as a bolus of 50 to 100 mg. followed by infusion at a rate of 2 to 4 mg. per minute. Quinidine and procainamide are quite useful in the treatment of supraventricular tachycardia in the WPW syndrome. These agents prolong the refractory period of the accessory pathway and may interrupt the reentry circuit. They are particularly useful in the treatment and prevention of recurrent atrial fibrillation. Quinidine sulfate, 200 to 400 mg. four times a day, or quinidine gluconate (Quinaglute), 324 mg. three times a day, has been considered the drug of choice for prevention of the atrial flutter and fibrillation. Propranolol, 10 to 40 mg. three to four times a day, is probably the most useful drug for the prevention of reciprocating supraventricular tachycardia with normal QRS complexes. Combined drug therapy, e.g., propranolol plus quinidine, is required in some patients who are refractory to a simple drug regimen. Direct current (DC) shock is very effective in terminating any type of tachyarrhythmia associated with the Wolff-Parkinson-White syndrome. It is particularly useful in urgent situations. In atrial tachycardia, atrial flutter, and fibrillation with extremely rapid ventricular response, DC cardioversion is the treatment of choice. When tachyarrhythmia associated with the WPW syndrome is refractory to drug treatment, pacemaker therapy, in a manner similar to that in atrioventricular nodal reentrant tachycardia, is indicated. When drug and pacemaker therapy fail, surgical interruption of the accessory pathway should be considered. Surgery should be done in medical centers that have wide experience in the electrophysiologic evaluation and surgery of these patients.

Tachycardia-bradycardia Syndrome

The tachycardia-bradycardia syndrome is usually seen in patients with the sick sinus node syndrome. The sick sinus syndrome is characterized by one or more of the following: (1) persistent severe sinus bradycardia; (2) episodes of sinus arrest and sinoatrial block; and (3) atrial fibrillation, often with slow ventricular response and often unresponsive to cardioversion.

In some patients with sick sinus syndrome episodes of paroxysmal atrial tachycardia, flutter, or fibrillation occur. These episodes may be followed by sinoatrial block or sinus arrest, resulting in Stokes-Adams attacks. The treatment of choice initially is a permanent pacemaker. The ventricular pacemaker is more widely used, although an atrial pacemaker may be more appropriate in patients without atrioventricular block. The tachycardia may be suppressed in some patients following the insertion of the pacemaker, but most patients require drug therapy. Following pacemaker insertion, antiarrhythmic agents such as digoxin, propranolol, and quinidine can be used to control the tachycardia without fear of producing cardiac standstill.

Ventricular Tachycardia

Ventricular tachycardia consists of a run of three or more consecutive premature ventricular beats. The ventricular complex is wide and bizarre, at a rate of usually 100 to 250 and often 150 to 200 per minute. The rhythm is regular, and sinus P waves independent of the ventricular complexes may be seen. The retrograde activation of the atrium causing a P wave after each QRS complex may occur occasionally. The ventricular tachycardia is usually a life-threatening arrhythmia and is seen in patients with serious organic heart disease. It is a fairly common arrhythmia in acute myocardial infarction. Coronary artery disease, cardiomyopathy, valvular heart disease, and a balloon mitral valve can be associated with this arrhythmia. It may be caused by intoxication with cardiac drugs such as digitalis, quinidine, and procainamide. Intoxication with phenothiazines and the tricyclic antidepressants may be associated with this arrhythmia. Paroxysmal ventricular tachycardia can occur occasionally in patients without organic heart disease.

In a diseased heart ventricular tachycardia often produces a rapid deterioration of the cardiac function, requiring emergency treatment. In these situations DC countershock is the treatment of choice. Diazepam (Valium) is usually given intravenously to produce amnesia and 200 to 400 joules are recommended to convert the arrhythmia. If the situation is less urgent lidocaine

(Xylocaine), 75 to 100 mg., is administered as a bolus intravenously and may be repeated in 2 to 3 minutes. If ventricular tachycardia persists, DC countershock is applied. Following cessation of the ventricular tachycardia infusion of lidocaine (Xylocaine), 2 to 4 mg. per minute, is the treatment of choice for suppression of this arrhythmia. Intravenous procainamide (Pronestyl) may be used for those patients who do not respond to the intravenous lidocaine. It may be given intravenously in increments of 50 to 100 mg. every 5 minutes until the tachycardia is terminated or a total of 1 gram is administered. This is followed by an intravenous infusion of 1.5 to 5 mg. per minute in order to maintain an adequate blood level. Recently, intravenous disopyramide phosphate (Norpace) has been used for the treatment of refractory ventricular tachycardias. A bolus of 2 mg. per kg. body weight, over 5 minutes, followed by an intravenous infusion of 20 to 40 mg. per hour is recommended (the intravenous use of disopyramide is not listed in the manufacturer's official directive). Intravenous propranolol (Inderal), 0.5 to 1 mg. every 5 minutes to a total of 3 mg., may also be used in refractory ventricular tachycardias. For long-term suppression therapy of this arrhythmia several oral antiarrhythmic agents are available. Quinidine sulfate, 200 to 400 mg. four times a day, or quinidine gluconate (Quinaglute), 324 mg. three times a day, is usually used first. The dosage should be adjusted to reach the therapeutic plasma level (1 to 6 micrograms per ml.). Disopyramide phosphate (Norpace), 300 mg. initially and 150 to 200 mg. four times a day, is used increasingly for the suppression of ventricular arrhythmias. Several pharmacologic actions of this drug are similar to quinidine, and it has been shown to be as effective as quinidine in reducing ventricular ectopic activity. This drug is particularly useful when the patient has intolerance to quinidine. Procainamide (Pronestyl), 250 to 500 mg. every 4 hours, may be used for the suppression of the ventricular tachycardia. We tend to avoid long-term use of this agent, as not uncommonly it produces a lupus-like picture. The therapeutic plasma level of procainamide is 4 to 8 micrograms per ml. Propranolol (Inderal), 10 to 40 mg. four times a day, is also a useful agent for suppression of the ventricular tachycardia. Digitalis may be useful in some patients with ventricular tachycardia. Phenytoin (Dilantin), 300 to 400 mg. per day, may be used as an adjunct for suppression of ventricular tachycardia (this use of phenytoin is not listed in the manufacturer's official directive). In patients with refractory ventricular tachycardia the combination of digitalis, propranolol, and quinidine seems to be the most effective. If the ventricular tachycardia is caused by digitalis the drug should be discontinued, and if hypokalemia is present, it should be corrected. Infusion of potassium chloride, 40 to 160 mEq. in 24 hours, is used for this purpose. Intravenous phenytoin (Dilantin) is an effective agent in the treatment of digitalis-induced ventricular tachycardia (this use of phenytoin is not listed in the manufacturer's official directive). It is given as a bolus, 50 to 100 mg. over 1 to 2 minutes every 5 minutes, until the arrhythmia is terminated or a total of 1 gram is given. Infusion of lidocaine (Xylocaine) is also effective. It is given as a 100 mg. bolus followed by infusion at a rate of 2 to 4 mg. per minute. Propranolol and procainamide can also be used. Countershock should be avoided. Interruption of the arrhythmia by intracardiac pacing is a fairly safe and effective treatment in this situation.

In patients with ventricular tachycardia refractory to drug treatment who can be considered for surgery, coronary angiography and left ventriculography should be performed. If a left ventricular aneurysm or coronary artery disease is present, surgical treatment should be considered.

In ventricular tachycardia resistant to drug treatment, chronic overdrive pacing (atrial or ventricular) may be used. The minimal effective rate should be determined by temporary pacing and is usually 70 to 110 per minute. In ventricular tachycardia associated with a high degree of atrioventricular block a ventricular pacemaker should be inserted prior to administration of the antiarrhythmic agent.

CONGENITAL HEART DISEASE
method of
JILL H. MORRISS, M.D.,
and DAN G. McNAMARA, M.D.
Houston, Texas

Congenital defects of the heart continue to occur at a remarkably constant rate of 7 per 1000 live births. We can estimate that approximately 25,000 infants with congenital heart disease are born each year in the United States. Since the occurrence rate in offspring of adult persons who have congenital heart disease is about 3 per cent, it is possible that the incidence of congenital heart disease will increase slightly as more patients survive and reproduce.

Initial recognition of congenital heart disease often presents more difficulty for the primary physician than does the actual medical treatment. Only about 20 per cent of infants with congenital heart disease can be easily recognized in the first week of life. Furthermore, many physicians who recognize that heart disease is present feel uncertain concerning the clinical estimation of the severity of the defect.

An estimated one half of newborns with congenital heart disease have a benign defect. In the other half of patients who have functionally important heart disease, the natural mortality in the first year is high for the untreated patient. With modern techniques, expertly applied, physicians can anticipate an 80 per cent survival rate during the first year of life for these critically ill infants.

Surgical treatment remains an important form of management for congenital heart disease; however, early case detection and application of modern medical management are necessary to enable surgical therapy.

It behooves clinicians to be better informed about the care of patients with important congenital heart disease and to avoid over-treatment and over-concern for the patient with a benign defect.

Assuming that a correct diagnosis has been made, the recommendations in this chapter are confined to therapy. New developments in the management of congenital heart disease are emphasized; less attention is directed to standard, well accepted methods, unless the conventional treatment regimen requires mention in light of new knowledge.

Cyanosis

The term "cyanotic congenital heart disease" implies that the low arterial oxygen saturation (hypoxemia), responsible for the blue color of the mucous membrane and nail beds, is due to right-to-left intracardiac shunting. However, cyanosis in the patient with congenital heart disease may sometimes result from pulmonary edema (ventilation-perfusion imbalance), or from low cardiac output (increased oxygen extraction by the tissues). Management of the cyanotic patient must therefore be based upon the pathophysiology of the cyanosis.

Cyanosis Associated with a Paroxysmal Hypoxemic Attack ("Spell"). Hypoxemic spells usually occur in the very young patient with tetralogy of Fallot or any of the anomalies with a ventricular communication and pulmonary stenosis. These episodes of tachypnea, dyspnea, cyanosis, and weakness or loss of consciousness sometimes have been mistaken for central nervous system seizures. The immediate differentiation is critical to the recovery of the patient. For instance, anticonvulsant medications such as diazepam (Valium) could have the adverse effect of lowering systemic arterial resistance in the patient with tetralogy of Fallot with further potentiation of the right-to-left shunt. Once the nature of the "spell" is recognized as resulting from severe hypoxemia, treatment must be prompt to be life-saving:

1. Force the infant into a knee-chest position attempting to find the position most comfortable for the infant, either prone or upright.

2. Administer oxygen by face mask (counter-productive if the infant is unduly disturbed by the therapy).

3. Avoid feeding and aspirate contents of a dilated stomach.

4. Morphine sulfate, 0.04 mg. per kg. per dose, subcutaneously, repeated every 5 minutes for two or three doses if there is no improvement.

5. For life-threatening spells resistant to the above therapy; propranolol (Inderal),* 0.01 to 0.15 mg. per kg. intravenously slowly over 5 minutes. Prostaglandin (PGE_1), 0.1 microgram per kg. per minute has been used in newborn infants less than 2 weeks of age to promote patency of the ductus arteriosus when the infant is in the cardiac catheterization laboratory with a means to infuse the drug by catheter near the patient ductus arteriosus; current use of prostaglandins for this purpose is restricted to an investigational protocol. Immediate surgery for either definitive intracardiac repair of the defect or a palliative systemic-to-pulmonary artery anastomosis in very small patients is required.

Cyanosis Associated with Pulmonary Edema. 1. Place the patient in an upright position.

2. Administer oxygen by mask.

3. Morphine sulfate, 0.04 mg. per kg. per dose, subcutaneously, intramuscularly or intravenously, and repeat in 5 minutes if respiratory distress persists.

4. Furosemide (Lasix), 1 mg. per kg. per dose intravenously or intramuscularly.

5. Prepare for heart catheterization.

6. Do not feed. Place nasogastric tube to empty stomach distended with gas or fluid.

7. Assisted ventilation through endotracheal tube if clinical response to above measures is unsatisfactory.

Cyanosis Secondary to Inadequate Mixing Between the Two Circulations (As in Transposition of the Great Arteries or Total Anomalous Pulmonary Venous Return). 1. Diuretic therapy with furosemide while preparations are made for cardiac catheterization if pulmonary edema with obstruction to pulmonary venous return exists.

2. Rashkind balloon atrial septostomy during cardiac catheterization.

---

*This use of propranolol is not listed in the manufacturer's official directive.

3. General supportive measures for the critically ill infant during transportation to a cardiac center, or while awaiting heart catheterization or surgical treatment.

Maintain body temperature at 36°C. (97°F.) (core temperature) or 36.5°C. (98°F.) (skin temperature) to protect against temperature extremes which create excessive oxygen demand.

Maintain blood sugar; serum glucose levels below 30 mg. per dl. (100 ml.) require treatment with maintenance fluid of $D_{10}W$ or $D_{20}W$ beginning at a rate of 100 ml. per kg. per 24 hours.

Transfuse to maintain hematocrit in the range of 40 to 50 per cent; whole blood at 10 ml. per kg. or packed red cells at 5 ml. per kg. may be safely given over 2 to 3 hours with the amount of transfusion based on actual and desired hemoglobin values. A transfusion of 2 ml. per kg. of packed cells is estimated to raise the hemoglobin by 1 gram per dl.

Carefully administer sodium bicarbonate in an attempt to correct metabolic acidosis and stabilize infant's pH above 7.20. Give small doses slowly to avoid intracranial hemorrhage. Calculate bicarbonate to be administered as follows:

$$\text{mEq. } HCO_3^- =$$

$$\frac{|\text{actual base excess} - \text{desired base excess}|}{6}$$

$$\times \text{ weight (kg.)}$$

Obtain actual base excess from Siggaard-Anderson nomogram using the patient's P_{CO_2} and pH values. The desired base excess takes into consideration the shift in bicarbonate at elevated P_{CO_2} values and its inclusion makes overcorrection less likely. To estimate the desired base excess for newborn infants:

Pa_{CO_2} (mm. HG)	"Desired Base Excess" to Use in Calculation
30	−3
40	−4
50	−5
60	−6
70	−7
80	−8

For example:

pH	7.15
Pa_{CO_2}	20
Hgb	15 grams per dl.
Wt	3 kg.

Base excess (nomogram) – 10 (negative value indicates a deficiency of buffer base)

Desired base excess   −2

$$\text{mEq. } HCO_3^- = \frac{|(-10) - (-2)| \times 3}{6}$$

$$\text{mEq. } HCO_3^- = 4 \text{ mEq.}$$

Half of the calculated bicarbonate may be given slowly over 20 minutes and the remainder given over the next 1 to 2 hours to avoid rapid increases in plasma osmolality.

Cyanosis Secondary to Congenital Heart Disease Unassociated with "Spells", Pulmonary Edema, or Respiratory or Circulatory Distress. 1. Treatment of the cyanosis per se may be unnecessary.

2. Referral to a pediatric cardiology center to establish definitive diagnosis.

Cyanosis with Excessive Polycythemia When Correction or Palliation of the Underlying Defect is Not Available. 1. Phlebotomy. Removal of whole blood with volume replacement is therapeutic and safe in selected cases. Phlebotomy is performed if the spun hematocrit exceeds 70 per cent or is between 65 and 70 per cent and the patient is symptomatic (headaches or extreme fatigue with ordinary activity). An attempt is made to lower the hematocrit to 55 per cent. The total blood volume in the polycythemic patient is estimated to be 100 ml. per kg. rather than 65 to 80 ml. per kg. A sample calculation follows:

x = volume of blood to be removed
actual hematocrit (Hct) 75 per cent
desired hematocrit (Hct) 55 per cent

$$x = [\text{wt. (kg.)} \times \text{blood volume (100 ml./kg.)}]$$

$$\times \frac{\text{actual Hct} - \text{desired Hct}}{\text{actual Hct}}$$

$$x = [(30)\,(100 \text{ ml./kg.})] \times \frac{75-55}{75}$$

$$x = 800 \text{ ml.}$$

Replacement of 80 per cent of the volume removed is done with a colloid solution; 50 ml. of salt-poor albumin is added to 200 ml. of Ringer's lactate and this solution is used to replace the patient's blood as it is slowly removed.

Cyanosis Accompanying "Persistence of the Fetal Circulation." This entity is thought to be the result of prolonged elevation of pulmonary vascular resistance and right-to-left shunting through fetal pathways such as the foramen ovale and ductus arteriosus.

1. Establish diagnosis with cardiac catheterization.

2. Digoxin and furosemide (Lasix) if congestive heart failure coexists (see doses in Table 1).

3. Tolazoline (Priscoline), 1 to 2 mg. per kg. infused over 10 minutes, preferably into the pulmonary artery followed by a continuous infusion of 1 to 2 mg. per kg. per hour intravenously.

4. Ventilatory support with endotracheal tube and mechanical assistance.

Congestive Heart Failure

Predominant Left-sided Heart Failure with Acute Distress. Many malformations of the heart

TABLE 1. **Digoxin (Lanoxin)—Total Digitalizing Dose (TDD) for Infants and Children**

Oral: 0.05 mg./kg./TDD divided ½, ¼, ¼
IM: 0.04 mg./kg./TDD divided ½, ¼, ¼
IV: 0.03 mg./kg./TDD divided ½, ¼, ¼
Divide TDD and give half of TDD initially, followed in 6 to 8 hours by the next one fourth of TDD and in 12 to 16 hours by the last one fourth of TDD.
Maximum TDD is 1.0 mg. (1000 micrograms)

FOR PREMATURE INFANTS
Oral: 0.02 mg./kg./TDD divided ½, ¼, ¼
Parenteral: 0.015 mg./kg./TDD divided ½, ¼, ¼

MAINTENANCE DOSE
Give one fourth to one third of the TDD per day in two divided doses. Begin maintenance 12 to 24 hours after the last digitalizing dose.

---

present with manifestations of pure or predominant left-sided failure and pulmonary edema. These defects include left heart obstructive lesions, transposition of the great arteries, truncus arteriosus, ventricular septal defect, patent ductus arteriosus, and left ventricular congestive cardiomyopathy. Tachypnea or more obvious signs of labored breathing are associated with elevated pulmonary venous pressure while liver enlargement, distended neck veins and peripheral edema may be absent. Supportive treatment can be carried out *before* the specific anatomic diagnosis is made so that cardiac catheterization carries less risk.

1. Place infant in a semi-upright position.

2. Furosemide (Lasix), 1 mg. per kg. per dose, intramuscularly or intravenously slowly repeated in a half hour if diuresis has not occurred.

3. Do not feed, and empty distended stomach via nasogastric tube.

4. Digitalize (see Table 1), particularly if ventricular dilatation is present.

5. Morphine sulfate, 0.04 mg. per kg. subcutaneously, intramuscularly or intravenously, is given for labored, distressed breathing.

6. Assisted ventilation via endotracheal tube if improvement has not occurred.

7. Maintain body temperature (core temperature 36°C. [97°F.] or skin temperature 36.5°C. [98°F.]).

8. Check for and correct acidemia and hypoglycemia.

9. In addition to digitalis, give other inotropic agents if dilated poorly contracting left ventricle is confirmed by echocardiogram. Dopamine (Intropin) infusion is begun at 2 micrograms per kg. per minute when oliguria but no hypotension is present; increase to 5 to 10 micrograms per kg. per minute when both oliguria and hypotension coexist. *Do not add to fluid containing sodium bicarbonate,* since dopamine is inactivated in alkaline solutions. High doses may result in tachycardia, excessive vasoconstriction, and reduced blood flow. Dopamine currently is preferred over isoproterenol as it has less chronotropic effect and is unique in selectively dilating renal vessels. Unlike isoproterenol, however, it causes pulmonary vasoconstriction; thus, use cautiously, if at all, in patients with known pulmonary hypertension.

Chronic Left-sided Heart Failure Without Acute Distress. 1. Daily maintenance diuretic therapy: Furosemide (Lasix), 1 mg. per kg. per dose orally usually once or twice daily, but may be given four times daily in refractory cases. Discontinue diuretics if food intake is poor, or if fluid losses from vomiting or diarrhea occur.

2. Daily maintenance digoxin (Lanoxin) dose (see Table 1).

3. Dietary salt restriction: By restricting added table salt, the average diet containing 6 to 15 grams salt daily can be reduced to 4 to 7 grams and further reduced to 3 to 4 grams by eliminating salt during cooking. Diets containing less than 2.5 grams salt (1000 mg. sodium) are unpalatable. Salt substitutes are available and may be selected on the basis of the patient's taste preference. Listed below in order of decreasing sodium content are nutritional products suitable for infants:

Cow's milk	25 mEq./L.
Evaporated milk	18 mEq./L.
Similac	13 mEq./L.
Enfamil, SMA	11 mEq./L.
Similac	7 mEq./L.
Lonalac	1 mEq./L.

It is preferable to avoid extremely low sodium intake concurrent with diuretic therapy. Allow normal formula intake without severe salt restriction and liberalize diuretic therapy if necessary.

Predominant Right-sided Heart Failure Secondary to Right Ventricular Outflow Obstruction. 1. Avoid digitalis therapy.

2. Diuretic therapy is controversial, as administration may reduce necessary filling volume.

3. Remove cause promptly by operation, if feasible.

Coexisting Left and Right Heart Failure. Use therapy as outlined under predominant left heart failure.

Left-to-Right Shunt with Congestive Heart Failure in Premature Infant with Patent Ductus Arteriosus (PDA). 1. Establish diagnosis with physical examination and supportive laboratory data including echocardiogram; cardiac catheterization is risky and rarely necessary in these ill neonates.

2. Restrict fluid intake to 70 ml. per kg. per day.

TABLE 2. **Dosage Schedules** (See text for additional details)

DRUG	USAGE	DOSE	HOW SUPPLIED	REMARKS
Dopamine (Intropin)	Positive inotropic agent, "shock"	3–5 microgram/kg./min. IV up to 5–10 micrograms/kg./min. IV	Intropin 40 mg./ml. (5 mg. vial)	Inactivated in alkaline solutions; unfavorable pulmonary vasoconstriction; high doses—tachycardia, reduced renal blood flow
Furosemide (Lasix)	Potent diuretic	1 mg./kg./dose, orally IM, IV	Injectable 10 mg./ml. Liquid 10 mg./ml. Tablet 20 mg., 40 mg.	Discontinue if anorexia, vomiting, diarrhea, or other reason for low serum potassium
Indomethacin* (Indocin)	Pharmacologic closure of PDA	0.1 mg./kg./dose orally by nasogastric tube; repeat q8h × 2	Capsule, 25 mg.	Contraindications: hyperbilirubinemia, bleeding tendency, reduced renal function. Not approved for neonatal use
Isoproterenol (Isuprel)	Positive inotropic agent "shock"	IV-0.05-0.1 microgram/kg./min. up to 0.5 microgram/kg./min. Intracardiac 0.02 mg. (0.1 ml.)	Isuprel HCl sterile solution 1:5000 0.2 mg./ml.	Tachycardia limits use of high doses
Morphine sulfate	Sedation	0.04 mg./kg./dose SC, IM, IV	Injectable 10 mg./ml. or 30 mg./ml.	Dilute usual commercial preparation, 1 ml. (10 mg.) with 9 ml. water to be able to administer small doses more accurately
Propranolol (Inderal)	Hypercyanotic spells	Orally 1–4 mg./kg./day in 4 divided doses; IV 0.01–0.15 mg./kg. slowly over 5 min.	Liquid (investigational) 10 mg./ml. Tablet 10 mg., 40 mg., 80 mg. Injectable 1 mg./ml.	Intravenous use reserved for life-threatening situations
Prostaglandins (PGE₁)	Promote patency of PDA	Infusion: 0.1 microgram/kg./min. at site of PDA		Investigational use only at present. Drug is kept refrigerated
Tolazoline (Priscoline)	Pulmonary vasodilatation	1 mg./kg./dose infused into the pulmonary artery over 10 min., followed by 1–2 mg./kg./hour IV	25 mg./ml. (10 ml. vial)	Not selective for pulmonary circuit; systemic hypotension can occur

*This use of this agent is not listed in the manufacturer's official directive.

3. Diuretic therapy: furosemide (Lasix), 1 mg. per kg. per dose; with concomitant fluid restriction, large doses may not be necessary.

4. Digoxin (Lanoxin) (see Table 1) for premature dosage schedule. The need for digitalis in these patients is debatable, since contractility already may be optimal and, in fact, increased. In most centers, digitalis is used, but the dosage should be at a low level.

5. Trial at pharmacologic closure with indomethacin (Indocin). In vivo studies have demonstrated that the ductus can be constricted or closed by inhibiting prostaglandin synthesis with "prostaglandin inhibitors" such as indomethacin. Several clinical trials confirm the feasibility of this method. This treatment is reserved for symptomatic infants with inadequate response to medical therapy who would be considered candidates for surgical closure of the ductus. Indomethacin must not be given if hyperbilirubinemia is present (total bilirubin > 10 mg. per dl.). The drug is also contraindicated if there is a bleeding tendency or if there is reduced renal function manifest by decreased urine output, high blood urea nitrogen (BUN) or serum creatinine. Informed parental consent should be obtained, since indomethacin has not been approved for general use in the neonate. Initial dose of indomethacin is 0.1 mg. per kg.

orally by nasogastric tube; repeat in 6 hours if no clinical response; repeat in 12 to 14 hours if ductal closure has not occurred.

The contents of the smallest capsule (25 mg.) must be separated and weighed by the pharmacist to provide the small doses. Occasionally, the ductus will not be closed with this regimen or will reopen and retreatment is necessary. Treatment may not be successful after 3 weeks of postnatal age.

6. Surgical ligation of the patent ductus arteriosus (PDA) should be performed in the symptomatic neonate when there has been no response to medical management; this approach is used if the patient is not a candidate for pharmacologic closure of the ductus or if pharmacologic closure has failed.

Rhythm Disturbances of the Heart

Sinus Bradycardia. 1. Document mechanism of slow rate with electrocardiogram (ECG) to exclude second or third degree block.

2. Seek underlying cause for excessively slow sinus rates, i.e., hypothermia, drugs, cerebral, pulmonary, metabolic, or electrolyte disorders; treat underlying cause.

3. Atropine sulfate, 0.005 to 0.02 mg. per kg. per dose subcutaneously, to decrease vagal tone and increase heart rate; a failure of sinus rate to increase after atropine may imply sinus node damage or acidemia.

4. Arrange for cardiac pacing if symptomatic (Stokes-Adams attacks, low blood pressure, lethargy, or congestive heart failure).

Sinus Tachycardia. 1. Document sinus tachycardia with ECG.

2. Investigate cause such as fever, anemia, exercise, drugs or thyrotoxicosis.

3. Manage precipitating cause.

4. Digitalis should not be used to slow the rate of sinus tachycardia.

Paroxysmal Atrial Tachycardia. 1. Document type of supraventricular dysrhythmia with ECG. Paroxysmal atrial tachycardia (PAT) is more common in pediatric age group than atrial fibrillation or atrial flutter. Newborns and older infants with PAT generally have rates in excess of 220 beats per minute, distinguishing this from sinus tachycardia.

2. Digitalization (see Table 1) can be used for treatment of less severely ill patients with digitalizing doses separated by shorter intervals of 4 to 6 hours.

3. Give phenytoin (Dilantin), 5 mg. per kg. intravenously over 10 minutes, if cardioversion follows digitalis administration since there is a risk of postconversion dysrhythmias in this setting.

4. Oral maintenance digoxin is given for 6 to 12 months after a single documented episode of PAT in infancy.

5. Add propranolol, 1 to 4 mg. per kg. per day orally in four divided doses, if tachycardia is not controlled with satisfactory serum levels of digoxin alone.

6. If arrhythmia is not controlled or worsens on digoxin therapy alone, intracardiac electrophysiology should be performed to further direct therapy.

7. Eyeball pressure may damage the eye and is unsafe in infants and children for conversion of PAT.

8. Carotid massage is usually an ineffective method of treatment. The induction of emesis and facial ice water submersion has been recommended by some but is not used by the authors.

Congenital Complete Atrioventricular Block. The clinical features and the indications for treatment of congenital atrioventricular block in the infant differ from that in the older child, or in the adult who has acquired atrioventricular block. The only specific treatment that is effective is electrical ventricular pacing. While a temporary chronotropic effect may be effected by some drugs, such as atropine and isoproterenol, their side effects, variable action, and ultimate ineffectiveness render such treatment impractical.

1. Management in infancy. Indications for surgical placement of a permanent ventricular pacemaker include any one or combination of the following:

Ventricular rate of less than 50 beats per minute in the awake, resting state. During sleep, a rate of 40 beats per minute may be well tolerated by the patient.

Unresponsiveness of the ventricular rate to a test injection of atropine in a dose of 0.005 to 0.02 mg. per kg. per dose subcutaneously or intravenously.

An atrial rate sustained at greater than 150 beats per minute with slow ventricular rate.

Cardiac enlargement and other signs of congestive heart failure.

Signs of low cardiac output: skin pallor, lethargy, syncope (rare in infancy), and oliguria.

An associated structural defect of the heart which is hemodynamically important. Approximately 40 per cent of neonates with congenital complete atrioventricular block have an associated heart defect.

Demonstration by intracardiac electrophysiologic studies of block *distal* to the bundle of His. Block *within* the His bundle may also be an indication for permanent pacing.

2. Management in childhood. Indication for permanent ventricular pacing includes:

A ventricular rate less than 40 beats per minute in the awake, resting state.

Failure of the ventricular rate to increase with exercise. If the child is unable to exercise, atropine, as above, may be used for testing of the rate response.

The last four indications under "management in infancy" are the same for the child as for the infant.

3. Temporary transvenous ventricular pacing for complete atrioventricular block.

During anesthesia, in severe infection or unusual periods of transient stress, temporary pacing may be indicated for the patient whose atrioventricular block is otherwise well tolerated.

Temporary pacing is used for the patient in whom a permanent pacemaker is to be inserted while the patient is awaiting surgery, during induction of anesthesia, and during surgery.

4. The use of digitalis for congestive heart failure in the patient with complete atrioventricular block.

Since severe digitalis toxicity may cause complete atrioventricular block, many physicians are reluctant to use this drug in patients with any form of complete atrioventricular block. If congestive heart failure accompanies complete heart block, however, the inotropic effect of digitalis may be useful on a temporary basis. If congestive heart failure is present, the use of electrical pacing is the best therapy with digitalis then added if congestive heart failure persists.

Premature Ventricular Contractions (PVCs). 1. No treatment is required for PVCs with all of the following characteristics: unifocal, fixed coupling, occur singly, disappear with exercise, unassociated with structural heart disease, and unaccompanied by a prolonged Q-T interval on electrocardiogram.

2. Treatment of PVCs is necessary if they are multifocal, occur in runs of two or more beats, and persist or increase with exercise.

If the ominous type of PVCs are unassociated with a dilated heart, treatment may begin with quinidine gluconate, 10 to 30 mg. per kg. per day orally in two to three divided doses, or propranolol (Inderal), 1 to 4 mg. per kg. per day orally in four to six divided doses. Physical activity is limited to exclude strenuous competitive athletics.

If ominous PVCs are associated with a dilated heart or congestive heart failure, treatment of the heart failure may result in a decrease or disappearance of the PVCs. Digitalis may be used for the treatment of the congestive failure in spite of the PVCs, but diuretic therapy alone can be used if there is concern that the PVCs will increase with digitalis therapy. In the setting of a dilated heart with PVCs, quinidine and propranolol should be avoided. Effort is made to suppress the ectopic

beats with phenytoin, 2 to 7 mg. per kg. per day orally in two divided doses. (This use of phenytoin is not listed in the manufacturer's official directive.)

3. Treatment of PVCs associated with a prolonged Q-T interval (such patients are susceptible to attacks of ventricular tachycardia and fibrillation).

Give propranolol (Inderal), 1 to 4 mg. per kg. per day orally in four to six divided doses.

Avoid strenuous exercise.

Consider left stellate ganglion block or ablation for resistant cases.

4. Treatment of PVCs associated with left ventricular hypertrophic cardiomyopathy.

Propranolol (Inderal), 1 to 4 mg. per kg. per day orally in four to six divided doses.

Surgical treatment for relief of left ventricular outflow obstruction sometimes is of value for relief of elevated left ventricular pressure but does not appear to influence the tendency to PVCs.

5. Treatment of PVCs associated with mitral valve prolapse and left ventricular dyskineses.

Propranolol (Inderal), 1 to 4 mg. per kg. per day orally in four to six divided doses or

Quinidine gluconate, 10 to 30 mg. per kg. per day orally in two to three divided doses.

Mitral valve annuloplasty has been reported to be beneficial in a few patients, but this has not yet been confirmed to be a generally effective treatment.

Ventricular Tachycardia. 1. Deliver a single sharp blow to the chest when ventricular tachycardia is sustained.

2. Synchronized electrical cardioversion with 1 watt-sec. per lb.

3. Lidocaine, 1 mg. per kg. per dose intravenously, given while preparations are made for electrical cardioversion and repeated if necessary, or given by continuous infusion, 0.01 to 0.05 mg. per kg. per minute, not exceeding 1.5 mg. per kg. per hour.

4. For chronic control of recurrent ventricular tachycardia when the underlying cause of the arrhythmia cannot be removed: propranolol, 1 to 4 mg. per kg. per day orally in four divided doses.

5. Additional drug therapy with quinidine, phenytoin, or procainamide may be necessary.

6. Digitalis is usually contraindicated in ventricular tachycardia, since it may increase myocardial irritability. As an exception, when a dilated heart contributes to the propensity for ventricular arrhythmias, digitalis may be combined with one of the above mentioned antiarrhythmic agents.

Cardiopulmonary Arrest

No audible heart beat and an imperceptible pulse imply cardiac arrest. These findings occur with either ventricular asystole, ventricular fibrillation, or ineffective ventricular contraction despite persistence of QRS complexes on the ECG. Whatever the mechanism of cardiac arrest, prompt ventilation accompanied by external cardiac compression is required. The decision for giving specific drugs and for the use of electrical shock is best guided by the ECG. The method of resuscitation is as follows:

1. Ventilation. Clear the airway. Give mouth-to-mouth breathing. When personnel and equipment become available, oxygen administration and endotracheal intubation may be required. During mouth-to-mouth breathing, the patient's nostrils must be occluded with one hand while the other hand depresses the stomach to prevent inflation. In the infant, the resuscitator's mouth will cover the nostrils. Monitor breath sounds with a stethoscope to assure bilateral ventilation.

2. External cardiac compression. Place the patient on a firm surface. With the heel of the hand placed over the midsternum, compress the heart briskly between the anterior and posterior chest walls sufficient to produce a palpable pulse. For an infant, exert pressure on the sternum with two or three fingers keeping in mind that the ribs are fragile and the liver is easily injured. Sudden release of pressure allows better venous filling of the heart. Have an assistant monitor the peripheral pulse continuously to assure adequate effect of cardiac compression. Have assistant secure intravenous route while proceeding with resuscitation.

3. Restoration of heart action. Spontaneous reversion to sinus rhythm may result from the aforementioned measures. Obtain ECG to determine type of cardiac arrest (ventricular fibrillation vs. asystole).

Electrical countershock is indicated when ventricular fibrillation fails to convert after ventilation and massage. Defibrillator paddles are placed so that the electrical current passes through the greatest diameter of the heart, either from the base to the apex of the heart or across the anterior-posterior diameter of the chest. Liberal application of electrode paste beneath the paddles ensures good electrical contact and minimizes skin burn. The electrical output for defibrillation varies with the child's size and is recommended to be 1 watt-sec. per lb. If the heart is not defibrillated with the initial energy dose, the output is doubled. If the defibrillation is successful but not sustained, do not increase the energy dose but precede the next defibrillation attempt by correcting acidemia with sodium bicarbonate.

For asystole, deliver sharp blow to the precordium. Correct acidemia with sodium bicarbonate. A single electrical shock delivered from a defibrillator in the energy dose above may initiate contrac-

tion. Intracardiac epinephrine, 1 to 3 ml. of 1:10,000 solution, can be delivered. Commercially available epinephrine is 1:1000 and must be diluted to obtain a 1:10,000 solution. Use calcium if asystole continues, 1 ml. of 10 per cent calcium gluconate by intravenous route or direct intracardiac injection.

Direct cardiac massage via thoracotomy is indicated only with suspected cardiac tamponade, chest wall injuries, or intrathoracic hemorrhage.

Maintain blood pressure. Sustain blood pressure with inotropic support of the circulation if necessary.

Isoproterenol (Isuprel) may be the agent of choice in patients who have elevated pulmonary vascular resistance. Dilute 4 mg. in 500 to 1000 ml. of intravenous fluid and administer as a constant controlled drip while heart rate and blood pressure are monitored. A proper rate for infusion is 0.005 to 0.1 micrograms per kg. per minute up to 0.5 micrograms per kg. per minute.

Dopamine (Intropin) is less likely to accelerate the heart rate when compared to isoproterenol and is unique among sympathomimetic amines in that it selectively vasodilates renal vessels and increases renal blood flow until large doses are reached. The major objection to its use is that, unlike isoproterenol, it causes pulmonary vasoconstriction. It cannot be given with sodium bicarbonate as it is inactivated in alkaline solutions. Begin dopamine at an infusion rate of 2 micrograms per kg. per minute and increase gradually, if necessary to 5 to 10 micrograms per kg. per minute. Monitor heart rate and blood pressure, because high doses may result in unfavorable tachycardia and excessive vasoconstriction. Avoid doses of dopamine in excess of 20 micrograms per kg. per minute, which may result in reduced renal blood flow.

General Problems

Immunization Schedules. Routine immunizations are recommended for all patients with congenital heart disease. If interruption of the suggested schedule is necessary due to hospitalization or illness, it is unnecessary to restart the series.

Physical Activity. Young children (2 to 10 years) with congenital heart disease will usually set their own limits with respect to physical activity and should not be held back from normal crawling and walking. Parental restriction of activity may be necessary when children reach the ages when competitive athletics are offered. It is important for parents to discuss the physical education program with the school personnel. A physician's statement that the child should be permitted to rest when he becomes fatigued may allow a child a certain amount of participation without focusing undue attention on the child's "differences." We are strict about prohibiting participation in competitive sports for patients with severe left or right ventricular obstructive lesions, as well as any patient with a large dilated heart. Patients with aortic stenosis and hypertrophic cardiomyopathy are particularly at risk.

Prophylaxis Against Bacterial Endocarditis. Antibiotic prophylaxis to prevent endocarditis is recommended for all patients with structural abnormalities of the heart at times when transient bacteremia is known to occur in association with dental or surgical manipulations. Antibiotics are selected depending on the operative site (Table 3) to eliminate the organisms most likely to be causative. For dental work, including cleaning, drilling, extractions, and initial application of orthodontic devices, penicillin is recommended. There is no evidence to suggest that dental prophylaxis need be observed when primary teeth are spontaneously lost. Attention to good dental hygiene is to be encouraged in all children with congenital heart disease; some cyanotic children have defective enamel and appear to have a higher incidence of dental caries.

There is no role for continuous antibiotic prophylaxis to "minimize infections" as this practice invites emergence of resistant strains of bacteria.

Patients who have prosthetic heart valves are at unusually high risk for development of bacterial endocarditis and should receive a parenteral combination of penicillin plus streptomycin for dental manipulations and upper respiratory tract surgery. Patients with rheumatic valve disease who receive rheumatic fever penicillin prophylaxis should have erythromycin or streptomycin added when dental procedures are undertaken.

Anesthesia. General anesthesia can be tolerated by most patients with congenital heart disease if expertly performed for indicated procedures; however, many of these patients cannot tolerate either hypoxia from improper ventilation or hypotension from certain anesthetic agents.

It is advisable to monitor an intraoperative electrocardiogram and blood pressure.

The choice of an anesthetic agent is influenced by the nature of the cardiac defect. Agents that lower systemic resistance significantly, such as halothane, thiopental (Pentothal), and spinal anesthetics, are given with greater risk to patients with tetralogy of Fallot; whereas either cyclopropane, with its adrenergic effects, or nitrous oxide may be used more safely.

Anesthetic risk is high in patients with cardiomegaly and in patients with pulmonary hypertension. Cyclopropane and ether increase pulmonary vascular resistance and may be particularly hazardous in the latter category of patient.

Preoperatively, precautions against bacterial endocarditis are begun, and particular care is given to intravenous lines in cyanotic patients who are jeopardized by even small quantities of air in the tubing. Because intracardiac right to left shunting is possible in such patients, air bubbles may directly reach the systemic circuit.

Education and Rehabilitation. Constant effort must be made by both parents and teachers to provide every opportunity for normal emotional and intellectual development. Similarities to contemporaries rather than differences require emphasis. Mentally normal children with cardiac malformations have no place in classes for the handicapped or "special" classes. Vocational guidance is important in helping patients with congenital heart disease live full and useful adult lives.

TABLE 3.　**SBE Prophylaxis**

Penicillin V = phenoxymethyl penicillin
For dental work
For orotracheal intubation
For surgery of upper respiratory tract
  Oral: Children >60 lb.
    Penicillin V, 2.0 grams orally 30 minutes to 1 hour prior to procedure followed by 500 mg. orally every 6 hours for 8 doses
    Children <60 lbs.
    Penicillin V, 1.0 gram orally 30 minutes to 1 hour prior to procedure followed by 250 mg. orally every 6 hours for 8 doses
    For penicillin allergy, erythromycin is substituted: Erythromycin, 20 mg. per kg. orally 1.5 to 2 hours prior to procedure followed by 10 mg. per kg. every 6 hours for 8 doses
  Parenteral: Aqueous penicillin G, 30,000 units per kg. (up to 600,000 units) mixed with procaine penicillin G, 600,000 units intramuscularly 30 minutes to 1 hour prior to procedure to be followed by appropriate oral antibiotic therapy above
For genitourinary surgery
For gastrointestinal surgery
  Children: Ampicillin, 50 mg. per kg. intramuscularly or intravenously 30 minutes to 1 hour prior to procedure plus either:
    streptomycin, 20 mg. per kg. intramuscularly, or gentamicin, 2.0 mg. per kg. intramuscularly or intravenously
    Give initial doses 30 minutes to 1 hour prior to procedure and repeat each every 8 hours for two additional doses

CONGESTIVE HEART FAILURE

method of
DAVID Z. MORGAN, M.D.,
and CARL E. HELTNE, M.D.
Morgantown, West Virginia

Congestive heart failure may be an acute event or a chronic state. Left ventricular failure may present dramatically with sudden transudation of fluid into the pulmonary alveoli, producing marked pulmonary congestion. In contrast, congestive heart failure may present insidiously with only exertional dyspnea or nocturnal cough and minimal physical findings. In these patients the chest radiograph may be helpful by revealing Kerley B lines, which are intralobular accumulation of edema fluid appearing as short, straight lung markings in the costophrenic angles, as well as dilation of pulmonary veins.

The chronic state of congestive heart failure may be mild, moderate, or severe when the heart as a pump is no longer able to meet the demands placed upon it. The degree of severity is usually characterized by the underlying cause of the failure and the success of therapy in making the patient comfortable and able to renew and maintain daily activities.

The pathophysiologic basis for this syndrome is an abnormality of myocardial fiber shorting, the determinants of which are preload, contractility, and afterload. Preload determines the fiber end-diastolic length and thus is an expression of the end-diastolic pressure and end-diastolic volume of the ventricle. Systemic and pulmonary congestion are manifestations of an increased preload. Contractility is an expression of the heart's intrinsic inotrophy, which is independent of volume loading. Afterload is equivalent to left ventricular systolic impedance and is quantified as systemic vascular resistance. In congestive heart failure the reduction of the effective forward cardiac output leads to a compensatory increase in systemic vascular resistance in order to maintain arterial pressure. This results in increased resistance to ejection and causes further reduction in cardiac output. With an appreciation of these determinants of ventricular function as well as the critical importance of heart rate and rhythm, one can formulate a physiologic approach to the treatment of congestive heart failure.

It must be remembered that the term "congestive heart failure" describes an altered physiologic state that can be the end result of conditions which impair the function of the left ventricle, such as prolonged hypertension, coronary artery disease, valvular heart disease, myocardiopathy, or certain forms of congenital heart disease.

The same clinical constellation of findings may be produced by an increase in left atrial pressure, such as by mitral stenosis; by extra-cardiac reasons, such as cardiac tamponade; or even by noncardiac causes, as for example, volume overload associated with injudicious blood and fluid replacement during and following a surgical procedure.

It is thus extremely important to attempt to arrive at a precise diagnosis of the cause. Such measures as reducing the volume overload with diuretics, and increasing the contractile state of the myocardium with digitalis are common to the management of most forms of congestive heart failure. Nevertheless, specific causes may require special therapy, such as the management of persistent hypertension or measures to improve pulmonary function for right heart failure accompanying chronic respiratory disease.

The physician should also be alert to those things that may precipitate congestive heart failure or worsen the status of a treated patient. This list includes, among others, acute myocardial infarction, excessive salt intake, severe physical or emotional stress, pulmonary embolism, infections, including bacterial endocarditis, arrhythmias, pregnancy, and thyrotoxicosis.

Basic Therapeutic Regimen

Reduction of Work Load. Some reduction in activity is usually needed, but strict bed rest should be avoided except in moderate or severe congestive heart failure. The severely disabled patient will require hospitalization. Sitting in a bedside chair approximately 15 minutes to an hour twice a day should be encouraged, and there should be a footboard at the end of the bed to allow leg exercises. For those patients in mild relapse and those convalescing from heart failure we recommend a nap each day after lunch.

Oxygen. Oxygen is indicated in the very dyspneic patient; 4 to 5 liters per minute through nasal prongs is well tolerated. If the underlying problem is chronic obstructive lung disease, Venturi masks, which deliver lower concentrations of oxygen, should be used.

Diet. When the patient is initially hospitalized the diet may include 1000 calories and 1 gram of sodium per 24 hours. When improvement occurs, the diet may be increased to 1200 to 1500 calories with a 2 gram sodium restriction over a 24-hour period. Extremely rigid salt restriction is usually not necessary with the efficacy of present-day diuretics. The physician should have some knowledge of the content of sodium in the water that the patient drinks, which in some areas may be as high as 35 mg. per dl. (100 ml.). One should be aware that some home water softeners add an excessive amount of sodium to the water supply. Administration of nonsteroidal anti-inflammatory agents and estrogens may also result in sodium and fluid retention. If the patient uses an antacid, it should be one with a low sodium content.

Other Measures. The correction or alleviation of problems that add an additional burden to the failing heart is mandatory.

Control of hypertension is of utmost importance in the reduction of the work load of the heart.

Pulmonary thromboembolism is a frequent complication of congestive heart failure and anticoagulant therapy may be indicated prophylactically in those with a history of thromboembolism or in the very immobile patient, such as the grossly obese.

Most patients will be committed to the continued use of medications and frequent visits to the physician once congestive heart failure has occurred. The physician is obligated to relieve the psychologic impact of this in every way possible, including honest explanations to the patient and family. Many patients will be able to return to their usual employment, and the physician can often help the employer plan a suitable work load within the patient's capability.

Use of Digitalis

Digoxin is the most widely used digitalis preparation because its serum half-life is less than three days, thus digitalis toxicity can be reversed more readily.

Therapeutic levels are achieved within one hour of oral administration by absorption of about 65 per cent from the small intestine.

The kidneys normally excrete almost all the digoxin, except for a small stool loss from bile excretion. Renal clearance approximates the creatinine clearance rate, but shows a wide variability. About one third of the body's digoxin is excreted per day. Digoxin may be initiated by an oral loading dose which should not exceed three times the desired maintenance dose. For example, if the desired maintenance dose is 0.25 mg. daily, the loading dose should not exceed 0.75 mg.; on the other hand, if the urgency is less, digoxin may be initiated by a daily maintenance dose. Steady-state serum concentraions will be achieved in less than one week with the same serum level as if a loading dose had been given. Most patients with mild, and many with moderate severity, can be treated on an outpatient basis by initiating therapy with maintenance digoxin, usually 0.25 mg., and appropriate diuretic therapy.

There are several important principles which must guide the use of digoxin:

1. Digoxin is not fat-soluble, and therefore the dose need not be increased in the obese patient.

2. Elderly patients have a decreasing creatinine clearance (not directly reflected by serum creatinine levels) and require significantly lower dosages of digoxin. The maintenance dose for patients in their 60s and 70s is often 0.125 mg., especially if the glomerular filtration rate is below 50 ml. per minute.

3. Oral administration is the preferred route unless some urgency exists to achieve a therapeu-tic serum level. In this circumstance the initial intravenous dose should be 25 to 30 per cent less than the usual oral loading dose, usually 0.5 mg. The physician may then repeat doses of 0.25 mg. every 2 to 4 hours, depending on clinical response. Intramuscular injections are best avoided because of an erratic absorption from this site.

4. Clinical judgment, not laboratory values, remains the major determinant in the use of digitalis.

Digitalis effect, primarily S-T and T wave changes on the electrocardiogram (ECG), signifies neither full digitalization nor digitalis toxicity.

The heart rate is not always useful as a guide in determining whether to increase or withhold digitalis. Some patients with a bradyarrhythmia may actually require more digitalis and a tachyarrhythmia may be a manifestation of digitalis toxicity.

Management of Digitalis Intoxication. The common manifestations of digitalis intoxication are gastrointestinal—anorexia, nausea, and vomiting. The most serious problem is the development of arrhythmias. Almost any arrhythmia can occur, although certain arrhythmias may suggest digitalis toxicity, including ventricular bigeminy, atrial tachycardia with block, and the regularization of atrial fibrillation.

The first and most important principle in treatment is to discontinue digitalis and to reassess the clinical status carefully.

Diuretic-induced hypokalemia is a common cause of increased ventricular irritability in association with digitalis intoxication and may be corrected by the intravenous administration of 40 mEq. of KCl in 50 ml. of 5 per cent dextrose in water over 1 to 2 hours. Potassium chloride may also be given orally, 2.0 grams every 2 to 4 hours, until the deficiency is corrected.

Specific drug therapy of digitalis-induced serious ventricular arrhythmias include the following:

1. Lidocaine may suppress ventricular irritability when given in a bolus of 50 to 100 mg. followed by an infusion of 1 to 5 mg. per minute.

2. Phenytoin sodium (Dilantin) is said to be rather specific for digitalis-induced ventricular tachycardia. This may be given in dosages of 100 to 150 mg. intravenously, not exceeding 50 mg. per minute to a total of 750 mg. If successful, maintenance dosages may be maintained at 300 to 600 mg. per day. Despite the advocacy of this drug by many, it must be remembered that this is not a Food and Drug Administration approved indication at this time in the United States.

3. Procainamide (Pronestyl) may be effective in digitalis-induced ventricular arrhythmias. Intravenously, it may be given under ECG and

blood pressure monitoring at the rate of 50 mg. per minute, to a total of 1.0 gram. The intramuscular or oral maintenance dose is 50 mg. per kg. total daily dose, given at three-hour intervals.

4. Propranolol (Inderal) may be given up to 3.0 mg. intravenously under ECG and blood pressure monitoring at the rate of 1.0 mg. per minute. If necessary, this dose may be repeated after 2 minutes and then not given again in less than 4 hours.

Less urgent ventricular irritability caused by digitalis may be treated with some of these agents (Dilantin, Pronestyl and Inderal) by the oral route. In addition, disopyramide phosphate (Norpace) is often effective at 400 to 800 mg. per day in divided doses.

The physician should be very familiar with the agent selected, and when used for urgent problems parenterally, the clinical status and ECG should be carefully monitored. Many of these drugs increase AV block and should not be used when that is the underlying rhythm.

Finally, cardioversion may be necessary in treating ventricular arrhythmias unresponsive to medication. A temporary pacemaker may be required in the management of third degree blocks or marked digitalis-induced brachycardia.

Diuretics

These agents reduce intravascular volume and thus reduce *preload*. Some potent diuretics such as furosemide (Lasix) and ethacrynic acid (Edecrin) act within approximately 10 minutes of their intravenous administration, dilating systemic veins, transiently pooling blood and reducing the pulmonary wedge pressure. A peak diuretic effect occurs in approximately 30 minutes. Weight loss produced by a diuretic should be gradual and not exceed 0.5 to 1 kg. per day.

Thiazides. Many patients with congestive heart failure will respond to thiazides and related sulfonamide compounds such as hydrochlorothiazide, chlorothiazide, and chlorthalidone. The physician should become familiar with one preparation such as hydrochlorothiazide, which is used in a dosage of 25 to 200 mg. daily. The usual dose is 50 mg. each morning.

Loop Diuretics. If the patient fails to respond to the less potent diuretics, then one should use furosemide or ethacrynic acid. Both of these have diuretic effects in common, even though they are unrelated chemically. They are potent and rapidly active. Both of these agents are effective in the presence of electrolyte imbalance and renal insufficiency. Occasionally, one will be effective when the other is not. The usual oral dose for furosemide is 40 to 80 mg. per day. The usual oral dose for ethacrynic acid is 50 to 100 mg. per day.

Either agent may be given intravenously. If the patient becomes refractory to these agents, one may add a thiazide, or spironolactone (25 mg. 4 times daily), or triamterene (100 mg. 3 times daily).

Potassium-sparing Diuretics. Spironolactone (Aldactone) is a competitive antagonist of aldosterone and thus interferes with its action at the distal tubule and thereby lessens the reabsorption of sodium and chloride and reduces the loss of potassium. Triamterene acts directly on tubular transport and is independent of aldosterone. Potassium excretion is reduced by an inhibition of potassium secretion at the distal tubule. These agents are rarely effective alone. They can be useful adjuncts to thiazide or loop diuretic therapy. Potassium supplements must not be given when these agents are used.

Complications of Diuretic Therapy. In elderly patients or those with renal insufficiency, excess loss of body water and sodium may lead to malaise and asthenia, orthostatic hypotension, and even postural syncope. In time, oliguria and azotemia may result. Hypokalemia and hypokalemic hypochloremic alkalosis are universal risks with any potent diuretic. It is essential, until a stabilized regimen is established, to monitor serum electrolytes and blood urea nitrogen (BUN) frequently. Hypokalemia and hypokalemic hypochloremic alkalosis may be treated by potassium chloride supplements, usually 5 ml. of 20 per cent KCl or 10 ml. of 10 per cent KCl one to four times a day in tomato or orange juice. Spironolactone or triamterene in the dosages of 25 mg. orally four times daily or 100 mg. orally three times daily respectively may be used to prevent hypokalemia. Tablets containing KCl in a wax-matrix may be better tolerated by some patients than the oral liquid preparation. Potassium supplements and potassium sparing diuretics should not be used together.

Hypomagnesemia may also occur with prolonged use of diuretic agents. This is mild and asymptomatic in the vast majority of patients, but symptomatic hypomagnesemia has been reported and even mild hypomagnesemia is of significance in patients receiving cardiac glycosides.

Vasodilator Therapy

Much interest has focused on vasodilators in the management of congestive heart failure. The altered performance of the myocardium results in congestion and an increased cardiac filling pressure (preload). The decrease in forward flow causes, by virtue of increased systemic vascular resistance, impedance to ventricular ejection (afterload).

Vasodilators as a group have two main actions: (1) venodilation and (2) reduction of left ventricular ejection impedance. Venodilation by virtue of an increased venous capacitance allows redistribution of intravascular volume from the central to the peripheral reservoirs and produces (1) a decrease in intracardiac volume, (2) a decrease in cardiac filling pressure, and (3) a decrease in pulmonary wedge pressure. All of these responses are reflected as a decrease in preload.

Left ventricular ejection impedance is reduced by either an increase in compliance in the large arteries or relaxation of the arteriolar resistance vessels.

Nitrates and nitrites act primarily on the venous side of circulation and produce a reduction in left ventricular filling pressure. The two principal agents are nitroglycerin and isosorbide dinitrite (Isordil). Nitroglycerin may be administered sublingually with a duration of an action of approximately 15 to 20 minutes. The skin ointment has a demonstrable hemodynamic effect for 4 to 6 hours. Some patients with severe chronic congestive heart failure do not show any significant hemodynamic response to nitroglycerin ointment.

Isosorbide dinitrite may be administered sublingually or orally. The duration of action when given sublingually or chewed is approximately 2 to 3 hours. The oral route has significant hemodynamic effects, which may be demonstrated up to as long as 4 to 6 hours after administration of dosages ranging from 20 to 80 mg.

Drugs that result in a decrease in left ventricular ejection impedance are phenoxybenzamine and hydralazine. Hydralazine is the most widely used agent. This agent may reduce arteriolar impedance in patients with congestive heart failure with a resultant decrease in systemic vascular resistance and increased forward cardiac output. This may mildly decrease blood pressure and has little, if any, effect on the heart rate. Its effect is potentiated if given with meals. The hemodynamic effects are readily demonstrable at 45 minutes and the duration of action is sustained for at least 6 hours. An appropriate starting dose is 75 mg. with close monitoring of heart rate and blood pressure response. With desired response, a dose of 100 mg. may be given at 6 to 8 hour intervals. (This dose may be higher than that listed in the manufacturer's official directive.)

Drugs that cause both venous and arteriolar dilation are nitroprusside, phentolamine, and prazosin.

Nitroprusside must be carefully titrated by intravenous drip. The recommended dose ranges from a starting dose of 15 micrograms per minute to a maximum of approximately 400 micrograms per minute. Hemodynamic monitoring is essential in the proper safe use of this agent.

Phentolamine, an alpha-adrenergic blocking agent with direct smooth muscle relaxing properties has the distinct disadvantage of producing tachycardia and thus increasing myocardial oxygen consumption. It is therefore of limited usefulness.

Prazosin is given orally and produces arteriolar vasodilation by a functional blockage of postsynaptic alpha-adrenergic receptors rather than by direct relaxation of arteriolar vascular muscle. The specificity of postsynaptic receptors probably accounts for the failure of this agent to produce tachycardia.

Complications of Vasodilator Therapy. Although vasodilator actions may produce beneficial hemodynamic effects in patients with acute or chronic heart failure, the potential complications of vasodilators should not be overlooked. Unexpected hypotension is a potential hazard and may occur with any vasodilator agent. A modest reduction in blood presure is observed in most patients without ill effect. A marked reduction in arterial pressure in patients with coronary artery disease may be hazardous.

There are also specific complications with each vasodilating agent. Cyanide poisoning is a potential lethal complication of nitroprusside therapy. This is extremely rare because of the rapid conversion of cyanide to thiocyanate. Thiocyanate concentrations may obtain toxic levels manifested by muscular weakness, nausea, epigastric discomfort, hypothyroidism, convulsions, muscle twitching, hiccups, and psychosis. If nitroprusside is to be used for prolonged periods at high dosages, serum levels of thiocyanate should be monitored. If the serum concentration exceeds 6 mg. per dl., the infusion should be discontinued.

Headache and postural hypotension are the two major complications of the use of nitrates. These complications are rare in patients with congestive heart failure. Bradycardia and marked hypotension occasionally occur in patients with an acute myocardial infarction. Therefore, small doses should be used initially.

Hydralazine may result in nausea, vomiting, and headache at the initiation of therapy, but these manifestations disappear with continued use. Fluid retention and weight gain may occur in some patients despite hemodynamic improvement. This may be treated with an increase in the diuretic dose. Tachycardia is extremely rare. Peripheral neuropathy secondary to pyridoxine deficiency may occur.

The most serious complication of hydralazine therapy is the development of drug-induced lupus erythematosus. This syndrome is seen in approximately 10 to 20 per cent of the patients who are receiving more than 400 mg. per day for an extended period.

Clinical Application of Newer Concepts

Emergency treatment of acute pulmonary edema should be started while studies for its cause are initiated. Chest x-ray and electrocardiogram are indicated in addition to the history and physical examination. The patient should have the head and trunk elevated approximately 60 to 90 degrees from the horizontal position. This reduces preload. Morphine, 4 to 6 mg. intravenously, should be given. This agent calms the patient and decreases the venous return to the right side of the heart. Oxygen is usually given at a rate of 6 to 8 liters per minute by nasal cannulae, but 100 per cent oxygen by face mask, if tolerated, is more effective. Furosemide (Lasix), 40 to 80 mg. intravenously, is very effective. This lowers preload by venodilation within 5 to 15 minutes after injection and has a diuretic effect that peaks at approximately 30 minutes.

Sublingual nitroglycerin in the patient with pulmonary edema who is normotensive or hypertensive is effective in reducing pulmonary venous congestion. One can give 0.4 to 0.8 mg. of nitroglycerin sublingually and monitor the blood pressure and symptomatic response. If this is effecitve, isosorbide dinitrate (Isordil) may be used in a dose of 5 to 10 mg. sublingually every 3 to 4 hours.

Nitroprusside, which reduces pulmonary congestion, decreases systemic vascular resistance, and increases cardiac output, is also an effective agent in patients with pulmonary edema, especially if they are hypertensive. Dosages are increased every 5 minutes from the starting level of 15 micrograms per minute until the patient improves or hypotension occurs.

Nitroprusside has been advocated in the care of the patient who has sustained an acute myocardial infarction with pump failure. One approach to persistent hypotension is the use of a titratable inotropic agent such as dopamine and a vasodilator agent such as nitroprusside. These patients will require hemodynamic monitoring.

Patients who present with refractory heart failure should be hospitalized initially. This in itself is often helpful. Careful consideration should be given to possible precipitating factors. If after vigorous therapy the patient's weight remains stable and the blood urea nitrogen (BUN) continues to rise due to diuretics and fluid retention, then one should consider the addition of vasodilator therapy to the therapeutic regimen. Hydralazine is currently the most studied of the effective agents. One should begin with a dose of 75 mg. every 6 hours and carefully watch blood pressure and heart rate. The dose may be increased to 100 mg. every 6 hours. (This dose may be higher than that listed in the manufacturer's official directive.) Oral isosorbide dinitrate may be used starting at a dose of approximately 20 mg. orally four times daily or every 6 hours and increasing to a maximum of 80 mg., with careful monitoring of blood pressure and symptoms of orthostatic hypotension.

It is important to follow these patients closely. They should weigh themselves each morning and report any weight gain over a 5 pound limit. They need frequent medical attention to ensure compliance and satisfactory progress.

With careful patient selection, vasodilator therapy may prove to be a useful treatment adjunct in the management of patients with congestive heart failure.

INFECTIVE ENDOCARDITIS

method of
MARVIN J. TENENBAUM, M.D.,
and GORDON L. ARCHER, M.D.
Richmond, Virginia

Antimicrobial therapy can cure 80 per cent of patients who have infective endocarditis, a disease that is uniformly fatal if left untreated. However, patients still die unnecessarily because of delays in diagnosis and inappropriate therapy. A rational approach to the therapy of the patient with infective endocarditis can be outlined, but it must be emphasized that treatment must ultimately be *individualized* for each patient and for each infecting organism.

General Principles of Therapy

The effectiveness of antimicrobial therapy depends upon selecting a therapeutic regimen which includes all of the following:

Bactericidal Antimicrobials.　With rare exception, bacteriostatic antibiotics *have no place* in the therapy of infective endocarditis. The infected vegetation is composed of a mass of fibrin and platelets in which colonies of bacteria are buried. There are no capillary networks to supply leukocytes to the areas of bacterial multiplication, and the platelet-fibrin matrix provides a barrier to the migration or chemotaxis of phagocytes from part of the vegetation to another. Thus, there are no host factors that can eradicate bacteria, which are inhibited but not killed; relapse will predictably follow the cessation of bacteriostatic therapy.

High Serum Bactericidal Activity. Colonies of bacteria are buried deep in the platelet-fibrin matrix of the vegetation. Antimicrobial activity in the serum must be sufficiently high so that bactericidal activity can penetrate passively from the cardiac blood bathing the vegetation to all areas containing metabolically active microorganisms. The dilution of the patient's serum that kills his own infecting organism (serum bactericidal test) should be kept at 1:8 or greater at the peak of antimicrobial activity and should be at least 1:2 to 1:4 at the point of lowest activity, usually just before the next dose. High doses of antimicrobials must usually be administered at short intervals to achieve these titers.

Parenteral Antimicrobials. Although some investigators have successfully used combinations of oral and parenteral antimicrobial agents, serum levels produced by the administration of oral drugs are too variable for these agents to be used for routine therapy. They may be indicated in special cases and used only when constant and accurate monitoring of serum bactericidal activity is available.

Prolonged Therapy. In general, a minimum of 4 weeks of therapy is required to treat infective endocarditis, particularly if a single antibiotic is used. Therapy should never be for less than 2 weeks, and for some organisms 6 weeks may be required.

Monitoring and Follow-up. Serum bactericidal activity should be monitored at regular intervals, particularly if there is a change in antibiotics or a reduction in dosage during therapy. In addition, the patient must have regular follow-up examinations for 3 months after the completion of therapy, as most patients who relapse will do so within this time period. Although patients with endocarditis usually respond symptomatically within 72 hours of the start of therapy, this early response will not predict those patients who are going to relapse; only careful follow-up will accomplish this.

Blood Culturing

The most important aspect of the diagnosis of infective endocarditis relevant to therapy is obtaining and identifying the causative organism. Endocarditis is an intravascular infection with constant access to the blood, and, therefore, the presence of bacteremia identified by blood culturing is the hallmark of this disease. The proper collection of *blood cultures* is of utmost importance and the following details should be observed.

1. Since the bacteremia of infective endocarditis is continuous, the timing of blood culture collections is not critical; they can all be obtained in the first hours after admission.

2. The optimum number of specimens to be collected is 3 to 5. This number of cultures will allow the diagnosis of 98 per cent of the cases of endocarditis and will include enough samples so that skin contaminants can be distinguished from organisms present in the blood. Additional cultures merely add to the patient's discomfort and hospital cost. More blood cultures can be obtained in the small group of patients whose cultures are negative after 48 hours of incubation. Delaying therapy for this length of time will be of no consequence to those patients with a chronic or subacute disease.

3. Every blood culture should be obtained from a separate venipuncture site, which is freshly prepared with 70 per cent alcohol followed by 1 to 2 per cent tincture of iodine or an iodophor. It is wise for the phlebotomist to prepare his palpating finger as well.

4. Ten to 20 ml. of blood should be obtained from each venipuncture and inoculated into each of two blood culture bottles so that the ratio of blood to broth is 1:10. There is some evidence that the culturing of a large volume of blood (10 ml.) increases the recovery rate of some microorganisms. One bottle should be vented and the other left unvented so that both obligate aerobic and anaerobic organisms can be recovered.

5. The laboratory should be instructed to save all organisms recovered from blood cultures for 4 weeks so that antibiotic susceptibility testing (tube-dilution studies) and serum bactericidal tests can be performed as needed.

6. Cultures negative after 48 hours should be incubated for 3 weeks at 35 to 37°C. The use of special media or lower incubation temperatures may be necessary for the recovery of thiol-dependent streptococci, yeasts, filamentous fungi, meningococci, or cell wall defective bacteria. There may be some advantage to adding penicillinase to blood culture bottles in patients who have recently received penicillin. Any added penicillinase should be carefully tested for sterility.

Specific Therapeutic Recommendations

Antibiotics of choice, alternate regimens, and dosing schedules are outlined in Table 1. The following specific data are important in choosing therapy.

Streptococcal Endocarditis (60 to 80 per cent of cases)

1. *Penicillin-sensitive streptococci* (MIC < 0.1 microgram per ml.). For therapeutic purposes it is important to know only if the causative streptococcus is exquisitely, moderately, or not at all susceptible to penicillin G. The identification of strep-

tococci by hemolysis, Lancefield grouping, and species will not always give an indication of penicillin susceptibility; only tube-dilution susceptibility studies of each isolate will do this. As to which is the best therapy of penicillin-sensitive streptococcal endocarditis is debated but either of the following regimens is acceptable:

    a. High-dose aqueous penicillin G alone by either intravenous bolus or continuous intravenous infusion for four weeks.

    b. Procaine penicillin G plus streptomycin for 2 weeks followed by 2 weeks of penicillin G alone. High-dose aqueous penicillin G can be given in place of procaine penicillin G as in (a).

Penicillin G plus streptomycin for only 2 weeks may be as effective as the combination plus an additional two weeks of penicillin G. However, at the present time the data are insufficient to recommend this course of therapy. Since susceptibility of penicillin-sensitive streptococci to alternative antibiotics (cephalosporins, vancomycin, and clindamycin) is variable, therapy in penicillin-allergic patient should be guided by susceptibility studies.

2. *Penicillin-resistant streptococci* (MIC > 0.1 microgram per ml.). A *single* antibiotic should *not* be administered to patients infected with penicillin-resistant streptococci—a combination of a penicillin plus an aminoglycoside is necessary for cure. Enterococci are resistant to the bactericidal action of *all* penicillins (including ampicillin) and require 6 weeks of therapy with a penicillin (high dose) plus streptomycin or gentamicin (if the isolate is highly streptomycin resistant). We begin the patient on penicillin plus streptomycin and only substitute gentamicin for streptomycin if serum bactericidal titers are not adequate. Therapy for the penicillin-allergic patient is vancomycin plus an aminoglycoside. Penicillin desensitization may have to be attempted if the vancomycin regimen fails. Cephalosporins *have no place* in the therapy of enterococcal endocarditis. Patients on long-term penicillin prophylaxis for rheumatic fever should be treated as if they are infected with a penicillin-resistant streptococcus until sensitivity studies are returned.

Staphylococcal Endocarditis (10 to 30 per cent of cases)

1. *Staphylococcus aureus.* Therapy for suspected *S. aureus* endocarditis should be begun *immediately* when the diagnosis is suspected without waiting for blood culture results. We begin treatment with a semisynthetic penicillin alone in high dose, but we will add gentamicin if the patient is extremely toxic on admission, does not show improvement in 48 to 72 hours, or has low serum bactericidal titers on one drug. The combination is more effective than the single antibiotic experimentally, but this has yet to be documented clinically; patients with *S. aureus* endocarditis often respond slowly on any regimen. Cephalosporins and vancomycin are effective alternative drugs and clindamycin has been used successfully in treating tricuspid endocarditis. Penicillin G should be used *only* if tube dilution studies show the minimum *bactericidal* concentration to be < 0.1 microgram per ml.

2. *Staphylococcus epidermidis* and *micrococci.* Susceptibility testing is extremely important in devising therapy for endocarditis caused by these organisms. Most infections occur on prosthetic heart valves and the majority of organisms are resistant to semisynthetic penicillins and multiple other antistaphylococcal antibiotics. Initial therapy should always include at least two antibiotics. We use a cephalosporin or vancomycin plus gentamicin. The addition of rifampin has been effective in particularly refractory cases.

Gram-negative Rod Endocarditis (1 to 4 per cent of cases)

1. *Aerobic bacilli.* Intravenous drug abusers, patients with prosthetic heart valves, and alcoholics are the most commonly infected persons. Prolonged (6 weeks), high-dose, combination therapy is mandatory; it may be necessary to administer aminoglycosides in toxic doses to achieve cure.

2. *Anaerobic bacilli. Bacteroides fragilis,* the anaerobic bacillus that most commonly causes endocarditis, is usually penicillin-resistant. Clindamycin or carbenicillin have been effective, but treatment is usually difficult. Metronidazole has afforded dramatic cures in cases of *Bacteroides* sepsis, but the parenteral form of the drug and its use in this condition are investigational.

Endocarditis Caused by Miscellaneous Bacteria (1 to 5 per cent of cases)

1. *Hemophilus* sp. endocarditis caused by ampicillin-susceptible organisms should be treated with 12 to 20 grams of ampicillin per day for 4 to 6 weeks. The therapy for ampicillin-resistant *Hemophilus* sp. endocarditis is not clear but should probably include multiple antibiotics.

2. *Neisseria* sp. endocarditis should be treated with penicillin alone; these organisms are usually exquisitely penicillin-sensitive.

3. *Corynebacterium* sp. ("diphtheroids") is an increasingly important cause of prosthetic valve endocarditis. Vancomycin is one of the few antibiotics to which these organisms are uniformly susceptible.

TABLE 1.   Treatment Regimens for Infective Endocarditis*

ORGANISM	REGIMEN(S) OF CHOICE	ALTERNATE REGIMEN(S)	DURATION OF TREATMENT
A. Streptococci			
1. Penicillin-sensitive (MIC < 0.1 µg./ml.)	Aqueous penicillin G, 2.4 million units I.V. q. 3 h. *or* Aqueous penicillin G, 2.4 million units I.V. q. 3 h. (Procaine penicillin G, 1.2 million units I.M. q. 6 h.) *plus* Streptomycin 500 mg. I.M. q. 12 h.	Cephalothin, 2 grams I.V. q. 4 h. (Cefazolin, 1 gram I.M. or I.V. q. 4 h.) Vancomycin, 500 mg. I.V. q. 6 h. Clindamycin, 600 mg. I.V. q. 6 h.	4 weeks (penicillin or alternate drug alone) *or* 2 weeks, penicillin plus aminoglycoside Additional 2 weeks, penicillin alone
2. Penicillin-resistant (MIC > 0.1 µg./ml.)	Aqueous penicillin G, 3 million units I.V. q. 3 h. *plus* Streptomycin, 500 mg. I.M. q. 12 h. *or* Gentamicin, 1 mg./kg. I.M. or I.V. q. 8 h.	Vancomycin, 500 mg. I.V. q. 6 h. *plus* Streptomycin, 500 mg. I.M. q. 12 h. *or* Gentamicin, 1 mg./kg. I.M. or I.V. q. 8 h.	6 weeks (any regimen)
B. Staphylococci			
1. *Staphylococcus aureus* (MBC > 0.1 µg./ml.)	Nafcillin, 2 grams I.V. q. 4 h. (plus gentamicin, 1 mg./kg. I.M. or I.V. q. 8 h.) (any other semisynthetic penicillin)	Cephalothin, 2 grams I.V. q. 4 h. Vancomycin, 500 mg. I.V. q. 6 h. Clindamycin, 600 mg. I.V. q. 6 h.	6 weeks (any regimen)
2. *Staphylococcus aureus* (MBC < 0.1 µg./ml.)	Aqueous penicillin G, 3 million units I.V. q. 3 h.		
3. *Staphylococcus epidermidis* (methicillin-resistant)	Cephalothin, 2 grams I.V. q. 4 h. *plus* Gentamicin, 1 mg./kg. I.M. or I.V. q. 8 h. *plus* Rifampin, 600 mg. p.o. q. 12 h.	Vancomycin, 500 mg. I.V. q. 6 h. *plus* Gentamicin *plus* Rifampin	6 weeks (any regimen)
4. *Staphylococcus epidermidis* (methicillin-sensitive)	Nafcillin, 2 grams I.V. q. 4 h.	Cephalothin, 2 grams I.V. q. 4 h.	4 to 6 weeks
C. Gram-negative rods			
1. Aerobic bacilli			
a. susceptible enterobacteriaceae	Cephalothin, 2 grams I.V. q. 4 h. *plus* Gentamicin, 1.5–2 mg./kg. I.M. or I.V. q. 8 h.	Cephalothin or carbenicillin *plus* Amikacin 5 mg./kg. I.M. or I.V. q. 8 h. (for gentamicin or tobramycin resistant organisms)	6 weeks

*See text for explanations of regimens. The regimens listed are the choice of the authors; those in parentheses are acceptable regimens favored by others. All dosages are for adults with normal renal function. The suggested doses of some antibiotics in this table are higher than those stated in the manufacturer's official directive.

TABLE 1. **Treatment Regimens for Infective Endocarditis** *(Continued)*

ORGANISM	REGIMEN(S)	ALTERNATE REGIMEN(S)	DURATION OF TREATMENT
b. susceptible *Pseudomonas* sp.	Carbenicillin, 5 grams I.V. q. 4 h. *plus* Gentamicin or tobramycin, 1.5–2 mg./kg. I.M. or I.V. q. 8 h.		6 weeks
2. Anaerobic bacilli			
a. penicillin-sensitive	Aqueous penicillin G, 2.4 million units I.V. q. 3 h.	Cephalothin, 2 grams I.V. q. 4 h. Clindamycin, 600 mg. I.V. q. 6 h.	4 weeks
b. penicillin-resistant (i.e., *Bacteroides fragilis*)	Clindamycin, 600 mg. I.V. q. 6 h.	Metronidazole, 500 mg. p.o. q. 8 h. (500 mg. I.V. q. 8 h.)† Carbenicillin, 5 grams I.V. q. 4 h.	6 weeks
D. Miscellaneous bacteria			
1. *Hemophilus* sp.	Ampicillin, 2.5 grams I.V. q. 4 h.	Carbenicillin, 5 grams I.V. q. 4 h. *plus* Gentamicin, 1 mg./kg. I.M. or I.V. q. 8 h. (chloramphenicol, 1 gram I.V. q. 6 h.) According to susceptibility of organism	4 to 6 weeks
2. *Neisseria* sp.	Aqueous penicillin G, 2.4 million units I.V. q. 3 h.	Cephalothin, 2 grams I.V. q. 4 h. (Cefazolin, 1 gram I.M. or I.V. q. 4 h.) Penicillin-resistant organism: according to susceptibility data	4 weeks
3. *Corynebacterium* sp.	Vancomycin, 500 mg. I.V. q. 6 h.	According to susceptibility of organism	4 to 6 weeks
E. Fungi	Amphotericin B, 1 mg./kg. I.V. q. day *plus* Flucytosine, 150 mg./kg. p.o. q. day *plus* Surgical excision of valve or prosthesis	No effective alternative	6 to 8 weeks
F. Culture-negative endocarditis	As for penicillin-resistant streptococci		

†This use of metronidazole is investigational.

4. Therapy for other unusual organisms that may cause endocarditis should be devised on the basis of each isolate's antimicrobial susceptibility.

Endocarditis Caused by Yeasts and Filamentous Fungi (less than 1 per cent of cases)

Although a rare cause of endocarditis, these organisms are important because of their uniformly poor response to therapy. *Candida* sp. (yeast) and *Aspergillus* sp. (filamentous fungus) are the most common organisms involved. Therapy with amphotericin B and flucytosine should be begun and surgical removal of the infected natural or prosthetic valve should be performed after no more than 2 weeks of drug therapy. The antifungal agents should be continued for a minimum of 6 weeks postoperatively and the patient should be followed closely for at least 1 year postoperatively; patients have relapsed as long as 2 years following the end of therapy.

Culture-negative Endocarditis (5 to 15 per cent of cases)

Multiple blood cultures and serologies should be obtained in an attempt to make a specific diagnosis. If no causative agent can be identified, treatment should be as outlined for penicillin-resistant streptococcal endocarditis.

Surgical Therapy of Endocarditis. Surgery is important in the care of infective endocarditis in the folowing circumstances.

CONGESTIVE HEART FAILURE. Persistent or progressive heart failure during active endocarditis that does not respond to medical therapy is an indication for surgical removal of the infected valve and its replacement with a prosthesis. Heart failure is the most common complication of infective endocarditis and the most common cause of death. Severe heart failure on admission in a patient with aortic valve endocarditis or acute heart failure due to rupture or prolapse of the aortic valve are indications for emergency valve replacement regardless of the duration of prior antimicrobial therapy. Appropriate antibiotics should be continued for several weeks after valve replacement.

PERSISTENT INFECTION. This is uncommon but occurs in the following circumstances:

a. Gram-negative rod endocarditis. These organisms, especially *Pseudomonas aeruginosa,* are often only moderately or poorly susceptible to antibiotics, and valve removal is often necessary for cure.
b. Fungal endocarditis (see above).
c. Prosthetic valve endocarditis. Valve ring abscesses and dehiscence of the prosthesis are seen in early prosthetic valve endocarditis (within 2 to 3 months of surgery).

Surgery is often an emergency procedure in this setting.

RECURRENT EMBOLI. Indications for surgery in this setting are controversial. Major emboli can continue to occur after sterilization of vegetations and, therefore, antibiotic therapy may not prevent recurrent embolization. The association of more than one major embolic episode with echocardiographic evidence of large, shaggy valvular vegetations is probably indication for valve replacement.

Other Aspects of Therapy

ANTICOAGULATION. We feel that anticoagulation is contraindicated at all times in endocarditis because it is ineffective in preventing embolization from the vegetation and may convert a bland infarction to one that is hemorrhagic. If patients are taking anticoagulants to prevent thrombus formation on a prosthetic valve, the anticoagulant administration may not need to be stopped if prosthetic valve endocarditis develops.

MONITORING AND TREATING CARDIAC ABNORMALITIES. *Heart Failure.* The importance of early recognition of heart failure occurring during the course of antibiotic therapy has been mentioned. Some antibiotics (e.g., nafcillin, ampicillin, and carbenicillin) contain significant quantities of sodium that may contribute to volume overload. A reduced glomerular filtration rate secondary to nephrotoxic antibiotics (vancomycin and aminoglycosides) may also contribute to volume overload and heart failure.

Arrhythmias. The patient should be carefully observed, particularly in the first 2 weeks of therapy, for major rhythm disturbances. Complete heart block and ventricular tachyarrhythmias can be the result of myocardial or valve ring abscesses.

ALTERATION OF DOSAGE FOR DECREASED RENAL FUNCTION. The dosage of *all* antibiotics excreted by the kidneys must be reduced if renal insufficiency develops during therapy. These antibiotics include penicillin, ampicillin, cephalosporins, methicillin, oxacillin (but not nafcillin), vancomycin, and the aminoglycosides.

Antibiotic Prophylaxis of Infective Endocarditis

The recommendations outlined in Table 2 are the recommendations of the Committee on Prevention of Rheumatic Fever and Bacterial Endocarditis of the American Heart Association (Circulation, 56:139A, 1977). The following are important additional points.

Cardiac abnormalities which require prophylaxis include the following: (a) congenital heart disease (*except* secundum atrial septal defect); (b) rheumatic or other acquired valvular disease; (c) idiopathic hypertrophic subaortic stenosis; (d) mitral valve prolapse with severe insufficiency; and (e) prosthetic heart valves.

TABLE 2. **Antibiotic Prophylaxis to Prevent Bacterial Endocarditis***

PROCEDURE	REGIMEN(S) OF CHOICE	ALTERNATE REGIMEN(S)	DURATION
A. Dental procedures and surgery of the upper respiratory tract	1. *Aqueous crystalline penicillin G,* 1 million units I.M., *mixed with procaine penicillin G,* 600,000 units I.M., 30 minutes prior to procedure then *penicillin V,* 500 mg. p.o. q. 6 h. 2. *Penicillin V,* 2 grams p.o. 30 minutes prior to procedure then *penicillin V* 500 mg. p.o. q. 6 h. 3. *Aqueous crystalline penicillin G,* 1 million units I.M., *mixed with procaine penicillin G,* 600,000 units I.M. *plus* *streptomycin,* 1 gram I.M. 30 minutes prior to procedure, then *penicillin V,* 500 mg. p.o. q. 6 h.	1. *Vancomycin,* 1 gram I.V. over 30 minutes started 30 minutes prior to procedure, then *erythromycin,* 500 mg. p.o. q. 6 h. 2. *Erythromycin,* 1 gram p.o. 90 minutes prior to procedure, then *erythromycin,* 500 mg. p.o. q. 6 h.	8 doses of oral medication (48 hrs)
B. Genitourinary tract and gastrointestinal tract surgery or instrumentation	1. *Aqueous crystalline penicillin G,* 2 million units I.M. or I.V. *plus* *streptomycin,* 1 gram I.M., *or gentamicin,* 1.5 mg./kg. I.M., 30 minutes prior to procedure 2. *Ampicillin,* 1 gram I.M. or I.V. *plus* *streptomycin,* 1 gram I.M. *or gentamicin,* 1.5 mg./kg. I.M., 30 minutes prior to procedure	1. *Vancomycin,* 1 gram I.V. over 30 minutes *plus* *streptomycin,* 1 gram I.M.	1. If streptomycin is used with penicillin or ampicillin, give a similar dose every 12 hours for two additional doses 2. If gentamicin is used with penicillin or ampicillin, give a similar dose every 8 hours for two additional doses 3. With alternate regimen the same dose may be repeated in 12 hours
C. Cardiac surgery	1. *Cefazolin,* 1 gram I.M. or I.V. *plus* *gentamicin,* 1.5 mg./kg. I.M. or I.V. at time of surgery, followed by *cefazolin,* 1 gram I.M. or I.V. q. 6 h., *and* *gentamicin,* 1.5 mg./kg. I.M. or I.V. q. 8 h. 2. *Nafcillin,* 1 gram I.V. or I.M., *plus* *gentamicin,* 1.5 mg./kg. I.M. or I.V. at time of surgery, followed by *nafcillin,* 1 gram I.V. or I.M. q. 4 h., *and* *gentamicin,* 1.5 mg./kg. I.M. or I.V. q. 8 h.	1. *Vancomycin,* 1 gram I.V., *plus* *gentamicin,* 1.5 mg./kg. I.M. or I.V. at time of surgery, followed by *vancomycin,* 500 mg. I.V. q. 6 h., and *gentamicin,* 1.5 mg./kg. I.M. or I.V. q. 8 h.	No more than 48 hours (2 days) postoperatively

*These recommendations are based on those of the Committee on Prevention of Rheumatic Fever and Bacterial Endocarditis of the American Heart Association.

Procedures which do *not* require prophylaxis include the following: (a) cardiac catheterization and angiography; (b) upper gastrointestinal endoscopy (without biopsy); (c) uncomplicated vaginal delivery; (d) proctoscopy and sigmoidoscopy; (e) barium enema; and (f) pelvic examination, dilation and curettage of the uterus, and uncomplicated insertion or removal of intrauterine devices. The risk of side effects from antibiotics is greater than the very slight risk of endocarditis following these procedures.

In patients with prosthetic cardiac valves and in patients receiving monthly antibiotics to prevent recurrences of rheumatic fever, penicillin should *always* be combined with an aminoglycoside or, in the penicillin-allergic patient, vancomycin should be used.

HYPERTENSION

method of
LAWRENCE R. KRAKOFF, M.D.
New York, New York

Introduction

At present, the use of antihypertensive drugs in the treatment of systemic arterial hypertension represents the keystone in prevention of cardiovascular morbidity in the adult population. Despite the well-known correlation of a number of risk factors with future cardiovascular disease in prospective epidemiologic surveys and the likelihood that some of these risk factors are indeed causative agents, the only well-accepted intervention trials that virtually prove the efficacy of therapy are in the field of hypertension.

The Veterans Administration Cooperative Studies have made it clear that those with the highest level of pretreatment arterial pressure (diastolic $\geq$ 105 mm. Hg) will benefit from blood pressure reduction through a decreased frequency of dissecting and ruptured aneurysm, stroke—both cerebral hemorrhage and infarction, left ventricular failure and progression to the malignant phase of hypertension. A more recent long-term clinical trial carried out over 10 years by the United States Public Health Service evaluating treatment of mild hypertension (pretreatment diastolic pressure 90 to 104 mm. Hg) indicates that the rate of left ventricular hypertrophy, the rate of rise of arterial pressure and progressive retinopathy can be attenuated by antihypertensive drugs.

TABLE 1.   **Diagnostic Evaluation**

1. Overall risk profile
    a. Pretreatment arterial pressure
    b. Smoking history
    c. Serum lipids/lipoproteins
    d. Obesity—presence or absence of
    e. Diabetes—presence or absence of
    f. Family history of cardiovascular disease
2. Stage of cardiovascular disease
    a. Retinal findings
    b. Cardiac—coronary heart disease, ventricular dysfunction
    c. CNS—ischemic episodes, stroke
    d. Renal function
    e. Peripheral arterial occlusive disease
3. Etiology
    a. Renal causes
    b. Disorders of adrenal cortex or medulla
    c. Coarctation of aorta
    d. "Environmental," i.e., oral contraceptive pills, licorice
    e. Other
4. Pathogenetic mechanisms
    a. Renin-angiotensin vasoconstriction
    b. Sodium chloride/water retention
    c. Hyperadrenergic state
    d. Other

In neither of these American trials was compelling evidence produced to indicate that coronary heart disease was affected by antihypertensive therapy despite the background evidence that hypertension indeed accelerates the atherosclerotic process in the coronary arteries as well as elsewhere in the arterial tree. A recently published account of a large scale clinical trial in Sweden indicates that antihypertensive therapy may halve morbidity due to coronary heart disease. A principal difference between the American trials and the Swedish one was the drug program. The former relied on thiazide diuretics and reserpine, whereas in the latter study beta receptor blocking agents formed the mainstay of therapy.

The approach to management of hypertensive patients to be outlined will focus on the use of currently available therapeutic modalities to reduce arterial pressure: (a) in relation to the detectable mechanisms specifically related to the elevation of blood pressure where clinically possible and (b) in appreciation of the actions of antihypertensive drugs which are related to overall risk factors bearing on the pathogenesis of arterial pathology. In particular, emphasis will be placed upon the potential tradeoffs that may occur when oversimplified approaches are employed in the treatment of mild hypertension. Patients with this disorder face many years, even decades, of management. This should be plotted in the most rational manner with full attention to all the complexities of the present state of the art. This presentation will not cover the details of the diagnostic assessment of the hypertensive patient. In planning therapy, however, some aspects of the diagnostic approach cannot be overlooked. Table 1 summarizes the factors that should be considered in developing therapeutic strategy.

Therapy of the Hypertensive Patient

Nonpharmacologic Interventions. Long-term reduction of arterial pressure without the use of antihypertensive drugs remains to be established as a successful therapeutic modality. Nonetheless, short-term decreases in blood pressure have been produced by weight loss in the obese patient, meditation or relaxation techniques in selected patients, or reduction of diet salt intake. The obese patient with mild uncomplicated hypertension, ingesting a diet of 800 to 1200 calories coupled with an appropriate exercise program may reduce blood pressure even in the absence of diet salt restriction. It is not clear as to the best techniques for motivation to keep patients in such programs. However, the benefits of concurrent weight reduction and blood pressure control are obvious.

The current vogue for meditation, relaxation, or biofeedback techniques has led to great interest with regard to blood pressure reduction. When arterial pressure is indeed reduced concurrent with such approaches there is no reason to question the potential benefit. However, patients should be counseled that meditation, and other approaches may affect their "inner state" and yet result in little change in arterial pressure. To the extent that long-term cardiovascular risk is related to arterial pressure, such patients should be placed on antihypertensive drug therapy to normalize pressure. Reduction in diet salt content may lower blood pressure in the extreme situation when sodium intake is reduced to less than 20 mEq. per day. However, this is unaccepable or impractical for most patients. An attempt to maintain sodium intake to between 80 and 150 mEq. per day seems reasonable and can be achieved by having patients avoid the use of the salt shaker, salty foods, and preprocessed foods. Counseling by a nutritionist or dietician may assist in patient education, not only with regard to hypertension but also for other considerations as may be the case in patients with diabetes or hyperlipoproteinemia.

Another current vogue is to perceive exercise as a preventive modality for cardiovascular disease. Again, some patients with mild hypertension may have a reduction of arterial pressure when undergoing a sustained program of exercise such as jogging or bicycling. If the arterial pressure is reduced to normal, the therapy is beneficial. However, when the arterial pressure remains elevated despite the enhanced sense of well being that daily exercise often produces, patients should be well informed as to the real risk and the need for drug therapy.

Rationale for the Use of Antihypertensive Drugs. Reduction of arterial pressure through the use of antihypertensive drugs is effective with regard to blood pressure, safe in relative terms, and does indeed prevent cardiovascular morbidity. For patients with pretreatment diastolic blood pressures of 105 mm. Hg or greater, antihypertensive drug therapy can be considered mandatory. For those with pretreatment diastolic levels between 90 and 104 mm. Hg, indications for aggressive therapy are less clear, but often drug treatment is imposed (a) as the arterial pressure begins to show elevations such that diastolic pressure is consistently above 95 mm. Hg, (b) in the presence of advanced retinopathy, cardiomegaly by electrocardiographic or radiologic criteria, renal disease, diabetes, or evidence of other risk factors which are not reversible and (c) in the presence of a family history suggesting a high degree of likelihood that the blood pressure will become further elevated with time.

In young patients with labile blood pressure or those with borderline elevations in whom reversible other risk factors are present, such as smoking or obesity, the withholding of antihypertensive drugs for varying periods of time may permit the establishment of a more appropriate baseline against which to assess the eventual effects of drug treatment.

Selection of antihypertensive agents should be undertaken with the following features in mind: (a) pathogenetic mechanisms accounting for the blood pressure elevation when these are already determined by such procedures as hormone profiling or are to be analyzed by the results of therapy, (b) associated risk factors and complicating events that will affect the choice of agents to be employed, and (c) general medical status of the patient which might affect the action of antihypertensive agents or anticipated adverse reactions. The urgency with which blood pressure reduction is sought will vary in relation to (a) the level of arterial pressure prior to therapy, and (b) the presence of imminent cardiovascular damage as reflected by more severe grades of hypertensive retinopathy, evidence of progressive cardiac, central nervous system (CNS), or renal dysfunction, i.e., evidence of the malignant phase and special circumstances in which screening studies indicate the likelihood of pheochromocytoma, acute glomerulonephritis, or other diseases in which the need for urgent therapy is apparent.

Conditions in which antihypertensive therapy should be considered as an urgent or emergent measure are listed in Table 2. The choice of such therapy will be related to the specific cause that is most likely, e.g., pheochromocytoma should be managed by alpha and occasionally beta receptor

TABLE 2. **Indication for Emergency Control of Arterial Pressure**

1. Hypertensive encephalopathy
2. Malignant hypertension
   (retinal hemorrhage, exudate with or without papilledema)
3. Dissecting or expanding aneurysm
4. Acute left ventricular failure due to hypertension
5. Subarachnoid or brain hemorrhage
6. Pheochromocytoma
7. Monoamine oxidase inhibitor—tyramine syndrome
8. Clonidine withdrawal syndrome
9. Toxemia of pregnancy

blocking agents, whereas the malignant phase of hypertension when related to chronic renal disease may require vigorous diuretic therapy and dialysis.

For more moderate types of hypertension the therapeutic decision tree as given in Figure 1 provides a rationale in which age, expected pathogenetic mechanisms, and adverse reactions to currently available antihypertensive therapy form the basis for decision making. As indicated, patients under 60 years old without contraindications should be considered candidates for beta receptor blocking agents as the initial medication for blood pressure reduction. This is based upon the observation that most hypertensive patients in this age group have either normal or elevated plasma renin activity. (This may not be the case for black populations, in which a greater percentage of low renin hypertension may be present at an earlier age. Careful pathophysiologic studies should resolve the question as to whether the patient's ethnic origin should be a consideration in initial choice of antihypertensive agent.) In those patients 60 years of age or more, a greater prevalence of low renin hypertension is well documented and indicates that diuretic drugs offer greater therapeutic efficacy. When diuretics fail to

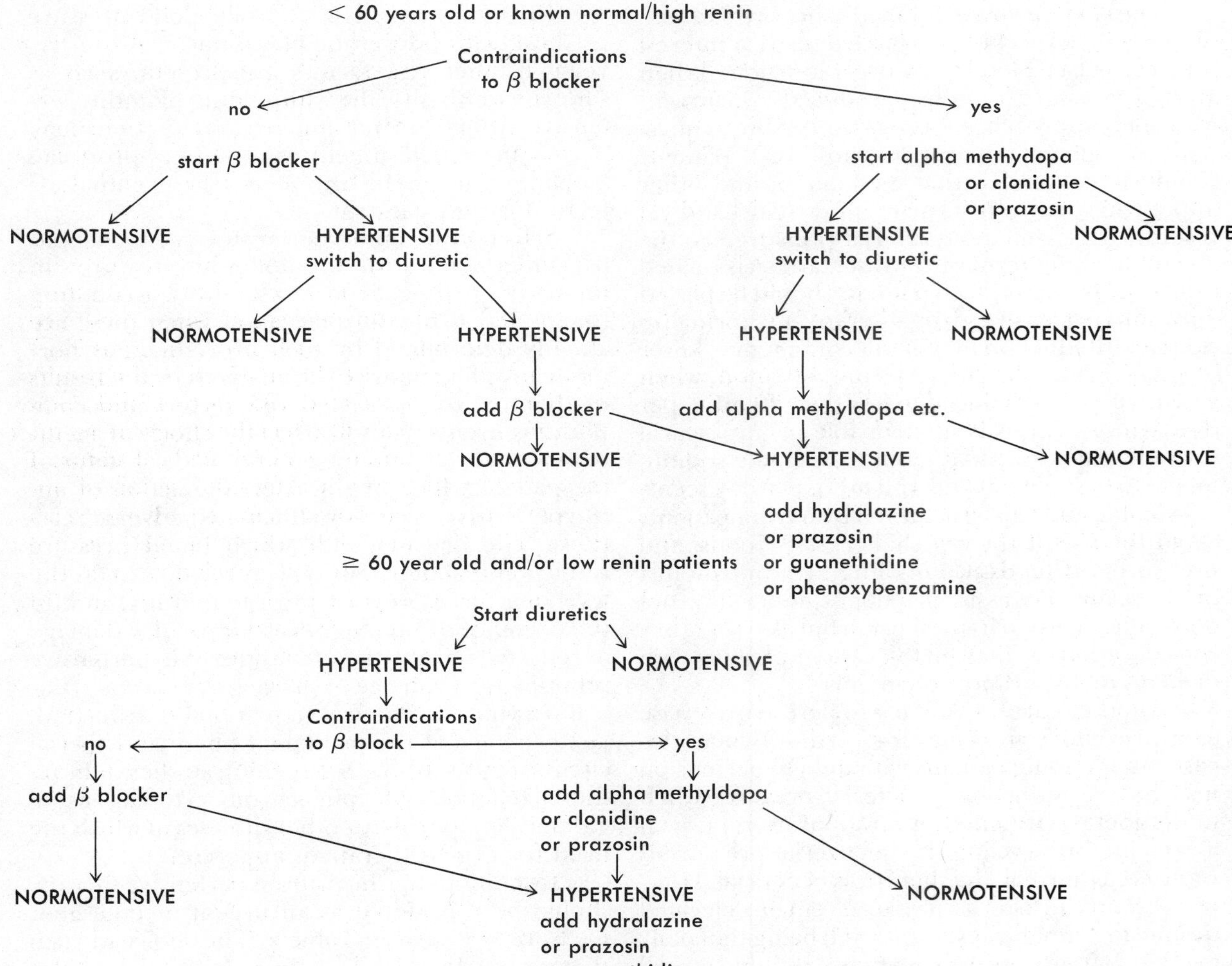

Figure 1. Treatment Scheme for Mild-moderate Hypertension

normalize arterial pressure in this older group of subjects, these agents should not be abandoned, as age related propensities for decreased cardiac and renal function in older subjects might make them more susceptible to adverse reactions to beta blocking agents when given alone. It is preferable, in the absence of contraindications, to add beta blocking drugs and observe the response in arterial pressure. It is reasonable to taper and discontinue diuretic agents if a successful antihypertensive response is observed with beta blocking drugs in the presence of a normal heart, even in older patients. In younger patients, the use of beta blocking drugs alone may normalize arterial pressure in a high percentage of subjects. When these drugs are contraindicated by the patient's history, antiadrenergic therapy such as alpha methyldopa, clonidine, or prazosin may normalize pressure and reduce plasma renin activity. A cardioselective beta receptor blocking drug, metroprolol (Lopressor), has been recently approved in the United States for treatment of hypertension. The principal difference between this drug and propranolol is relative specificity of blockade for B_1 receptors with metoprolol. Thus, metoprolol can be considered (cautiously) in patients with bronchial asthma or obstructive lung disease which are contraindications to the use of propranolol. It should be borne in mind that specificity for β_1 receptors is relative so that high doses of cardioselective beta blockers will produce nonspecific beta receptor blockade. As indicated in Figure 1, the young patient who fails to respond to beta receptor blocking drugs may then receive a trial of diuretic therapy. It is suggested that comparing the responses of the patient to these two approaches will, in effect, provide a form of hormone profiling as would be predicted by pretreatment measurement of plasma renin activity in relation to sodium balance.

Perhaps 30 to 50 per cent of patients fail to respond to a single form of therapy with normalization of arterial pressure. The addition of other forms of antihypertensive medication addressed to those mechanisms buffering arterial pressure at levels above normal should result in normalization in perhaps 90 to 95 per cent of all patients. The use of propranolol to inhibit renin production in patients remaining hypertensive on diuretic agents is well established and effective. When beta blockade is contraindicated, alpha methyldopa, clonidine, or prazosin may function well as alternate choices. In those few subjects who remain hypertensive despite two-drug therapy, the addition of either direct-acting vasodilator drugs such as hydralazine or those agents that inhibit sympathetic nervous system mediated vasoconstriction via the alpha receptor should be chosen.

Refractory Hypertension. The term refractory hypertension delineates those patients whose diastolic blood pressure cannot be reduced to below 105 mm. Hg with conventional antihypertensive medication. The most likely cause of therapeutic failure is lack of patient adherence to the prescribed regimen so that the initial step is an attempt to determine whether or not compliance is the issue. Another consideration to be made is whether the choice of antihypertensive agents is rational in terms of the mechanisms that might be playing a role in sustaining the blood pressure elevation. Combining methyldopa with clonidine would employ two agents whose mechanisms of action are quite similar. Little additive effect is to be expected. A third possibility is that drug interaction is interfering with blood pressure reduction. The tricyclic antidepressants block the antihypertension action of guanethidine and bethanidine by inhibiting the uptake of these drugs at the sympathetic nerve terminal. Patients with refractory hypertension should have a thorough review of all of their medications, not just those prescribed for hypertension. The fourth consideration to be made is whether the underlying cause of the hypertension may account for its refractoriness to therapy. Some patients with renal artery stenosis, pheochromocytoma, Cushing's syndrome may be extraordinarily refractory to antihypertensive medication, particularly when these medications are not chosen specifically to counteract the pathogenetic mechanisms that account for the blood pressure elevation. Hyperangiotensinemia of severe renal artery stenosis may counteract the effect of all conventional antihypertensive drugs so that only specific angiotensin II antagonists or inhibitors of the converting enzyme such as SQ 20881 or SQ 14225 (Captopril) will be effective in lowering arterial pressure. Similarly, the extraordinary vasoconstriction sometimes observed in pheochromocytoma may respond only to alpha receptor blocking agents such as phentolamine or phenoxybenzamine. There still remain those patients without such rare causes who are indeed compliant but fail to respond adequately to conventional antihypertensive drugs. The use of newer agents remaining in the investigative stage such as Minoxidil (Upjohn) offers promise in this regard.

The Antihypertensive Drugs. The spectrum of useful drugs that lower arterial pressure is a broad one and expanding at the present time. This spectrum now includes: (a) drugs with which action may occur within the central nervous system (CNS) in modulating sympathetic tone, (b) those which act upon the neurones of the peripheral sympathetic nervous system (SNS), (c) drugs which compete for adrenergic receptor sites, (d) agents which inhibit the action of the renin-angiotensin system, (e) a variety of diuretics, including spironolactone, which specifically inhibits the action of aldosterone, and (f) vasodilators which affect the vascular smooth muscle of the arteriole. It has become apparent that most antihypertensive drugs given by mouth can be prescribed once or twice daily, maximizing convenience for the patient and assisting in achieving optimal compliance.

Antiadrenergic Drugs. An array of drugs with antiadrenergic properties extends from those whose action is confined within the central nervous system in modulating sympathetic tone to those whose primary action is at receptor sites in effector organs. Table 3 displays the major antiadrenergic drugs, their principal site of action, dose range, and more common adverse reactions. Only those drugs that can be given by mouth are presented. Agents for parenteral use in emergency situations are dealt with elsewhere. Several comments should be made regarding specific agents. Propranolol is listed as a nonspecific beta receptor blocking drug. Its renin-lowering properties may well result from this action. A central action has been suggested for propranolol and may account in part for its ability to lower arterial pressure when given in very high doses even to low renin hypertensive patients. Other β blockers, alpha methyldopa, clonidine, and reserpine have documented renin-lowering properties. The evidence with regard to guanethidine is much less clear. In several studies, guanethidine administration and resultant reduction in arterial pressure was associated with an increase in plasma renin activity. Prazosin is listed as having alpha receptor blocking properties. However, its mechanism of action is more complex, involving direct vasodilation, perhaps in part mediated through alterations in metabolism of cyclic nucleotides. The alpha receptor blocking drugs phentolamine and phenoxybenzamine are ordinarily employed only for the management of pheochromocytoma. However, phenoxybenzamine has been combined with beta receptor blockers in the management of other hypertensive states and provides a rationale for the development of drugs such as labetalol, which combines properties of both alpha and beta receptor inhibition.

Diuretics. The principal diuretics employed in antihypertensive therapy are listed in Table 4. These are classified according to familiar pharmacologic criteria, and examples from each of the categories are given rather than an exhaustive list.

TABLE 3. Antiadrenergic Drugs

DRUG	SITE AND MECHANISM OF ACTION	DOSE RANGE	ADVERSE REACTIONS
Reserpine (Serpasil)	CNS and peripheral SNS Depletes catecholamines	0.1–0.5 mg./day	Depression, nasal congestions, gastric hyperacidity, lethargy, impotence
Alpha methyldopa (Aldomet)	CNS and peripheral SNS False transmitter Central agonist	250–2000 mg./day	Transient sedation, hepatitis, positive Coombs' test, impotence
Clonidine (Catapres)	CNS α agonist	0.1–1.2 mg./day	Sedation, dry mouth, constipation, rebound hypertension
Guanethidine (Ismelin)	Peripheral SNS, depletes norepinephrine	10–200 mg./day	Orthostatic hypotension, retrograde ejaculation, diarrhea. Action blocked by tricyclic antidepressives
Receptor Blockers			
Phenoxybenzamine (Dibenzyline)	Peripheral α blocker	10–100 mg./day	Tachycardia, orthostatic hypotension, retrograde ejaculation
Phentolamine (Regitine)	Peripheral α blocker	100–300 mg./day	Diarrhea, tachycardia, orthostatic hypotension
Propranolol (Inderal)	Peripheral nonspecific β blocker	20–640 mg./day	Congestive heart failure, bradycardia, heart block. Contraindicated in obstructive pulmonary disease, diabetes requiring insulin
Metoprolol (Lopressor)	Selective (β_1) β blocker	100–450 mg./day	Congestive heart failure, heart block
Prazosin (Minipress)	Peripheral α blocker ?other antiadrenergic action	3–15 mg./day	First dose orthostatic hypotension, fatigue

SNS: Sympathetic nervous system
CNS: Central nervous system

TABLE 4. **Diuretic Agents**

THIAZIDE AND THIAZIDELIKE DIURETICS	DOSE RANGE
Hydrochlorothiazide (HydroDIURIL, Esidrix, Oretic)	25–150 mg./day
Chlorthalidone (Hygroton)	50 mg. three times weekly to 100 mg./day
LOOP DIURETICS	
Furosemide (Lasix)	20–400 mg./day
Ethacrynic Acid (Edecrin)	25–200 mg./day
POTASSIUM SPARING DIURETICS	
Spironolactone (Aldactone)	25–400 mg./day
Triamterene (Dyrenium)	100–200 mg./day

When given alone, antihypertensive effects may be observed with rather small doses of diuretic agents. This is especially true for the longer acting thiazidelike drugs such as chlorthalidone. In compliant patients these diuretics often cause hypokalemia. Potassium supplementation with liquid potassium chloride preparations or microcrystals in wax (Slow K) may or may not restore serum potassium levels to normal. The use of potassium-sparing diuretic agents such as spironolactone or triamterene may be effective therapy when given alone or as adjunctive measures when combined with the thiazide-type diuretics. Potassium supplementation should not be given with a potassium-sparing diuretic, as significant and occasionally fatal hyperkalemia has been reported in such circumstances. When renal insufficiency is present, as reflected by serum creatinine concentrations of 2.0 mg. per dl. (100 ml.) or greater, more diuretic potency is required, and the agents of choice are the loop active drugs, furosemide, or ethacrynic acid.

Common adverse reactions to diuretics are well described and need little comment. Disturbances in serum potassium have already been discussed. Hyperuricemia, not an infrequent finding in untreated hypertensive patients, may also be caused by diuretic use and may cause typical attacks of gout. When hyperuricemia is excessive (serum uric acid > 12 mg. per dl.) or causes symptoms, therapy is to be warranted in the form of allopurinol (Zyloprim), 100 to 300 mg. per day, or probenecid (Benemid), 500 mg. three to four times daily. A uricosuric diuretic with antihypertensive properties (ticrynafen) is now in clinical trial and may prove to be valuable for management of such problems.

Chronic use of the thiazidelike diuretics has been reported to cause sustained elevations of serum lipids albeit to a small degree. Thiazide-induced glucose intolerance is a well described phenomenon but an uncommon event. Taken together, however, such adverse reactions may alter the patient's risk factor profile in a less than favorable direction. That is, reduction in blood pressure is offset by increased serum lipids and carbohydrate intolerance. Perhaps this risk trade-off explains the failure of diuretic based antihypertensive treatment schemes to reduce morbidity due to coronary heart disease.

Vasodilator Drugs.   Hydralazine remains the one approved drug for use by mouth whose mechanism of action is confined to arteriolar vasodilation. When given alone this drug causes an increase in heart rate, increased plasma renin activity, and a tendency for fluid retention. Consequently, the role of hydralazine has changed over the years so that it is most often combined with propranolol in order to control heart rate and renin secretion and a diuretic drug for maintenance of stable fluid balance in the management of severe hypertension. Hydralazine may be started at a dose of 10 mg. twice daily and progressively increased to 200 mg. twice daily. (This dose of hydralazine may be higher than that listed in the manufacturer's official directive.) The appearance of a lupuslike syndrome with positive antinuclear antibody (ANA) tests may occur in patients treated with high doses of hydralazine for prolonged periods of time. When symptoms are absent, but the ANA turns positive, the choice of whether or not to discontinue hydralazine should depend upon the effectiveness of the drug in the particular patient involved and the availability of alternative therapy. Prazosin (Minipress) has both vasodilator and alpha receptor blocking properties. In some patients it may function as a successful substitute for hydralazine. When given alone or in combination with a diuretic, prazosin may reduce arterial pressure effectively and without the usual tachycardia and increase in plasma renin activity that accompanies the use of a more pure vasodilator. This has given rise to the speculation that prazosin may have additional antiadrenergic activity.

Attention has been directed to first dose hypotension with prazosin. Orthostatic syncope occurring shortly after the first dose of this medication or upon an increase in dosage has been reported. It is suggested that when patients receive their first dose of prazosin or upon the first occasion of an increased dose, this be taken at bedtime. Thereafter, the medication is usually given three times daily. The initial dose is 1 mg. three times daily.

The much more potent pure vasodilator drug, Minoxidil, is available on an emergency use protocol by the Upjohn Company for the management of severe hypertension that is uncontrollable by conventional agents, Minoxidil is almost invariably given in combination with propranolol and a diuretic. Its use in controlling the most refractory hypertensive patients has been well documented and should be considered when high doses of hydralazine have failed. Adverse reactions to be anticipated are fluid retention usually managed by adjustment of diuretic dosage and hair growth which may occasionally approach disfiguring proportions. Nonetheless, Minoxidil can be considered a lifesaving drug for a selected group of hypertensive patients.

Emergency Treatment of Hypertension

Rapid and controlled reduction of systemic arterial pressure is warranted for several medical emergencies as indicated in Table 2. Parenteral medications are justified because of the speed of their action, but require a setting of an intensive care unit in which there is provision for minute to minute monitoring of vital signs and the rate of infusion. The patient with malignant hypertension that is otherwise uncomplicated can be managed by oral medications. The combination of propranolol and hydralazine is quite effective in such patients. Diuretics may be added if there is clear-cut evidence of fluid retention, i.e., weight gain and peripheral edema. Such is most often the case when there is a background of chronic renal disease. Often the patient with malignant hypertension presents with evidence of weight loss and is actually underhydrated. Diuretics are contraindicated in such circumstances and patients should be managed by antiadrenergic and vasodilator drugs. Such patients usually have elevated plasma renin activity levels and benefit from drugs that inhibit the action of the renin-angiotensin system.

Drugs that are ordinarily used in the management of hypertensive emergencies are listed in Table 5. A wide spectrum of actions is represented and allows for considerable choice in achieving the therapeutic goal. In pheochromocytoma, the monoamine oxidase inhibitor—tyramine syndrome, and clonidine withdrawal alpha adrenergically mediated vasoconstriction is the cause of hypertension. When parenteral therapy is required the agent of choice is phentolamine. When dissecting aneurysm is the problem, the blood pressure should be reduced without increasing left ventricular contractility. Antiadrenergic agents that inhibit catecholamine action upon the heart are preferable. Trimethaphan should be strongly considered and intravenous propranolol may be valuable.

TABLE 5. **Drugs for Hypertensive Emergencies**

	ROUTE OF ADMINISTRATION	DOSE RANGE	ADVERSE REACTIONS	COMMENT
Nitroprusside (Nipride)	I.V. infusion	0.5–8 μg./kg./min. titrate with BP Solution: 100 mg. nitroprusside in 1 L D5W	Methemoglobinemia, thiocyanate or cyanide toxicity, acidosis	Decomposition by light protection from toxicity by hydroxy cobalamin
Trimethaphan (Arfonad)	I.V. infusion	1–15 mg./min. (2 grams/L solution)	Obstipation, urinary retention	More effective in partial upright position
Diazoxide (Hyperstat)	I.V. bolus (rapid)	100–600 mg.	Hyperglycemia, tachycardia, Na and H_2O retention	Give rapidly, over 10–30 seconds
Phentolamine (Regitine)	I.V. bolus/infusion	1.0–5.0 mg. by bolus infusion, 0.1 mg. per minute or more.	Tachycardia	
Propranolol (Inderal)	I.V. infusion	1 mg. over 10–15 min. (give in small increments of 0.1 to 0.2 mg. to total of 1 mg.)	Congestive heart failure, bradyarrhythmias, bronchospasm	Can repeat slowly IV if first 1 mg. dose is well tolerated
Hydralazine (Apresoline)	I.M., I.V. bolus (slow)	5–50 mg.	Tachycardia, Na and H_2O retention	
Furosemide (Lasix)	I.V. bolus (slow)	40–120 mg.	Hearing loss, hypokalemia, hyponatremia, hyperreninemia, volume depletion	Higher doses may be needed in renal insufficiency
Ethacrynic acid (Edecrin)	I.V. bolus (slow)	25–200 mg.*	See Furosemide	See Furosemide
Alpha methyldopa (Aldomet)	I.V. bolus (slow)	250–1000 mg.	Somnolence, hepatitis, salt and water retention	Slow onset of action

*Dose may be higher than that listed in the manufacturer's official directive

When left ventricular decompensation is present, reduction of afterload through the use of vasodilators is warranted. If there is evidence that activation of the renin-angiotensin system is the cause, propranolol may be helpful, but should always be employed with caution in the presence of cardiac failure. Although this drug inhibits renin secretion, renin has a long half-life in the circulation. It thus may take hours for this effect to become apparent. Newer agents, still in developmental phases, such as saralasin or the converting enzyme inhibitors, may prove especially valuable in such circumstances because of their rapid action. In managing such patients one should consider whether the cause of left ventricular decompensation is increased afterload alone or whether intramyocardial disease such as acute infarction is not also playing a role and formulate the therapeutic approach accordingly.

Once the acute emergency situation has passed, most patients should be placed on medications that can be given by mouth. Reasons for continuing parenteral therapy are inability of the patient to take oral medications or the continued need for minute to minute control of blood pressure.

Toxemia of pregnancy represents a special circumstance in which the choice of medications should be undertaken with recognition that there are two patients involved, mother and fetus. The management of preeclampsia is controversial at the present time, with a trend towards avoiding the use of diuretic agents. In the eclamptic state, where there is an acute rise in arterial pressure, central nervous system (CNS) changes, and reduced urine output, magnesium sulfate is still employed and hydralazine may be useful. Prevention remains a better course now that it is possible to assess fetal age and maturation with precision, and patients should be delivered at the earliest possible date consistent with the well being of the neonate.

The clonidine withdrawal syndrome deserves some comment. Cessation of clonidine therapy is occasionally accompanied by a rapid increase in arterial pressure to dangerously high levels. Evidence suggests that this is due to activation of the sympathetic nervous system with alpha receptor mediated vasoconstriction. Restoration of clonidine treatment will reduce the arterial pressure. However, if the patient cannot take medication by mouth, intravenous phentolamine may be necessary. Although this syndrome is a rare event, it has given rise to concern about the use of clonidine in patients who may be unreliable in their use of medications.

Significant elevations of arterial pressure may accompany subarachnoid hemorrhage and are often part of the clinical picture of intracerebral hemorrhage. It is believed that cautious reduction of arterial pressure is warranted in such patients. However, the risk of hypotension should be carefully considered, so that maximum control of the therapeutic situation is mandatory. Rapid-acting parenteral agents such as nitroprusside or trimethaphan camsylate (Arfonad) may be employed, but infusion rate must be controlled on a minute to minute basis in relation to the monitoring of arterial pressure. Reduction of diastolic pressure to the 90 to 100 mm. Hg range is a reasonable therapeutic goal.

Summary

Management of the patient with arterial hypertension cannot be oversimplified because the setting in which hypertension occurs varies with each patient. Selection of the appropriate therapeutic strategy depends upon a diagnostic assessment that takes into account the overall risk factor profile, stage, i.e., cardiovascular, central nervous system, and renal function, etiologic and pathogenetic factors. Selection of initial and subsequent therapeutic modalities should take into account the diagnostic aspects as mentioned, the clinical pharmacology of drugs to be employed, and realistic goals for therapy. The array of drugs already available for emergency and chronic treatment of hypertension indicates that considerable individualization is possible in order to achieve the most favorable benefit to adverse reaction status for each patient under treatment.

ACUTE MYOCARDIAL INFARCTION

method of
THOMAS R. GRIGGS, M.D.
Chapel Hill, North Carolina

More than half the patients who die from myocardial infarction do so within the first 2 hours after the onset of symptoms. Almost all of these die because of sudden ventricular fibrillation. Prevention or reversal of the ventricular fibrillation is possible in a sizable group of patients if advanced life support is quickly available. Therefore, the practical goals in management of acute myocardial infarction must include patient education about the early symptoms of myocardial infarction, information to the public on the methods of summoning emergency medical care, and either quick transportation of advanced life support personnel and equipment to the patient or transportation of the patient to a life support facility. Subsequent care is aimed at making the patient comfortable, managing the complications, and reambulation, all with the precaution of careful monitoring.

Prehospital Treatment

When a patient has chest pain suggesting myocardial infarction or unstable angina pectoris, emergency medical care should be made available as quickly as possible. In communities where mobile advanced life support is provided, the responding professional or paraprofessional personnel should institute resuscitation if needed. Modern equipment allows initial assessment of electrocardiogram using paddles on the defibrillator as leads. If ventricular fibrillation is detected in an unresponsive, pulseless patient, defibrillation should be performed by certified technicians on standing orders and without direct consultation. Subsequent resuscitation is done as described elsewhere in this book. A physician or special nurse should be consulted via radio. If the patient is responsive or has been successfully resuscitated, the technicians should establish cardiac monitoring. An intravenous line should be established using an indwelling catheter. If the patient has no allergic history and is in normal sinus rhythm, lidocaine should be given as an intravenous bolus of 70 to 100 mg. If adequate control of flow rates can be maintained, a solution of lidocaine can be administered at 2 to 3 mg. per minute thereafter. In our experience, this control is difficult in an ambulance, so we prefer to repeat 25 mg. doses at 10 to 20 minute intervals. Intramuscular administration of lidocaine is effective, but the onset of the effect of the drug is delayed. If the patient is bradycardic, blood pressure and mental status should be monitored closely. Atropine should be administered only if the bradycardia is associated with hypotension, obvious heart failure, altered mental state, cold, clammy skin, or frequent premature ventricular contractions. The dose of atropine is 0.5 mg. intravenously. This can be repeated after 10 minutes if the response is inadequate. We do not routinely administer atropine to patients with bradycardia who are otherwise stable. Chest pain can be safely treated in the prehospital situation with morphine, 5 to 10 mg. intravenously or subcutaneously. Occasionally, patients will develop hypotension after administration of morphine. This hypotension is almost always the result of inadequate left ventricular filling pressures resulting from the effects of the morphine and can be reversed by raising the legs and administering fluid. Nitroglycerin is not routinely used in the prehospital management of acute myocardial infarction. One or two sublingual tablets may be of benefit, however, in the patient with hypertension or pulmonary edema complicating acute myocardial infarction. Like morphine, the nitroglycerin can lower blood pressure and cardiac output, at least partially by decreasing left ventricular filling pressures. Hypotension resulting from these effects of nitroglycerin should be treated by raising the legs and infusing fluid.

Hospital Management

The patient's initial evaluation and in-hospital disposition should move along rapidly. Long delay in an emergency room while numerous electrocardiograms and blood studies are obtained places the patient at high risk and should be avoided. Electrocardiographic monitoring is begun immediately, and a secure intravenous catheter is placed. During the initial evaluation process the patient should be attended by a trained person who has immediate access to advanced life support equipment and medications. The optimal method for handling the admission process for a patient with acute myocardial infarction is to have the mobile intensive care technicians transfer care of the patient directly to the coronary care unit physicians and nurses.

After admission to the coronary care unit the patient should undergo a complete history and physical examination. The aim of this assessment is manifold, but two major goals are obvious. First, an effort should be made to establish the exact cause of the chest pain. Causes of chest pain such as pulmonary embolus, dissecting aortic aneurysm, or pericarditis must be considered in every patient. Second, the assessment should provide information about the effects of the myocardial infarction on peripheral circulation and on the heart itself. To gather this information, the physician must note the quality of the breath sounds, the state of the peripheral circulation, and the presence of such cardiac abnormalities as gallop sounds, murmurs, pericardial friction rubs and abnormal precordial pulsations. As the care plan is designed, therefore, the physician is aware of the presence or absence of such complications as low output syndrome, congestive heart failure, pericarditis, or cardiac structural problems such as papillary muscle dysfunction. In fact, the subsequent care of the patient will depend upon the number and magnitude of these complications.

Management of the Uncomplicated Myocardial Infarction

Relief of Pain. Narcotic agents, especially morphine, are the preferable analgesic medications for treatment of the pain of myocardial infarction. As patients vary greatly in their response to analgesic administration, no single dosage schedule can be outlined. A good method for treating the pain is to administer an initial 5 to 10 mg. intravenously, then to titrate subsequent doses to the pain by administering 2 to 5 mg. at 10 to 20 minute intervals until the pain is controlled. Meperidine (Demerol) can be used similarly in initial doses of 75 mg. and subsequent doses of 10 to 25 mg. The patient must be constantly attended during this procedure. As noted, an occasional patient will become hypotensive after narcotic administration. This can usually be quickly reversed by raising the feet or administering fluid. Inadvertent depression of respiration and sensorium by administration of a narcotic analgesic should be avoided. This complication can be managed for a short time by stimulating the patient to talk. Definitive reversal of the effects of narcotic excess can be accomplished by giving 0.4 mg. naloxone intravenously.

Sedation. Sedation is used in myocardial infarction to allay anxiety and to help the patient rest. A minor tranquilizer such as diazepam (Valium) in doses of 2.5 to 5 mg. two or three times per day is sufficient for this purpose. Heavy sedation in patients with myocardial infarction has not been shown to be of benefit. Further, sedation in a patient who is accustomed to being in control of his or her environment is sometimes anxiety-producing. Therefore, sedation should be chosen for each patient on an individual basis.

Oxygen. Oxygen has traditionally been administered to patients with acute myocardial infarction, and recent evidence supports this practice. Routine administration should be by face mask or nasal cannula at a flow rate of 4 liters per minute. Patients with pulmonary disease or with complicated myocardial infarction of any sort should have frequent measurement of arterial blood gases, and oxygen administration should be regulated according to the results of those measurements.

Activity. Early ambulation is a relatively modern innovation in the care of patients with myocardial infarction and is credited with a decrease in the incidence of thromboembolic complications in these patients. Patients with uncomplicated myocardial infarction can sit in a chair on the day following the infarction. Progressive ambulation is started at about 5 days after the infarction. Patients with an uncomplicated course can be discharged to close home follow-up at 10 to 14 days. Patients with continuing chest pain, congestive heart failure, dysrhythmias, or other complications are ambulated and discharged on a slower, individualized schedule. Many hospitals now have a team of specially trained paraprofessional personnel, including physical therapists, nurses, social workers, dieticians, and occupational therapists, who provide education and direction to the patient during the hospital phase of his myocardial infarction care. This is done on the prescription of the patient's physician, but it allows for some standardization of the approach to the hospital management of myocardial infarction.

Bowel Movements. Since the bedside commode is less stressful for most patients to use than is the bedpan, we allow any stable patient to use the commode. Transfer of the patient from the bed to the commode is done by the nursing personnel, and the patient is constantly monitored. Stool softeners such as dioctyl sodium sulfosuccinate (Colace) or mild laxatives are ordered routinely during the patient's coronary care unit stay.

Diet. A light diet is usually given for the first few days after a myocardial infarction. Very cold and very hot food and drink are routinely excluded. Some patients require salt restriction. All coronary care unit diets should be low in saturated fat and cholesterol.

Anticoagulation. The use of anticoagulation in the secondary prevention or palliation of myocardial infarction remains controversial after many years of debate. Recent retrospective reviews have raised this issue again, and some reputable authorities feel strongly that all patients with myocardial infarction should be given anticoagulants. Additionally, there is general agreement based upon prospective, controlled studies that anticoagulation reduces the thromboembolic complications of myocardial infarction. These complications are primarily the result of deep venous and left ventricular mural thrombosis. Patients with congestive heart failure, shock, large myocardial infarctions or history of previous thromboembolic disease constitute a group at high risk of developing these complications after acute myocardial infarction, and should therefore be given anticoagulants. Heparin is given by constant intravenous infusion in doses sufficient to prolong the clotting time to 20 minutes or the activated partial thromboplastin time to 1.5 times control. This usually requires an infusion of 1000 units per hour. If a coumarin agent is started simultaneously, heparin can be stopped at the time of discharge from the coronary care unit. We give anticoagulants to high risk patients for extended periods. In the remainder, the anticoagulation is discontinued when the patient is ambulatory. Anticoagulation is withheld from any patient with active bleeding and from patients with pericardial friction rubs.

In recent years "low-dose" heparin has been shown to reduce the incidence of deep vein thrombosis in patients with myocardial infarction.

However, this approach has not been proved to reduce the embolic complications of the thrombosis. Similarly, no effect of "low dose" heparin on development or embolization of left ventricular mural thrombosis has been shown. "Low-dose" heparin therapy is, therefore, used only in patients with low risk of thromboembolism or in those in whom there is a relative contraindication to full dose anticoagulation.

Finally, a recent multicenter study has shown that sulfinpyrazone (Anturane), an agent that inhibits platelet function, reduces mortality among patients with recent myocardial infarction. In this study, the agent was started after the acute phase of the myocardial infarction. There are no data to indicate that the use of antiplatelet agents is of benefit in the acute management of myocardial infarction.

Management of Complications

Continuing Pain. In most cases the pain of myocardial infarction will subside within 24 hours. In those situations in which pain continues, the cause of the pain may be continuing myocardial ischemia or extension of infarction, pericarditis, or noncardiac. If the pain is thought to be from myocardial ischemia and is not easily controlled with nitroglycerin, we consider the addition of propranolol, starting at 20 mg. four times per day. This medication can be added only if the patient is felt to have little or no left ventricular dysfunction. The accurate assessment of ventricular function in this situation may occasionally require insertion of a Swan-Ganz catheter and measurement of left ventricular filling pressures and cardiac output.

Hypertension. Hypertension in the acute phase of myocardial infarction is usually the result of sympathetic nervous system activity. Usually, the hypertension will subside within a few hours with no specific treatment. If it does not, furosemide (Lasix) can be administered in a moderate dose intravenously. If this is not effective, a nitroprusside (Nipride) infusion should be started. The nitroprusside is prepared as a solution in dextrose 5 per cent in water. Since the solution decomposes in light, the bag or bottle should be protected with an opaque wrapper. Additionally, the solution is unstable and must be used within 4 to 6 hours of preparation. The solution is prepared by adding one vial (50 mg.) to 250 or 500 ml. of D_5W. With either concentration of drug, the blood pressure can be altered with very small changes in infusion rate. This creates a significant hazard which dictates the absolute necessity to monitor the blood pressure constantly during the use of this medication. While the average dose is 200 to 400 micrograms per minute, the range is broad. For practical purposes, the dose should be carefully titrated to the desired blood pressure. The only safe method for accomplishing this degree of control, especially for the nurse or physician who is not experienced with the use of nitroprusside, is with constant blood pressure monitoring through an indwelling catheter. The nitroprusside can usually be withdrawn over a few days while oral antihypertensive agents are being added.

Dysrhythmias. Dysrhythmia of some sort complicates almost every myocardial infarction. Additionally, the myocardial infarction or its sequelae can create virtually any dysrhythmia. Consequently, the care of the patient with myocardial infarction can be effectively accomplished only with the aid of constant electrocardiographic monitoring, especially during the early phases, and with special attention to the need for early diagnosis and management of dysrhythmia.

SINUS TACHYCARDIA. Sinus tachycardia occurs in about one third of patients with myocardial infarction, probably in response to catecholamine release or heart failure. A few patients have persistent sinus tachycardia. In these it is important to identify the cause of the tachycardia if possible. Common causes such as anemia, fever, thyrotoxicosis, or medication effect should be ruled out. An attempt should also be made to determine if there is some degree of heart failure or relative hypovolemia. Some patients may require pulmonary artery catheterization so that this assessment can be made. In the few patients who have none of these treatable causes for the tachycardia and who have sustained heart rates of 120 or greater, propranolol should be administered orally starting with doses of 10 mg. four times per day.

SINUS BRADYCARDIA. Sinus bradycardia is seen in about 40 per cent of patients with acute myocardial infarction. This rhythm is more common in patients with inferior myocardial infarction than in those with anterior infarctions. In most cases the bradycardia is uncomplicated and short-lived. Only those patients with sinus bradycardia associated with hypotension, heart failure, or ventricular ectopy should be treated. The management of these patients should begin with atropine, 0.5 mg. intravenously followed by a second dose in 10 minutes if the patient fails to respond. Only rarely will ventricular pacing be required to improve a low output state associated with sinus bradycardia.

Ventricular Dysrhythmias. PROPHYLAXIS. Approximately 10 per cent of patients with myocardial infarction will sustain ventricular fibrillation during the first 24 hours of their hospitalization. Many of the cases of sudden ventricular fibrillation occur without warning in spite of the fact that the patients are constantly monitored. The incidence of sudden ventricular fibrillation can be significantly reduced if the patient is treated prophylactically with lidocaine. The effective dose of lidocaine is an initial intravenous injection of about 1 mg. per kg. followed by an infusion of 3 mg. per minute. The infusion rate should be halved in patients with low cardiac output or liver disease. Infusions at these rates can result in side effects in a substantial proportion of patients. Maximum therapeutic benefit with fewer side effects can be achieved if the dose of lidocaine is adjusted to maintain plasma levels between 2 and 5 micrograms per ml.

VENTRICULAR ECTOPY. Ventricular premature beats are a common accompaniment of acute myocardial infarction. The beats are usually caused by reentry of an electrical impulse that is slowed during conduction through ischemic or infarcted myocardium. It must be remembered, however, that patients with myocardial infarction may well have ventricular ectopy for a number of reasons, and that treatable causes such as digitalis excess, hypoxia, or electrolyte imbalance must be sought in every patient. The ectopy is dangerous because premature depolarization of the ventricle during the vulnerable period of the conduction cycle can result in ventricular tachycardia or fibrillation. Therefore, suppression of the ectopy is indicated if the extra beats are as frequent as 5 per minute or if they are multifocal or occur in pairs or triplets. In many cases the use of prophylactic lidocaine will reduce the number of premature contractions to a satisfactory level. However, in those patients with overt ectopy that fails to respond to lidocaine infusion, procainamide can be used. A loading dose is administered by injecting 100 mg. intravenously at 5 minute intervals until the ectopy subsides or a total dose of 1 gram has been achieved. A constant infusion is then begun at a rate of 20 to 50 micrograms per kg. per minute. Alternatively, the loading and maintenance doses can be given orally. The maintenance dose is usually 250 to 500 mg. every 4 hours. Doses should be reduced in the presence of liver or renal dysfunction. Maintenance doses should be adjusted to maintain the plasma level between 4 and 8 micrograms per ml.

Other medications used in the treatment of ventricular ectopy or recurrent ventricular tachycardia in acute myocardial infarction include propranolol, quinidine, and phenytoin. Propranolol may be especially useful in the patient with ongoing myocardial ischemia. It is used in oral doses starting at 20 mg. every 6 hours. In some circumstances much more is required. Propranolol is contraindicated in the face of congestive heart failure and severe bronchospasm. In an emergency, intraveous propranolol can be administered in doses much smaller than oral doses.

A common method is to administer 1 mg. of propranolol every 5 to 10 minutes until the dysrhythmia is controlled or until a total of 5 mg. has been administered. Quinidine is given in a dose of 10 mg. per kg. initially, followed by a maintenance dose of 200 to 300 mg. every 4 to 6 hours. The dose should then be adjusted to sustain a blood plasma level of 2.5 to 5 micrograms per ml. Quinidine has been associated with a number of dangerous side effects including sudden death. This fact plus the inability to use it parenterally reduce its usefulness in patients with acute myocardial infarction. Phenytoin (Dilantin) is used in doses similar to those described for procainamide. Phenytoin seems to be especially useful in the suppression of ventricular ectopy associated with digitalis intoxication. (This use of phenytoin is not listed in the manufacturer's official directive.)

Ventricular ectopy that continues in spite of maximal drug therapy with a variety of agents is one of the most trying challenges that faces the physician caring for patients with heart disease. These situations require careful clinical judgment and a constant awareness that the potential risks of each of these agents will at some point outweigh the benefits of the agent.

VENTRICULAR TACHYCARDIA AND FIBRILLATION. The reason for treating ventricular ectopy, again, is to prevent ventricular tachycardia and fibrillation. When this effort is not successful, quick, decisive action is required for the patient to be saved. In the case of ventricular fibrillation, immediate defibrillation is needed. If this cannot be achieved immediately, artificial ventilation and closed chest cardiac massage must be performed. It is of key importance that the patient be defibrillated as quickly as possible, since chances of recovery decrease dramatically as the delay before defibrillation lengthens. If initial efforts at resuscitation fail, airway management and drug administration should progress as described in another section of this volume.

Ventricular tachycardia is a serious, life-threatening dysrhythmia that usually is accompanied within minutes by hypotension and ventricular fibrillation. A few patients might appear relatively stable over a prolonged period of time, however. The patient who is hypotensive from ventricular tachycardia should be treated with DC cardioversion. In a few patients conversion can be accomplished with a gentle thump to the chest with the side of the fist. It is reasonable for trained personnel to attempt "thumpversion," but this technique, if improperly employed, can cause flail chest and other dangerous trauma. Certainly, DC cardioversion should not be delayed while repeated attempts to convert the patient with a thump are employed. Patients with ventricular tachycardia who are reasonably stable can be treated with a 50 or 100 mg. bolus of lidocaine. Of course, consideration must always be given to the possibility that such patients have a supraventricular tachycardia mimicking ventricular tachycardia because of aberrant conduction. It is sometimes appropriate to attempt to make this distinction by inserting a transvenous pacing wire and recording intra-atrial and intraventricular electrocardiograms. The wire can also be used then to overdrive suppress either atrial or ventricular tachycardia and thereby to convert the patient to normal sinus rhythm. Finally, some patients with recurrent ventricular tachycardia unresponsive to aggressive medical therapy can be controlled with constant pacing at a rate of 90 beats per minute or faster.

Conduction Blocks. Injury to the conduction system of the heart with myocardial infarction occurs in two basic situations. First, inferior myocardial infarction can be complicated by ischemia or injury to the atrioventricular node. Second, with extensive anterior infarction, the ventricular conduction tissue can be injured or infarcted. When the atrioventricular node is involved in inferior infarction, Mobitz type I (Wenckebach) second degree heart block or complete heart block can result. This type of block is usually temporary. Further, because of the proximal location of this block in the conduction system, the escape heart rate is usually adequate, and severe hemodynamic distress does not occur. Therefore, the patient with inferior infarction and associated heart block requires no specific therapy as long as he is stable and has an adequate heart rate. Indications for pacing in the patient with inferior infarction are: (1) a heart rate of less than 40 beats per minute, (2) hypotension, loss of consciousness or congestive heart failure, (3) bradycardia associated with ventricular ectopy, and (4) evidence of atrioventricular node dysfunction in the presence of bundle branch block.

In the patient with anterior infarction, the existence of conduction system damage implies extensive infarction and is frequently associated with heart failure or low output syndrome. In these patients heart block can occur suddenly without warning and escape heart rates may be inadequate to sustain life. Therefore, the physician must be alert to the development of any conduction disturbance in the patient with anterior infarction. Evidence of conduction system disease includes bundle branch block, left anterior or posterior fascicular block, which are manifest respectively as extreme left or right axis deviation, or combinations of right bundle branch and left fascicular blocks. A pacemaker should be placed prophylactically in patients with anterior infarction who develop second degree heart block, complete heart block, right bundle branch block, new left

bundle branch block, right bundle branch block with right or left axis deviation, or alternating bundle branch block.

The use of temporary pacing in patients with myocardial infarction requires experience and skill and is not without risks. Prolonged use of medications, such as atropine or isoproterenol, however, is an inadequate substitute for pacing and should be done only as emergency life support for patients who are being transported to a facility where pacing can be performed.

Atrial Dysrhythmias. Atrial fibrillation and atrial flutter are commonly seen among patients with acute myocardial infarction. These dysrhythmias may be caused by pericarditis, left ventricular dysfunction with atrial hypertension, or atrial infarction. If the ventricular rate in response to the atrial tachycardia is rapid, the patient's myocardial ischemia may be increased or congestive heart failure may develop. Management, therefore, is aimed at slowing the ventricular rate. If the patient with atrial fibrillation is stable, slowing can be accomplished by administration of digitalis. If the patient has had no digitalis within the recent past, he or she should receive 0.75 mg. of digoxin intravenously followed by 0.25 or 0.125 mg. every 2 to 3 hours until the average ventricular rate is less than 100 beats per minute. If the patient is having continuing chest pain or is in congestive heart failure, DC cardioversion should be undertaken, starting with 100 joules of delivered energy. Anesthesia can be provided in this situation with 10 mg. of diazepam administered intravenously. Control of the ventricular rate in the patient with atrial flutter is less predictable than in the patient with atrial fibrillation. Although digitalis or quinidine therapy can be attempted, the physician should monitor the patient's condition carefully and provide DC cardioversion if there is a question about the patient's stability. In some circumstances, atrial flutter will convert if the atrium is paced to a rapid rate.

Power Failure. Some degree of ventricular dysfunction occurs with every myocardial infarction. This becomes clinically apparent in about half the patients admitted to a coronary care unit. The clinical presentation of the ventricular dysfunction can range from mild pulmonary congestion to shock, depending upon the degree of damage to the ventricular myocardium and hemodynamic factors such as volume status, activity of the autonomic nervous system, and medications. Proper assessment of the myocardial function and hemodynamic parameters is important if optimal management of the power failure syndrome is achieved. In most cases this can be achieved by routine physical examination and x-ray techniques. In some circumstances, however, these techniques may be too inaccurate to be reliable and special measures using Swan-Ganz pulmonary artery catheters and intra-arterial catheters may be needed. In all cases assessment should provide an estimate or measurement of the major determinants of cardiac output. These include preload, afterload, contractility, and heart rate. Preload is, for practical purposes, the left ventricular diastolic pressure. According to the Starling law of the heart, increasing this pressure, up to a point, will increase the force of ventricular emptying. Very high filling pressures, on the other hand, cause pulmonary edema. Afterload refers to the impedance to ventricular emptying. Afterload is best stated as systemic vascular resistance. In man, systemic vascular resistance is equal to the difference between mean aortic and right atrial pressures times a constant factor of 80 divided by the cardiac output in liters per minute. The normal values for systemic vascular resistance are 800 to 1200 dynes-seconds-centimeters -5. The state of contractility of the myocardium is the ability of the ventricle to contract. In myocardial infarction, the contractility is decreased because of loss of contracting units of muscle. Agents such as digitalis and dopamine increase contractility to varying degrees, but always with an increase in oxygen consumption by the myocardium.

The most common manifestation of power failure in the patient with myocardial infarction is pulmonary congestion or edema reflecting a high preload state. In this situation the patient will usually have moist pulmonary rales, gallop heart sounds, and x-ray evidence of pulmonary congestion. Because the ventricular damage is predominantly left ventricular, it is very common for the patient in pulmonary edema to have no cervical venous distension and normal central venous pressure measurements. The therapy for such a patient is aimed primarily at reduction of the pulmonary congestion. This can usually be accomplished with the intravenous use of a potent diuretic such as furosemide. A dose of 20 to 80 mg. is usually sufficient. In this situation furosemide provides some immediate venodilatation as well as the later diuretic effect. It should be remembered that patients with myocardial infarction require a higher preload than do patients with normal hearts. Therefore, diuretic therapy for heart failure may cause hypotension. This problem should respond to leg raising or fluid infusion.

The use of digitalis to increase the state of contractility in patients with pulmonary congestion is controversial. Most authorities feel that the benefit is minimal in patients with no cardiomegaly and that the augmentation in myocardial oxygen consumption that occurs with use of digitalis does not justify the potential benefit of the medicine. We usually withhold the use of digitalis until 48 hours after the acute event. Patients with ongoing evidence of pulmonary congestion are digitalized carefully at that time.

Some centers have reported good results with use of vasodilators for afterload reduction in treatment of patients with congestive heart failure after myocardial infarction. Except for the use of nitroglycerin in some patients with acute severe pulmonary edema, this method of therapy should be undertaken only in those patients who can be monitored closely via pulmonary and systemic arterial catheters.

Most patients with heart failure complicating acute myocardial infarction will improve with bed rest and moderate doses of an intravenous diuretic, as described above. A few, however, will continue to show signs of increasing pulmonary congestion. Other patients will present with or develop signs of low output syndrome with hypotension, cool, clammy skin, altered mental status, and oliguria. We advocate the use of invasive monitoring in these situations. The added assessment capability that these devices offer frequently affects the forms and magnitude of therapy in these very ill patients; and we feel that outcome is improved. For instance, patients with low output syndrome may have pulmonary rales because of chronic lung disease rather than pulmonary congestion. Accurate determination of this fact would cause the physician to use volume infusion in a situation in which he would use diuretics if he had only the diagnostic information from his physical examination. Many other examples are possible.

Whether or not invasive monitoring is available, the management of the patient with power failure syndrome should be aimed at providing optimal ventricular preload, afterload, contractility, and contraction rate. As noted, if pulmonary congestion is present, this should be treated with diuretics. However, if congestion is not obvious, the adequacy of the preload should be tested with leg raising and an infusion of dextran 70 in 50 ml. boluses until a total of 500 ml. has been infused or the patient is improved. If the pulmonary artery diastolic or wedge pressure is known, volume should be infused to raise the filling pressure to 18 to 20 mm. Hg. If the patient with low output state fails to respond to volume infusions, an inotropic agent should be added. The first choice agent for this purpose is dopamine. It should be administered at 2 to 10 micrograms per kg. per minute with the dose titrated to bring the mean blood pressure to 70 mm. Hg or the systolic blood pressure to 90 mm. Hg. If higher doses are needed for this result, the prognosis is poor. If proper monitoring is available, the physician may wish to reduce the amount of dopamine needed by carefully lowering the afterload with an agent such as nitroprusside. Care should be taken to maintain systemic pressures above a mean of 70 mm. Hg. The goal of this therapy is to lower systemic vascular resistance to normal levels and thereby to allow the cardiac output to improve. If this is successful, the blood pressure may fall very little. Most patients can be withdrawn from inotropic or vasodilator therapy after 5 to 7 days.

Patients who do not respond to pharmacologic adjustment of preload, afterload or ventricular contractility have a very poor prognosis. In some centers where sophisticated diagnostic and surgical capabilities are available, a few of these patients may be saved by use of the intra-aortic balloon counterpulsation device.

Miscellaneous Complications. MECHANICAL PROBLEMS. A small number of patients with acute myocardial infarction will develop severe mitral regurgitation because of papillary muscle dysfunction or rupture. Others will develop ventricular septal defect. The prognosis for these patients is obviously quite poor, but some can be dramatically improved if surgical replacement of the mitral valve or correction of the ventricular septal defect can be undertaken. Mortality in this group is improved if the surgery can be delayed for several weeks or months after the acute infarction.

PERICARDITIS. A pericardial friction rub will be heard in most patients with myocardial infarction if a diligent effort is made to listen frequently. Usually this rub is fleeting and associated with no complications. A few patients, however, will develop chest pain with the rub and fewer still will have a pericardial effusion. Some of these patients will also have fever. Treatment of the pain and effusion is usually done with aspirin, 600 mg. every 4 hours. Some physicians prefer to use indomethacin, 25 mg. three times per day. (This use of indomethacin is not listed in the manufacturer's official directive.) As noted above, anticoagulants should be discontinued in the face of symptomatic pericarditis.

CARE AND REHABILITATION AFTER MYOCARDIAL INFARCTION

method of
ROSEMARIE SALERNI, M.D.
Pittsburgh, Pennsylvania

The goals of any program for the care and rehabilitation of patients after an acute myocardial infarction are to (1) return the patient to as close to normal activity as possible, (2) minimize the chance of recurrence, and (3) educate both the patient and his family. These three goals are interrelated and must be individualized for each patient.

Physical Activity

In recent years, the trend in the management of the myocardial infarction patient has been toward early mobilization and return to greater degrees of physical activity than had been previously thought possible. Studies of early mobilization and discharge have shown no deleterious effects when patients are carefully selected, and such programs generally result in a greater percentage of patients returning to work and, for many, an earlier return. In addition, this approach will minimize the adverse effects of prolonged bed rest. The progressive increase in physical activity can be considered in four stages:

   I.   Acute—Coronary Care Unit
  II.   Intermediate—in hospital
 III.   Convalescence—at home
 IV.   Long-term rehabilitation

The rate at which patients can progress through these stages and the degree of physical activity attainable vary from patient to patient. Throughout the program, the patient's response to activity must be evaluated and adjustments made as necessary.

Stage I begins in the Coronary Care Unit after the patient has been stabilized, generally in 24 to 48 hours. He should be free of chest pain, uncontrolled congestive heart failure, shock, and uncontrolled arrhythmias. The low level of physical activity necessary for self-care (feeding, shaving, personal hygiene) can be performed by most patients without difficulty. The use of a bedside commode is actually less stressful and requires less energy expenditure than the use of a bed pan. Passive and active motion of the extremities can maintain muscle tone and decrease venous stasis. Activity progresses to sitting on the side of the bed, and then in a chair 2 to 3 times per day, for 15 to 30 minutes by the end of the stay in the Coronary Care Unit. For most patients, this is 4 to 6 days. The rate at which a patient progresses through this stage is guided by his response to effort. Adverse responses, which indicate the need to decrease the activity level, include: (1) recurrence of chest pain, (2) development of dyspnea or undue fatigue, (3) development of arrhythmias, (4) an increase in heart rate above 120 per minute, and (5) a decrease in systolic blood pressure of more than 20 mm. Hg.

Psychologic support during this phase of illness is extremely important. The apprehension and fear associated with an acute myocardial infarction can be increased by the "intensive care unit" setting, with significant restriction of physical activity, and isolation. Disorientation and actual psychiatric disorders that may occur in this setting can be minimized by maintaining contact with the outside world. A sympathetic nursing staff, as well as a window and radio in the room, provide outside contact. An explanation of the function of the Coronary Care Unit and its equipment, with an outline of expectations for at least the immediate hospital course, should be given early. Reassurance by the physician that the physical restrictions are temporary, coupled with the physical evidence of gradually increasing activity without untoward effects, can provide psychologic support for the patient, and diminish depression.

During Stage II, the remainder of the hospitalization, physical activity is further increased so that at the end of 2 to 3 weeks, the patient is ambulatory and able to perform those activities necessary for complete self-care at home. Increased physical activity begins with sitting in a chair for increasing periods of time. Bathroom privileges may be given with assistance at first, then alone as walking is increased. Supervised walking is instituted first 1 to 2 times per day in the room, then in the hospital halls, so that most patients are up as desired by the end of the second week, when they may be ready for discharge. Activity may include climbing down and up a stair toward the end of this period. Ideally, this increased ambulation is conducted while the patient is monitored by telemetry, at least during the initial increase in physical activity. As in Stage I, any abnormal response to activity indicates a need to reduce the activity level and to proceed more slowly. Absence of any adverse effect allows the patient to increase his activity daily.

As the heart rate response is related to the work load imposed, it is used as a means of defining the degree of physical exertion allowed. The patient should be instructed how to count his heart rate during activity. The reasons for this should be fully explained, without causing undue concern or preoccupation with the heart rate. The patient should be discharged with specific instructions as to the activities allowed at home, with a scheduled reevaluation appointment and tentative schedule for return to work.

During Stage III, the period of convalescence at home, the goal is for the patient progressively to increase his level of physical activity to the point at which he can return to work 6 to 12 weeks after the infarction. For most people, this is an energy expenditure of 4 to 6 METS, equivalent to walking 3 to 4 miles per hour. Those patients whose employment requires greater energy output

should have their functional capacity determined by graded exercise testing before their return to work. A gradual return to full employment, coupled with a physical conditioning program, may be required.

Physical activity at home can include most usual household tasks that do not require heavy lifting or extensive use of the arms. Isometric activities have a higher level of myocardial energy expenditure for the amount of work performed and should be avoided. Arm work also requires a higher energy expenditure. Specific increases in physical activity should be avoided immediately after meals. Walking is the usual physical activity prescribed. A gradual increase in distance and speed should be prescribed so that the patient can comfortably walk 1 to 2 miles per day by the end of 6 weeks. This may be divided into 2 or 3 sessions. The development of dyspnea, fatigue, or chest pain, as in the previous stages, indicates the need to decrease the activity level.

The aim of Stage IV is to further improve the cardiovascular functional status by physical conditioning. A program can be started 8 to 12 weeks postinfarction after graded exercise testing to determine the functional capacity. As in the previous stages, heart rate is used to prescribe activity. The maximum attainable heart rate, which may be the age-predicted maximum or the rate at which symptoms or electrocardiographic abnormalities occur, is first determined. A training effect requires regular exercise at 60 to 80 per cent of the exercise capacity, which is equivalent to 70 to 85 per cent of the maximum attainable heart rate. Exercise sessions 3 to 5 times per week for a minimum of 20 to 30 minutes, with warm-up and cool-down periods at lower activity levels are sufficient to produce a training effect. If available, a supervised program is preferable, at least at the onset of the training program. Reevaluation by repeat exercise testing should be performed at about 6 weeks into the program. The activity level can be maintained or readjusted at that time.

Education

Education of the patient and family takes place throughout the period of rehabilitation and begins during his stay in the Coronary Care Unit. An explanation of the reasons for a coronary care unit, the disease process, and what to expect in the future, are appropriate early in the course of the hospitalization. Immediate plans for increasing physical activity with the necessity of patient cooperation, especially in reporting any difficulty such as fatigue, dyspnea, recurrent pain, or dizziness, should be discussed. The emphasis should be on the temporary nature of the restrictions imposed and that the goal is to return the patient to his previous level of activity and employment. This should be made clear to the family as well, as they may tend to be overprotective of the patient, especially after he returns home.

Although many patients can return to their previous employment, some, because of the severity of the infarction and degree of functional impairment, are unable to do so. Others may require longer than the usual 6 to 12 week convalescent course to be able to engage in the required amount of physical exertion for their jobs. Job counseling and retraining may be required for such patients.

A major part of the rehabilitation program should concern identification of and education about risk factors and their modification. These include weight and lipid control, generally by diet; control of hypertension; control of any other associated disease; and cessation of smoking. Modification of the diet to control weight or cholesterol and triglycerides should include the family, not just the patient, since any dietary modification may be more easily adhered to if all family members are involved.

The patient should be aware of any medications he is taking by name, and the reason they have been prescribed, as well as the more common potential side effects.

Special Considerations

As noted, patients whose previous employment requires high level energy expenditure may not be able to return to this type of employment. Retraining may be necessary. Some may be considered for coronary angiography, as knowledge of the anatomy, i.e., whether single vessel disease is present or not, can be considered in the decision about employment. The use of beta blocking drugs in asymptomatic patients as a preventive measure has not been firmly established. The same may be said of anticoagulants and drugs that interfere with platelet function.

Those patients who have recurrent angina after infarction, those with persistent arrhythmias, and those with uncontrolled congestive heart failure may be considered for cardiac catheterization and possible surgical intervention.

Arrhythmias during the early stages of a myocardial infarction and their therapy are well known. More recent investigation suggests that the occurrence of late arrhythmias may define a subset of patients who are at risk for sudden death in the subsequent year. Holter monitoring to identify these patients before hospital discharge and therapy with antiarrhythmic agents has been suggested.

PERICARDITIS

method of
DEEB N. SALEM, M.D.
Boston, Massachusetts

The management of a patient with pericarditis may be divided into the treatment of (1) the underlying cause, (2) pericardial pain, (3) pericardial effusion, (4) constrictive pericarditis, and (5) arrhythmias.

Underlying Cause

The percentage of occurrence of any underlying cause of pericarditis varies greatly with the make-up of the patient population being cared for. It should be noted that almost every disease process may, at some time, involve the pericardium.

Acute idiopathic pericarditis is probably the most common presentation of clinically recognized pericardial disease. In this condition (as in viral, postmyocardial infarction, and postpericardiotomy pericarditis), the therapy is nonspecific; see below.

Uremic pericarditis can often be avoided by the use of periodic hemodialysis or peritoneal dialysis in a patient with severe renal failure. Furthermore, the development of pericarditis in a patient with uremia is treated by the initiation of an adequate dialysis program. There are some patients with uremic pericarditis who may continue to be symptomatic after dialysis and thus may require the measures described below.

Purulent (pyogenic) pericarditis is most frequently due to staphylococcal or gram-negative aerobic bacilli. Treatment consists of (1) surgical drainage and (2) systemic antibiotics. Cultures should be obtained from sputum, pleural fluid, blood, and pericardial fluid. A Gram stain of aspirated effusion may help in choosing antimicrobial therapy while culture results are pending. Treatment with methicillin, 12 grams per day intravenously, and gentamicin, 4 to 6 mg. per kg. in divided doses, may be given until culture and sensitivities are available. (This dose of gentamicin may be higher than that listed in the manufacturer's official directive.) Antibiotic dosages are in the "high range" because of the life-threatening nature of the disease.

Tuberculous pericarditis requires (1) prolonged treatment with antituberculous chemotherapy and (2) measures such as pericardiectomy and pericardial aspiration when hemodynamic compromise is present. Pending sensitivity testing, treatment should be initiated with isoniazid, 5 to 8 mg. per kg. per day (pyridoxine should be given concomitantly to help avoid neurotoxicity), ethambutol, 15 mg. per kg. per day, and streptomycin, 1 gram intramuscularly per day. The streptomycin dosage is decreased (or discontinued) after the acute stage, which often lasts two to three months. Although not universally accepted, many feel that corticosteroids (i.e., prednisone, 80 mg. daily in divided doses) are of some benefit to the patient with effusive tuberculous pericarditis. Surgery may be performed in the presence of active disease and is indicated when severe constriction is present. The role of surgery for tuberculous effusion is still not clear.

Neoplastic pericarditis is managed by appropriate therapy for the underlying malignancy. Pericardiocentesis, radiotherapy, pericardial surgery, and intrapericardial drug therapy (e.g., nitrogen mustard or thiotepa) all have a role in managing these patients.

Traumatic pericarditis, which may be due to blunt as well as penetrating trauma, is managed by close observation for bleeding or tamponade. It should be remembered that closed cardiac massage and electrical cardioversion are potential causes of "traumatic" pericarditis.

Pericardial Pain

Pericardial pain may be very mild and require little or no treatment, or it may be severe enough to require the use of morphine or meperidine. The analgesic and anti-inflammatory properties of aspirin (600 mg. every 4 to 6 hours) and indomethacin (25 to 50 mg. every 6 hours) (this use of indomethacin is not listed in the manufacturer's official directive) have made these agents very helpful in treating pericardial pain. It should be noted that, because of its effect on platelet function, aspirin may be contraindicated in forms of pericarditis where there may be a risk of intrapericardial hemorrhage (e.g., postmyocardial infarction, post-trauma, and postpericardiotomy syndromes). Corticosteroids (e.g., prednisone, 60 to 80 mg. per day) may often have a dramatic effect on the resolution of pericardial pain and effusion. It has recently been shown that steroids will cause a more rapid decrease in antiheart antibodies than salicylates. Rarely, pericardial surgery may be required to alleviate severe pain when all other measures fail.

Pericardial Effusion

The adverse hemodynamic effects of pericardial effusion are related to (1) the rate of fluid accumulation, (2) the compliance (distensibility) characteristics of the pericardium or underlying myocardium or both, and (3) the intravascular fluid volume. Large amounts of pericardial effusion that develop over a long period of time may be totally asymptomatic (e.g., in myxedema), while much smaller amounts of fluid accumulating rapidly can cause cardiovascular collapse and death (e.g., acute intrapericardial hemorrhage).

Clinical evidence of cardiac tamponade or pericardial infection should be present to justify pericardial aspiration as a form of *therapy*. Pericardiocentesis may also be performed for *diagnostic* purposes and, occasionally, for the instillation of antitumor therapy. In an emergency, pericardiocentesis may have to be performed under suboptimal conditions as a lifesaving maneuver, but most often there is time to transfer the patient to areas equipped with the proper monitoring and resuscitation equipment (e.g., cardiac catheterization laboratory or intensive care unit).

Prior to the procedure, the patient may be premedicated with intramuscular diazepam; atropine, 0.6 to 1.0 mg. subcutaneously or intravenously, may be employed to prevent or treat vagal reactions. Utilizing standard aseptic technique, the site of aspiration is cleansed, draped, and infiltrated with subcutaneous lidocaine. Although a variety of sites have been used for pericardiocentesis, the angle between the xiphoid process and left costal cartilage seems to be preferred by many cardiologists and surgeons. The patient is positioned in a head-up posture (45 to 60 degrees) and an 8 cm. long 18 or 16 gauge needle is connected to a large syringe via a three-way stopcock; sterile tubing is connected to the stopcock in order to allow for collection of large volumes of fluid. The needle may be connected to the V-lead of the electrocardiogram *only* if it is certain that the machine is properly grounded (current leaks, particularly when the needle is covered by a plastic sheath, may induce ventricular fibrillation).

The needle is advanced slowly at a 30 to 45 degree angle to the skin, moving posteriorly towards the right sternoclavicular joint or the left shoulder. The pericardium is usually found at a depth of 2 to 4 cm. and a "give" is often (but not always) felt when the pericardial space is entered. If the needle is attached to the V-lead of the electrocardiogram, ST segment elevation usually develops when the epicardium is touched, signaling that the needle should be withdrawn slightly. Once in the pericardial space, a clamp may be attached to the needle at the skin or, if a plastic sheath is present, the needle may be removed. Often the removal of the first 50 ml. of fluid may yield dramatic improvement (i.e., increased blood pressure and decreased central venous pressure). When bloody fluid is encountered, its hematocrit should be compared to a simultaneously obtained venous hematocrit. Samples should be sent for appropriate laboratory examinations.

It should again be emphasized that pericardiocentesis is the treatment of choice for cardiac tamponade, but temporary cardiovascular support can be obtained by inotropic agents (e.g., isoproterenol [Isuprel] or dopamine) or volume expansion or both.

Recurrent tamponade may be treated with repeat aspiration or the positioning of an indwelling catheter for 24 to 48 hours or both. Chronic tamponade may necessitate surgical intervention (e.g., a pericardial window or pericardiectomy).

Constrictive Pericarditis

Constrictive pericarditis may be the end stage of almost all forms of pericardial disease. It may present without any previous history of acute pericardial inflammation. Medical management is usually of temporary benefit and pericardiectomy should be performed once the diagnosis is established. Preoperative management includes digitalis, salt restriction, and diuretics. It should be emphasized that overdiuresis must be avoided, since low "filling pressures" may severely depress cardiac output in constrictive pericarditis.

When available, a thermodilution cardiac output Swan-Ganz catheter may be very helpful in the medical management of severely ill patients with constrictive pericarditis and cardiac tamponade.

Recently, there have been reports of significant pericardial constriction without overt manifestations ("occult constrictive pericardial disease"). This entity is said to be diagnosed in the cardiac catheterization laboratory after rapid volume expansion. Nonspecific symptoms of fatigue, dyspnea, and chest pain have been reported to improve after pericardiectomy in a small series of patients. It remains to be seen whether these early reports will be substantiated in larger studies.

Arrhythmias

Cardiac arrhythmias are commonly seen in patients with acute pericarditis. They may be due to underlying myocardial disease, electrolyte disturbances, or cardiac tamponade. Whatever their cause, arrhythmias may be poorly tolerated in patients with pericardial disease. Digitalis is generally effective in treating supraventricular arrhythmias, while ventricular arrhythmias may require lidocaine. Theoretically, procainamide, because of its tendency to cause a lupuslike reaction, should be avoided in allergic forms of pericarditis. Myocardial depressants such as propranolol may also be quite hazardous in pericardial disease.

DEGENERATIVE ARTERIAL DISEASE

method of
JONATHAN B. TOWNE, M.D.
Milwaukee, Wisconsin

Acute Ischemia

Acute ischemia of the extremity is the most serious and urgent complication in patients with degenerative arterial disease. A carefully performed physical examination is most important, as it quantitates the severity of the ischemia and locates the site of arterial obstruction. On inspection, the extremity is pale, occasionally cyanotic, with collapsed pedal veins and pale or blanched nail beds. When only one extremity is involved, comparison of the warmth and color of the unaffected extremity to the symptomatic extremity aids the diagnosis. The absence of hair on the extremity, the thinning of skin, and the presence of ulcers or localized areas of gangrene indicate that progressive arterial occlusive disease is the cause of the ischemia rather than embolic disease. The interdigital spaces should be carefully examined, since they are sites of early gangrene, especially in diabetics. The presence of edema will alert the examiner to possible infection. The presence of ischemic rubor can be confusing. In the ischemic foot, maximal vasodilation causes pooling of blood when the foot is in a dependent position, resulting in a characteristic cyanotic red color. This is easily distinguished from a normal extremity or one with venous insufficiency by elevation, which causes the color to disappear rapidly with the development of a pale, ischemic color characteristic of poor arterial inflow.

Palpation of pulses will localize the level of obstruction. Absence of a femoral pulse indicates involvement of the aortoiliac segment, while absence of the popliteal pulse demonstrates involvement of the superficial femoral artery. The pulses should always be compared with the asymptomatic extremity. The warmth of the extremity should be ascertained by examining with the dorsum of the hand, since the level and degree of coolness is directly proportional to the severity of the ischemia. Comparison with the asymptomatic extremity aids in this determination. Capillary fill time is a good estimation of arteriolar flow and is measured by placing mild pressure on the skin and noting the time it takes for color to return. Normal value is less than two seconds. Evaluation of the status of sensation in the affected extremity is most important. Inability to detect touch and pain are important indicators of severe ischemia. The only exception is the patient with diabetes mellitus who has peripheral neuropathy. With the sensory and neurologic examination, muscle function of the involved extremity should be tested. The intrinsic muscles of either the hand or the foot are tested by abduction and adduction of the fingers or asking the patient to wiggle his toes. The presence of anesthesia and muscle paralysis in the extremity indicates severe ischemia, which will result in irreversible ischemia with tissue loss if not corrected in a short period of time. Immediate vascular surgical consultation in this instance is mandatory.

The use of the Doppler can be helpful in making the diagnosis of acute arterial ischemia by aiding in the detection of pulses and measuring the arterial pressure in the foot. A patient with a pressure of less than 40 mm. Hg at the ankle is in a limb-threatened category. The two principal differential diagnoses are embolic disease and acute thrombosis secondary to obstructive arterial occlusive disease. The origin of emboli is often the left atrium in patients with atrial fibrillation and the left ventricle in patients with recent myocardial infarctions. Emboli can also originate from ulcerative atheromatous plaques in any portion of the aorta. Abdominal aortic and iliac aneurysms as well as popliteal aneurysms can also shower the distal circulation with emboli. Clinical findings that favor embolism as the cause of the ischemia are the involvement of only one leg with all pulses present in the unaffected extremity, absence of history of intermittent claudication, and absence of findings of occlusive disease elsewhere in the body, which may be manifested by differential in arm blood pressure or the presence of bruits anywhere in the vascular system. Once the diagnosis of embolism is made, the location is determined by examination of pulses. Most often only one leg is affected, but occasionally an aortic saddle embolus will obstruct both iliac arteries, resulting in absence of both femoral pulses with profound ischemia of both legs. Patients with acute ischemia are given 5000 units of heparin intravenously immediately and scheduled for angiography. Angiography will determine the extent of the thrombosis, the patency of the renal arteries, and the status of visceral arteries. Following arteriography, the patient should have an embolectomy. If the patient is in poor medical condition, which may be a relative contraindication to general or regional anesthesia, embolectomy can be done with local anesthesia, as it usually involves only dissection of the common femoral artery in the groin on the involved side and extracting the embolus with a Fogarty balloon catheter. Anticoagulation is continued in the postoperative period initially with heparin and subsequently with warfarin. A vigorous search for the source of the emboli should be done in the postoperative period. If the patient is in atrial fibrillation, cardioversion should be considered. If the patient has a ventricular aneurysm, he should be evaluated for repair. All abdominal aortic, iliac, and popliteal aneurysms that shower the distal circulation with emboli should be resected if the patient can tolerate the surgery.

The other common cause of acute arterial ischemia is arterial occlusion secondary to atherosclerosis. These patients may also present with acute ischemia; however, they often have signs and symptoms that indicate the presence of widespread arterial occlusive disease. It is important to determine the severity of the ischemia in these patients with rest pain or acute limb ischemia secondary to chronic arterial occlusive disease. If the patient only has mild or moderate rest pain or has an ischemic ulcer, it is best to admit him to the hospital for a complete evaluation, which includes arteriography, evaluation of his heart, and a general medical evaluation with the idea of proceeding to an elective operation when the patient is in the best possible condition. If the patient has severe ischemia that precludes a more routine work-up, he should be given 5000 units of heparin and scheduled for an emergency angiogram. Urgent vascular reconstruction should be performed if a bypassable lesion is identified on the angiograms. One relatively uncommon but very dramatic clinical syndrome is acute aortic thrombosis. This fatal complication is often associated with the low cardiac output syndrome secondary to myocardial insufficiency and presents with severe ischemia involving both lower extremities and occasionally ischemia of the perineum manifested by cyanosis of the scrotum and perineal structures as well as ischemia of the gluteal region and the lower abdominal wall distal to the umbilicus. This thrombosis usually extends to but does not involve the renal arteries. However, in the presence of preexisting renal artery stenoses, the thrombosis may occasionally extend proximal to the renal arteries. Heparinization and immediate angiography are necessary. If the renal arteries are angiographically free of embolic disease and the patient is in dire medical straits, flow can be restored to the lower extremities with an axillary femoral and femoral-femoral graft, which these patients easily tolerate.

Another unusual and dramatic presentation of acute ischemia is the "blue toe syndrome." The patient has excruciating pain, most often in one toe or in several toes, accompanied by cyanotic discoloration of the involved digits despite palpable pedal pulses. Atheromatous embolization from an ulcerated plaque proximal in the arterial stream is the cause. The emboli occlude digital arteries but are usually too small to occlude the more proximal dorsal pedal or posterior tibial arteries. This results in ischemia of a solitary or two adjacent digits with normal flow to the rest of the foot. This syndrome should not be confused with gout or other arthritides. Treatment is symptomatic, with the addition of salicylates to cause inhibition of platelet aggregation. The toe, over the next 2 to 3 weeks, will gradually regain normal arterial supply through collateral flow. This syndrome is a harbinger of an ulcerated plaque in the proximal arterial system that should be evaluated with arteriography and repaired to prevent further episodes of embolization.

Chronic Ischemia

Patients more frequently present with more chronic forms of vascular occlusive disease. Intermittent claudication is the most common type of chronic occlusive disease encountered. In evaluation, it is important to obtain a good history determining such contributing factors as smoking, diabetes mellitus, coronary artery disease, hypertension, and various types of hyperlipidemia. There are two forms of claudication: gluteal claudication, primarily involving the buttock, and calf claudication, which affects the leg. Buttock claudication usually is indicative of severe diffuse arterial occlusive disease in both hypogastric arterial systems, while calf claudication usually indicates occlusive disease involving either the ipsilateral aortoiliac or femoral-popliteal segment. Physical findings in these patients usually demonstrate a lack of pedal pulses in the involved leg. The degree of ischemia can be quantitated by obtaining Doppler ankle-brachial index, by treadmill exercise, and by determining the ankle pressure response to reactive hyperemia. Occasionally, a patient will give a classic history of intermittent claudication but when examined will have palpable pedal pulses. The physician must be aware of the possibility of latent aortoiliac occlusive disease with high-grade stenosis but not complete occlusion of any vessel. This is easily determined by walking the patient for 50 to 100 yards and then reexamining the pulses. With latent aortoiliac occlusive disease, the pulses will disappear with modest exercise. Initial treatment for patients with intermittent claudication consists of the patient's stopping smoking, losing weight, and being instructed in foot care such as avoiding extremes of temperature and avoiding injury by adequate protection. An exercise program is valuable. Since it may promote the development of collateral circulation, the patient is instructed to walk to the point of claudication several times a day. Following an occlusion of an artery, the collateral circulation of the leg will increase for up to 6 months. Angiography should be reserved only for those patients who are candidates for reconstructive procedures. An operation is indicated in intermittent claudication only if it is felt that the ability to walk long distances is necessary to maintain livelihood or if claudication is rapidly progressing to rest pain. Patient education is the most important aspect of care. Once the patient understands his limitations as well as the need for optimum leg and foot care, he usually does quite well. The operative procedure generally depends on the location of the occlusive process. Aortofemoral bypass is usually performed for aortoiliac occlusive disease and femoral-popliteal bypass for superficial femoral block.

Patients who have severe chronic arterial insufficiency of the leg resulting in rest pain, ischemic ulcers, or localized areas of gangrene are in a limb salvage category. If the arterial inflow into the foot is not increased, a major amputation will be required. Any of these symptoms are indications for further evaluation. If there is infection in the extremity associated with the ischemic ulcers or gangrene, the patient should be admitted immediately and started on intravenous antibiotics. All patients in the limb salvage category should undergo an extensive work-up, including careful evaluation of cardiac and pulmonary status. If arteriography demonstrates obstructive disease remedial by a vascular reconstructive procedure, the patient should be scheduled for the appropriate operation. If there is no bypassable disease, as is often seen in diabetics with small vessel disease, an amputation will be necessary. The level of the amputation is the most distal amputation that will heal. In general, a below-knee amputation can be done if there is at least 70 mm. Hg arterial pressure at the popliteal fossa.

Buerger's disease (thromboangiitis obliterans) is an arterial disease that involves primarily medium and small arteries of both the upper and lower extremities that almost exclusively affects young males who smoke. These patients often have recurrent episodes of superficial thrombophlebitis. The diagnosis is confirmed on arteriography, where classic findings of segmental arterial occlusion are noted. The primary treatment of Buerger's disease is cessation of smoking. If the patient can abstain from tobacco, he is often able to get by without amputation. Ulceration of tips of digits is managed with debridement and antibiotics if local infection is present. Occasionally, sympathectomy helps in selected patients. If the patient continues to smoke, he will ultimately need major bilateral amputations.

A significant problem in the evaluation of the ischemic extremity is the treatment of the patient with acute infection in the ischemic foot. These patients should be immediately admitted to the hospital and Gram stains obtained from the purulent exudate to determine the type of antibiotic coverage. If the Gram stain demonstrates mostly gram-positive cocci, intravenous penicillin and methicillin should be instituted. If gram-negative rods are seen, an aminoglycoside and clindamycin should be started. The patient should be at absolute bed rest with the legs horizontal. Tetanus prophylaxis is indicated. The foot should be carefully examined for a plantar space abscess. Following 12 to 18 hours of intravenous antibiotic administration, all necrotic tissue should be debrided and the wound left open. It is important to open all involved fascial spaces. Following resolution of the infection, definitive amputation and reconstruction of the foot should be performed.

Abdominal aortic aneurysms are one type of degenerative arterial disease requiring judgment for optimum care. Usually they are asymptomatic and found on routine physical examination. A definitive diagnosis can be obtained with a sonogram that outlines the aorta and clearly demonstrates the aneurysm. The distal aorta normally measures 2.5 cm., and anything over 3.5 cm. is considered aneurysmal. Following the diagnosis of an aneurysm, the patient should be evaluated for surgical risk. In a good risk patient, an elective resection of the aneurysm is indicated.

The presence of a symptomatic abdominal aortic aneurysm is an emergency. The symptoms of an acutely expanding or ruptured aneurysm consist of back pain, shock, abdominal pain, syncope, Grey-Turner sign of the left flank, discoloration of the scrotum, genitourinary symptoms that mimic renal colic, or ureteral calculi. The patient should be admitted to the operating room immediately, have several large intravenous lines inserted, have blood sent for type and crossmatch, and have a pneumatic antishock suit applied to the abdomen and both lower extremities. Immediate celiotomy is necessary to control the hemorrhage. Occasionally, a patient will present with vague abdominal pain and because of his body habitus, an aneurysm is not palpable. If an aneurysm is suspected, a cross-table lateral film of the abdomen will often demonstrate calcification of the aneurysmal wall. If available, an emergency sonogram should be obtained in all questionable cases. Although abdominal aortic aneurysms are more common, iliac artery aneurysms occasionally occur and present with the same symptoms as abdominal aortic aneurysms. Patients can also have femoral or popliteal aneurysms. Femoral aneurysms rarely present as an emergency, although if neglected can occasionally expand large enough to rupture. Because of their relatively superficial location in the groin, medical help will usually be sought before the aneurysm becomes

large. Popliteal artery aneurysms often cause problems by either acutely thrombosing or showering the distal arterial system with emboli. Their embolic potential is much greater than the potential for rupture. Any patient with a popliteal or femoral artery aneurysm should be examined carefully for an abdominal aortic aneurysm, as there is a very high degree of coexistence of multiple aneurysm. An occasional patient will be seen who has a false aneurysm that is usually related to trauma, most often penetrating wounds in the vicinity of major vascular structures. These are rarely emergencies but should be resected electively to prevent enlargement with nerve compression and the risk of eventual rupture.

Vasospastic diseases are relatively uncommon in clinical practice. The most common is Raynaud's disease, which consists of intermittent attacks of vasospasm, aggravated by cold or anxiety. It is important to distinguish between the patient with Raynaud's phenomenon and the patient with Raynaud's disease, which is a diagnosis of exclusion. In Raynaud's phenomenon, symptoms of arterial vasospasm are more common in both upper extremities and are secondary manifestations of other disease processes, most notably collagen vascular disease such as scleroderma, lupus erythematosus, rheumatoid arthritis, and dermatomyositis. The Raynaud's phenomenon is also seen in Buerger's disease and in nerve injury such as carpal tunnel syndrome, thoracic outlet syndrome, and traumatic nerve injury. Occasionally, patients with cryoglobulinemia, macroglobulinemia, and cold agglutinins will have Raynaud's phenomenon. In its end stage there is necrosis of the fingertip from prolonged vasospasm. Evaluation should include LE prep, ANA, complete blood count (CBC), platelet count, cold agglutinins, sedimentation rate, serum protein electrophoresis, and barium swallow. If the patient's symptoms are mild, they do well by protecting their hands with gloves and avoiding smoking. If this is insufficient, they may be started on phenoxybenzamine, 10 mg. per day orally, and the dosage is slowly increased at five-day intervals to a maximum of 10 mg. orally three times daily. Also, guanethidine, 10 to 30 mg. per day orally, can be used. (This use of guanethidine is not listed in the manufacturer's official directive.) In an occasional patient who develops rather severe Raynaud's disease with necrosis of the fingertips, a dorsal sympathectomy is recommended.

Another vasospastic syndrome that should be considered is ergotism, which can present with rather marked vasospasm. The diagnosis is primarily obtained by the history of a patient taking ergot-type drugs who has significant vasospasm. Treatment is discontinuation of ergot drugs. If the ischemia is severe, heparin administration and intravenous administration of low molecular weight dextran are indicated. In the rare case of limb-threatening ischemia, intra-arterial tolazoline and intravenous papaverine are helpful.

MASSIVE DEEP VENOUS THROMBOSIS OF THE LOWER EXTREMITIES

method of
DONALD SILVER, M.D.
Columbia, Missouri

Massive thrombosis of the lower extremity usually presents with marked edema of the entire lower extremity and a burstinglike pain. The thrombosis frequently involves the superficial and deep femoral, superficial saphenous, and iliac venous systems and occasionally extends into the inferior vena cava. The limb usually appears edematous and cyanotic, although if arterial inflow becomes restricted by the increased tissue pressure and venous hypertension the limb may become pale. The diagnosis, which is usually suspected from the history and physical examination, can be confirmed by Doppler study or with the plethysmograph and is established with a phlebogram.

The goals and management of massive thrombosis include: (1) stopping the thrombotic process, (2) restoring venous patency, (3) preventing pulmonary embolism, and (4) minimizing the sequelae of the venous hypertension.

General Measures. All patients with significant deep venous thrombosis should be hospitalized and placed at bed rest with the lower extremities elevated at least 20 degrees above the pelvis and right atrium. The level of elevation is increased when massive edema is present. Large amounts of fluid may be lost into the edematous limbs, and several liters of balanced salt solution and blood may be necessary to maintain an adequate blood volume and hematocrit. Soft bulky protective dressings are placed around the feet and lower legs. The distal portions of the feet should be exposed to permit an evaluation of arterial perfusion.

Anticoagulation. Heparin remains the anticoagulant of choice with large amounts being required to stop (as opposed to prevent) the thrombotic process. I usually give 300 to 500 units per kg. of body weight of heparin intravenously as a priming dose and follow this with a continuous heparin infusion of, usually, 1000 units per hour. The heparin infusion is regulated 16 to 20 hours after the priming dose to maintain an activated partial thromboplastin time (APTT) of 80 to 90 seconds. Hemorrhage has not been a problem when the APTT has been maintained in this range. The heparin infusion is continued 10 to 14 days or longer if symptoms of inflammation and edema persist.

The patient is allowed out of bed with the lower extremities wrapped with elastic wraps when the pain has subsided. The patient is allowed to walk or sit with his legs elevated, but may not stand stationary nor sit with the legs dependent. When the edema has subsided the patient is fitted for full length heavy elastic stockings (the custom made stockings of the Jobst Company, Toledo, Ohio, meet these criteria).

During the last few days of the heparin infusion the patient is taught to give himself injections and is maintained on heparin at home, 5000 units subcutaneously every 8 hours for three months. After three months, if there are no signs of recurrent thrombosis, the heparin is stopped.

Prothrombinopenic Agents. The prothrombinopenic agents do not have a role in the early management of deep venous thrombosis because of the delay of onset of the anticoagulant effect. The agents are frequently utilized for 3 to 6 months after the initial 14 days of intensive heparin therapy, with warfarin being the most commonly utilized prothrombinopenic agent.

If warfarin is to be utilized, it is usually begun on the seventh day of heparin therapy at approximately 10 mg. per day. By the fourteenth day of heparin therapy the prothrombin time (PT) is usually prolonged to twice the control time and heparin is stopped. The dose of warfarin required to maintain the prothrombin time (PT) twice the control time, usually 2.5 to 7.5 mg. per day, is determined and the patient maintained on that dosage for 3 to 6 months. The PT should be determined at least weekly for the first month and then at least every 2 weeks for the remainder of the anticoagulant period to avoid excessive anticoagulation with its threat of bleeding.

Fibrinolytic Agents. Adequate doses of heparin will stop thrombosis and permit fibrinolysis and recanalization to occur. However, most often these processes occur slowly and the veins are permanently damaged with loss of their valves. The fibrinolytic agents, urokinase and streptokinase, offer the possibility of rapid lysis of the thrombus with preservation of venous walls and valves. The fibrinolytic agents are contraindicated in the early postoperative or postpartum periods, in children, in hypertensive patients, or in patients with bleeding disorders, after trauma, in patients with renal or hepatic insufficiency, and in patients with recent strokes.

My preferred fibrinolytic agent is urokinase. Urokinase is usually given as a 2000 units per pound (4,400 units per kg.) priming dose in 10 to 15 minutes and is followed by 2000 units per pound per hour for 12 hours. A heparin infusion is begun after the urokinase infusion to prevent rethrombosis and is usually continued 7 to 10 days. If the thrombosis lyses and the precipitating cause for the thrombosis has been eliminated, long-term anticoagulation is not necessary. However, most often some of the thrombus persists and the patient is maintained on heparin (or warfarin) for 3 to 6 months.

Surgery. At present, surgery is rarely indicated in the management of lower extremity deep thrombosis because most patients respond to nonoperative management and because thrombectomy usually fails to restore completely the patency of the venous system or preserve valve function. However, thrombectomy may become necessary when the venous stasis becomes so pronounced that tissue perfusion is altered and ischemic changes occur and persist despite elevation of the limb and the utilization of heparin or urokinase. Thrombectomy is also utilized in the management of the patient who presents with an acute, i.e., less than 24 hours old, massive iliofemoral thrombosis, and if the patient has not had previous episodes of thrombophlebitis. In these rare patients the surgeon attempts to remove the obstructing thrombosis before the secondary and tertiary venous channels become occluded. Heparin therapy is begun at the time of thrombectomy, if not before, and is continued for 10 to 14 days, after which the patient is usually maintained on subcutaneous heparin or warfarin for 3 to 6 months.

Pulmonary Embolism. The most serious sequela to deep venous thrombosis of the lower extremity is pulmonary embolism. More than 50 per cent of patients with deep venous thrombosis develop perfusion defects in their lung scans. Fortunately, many of these emboli are small and of little clinical consequence. The anticoagulant or fibrinolytic schedule for pulmonary embolism is the same as that outlined for deep venous thrombosis. Additional minor embolizations are not uncommon during the first few days of therapy. These emboli are usually quickly lysed and are of little clinical consequence. If anticoagulants are contraindicated or significant recurrent pulmonary embolism occurs while the patient is "adequately" anticoagulated, vena caval interruption is indicated.

Before interrupting the vena cava one should obtain a phlebogram and an inferior venacavogram to be certain that the emboli have arisen in the venous system inferior to the level of the renal veins. The vena cava may be "interrupted" by the transvenous placement of intracaval devices, the placement of clips around the cava, the creation of a suture grid across the cava, or by ligating the inferior vena cava. If ligation is performed, the gonadal and other large retroperitoneal veins are also ligated. Heparin is begun postoperatively and is continued for 7 to 10 days, after which the patient remains on a less intensive regimen of anticoagulation for 3 to 6 months. Elevation of the foot of the bed, elastic stockings, early ambulation, and avoiding positions of stasis are important components of the postoperative care.

Experience with a large number of patients with pulmonary embolism has indicated that most patients with pulmonary embolism can be managed nonoperatively.

Sequelae to Deep Venous Thrombosis. Only rarely is patency of the deep venous system completely restored by heparin, urokinase, or surgery. Most patients have some degree of venous insufficiency after a deep venous thrombosis. These patients are told that they must spend the remainder of their life protecting their legs against the complications that occur from the absence of valves, i.e., the markedly increased venous pressure in the distal leg with standing and the resultant poor tissue perfusion. These patients are requested to sleep with the foot of the bed elevated, put on elastic stockings upon rising and remove them when retiring, avoid positions of stasis, practice good hygiene, and promptly treat all infections of the involved extremity.

If these measures are utilized, postphlebitic complications are rare. If they are not utilized, secondary varicose veins, stasis dermatitis and stasis ulcerations will occur. Most often the dermatitis and ulcerations will heal with bed rest, elevation, compresses, and antibiotics if cellulitis is present. Stripping and ligation of secondary varicose veins is rarely indicated, because the veins contribute only minimally to the dermatitis and ulceration and because the varicosities usually reoccur after stripping.

If the ulceration is refractory to treatment, or if it recurs frequently, surgical therapy is recommended. A 90 per cent long-term "cure" of these ulcers can be achieved by interrupting the communications between the deep and superficial veins, removing the subcutaneous tissue from the ankle to the knee, and by applying a delayed split-thickness graft to the area of ulceration.

PRIMARY VARICOSE VEINS

method of
JERE W. LORD, JR., M.D.
New York, New York

Of all earth's mobile creatures, only the human animal, with his penchant for standing erect, is afflicted by this abnormal state. According to one authority, not one instance of varicosities has been observed in horses, dogs, cats, and other four-legged animals. The standing and sitting positions which occupy two thirds of the 24-hour day of man and woman are clearly the responsible factors. That all humans do not develop varicose veins is a tribute to the superior substance of the favored subjects' venous valves and walls from ankle to iliac region.

Hemodynamic Factors

Peripheral venous blood flow or venous pressure depends mainly on hydrostatic pressure. Investigators have repeatedly studied venous pressure at the ankle in normal persons and in those with varicose veins. In the resting, sitting and standing positions, the venous pressure at the ankle is equal to the hydrostatic pressure of a column of blood up to the level of the right atrium. In the standing position, the average mean venous pressure at the ankle is 87 mm. Hg in normal persons and about the same in patients with primary varicose veins. With muscular activity of the limb (as in walking), the pressure in the superficial venous system decreases to an average mean value of 22 mm. Hg in normal persons and to 44 mm. Hg in patients with simple incompetence of the long saphenous vein. In patients who have incompetence of a greater saphenous vein and a history of iliofemoral thrombophlebitis, this value is 77 mm. Hg.

These studies have been interpreted as follows: in normal persons, the fall in venous pressure at the ankle is due to the pumping action of the muscles (venous or muscle pump) and to the competence of the valves in preventing reflux of blood into emptied segments of veins during the period of muscular relaxation. In patients who have uncomplicated primary varicose veins, the valves are unable to prevent the return flow of blood during muscular relaxation, and venous pressure returns quickly to the hydrostatic level. The relatively small drop in the venous pressure at the ankle in patients with varicose veins and a history of iliofemoral thrombophlebitis suggests that there is interference with the outflow of venous blood from the leg in this condition. The actual genesis of this finding, however, has not been satisfactorily explained.

When proper venous drainage of the limb is disturbed by the presence of incompetent veins and valves, the equilibrium of the osmotic pressure mechanisms responsible for extravascular fluid transit becomes altered and edema develops. Other conditions that commonly upset these balanced factors include (1) alteration in capillary membranes resulting from heat, toxins, or hypoxia; (2) variation in osmotic pressures, as in edema due to hormonal, renal, hepatic, or nutritional disorders; and (3) obstruction of lymphatic channels caused by inflammation or tumor.

Particular attention should be given to edema caused by a change in intravascular pressures, principally of the venous pressure. If this process of accumulation of abnormal amounts of extravascular fluid is allowed to persist, subcutaneous fibrosis and skin atrophy may occur and lead to the "stasis syndrome" and eventual ulceration of the skin above the medial aspect of the ankle. The importance of elevation of the limb, application of elastic bandages before arising, and eventual eradication of the underlying incompetent veins in order to avoid the crippling sequelae of edema formation cannot be overemphasized.

Therapy

Patients with varicose veins exhibit a varied clinical picture. At one end of the spectrum there are slightly dilated veins, often with spider capillary bursts, so-called telangiectasia, whereas at the other end there are huge nests of varicosities stemming from an incompetent greater saphenous vein, lesser saphenous vein, or both. Selection of patients for sclerotherapy vs. operative intervention rests on the determination of the competency of the valves of the greater and lesser saphenous veins. The tourniquet test, employing a soft rubber tubing applied to the midthigh of the elevated leg with the patient in the recumbent position, yields definitive information concerning the competency of the valves of the greater saphenous and of communicating veins. On assuming the erect position, rapid filling of the varicosities with the tourniquet in place indicates incompetent communicating veins. If there is no filling of the veins on standing until the tourniquet is released, then the communicating veins are competent and the valves of the greater saphenous are incompetent. Last, if the filling of the varicosities in the lower leg takes the same time whether or not the tourniquet is in place, it may be concluded that the valves are functioning well.

It has been my practice to employ sclerotherapy for smaller varicosities with competent valves and to operate on those with incompetent valves of one or more of the three systems.

Sclerotherapy

There are several sclerosing agents on the market, some of which may cause allergic reactions. For the past several years I have used sodium tetradecyl sulfate (Sotradecol) in a 1 per cent solution. On a rare occasion there has been a systemic allergic response that has been controlled by a hypodermic injection of 0.5 ml. of 1:1000 solution of epinephrine. It is wise to have a sterile vial of this agent handy. Further, if there is extravasation of the sclerosing solution into the perivenous tissues, a slough may sometimes develop. This can usually be prevented by the prompt injection of 1 to 2 ml. of a 1 per cent solution of procaine into the subcutaneous region around the injected vein. The injection should be discontinued immediately on viewing filling outside the vein, or if the patient complains of a burning sensation. Procaine is injected promptly, as noted above. No matter how careful and how skilled the physician is, an occasional slough will occur. This may be due to a perfectly performed injection, but after the patient leaves the office, the pressure dressing applied immediately following the injection may loosen. Some of the injected fluid may leak through the needle puncture site and cause a so-called "leak" ulcer. Usually these ulcers will heal in 2 to 4 weeks and leave a small scar resembling a vaccination mark. I have had 5 ulcers develop in approximately 15,000 injections. The last of these ulcers appeared in a pregnant woman and did not heal until 2 weeks following delivery of her baby. With exceptions, I believe that it is unwise to inject varicosities during pregnancy for two reasons: first, the injections are not usually effective, and second, the varicosities will usually recede significantly following delivery. In this case, the patient was unaware of the fact that she was 5 months pregnant, and it was not until the ulcer developed 3 weeks later that she visited a gynecologist and learned of her gravid state.

Two methods of injection are practiced and have their proponents.

The *full vein technique* has the patient sitting or standing. In recent years I have drawn into a 2 ml. syringe with a 26 sized needle, 0.5 ml. of 1 per cent solution of sodium tetradecyl sulfate (Sotradecol) and 1.5 ml. of air. During the injection the air displaces blood from the small varicosity, and the fluid follows to irritate the endothelium, which is then compressed immediately on withdrawing the needle by 4 or 5 pieces of 2 inch gauze. This is held in place by a single encircling strip of half-inch adhesive tape. A 3 or 4 inch elastic bandage is then applied from the ankle to above the site of the injection and left in place for 36 hours unless the patient notices discomfort. If so, the bandage is removed promptly. Longitudinal strips of adhesive help prolong the proper application of the elastic bandage. After removal of the elastic bandage, wetting of the adhesive tape in a tub or shower facilitates its removal without an accompanying piece of skin.

The *empty vein technique* is more effective, as there is little or no blood to displace. However, the chances of extravasation are greater as the needle may pierce both sides of the vein. Pressure is applied as in the full vein technique.

For the injection of telangiectatic venules and spiders, a "tuberculin" syringe with a 1 ml. capacity is attached to a number 30 needle and filled with 0.2 ml. of sodium tetradecyl sulfate (Sotradecol) and 0.8 ml. air. By means of glasses with a 2.5 magnifying lens used for operative procedures on small arteries, it is possible to inject these tiny vessels with a measure of success.

Regardless of how skilled and experienced the sclerotherapist is, all patients should be warned that following an occasional injection a permanent yellow streak may develop.

Surgical Therapy

The results of surgical treatment will depend as much on the preoperative determination of deficient venous systems as on the completeness of the surgical procedure. Since it is quite impossible to describe all the venous patterns, it is essential that all involved veins, and especially sites of incompetent perforators, be carefully marked preoperatively. An indelible pencil may be used for this purpose. The veins should be marked with the patient standing and before preoperative medication has been administered so that the patient can be fully cooperative and in no danger of falling. Common causes of poor results after high ligation and stripping include failure to ligate all tributaries of the long saphenous vein at the saphenofemoral junction, failure to ligate incompetent perforators, and incomplete stripping of varicose veins. Accurate marking is essential. Once the patient is horizontal or in a slight Trendelenburg position, the involved veins collapse and become difficult to identify.

The saphenofemoral junction is exposed by an oblique incision parallel to and just below the flexion crease of the groin. The femoral arterial pulsation should be palpated as a guide and the deeper dissection should be kept medial to it. The long saphenous vein courses along the border of the adductor longus muscle, whose bulging border can be easily palpated when the knee is flexed and the hip is externally rotated. The saphenous vein is located and transected between clamps. The proximal end is dissected upward, with ligation and division of all tributaries en route. Adequate exposure of the saphenofemoral junction with the fossa ovalis is essential to ensure ligation of all tributaries in this area and to prevent injury to the common femoral vein. The saphenous vein is ligated and transfixed 2 to 4 mm. from the femoral vein. The dissected vein is removed; by means of an extraluminal stripper the greater saphenous vein is removed from the groin to the previously marked lowest major varicosity. I do not like the "giant strip" from ankle to groin. When the stripper passed distally encounters a branch that causes significant impedance to further passage, a transverse incision is made over the ring of the stripper and the branch or branches are ligated and divided. Usually three to four such incisions are made in the thigh to include ligation of all major branches and perforators. Below the knee stripping is continued with excision of all previously marked varicosities.

When the lesser saphenous vein is involved, external rotation of the thigh and leg with moderate flexion of the knee joint will then permit adequate exposure of the popliteal space and the previously marked level for a transverse incision at the site of penetration of the lesser saphenous vein through the deep popliteal fascia. Ligation and transfixion of the vein are made deep to the fascia, but no attempt is made to dissect it to the popliteal vein. No difficulty has been recognized in my patients postoperatively with this technique. Great care is taken to avoid injury to the common peroneal nerve, which is located laterally in the popliteal space. Stripping of the lesser saphenous vein is performed in similar fashion to the technique for the greater saphenous vein.

Avoidance of Complications

Complications associated with the operation range in severity from single areas of ecchymosis to catastrophic instances of ligation and even stripping of the femoral artery that result in loss of the limb. Complications may be considered peculiar to three stages of the operation. These include: (1) complications during the performance of high ligation of the vein, (2) complications peculiar to stripping and (3) wound complications.

During high ligation and exposure of the saphenofemoral junction, the femoral vein is vulnerable to injury. Care should be exercised that the anterior wall of the femoral vein is not "tented" and therefore apt to be included in the placement of the high ligature. The ligature should not be placed flush with the femoral vein, but at a point 2 to 4 mm. distally; a small stump of the long saphenous is allowed to remain.

Careless dissection in this region may lead to laceration of the femoral vein and result in severe hemorrhage. In this emergency, it is important to remember a few basic principles involved in arresting "blind" hemorrhage. Frantic swabbing and suction will not stop the bleeding, and blind attempts to clamp the bleeding point may cause further laceration. Apply firm pressure with a large sponge; increase the Trendelenburg tilt of the table, and wait patiently until the bleeding is arrested. This will provide time for the preparation of vascular clamps and 5–0 arterial sutures. Thereafter, if the source of the bleeding is found to be a small vein, deliberate clamping of the bleeding point and ligation can be performed under direct vision. If the femoral vein is found to be lacerated, the vein must be exposed by incising the deep fascia. The vein is clamped above and below the laceration with vascular clamps, and the rent is closed with a 5–0 arterial suture.

Injury to the femoral artery during the high ligation procedure is difficult to comprehend and is unpardonable. Positive identification of the long saphenous vein is imperative before the structure is divided. Palpation of the structure for any sign of pulsation should be routine.

The superficial inguinal nodes surround the saphenofemoral junction and may be injured easily. Injury may be avoided by performing all dissection in the vertical plane, close to the vein, and by "pushing the surrounding anatomy away." If the lymphatics are injured, ligation of severed structures is mandatory. This will prevent postoperative lymphorrhea. During the stripping state of the procedure, hematomas can be avoided by the use of the Trendelenburg position, further elevation of the extremity, and properly applied compression.

Neuritis due to trauma to the saphenous and sural nerves, leading to paresthesias and numbness, is a fairly common but transient complication.

Wound complications associated with varicose vein surgery are similar to those associated with any surgical wound. They may be avoided by strict adherence to the principles of aseptic technique, good hemostasis, and gentle handling of tissues.

Postoperative Program

During the immediate postoperative period, primary attention is directed toward minimizing traumatic phlebitis and venous thrombosis that may be incited by the operative procedure. The patient is allowed to stay in bed on the day of operation, but "ambulation in bed" is encouraged and lavatory privileges are permitted. The foot of the bed is elevated on 6-inch blocks and flexion of the knee is discouraged.

On the first postoperative day, the patient is instructed to walk to tolerance and to lie down on his bed as desired. Sitting with the knees flexed is not allowed.

Sutures are removed on the fifth to seventh day after operation. Elastic bandage support of the lower legs is continued for 2 to 3 weeks to discourage the development of edema and lymphatic stasis.

It is important to reexamine the patient at frequent intervals during the early postoperative period so that edema, cellulitis, hematomas and wound infections can be detected early and proper therapy instituted.

In the later postoperative period, reexaminations are required to identify persistent varicosities and to detect any new ones which may develop. Suitable sclerosing therapy can then be given as an adjunct to an adequate operation.

SECTION
4

The Blood and Spleen

BONE MARROW FAILURE
(Aplastic Anemia)

method of
VIRGIL LOEB, JR., M.D.
St. Louis, Missouri

Anemia due to bone marrow failure has been variously designated as hypoplastic anemia, aplastic anemia, aregenerative anemia, and refractory anemia. None of these terms is completely satisfactory; the phrase bone marrow failure best describes the basic defect common to a spectrum of hematologic disorders. The designation can be applied where there is failure of the bone marrow to produce an adequate number of any of the normally formed elements of the blood, so that anemia, leukopenia, thrombocytopenia, or any combination of the three results. Furthermore, the hematopoietic precursors in the marrow are usually decreased and will not respond to administration of known hematinics. Functional impairment of the marrow may be acute or chronic, it may be secondary to known bone marrow depressants or of unknown cause, and may be absolute or relative to other changes in the hematopoietic equilibrium.

In order to develop a rational treatment strategy for any disease it is important to understand cause and pathogenesis; unfortunately, little is known about these factors in primary bone marrow failure, and even the differential diagnosis may remain obscure. Whereas most cases of aplastic anemia are undoubtedly due to an acquired disorder of the hematopoietic stem cells, there is evidence suggesting that unspecified autoimmune reactions as well as changes in the marrow stroma or microenvironment may occasionally be responsible for failure of marrow function. Although inadequate production (hypoproliferation) characterizes all forms of marrow failure, accelerated destruction of red cells, white cells, and platelets may play a secondary role in increasing the peripheral cytopenia. The following is a simplified classification of clinical varieties of bone marrow failure:

1. Primary or idiopathic marrow failure
2. Acquired marrow failure due to extrinsic factors
   a. Ionizing irradiation
   b. Chemical agents and drugs
   c. Infectious agents
      i. Viral, e.g., hepatitis
      ii. Bacterial, e.g., miliary tuberculosis
3. Acquired marrow failure due to infiltrative disease
   a. Leukemia, lymphoma, myeloma
   b. Metastatic neoplasms
   c. Granulomatous and storage diseases
   d. Myeloproliferative diseases
4. Congenital/familial marrow failure
5. Miscellaneous, e.g., paroxysmal nocturnal hemoglobinuria, pure red cell anemia associated with thymoma, chronic inflammatory or metabolic disease

In a compendium emphasizing treatment methods, it is most important to consider the possibility that disease may result as a consequence of exposure to potentially toxic drugs and chemicals. The role of environmental factors as well as therapeutic agents in the causation of bone marrow failure is difficult to assess. The number of affected persons is usually small in proportion to the population exposed. Additionally, many of the suspected agents fail to induce marrow depression in the experimental animal. Since a cause and effect relationship between a given chemical and bone marrow failure can be confirmed only by reexposure of the affected persons following recovery to the suspected offending factor, such proof is rarely available in human beings. Although the evidence implicating most drugs is therefore essentially circumstantial, sufficient observations have been made with certain agents to justify identification as potential bone marrow toxins. In many cases patients are exposed to a variety of chemicals, any one of which might be incriminated as the causative agent. The most commonly reported compounds associated with aplastic anemia are chloramphenicol, phenylbutazone, mephenytoin, gold salts, benzene, and several insecticides and pesticides. Other drugs are more prone to cause leukopenia, agranulocytosis, thrombocytopenia, or any combination of these. Ionizing irradiation and many drugs used in cancer chemotherapy invariably cause bone marrow depression, provided there is sufficient exposure.

That some persons may experience prolonged contact with these agents and suffer no obvious ill effects cannot be denied, but the occurrence of bone marrow failure under such conditions is great enough to demand caution in therapeutic use or in occupational exposure. Sound medical principles often justify the prescription of potentially toxic compounds in a variety of clinical situations. Under these circumstances, awareness of the potential risk and alertness for early signs of bone marrow failure may avert a serious and possibly fatal complication of therapy. Unfortunately, it is not always possible to maintain adequate surveillance in order to avoid bone marrow suppression and the risk of such treatment may have to be accepted, providing no other therapeutic approach is available.

Treatment

Treatment of acquired bone marrow failure secondary to infiltrative diseases (myelophthisic anemia) is beyond the scope of this discussion. As there is no specific therapy available to reverse the functional defect in primary marrow failure or in failure secondary to extrinsic marrow damage, the fundamental treatment objective must be to provide appropriate and necessary support to the patient while anticipating spontaneous recovery. It follows that one of the most important requisites to minimize continuing myelosuppression is the need to ascertain the causative factor if possible. If a temporal relationship between exposure to a suspected offending agent and changes in the peripheral blood can be established, further contact can usually be avoided. In most cases, however, it is difficult to incriminate a specific factor. As noted previously, individual susceptibility varies considerably, and one person exposed to a marrow toxin may develop aplastic anemia, whereas his associates similarly exposed are unaffected. Any history of exposure to a potential toxin in a patient with bone marrow failure is sufficient reason to be suspicious of the particular substance and further contact with all such agents must be avoided.

Treatment of Anemia

Transfusions are usually the mainstay of any program for the treatment of bone marrow failure. Hemoglobin levels need not be maintained above 7 or 8 grams per dl. (100 ml.), since most patients with this disease are restricted in their activities and remain quite comfortable in this range. Patients requiring more than three or four transfusions per month to maintain a suitable level of hemoglobin are usually bleeding or have a hemolytic component to the anemia. As time goes on, patients with impaired marrow function often require transfusions with increasing frequency, particularly if splenomegaly from iron overload or extramedullary hematopoiesis develops. The use of packed red blood cells from which the plasma and buffy coat have been removed is to be encouraged. Overloading of plasma volume and sensitization to white blood cells and platelets occur frequently with administration of whole blood, particularly in those patients with chronic bone marrow failure who require prolonged blood replacement. As the effective survival time of transfused red blood cells decreases with length of storage in the blood bank, it is preferable to use blood obtained from a donor within the preceding 5 days. Care must be exercised with respect to sterility and technique of venipuncture. In general, it is most satisfactory to administer 2 or even 3 units of packed red blood cells at one time in order to conserve the patient's veins and to allow the maximal interval between visits to the hospital or physician's office. It must be emphasized, however, that anemia itself may be a stimulus to erythropoiesis, and maintenance of the hemoglobin level above that required to prevent symptoms of hypoxia is usually unnecessary. Careful attention to complete blood grouping of patient and donor together with optimal cross-matching technique will tend to minimize the inevitable danger of isosensitization.

Treatment of Bleeding

Since death associated with bone marrow failure usually occurs from hemorrhage or infection, treatment of these two complications is of prime importance. The administration of freshly drawn whole blood (within 4 hours after phlebotomy) or platelet-rich plasma can be of some help in the management of bleeding due to thrombocytopenia. Where available, the use of platelet concentrates appropriately prepared and stored under optimal conditions can have a major impact on the bleeding tendency particularly if the level of circulating platelets falls below 20×10^9 per liter. Although formulae are available to calculate theoretical incremental platelet rise in the circulating blood of a recipient of 1 unit of platelet concentrate, there is considerable variation in effective yield, depending upon prior isosensitization, presence of fever or infection or both, technique of procurement and administration, etc. In general, adults will require the transfusion of 6 to 10 units of platelet concentrate two or three times weekly in order to maintain a level of platelets sufficient to prevent spontaneous bleeding. However, it must be emphasized that some patients with thrombocytopenia secondary to marrow failure may tolerate platelet levels considerably lower than 20×10^9 per liter without significant hemorrhage. Blood component transfusion therapy should be used judiciously with consideration of individual need rather than according to preconceived rules of thumb. Additionally, the physician must recognize that there is a limited period of usefulness of platelet transfusion therapy, since effectiveness is invariably lost as sensitization develops with increasing numbers of transfusions. More specific information is available in the article on Therapeutic Use of Blood Components (p. 323).

It has often been observed that corticosteroids such as prednisone may decrease the tendency towards spontaneous bleeding in patients with thrombocytopenia secondary to bone marrow failure. The administration of 20 or 30 mg. of prednisone daily may ameliorate capillary oozing and purpura for a while, even though there is no rise in the level of circulating platelets. In general, it is best to maintain such patients on as small a dose as possible, and it may be preferable to administer the drug on a 48 hour schedule, such as 50 mg. of prednisone given at one time every other morning. This technique of administration tends to minimize the side effects of corticosteroid therapy while preserving whatever antihemorrhagic effect it may have. Long-term use of steroids should be avoided, however, whenever possible.

Other helpful measures to minimize spontaneous bleeding include avoiding salicylates, suppressing excessive menses with appropriate hormonal manipulation, and using water-jet tooth cleaning rather than a stiff brush.

Treatment of Infections

Patients with bone marrow failure frequently develop infections of a serious nature. Unnecessary exposure to infection must be avoided, and patients should be instructed to report to their physician if unexplained fever, sore throat, or other stigmata of infection are present. In those patients receiving prednisone therapy it may be extremely difficult to detect the presence of bacterial disease, and appropriate cultures should be obtained upon suspicion. The tendency to administer "prophylactic" antibiotics is to be deplored, since the development of infections with resistant organisms or latent fungal superinfections or both is almost inevitable. In general, it is best not to administer intramuscular therapy of any type in order to avoid the possibility of cutaneous infection or hematomas. When a bacterial organism is isolated, antibiotic sensitivities should be obtained so that appropriate therapy can be instituted promptly. Aggressive and sustained intravenous treatment is essential in order to combat sepsis in the absence of sufficient granulocytes. It is good practice to administer as few drugs as possible to patients with bone marrow failure, and patients should be cautioned against the use of any medication not specifically prescribed by the physician. If unexplained fever occurs and sound clinical judgment makes infection a likely probability, treatment with bactericidal broad-spectrum antibiotics such as gentamicin and cephalothin or carbenicillin can be initiated until the results of appropriate cultures and sensitivities are available. Prophylactic isoniazid should be administered in a dosage of 300 mg. daily if long-term corticosteroid therapy is anticipated. The role of white blood cell transfusions in treating infections associated with granulocytopenia is not sufficiently well defined nor are techniques adequately refined to recommend this procedure for routine use other than in appropriate research settings. However, granulocytes harvested with continuous-flow centrifugation or with filtration leukophoresis may provide a valuable adjuvant to antibiotic therapy.

Hormonal Stimulation of Bone Marrow Function

The impact of male hormones on the treatment of bone marrow failure is difficult to assess. Although there are occasional enthusiastic reports and examples of substantial benefit, controlled and randomized clinical trials using different dose schedules and types of androgens have provided unconvincing evidence of therapeutic success. Testosterone is frequently effective in children with marrow failure, particularly of the congenital/hereditary type, but the results in adult patients have been disappointing. Other anabolic androgenic steroids may be somewhat more effective, although the responses are inconsistent. Optimal oral doses have not been defined but it is reasonable to administer 2 to 3 mg. per kg. body weight daily of oxymetholone or 30 to 50 mg. daily of fluoxymesterone* or methandrostenolone.* Parenteral androgens are usually administered as nandrolone dacanoate, 150 to 300 mg. intramuscularly weekly or testosterone enanthate,* 300 to 600 mg. intramuscularly weekly. Oral therapy is preferred, since the intramuscular route may be associated with hematomas and skin infection. Hepatotoxicity is occasionally seen with any an-

---

*This use of these agents is not listed in the manufacturer's official directive. Doses recommended may also be higher than those listed in the manufacturer's official directive.

drogen, particularly those compounds containing a methyl group in the C17 position (oxymetholone and methandrostenolone), but this is usually mild. Acne and hirsutism may be annoying to female patients. Clearly, the potential liabilities of androgen treatment must be weighed against the possible benefit that might be achieved in patients with bone marrow failure. Treatment may have to be administered for 4 to 6 months before evidence of therapeutic benefit is observed, but prolongation beyond this time in the absence of response cannot be justified. Early improvement may be manifested by a decrease in transfusion requirement alone; a rise in hemoglobin level often lags behind, and platelets and white blood cells may never reach normal levels.

Many hematologists combine corticosteroid (prednisone) therapy with androgens in an attempt to achieve enhanced bone marrow stimulation. Although there is no convincing evidence that concomitant adminstration potentiates the therapeutic response observed with androgen alone, there may be supportive benefit, particularly when spontaneous bleeding is a clinical problem (see above) or when there is a hemolytic component to the anemia. Caution must be exercised to avoid the deleterious side effects of prednisone; doses of 20 to 30 mg. daily or 50 mg. on alternate days are probably optimal for short periods of time.

Splenectomy

For those patients in whom significant hemolysis is associated with splenomegaly or where there is evidence of selective sequestration of red blood cells in the spleen, splenectomy may be of benefit. The dangers of surgery in patients with bone marrow failure, particularly when there is an associated thrombocytopenia, cannot be overemphasized, but if the patient requires transfusions with increasing frequency in the absence of blood loss, consideration should be given to the removal of the spleen. The criteria for recommending splenectomy are difficult to delineate, and the decision must be influenced by the surgical risk and complications to be anticipated. There is some evidence that under certain conditions the spleen may actually inhibit bone marrow function, and in those patients who have responded to prednisone therapy but who cannot tolerate continued use of the drug, splenectomy may result in improvement in the peripheral blood counts. In general, however, splenectomy should be considered only when the patient has failed to respond to more conventional treatment and then only after thorough deliberation and clinical evaluation.

Bone Marrow Transplantation

Although still recognized as an experimental procedure, it is becoming increasingly clear that under appropriately selected circumstances bone marrow transplantation can achieve cure of aplastic anemia. A major deterrent to successful engraftment is donor-host histoincompatibility; this is not a problem where an identical twin is available as a source of marrow. Otherwise, HLA-identical siblings can serve as potential donors, providing the recipient-patient is "immunosuppressed" with aggressive chemotherapy or total body irradiation. The clinical effectiveness of this therapeutic approach is improving rapidly, although the technique is still fraught with considerable complexity and risk. Its exact role in the treatment of aplastic anemia is being defined in those several centers where adequate facilities and skills are available to carry out the necessary research. Of practical importance at the present time is the need for awareness on the part of practicing physicians of the availability of this procedure so as to maximize the opportunity for successful treatment in the future.

Pure Red Cell Anemia

This unusual form of bone marrow failure is occasionally observed in association with the presence of a thymoma in the upper anterior mediastinum. Since removal of the tumor may result in improved or normal erythropoiesis, it is important to examine patients with pure red cell anemia carefully for possible thymoma with chest x-rays, tomograms, and computerized tomography (CT) scans. Some patients with this hematologic disorder will demonstrate immune inhibition of erythropoiesis and may respond to immunosuppressive therapy.

Prognosis

It is commonly said that 50 per cent of patients with bone marrow failure will live for at least 2.5 years after developing their disease and that 40 per cent will live for more than 4 years. Yet it seems clear that survival depends to a considerable degree upon the severity of the marrow hypoplasia in the early stages. Those patients with less severe cytopenia usually respond better to hormonal therapy and live longer than those with more fulminant onset and profound aplasia. Overall response rates suggest that anemia can be corrected in approximately half the patients who receive aggressive hormonal and supportive therapy but that only one third will develop increased numbers of circulating white blood cells and one fourth show improvement in the platelet count.

ANEMIA DUE TO IRON DEFICIENCY

method of
EDWARD R. EICHNER, M.D.
Oklahoma City, Oklahoma

Iron deficiency is the most common cause of anemia worldwide. For infants, adolescents, and menstruating or pregnant women the most common cause of iron deficiency is the combination of normal iron losses plus increased physiologic needs for iron that exceed the limited ability of the body to absorb iron from diets often marginal in iron. In adult men and postmenopausal women, however, the most common cause of iron deficiency is blood loss, usually from the gastrointestinal tract. Bleeding in excess of 5 ml. per day will exceed the limited capacity of the intestinal mucosa to absorb dietary iron. In an adult man or older women eating a normal diet, iron deficiency anemia equates with blood loss and demands a search for the underlying lesion. This adage has been strengthened by the recent epidemiologic finding that the incidence of carcinoma of the colon arising on the "silent" right side has increased from 20 to 40 per cent.

Rare causes of iron deficiency include trapping of blood in the lung (idiopathic pulmonary hemosiderosis), the loss of hemosiderin-hemoglobin in the urine with intravascular hemolysis (paroxysmal nocturnal hemoglobinuria, heart-valve fragmentation of red cells), malabsorption of iron (diseases of the upper small intestine), and lifelong fad diets almost devoid of iron. Chronic aspirin therapy can, in some subjects, eventually cause iron deficiency anemia from the daily gastrointestinal loss of blood in amounts too small to produce guaiac-positive stools.

Oral Iron Therapy

The treatment of choice for almost all patients is oral iron therapy. The most effective and least expensive preparation for adults is ferrous sulfate as a 300 mg. tablet (contains 60 mg. of elemental iron), which rapidly disintegrates to release easily absorbable divalent iron in the stomach or duodenum. Several other ferrous salts are also satisfactory, but ferrous sulfate is the preparation of choice. For infants and children, the treatment of choice is the administration of a concentrated solution of ferrous sulfate (125 mg. of ferrous sulfate and 25 mg. of elemental iron per ml.) or ferrous sulfate syrup (40 mg. of hydrated ferrous sulfate and 8 mg. of elemental iron per ml.), in a dose of 5 mg. of elemental iron per kg. body weight per day.

Oral iron for adults is usually given as one ferrous sulfate tablet 3 times daily with or immediately after meals. To minimize gastrointestinal intolerance, begin with 1 tablet with dinner for 2 days, then add 1 tablet with lunch for another 2 days, and then add 1 tablet with breakfast. Although it has been reliably shown that iron therapy causes minor side effects (abdominal discomfort, nausea, diarrhea, constipation) more often than does a placebo, such side effects are tolerated by almost all patients, especially if the physician makes little of them. Gastrointestinal side effects vary directly with the amount of iron absorbed, and thus are less with ferrous gluconate (contains only 37 mg. of elemental iron per tablet) and far less with enteric-coated or delayed release preparations, which *should not be used* because they disintegrate unpredictably and usually fail to deliver their iron to the effective absorptive sites. Likewise, although large doses of ascorbic acid increase iron absorption, they increase side effects, may cause false-negative stool occult blood tests, and do not enhance the therapeutic effectiveness of ferrous sulfate. There is no advantage in tablets which combine ferrous sulfate with vitamin C, other vitamins, cobalt, molybdenum, or any other agent.

Patients who eat starch or clay should be encouraged to stop. Starch may, and some clays definitely do, impair absorption of iron. Further, starch eating provides empty calories, causes parotid enlargement, and can cause starch gastroliths, while clay eating can cause either hypokalemia or, in patients with chronic renal disease, life-threatening hyperkalemia. Pagophagia is a consequence, not a cause, of iron deficiency and will abate soon after iron therapy is begun.

In the final analysis, a prompt reversal of the anemia by iron confirms the diagnosis of iron deficiency anemia. The maximal reticulocyte response usually occurs 7 to 12 days after iron is begun. There is little rise in hemoglobin during the first week or so, but thereafter the rise should be 0.7 to 1 gram per dl. (100 ml.) per week in cases of severe anemia. As the hemoglobin rises, the rate of rise slows, but the anemia should be fully corrected within 2 months. Efficiency of absorption of iron falls as the hemoglobin rises, so oral iron therapy should be continued for 6 to 9 months after the hemoglobin is normal to replenish the normal body iron stores of 500 to 1000 mg. Prolonged oral iron therapy (many years) can rarely cause hemochromatosis.

A subnormal response to oral iron therapy calls for reassessment of the diagnosis. For example, the anemia of chronic disease, shown to be the most common anemia of hospital patients, does not respond to iron. Sideroblastic anemias and thalassemia minor have also been mistaken for iron deficiency anemia. Beta-thalassemia minor may coexist with iron deficiency and be masked because the diagnostic elevation of hemoglobin A_2 is missing in the face of iron deficiency. If the diagnosis of iron deficiency anemia is correct, a subnormal response to oral iron suggests the following complications: continued blood loss; underlying infection, inflammation, renal disease, liver disease, or malignancy; insufficient intake of ferrous sulfate tablets or intake of enteric-coated tablets by mistake; or, very rarely, malabsorption of iron.

Iron tablets, which resemble candy, are the second most frequent cause of serious poisoning in children, with 2000 cases annually, a mortality rate up to 45 per cent in untreated cases, and deaths having occurred with as few as 12 tablets. Acute iron intoxication, characterized by vomiting, diarrhea, melena, shock, coma, convulsions, metabolic acidosis, and bleeding, has also been seen rarely in adults who attempt suicide. Iron preparations should be kept away from children and should be in "child-proof" containers. The case has recently been made for reducing the dosage contained in standard iron tablets. Smaller tablets would mean somewhat slower repair of iron deficiency in patients but would be worthwhile if such smaller tablets meant an end of accidental, fatal poisonings of children.

It is important to remember that anemia is a sign, not a disease, and that successfully treating iron deficiency anemia does not treat the underlying cause, which in many instances is curable if found early. An example is carcinoma of the colon.

Parenteral Iron Therapy

Parenteral iron therapy is rarely required, and there are increasing reasons not to use it. It is sometimes given to avoid blood transfusions in the patient with irremediable, diffuse gastrointestinal tract bleeding from hereditary telangiectasia in whom the blood loss maintains negative iron balance despite maximal oral doses of iron. Three rare indications for parenteral iron therapy are (1) patients whose gastrointestinal disease (gastritis, enteritis) prevents their tolerating oral iron in any effective dose; (2) patients with documented malabsorption of ferrous sulfate; and (3) patients who cannot be relied upon to take oral medication.

Parenteral iron is overused. It does *not* stimulate erythropoiesis in normal, nonanemic subjects. It does *not* accelerate the reversal of anemia; studies with identical twins and with matched groups of iron deficient patients have shown identical response rates with parenteral versus oral iron therapy. Parenteral iron therapy is expensive and uncomfortable. The body does not use parenteral iron efficiently; phlebotomy studies have shown that up to 35 per cent injected remains, apparently inert and unusable, in the reticuloendothelial storage cells. Parenteral iron has caused fatal anaphylactic reactions. Intravenous iron can exacerbate rheumatoid arthritis and ankylosing spondylitis, while intramuscular iron stains the skin and occasionally causes severe delayed reactions with fever, sterile abscesses, and

regional lymphadenitis. Most important, subcutaneous or intramuscular iron dextran causes sarcomas in rodents, and a recent epidemiologic study from Britain strengthened the possible link in man between parenteral iron and sarcoma when 4 of 90 patients with sarcoma of the buttock were found to have received intramuscular iron.

Iron dextran (Imferon) is the most widely used parenteral preparation. It contains 50 mg. of elemental iron per ml. and may be given either intramuscularly or intravenously, after a 0.5 ml. dose to test for anaphylaxis. The proper technique for "Z track" intramuscular injection into the buttock is given in the package insert, as is a table for picking the correct dose. The total dose to be given can also be calculated as follows: hemoglobin deficit in grams per dl. $\times$ body weight in pounds = mg. of elemental iron necessary to correct the anemia, plus 1000 mg. of iron to replenish body stores. Iron dextran is usually given in doses of 2 to 5 ml. intramuscularly daily until the desired goal is reached, but it also can be given undiluted intravenously in doses of 2 ml. per day at a rate not exceeding 1 ml. per minute. It has also been given intravenously in a total-dose infusion, diluted in 250 to 1000 ml. of isotonic saline; however, this procedure is not yet approved in the United States.

It should be reiterated that there are few indications for parenteral iron, and, in light of the concerns about severe reactions, ultimate risk of sarcoma, and unknown long-term consequences of the fraction remaining inert in storage cells, it should be avoided whenever possible. Because of the risk of sarcoma, a recent *Medical Letter* has suggested the preferred route of administration of *iron dextran* is by slow intravenous administration, after a minute test dose.

Blood Transfusion

Blood transfusion is rarely necessary in the treatment of iron deficiency anemia. Iron deficiency anemia develops very gradually and plasma volume rises to maintain normal blood volume as red cell mass falls. Thus, hypovolemia is not a problem, and whole blood is never required, because the only indication for whole blood in clinical medicine is severe hypovolemia and shock from massive hemorrhage. The only situation in which transfusion should be considered for iron deficiency anemia is the elderly patient with a severe reduction in hemoglobin and consequent tissue hypoxia who develops angina, congestive heart failure, or cerebral dysfunction. For this patient, 1 or perhaps 2 units of packed red cells, given over 6 to 12 hours, perhaps with a diuretic, should increase the red cell mass enough to relieve the consequences of tissue hypoxia without increasing the blood volume enough to precipitate pulmonary edema. The majority of patients with even severe iron deficiency anemia, however, do not need blood transfusion, and the hazards of transfusion in such patients far outweigh any putative benefit.

HEMOLYTIC ANEMIA—IMMUNE

method of
BRUCE C. GILLILAND, M.D.
Seattle, Washington

The treatment and prognosis of immune hemolytic anemia depend on arriving at the correct diagnosis, which is largely based on serologic manifestations. Most patients with immune hemolytic anemia have a positive direct antiglobulin test. Three patterns of red cell coating are observed: IgG, IgG plus complement, or complement alone. In a few patients, IgM and IgA may also be detected with or without the presence of IgG. The complement component on the red cell most readily detected by the direct antiglobulin test is C3, which is mainly in the form of C3d (alpha 2D).

The autoantibodies responsible for these patterns of red cell sensitization are divided into warm type, cold type, and drug related. Warm type autoantibodies react optimally with the red cell at 37°C. (99°F.) and usually require a direct antiglobulin test for their demonstration. Cold type antibodies bind optimally at 0 to 4°C. and directly agglutinate red cells at reduced temperatures. The antibodies in drug-induced hemolytic anemias are most often IgG and behave as warm type antibodies.

Warm Type Autoimmune Hemolytic Anemia

Autoimmune hemolytic anemia due to warm type autoantibodies occurs in an idiopathic form or associated with other disorders such as systemic lupus erythematosus, lymphomas, or chronic inflammatory disorders. The direct antiglobulin test may show any of the above three patterns of red cell coating. Free autoantibody may be present in the serum and is detected by indirect antiglobulin test. Red cells showing only complement by conventional direct antiglobulin testing and where cold agglutinins cannot be implicated may have small amounts of cell bound IgG antibody detectable by more sensitive quantitative techniques. Thus, complement alone pattern in this circumstance is an extension of the IgG plus complement pattern with the amount of IgG being below the threshold of the usual direct Coombs' test.

A small number of patients (2 to 4 per cent) have all the clinical features of immune hemolytic anemia except for a positive antiglobulin test. Many of these patients can be shown by more sensitive quantitative techniques to have antibody on the red cell that falls below the level required for detection by the usual direct antiglobulin test.

The mechanism for destruction of IgG coated red cells with or without complement is usually by erythrophagocytosis, a process that produces spherocytes. The spleen plays a major role in the destruction and removal of IgG coated red cells. Red cells heavily coated with IgG antibodies are also destroyed in the liver.

Steroid Therapy. Glucocorticoids in doses equivalent to 40 to 60 mg. of prednisone produce marked improvement in the majority of patients. A favorable response is manifested by a decrease in red cell destruction within a few days, followed by a gradual increase of hematocrit and hemoglobin within the next 10 to 14 days. Prednisone is then reduced by 10 mg. decrements at 5 to 7 day intervals until 40 mg. is reached, at which point 5 mg. decrements are made at the above intervals. The tapering of steroids may take several months, and some patients may continue to require 5 to 15 mg. per day for suppression of disease. Some patients may reach a compensated hemolytic state that does not require prednisone, while others may go on to complete remission after several months or even years of treatment. Patients who are refractory to 40 to 60 mg. may respond to 80 to 120 mg. per day. If a patient does not show a satisfactory response to high doses of prednisone in 3 to 4 weeks, splenectomy or other forms of therapy should be contemplated. Cushingoid features in patients on less than 10 mg. of prednisone per day are usually mild and well tolerated. These features may be minimized by alternate therapy, especially in those patients requiring daily doses greater than 10 mg. of prednisone for suppression. Alternate day steroids should not be considered until the patient's hematologic picture is stabilized. In preparation for alternate day steroids, prednisone is given daily as a single morning dose. The patient is then gradually shifted to alternate day program by increasing the prednisone by 5 mg. on one day and reducing it by 5 mg. on the next day. The dose changes are made at intervals of approximately 5 to 7 days until the patient is on a single morning dose one day and none the next.

The direct Coombs' test remains positive during the first weeks of therapy. Serum (free) autoantibody, when present, usually disappears and is usually followed by a decreased titer of the direct Coombs' test. The Coombs' test remains positive in some patients even though the hematologic picture is stabilized.

Splenectomy. Splenectomy is considered when (1) little or no response to an adequate trial of steroids occurs, (2) large doses of prednisone are required for suppression of the disease, and (3) serious steroid complications develop. The purpose of splenectomy is to reduce the rate of red cell destruction. Later decreased antibody production may occur. Splenectomy often enables the patient to reduce or eventually stop prednisone. Splenectomy may be beneficial even though an increased splenic uptake of chromium-51 is not demonstrated. The benefit of splenectomy outweighs in most patients the possibility of an increased susceptibility to pneumococcal infection.

Immunosuppressive Therapy. Immunosuppressive drugs may be effective in the treatment of immune hemolytic anemia; however, they should be reserved for those patients refractory to steroids or splenectomy or both because of their potential toxicity. A favorable response to an immunosuppressive drug in a patient who is on high doses of prednisone will permit reduction of the steroid dose to an acceptable level. These drugs suppress destruction of red cells by the reticuloendothelial system and eventually decrease antibody synthesis. Commonly used cytotoxic drugs include cyclophosphamide (Cytoxan), in an adult dose of 75 to 150 mg. per day (1 to 2 mg. per kg. per day), azathioprine (Imuran), 75 to 150 mg. per day (1 to 2 mg. per kg. per day), and chlorambucil (Leukeran), 4 to 6 mg. per day. These and other immunosuppressive drugs have not been approved for use in the treatment of immune hemolytic anemia by the Food and Drug Administration. Their beneficial effects may be compromised by suppression of bone marrow function as well as other toxic effects including increased susceptibility to infection, hemorrhagic cystitis, sterility, thrombocytopenia, or leukopenia. If improvement occurs, the drug dose is reduced to the lowest possible level required for suppression of the disease. It is advisable to check the hematocrit, white blood count, and platelet count once a week. The decision to maintain a patient on long-term therapy must depend upon the severity of the hemolytic disease or underlying associated disorder.

Transfusion Therapy. Transfusion is reserved for patients with life-threatening anemia because of the increased risk of receiving incompatible blood, owing to the difficulties in cross-matching. Most patients can tolerate hematocrits in the range of 25 to 30 per cent, the exception being patients with cerebrovascular insufficiency or severe heart disease who may require careful transfusion of packed red cells. One of the problems in finding compatible blood is in identifying alloantibodies when autoantibodies are present in serum. If time does not permit an adequate search for alloan-

tibodies, then Rh phenotype-identical blood can be given. There is still the possibility of transfusion reaction occurring secondary to alloantibodies of other blood groups such as anti-K, anti-Fy^a, and others. In most instances, packed cells are preferred, especially in older patients, since the plasma volume in hemolytic anemia is usually normal. The transfused red cells are usually destroyed at the same rate as the patient's own cells.

Cold Type Autoimmune Hemolytic Anemia

Immune hemolytic anemia of the cold antibody type is divided into acute cold agglutinin disease (associated most often with mycoplasma pneumonia, or infectious mononucleosis), chronic cold agglutinin disease (associated with benign or malignant lymphoproliferative disease), and paroxysmal cold hemoglobinuria. The direct antiglobulin test shows only complement on the red cell; however, the test might be weakly positive or negative for complement due to the lack of a good antiglobulin serum or to the low density of complement on the surviving red cells. In acute disorders, the IgM cold agglutinin is polyclonal, while in the chronic disorder, the IgM is monoclonal. High titers of cold agglutinins (1:1000 or greater) are usually found in association with hemolytic anemia. Occasionally, hemolytic anemia occurs with low titers in the range of 1:100. In any event, the cold agglutinin must have the ability to fix complement to the red cell at the temperatures encountered in vivo, as the mechanism for the red cell damage in these disorders is mainly through complement hemolysis. Thus, cold agglutinins that are pathologic will have a thermal amplitude of 30 to 32°C., temperatures that are attainable in the extremities.

Paroxysmal cold hemoglobinuria is an uncommon disorder occurring in a chronic intermittent form associated with congenital syphilis or in an acute transient form most likely associated with viral infections. The cold hemolysin is termed the Donath-Landsteiner antibody, which is an IgG immunoglobulin and reacts with red cells at reduced temperatures to fix complement to the red cell.

General Measures. Cold exposure in patients often produces exacerbations of hemolysis. Prolonged cold exposure to an extremity may also lead to vascular thrombosis or even gangrene. The patient's home should be well heated and the patient should dress warmly when outdoors to protect hands, feet, and face. It is also recommended that ice packs or cold baths that are often used to reduce temperature in febrile children not be given to patients with an acute febrile illness, for example, infectious mononucleosis, unless cold antibodies have been excluded.

Therapy. Patients with cold agglutinin disease usually have little or no response to glucocorticoids, thus pointing out the importance of identifying the type of autoimmune disease. In acute cold agglutinin disease, the hemolytic anemia is usually short-lived, the only treatment required being that of the underlying disorder, cold avoidance, and transfusion only if the hematocrit falls to a dangerous level.

Patients with chronic cold agglutinin disease may maintain a compensated state at long intervals by cold avoidance. If the disease cannot be controlled then an alkylating agent such as chlorambucil (Leukeran) 4 to 6 mg. per day may be effective. (This use of chlorambucil is not listed in the manufacturer's official directive.) This results in a reduction of the IgM cold agglutinins and a decrease in the hemolysis. The beneficial effect of this drug, however, may be compromised by depression of bone marrow function. It is advisable to perform complete blood counts weekly. Even though the mode of red cell destruction in cold type antibody disease is intravascular hemolysis, some patients may benefit from splenectomy. A trial of prednisone for 2 to 3 weeks might be tried in patients refractory to other forms of therapy based on reports of favorable response in some patients. Plasmapheresis has only a short-term effect in reducing the level of cold agglutinins and is technically difficult, as the removed blood must be kept warm to prevent hemagglutination.

Transfusion. Transfusion, again, should be limited to those patients with severe degrees of anemia. Cross-matching is hindered by the cold agglutinins, which mask the presence of alloantibodies in the serum. If transfusion is necessary, blood should be given as packed red cells, and passed through a warming coil. In most instances, the transfused cells are destroyed at approximately the same rate as the patient's own cells. In some patients with chronic cold agglutinin disease, however, transfused red cells are destroyed at a faster rate than the patient's, as the patient's own red cells are protected from further complement lysis by being coated with inactive complement components which sterically block cold agglutinins from binding to the cell and activating more complement. Packed red cells are also preferred to whole blood, as whole blood might furnish complement components that have been reduced in the patient with active hemolytic anemia.

Drug-Induced Hemolytic Anemia

Several drugs produce a positive direct antiglobulin test and in some instances a hemolytic anemia. Unless a careful history is taken, drug-induced hemolytic anemia may not be suspected, because the clinical picture is identical to that seen with idiopathic immune hemolytic anemia. It is important to recognize drug-induced hemolytic anemia, because stopping the drug will usually lead to cessation of the increased red cell destruction. Four mechanisms are recognized: (1) Hapten type. Patients receiving penicillin may develop IgG antibodies specific for a penicillin metabolite. Hemolytic anemia occurs when these antipenicillin antibodies react with penicillin metabolite firmly bound to the red cell membrane. A dose of 10 to 20 million units of penicillin per day is needed to provide sufficient coating of drug on the red cells for antibodies to react. The direct Coombs test usually shows IgG on the red cell. (2) Immune complex or innocent bystander type. Drug-antidrug immune complexes may develop in patients receiving quinidine, quinine, or phenacetin. These complexes reversibly adsorb to the red cell and bind complement resulting in complement-mediated red cell destruction. The clinical presentation is usually acute intravascular hemolysis and hemoglobinuria followed at times by renal failure. The direct antiglobulin test is positive with only an anticomplement antiserum. (3) Autoimmune type. Alpha methyldopa (Aldomet) produces a positive direct antiglobulin test in 10 to 25 per cent of patients taking the drugs for 6 months or longer. Less than 1 per cent of these patients will develop hemolytic anemia. The antibodies are of the IgG type and have specificity for antigens closely related to the Rh system. Hemolytic anemia disappears within a few weeks after stopping the drug; however, the antiglobulin test may remain positive for as long as 18 months. L-dopa and structurally unrelated mefenamic acid produce a similar picture. Corticosteroid therapy may be beneficial in suppressing red cell destruction during the initial period of drug withdrawal. (4) Nonimmune type. Cephalothin alters the red cell membrane to cause uptake of plasma proteins including immunoglobulins. Hemolytic anemia is extremely rare by this mechanism. Cephalothin, however, might lead to hemolytic anemia through the hapten type mechanism.

General Comments

The need for hospitalization and reduction of activities depends on the severity of anemia or any associated disease. The underlying disease should be appropriately treated which, in some instances, results in improvement of the hemolytic anemia. Prompt treatment of intercurrent infection is important because viral or bacterial infection may cause exacerbation of anemia by increasing red cell destruction, depressing bone marrow response, or both. Because of increased red cell production, folic acid, 1 mg. three times daily, is recommended to assure an adequate bone marrow response.

HEMOLYTIC ANEMIA—NONIMMUNE

method of
ORLANDO J. MARTELO, M.D.
Cincinnati, Ohio

Hemolytic anemia refers to the premature destruction of red cells. It can occur in the extravascular or in the intravascular system. The hemolytic anemias may be classified as follows: (1) Intracorpuscular defects: Usually these anemias are hereditary and the abnormality is due to either membrane, metabolic defects, or hemoglobinopathies. (2) Extracorpuscular defects: These anemias are usually acquired and they may be classified as immune hemolytic anemias and nonimmune hemolytic anemias. The nonimmune hemolytic anemias are the subject of this discussion.

The causes of nonimmune hemolytic anemias are: (1) microangiopathic hemolytic anemia; (2) traumatic cardiac hemolytic anemia; (3) march hemoglobinuria; (4) hemolytic anemia due to infections; (5) hemolytic anemias due to chemical and physical agents; (6) spur cell anemia, and (7) hereditary spherocytosis and related disorders.

Microangiopathic Hemolytic Anemia

Hemolysis is usually intravascular and it is characterized by the presence of abnormal red blood cells in the form of schistocytes or helmet cells. Usually the hemolytic anemia results from an abnormality of the vascular endothelium of arterioles. Intravascular coagulation may be associated.

Treatment. The treatment of microangiopathic hemolytic anemia is largely dependent on the underlying disease. Thrombotic thrombocytopenic purpura may necessitate splenectomy and large doses of steroids (100 to 1000 mg. of prednisone per day) and antiplatelet drugs. There is recent evidence that exchange transfusion may be beneficial in patients with thrombotic thrombocytopenic purpura. Malignant hypertension should be treated with antihypertensive agents. Vascular abnormalities such as cavernous hemangiomata may need irradiation or removal of the hemangioma. Overwhelming infections will require the appropriate antibiotic. Microangiopathic hemolytic anemia in association with widespread metastatic malignant disease is usually unresponsive to all therapy unless the underlying malignant disease is brought under control.

Traumatic Cardiac Hemolytic Anemia

The shortened red cell survival results from traumatic rupture of red cells in the intravascular system. The majority of cases of cardiac traumatic hemolytic anemia are the result of hemolysis occurring on a prosthetic aortic valve (10 per cent of patients). Hemolytic anemia may be in a compensated state. It may also occur following insertion of a prosthetic patch in the repair of an endocardial cushion defect (ostium primum defect). Rarely, an immune hemolytic anemia has been reported in association with cardiac prosthetic devices. The severity of anemia in these patients varies. In severe calcific aortic stenosis, a moderately shortened red cell survival may be found. In some patients the hemolysis may be severe and may appear as a syndrome of intravascular hemolysis. Thus, one may find anemia with abnormalities of the red cell morphology (helmet cells, schistocytes, microspherocytes) and the evidence of intravascular hemolysis such as free plasma hemoglobin, absence of haptoglobin, hemoglobinuria, and hemosiderinuria.

Treatment. The treatment of this anemia depends on the severity. In cases due to cardiac prosthesis, the severity may necessitate reoperation and replacement. Persistent hemosiderinuria, as a result of intravascular hemolysis, may lead to depletion of iron stores. Treatment of iron deficiency may be required. Transfusion of red blood cells may be necessary in those instances in which bone marrow reserves cannot compensate for the shortened red cell survival. Corticosteroids are usually not indicated except in rare instances of immune hemolytic anemia.

March Hemoglobinuria

This type of traumatic hemolytic anemia has been reported following certain types of exercises. It usually involves long distance running on hard surfaces. Rarely, it may be found in other activities such as karate and playing of drums. In this instance, hemolysis results from direct trauma of red blood cells in small blood vessels in the arms and legs. These patients may or may not show evidences of intravascular hemolysis and the anemia may or may not be compensated.

Treatment. The treatment of this form of hemolytic anemia is predominantly that of prevention. Using certain rubberized insoles in the shoes in long distance runners may be of help. Renal failure resulting from hemoglobinuria may be prevented by alkalization of the urine.

Hemolytic Anemia Due to Infections

Malaria. Malaria is probably the most common cause of hemolytic anemia due to a microorganism. In this instance the hemolytic anemia is due to a direct destruction of parasitized red cells. Destruction occurs both intravascularly and extravascularly.

TREATMENT. The treatment of the hemolytic anemias which result from malaria is that of the underlying disease. (See malaria, p. 37.)

Bartonellosis. *Bartonella bacilliformis* is a flagellated bacillus that can produce an acute severe hemolytic anemia. This type of infection occurs frequently in Peru, where it is transmitted by a sandfly and probably by other arthropods. The disease is also called Oroya fever. Aside from systemic symptoms such as myalgias, fever, and chills, an acute extravascular hemolysis may be present. Diagnosis is usually made by examination of a Wright-stained blood smear.

TREATMENT. Oroya fever responds dramatically to a number of antibiotics including tetracycline and chloramphenicol. Chloramphenicol, in a dosage of 2 grams per day for 7 days, is probably the preferred form of treatment because *Salmonella* infections frequently are found in association with bartonellosis. Transfusions of red blood cells may be needed in certain severe cases of hemolysis. Insect repellent should be used in endemic areas to prevent the bite of the infecting sandfly.

Clostridium Welchii Infection (C. perfringens). This type of septicemia occurs frequently after incomplete abortions induced under nonsterile conditions. The organisms damage the endometrium and gain access to the blood stream.

TREATMENT. Therapy for septic abortion from *C. perfringens* consists of antibiotics and uterine curettage. The role of hysterectomy in this situation is controversial.

Hemolysis Due to Other Bacterial Infections. In a few cases of hemolytic anemia, other bacterial infections have been encountered. Other organisms responsible have been streptococci, staphylococci, pneumococci, and meningococci.

Hemolytic anemia has also been reported in association with some gram-negative bacillary infections. Evidence of acute intravascular hemolysis has been reported in patients with typhoid fever and cholera.

Hemolytic Anemias Due to Chemical and Physical Agents

Patients who have defects in the hexose monophosphate shunt pathway are especially vulnerable to drug-induced oxidative injury to hemoglobin. Certain oxidant drugs result in oxidization and denaturation of hemoglobin with precipitation of the degraded hemoglobin in clumps called Heinz bodies. These bodies adhere to the red cell membrane, leading to decreased deformability of red cells and increased membrane leakiness of cations.

The drugs which have commonly been implicated in causing hemolysis in glucose-6-phosphate dehydrogenase (G-6-PD) deficiency are as follows: (1) antimalarials, (2) analgesics, (3) sulfonamides, (4) nitrofurans, (5) the sulfones, and (6) other drugs such as vitamin K, methylene blue, and ascorbic acid. Infections have also been implicated in producing hemolysis in patients with G-6-PD deficiency. Presumably, in this instance, generation of superoxide and hydrogen peroxide from macrophages-bacterial interaction results in damage to red cells.

Other chemicals that may lead to hemolysis by nonoxidative mechanisms include arsine, copper sulfate, lead, chloramine, chlorates, and hydroxyamines. The accidental infusion of distilled water (<0.5 liter) into the blood stream during transurethral resection of the prostate may result in massive intravascular hemolysis.

Hemolytic anemias have also been reported in patients with burns. Hemolysis may be intravascular. Presence of hemolysis is related to the percentage of burned body surface. The hemolysis in cases of thermal injury probably results from a direct effect of temperature on erythrocytes of tissues burned. The treatment of these patients consists of the general management of burned patients. Besides this, certain measures such as hydration, transfusion of red cells, and osmotic diuresis should be provided in those patients with acute intravascular hemolysis to prevent acute renal failure.

Hemolytic Anemia Resulting from Abnormal Lipid Composition of Red Cells

Two types of morphologic abnormalities of red cells may be associated with abnormal lipid composition of the red cells—target cells and acanthocytes.

Patients with liver disease and biliary obstruction often have circulating target red cells. These red cells accumulate excess cholesterol and phospholipid from the abnormal serum lipoproteins. Specific treatment is rarely indicated for the treatment of this type of disorder since it is associated with little clinical morbidity.

Acanthocytes, or spur cells, may also occur in patients with severe hepatocellular disease and in patients with vitamin E deficiency and abetalipoproteinemia. The treatment of this type of severe hemolytic anemia is that of the underlying hepatocellular disease. Splenectomy may be of value in certain patients who may be able to tolerate the procedure. Vitamin E supplements will be indicated in those patients who develop this deficiency due to a malabsorptive process. The recommended dietary allowance for vitamin E in adults is 12 to 15 I.U. per day.

Hereditary Spherocytosis and Related Disorders

Hereditary spherocytosis (HS) is a relatively common hemolytic anemia that affects about 20 per 100,000 population in the United States. The disease is inherited as an autosomal dominant.

The underlying defect in hereditary spherocytosis is a poorly understood membrane abnormality that leads to increased osmotic fragility of red cells. The defective red cell membrane is abnormally permeable to sodium. To compensate for this increased leakage of sodium into the cell, the cell increases its metabolism for sodium extrusion but this requires more adenosine triphosphate for energy. Favorable conditions for more adenosine triphosphate generation are not found in organs such as the spleen, through which the cell must navigate. As the result, the cells are destroyed prematurely in the spleen.

The treatment of choice for hereditary spherocytosis is splenectomy, which halts the shortened red cell survival but not the underlying membrane abnormality. Splenectomy may increase susceptibility of some of these patients to sepsis with pneumococci and other organisms. Therefore, this procedure should be avoided in children less than 4 years of age.

Hereditary elliptocytosis is a similar disorder that leads to a mild hemolytic anemia and reticulocytosis. Overt hemolysis is rare. The hemolytic anemia is predominantly in the extravascular system. This disease is also thought to be due to a membrane defect. These patients have also been reported to benefit from splenectomy.

Patients with low serum phosphorus (less than 0.1 mg. per dl.) may also show a severe spherocytic hemolytic anemia with reticulocytosis. In this case the hemolysis results from increased rigidity of the red cells. The treatment of choice is the use of parenteral phosphate administration.

MACROCYTIC (MEGALOBLASTIC) ANEMIA

(Other than Pernicious Anemia)

method of
MARIA DA COSTA, M.D., and
SHELDON P. ROTHENBERG, M.D.
New York, New York

The proper management of a patient with megaloblastic anemia requires (1) the determination of the specific cause (of the anemia) and institution of specific therapy; and (2) the identification and correction, if possible, of the underlying mechanism(s) responsible for the disorder.

Megaloblastic anemia occurs whenever there is impairment of DNA synthesis and disordered replication of hematopoietic cells. The resulting morphologic changes, recognized as megaloblastic maturation, affect the erythroid, myeloid, and megakaryocytic cell lines and produce corresponding abnormalities in the peripheral blood cells, viz., anemia with macrocytosis, leukopenia with hypersegmented polymorphonuclear leukocytes, and thrombocytopenia with abnormal platelets. These features are common to all megaloblastic anemias regardless of the cause.

Though more than 95 per cent of megaloblastic anemias are due to either vitamin B_{12} or folic acid deficiency and are easily corrected by replacing the deficient vitamin, the specific cause of the anemia must be established, not only to identify the small percentage of cases not caused by either of these vitamin deficiencies, but because failure to institute specific therapy may be harmful to the patient. Thus, the anemia of vitamin B_{12} deficiency may respond to pharmacologic doses of folic acid, but the neurologic symptoms will progress and ultimately be irreversible unless vitamin B_{12} is administered. The mechanism of the deficiency is determined in order to correct it if possible, and if not, to ensure that the patient receives life-long treatment.

Knowledge of the physiology and metabolism of these vitamins is necessary to understand the clinical manifestations of the deficiency states and appropriately investigate the causative mechanisms.

Vitamin B_{12}, or cyanocobalamin, is synthesized by microorganisms which are the sole source of the natural vitamin. Animals depend on microbial synthesis for their supply of vitamin B_{12}, which is completely absent from the plant-life kingdom. Dietary sources of vitamin B_{12} are meat, particularly organ meats, shellfish, fish, and, to a lesser extent, milk and milk products.

The minimal daily requirement of vitamin B_{12} is 0.1 microgram in normal subjects. The recommended daily intake (FAO/WHO) is 2 micrograms for normal adults and 3 micrograms daily during pregnancy and lactation. Total stores of the vitamin are 2000 to 5000 micrograms and there is an obligatory daily loss of 0.1 to 1 microgram per day. The average western diet contains 5 to 30 micrograms of vitamin B_{12}, of which 2 to 5 micrograms are absorbed so that nutritional vitamin B_{12} deficiency does not occur unless there is severe restriction of animal products.

Ingested vitamin B_{12} is cleaved from its polypeptide linkages by peptide digestion in the stomach, and the free vitamin is coupled to intrinsic factor (IF) secreted by the parietal cells of the stomach. The IF-B_{12} complex must then transit the entire small intestine to reach the terminal 100 cm. of the ileum, where absorption occurs. In the presence of calcium ions and at a pH greater than 6.0, the IF-B_{12} complex attaches to specific receptors on the ileal mucosa. Somewhere during the transepithelial transport, the vitamin B_{12} separates from the IF and enters the portal blood, where it is bound primarily to a carrier protein called transcobalamin II. This transport protein is necessary to affect delivery and uptake of vitamin B_{12} by all tissues and cells. Any abnormality in this complex mechanism of intestinal transit, mucosal absorption or plasma transport could result in vitamin B_{12} deficiency.

Thus, the major causes of vitamin B_{12} deficiency are:

1. Dietary insufficiency. This is rare except in vegans or when intake of animal protein is very limited.

2. Malabsorption of vitamin B_{12}. This may be due to lack of gastric intrinsic factor, which may be secondary to atrophic gastritis and gastric atrophy which results in the classical addisonian pernicious anemia; surgical gastrectomy or infiltrative diseases of the stomach mucosa; or congenital lack of intrinsic factor secretion or the secretion of an abnormal intrinsic factor with otherwise normal stomach function.

It may also be caused by diseases affecting the terminal ileum, such as regional enteritis, ileal tuberculosis, or other granulomatosis or infiltrative disease of the terminal ileum; tropical or nontropical sprue; or ileal resection or ileal bypass surgery.

Rare causes of vitamin B_{12} deficiency are lack of IF-B_{12} receptors on the ileal mucosa (speculative); chronic pancreatic insufficiency; acid pH in the ileum, as may occur in the Zollinger-Ellison syndrome; and congenital or selective malabsorption of vitamin B_{12} with normal IF secretion (Imerslund-Gräsbeck syndrome).

3. Competitive utilization of vitamin B_{12} in the intestine by fish tapeworm (*Diphyllobothrium latum*) infestation or bacterial overgrowth (blind loop syndrome, intestinal diverticuli and strictures).

4. Congenital absence of transcobalamin II.

5. Drugs which depress vitamin B_{12} absorption, such as *para*-aminosalicylic acid (PAS) or colchicine.

Folic acid, unlike vitamin B_{12}, is present in nearly all natural foods. Sources rich in folate are yeast, liver, green vegetables, and fresh fruits. The naturally occurring food folates occur as polyglutamates and must be deconjugated to mono- and diglutamates by intestinal carboxypeptidase before they can be absorbed. The folates are highly susceptible to oxidative destruction and prolonged boiling or canning may destroy 95 per cent of the folate content of food.

The minimal daily requirement of folate is 50 micrograms for adults. This requirement is increased whenever there is an increase in the metabolic rate or when cell turnover is increased as in hemolytic anemias, or during periods of rapid body growth. Total body stores are approximately 10 to 15 mg., and these may be depleted in 12 to 20 weeks when folate intake is inadequate. The recommended daily intake of folate is 200 micrograms in adults, 100 micrograms in children, and 400 micrograms during pregnancy and lactation. The average diet contains 500 micrograms of available folate.

Folate is absorbed primarily in the proximal third of the small intestine after deconjugation of the polyglutamates by enzymes closely associated with the epithelial mucosa.

The major causes of folate deficiency are:

1. Nutritional: inadequate diet due to poverty, ignorance, and improper preparation of food; chronic alcoholism; or increased requirements as with pregnancy, lactation, infancy, increased cell turnover as in chronic hemolysis, myeloproliferative disorders, malignancies, and skin diseases.

2. Malabsorption: tropical sprue; nontropical sprue; specific congenital malabsorption for folates (rare); drugs or chemicals that may interfere with intestinal absorption (alcohol, phenytoin [Dilantin], barbiturates, cycloserine, oral contraceptives).

3. Antifolate drugs (such as methotrexate, triamterene, trimethoprim).

Rare causes of megaloblastic anemia not due to vitamin B_{12} or folic acid deficiency are:

1. Inborn errors: hereditary orotic aciduria or formimino transferase deficiency.

2. Drugs that inhibit other pathways of DNA synthesis or drugs that alter the structure of DNA, such as the chemotherapeutic agents used to treat cancer.

3. DiGuglielmo's syndrome, refractory anemia, and sideroblastic anemias (some may have associated folate deficiency because of increased turnover).

It should be appreciated that the overwhelming majority of megaloblastic anemias are due to vitamin B_{12} or folate deficiency, and when the diagnosis of megaloblastic anemia is confirmed by the characteristic peripheral blood and bone marrow changes, the patient should be evaluated for one or both of these deficiencies.

The simplest way to establish the deficiency is to obtain blood levels of the vitamins; however, several clinical signs and symptoms make one or other deficiency more likely. Thus, the additional presence of central nervous system neurologic defects, such as posterior and lateral column lesions, is pathognomonic of vitamin B_{12} deficiency. Minimal symptoms associated with moderate or severe anemia are more likely to be due to vitamin B_{12} deficiency because it takes several years to deplete the body stores of vitamin B_{12} and the anemia, therefore, develops slowly. With folate deficiency, the patient is frequently more symptomatic for the same degree of anemia, which develops more rapidly and is usually associated with an obvious underlying disease process.

Serum vitamin B_{12} of less than 200 picograms per ml. by radioisotope dilution assay and less than 100 to 150 picograms per ml. by microbiologic assay is usually diagnostic of vitamin B_{12} deficiency.

A low serum folate may not, however, indicate folate deficiency. Serum folate is more sensitive to dietary intake and may decrease before tissue stores are depleted. Normal serum folate is greater than 4 nanograms per ml. and red cell folate is greater than 140 nanograms per ml. Decreased red cell folate is usually diagnostic of folate deficiency except in vitamin B_{12} deficiency when the red cell folate may also be low. In this instance, however, the serum folate is usually normal or high unless there is concomitant folate deficiency.

When vitamin B_{12} deficiency is diagnosed by its clinical manifestations and confirmed by a low serum vitamin B_{12} concentration, the next step is to determine the cause of the deficiency. Addisonian pernicious anemia is the most frequent of the vitamin B_{12} deficiencies.

If vitamin B_{12} deficiency is not caused by pernicious anemia, other causes must be sought. These are often quite obvious from the history and physical examination, and radiologic examination of the stomach and small bowel will very often disclose the mechanisms for the impaired absorption. If an anatomic lesion is not present and a Schilling test confirms the presence of malabsorption not corrected by intrinsic factor, further evaluation for a malabsorption syndrome including an intestinal biopsy may be necessary.

When vitamin B_{12} deficiency is diagnosed, treatment consists of (1) administration of vitamin B_{12} to provide the daily requirements of 1 to 3 micrograms; (2) replenishment of the total stores which contain 2.5 to 5.0 mg.; (3) correction of the cause of the deficiency; and (4) maintenance of therapy for the life of the patient if the cause of the malabsorption cannot be corrected.

Except in dietary vitamin B_{12} deficiency, therapy consists of parenteral vitamin B_{12} administration. Many regimens are used to treat vitamin B_{12} deficiency. A patient with vitamin B_{12} deficiency will partially respond hematologically to as little as 0.1 microgram of vitamin B_{12} daily with a reticulocyte response evident in 5 to 6 days. This is the final proof that the patient is indeed vitamin B_{12} deficient and this therapeutic response may also be used as a test for vitamin B_{12} deficiency in patients in whom no other studies are available.

When treating the patient, it must be remembered that vitamin B_{12} not bound to serum transcobalamin is rapidly excreted in the urine, hence frequent doses must be administered initially to saturate tissue stores. In practice, we recommend (1) 1000 micrograms of vitamin B_{12} injected intramuscularly daily or 2 to 3 times a week as convenient for a total of 10 to 14 doses. If neurologic symptoms are present, this initial intensive therapy is prolonged for 3 or 4 weeks; and (2) 1000 micrograms of vitamin B_{12} is given intramuscularly at 1 to 3 month intervals for the lifetime of the patient. This depends on the discretion of the physician and the reliability of the patient to return for therapy. Thirty micrograms of retained vitamin B_{12} per month is all that is theoretically required to maintain normal stores of this vitamin.

Children with congenital transcobalamin II deficiency require frequent injections of 1000 micrograms (approximately weekly).

Intestinal diseases such as sprue syndromes or regional ileitis should be appropriately treated.

Folate deficiency is treated by the administration of folic acid. Anemia due to folate deficiency will respond to 50 micrograms of folic acid with a reticulocyte response, and this can be used as both a diagnostic and therapeutic measure. We recommend parenteral folic acid only initially to replete tissue stores, and this requires a total retained amount of 10 to 15 mg. Parenteral folic acid is then seldom required, even in malabsorption, because the synthetic folic acid, which is available commercially for treatment, is a monoglutamate, and even in the presence of intestinal malabsorption it can be sufficiently absorbed to maintain the remission. Where the compliance of the patient to continued oral medication is poor, we have used monthly folic acid injection (10 to 15 mg.) to prevent recurrence of the deficiency.

If stores are to be replenished by oral therapy alone, we recommend 5 mg. daily given for 2 to 3 months after the anemia is corrected. Maintenance therapy then requires a daily supplement of 0.5 to 1.0 mg. This supplement may be given where there is increased need for folate as occurs in pregnancy, lactation, infancy, and where dietary intake is only marginally adequate. If the nutritional or intestinal disorder that resulted in the folate deficiency is corrected, life-long therapy with supplemental oral folic acid will not be required.

If vitamin B_{12} deficiency has not been excluded as the cause of the megaloblastic anemia, the patient should be treated with no more than 200 micrograms of folic acid daily because vitamin B_{12} deficiency, which responds to pharmacologic doses of folic acid, will not respond to this dose, while there will be a complete therapeutic response in folic acid deficiency.

Blood transfusions are indicated only if anemia is producing symptoms of hypoxia in a vital organ system, e.g., angina, dyspnea, or cerebrovascular insufficiency. Packed red blood cells should be used to raise the hematocrit sufficiently to correct the symptoms. If the patient is in congestive cardiac failure, the packed erythrocyte transfusion should be accompanied by phlebotomies of an equal volume of blood to decrease plasma volume and prevent further circulatory overload.

It may occasionally be necessary to treat a patient with a megaloblastic anemia who is critically ill with pancytopenia, using a combination of vitamin B_{12} and folic acid, before the cause of the megaloblastosis can be determined. Such emergency therapy is indicated if the patient is leukopenic (WBC is less than 3000 per cu. mm.) and has a serious infection or if there is thrombocytopenia (platelet count is less than 50,000 per cu. mm.) with associated bleeding or both. Severe symptomatic anemia alone can be treated with packed cell transfusions and specific therapy can then await the diagnosis. When immediate therapy is necessary, blood samples should first be obtained for vitamin B_{12} and folic acid assays, and then the patient is treated with parenteral vitamin B_{12} (1000 micrograms) and folic acid (15 mg.). There should also be appropriate treatment of any associated illness. This will be sufficient to affect a remission of the megaloblastosis, and further administration of either or both vitamins can then be continued after the results of the diagnostic studies have been obtained.

The treatment of megaloblastic anemia other than vitamin B_{12} and folic acid deficiency depends on the cause. The clinical manifestations of hereditary orotic aciduria responds to oral uridine or cytidine or both.

The megaloblastosis of DiGuglielmo's syndrome, refractory anemia and sideroblastic anemias do not specifically respond to vitamin B_{12} or folic acid unless there is also concomitant deficiency of either vitamin that can be demonstrated by serum and red cell assays.

PERNICIOUS ANEMIA AND OTHER FORMS OF VITAMIN B₁₂ DEFICIENCY

method of
JACK METZ, M.D.
Johannesburg, South Africa

The vast majority of the megaloblastic anemias are the result of deficiency of either vitamin B_{12} or folate. Pernicious anemia is a form of megaloblastic anemia resulting from vitamin B_{12} deficiency, and all the clinical features of the disease can be ascribed to deficiency of this vitamin. Administration of vitamin B_{12} is complete therapy for the *uncomplicated* disease. As the underlying cause of the vitamin B_{12} deficiency cannot be corrected, therapy is life-long, and the patient should be informed that therapy must never be stopped.

It is of paramount importance that steps be taken to enable the nature of the anemia to be established before instituting therapy. This includes the drawing of blood samples for blood count and assay of vitamin B_{12} and folate levels, and obtaining a bone marrow aspirate. Ideally, specific therapy should be delayed until the blood levels of vitamin B_{12} and folate are known, and with modern radioisotope dilution techniques the results of such assays need not delay therapy for more than a day or two. However, in the severely anemic patient, particularly if elderly, and in patients with cardiac decompensation, treatment is begun immediately after obtaining blood and marrow samples. Situations requiring immediate therapy are discussed below in greater detail.

Vitamin B₁₂ Therapy

The aim of therapy is to restore the blood picture and vitamin B_{12} nutrition to normal, and maintain this state throughout life. Repletion of vitamin B_{12} stores is achieved by administering relatively large doses of the vitamin in excess of those required to restore the blood picture to normal.

Available Preparations, Route of Administration, and Dosage. Hydroxycobalamin is preferred to cyanocobalamin because it is retained better in the body, and is thus more effective in restoring and maintaining vitamin B_{12} nutrition. However, hydroxycobalamin is not freely available in many countries, in which case cyanocobalamin is used. Depot preparations of vitamin B$_{12}$ have little real advantage, and liver extracts and combinations of vitamin B$_{12}$ and intrinsic factor, have no place in therapy.

Vitamin B$_{12}$ should be given by injection, rather than by mouth, because of greater reliability and less cost. Only in patients who refuse injections, develop sensitivity reactions to the injected vitamin, or have an unrelated bleeding disorder is the oral route justified.

There is much latitude in the dosage of vitamin B$_{12}$, but it is better to err towards doses in excess of body needs than to run the risk of treating with suboptimal doses. In practice, a single regimen is employed for *all* patients. The following regimen fulfills the aims of therapy.

Vitamin B$_{12}$, 1000 micrograms by intramuscular injection 3 times per week for 2 weeks, followed by maintenance therapy of 500 micrograms every 2 months, for life. The total of 6000 micrograms vitamin B$_{12}$ administered during the initial 2 weeks of therapy contributes significantly towards the repletion of body stores and is more than adequate to induce hematologic remission. In patients who cannot attend regularly for injections, maintenance can be given as six injections of 1000 micrograms of vitamin B$_{12}$ spread over a 2-week period once per year. In the rare pernicious anemia patient in whom vitamin B$_{12}$ must be given orally, initial dosage should be 1000 micrograms per day, followed by maintenance therapy of 300 to 500 micrograms daily.

Monitoring the Response to Therapy. In the patient with pernicious anemia in relapse, treatment with vitamin B$_{12}$ produces an increase in well-being before hematologic changes are recognizable. The serum iron value falls within the first 48 hours, and the bone marrow becomes normoblastic by day 3. Reticulocytes reach a peak by day 5 to 7 and the hemoglobin and red cell count returns to normal within 6 to 12 weeks of commencing therapy.

It is essential that the initial response to treatment is monitored as follows:

1. Daily reticulocyte counts for the first 10 days.

2. Daily determinations of serum potassium for the first 4 days. In some patients, hypokalemia occurs in the first few days after instituting vitamin B$_{12}$ therapy. Potassium in a dose of 40 mEq. per day should be administered promptly to patients manifesting hypokalemia. Patients receiving diuretics for cardiac decompensation, should be given potassium supplements prophylactically during the first few days of vitamin B$_{12}$ treatment.

3. Weekly determination of the hemoglobin concentration and red cell count until these values return to normal.

Absence of reticulocytosis and failure of the hemoglobin value and red cell count to rise after adequate vitamin B$_{12}$ therapy is usually the result of incorrect diagnosis. A suboptimal response, i.e., poor reticulocytosis, and failure of the hemoglobin value and red cell count to reach normal levels are usually indicative of the presence of accompanying disease such as infection, renal disease, thyroid disease, malignant disease (particularly carcinoma of the stomach), rheumatoid arthritis, cardiac failure, or iron deficiency.

Once hematologic remission has been achieved, all patients should undergo tests of vitamin B$_{12}$ absorption (Schilling test with and without intrinsic factor) to confirm the diagnosis of pernicious anemia or reveal some other cause of vitamin B$_{12}$ deficiency.

Careful supervision of maintenance therapy must be exercised throughout the patient's life. The hematocrit and neurologic status are checked at 4-month intervals, as are any symptoms that may herald the development of carcinoma of the stomach. In the rare patient receiving vitamin B$_{12}$ by mouth, closer supervision is required.

Patient with Cardiac Decompensation

Although the megaloblastic anemias are eminently treatable diseases, there remains an appreciable mortality. In hospitalized patients the mortality is of the order of 4 per cent, and in severely anemic patients (hematocrit less than 25 per cent) the figure may be as high as 14 per cent. The mortality rate is directly related to age. More than half the fatalities occur within one week of hospitalization, and one third are sudden and unexpected. More than three quarters of fatal cases show evidence of congestive cardiac failure. In patients with evidence of cardiac decompensation, conventional therapy for cardiac failure is instituted. When anemia is severe, the cardiac decompensation may be aggravated by the low level of hemoglobin, and blood transfusion may be lifesaving. Blood transfusion is a hazardous procedure in the severely anemic patient, for it may readily induce circulatory overload with a fatal outcome. Fortunately, in most patients with pernicious anemia blood transfusion is unnecessary and should be avoided.

Severe anemia per se is not an indication for transfusion, but the presence of circulatory collapse, cardiac failure with pulmonary congestion and dyspnea at rest, or severe intractable angina are situations requiring immediate transfusion. The patient should be propped up in bed and a diuretic (furosemide 40 mg.) administered. Packed cells (never whole blood) in a volume not exceeding 250 ml. should be administered *slowly* over a period of 4 to 6 hours. If there is severe congestive failure, some 100 ml. blood should be withdrawn from the other arm, so that the patient receives a partial exchange transfusion. During the transfusion, signs of circulatory overload such as increase in jugular venous pressure, restlessness, cough, and moist sounds at the lung bases are monitored.

In severely anemic patients with cardiac decompensation or with bleeding or severe thrombocytopenia the institution of vitamin therapy cannot wait for the establishment of the nature of the underlying deficiency. Immediate therapy should consist of vitamin B_{12} 1000 micrograms by injection, and folic acid 15 mg. by mouth. The latter is given in case the megaloblastic anemia of undiagnosed cause is due to folate and not vitamin B_{12} deficiency. Folic acid *alone* should never be administered to a patient with megaloblastic anemia in whom the underlying deficiency has not been established. However, there is no evidence that folic acid is harmful to patients with vitamin B_{12} deficiency when administered together with adequate doses of vitamin B_{12}.

In pernicious anemia, leukopenia and thrombocytopenia are common. Occasionally, the thrombocytopenia is so profound that bleeding ensues, and in these patients platelet transfusions should be given as a matter of urgency.

Patients with Subacute Combined Degeneration of the Spinal Cord

In patients with neurologic complications, physiotherapy should be given, and the patient gotten out of bed as soon as the physical condition permits. Higher doses of vitamin B_{12} have been administered to patients with neurologic complications, but there is no evidence that such doses are more effective than those cited in the regimen for uncomplicated pernicious anemia. The response of the neurologic complications to vitamin B_{12} therapy is inconstant and unpredictable and is related to the duration of the process. In all patients the progress of the neurologic disease is arrested; almost all patients show some improvement, but response to therapy is usually very slow. Improvement may continue for months, but little further improvement can be anticipated after 6 months' therapy.

Patients with Infection

Pulmonary or urinary infection is not uncommon in patients with pernicious anemia. In one third of fatal cases of megaloblastic anemia, pneumonia is found at autopsy. These infective complications should be treated with suitable antibiotics, but sulfamethoxazole-trimethoprim preparations are contraindicated in patients with untreated vitamin B_{12} deficiency, due to the antifo-

late activity of the latter drug. Higher doses of vitamin B_{12} are required by patients with active infection.

THALASSEMIA

method of
RICHARD D. PROPPER, M.D.
Boston, Massachusetts

The thalassemias are a group of inherited disorders of hemoglobin synthesis characterized by defects in the rate of synthesis of one or more of the globin chains. To understand the thalassemias, it is necessary to grasp the ramifications of the globin chain synthesis imbalance. In the production of normal red cells approximately equal numbers of alpha and nonalpha ($\beta + \delta + \gamma$) globin chains are produced. Subsequent incorporation of the heme moiety to produce hemoglobin yields a normal well-hemoglobinized homogeneous red cell. An imbalanced decrease in either alpha or nonalpha chain synthesis has two ramifications. First, there are fewer completed complimentary pairs of globin chains produced per cell, which leads to a decrease in intracellular hemoglobin concentration. If the defect is severe enough, the developing red cell destructs while still in the bone marrow, leading to tremendous ineffective erythropoiesis. Even cells that have enough hemoglobin to survive intramedullary maturation are still poorly hemoglobinized by normal standards. In addition, these red cells are further handicapped because the unbalanced chain synthesis has led to a relative excess of one of the globin chains. These chains, unable to find a complimentary chain with which to pair, eventually form aggregates with themselves. These aggregates are variably soluble and often produce large intracellular inclusions, which are pathologic in and of themselves. They may attach to the cell membrane and cause a decrease in deformability; they may act as an oxidant stress and cause irreversible membrane damage; they may mediate reticuloendothelial destruction of the cell in the spleen.

The basic pathophysiology of the thalassemias relates to the interaction of these various parameters. The beta thalassemias, so called because of the decreased synthesis of a gene product (β^+) or the complete absence of synthesis of a gene product (β^0), can be divided into the heterozygous state (thalassemia minor) and the homozygous state (thalassemia major). The heterozygous state, as is true in most genetic disorders, is a non-disease, being limited to a mild asymptomatic hypochromic microcytic anemia. It is most easily differentiated from mild iron deficiency anemia by its hemoglobin electrophoretic pattern, which usually demonstrates a pathognomonic increase in hemoglobin A_2 to a level of 3 to 5 per cent of total hemoglobin (twice normal). The homozygous condition is referred to as Cooley's anemia archaically or beta thalassemia major and will be addressed here.

The alpha thalassemias have received less acclaim, primarily because of their genetics and the lethal presentation of the pure homozygous state. There seem to be four loci for the alpha gene, at least in Caucasians, and therefore a more significant genetic defect is needed to produce overt pathology. One- and two-gene product defects are compatible with life and generally lead only to mild anemia. The homozygous state, on the other hand, leads to hydrops fetalis in the neonate and a nonviable infant. The rare three-gene deletion produces hemoglobin H disease, a severe, often transfusion-dependent anemia. The alpha-thalassemias are of clinical importance in this country primarily because they usually present as hypochromic microcytic anemias which are easily confused with iron deficiency anemia.

Historical Pathophysiology of Beta-Thalassemia Major

Thalassemia major can be detected in utero but classically presents in the young infant only when the normal physiologic anemia of the newborn fails to resolve at age 3 months and actually continues to become progressively more severe. In the untreated patient, hematocrits may fall to 8 or 9 per cent, or even lower, before stabilizing. The spleen and liver enlarge and the medullary cortices of the marrow-containing bones expand tremendously as the marrow strains to compensate for the severe anemia. The cells that do manage to survive long enough to reach the circulation represent the cream of the crop and yet are markedly hypochromic and microcytic, often nucleated, and contain numerous inclusion bodies. As a result, red-cell lifespan can often be measured in hours, and the anemia persists despite the marked marrow erythropoiesis. The anemia, therefore, evokes two sets of reactions. The first is merely an accentuation of the normal physiologic response to anemia, namely marrow expansion and increased gastrointestinal absorption of iron. The gross marrow expansion and concurrent thinning of the cortices cause marked deformity of the bones and a propensity for pathologic fractures. In addition, the increased metabolic requirements of the marrow are insatiable and are met by a shunting of blood to this organ that can amount to as much as 40 per cent of the total cardiac output. This increase in cardiac work load compounds the myocardium's already limited ability to cope with the severe anemia and often leads to severe congestive heart failure. In addition, most thalassemic patients develop a high degree of hypersplenism over time, as the spleen is called upon excessively to remove abnormal red cells from the circulation. This, in turn, accentuates the anemia and the vicious cycle usually proves fatal in the untreated patient before age 7. The stunting of growth and severe infections that historically accompany the disease are probably secondary to the decreased level of activity and to the chronic hypoxia which are characteristics of this disease.

The excessive gastrointestinal absorption of iron that accompanies the severe anemia may reach 8 to 10 mg. per day and will, in itself, cause problems in patients fortunate enough to live into their teens.

Historically, treatment has consisted of intermittent transfusions of whole blood or packed red cells to ameliorate the problems associated with the severe anemia. However, the therapy itself inadvertently hastens the development of severe iron overload. As iron is deposited in excess throughout the body, endocrine failure ensues. It is manifested most frequently by diabetes mellitus and hypoparathyroidism or by delay or absence of development of secondary sexual characteristics. Iron deposition in the liver characteristically leads to hepatic fibrosis and eventually can even cause cirrhosis. However, the slowly progressive liver pathology is usually overshadowed by the onset of severe cardiac problems. Death is usually cardiac in nature, either secondary to resistant congestive failure or intractable arrhythmia. Life expectancy, until recently, has ranged from 14 to 22 years.

Treatment

The treatment of thalassemia major has, historically, focused on maintenance of hematocrits at levels that permitted relatively normal functioning for 15 to 18 years. Recently, advances on a number of fronts have dramatically altered therapeutic regimens and attempts at totally controlling the overt pathology are encouraging enough to begin to think in terms of a prolonged life expectancy. The therapy discussed here is not yet universally accepted as optimal, but most experts agree that it should be employed wherever practical. The therapy demands: (1) a supertransfusion regimen to persistently inhibit intrinsic hematopoiesis, (2) control of iron overload with chronic subcutaneous deferoxamine chelation, (3) splenectomy when indicated to reduce hypersplenism, and (4) control of infections in splenectomized patients.

Supertransfusion. Supertransfusion, the maintenance of hematocrits above 36 per cent at all times, has replaced the old "high" transfusion regimen (maintenance of a *mean* hematocrit of 33 per cent) as the regimen of choice. The advantages of this regimen are numerous. First, continual maintenance of hematocrits in the normal range permits normal daily functioning and activity level as well as normal growth and development in the early years. Bony pathologic changes are completely avoided, as there is no stimulus for marrow expansion. This leads to normalization of blood volume, which in turn decreases cardiac work and, not surprisingly, transfusion requirements. In addition, it has been demonstrated that maintenance of normal hematocrits has a direct effect on decreasing the rate of gastrointestinal iron absorption to normal, further helping to ameliorate the problems associated with iron overload. To effect these changes, a transfusion schedule of approximately 1 unit of washed frozen packed cells for each 5 years of age every 4 to 5 weeks is required. One can demonstrate that such a regimen is actually more "iron-sparing" than less vigorous regimens and is associated with maintenance of an entirely "normal" life style. Present research is focusing on methods of obtaining units of primarily young red cells ("neocytes") from normal donors in order to increase mean red cell survival and further decrease transfusion requirements. Supertransfusion alone will decrease net daily total iron accumulation to less than 16 mg. per day. When neocytes become generally available, daily iron accumulation will decrease further to 9 to 10 mg. per day.

Chelation Therapy. Since man has no mechanism for excreting excess iron, chelating agents must be used to prevent potentially toxic siderosis. Deferoxamine B, a relatively specific and nontoxic agent given intramuscularly has been used sporadically in various regimens for 16 years. However, it is now fairly well established that a continuous infusion of 20 to 60 mg. per kg. over 10 to 12 hours daily by means of a small portable infusion pump effects excretion of 15 to 60 mg. per day of iron, depending upon the patient's age and iron stores. All patients over the age of 5 years reported to date on this regimen are in net negative iron balance. Although this regimen will undoubtedly prevent many of the sequelae of siderosis if begun early enough, whether or not it is capable of dramatically improving the clinical condition of patients with already severe iron overload is still not known. The drug is usually diluted in sterile water to 3 or 5 ml. and given via a small 27 gauge butterfly needle into the subcutaneous tissues of the anterior abdominal wall. All of our patients over 6 years of age mix their own medicine, insert their own needles, and place the disposable syringes correctly in their pumps. The only side effects reported are transient pruritus, rubor, and slight swelling at the puncture site, which are probably due more to mechanical trauma than to the drug. Adding 1 mg. of hydrocortisone per ml. of deferoxamine solution usually cures the problem.

Although it has been shown that a dramatic augmentation in iron excretion can be effected in ascorbic acid–depleted patients by the administration of as little as 100 mg. of oral vitamin C daily, there have been some questions raised concerning the potentially toxic effects that might result from a combination of ferric iron and ascorbic acid vis-a-vis free radicals. The problem is obviated, of course, as long as deferoxamine is around to bind any stray iron molecules, but until the jury is in, some discretion should be used in recommending supplemental ascorbic acid.

Splenectomy. Two points need to be evaluated when considering indications for splenectomy. First, and foremost, is the development of hypersplenism, with its excessive destruction of red cells and the coincident increase in transfusion requirement. When a lower than expected rise in hematocrit regularly follows transfusion of packed red cells, splenectomy is probably indicated. In a patient who shows no overt evidence of hypersplenism, the actual effect of the spleen on the overall body iron status is not known. Since the spleen stores iron in its reticuloendothelial cells, it functions as both a culprit (increasing red cell destruction and iron release) and a hero (storing the released iron in a seemingly nontoxic pool). It is known that iron does travel from one storage pool to another. However, the exact role of the spleen in the overall iron-transport schema still remains to be determined. If the spleen acts primarily as a sump for excess iron, then premature removal might prove detrimental. On the other hand, the splenic iron may be the most readily available for chelation, and hence the beneficial effects of aggressive chelation therapy may be markedly diminished or even aborted by preferential removal of iron from this iron pool. In general, most thalassemic patients become hypersplenic by 5 to 6 years of age and require splenectomy to minimize transfusion requirements. Splenectomy at that age has not yielded any problems with increased morbidity or mortality in our hands, but the historical considerations of overwhelming pneumococcal, *Hemophilus influenzae,* and meningococcal infections must always be foremost in the mind of the attending physician. Our patients have all been immunized with the new pneumococcal vaccine postsplenectomy and, in addition, have been placed on penicillin, 125 mg. orally twice daily, indefinitely. Illnesses accompanied by high fevers and unexplained foci are treated aggressively with parenteral ampicillin until culture results are known. Hematologically, splenectomy immediately increases red cell survival. In addition, evidence of extramedullary hematopoiesis becomes more obvious when hematocrits are not maintained sufficiently high. These include development of a peripheral smear with numerous thalassemic-appearing red cells, of which many are nucleated, thrombocytosis of often to over 1 million and leukocytosis with a normal differential.

Thalassemia Intermedia

Thalassemia intermedia is a condition in which patients demonstrate most of the pathologic changes associated with thalassemia major, except that they are able to maintain hematocrits between 20 and 30 per cent without transfusion. Historically, it was crucial to identify this population because they had an increased prospect for long-term survival and often had better sexual maturation and reproductive capacity than their transfusion-dependent counterparts. As a result, differentiating patients with thalassemia intermedia and coincident hypersplenism from those with thalassemia major was critical. It was thought that the difference in prognosis between the two forms of the disease was sufficient to permit patients with thalassemia intermedia to remain untransfused, despite the fact that this maneuver markedly limited their overall functioning. Characteristically, it was usually easy to identify these patients because they (1) presented relatively late in infancy (18 months), (2) had a moderately low hematocrit unresponsive to parenteral or oral iron supplementation (24 to 30 per cent), (3) reticulocytosis of greater than 4 per cent, (4) hyperbilirubinemia to 1.5 to 2 grams per dl. (100 ml.), and (5) a thalassemic-appearing peripheral blood smear.

This group represents 2 to 10 per cent of the total thalassemia population and is an extremely heterogeneous group. Some patients are delta-beta⁰, beta⁰ double heterozygotes who are able to compensate for their anemia by dramatically increasing their intrinsic fetal hemoglobin production. Those cells having enough fetal hemoglobin to avoid intramedullary destruction are released into the circulation. As a result, hemoglobin electrophoretic patterns of the peripheral blood from such patients often demonstrate a pattern of fetal hemoglobin that approaches 100 per cent of the total hemoglobin concentration. On the other hand, some of these patients are genetic representatives of one end of the thalassemia major spectrum. These patients have enough beta gene output (β^+) to produce enough well-hemoglobinized red cells to maintain a hematocrit that is compatible with life. The tremendous expense that the body pays for this luxury, however, may not be worth the price. These patients are often the most thalassemic-appearing patients because of the tremendous marrow expansion and extramedullary hematopoiesis needed to maintain this low hematocrit.

With the new approaches to therapy described under treatment of thalassemia major, our present feeling is that, if at all possible, patients with thalassemia intermedia should be treated as if their disease were thalassemia major. In this way, we will probably be able to minimize the long-term sequelae. With the advances that are occurring in chelation therapy and transfusion, we are becoming more and more optimistic that we can prevent the ultimate manifestations of the toxic accumulation of iron. If this is true, then adequate transfusion therapy coupled with chronic chelation will decrease the overall incidence of pathologic sequelae and permit a more active and normal life style.

In patients in whom chronic transfusion is not feasible or desirable, two additional aspects of therapy should be considered. The first is the addition of daily oral folic acid (1 mg. per day) to the diet. Since the body is unable to store folate to any degree, the hyperproliferative, almost malignant turnover of the marrow often depletes normal folate stores. This, in turn, leads to a further accentuation of the ineffective component of hematopoiesis and ultimately leads to the development of a compound anemia. Oral supplementation with folic acid obviates this problem. The second aspect of therapy in the untransfused patient with thalassemia intermedia is the potential for the development of hyperuricemia and the sequela thereof. Again, it is the tremendous proliferative thrust of the bone marrow that leads to the excess of purine catabolism and resulting hyperuricemia. Adequate control may be obtained by adding allopurinol to the daily regimen and by placing the patient on a hypertransfusion regimen that inhibits intrinsic erythropoiesis.

SICKLE CELL DISEASE

method of
JEANNE A. SMITH, M.D.
New York, New York

Introduction

Sickle cell anemia, the most common form of sickle cell disease is an inherited disorder of hemoglobin structure caused by an amino acid substitution on the beta chains of hemoglobin. The disorder is inherited as an autosomal recessive. A gene for sickle hemoglobin must be inherited from each parent. Inheritance of a sickle gene from one parent and a normal hemoglobin gene from the other results in the carrier state known as sickle cell trait. *This latter condition is not associated with anemia, painful crises, or other complications and has virtually no clinical significance.*

The gene for sickle hemoglobin is found in several ethnic groups, most commonly among those of African ancestry. The gene also occurs in certain parts of the Mediterranean, India, the Arab world and elsewhere. Other disorders of hemoglobin such as hemoglobins C, D, and O Arab and the α and β thalassemic disorders of hemoglobin production occur in the same geographic areas as sickle hemoglobin, and the inheritance of a sickle gene from one parent and a gene for one of the other disorders from the other results in a disease state that may be quite similar to the homozygous SS state. Collectively, these disorders (SS, SC, SD, S β thalassemia, etc.) are known as sickle cell disease.

The disease results from the relative insolubility of hemoglobin S particularly at low oxygen tensions. The hemoglobin thus has a tendency to precipitate within the red cells and through a process of gelation and the formation of tactoids (crystals) produce distortion of the cell shape (sickling) and rigidity. As a result of sickling, the red cells do not traverse the capillary bed with ease and may produce obstruction, tissue anoxia, and resultant necrosis. The red cell life span is shortened because the membrane damage that occurs during sickling results in increased mechanical fragility and phagocytosis by macrophages.

General Management

As the disorder is frequently identified within the first few years of life and many persons with sickle cell disease live well into adulthood, it is as important to recognize the need for general health maintenance and nutrition as to manage the specific complications of the disease. Persons with the disorder should be encouraged to lead as normal lives as possible, and to understand the nature of their disease so that they may cooperate with their physicians in its management.

Both patients and physicians should also understand that the disease has considerable variability in its severity and that not all patients will suffer all complications.

Management of Anemia

The hemolytic anemia varies in severity but usually does not require transfusion except under the following conditions:

Aplastic Crisis. Occasionally, particularly during severe infections, the rate of marrow red cell production will decrease, resulting in a low reticulocyte count and a rapid fall in hematocrit. Transfusion of packed cells to a level of 30 per cent is indicated.

Splenic Sequestration. In small children, and rarely in adults, a sudden fall in hematocrit associated with a shocklike state and increasing splenomegaly may occur. Rapid replacement of blood volume with packed cells is essential. Such a child should be managed with a chronic transfusion program for 2 to 3 years to prevent recurrence.

Preparation for Surgery. As sickling occurs at low oxygen tensions, the patient with sickle cell disease should be prepared for surgery by increasing the hematocrit and reducing the risk of intravascular sickling.

METHODS AVAILABLE FOR ADULTS. (1) Direct Transfusion: For either elective or emergency surgery, packed cells can be given to raise the hematocrit to between 30 and 35 per cent. Frozen, washed red cells if available are desirable as the risk of sensitization to red cell antigens is lessened. (2) Exchange Transfusion: For elective surgery it is preferable to use partial exchange transfusion, which may be accomplished over a period of 2 to 3

days by alternately transfusing the patient with packed cells and then removing blood by phlebotomy. This can be done using a 16 gauge needle implanted in a vein attached to a Y tube or an adapter with a side arm. After the third or fourth such exchange the percentage of S cells will be reduced significantly and the hematocrit increased, thus further lessening the chances of sickling.

METHODS FOR CHILDREN. (1) Direct transfusion of packed cells can be performed at the rate of 5 ml. per pound (11 ml. per kg.) to raise the hematocrit above 30 per cent.

(2) The exchange procedure outlined for adults can be used in older children.

Children can be prepared for surgery over a 10 to 15 day period by transfusion of packed cells every 3 to 4 days. This procedure will suppress production of sickle cells. Because of the short life span of the patient's erythrocytes, by the time of surgery the percentage of sickled cells will be low.

Management of Painful Crises

Painful crises may affect varying areas of the body, the head, chest, back, abdomen, joints, or long bones. Crises vary considerably in severity and duration and may mimic other disorders or be mimicked by other disorders.

Analgesia. Analgesics such as propoxyphene hydrochloride or acetaminophen or codeine-containing compounds may be useful for children or in the adult during a mild crisis. In many adults with severe pain, meperidine in doses of 50 to 100 mg. intramuscularly, may be required every 4 to 6 hours for several days. Promethazine hydrochloride, 25 mg., can be used with the meperidine to potentiate its effect. Dihydrocodeinone compounds may also be used. Up to 2.0 mg. per kg. of meperidine (Demerol) can be used in children.

Hydration. Oral or intravenous fluids are essential. In mild crises the adult patient should be encouraged to consume 2 to 3 liters of the most palatable fluid daily with a reminder to include salty liquids. Hospitalized adults should receive a minimum of 4 liters of dextrose and saline solution daily. The addition of potassium and bicarbonate should be dictated by the individual patient's needs. In children the volume of fluid administered should be calculated on the basis of 2500 ml. per square meter per 24 hours.

Rest. Patients at home should be encouraged to rest in a quiet atmosphere. Emergency room patients, if at all possible, should be placed in a comfortable quiet place, as fatigue and anxiety are known to precipitate or aggravate painful crises.

Treatment of Associated Conditions. Viral and bacterial infections, including upper respiratory infections, bronchitis, bronchopneumonia, pneumonia, and genitourinary tract infections, are frequent precipitators or concomitants of crises. These should be sought and vigorously treated.

Transfusion. Transfusion is not necessary in the average crisis. Prolonged or very frequent crises will occur in the occasional patient and result in almost constant incapacitation. Some of these patients have responded well to a program of chronic transfusion so as to establish and maintain a percentage of hemoglobin S below 30 to 40 per cent. This will require transfusion every 4 to 6 weeks. Because of the attendant complications of hemochromatosis, hepatitis, and red cell antibody development, a chronic transfusion program should be used only in patients who are very severely incapacitated.

Management of Infections

In young children, sepsis, pneumonia, and meningitis represent the greatest threats to life. The most common bacterial pathogens are pneumococci, streptococci, *H. influenzae,* salmonella, and meningococci. Serious infections may occur in the first few months of life. The management of infection in infants and children under 5 years of age should include:

Parent Education. Parents should be instructed that the infant or child who appears lethargic, is febrile above 102°F. (38.9°C.), refuses to eat, or otherwise behaves in an unusual manner should be brought to the physician or emergency room immediately for evaluation.

Evaluation. In addition to a thorough physical examination in search of the site of infection, blood, throat, and other appropriate cultures should be obtained. Chest x-rays should also be done. In severely ill children lumbar puncture should be performed for examination of cell count, Gram stain, and culture.

Antibiotic Therapy. Early antibiotic therapy is essential in the severely ill child. Parenteral penicillin G, 150 to 200 mg. per kg. should be given every 4 to 6 hours until the source of infection is found and a need to switch to another antibiotic is identified or until the child is afebrile for several days. In instances of tonsillitis or otitis media, oral medication may be substituted after the bacteriologic diagnosis is made.

Hydration. Close attention should be paid to the state of hydration during infections, as painful crises may either accompany the infection or be precipitated by it. Glucose and saline solution, 2500 ml. per square meter per day, is recommended.

Transfusion. The transfusion of packed red cells in anemic patients with severe pulmonary or other types of infection may, by improving oxygen delivery, result in better management of the infection.

Prevention of Infection. Prophylactic penicillin has been used for the prevention of pneumococcal and streptococcal infections. It is particularly recommended in infants and young children who have experienced one or more episodes of severe infection. Penicillin VK or G may be used in a dosage of 125 mg. twice daily in infants, and 250 mg. twice daily in children over 1 year of age. Pneumococcal vaccine containing 14 serotypes has become available and has been shown to be effective in children over the age of 2 years. The duration of protection is presently not known, as sufficient experience with the vaccine is not available. The vaccine is *not recommended for children under 2 years of age.* Influenza vaccine is currently under clinical trial and may become available shortly for clinical use. The principles for management of children over 5 years of age are much the same, except that the frequency of life-threatening sepsis is much less and the occurrence of viral and mycoplasma infections much more frequent. It is therefore possible to await culture or Gram stain results except in those who appear acutely ill prior to the institution of antibiotic therapy.

In this age group and in adults fever may occur as a part of a painful crisis. It should be remembered that this is a diagnosis of exclusion and that prolonged fever, more than 48 to 72 hours, is suggestive of an undiagnosed infection.

Two other types of infection occur with increased frequency among patients with sickle cell disease: genitourinary tract infections and osteomyelitis. The diagnosis of pyelonephritis is made by history, urinalysis, and physical findings and should be treated in accordance with the results of bacteriologic cultures. Osteomyelitis may be present without any radiologic evidence of bone destruction and may present as a prolonged period (weeks) of fever and pain and swelling over a bone. Culture of aspirated material may be needed to establish the diagnosis.

Leg Ulcers. Ulcerations may develop over the medial or lateral malleoli in adolescents and adults. These are invariably superficial in nature, and, while they may be quite painful, do not involve the underlying bone or produce sepsis.

Conservative management with debridement of the ulcers with twice daily application of hydrogen peroxide followed by application of a lanolin and petrolatum (A and D) or bacitracin ointment covered by a sterile dressing may result in healing after several weeks. Dressings should always be moistened before removal is attempted.

The use of a zinc oxide (Unna) boot may be attempted if healing does not occur after several weeks. Care should be taken to avoid venous constriction when the boot is applied, and the patient should be instructed to remove it immediately if swelling occurs. The boot should be changed weekly.

Split thickness skin grafts or pinch grafts may be necessary for ulcers that fail to heal when these methods are tried.

Management of Neurologic Disorders

Cerebrovascular accidents occur in a small percentage of children and an even smaller percentage of adults with sickle cell disease. No characteristics have been identified that would allow identification of this group prior to the event. Management of these patients should include immediate institution of a chronic transfusion program as previously described, as recurrent strokes frequently occur. Vigorous physical rehabilitation programs are also essential.

Ophthalmologic disease has been described in children as young as 5 years of age. It is best detected by fluorescein angiography which should be performed ideally on a yearly basis. Fluorescein angiography must be performed whenever there is loss of visual acuity. Photocoagulation has shown promise in preventing retinal detachment when proliferative lesions are identified. Retinal detachment can also be managed by photocoagulation or retinal surgery in an attempt to preserve vision.

Management of Skeletal Disease

Hand Foot Syndrome. In infants and young children swelling and pain of the hands and/or feet may occur with sudden onset. This syndrome can be differentiated from osteomyelitis by the fact that it is symmetrical. Management includes vigorous hydration orally or intravenously and analgesics such as acetaminophen.

Adult Bone Syndrome. A similar episode of pain, swelling, and low grade fever may occur in older children and adults, particularly affecting the long bones and the knee, wrist, and ankle joints. Management again is with hydration. Restriction of weight bearing may be helpful.

Aseptic Necrosis. Older children and adults may be subject to gradual painful bone necrosis, usually occurring in the heads of the femur but occasionally in the humeral heads, spine, or other bones. Early radiologic manifestations may appear as bone cysts. Some of these have successfully been treated with bone grafts. When the lesion has progressed to the point of anatomic destruction, prostheses such as the Charnley may be used to replace the femoral head and acetabular cup.

Gout. The increased turnover of red cells in patients with sickle cell disease leads to hyperuricemia in many patients. In some instances classic gout has occurred. This can be managed with colchicine or other anti-inflammatory agents for the acute episode. The use of probenecid or allopurinol to prevent recurrence is recommended.

Other Arthropathies. It must be remembered that patients with sickle cell disease are as subject to other conditions affecting bone and joints as the general population and signs and symptoms of these should not be assumed to be due to sickle cell disease. When present, appropriate laboratory studies and management are indicated.

Management of Renal Dysfunction

Hyposthenuria. Inability to concentrate the urine is a defect acquired by patients with sickle cell disease. It is believed to be the result of damage to tubular epithelium as a consequence of recurrent episodes of intravascular sickling.

As a result of this defect the patient with sickle cell disease is continuously at risk of dehydration. Under normal circumstances thirst will result in compensation, but patients should be instructed to force fluids during episodes of fever, gastroenteritis, and other causes of fluid loss. Of particular importance is the potential loss of both fluid and salt during periods of high external temperature leading to heat stroke. All patients should be instructed to include salty fluids, such as broth, or bouillon in their fluid intake.

Hematuria. Painless gross hematuria occurs as an uncommon but recognized complication of both sickle cell disease and trait. It has been suggested that the relative anoxia of renal medullary tissue and the hypertonicity of medullary blood may promote sickling in vessels just below the pelvic mucosa. Microscopic or macroscopic papillary necrosis may occur and lead to bleeding from the engorged vessels.

It is important to recognize that patients with sickle cell disease are susceptible to all other disorders that can cause hematuria, and therefore thorough evaluation must include: (1) cultures for bacterial pathogens and *Mycobacterium tuberculosis,* (2) evaluation of urine sediment and 24 hour urine protein excretion, (3) intravenous urography, and (4) cystoscopy.

Experience has shown that many episodes of hematuria will cease within 1 week to 10 days. Recently, we have managed more prolonged episodes with sodium bicarbonate, 1500 mg. orally three to four times daily, and ethacrynic acid, 25 mg. three to four times daily, with cessation of bleeding after a few days. These drugs can then be tapered over a 1 week period.

A few patients will have more than one episode of gross hematuria. It is important to recognize that nephrectomy is contraindicated, as episodes, even if prolonged, will usually cease, and bleeding is as likely to occur from the other kidney. Patients with prolonged episodes of bleeding should be evaluated for iron deficiency, particularly if the patient is a female, and appropriate therapy given.

Nephrolithiasis. Renal calculi may be seen in the occasional patient but are unusual because of the hyposthenuria. Most frequently, these are uric acid stones and should be managed as in routine practice.

Pyelonephritis. The papillary necrosis also leads to an increased susceptibility to pyelonephritis, particularly among adult females. Such patients should be managed by vigorous treatment with the appropriate antibiotics according to the results of urine cultures and sensitivities. Patients with recurrent episodes of pyelonephritis should also be evaluated for congenital abnormalities of the urogenital tract and these corrected if found.

Renal Failure. Chronic renal disease may result from the consequences of intravascular sickling, infection, or diseases common to the general population; the management does not differ. End stage renal disease has been managed successfully in several patients by hemodialysis. Grafting or shunt procedures necessary for vascular access are tolerated well.

Priapism. Prolonged painful penile erections occur rarely in patients with sickle cell disease and trait. In many instances sedation and analgesia will result in remission. Drainage of the corpus cavernosum has been advocated by some, but infection and loss of tissue has been reported. Exchange transfusions have also been recommended.

Management of Gastrointestinal Disease

As in most chronic hemolytic states, gallstones are common in sickle cell disease and are probably present in most patients by the time they reach adulthood. These stones *may or may not* result in clinical disease.

Episodes of abdominal pain are a common manifestation of sickle cell disease. It is therefore essential to determine whether the patient who has stones has pain as a result of cholecystitis or as a result of painful crises, prior to a decision as to management. The evaluation should include: (1) careful physical examination, (2) liver enzymes (alkaline phosphatase, serum glutamic oxaloacetic transaminase [SGOT], serum glutamic pyruvic transaminase [SGPT]) on more than one occasion, and (3) intravenous cholangiography.

Emergency surgery should be avoided unless the evidence for gallbladder disease as a cause of abnormal liver function or pain is excellent. A rising bilirubin may be due to sickle cell hepatopathy (see below) or hepatitis. In these instances surgery is contraindicated. Management of stones which have resulted in obstruction, empyema or other significant disease is, of course, surgical; the patient should be prepared for surgery as previously described.

Liver Disease. Many patients with sickle cell disease have an enlarged liver with no evidence of abnormal liver function. The hepatomegaly is most probably due to the surrogate role of the liver in disposing of damaged cells in the absence of a functional spleen and possibly to extramedullary hematopoiesis.

The patient with deranged liver function studies presents a particular problem. The differential diagnosis should include: (1) presence of congestive heart failure, (2) presence of post-transfusion hepatitis or hepatitis of other cause, and (3) presence of obstructive liver disease secondary to cholelithiasis.

In the rare patient none of these disorders can be diagnosed. In these instances it is believed by some that the underlying disorder is sickle cell disease hence the term "sickle cell hepatopathy," for which there is no specific therapy. In some patients episodes of severe hyperbilirubinemia (50 mg. per dl. [100 ml.]) may occur and spontaneously revert to normal without sequelae. Liver biopsies in some of these patients have shown only nonspecific changes. Exchange transfusion, as previously described, could theoretically be of benefit in patients with prolonged or repeated episodes.

Management of Cardiopulmonary Disease

Acute Chest Syndrome. The sudden onset of pleuritic chest pain, shortness of breath, and tachycardia with or without fever may be a presenting complaint. Such patients frequently have negative or equivocal x-rays and negative bacterial cultures. Lung scan may reveal an area of poor arterial perfusion. The pathogenosis of vascular obstruction in sickle cell disease is believed to be in situ sickling rather than embolic phenomena. Anticoagulation is therefore generally not indicated. The patient should be managed with supportive care including oxygen therapy. Repeated episodes may be an indication for transfusion.

Respiratory failure and cor pulmonale are uncommon sequelae of sickle cell disease, occurring in patients who have had multiple episodes of infection or pulmonary infarction or both. The management is no different from other causes of respiratory failure. Congestive failure may be the presenting manifestation of worsening anemia, and may improve only when transfusion of packed cells improves oxygen delivery to the myocardium.

Management of Pregnancy

Many women with sickle cell disease have conceived and delivered healthy children. The two essential factors these women appear to have in common is good prenatal care and good obstetrical care. These women should be instructed to report early in pregnancy, so that adequate follow-up can be achieved to ensure a successful outcome.

The patient should be seen at monthly intervals during the early trimesters and at least biweekly after the twenty-sixth week. Examination at each visit should include a hematocrit in addition to routine obstetrical evaluation.

In addition to multivitamins and iron, folic acid, 1 mg. daily, should be given to prevent the development of megaloblastic anemia.

Intercurrent illness should be managed as previously described. Occasional patients will suffer from recurrent painful crises. It may be advisable to transfuse such patients, but this should be done with awareness of the risks involved. Either the direct or exchange method can be used. Subsequent direct transfusions will need to be given at 4 to 6 week intervals for the duration of pregnancy.

Labor and Delivery. Vaginal delivery utilizing a minimum of analgesia and anesthesia, with attention to good oxygenation is the method of choice. Postpartum transfusion may be indicated based on blood loss at the time of delivery. Decisions as to cesarean sections should be made, if possible, well in advance to allow for transfusions in the proper preparation of the patient for surgery.

Antisickling Agents

To date no agent has been found that will prevent in vivo sickling without producing severe toxic effects. Several new agents are currently under study, but none are yet at the stage of readiness for clinical trials.

NEUTROPENIA

method of
PAUL A. CHERVENICK, M.D.
Pittsburgh, Pennsylvania

Neutropenia refers to a decrease in the number of neutrophils that circulate in the blood. In whites the normal range is between 1800 and 7200 per cu. mm.,
while in the black population the lower limit is somewhat less at approximately 1400 per cu. mm. Neutrophils are produced in the marrow, where they remain for 6 to 10 days before entering the circulation. Upon entering the circulation, neutrophils are divided nearly equally between cells that circulate (circulating pool) and those which marginate along vessel walls (marginal pool) with free exchange between the two. Neutrophils spend only a short time in the blood (approximately 10 hours) before entering tissues, where they perform their function of phagocytosis and killing of microorganisms.

There are a number of circumstances in which neutropenia is observed. Neutropenia may be seen following the administration of a variety of drugs or following irradiation, and it may occur in association with a variety of disease including infections, various hematologic disorders, and in diseases associated with splenomegaly. In addition, neutropenia occurs as a congenital disorder and, in other instances, as an idiopathic acquired abnormality. In all these situations neutropenia results from either decreased production, increased destruction or a combination of these processes.

Drugs and physical agents are probably the most common cause of neutropenia. Agents such as antitumor drugs, which are toxic to the marrow, regularly produce neutropenia that is dose related. Included in this group are agents such as cyclophosphamide, chlorambucil, methotrexate, doxorubicin, daunomycin, the nitrosoureas, and 5-fluorouracil, as well as many others. Radiation and certain chemical solvents such as benzene behave in a similar manner. With other agents, neutropenia is unpredictable and occurs idiosyncratically in an occasional patient. Some of the more common compounds in this group are the phenothiazines, sulfonamides, analgesics, antithyroid drugs, gold compounds, certain antimicrobial agents, diuretics, and sedatives. The exact mechanism for the neutropenia is unknown, but certain compounds such as aminopyrine act as a haptene and stimulate the formation of antineutrophil antibodies. Other drugs such as the phenothiazines act by interfering with DNA synthesis in neutrophil precursors.

Hematologic diseases such as acute leukemia and aplastic anemia are nearly always associated with neutropenia some time during the course of the illness. In patients with leukemia, neutropenia results from suppression of normal neutrophil production by the leukemic cell population or from chemotherapy given in an attempt to induce a remission in the disease. In aplastic anemia, neutropenia in addition to anemia and thrombocytopenia result from a defective pluripotent stem cell. Patients with vitamin B_{12} and folic acid deficiency are often observed to have a mild neutropenia that is associated with large and hypersegmented neutrophils.

Infections caused by various microorganisms may be associated with neutropenia. It occurs commonly with viral infection such as measles, infectious mononucleosis, or influenza. It is usually mild in degree but on occasion may be severe, and disappears with recovery from the disease. With bacterial infections neutrophilia rather than neutropenia is the expected response. However, in overwhelming infections neutropenia may occur. This results from depletion of the neutrophil reserve because of the marked increase in utilization of neutrophils, a situation associated with a poor prognosis.

Diseases in which *splenomegaly* is present are often accompanied by neutropenia. Thus, it occurs in rheumatoid arthritis with splenomegaly (Felty's syndrome), and systemic lupus erythematosus as well as in less common disorders such as Gaucher's disease. It is also observed in congestive splenomegaly associated with portal hypertension in patients with cirrhosis or in disorders such as idiopathic myelofibrosis. The neutropenia in these disorders is most likely due to trapping and destruction of neutrophils by the enlarged spleen. In certain patients with Felty's syndrome, antineutrophil antibodies have been demonstrated in their serum.

Congenital neutropenia may be expressed in a variety of forms. A common form of congenital neutropenia is that which occurs due to maternal antibodies being formed against fetal neutrophils. This occurs transiently, and the neutropenia disappears within several weeks following birth. An autosomal dominant inherited form with a variable degree of neutropenia is associated with a normal life span. Severe infections are uncommon. A severe form of neutropenia inherited as an autosomal recessive (Kostmann type) is associated with severe infections and death usually occurs within the first few years of life.

Cyclic neutropenia is a rare disorder, most likely due to an abnormal stem cell. Neutropenia occurs at 3 week intervals and is often associated with fever and oral ulceration but severe infections are uncommon.

Acquired idiopathic neutropenia without any recognizable underlying disease occurs infrequently and is seldom associated with severe infections unless the neutrophil concentration is less than 1000 per cu. mm. A "chronic benign" form exists that is due to decreased production of neutrophils. A number of such patients are diagnosed early in life and may well represent a congenital form of the disease. In a portion of these patients, a remission of the disease occurs with increasing age. In other patients, the neutropenia is due to increased destruction of neutrophils, presumably due to antineutrophil antibodies.

Other causes of neutropenia include *pseudoneutropenia*, which results from a shift of neutrophils from the circulating to the marginal pool. The number of marginated cells can be determined by injecting epinephrine and counting the number of cells that enter the circulating pool. *Immunoglobulin deficiencies* and *pancreatic* insufficiency may, on occasion, be associated with neutropenia.

Approach to the Treatment of Neutropenia

Unless a treatable disease or toxic agent is identified as the cause, little can be done to alter the neutropenia. Therefore, in most instances, therapy is directed toward the treatment of infections. The milder forms of neutropenia pose no problem, and it is mainly when neutrophils are less than 500 per cu. mm. that life-threatening infections are likely to occur. When a drug or chemical toxin is suspected as the cause, these should be discontinued promptly and in most cases one can expect the neutrophils to return within 1 week. After chemotherapy with antitumor agents, the neutropenia may persist for longer periods of up to 2 weeks.

Antibiotics should not be given as prophylaxis but only in patients with proven or suspected infections. After appropriate cultures are obtained patients should receive broad-spectrum antibiotics to cover infections due to gram-positive and gram-negative organisms. Initial treatment usually includes cephalothin (2 grams intravenously every 4 hours) and gentamicin (1 mg. per kg. intravenously every 8 hours). Carbenicillin may also be used, especially in place of gentamicin in patients with renal disease. Further adjustments in antibiotic coverage are dictated by the results of microbial cultures and sensitivity studies.

Neutrophil transfusions are of benefit when transfused into patients with proven severe infections, such as those which occur in patients with acute leukemia who are receiving induction therapy or following bone marrow transplantation. Neutrophils are collected from normal donors. Family members are preferred as donors, since patients who are matched at two or more of the four HL-A loci have a greater number of circulating neutrophils. This procedure is time-consuming and expensive and is not a service provided by all blood banks at the present time.

Corticosteroids have been used to treat neutropenia but with little benefit. Steroids will increase blood neutrophils but this results from impaired migration of cells from the blood to the tissues, a situation that would only add to the severity of an infectious process. Steroids should not be used except where the neutropenia is due to antineutrophil antibodies. In certain patients with cyclic neutropenia, the administration of steroids has interrupted the cycling pattern.

Lithium carbonate given to normal persons results in an increase in blood neutrophils. This is in part due to an increase in colony stimulating factor (CSF), a glycoprotein that stimulates the proliferation of neutrophil progenitor cells. Lithium has been given to patients with neutropenia of various causes. The results have been variable and its ability to alleviate neutropenia has not been conclusively demonstrated.

Splenectomy has been performed in patients with most forms of neutropenia but only occasionally has it been of benefit. Those who have improved have had cellular marrows and an enlarged spleen such as occurs in certain patients with Felty's syndrome. Splenectomy should not be performed for neutropenia alone except in patients with recurrent and severe infections.

Marrow transplantation is the treatment of choice in patients with aplastic anemia who have a sibling that matches for the four major histocompatibility loci. Autologous marrow transplantation is being used as a means to reduce the period of neutropenia following intensive chemotherapy with antitumor agents, but its real value is yet unknown.

HEMOLYTIC DISEASE OF THE NEWBORN
(Erythroblastosis Fetalis)

method of
LILLIAN BLACKMON, M.D.,
and WENDELL F. ROSSE, M.D.
Durham, North Carolina

Hemolytic disease of the newborn (erythroblastosis fetalis) is a syndrome of newborn infants characterized by the immunologic destruction of the red cells by alloantibodies (isoantibodies) transferred across the placenta from the mother. These alloantibodies arise in the mother either due to previous sensitization by natural products (natural antibodies), in the case of ABO blood group incompatibilities, or by prior pregnancies or transfusions with red cells containing antigens that her red cells lack. When the red cells of the fetus exhibit the antigen to which such antibodies are directed, destruction of fetal red cells may ensue. The degree of destruction may be very mild, being observed only after birth, or may be very severe and result in fetal death due to anemia.

The most common antigen-antibody system involved is the Rh_0 (D) system. In this case, the sensitization is usually by previous pregnancy as it is uncommon in the first pregnancy. The mother is Rh (D) negative, but has previously borne Rh positive children and, at the time of their birth, sufficient red cells were transferred to the mother to elicit an antibody response. During the pregnancy in question, the titer of antibody increases and antibody is transferred across the placenta to react with the Rh positive cells in the fetus. Sufficient antigen-antibody interaction within the groups A and B can occur, particularly when the mother is group O. Hemolytic disease of the newborn due to other antigens (Kell, Duffy Kidd) is rare.

Evaluation and Treatment

Figure 1 presents an approach to the laboratory evaluation in schematic form. Once an infant has been identified as having an isoimmunization from the cord blood studies, management is focused on the two major manifestations, anemia and hyperbilirubinemia. Figure 2 diagrams the chain of options for treatment, utilizing the cord hemoglobin and bilirubin values as branching factors. In severe disease, coagulopathies and metabolic disturbances are frequent, necessitating careful monitoring both clinically and by laboratory studies. Basically, treatment can be divided into

three phases, which are distinct in time—birth to 24 hours, first week, after first week.

The problems immediately encountered at birth are related to the cord hemoglobin level. Those infants with severe intrauterine disease, as reflected by anemia at birth, are more likely to become severely asphyxiated during labor and delivery and thus, to require resuscitation at birth. A major advance in management of Rh isoimmunization in pregnancy has been the utilization of amnionic fluid pigment analysis to determine the severity of fetal involvement. The level of pigment as determined by the $\Delta OD450$ has been shown to correlate best with fetal cord hemoglobin and the risk of intrauterine fetal demise. Delivery by planned cesarean section is advocated by most authorities when the value is clearly in the zone of greatest risk for fetal demise. Certainly, intrauterine electronic fetal heart rate monitoring should be employed if a woman with a severely involved fetus is to be allowed to labor.

Beyond vigorous and thorough resuscitation immediately at birth, the next problem to resolve is the correction of the anemia, as this greatly impedes the cardiorespiratory adaptation necessary for survival. An immediate one-volume exchange transfusion with freshly drawn, heparinized, super-packed (hematocrit >75) cells allows for correction of the deficit in oxygen carrying capacity with minimal alteration in the circulating blood volume and stress on the cardiovascular system. Ventilatory support may be required for the severely sick infant during the initial hours. If the infant is also hydropic (low serum albumin with edema), the management is further complicated by the need to mobilize the edema fluid without precipitous overload of the circulation. No single therapeutic approach to the latter has been found superior.

The overwhelming majority of infants with erythroblastosis fetalis do not present with severe anemia and its consequences. Rather, they are identified by blood group incompatibility with the mother and the presence of antibody in the cord blood. Their management is determined by the presence of hyperbilirubinemia. Traditionally, cord blood values reflecting a mild anemia (hemoglobin 12 to 14 grams per dl. [100 ml.]), isoimmunization (positive direct Coombs' test), and hyperbilirubinemia (an indirect acting bilirubin of >3.5 to 4 mg. per dl.) were indications for immediate exchange transfusion. Dunn found early exchange transfusion, using these indications, did not decrease the number of exchange transfusions required for a given infant. Thus, immediate exchange transfusion in the early hours of life does not seem to offer any advantage and has the distinct liability of stressing the newborn during the

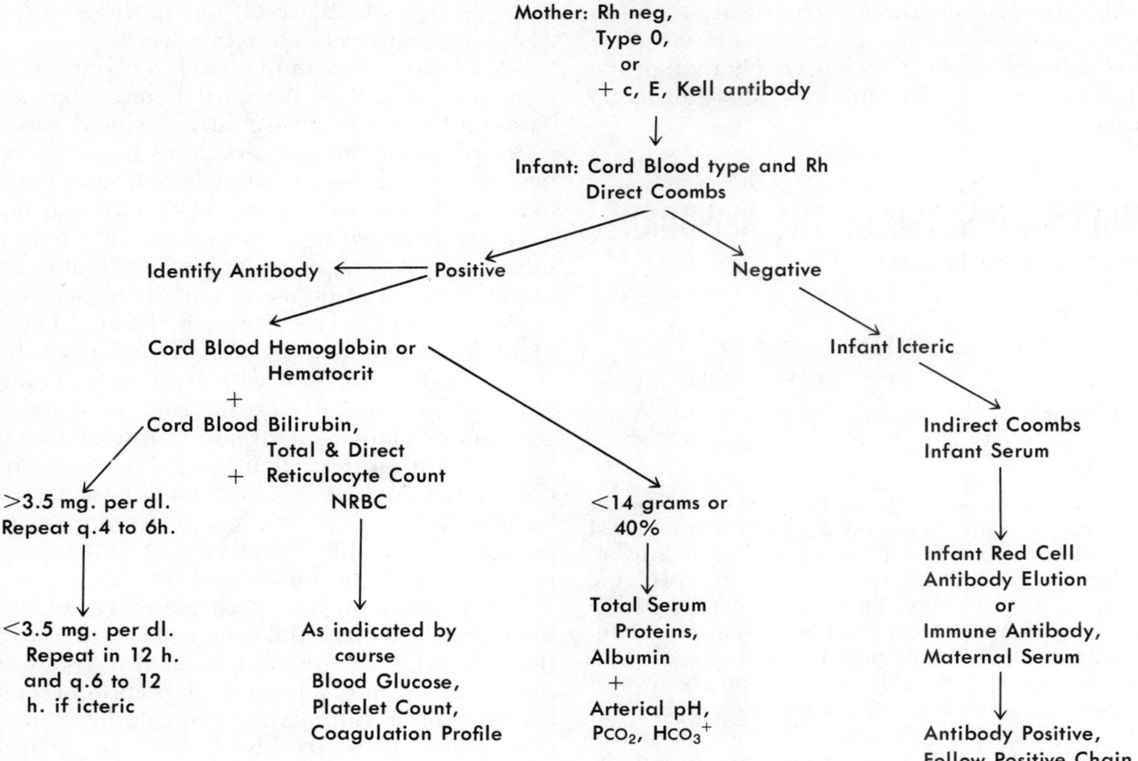

Figure 1.   Laboratory evaluation of erythroblastosis fetalis.

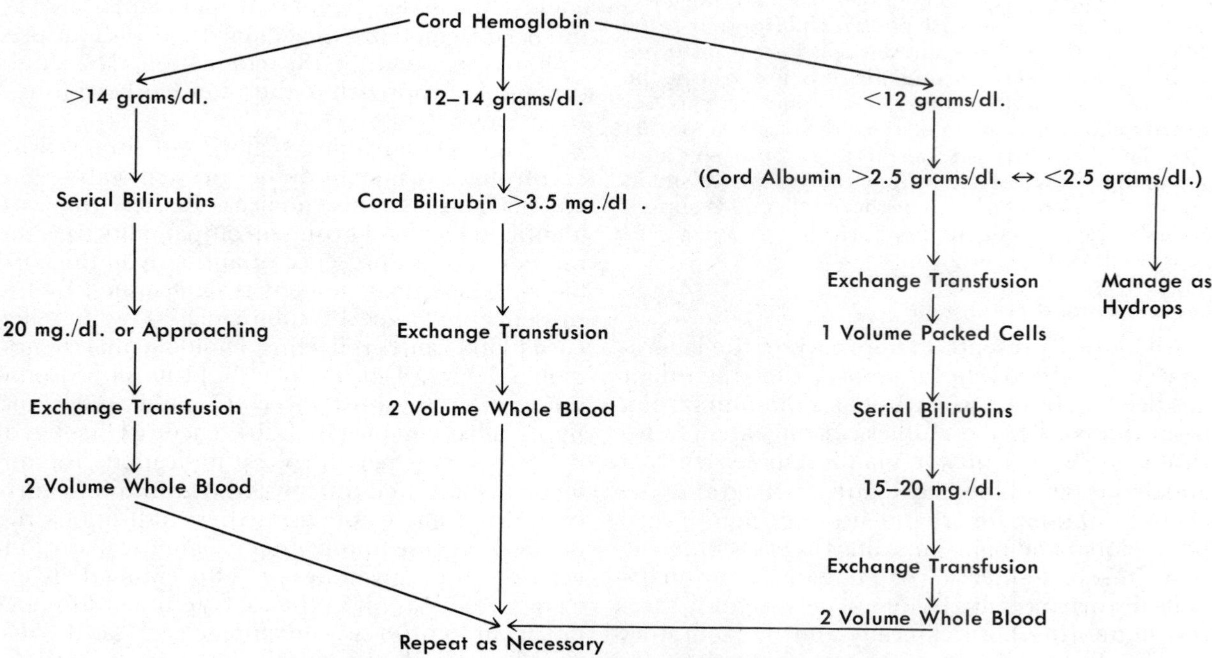

Figure 2.   Proposed Approach to erythroblastosis fetalis.

critical period of cardiovascular and respiratory adjustment to the extrauterine environment.

Exchange transfusion utilizing fresh adult blood decreases the serum bilirubin level, removes antibody coated cells and provides donor albumin with available binding sites. The most commonly used indication for exchange is a serum indirect acting bilirubin of 20 mg. per dl. although measurement of the "free" bilirubin would be more appropriate. Attempts to estimate this, primarily by measuring available albumin binding capacity, have not proved clinically practical, as yet. In infants with abnormalities known to reduce albumin binding (↓ pH, ↓ serum albumin, ↑ free fatty acids) or to alter the blood brain barrier (hypoxemia, hypoglycemia, hypotension), exchange transfusion at lower bilirubin levels, 10 to 15 mg. per dl., is probably indicated.

The choice of donor blood for exchanging involves a number of issues. The donor blood group and type should be compatible with mother and infant and must never contain the sensitizing antigen. Group O, Rh negative blood is always a suitable choice. Particular attention should be paid to identifying the specific antibody in the infant when there is both major group and Rh incompatibility.

The next two issues are interrelated, the type of anticoagulant and the shelf age of the donor unit. Acid, citrate, dextrose (ACD) anticoagulated blood is contraindicated because of its acid load and the decreased 2, 3-DPG concentration. Citrate, phosphate, dextrose (CPD) anticoagulant is less acid than ACD, and does not affect the 2,3-DPG level. Both facts are exaggerated by increasing shelf age. The citrate of both ACD and CPD has significant risks and disadvantages. Direct myocardial toxicity is reported from bolus injections of citrate. A rebound alkalosis occurs 8 to 12 hours following exchange. Calcium is bound by the citrate, decreasing the ionized fraction. However, no serious physiologic disturbance resulting from the decreased ionized calcium has been documented. Nevertheless, calcium has been infused with citrated blood exchange transfusions and is still recommended by some. Donor blood drawn in heparin anticoagulant has the least metabolic derangement but must be used within 48 hours of drawing. No controlled clinical trial has verified the supremacy of heparinized blood for exchange transfusion; however, with sick infants it would appear to be the better option because of the lesser biochemical stress to the infant. Irrespective of the anticoagulant used, blood that is more than 72 hours from collection should not be used because the serum potassium increases as the red cells age.

A two volume exchange (2 × blood volume [0.09 to 0.10 × body weight in kg.]) provides adequate efficiency of removal of excess bilirubin and sensitized red cells. The preferred technique includes cannulizing an umbilical vessel aseptically, usually the vein, and alternating withdrawal and infusion of an increment of blood, usually 5 to 10 per cent of the calculated blood volume. Careful monitoring of vital signs is necessary, and marked fluctuations are avoided by slowing the rate of the exchange.

The use of salt-poor albumin as an adjunct to the donor blood for exchanging has been advocated as a means of increasing the mass of bilirubin removed. Three methods have been proposed— removal of donor plasma from the unit and instillation of an equal volume of 25 per cent pooled albumin; pretreatment of the infant 1 to 2 hours prior to exchange with 1 gram of albumin per kg. body weight; and intermittently exchanging an aliquot of 25 per cent pooled albumin during the exchange transfusion. The latter is probably the most effective in promoting bilirubin removal. However, the spacing of the albumin replacement should be earlier in the exchange to avoid an undesirable reduction in hematocrit at the end of the exchange.

Repeat exchange transfusions are frequently required when there is severe hemolysis and hyperbilirubinemia. In general, the postexchange serum indirect-acting bilirubin is decreased to 50 per cent of the preexchange concentration. A rebound increase always occurs within 2 to 4 hours, reflecting mobilization of bilirubin from tissue sites. The magnitude of the rebound varies, but an increase of greater than 50 per cent of the postexchange level is worrisome. An increase to exchange level (greater than 15 mg. per dl.) within 6 to 8 hours should raise the question of an incompatible cross-match, as such rapid rises are not usually seen, even with severe isoimmunization. An occasional infant may require repeat exchange transfusion after age 5 days, but this is not common.

Phototherapy, light treatment to the skin to produce photodegradation of bilirubin, is controversial in the management of hyperbilirubinemia from isoimmunization. It offers a method for elimination of bilirubin without mortality or significant morbidity risks. The major argument against its use is that serious anemia from ongoing hemolysis may develop in the early weeks; thus, close follow-up of the infant is required. In infants with severe hemolysis, phototherapy probably does not limit the accumulation of bilirubin significantly. However, in milder cases exchange transfusion may be avoided with its use. As there is an established mortality risk (1 to 2 per cent) with exchange transfusion, it would seem advisable to avoid this whenever possible.

Infants with isoimmunization may develop

an anemia in the early postnatal weeks. Close surveillance to assure normal postnatal growth and absence of decompensation and to assess the anemia is necessary through age 6 to 8 weeks. It is probably advisable to withhold transfusion to treat the anemia if growth is adequate and the infant maintains sufficient cardio-respiratory compensation.

Treatment with iron during the recovery period is indicated only for those infants who are likely to have decreased stores—preterm infants of less than 36 weeks gestation and infants who have had multiple exchange transfusions reducing the hemoglobin level (less than 14 to 16 grams per dl.). If the abnormal hemoglobin level is low secondary to hemolysis alone, and the infant is term, there is probably no deficiency in iron stores.

Prevention. Hemolytic disease of the newborn due to the Rh antigen may be prevented by preventing the sensitization of the mother. This is done by the administration of a dose of hyperimmune anti Rh (anti D) globulin within 72 hours of parturition. In Rh negative women this antibody destroys the Rh positive cells that have entered her circulation during labor and delivery. Thus, sensitization does not occur and hemolytic disease of the newborn does not occur in subsequent pregnancies. This technique will not prevent hemolytic disease of the newborn due to any other antigen-antibody system. Furthermore, it is without value if the serum of the mother already contains demonstrable anti Rh_0 (anti D) antibodies prior to the administration of the hyperimmune globulin. This preventative treatment should be given for all pregnancies and abortions, therapeutic or spontaneous, of Rh negative women.

HEMOPHILIA AND ALLIED CONDITIONS

method of
PETER H. LEVINE, M.D.
Worcester, Massachusetts

Hemophilia A is an X-linked recessive bleeding disorder attributable to decreased blood levels of procoagulant factor VIII. This disorder accounts for approximately 80 per cent of the hemophilias and affects between 10 and 20 males per 100,000 in the United States. Hemophilia B, also an X-linked recessive disease, accounts for almost all other true hemophilias and is due to decreased levels of procoagulant factor IX. Much less common is factor XI deficiency, an autosomal recessive disorder sometimes referred to as hemophilia C.

Von Willebrand's disease is a variable and complex bleeding disorder, which appears to be at least as common as true hemophilia. The factor VIII molecule is normally found not only in plasma but also on the platelet membrane and is necessary for platelet adhesion to certain surfaces. The ability of the factor VIII molecule to mediate this and other platelet functions is referred to as von Willebrand factor activity (or ristocetin cofactor activity, after one of its laboratory assays). In hemophilia A, low factor VIII procoagulant levels are due to a qualitative disorder in the VIII molecule; when the molecule is measured by immunologic methods, VIII antigen is found to be present in normal amounts.

Because hemophilic plasma has normal von Willebrand factor activity despite its low level of factor VIII procoagulant activity, hemophiliacs have normal platelet function and normal bleeding time tests. In von Willebrand's disease, the ratio of VIII procoagulant level to VIII antigen level is approximately 1; i.e., there is a true decrease in VIII synthesis. For this reason, von Willebrand factor activity is also decreased, yielding prolonged bleeding time tests as well as low VIII levels. The ability to measure von Willebrand factor and VIII antigen have greatly aided in the diagnosis of von Willebrand's disease, but the variability of this syndrome, its fluctuating laboratory values from day to day, and the technical difficulty of the assay systems continue to confound the most skillful specialists in hemostasis.

Treatment

The treatment for each of these disorders is unique to that disorder, and generally ineffectual for the others. "A unit of fresh frozen plasma" is no longer acceptable treatment for bleeding due to any of these conditions, unless the disorder is unusually mild and the bleeding is trivial. For these reasons, adequate treatment requires a precise diagnosis, including: (a) identification of the deficient factor (or factors); (b) precise quantitation of the factor level to allow accurate prognosis and for calculation of replacement doses; and (c) determination of the presence or absence of an acquired inhibitor antibody against factor VIII or IX in patients with hemophilia A or B.

Hemophilia A

The clinical hallmark of classic hemophilia is frequent bleeding into muscles and joints; most such episodes are not due to identifiable external trauma. Easy bruising and severe postoperative hemorrhage are also found. Gastrointestinal and central nervous system bleeding are rare, the latter often occurring only in the setting of uncontrolled hypertension.

Severity. The frequency and severity of bleeding may be predicted from the factor VIII procoagulant level. A factor VIII level of 100 per cent is defined as the amount found in fresh frozen plasmas obtained from many normal donors and pooled together. In more recent terminology, such reference plasma is defined as containing 1.0

units of factor VIII per ml. Thus, a moderately severe hemophiliac with a factor VIII level of 2 per cent of normal can also be said to have a factor VIII level of 0.02 unit per ml. of plasma. The factor VIII level in a normal person on a given day may range between 50 and 200 per cent (0.50 to 2.00 units per ml.).

Patients with factor VIII levels of equal to or less than 1 per cent of normal ($\leq$0.01 unit per ml.) will have hemorrhages requiring therapy three to four times per month on the average, although the range is large and the episodes irregularly spaced. Such patients are classified as severe hemophiliacs. Patients with factor VIII levels of greater than 5 per cent of normal ($>$0.05 unit per ml.) are considered mild hemophiliacs and usually hemorrhage only with trauma or at surgery. Occasional "spontaneous" hemarthrosis may occur in such patients, especially in joints damaged by previously undertreated hemorrhage. Patients whose factor VIII levels fall between these two ranges are considered moderately severe, and their clinical picture falls somewhere between the two extremes. If such patients have had multiple untreated or suboptimally treated hemarthroses with subsequent joint damage, the anatomic instability of these joints will cause frequent and severe bleeding, and the patient will thus appear clinically more severe than the factor VIII assay would suggest.

Hemarthrosis. The majority of hemorrhages requiring therapy will be joint hemorrhages. The knees, ankles, elbows, hips, and shoulders are the most common sites for bleeding. The long-term sequelae of recurrent hemarthroses have, in the past, produced the major long-term disability, deformity, pain, expense, and social and vocational problems of hemophilia. Each episode of bleeding into the joint sets up a synovial inflammatory process that may become chronic if repeated hemorrhages are inadequately treated. This chronic synovitis leads to: (a) increasing proliferation of the inflamed synovium, whose intensely vascular nature sets up a viscious cycle of more frequent hemorrhage and more active inflammation; (b) destruction of cartilage and eventual resorption of bone, with cyst formation; (c) anatomic joint instability, making hemorrhages more frequent in the involved joint and in neighboring joints and muscles; and (d) pain, with subsequent disuse atrophy of local muscle groups, making joint instability worse.

In the early stages of hemorrhage patients can often recognize an "aura" that joint hemorrhage has begun. A few hours later, discomfort and mild limitation of motion may occur. In another several hours, pain and swelling will be found, along with increased cutaneous warmth and early discoloration. When any of these physical findings are present, the hemorrhage is far advanced and the process of synovitis will begin; the patient or the physician has waited too long before instituting therapy. *Unlike most conditions in medical practice, hemophilia should be treated at the earliest symptoms suggestive of joint hemorrhage, long before the development of any physical findings.* Only in this way can the long-term disabling sequelae be prevented.

The keystone of therapy in hemophilia is to provide the patient with access to immediate and adequate correction of his hemostatic defect at the earliest symptom suggestive of hemorrhage. For the majority of severe and moderately severe hemophiliacs, the achievement of this goal is via a combination of intensive education of the patient and his family plus the institution of a carefully supervised home therapy program.

The Self-therapy Program. Except for some patients with inhibitor antibodies, highly unreliable or unstable patients, or children less than 3 years of age, most patients are candidates for self therapy, often with the support of family members or close friends. All suitable candidates should first undergo an initial detailed history and physical examination, and a battery of appropriate laboratory and radiographic studies. The patient and his family are seen by two physicians, who independently attempt to identify family members with the greatest potential competence, and these members are selected for further training. Since hemophilia treatment centers now exist in all areas of the United States and Canada, such training now usually takes place at a major hemophilia center. The day to day supervision of the patient may often be provided by a physician in the patient's immediate geographic vicinity, with subsequent yearly visits to the center for long-term evaluation and comprehensive care.

At most centers, all patients and selected family members receive an individual half-day course on the pathophysiology, diagnosis, and therapy of hemophilia. Patients are taught the possible symptoms and signs of some of the major lesions of hemophilia, such as intracranial bleeding and psoas hematoma. They are taught how much factor VIII to give for various types of bleeding. The patient and his family are then taught intravenous technic and family members perform several venipunctures on each other. Special attention is also paid to the indications for making contact with their physician or the hemophilia center. These include the occurrence of any major hemorrhage (Table 1) or failure of a minor hemorrhage to resolve with two infusions at home.

The first several infusions are made under observation. If the patient demonstrates proficiency in self-infusion and a good grasp of basic principles, he is then allowed maximum independence. Replacement supplies of lyophylized factor

TABLE 1. **Typical Initial Doses of Replacement Products for Hemophilia A and B**

INDICATION FOR REPLACEMENT	HEMOPHILIA A (UNITS VIII/KG.)	HEMOPHILIA B (UNITS IX/KG.)
I. *Mild Hemorrhage*	15	20
A. Early joint or muscle bleeding		
B. Severe epistaxis		
C. Gingival or dental bleeding unresponsive to epsilon aminocaproic acid		
D. Hematuria		
II.* *Major Hemorrhage*		
A. Advanced joint or muscle bleeding		
B. Neck, tongue or pharyngeal hematoma		
C. Head trauma, without neurologic deficit		
D. Severe physical trauma, no evidence of bleeding		
E. Severe abdominal pain		
F. Gastrointestinal hemorrhage		
III.* *Life Threatening Lesions*		
A. Intracranial hemorrhage		
B. Surgery		
C. Major trauma with bleeding		

*For category II, subsequent doses will usually be required; for category III, one to several weeks of maintenance of minimum levels will be mandatory.

VIII concentrate, needles, and syringes sufficient for several months of infusions are sent by mail upon receipt of satisfactory written records. All patients carry an introductory letter from the center, which validates their diagnosis, their training in self-infusion, their authorization to carry needles and syringes, and which gives instructions for reaching hemophilia center personnel on a 24 hour basis.

Patients are instructed to raise their factor VIII level to 30 per cent at the first suggestion of joint or muscle hemorrhage. Prophylactic infusions are used for brief periods in occasional patients, as part of a therapy program for recurrent monarticular hemarthrosis, or when a child is mastering a new physical activity such as bicycle riding.

All patients attend twice yearly comprehensive evaluation sessions as a minimum mandatory requirement for continuation of the program. At this comprehensive clinic, a decision is made whether interim visits will be necessary during the ensuing year, and whether changes in supportive health care measures are required. During the course of each evaluation, every patient is personally interviewed and examined by a hematologist and an orthopedic surgeon. He is also seen by a nurse practitioner, a medical social worker, a psychologist, an oral surgeon, a physical therapist, a vocational counselor, and, when indicated, by a genetic counselor.

Patients who are excluded from the home therapy program still go through the education sessions and attend the comprehensive health evaluations. However, those patients who are highly unreliable or unstable, those who are very mild and therefore infrequently treated, and certain patients with inhibitor antibody against factor VIII are not placed on a home therapy regimen. Children under 3 years of age are placed on a modified type of home therapy in which their parents are fully instructed and keep factor VIII concentrate at home, but the venipuncture is performed by a health professional.

It should be emphasized that the least important aspect of self-therapy is the teaching of venipuncture. The program achieves its dramatic results via patient education plus the systematic application of the skills of a variety of appropriate medical personnel who can address (and usually prevent) the long-term problems of this lifelong disease.

Factor VIII Replacement. The half life of factor VIII in vivo is between 8 and 12 hours. Although the minimum plasma level necessary to achieve hemostasis will depend on the location, severity, and duration of hemorrhage, a level of 30 per cent (0.30 unit per ml.) is generally sought for most acute hemorrhages. Early bleeding into muscles or joints will be arrested by a single infusion to this level in 95 per cent of episodes.

For far advanced joint or muscle bleeding or for other major episodes (see Table 1), a factor VIII level of 50 per cent should be achieved. For categories II and III in Table 1, maintenance programs will be required, as will be outlined below.

The therapeutic material will contain a certain number of factor VIII units. One unit is equivalent to the factor VIII found in 1 ml. of pooled fresh frozen plasma. For factor VIII, the replacement formula is as follows:

Each unit of F. VIII infused per kg. of body weight yields a 2 per cent rise in plasma VIII level (i.e., 0.02 unit per ml.)

To achieve a 50 per cent level in vivo, in a 70 kg. man with an advanced hemarthrosis would thus require 25 × 70 kg., or approximately 1750 units of factor VIII, assuming a starting point of essentially zero per cent factor VIII. This calculation demonstrates why fresh frozen plasma cannot be used in hemophilia; it would require 1750 ml. of this material just to achieve the initial desired level, and volume overload would likely result.

If a given minimum level is to be maintained over several days, this can be achieved by: (a) giving an initial infusion to twice the desired minimum; (b) giving one half this dose every 12 hours, assuming a 12 hour half life, and (c) performing factor VIII assays every several days for more precise dose adjustments. For example, a 50 kg. boy has an extensive laceration, requiring that he be kept at levels above 30 per cent factor VIII until healing is complete. An initial infusion is given to the 60 per cent level, via 30 × 50 kg., or 1500 units of factor VIII. He then receives 750 units every 12 hours thereafter for 7 to 10 days.

Replacement Source. Fresh frozen plasma is no longer used for the treatment of hemophilia because one cannot achieve or maintain adequate dose levels without danger of circulatory overload.

Wet-frozen cryoprecipitate was the product of choice several years ago and is still used as such in some centers. It should be preferentially used when the patient has mild hemophilia and seldom requires exposure to blood products, in order to minimize the risk of hepatitis. For patients with moderately severe or severe hemophilia, their plasma product requirements will be such that clinical or subclinical hepatitis appears to be as frequent with cryoprecipitate as with commercial concentrates, according to several recent studies.

Cryoprecipitate results when fresh frozen plasma is slowly thawed at 4°C. Each bag of cryoprecipitate, at a volume of 10 to 40 ml. per bag, will contain factor VIII, which varies from between 20 and 150 units. The average bag from the average blood center, in my experience, should be assumed to contain approximately 70 units, for purposes of calculation. Only if the blood center institutes meticulous quality control and performs frequent assays on its products can one count on higher levels. Thus, the hemophiliac who requires 1500 units of factor VIII should receive 21 bags of cryoprecipitate.

The disadvantages of cryoprecipitate include its inconvenience for home use, need for storage at very low temperatures, low preparation time, and, most importantly, the unreliability of its factor VIII content. We now restrict the use of this material to mild hemophiliacs, and patients with von Willebrand's disease.

There are now available at least eight different commercial factor VIII concentrates, made from large pools of normal plasma, and sold in lyophilized form. When reconstituted, one can administer 1000 units of factor VIII in 30 to 100 ml. volume, depending on the product used; each vial is labelled with the number of units contained, and such figures are quite accurate.

These products not only allow accurate dose calculations, but are convenient for home use, stable at home refrigerator temperatures for months to years, stable at room temperature for weeks to months, and can be rapidly prepared for self-administration. The major disadvantage is cost; current prices are in the range of $0.07 to $0.12 per factor VIII unit ($17.50 to $27.50 per 250 unit vial) wholesale cost. These materials have made early and intensive home therapy possible, however, and thus overall costs of health care have greatly declined for patients treated with these materials.

Side Effects of Replacement Therapy. Occasional patients develop allergic reactions to cryoprecipitate, usually manifest as urticaria, pruritus, or low grade fever. Rarely, bronchospasm or serious anaphylactoid reactions have been reported.

Allergic reactions to concentrate are quite infrequent and very mild; changing to a different lot number of the product for subsequent infusions is probably warranted in this setting; subsequent reactions are rare. As with any plasma product, reactions lasting more than a few minutes may be ameliorated with low-dose antihistamine therapy. One life-threatening reaction to concentrate has been reported. It is important to note that patients who have had severe reactions to cryoprecipitate usually do not react to concentrate.

With infusion of large doses of factor VIII concentrate, usually in the setting of surgery or major trauma, recipients may develop severe hemolytic anemia. This infrequent side effect occurs only in recipients with Type A or B erythrocytes, and appears to be due to high titers of anti-A or anti-B antibodies in the concentrate. If transfusion is necessary, type O cells should be given. The process resolves as the dose of concentrate is decreased.

The major side effect of either cryoprecipitate or factor VIII concentrate is hepatitis, which may be either A, B, or non-A non-B type. Hemophiliacs also have high titers of cytomegalovirus antibody, and this or other viruses may also contribute to liver dysfunction. In most series, the great majority of treated hemophiliacs will have plasma levels of hepatitis B surface antibody, and a significant minority (2 to 5 per cent) will carry hepatitis B surface antigen. Presumably because of prior extensive plasma product exposure from early in life, the incidence of overt clinical hepatitis in moderately severe or severe hemophiliacs who receive pooled commercial concentrate is very low. (When factor VIII or IX concentrates have been given to nonhemophiliacs, the hepatitis incidence has been large.) The majority of treated hemophiliacs have persistent mild elevations of serum transaminases; this finding is independent of type, source, or dose of replacement product and is of uncertain significance.

The development of inhibitor antibody occurs only after exposure to factor VIII, but is not related to the source of the replacement product or to frequency or intensity of exposure. Recent data suggests that there may be a familial predisposition to the development of this dreaded complication.

Surgery in Hemophilia. Elective and emergency surgery in the hemophiliac is a challenge to the physician. The following general requirements should be met before surgery is undertaken:

1. A hematologist and diagnostic coagulation laboratory are available.

2. The surgeon is familiar with the handling of a patient with a coagulation disorder.

3. There is a blood bank capable of providing adequate supplies of appropriate replacement material.

4. There is an appropriate rehabilitation team for postoperative management.

5. No inhibitor is present; this should be rechecked a few days before surgery.

As orthopedic, general, oral, and other kinds of surgery become increasingly commonplace in the hemophiliac, certain guidelines require reemphasis. Both physician and patient should consider the following points in an orderly and systematic manner before surgery is undertaken.

1. Will the lesion recur postoperatively? If the lesion developed because of suboptimal medical control of hemophilia, it may well recur. This principle is of special importance with respect to orthopedic surgery in hemophilia. Orthopedic surgery will often fail when the patient has demonstrated unreliability in adhering to a conservative regimen. For this reason, elective orthopedic surgery should be preceded by a period of intensive nonsurgical management. This will emphasize to the patient the importance of basic medical principles (immediate infusion at the first sign of hemorrhage, appropriate physical therapy, etc.). It will also test the patient's ability to adhere to the regimen.

2. The patient should avoid antiplatelet medication before and after surgery. Aspirin, and aspirin-containing medications such as Darvon Compound, Empirin, and Percodan, can inhibit platelet function for 5 to 7 days. Other drugs, including phenylbutazone, phenacetin, and in-

domethacin should probably be avoided as well, for similar reasons.

3. Schedule the surgery for Monday or Tuesday. This allows the best availability of laboratory services for factor assays and the best access to consultants during the first few days after surgery.

4. Check the supply of replacement therapeutics. Calculate the expected dose of material needed for a period of at least 2 weeks, multiply by 2, and notify the blood bank or pharmacy of your need. Ask them to confirm the arrival of the material; do not proceed with surgery until such confirmation has been received.

5. Consider multiple procedures. Because of the great expense of hospitalization and replacement therapy, it makes sense to perform minor procedures such as dental extractions and excision of cutaneous lesions at the same time as major ones. These should be performed a day or two prior to the major surgery in some patients. For example, oral surgery with its transient bacteremia might increase the risk of osteomyelitis if done on the same day as elective orthopedic surgery.

6. Schedule a preoperative conference between the patient, his family, the surgeon, and the pediatrician or internist. This can often be conveniently done on the day of admission to the hospital. The benefits of such planned communications are obvious. Many patients or family members or both may have an unstated fear of fatal bleeding and will respond dramatically to reassurance on this issue.

7. In the order book should be written: "Hemophiliac: intramuscular medications contraindicated;" "Patient may not be given aspirin in any form including Darvon Compound, Empirin, or Percodan;" "Avoid prescription of any compound medicine to avoid unnoticed aspirin;" and "Joint or muscle pain may indicate hemorrhage—notify physician at once for possible coagulation factor infusion." These same instructions should be taped to the cover of the patient's chart holder to ensure their being seen by all house officers, medical students, medical consultants, and nursing staff.

For major surgery, the factor VIII level should be brought to the 80 to 100 per cent range, just prior to the surgery, and then kept at above 30 per cent for 10 to 14 days. For extensive orthopedic surgery, 4 to 6 weeks of replacement may be required. For example, in a 50 kg. boy who will require major surgery to achieve an 80 per cent factor VIII level, give 40 units per kg., or 2000 factor VIII units (e.g., 30 bags of cryoprecipitate averaging 70 units per bag, or 8 vials of factor VIII concentrate averaging 250 units per vial). Twelve hours later, his factor VIII level will have fallen to approximately 40 per cent. One could then give

1000 factor VIII units every 12 hours to keep him in the desired range.

These theoretical calculations must be checked at least every third day (preferably daily for the first few days) by performance of factor VIII assays on the patient's plasma. In the best of hands, and especially when cryoprecipitate is the therapeutic material, there is considerable error in these estimates. Doses should be adjusted according to the actual levels observed in vivo. For minor surgery half as much therapy may suffice but will still need to be maintained for 7 to 10 days. Precise regimens should be designed in advance of surgery by the appropriate medical consultant.

In oral surgery, the concomitant use of epsilon aminocaproic acid (Amicar) reduces further the amount of factor VIII needed. When Amicar is given at full therapeutic doses, either intravenously or orally, a single factor VIII infusion of 40 units per kg. just prior to the oral surgery is often sufficient. In some patients, if oozing occurs, another such infusion may be needed at intervals of once every other day. Amicar is not recommended for other forms of surgery, in which it appears to be without effect and could conceivably be a potentiator of postanesthesia deep venous thrombosis.

Inhibitor Antibody. Between 10 and 20 per cent of hemophiliacs will develop an inhibitor antibody at some time in their course, usually during infancy or childhood, and usually within the first hundred exposures to plasma products. The antibody results in the very rapid clearance of infused factor VIII procoagulant activity from the plasma such that no significant increase in circulating factor VIII can usually be measured, even after infusions of large doses. Bleeding can no longer be reliably controlled, and elective surgery should not be considered in such a patient.

Inhibitor antibodies in hemophiliacs have a highly unpredictable natural history. At times, very low titer and clinically weak antibodies, which are easily neutralized by factor VIII, will be found not to undergo anamnestic rises in titer after multiple challenges, later to become unexpectedly high in titer. Other patients will develop rising antibody titers after each exposure to factor VIII. Still other patients appear to have spontaneously lost their antibody despite multiple subsequent factor VIII challenges. The type of antibody response to factor VIII infusion and the patient's clinical response will dictate therapy. The therapy of patients with inhibitor ranges from total avoidance of all exposure to factor VIII in some centers to aggressive megadose factor VIII replacement in others. Factor IX concentrate, possibly because of its variable contamination with activated factor X, is thought to be efficacious by

some; it is usually given in large doses, such as 50 to 100 units of factor IX activity per kg. body weight. The use of immunosuppressives or corticosteroids has been abandoned in most centers, owing to lack of efficacy in this condition and to serious side effects.

In our own experience, patients with low titer antibodies which remain low in titer after repeated therapy often do well with standard but repeated doses of factor VIII concentrate. For those who fail to benefit, or have higher titers, factor IX concentrate is used; both groups of patients are often on home therapy, and bleeding is more likely to be arrested when treatment is applied at "aura" than if it is delayed.

A purposefully activated factor IX concentrate has recently been shown useful in certain inhibitor patients who are treatment failures, but this agent is still an experimental drug and is not generally available.

Because inhibitor patients depend on intensive and frequent use of all of the hemophilia center's comprehensive services (orthopedic, physiatric, psychiatric, social, financial) and because of their changing and complex replacement needs, all such patients should be followed, at least in part, at a major hemophilia center.

Hemophilia B (Christmas Disease)

From the point of view of the clinician, this disorder is indistinguishable from hemophilia A except by laboratory testing. All the comments made previously in the sections on severity, hemarthrosis, and self-therapy are applicable to this disorder. The mainstays of therapy remain patient education, early and intensive factor IX replacement when hemorrhage is suspected, and the application of periodic comprehensive evaluations as previously described. Factor IX is not found in either cryoprecipitate or factor VIII concentrate; these two materials are totally ineffective for the treatment of hemophilia B.

The half life of factor IX in vivo is between 20 and 24 hours. Although the plasma level necessary to achieve hemostasis will depend on the location, severity, and duration of hemorrhage, the minimum hemostatic level appears to be somewhat less than is needed for factor VIII. A minimum level of 20 per cent (0.20 unit per ml.) is generally aimed for most acute hemorrhages. Early bleeding into muscles or joints will be permanently arrested by a single infusion to this level in 95 per cent of episodes.

For more advanced joint or muscle bleeding, or for other major episodes (see Table 1) a factor IX level of 40 per cent should be achieved. For major trauma or surgery, initial levels of 60 to 80 per cent may be required, maintaining the level at above 40 per cent via repeated infusions for several days, and then at levels above 20 per cent for a total of 7 to 10 days. For major orthopedic surgery, considerably longer treatment periods may be needed.

The therapeutic material will contain a number of factor IX units. One unit is equivalent to the factor IX found in 1 ml. of pooled fresh frozen plasma. For factor IX, the replacement formula is as follows:

Each unit of F. IX infused per kg. of body weight yields a 1 per cent rise in plasma IX level (i.e., 0.01 unit per ml.).

To achieve a 20 per cent level in vivo, in a 70 kg. man with an early hemarthrosis would thus require 20 × 70 kg., or approximately 1400 units of factor IX, assuming a starting point of essentially zero per cent factor IX. Because factor IX has a significantly longer half life than factor VIII and because lower in vivo minimum levels appear necessary for hemostasis, fresh frozen plasma is still sometimes used in hemophilia B. For patients with moderately severe or severe disease, or for prolonged or major bleeding, factor IX concentrate is generally preferred, however.

If a given minimum level is to be maintained over several days, this can be achieved by methods similar to those described for factor VIII, except that the half life of 24 hours (as compared to approximately 12 hours for factor VIII) indicates the need for either lower or less frequent subsequent doses by a factor of 50 per cent. Factor IX assays should be monitored every few days for adequate control.

There are two commercially available factor IX concentrates at present. Both products contain factors II, VII, IX, and X, but because of the high hepatitis risk for persons not previously frequently exposed to blood products, these products should probably be used only for the treatment of hemophilia B. In addition to the allergic and infectious side effects listed for factor VIII concentrate, factor IX may also predispose to deep venous and other types of thrombosis. Such thrombosis has generally been associated with very large doses of factor IX given in the setting of general anesthesia and surgery, or in patients with clinically overt hepatic dysfunction. Some physicians recommend the addition of small doses of heparin to the factor IX concentrate or to the recipient in cases of large dose factor IX replacement for surgery. Thrombosis has not been recorded in the home therapy of routine acute hemorrhage in hemophilia B.

Inhibitor antibody against factor IX is exceedingly rare. There is no generally accepted efficacious therapy, treatment usually being reserved for severe episodes, and usually including large and frequent doses of factor IX concentrate.

Other Congenital Plasma Coagulation Factor Deficiencies

These nonsex-linked inherited deficiencies are very rare. Therapy is aimed at restoring in vivo levels of the missing procoagulant to the minimum hemostatic concentration at time of hemorrhage. Frequency of infusions will depend on half life. Table 2 shows the minimum hemostatic level and half life for each factor.

For fibrinogen (factor I) deficiency, the replacement material of choice is wet-frozen cryoprecipitate, which is rich in both factor VIII and fibrinogen. A starting dose of 4 bags per 10 kg. of body weight, with maintenance via 25 to 50 per cent of this dose every 48 hours according to plasma levels achieved, is generally sufficient.

For deficiencies of factors II, VII, or X, fresh frozen or stored plasma should be used. Starting doses should be in the range of 10 to 20 ml. per kg. Whereas subsequent maintenance of hemostatic levels can be achieved by daily infusions of 10 ml. per kg. in most patients with factor II or X deficiency, the short half life of factor VII dictates infusions of this amount of plasma every 12 hours in factor VII deficient patients. Because of the risk of hepatitis, commercial prothrombin complex concentrate should be used only in patients whose deficiency of factor II, VII, IX, or X is so severe that very frequent exposures to plasma products are necessary.

von Willebrand's Disease

Von Willebrand's Disease (vWD) is an autosomal defect for which the clinical manifestations include mucous membrane bleeding such as epistaxis, gingival oozing, gastrointestinal hemorrhage, and menorrhagia, as well as postsurgical blood loss. In severe cases only, joint and

TABLE 2. **Minimum Hemostatic Level and Biologic Half Life for the Less Frequently Encountered Congenital Coagulation Factor Deficiencies**

DEFICIENT FACTOR	MINIMUM HEMOSTATIC LEVEL (% OF NORMAL)	BIOLOGIC HALF LIFE (HOURS)
I	25–50 (50–100 mg./dl.)	72–96
II	20–40	48–72
V	10–20	15–24
VII	5–10	4–6
X	10–20	40–60
XI	10–20	40–60
XII	–	48–52
XIII	2–3	72–96

muscle bleeding may also occur, and the clinical picture may mimic hemophilia A. Most vWD patients have a mild or moderate hemostatic defect, and do not experience hemarthroses.

As noted in the introduction to this section, vWD differs from hemophilia A in that the decreased factor VIII procoagulant level of vWD is due to a true decrease in factor VIII synthesis. Thus, factor VIII antigen will also be decreased, unlike hemophilia A, in which it is normal. Because the factor VIII molecule also carries the von Willebrand factor (ristocetin cofactor), vWD patients will also have a defect in platelet function with prolonged bleeding time tests. For hemostasis, both factor VIII procoagulant activity and von Willebrand factor activity must be maintained at acceptable levels.

The vWD patient can apparently synthesize endogenous factor VIII procoagulant when given normal plasma, since factor VIII levels will be found to exceed those transfused, and will remain elevated longer than would be expected based on the known 8 to 12 hour half life of transfused factor VIII. Thus partial thromboplastin time (PTT) and factor VIII levels can easily be corrected with moderate amounts of plasma or cryoprecipitate. Unfortunately, however, the von Willebrand factor has a considerably shorter post-infusion half life than does factor VIII procoagulant, so that the prolonged bleeding time may sometimes only briefly be corrected by infusion therapy.

Because of these considerations, no uniform dosage recommendations for plasma products can be given for patients with vWD. Wet-frozen cryoprecipitate is the replacement product of choice, as it is rich in factor VIII procoagulant as well as the factor that stimulates endogenous factor VIII procoagulant synthesis, and also contains von Willebrand factor activity. Commercial factor VIII concentrates have not been well studied in vWD, have certain theoretical drawbacks for use in these patients, and probably should be avoided. If cryoprecipitate is not available, fresh frozen plasma can be used.

A reasonable starting replacement dose would be 1 to 2 bags of cryoprecipitate per 10 kg. of body weight per 24 hours. For fresh frozen plasma, 10 to 15 ml. per kg. per day can be tried. Ideal therapy will not only maintain the factor VIII level at above 30 per cent but will keep the bleeding time normal or only mildly abnormal. In practice, maintaining complete correction of bleeding time is often difficult and sometimes impossible to achieve.

For surgery, infusion therapy should probably be begun 24 hours preoperatively for optimum endogenous synthesis of factor VIII proco-

agulant, and to allow assessment of the effects of the infusion on the bleeding time. If the effect is transitory and the bleeding time rapidly returns to markedly abnormal, larger and more frequent doses of cryoprecipitate may be needed.

For gingival bleeding or hemorrhage accompanying dental extractions, epsilon aminocaproic acid is useful, as in hemophilia A.

Menorrhagia in females with vWD can be a serious problem. In mild or moderate cases, oral contraceptives are efficacious, possibly in part due to the ability of ovarian hormones to elevate the endogenous factor VIII level. Careful avoidance of aspirin-containing medications and other drugs that effect platelet function, and treatment of chronic iron deficiency are also indicated. In occasional patients, hysterectomy may eventually become necessary. Because of the elevated factor VIII procoagulant and von Willebrand factor levels seen during pregnancy, postpartum hemorrhage is usually not severe in vWD patients.

BLEEDING DISORDERS SECONDARY TO PLATELET ABNORMALITIES *

method of
JEANE P. HESTER, M.D.
Houston, Texas

Introduction

Bleeding disorders secondary to platelet abnormalities fall into two categories: bleeding disorders associated with quantitatively insufficient platelets in circulation and those with qualitative dysfunction in the presence of a normal level of circulating platelets.

Thrombocytopenic disorders can be categorized into essentially two groups: those associated with bone marrow dysfunction and those related to immunologic destruction with normal or increased numbers of bone marrow megakaryocytes.

Disorders associated with qualitative defects in platelets which inhibit their normal role in hemostasis include congenital disorders and acquired disorders related to leukemic processes or to drug usage.

Quantitative Disorders

Patient Population. Thrombocytopenia related to bone marrow dysfunction with depressed platelet production capacities is more likely to be

*Supported in part by grants CA11520 and CA19806 from the National Institutes of Health, Bethesda, Maryland.

associated with hemorrhagic risks than that associated with immunologically induced thrombocytopenia with increased platelet destruction. Decreased production is seen in patients with marrow replacement with neoplastic cell infiltration (leukemia or metastatic solid tumor) or marrow aplasia that can be drug-induced or of unknown cause and represents a primary aplasia or aplasia that is secondary to chemotherapy or radiotherapy regimens directed toward management of the neoplasia. Platelet component replacement may not be initiated until clinical evidence of hemorrhage occurs.

Gaydos and Freireich defined the quantitative relationship between platelet count and hemorrhage in patients with acute leukemia in the 1960s. The frequency and severity of hemorrhage clearly increased in patients with circulating platelet levels below 20,000 per microliter. While no absolute threshold existed, they observed that serious gross hemorrhage was rarely observed at levels greater than 20,000 per microliter, and that only 16 per cent of thrombocytopenic days were associated with hemorrhage at platelet levels greater than 20,000 per microliter. This is the level then at which component replacement is usually initiated.

Donor Selection. Short-term replacement utilizing single units of platelets from multiple donors can be effective. However, this has the immunologic disadvantage of exposing the recipient to multiple antigens. Long-term replacement is most effectively carried out with an HL-A compatible donor. Alloimmunization, in part, related to lymphocytes contained in concentrates collected by existing technology, continues to be a major barrier in long-term support of thrombocytopenic patients. There is no specific typing system to match donor recipient pairs as exists for red cell typing and crossmatching. The importance of the histocompatibility antigen system and its relevance to platelet transfusion was demonstrated in the late 1960s. Identification of donors, related or unrelated, who share all four HL-A antigens with no mismatched antigens with the patient, resulted in effective transfusion response. Because of the large number of HL-A antigens that are currently identified and the mathematical possibilities of pairing the antigens, the likelihood of finding unrelated HL-A identical donors will require establishment of large donor pools to support small numbers of patients. However, the utilization of donors who are less than compatible but who share at least two antigens (one haplotype) or have cross reactive HL-A antigens has provided an effective replacement for some patients.

Transfusion Product. The dose of cells transfused ranges from about 2.0 to 8.0 $\times 10^{11}$ platelets. As low as 2×10^{11} cells was identified in the 1960s as providing effective hemostasis. The variability in the yield is, in part, related to the technology used to collect the product, the expertise of operating the procedure, the volume of donor blood processed, and the height of the platelet count of the donor from whom the product is collected. Leukocyte and red cell contamination are also variable but should be minimized as much as possible. Preparation of lymphocyte-poor platelet concentrates have been shown to be effective in restoring transfusion response in patients refractory to transfusions from the HL-A identical donors suggesting that lymphocyte specific antigens as well as HL-A antigens may be playing an immunologic role in the transfusion response. Likewise, preparation of red cell free concentrates allows transfusions between ABO incompatible donor recipient pairs and expands the utilization of platelets collected from donors who are ABO incompatible with the recipient.

Patient Response. The quantitative relationship between the number of cells transfused and the expected rise in the recipient in terms of post-transfusion circulating platelet increment has not been clearly characterized. The increment varies directly with the cell dose transfused (a low increment results from a low cell dose) and inversely with the blood volume of the patient (for a given cell dose, donors with large blood volumes will have a lower increment).

The post transfusion increment, defined as the

$$\frac{\text{Post count} - \text{precount}}{\text{number cells transfused}} \times \text{BSA,}$$
$$\text{(or number units transfused)}$$

as reported by several investigators ranges from 26,000 units per square meter for donor-recipient pairs who are HL-A identical, to 12,000 units per square meter for donors who share two HL-A antigens (one haplotype) and about 1,000 units per square meter for patients receiving random platelet transfusions. The increments vary from 0 to $100,000/10^{11}$ cells per square meter indicating many variables are contributing to the increment. Fever, splenomegaly with sequestration, disseminated intravascular coagulopathy from infection or progranulocytic leukemia all reduce the post-transfusion increment regardless of the compatibility of donor-recipient pairs.

A variety of antibodies may be produced by the patient and include cytotoxic and agglutinating antibodies. Routine laboratory testing is not available to detect the presence or absence of such antibodies. The relationship between the precise number of transfusions received and the appearance of alloimmunization is unknown and related in part to the ability of the patient to mount an immune response. However, alloimmunization to platelet replacement has been seen in patients who have received 10 or more red cell transfusions.

A decrement, rather than an increment, post-transfusion may reflect alloimmunization. Replacement with random platelets should be abandoned and efforts made to identify a compatible donor.

If HL-A typing is not available, selection of a donor related as parent, sibling, or offspring offers almost a 75 per cent chance that at least one haplotype (two HL-A antigens) will be shared between the donor and recipient.

Replacement therapy then for long-term support is most effective if the donor shares both HL-A haplotypes, or at least one haplotype with the recipient. Single donor platelets offer some immunologic advantages to the patient by decreasing the number of antigens to which he is exposed. Platelet concentrates that contain only microscopic red blood cell (RBC) contamination permit transfusions between ABO incompatible pairs, and lymphocyte-depleted concentrates appear to have advantages through elimination of lymphocyte-specific antigens.

Replacement therapy may be used prophylactically or therapeutically in the event of hemorrhage. Successful intraoperative and postoperative replacement allows surgical procedures to be performed on the thrombocytopenia patient when necessary.

Thrombocytopenia Secondary to Increased Platelet Destruction

These disorders are, in general, characterized by thrombocytopenia in the presence of adequate, or increased megakaryocytes in bone marrow aspirates. Thrombocytopenia results from platelet destruction that exceeds the production capacity of the marrow. Some of these disorders are idiopathic thrombocytopenic purpura (ITP); some are related to administration of drugs, or they may be seen in association with lymphoma, chronic lymphocytic leukemia, lupus erythematosus, or disorders in which hypersplenism is a manifestation.

General measures that apply to all thrombocytopenic patients include: avoidance of trauma or strenuous activity that would induce or accentuate hemorrhage, and avoidance of aspirin, phenothiazines, or other drugs known to inhibit platelet function.

Specific measures usually involve discontinuation of any drugs that might be responsible for the immune thrombocytopenia and initiation of corticosteroid therapy. Prednisone, in doses of 60 to 100 mg. per day, is usually given until the platelet count normalizes, or for a 2 to 3 week trial period. If the platelet count normalizes, reduction in prednisone is carried out with careful monitoring of the platelet counts. Vincristine has been reported effective in some cases of ITP and could be given in conjunction with, or sequential to corticosteroid therapy. (This use of vincristine is not listed in the manufacturer's official directive.) Platelet replacement transfusions are not usually recommended for immune thrombocytopenia in the absence of hemorrhage, as transfused platelets are also destroyed and a post-transfusion increment may not be seen.

In the presence of life-threatening hemorrhage, platelet replacement should be initiated. Transfusion of 4 to 8 units of platelet concentrate, preferably single donor, followed by a 1 hour post-transfusion platelet count, will provide guidelines on whether or not additional platelet units are required. If an increment is obtained, or there is clinical evidence of hemostatic control, additional platelets are not transfused until reappearance of hemorrhage. When several transfusions of platelets are given simultaneously, it has been noted that a post-transfusion increment achieved with the first transfusion is abolished by the second transfusion. This is especially true in patients who may be alloimmunized from previous blood component transfusions.

Most adults with ITP require splenectomy for management of the thrombocytopenia. Remission of the disease is obtained in approximately two thirds of the patients. Platelet concentrates should be available for the intraoperative and immediate postoperative phase, but replacement may not be necessary for hemostasis once the splenic pedicle is ligated. For patients who may be alloimmunized from previous transfusion, HL-A matched donors are preferable. Immunosuppressive therapy has been used in management of patients who fail to respond to splenectomy and corticosteroids, or who require continuing maintenance therapy postoperatively. Azathioprine, 100 mg. per square meter of body surface area per day, or cyclophosphamide, 100 mg. per square meter per day, may be given. Blood counts, monitored 1 to 2 times weekly will allow dose adjustment should unacceptable myelosuppression appear. (This use of azathioprine and cyclophosphamide is not listed in the manufacturer's official directives.)

If a complete or good partial response is obtained, tapering of dose, then discontinuation of drugs can be carried out. Because of the increased occurrence of malignancies and opportunistic infections in patients receiving long-term immunosuppressive therapy, limitation in dose and duration of therapy is desirable.

Qualitative Disorders

Bleeding disorders manifested by a prolonged bleeding time and a normal peripheral blood count suggest a qualitative platelet function abnormality may be present. Abnormalities of platelet adhesion, aggregation or procoagulant activity or both have been described. An extensive overview of platelet function defects, possible mechanisms, and associated clinical diseases is discussed by Weiss (N. Engl. J. Med., *293*:531, 1975, and *293*:581, 1975).

Defects of Adhesion. Patients with von Willebrand's disease show a reduction in AHF, factor VIII, as well as impaired adhesion to subendothelium. In vitro platelet studies also show reduced aggregation response to ristocetin. There is evidence to suggest that some plasma factor may be decreased as plasma, cryoprecipitate, or fractions containing factor VIII correct the aggregation defect and shorten the patient's bleeding time.

Patients with the diagnosis of Bernard-Soulier (giant platelet) syndrome also appear to have defects in platelet adherence to subendothelial tissue. An aggregation defect to ristocetin is also manifested. As opposed to von Willebrand's disease, the aggregation defect is not corrected by transfusion with plasma. Some studies suggest these platelets cannot bind some of the clotting protein, notably factor V, VI, and VIII.

Defects of Aggregation. Platelets of patients with Glanzmann's thrombasthenia adhere normally to collagen, but do not aggregate in response to adenosine diphosphate (ADP), epinephrine, thrombin, or collagen. Clot retraction is also diminished. The cause of the defect is unknown but may reside in deficiencies in some of the platelet membrane proteins.

Investigators have also described patients whose platelets were aggregated by ADP but not by collagen. This impairment was attributed to a defect in the release of ADP.

There appear to be two categories of this defect. In one, ADP is present in normal amounts, but the mechanism for releasing it is defective. In the other there appears to be diminished platelet stores of ADP.

An example of diminished ADP release, in the presence of normal levels of ADP, is found in platelets from patients who have ingested aspirin. Aspirin appears to inhibit the conversion of arachidonic acid to the cyclic endoperoxidase that mediates the release reaction.

In the second category, storage-pool disease, there is usually a deficiency of ADP in the cytoplasmic dense granules. Additionally, there also appears to be a reduction in platelet calcium, serotonin, and dense granule content of these platelets.

A heterogenous population of patients may demonstrate storage pool defects. It may be seen in patients with oculocutaneous albinism (Hermansky-Pudlak syndrome), Wiskott-Aldrich syndrome, and thrombocytopenia with absent radius syndrome.

There also appear to be some abnormalities of hemostasis in patients with uremia and myeloproliferative disorders (essential thrombocythemia, polycythemia vera, chronic myelogenous leukemia, and myeloid metaplasia) that have been attributed to qualitative platelet defects of various types. Diminished response to one or more aggregating agents—ADP, collagen, epinephrine, serotonin, thrombin—has been reported in chronic myelogenous leukemia patients undergoing splenectomy. Platelet qualitative abnormalities appear to have contributed to postoperative hemorrhage in a few of these patients. Hemostasis could be restored, and hemorrhage controlled by prophylactic replacement with platelet concentrates from normal donors during the first 2 hour postoperative period.

DISSEMINATED INTRAVASCULAR COAGULATION (DIC)

method of
LAURENCE A. SHERMAN, M.D.
St. Louis, Missouri

Intravascular coagulation is a term applied when the coagulation mechanism is activated in excess of that necessary for hemostasis for injured blood vessels, and other disorders. Concomitant with activation of the coagulation system, the fibrinolytic system is also activated. The manifestations of intravascular coagulation are protean and, in part, depend on (1) the nature of inciting mechanisms and their severity; (2) the balance between consumption of various labile coagulation moieties and the ability of the body to increase their synthesis; (3) the body's capacity to "clear" activated coagulation species in the liver or reticuloendothelial system or both; (4) the compensatory mechanism of various circulating protease inhibitors which neutralize thrombin, factor Xa, and others; and (5) the relative degrees of thrombosis vs. fibrinolysis in various parts of the body. In certain instances, the consumption of coagulation moieties may so exceed production that effective hemostasis can no longer occur and the dominant clinical manifestation is bleeding. Conversely, various signs of thrombosis and ischemia may present. On occasion, intravascular coagulation may be truly disseminated, i.e., with multiple thromboses occurring throughout the body. Alternatively, the intravascular coagulation may be localized in certain organs such as the kidneys, but the process is sufficiently severe to have laboratory detectable abnormalities present in the peripheral blood similar to those found in the disseminated variety. Such abnormalities might include depression of platelets, fibrinogen, or Factor VIII, as well as the appearance of microangiopathic hemolytic anemia and various end products of coagulation or fibrinolysis or both. The latter include soluble complexes of fibrin and fibrinogen or degradation products or both, nonclottable fibrinogen/fibrin degradation products (FDP), fibrinopeptide A, platelet factor 4, and others. Although there is strong evidence for the presence of DIC when such test findings are present, other causes for the abnormalities should be excluded before accepting the diagnosis of DIC.

It is generally believed that intravascular coagulation occurs secondary to those diseases which can cause activation of the coagulation system by a variety of processes. In certain instances, the underlying disease is acute. This would include abruptio placenta, amniotic fluid embolus, crush injuries, certain septicemias, and other disorders. In such circumstances, the stimulus is often self-limited, as the abruptio placenta, or rapid medical therapy of the primary disease is available, as in septicemia. As a result, the secondary process of intravascular coagulation is limited and usually specific therapy of the coagulopathy is not required.

Other forms of intravascular coagulation may be chronic, such as that secondary to malignancies or vascular malformations. Rarely in chronic DIC, the primary disease may not be clinically manifest, as in occult neoplasms. Usually DIC does not occur with neoplasms unless the malignancy has metastasized. Effective therapy of the primary disease may not be available. Thus, occasionally, more specific therapy of the DIC may be required, *if* the coagulopathy is clinically severe.

Therapy

Therapeutic maneuvers in intravascular coagulation will fall into two categories: General supportive therapy includes improvement of abnormalities such as hypovolemia, anoxia, hypotension, and acidosis. These abnormalities can potentiate DIC. Also included in general therapy is hemostatic replacement therapy for instances of DIC when bleeding is present to such an extent as to be of serious immediate concern and one cannot wait for the return to normal levels of hemostatic components. Fresh frozen plasma is usually sufficient to treat depressed levels of the plasma coagulation factors. A few patients may have particularly striking depressions of fibrinogen levels. In such instances, cryoprecipitate may be used as a source of fibrinogen (0.15 gram per bag of cryoprecipitate). For patients with marked thrombocytopenia, platelet concentrates may be used. In general, unless the platelet count is below approximately 30,000 to 50,000, platelet concentrates are not necessary. If organic lesions such as recent trauma or surgery are present, hemostasis may not be achieved without higher platelet levels.

Specific therapy includes treatment of inciting mechanisms such as infection, dead tissue, or other mechanisms. Perhaps the most important aspect of the therapy of intravascular coagulation is to identify the inciting process and, if at all feasible, to remove the cause or to treat it with antibiotics, or other agents.

Anticoagulation is used in patients in whom the inciting mechanism is continuing, such as those with tumors, and in whom there is evidence of thrombi and ischemia in vital organs of the body such as the kidneys or the brain. There is some evidence that heparin therapy can be hazardous in patients with intravascular coagulation, particularly when given by intermittent bolus injections. Major bleeding can ensue. Therefore, it is best to administer heparin by continuous intravenous infusion. Some authors have advocated a starting dose of 100 units per kg. of body weight, followed by a dose of approximately one quarter to one third of the initial dose. If the patient's status is stable, it is frequently desirable to begin anticoagulation at a lower dose level than would ordinarily be used for the anticoagulation of routine thromboses. This is particularly true if the patient has a disease that can independently affect hemostatic components. For example, patients with DIC and acute leukemia can be expected to have their thrombocytopenia continue in spite of correction of the DIC and will have added risks from heparinization. In general, heparin is only occasionally used and its *overall* therapeutic effectiveness is uncertain.

Therapeutic anticoagulation in DIC is best monitored by selecting the particular laboratory test which, in the given patient, is most abnormal and in which the abnormality can only be attributed to the intravascular coagulation. When a patient has acute leukemia, it would be best to look for a rise in fibrinogen levels rather than in the platelet count. A patient with severe liver disease might not necessarily have a return to normal of the vitamin K–dependent clotting factors. Useful tests in monitoring therapy include decrease in fibrin degradation product levels, Reptilase clotting time, fibrin monomer complexes (protamine sulfate test, gel chromatography, and others), and, in the rare institutions in which it is available, fibrinopeptide A assays. A heparin level of 0.15 to 0.30 unit per ml. is desirable. If partial thromboplastin time (PTT) or other tests cannot be used because of the patient's abnormal hemostatic system, then heparin levels based on antithrombin III or protamine sulfate neutralization can be used.

For patients who have continuing subacute or chronic DIC, particularly with malignancies, truly satisfactory therapy of the DIC may not result with current drugs. In such patients, most clinicians have found that anticoagulation with coumarin derivatives is usually insufficient to control the clinical problems of intravascular coagulation. Similarly, antiplatelet agents such as dipyridamole, have been inadequate. Long-term heparin therapy, particularly when administered subcutaneously, may be effective, but the osteopenic effect of heparin is a concern. Severe complications such as collapsed vertebrae can occur and be difficult to differentiate from other complications such as metastases to bone. Anticoagulation in this group is a balance of relative risks in an individual patient.

HEMOCHROMATOSIS AND HEMOSIDEROSIS

method of
PHILLIP C. YOUNG, M.D.
New Orleans, Louisiana

Absorption of iron by the intestinal epithelium in man is regulated so as to replace that lost from exfoliation of cells of the skin or intestinal tract and, in women, additionally, to replace that lost with menstruation. The normal adult has a total body iron content of about 4 grams, of which 60 to 70 per cent is contained in hemoglobin. The average daily requirement of iron in an adult is 1 mg. and in females during the reproductive years, is 1.5 mg. Iron from the daily destruction of red cells is stored in the reticuloendothelial cells and is reused to synthesize more hemoglobin. Iron is bound to transferrin in the plasma and is transported to tissue stores and the bone marrow, where it is deposited as ferritin or aggregates of ferritin associated with carbohydrate and fat, called hemosiderin. Excess iron accumulates in the body in states where there is an increased absorption of iron from the intestine, where there is excessive iron in the diet, and in conditions of parenteral iron overload. Disorders of hepatic iron storage occur in which iron overload is associated with tissue damage, as in idiopathic hemochromatosis. In hemosiderosis excess iron accumulates in the liver and there may be no injury to the organ from the stored iron. Iron is absorbed by the hepatocyte in an amount proportional to the concentration of transferrin iron in the blood. An increased plasma iron is necessary for iron loading of parenchymal cells.

The serum iron level is increased above normal and the total iron binding capacity of the serum is saturated in conditions of iron overload. Ferritin levels are high and are a reliable indicator of body iron storage. Storage iron may be demonstrated within the liver, bone marrow, and intestinal epithelium. Liver function tests are poor indicators of the severity of the disease within the liver in hemochromatosis.

Treatment

In hereditary idiopathic hemochromatosis the body tissues slowly accumulate iron and the body may eventually contain between 20 and 60 grams of iron. This is in contrast to the normal body content of iron which is 4 grams. The continued absorption and accumulation of iron leads eventually to death from hepatic dysfunction and its complications or from cardiac failure. Removal of iron is most efficiently accomplished by venesection. Each 500 ml. of blood removed by phlebotomy removes from 200 to 250 mg. of iron. The removal of the blood stimulates rapid regeneration of the hemoglobin from existing iron supplies. Phlebotomies of 1 to 2 pints of blood weekly are continued for from 1 to 2 years until serum iron levels fall and remain depleted. At slower rates of removal there may be a tendency for the iron to reaccumulate, and with more rapid removal hypoalbuminemia and significant anemia may occur. Successful depletion of body iron storage is indicated by a low circulating hemoglobin concentration, a reduced reticulocyte response, and low serum iron values. Even with the decrease in serum iron, body iron stores may still be significantly large to require continued venesection at a slower rate. Iron stains of liver biopsy tissue and bone marrow confirm the effectiveness of the removal of tissue iron. Because of the increased absorption of iron in idiopathic hemochromatosis, venesection with removal of 500 ml. of blood at quarterly intervals will be necessary during the remainder of the individual's life. Depletion of tissue iron stores results in improved liver function, decrease in skin pigmentation, reduction in liver size, and often improvement in carbohydrate tolerance. The mean survival of phlebotomized patients is 8.7 years, whereas that of controls not phlebotomized is 4.9 years. Control of dietary iron is usually ineffective. Alcohol should be avoided, as it seems to increase the toxic effect of iron in the liver.

An iron chelating agent, deferoxamine mesylate (Desferal), may be used in those conditions where venesection is contraindicated. It is recommended for removal of iron in acute iron intoxication and in those patients with secondary iron overload from multiple transfusions. It is contraindicated in patients who have severe renal disease and anuria, as the chelated iron is excreted by the kidney. In conditions of acute iron intoxication the recommended dose is 1 gram of deferoxamine mesylate intramuscularly, followed by 0.5 gram every 4 hours for two doses. Subsequent doses of 0.5 gram at 4 hour intervals may be given, but a total dose of 6 grams should not be exceeded within a 24-hour period. Deferoxamine mesylate may be administered by vein but must be given by slow infusion and the rate should not exceed 15 mg. per kg. per hour. As iron chelating agents remove limited amounts of iron (15 to 21 mg. per day) they are less effective in depleting iron stores. For that reason venesection is recommended in the treatment of idiopathic hemochromatosis.

HODGKIN'S DISEASE: CHEMOTHERAPY*

method of
CHARLES A. COLTMAN, JR., M.D.
San Antonio, Texas

Introduction

There is unequivocal evidence that Hodgkin's disease is now curable with a high degree of frequency at all stages of the disease. The management of early staged (I and II) Hodgkin's disease, with curative intent, has developed over the past 20 years to the point at which expectations of high cure rates can be anticipated, not only in major treatment centers but also in the community setting. With the advent of MOPP chemotherapy, in excess of 50 per cent of patients with advanced disease (stage III and IV) are now living and free of disease with follow-up beyond 10 years. These advances in the management of Hodgkin's disease can be attributed to a number of important concepts being brought to bear on the patient with Hodgkin's disease. The multidisciplinary approach to each patient is of paramount importance. The close interaction of the hematopathologist, medical oncologist, surgical oncologist, and radiation oncologist, both at the outset and throughout the treatment course has allowed for precise definition of histologic type and staging as well as optimal choice of treatment modalities. This cooperative approach allows each patient to be appropriately treated, with curative intent, from the time of diagnosis.

Diagnosis

The patient with Hodgkin's disease characteristically presents with an enlarged lymph node, most often in the upper torso. The proper choice of biopsy site and lymph node is of considerable importance. Detailed pathologic studies show that lymph nodes adjacent to those bearing classical Hodgkin's disease may be normal or show only evidence of reactive hyperplasia. Invariably, the largest in a chain of nodes is that which is characteristically involved with the disease. Inguinal and femoral nodes often present ambiguous pathology because of their drainage of the lower extremity. Axillary nodes are often difficult to biopsy and an axilla that has been explored is never quite the same. If there is an alternative site, choose it. The fresh tissue should immediately be examined by touch preparation as well as properly fixed and sectioned.

The Rye modification of the Lukes and Butler classification has now been with us since 1966 and is well recognized by all pathologists as the proper classification to be used in tissue interpretation of Hodgkin's disease nodes (Table 1). In spite of the international use of the Lukes and Butler classification, there remains some confusion in interpretation of tissue. For example, when the average medical center pathologist's interpretation of tissue is compared with that of expert hematopathologists, there is an exceptional level of agreement in the histologic classification of nodular sclerosing Hodgkin's disease but considerably less agreement in the interpretation of mixed cellular Hodgkin's disease. When in doubt about the precise histologic classification, one should seek consultation from additional sources. The criteria for the diagnosis of Hodgkin's disease include a classic Reed-Sternberg cell, discovered in the milieu of Hodgkin's disease, characterized by a background of lymphocytes, eosinophils, plasma cells, and atypical histiocytes. The diagnosis of Hodgkin's disease in extranodal sites such as liver, bone marrow, and lung can be somewhat confusing and of extreme importance because of the impact on prognosis and management.

Staging

Historically, the most important prognostic factors in Hodgkin's disease have been stage and histology. Certainly the anatomic extent of the disease (stage) is of critical importance in predicting the outcome. Systemic symptoms, specifically weight loss, fever, and night sweats, have a very unfavorable implication as to the patient's prognosis, especially if subdiaphragmatic disease is present. The independent prognostic importance of histopathology, in a series of completely surgically staged patients, remains to be investigated.

Another important factor in prognosis is the age of the patient. The young adult has a tendency to have localized disease, more commonly mediastinal involvement, frequent infradiaphragmatic presentation, and more favorable histologic characteristics. On the other hand, the elderly, as well as the very young, frequently have disseminated disease at the outset, more frequent infradiaphragmatic presentation, and most commonly mixed cellular or lymphocyte depleted Hodgkin's disease histology.

The symposium on staging in Hodgkin's disease held in Ann Arbor, Michigan in April, 1971, reviewed the status of staging of Hodgkin's disease and the principles agreed upon at that conference are currently applicable. Table 2 shows the currently accepted staging classification of Hodgkin's disease. There are four variations from the previously applicable Rye classification of Hodgkin's disease. First, Stage I disease is involvement of a single lymph node region in contrast to one or more adjacent lymph node bearing areas. Second, patients with localized extralymphatic disease either alone (I_E) or in continuity with adjacent lymph node bearing disease (II_E, III_E) are considered to have essentially the same prognosis as that of patients with the same degree of lymphatic involvement as long as the extralymphatic involvement is localized and can be included within a reasonable radiotherapy port. Third, patients with splenic involvement are specifically identified by the subscript s (III_S), based on the concept that the spleen has more ominous prognostic significance than simply that of another lymphatic organ. Fourth, B symptoms include the presence of unexplained fever higher than 38°C. (100.5°F.), night sweats, or unexplained weight loss of more than 10 per cent of body weight over the past 6 months. Pruritus alone was considered no longer sufficient to include patients in the B prognostic category. While pruritus is often associated with the other symptoms, when it occurs alone it may not have an adverse prognostic influence.

---

*It is recommended that the administration of drugs listed in this article be under the supervision of a qualified physician experienced in their use. The manufacturer's official directive should be consulted for current dosage recommendations and other pertinent information before prescribing for patient use.

Table 1. Histologic Classification of Hodgkin's Disease

LUKES AND BUTLER	RYE MODIFICATION	FREQUENCE
Lymphocyte and Histiocyte Nodular or diffuse	→ Lymphocyte Predominant	Rare
Nodular Sclerosis	→ Nodular Sclerosis	Common
Mixed Cellularity	→ Mixed Cellularity	Common
Diffuse Fibrosis, Reticular	→ Lymphocyte Depleted	Rare

An important concept developed at the Ann Arbor Symposium was that of clinical versus pathologic staging. Participants in the Ann Arbor Symposium recognized that there would always be differences in the extent to which patients would be subjected to various staging procedures from one institution or group to another. They thus established the concept that each patient should have both a clinical stage (CS) and a pathologic stage (PS). Clinical staging (CS) was determined by history, physical examination, radiologic studies, isotope scans, laboratory tests of urine and blood, and the *initial* biopsy result. Table 3 shows the staging procedures required in the evaluation of the clinical stage of patients with Hodgkin's disease. Also listed are procedures required under certain conditions. If there are important therapeutic reasons to know more precisely the stage, additional tissue may be obtained for pathologic staging (PS) such as marrow biopsy and staging laparotomy. An initial detailed history and physical examination are the most important parts of precise clinical staging. These data, along with the necessary laboratory and x-ray procedures, need to be clearly and prospectively recorded on a standard form so that anyone in the future can clearly understand how the clinical stage was arrived at.

Table 2. Ann Arbor Staging Classification

Stage I	Involvement of a single lymph node region or of a single extralymphatic organ or site (I_E)
Stage II	Involvement of two or more lymph node regions on the same side of the diaphragm, or localized involvement of an extralymphatic organ or site (II_E) and of one or more lymph node regions on the same side of the diaphragm
Stage III	Involvement of lymph node regions on both sides of the diaphragm, which may also be accompanied by localized involvement of an extralymphatic organ or site (III_E) or spleen (III_S) or both (III_{SE})
Stage IV	Diffuse or disseminated involvement of one or more extralymphatic organs with or without associated lymph node involvement

Fever >38°C. (100.5°F.), night sweats, and/or weight loss >10 per cent of body weight in the 6 months preceding admission are defined as systemic symptoms and denoted by the suffix letter B. Asymptomatic patients are denoted by the suffix letter A. Biopsy-documented involvement of stage IV sites is identified by the following symbols: marrow = M+; liver = 11+; lung = 1+; pleura = P+; bone = O+; skin = D+.

It is important to recognize that clinical staging does require appropriate radiographic procedures. Thus, if a patient does not have a lymphogram he cannot be considered accurately clinically staged. Lymphography is also important in that it pinpoints nodes which the surgeon should biopsy at staging laparotomy, if that procedure is chosen. Finally, it is, if abnormal, an excel-

Table 3. Staging Hodgkin's Disease

REQUIRED EVALUATION PROCEDURES
1. Adequate surgical biopsy, reviewed by an experienced hematopathologist.
2. A detailed history recording the presence or absence of and duration of fever, unexplained sweating and its severity, unexplained pruritus, and unexplained weight loss
3. A careful and detailed physical examination; special attention to all node bearing areas, including Waldeyer's ring, and determination of size of liver and spleen
4. Necessary laboratory procedures:
   a. Complete blood count, including an erythrocytic sedimentation rate
   b. Serum alkaline phosphatase
   c. Evaluation of renal function
   d. Evaluation of hepatic function
5. Radiological studies include:
   a. Chest roentgenogram (PA and lateral)
   b. Intravenous pyelogram
   c. Bilateral lower extremity lymphogram
   d. Views of skeletal system to include thoracic and lumbar vertebrae, the pelvis, proximal extremities, and any areas of bone tenderness

PROCEDURES REQUIRED UNDER CERTAIN CONDITIONS
1. Whole chest tomography if any abnormality is noted or suspected on the routine chest roentgenogram
2. Inferior cavography to supplement equivocal lymphographic or pyelographic findings
3. Bone marrow biopsy (needle or open) in the presence of:
   a. An elevated alkaline phosphatase
   b. Unexplained anemia or other blood count depression
   c. Other evidence of bone disease (scan or x-ray)
   d. Generalized disease of stage III or greater
4. Exploratory laparotomy and splenectomy, if management decisions will depend on the identification of abdominal disease

USEFUL ANCILLARY PROCEDURES NOT REQUIRED FOR STAGING
1. Skeletal scintigrams*
2. Hepatic and spleen scintigrams*
3. Serum chemistries to include serum calcium and uric acid for overall management of patient
4. Estimates of the patient's delayed hypersensitivity of the tuberculin type
5. Gallium whole body scans*

*Cannot be used as evidence of Hodgkin's disease without biopsy confirmation.

lent tool for following the response to treatment. Examination of the bone marrow is an important consideration in determining the extent of the disease. Random bone marrow biopsy from a site not clinically involved by x-ray is extremely important under circumstances in which there is elevated alkaline phosphatase, evidence of peripheral cytopenia, other evidence of bone involvement by x-ray or scan or advanced (stage III or IV) disease. It is imperative that this examination be done by bone marrow biopsy rather than by aspirate.

A clear notation of pathologic staging (PS) was considered important because of the variable degree to which additional surgical staging procedures have been employed by various investigators. It has become necessary to distinguish such procedures because of subtle shifts from clinical stage to pathologic stage and thus most patients today see both clinical stage (CS) and pathologic stage (PS) for the designation of the extent of their disease.

Staging Laparotomy

There remains considerable debate concerning the usefulness of staging laparotomy in determining the extent of disease below the diaphragm. Accordingly, the Ann Arbor Symposium participants (Table 3) suggested "that exploratory laparotomy and splenectomy be required if management decisions will depend on the identification of abdominal disease." Staging laparotomy is not without its complications, and it is also clear that even a carefully done procedure in no way guarantees that the abdomen is free of disease. If the intent is to administer total nodal radiotherapy to all patients with stage I and II disease, then staging laparotomy is clearly not of value. If the extent of radiotherapy is to be tailored to the extent of the disease, then staging laparotomy is necessary. It does provide, in addition, some prognostic information. When the disease is confined to the upper abdomen, the overall prognosis is clearly better than in those patients who have disease that includes nodes throughout the para-aortic and iliac node chain. Another important consideration is the identification of disease in the portahepatic nodes that is found to be positive in a number of patients with upper abdominal disease. The usual inverted Y total nodal radiotherapy port does not encompass the portahepatis and, thus, if found to be involved at laparotomy and radiotherapy is the treatment of choice, an extension of the treatment port must encompass the involved area. It is clear that staging laparotomy should not be taken in a cavalier fashion. It should be done, in any institution, by the same surgical team on each occasion.

The use of laparoscopy as an aid to staging Hodgkin's disease has been studied by two groups. These techniques have been relatively safe and in fact confirm the results of staging laparotomy. The single most important drawback of this technique is the inability to safely evaluate splenic involvement. Even when multiple splenic biopsies are performed through the laparoscope, a procedure not without hazard, it is impossible to define the extent of Hodgkin's disease involvement in the spleen.

At the completion of clinical evaluation and whatever surgical staging is done, the precise clinical as well as pathologic stage should be determined and recorded.

Therapy

The accepted treatment of patients with stage I, II, and IIIA Hodgkin's disease is radiotherapy. The extent of the radiotherapy will depend primarily on the extent of surgical staging. Those patients who have undergone a complete staging laparotomy should have therapy directed at the extended field or total nodal field, depending on the extent of intra-abdominal involvement. In the absence of staging laparotomy all patients should receive total nodal irradiation. There are now data from a number of studies, which show that patients who have bulky mediastinal involvement that exceeds one third of the thoracic diameter are at high risk to develop extensions of their disease into extranodal sites in the lung. This problem can be avoided by the use of adjuvant chemotherapy. Although such patients, receiving adjuvant chemotherapy, have a longer relapse-free survival, the overall survival has not yet been demonstrated to be improved. Further data need to be collected concerning this matter.

There is debate concerning the proper management of patients with stage I_E and II_E Hodgkin's disease. The debate centers around whether generous radiotherapy ports alone, encompassing the extranodal sites, are effective in controlling disease or whether adjuvant chemotherapy will play an important role. Until the issue has been clearly solved, the use of radiotherapy alone, with ports sufficient to encompass the extra-nodal sites effectively, appears to be the treatment of choice.

Patients with advanced stage Hodgkin's disease (IIIB and IV) are candidates for intensive combination chemotherapy. The chance of complete response in previously untreated patients is approximately 80 per cent and the long-term survival is in excess of 50 per cent. There are several problems that remain to be solved in the management of advanced Hodgkin's disease. The first is that we have not yet reached a 100 per cent complete response rate in this disease; second, having achieved a complete response, in the first 3 years there is a high fraction of patients who recur. Those who recur do so in areas of prior bulky nodal disease. Combinations of noncross resistant combination chemotherapy or involved field radiotherapy or both, applied during remission induction or for early consolidation of complete remission, are techniques currently under study. At the present time, combination chemotherapy alone is the treatment of choice for patients with advanced Hodgkin's disease.

Combination Chemotherapy

The current standard treatment for patients with advanced Hodgkin's disease is MOPP combi-

DAYS	1	2–7	8	9	14	28
Drugs (mg./m^2)						
VCR	1.4		1.4			No
HN$_2$	6		6			Therapy
Procarbazine	100 ——————————————→					
Prednisone*	40 ——————————————→					

*Cycles 1 and 4 only.

Figure 1. MOPP—single cycle.

nation chemotherapy (Figure 1). Since the benchmark studies of DeVita and associates using this combination, a number of institutions and cooperative groups have documented that MOPP chemotherapy for advanced Hodgkin's disease represents the best available approach to the management of these patients in terms of complete response rate and survival. Approximately 40 to 50 per cent of patients treated with MOPP chemotherapy continue to remain free of disease in their initial complete remission while off all therapy up to 10 years.

Figure 1 illustrates a single cycle of MOPP combination chemotherapy, which is administered on a monthly basis. Vincristine and nitrogen mustard are given intravenously on days 1 and 8 of each of the monthly cycles of MOPP and procarbazine and prednisone are given orally for 14 days. Each cycle is repeated on day 29 and dosage adjustments are made in accordance with the data shown on Table 4. Scheduling of treatment is clearly much more important than dosage in any given cycle and thus retreatment of the patient on day 29 with a downward adjustment of dosage takes precedence over delaying treatment for one or several weeks.

Nausea and vomiting due to nitrogen mustard are important adverse side effects and occasionally become such an important psychologic barrier to treatment that patients will refuse to continue. Optimal use of antinausea medications, such as thiethylperazine maleate (Torecan), will be helpful in controlling this undesirable side effect. Procarbazine has monoamine oxidase inhibitor activity and thus use of alcohol or other narcotics should be avoided during these times. Alopecia is a common and reversible complication. Neuropathy is a frequent complication of vincristine in the doses outlined. The neurotoxicity is almost universally reversible and should not be considered an indication for discontinuation. Dose modification in patients who develop severe foot drop or other complications is preferable to discontinuation of the drug. All of the problems of neurotoxicity are amplified in the elderly patient.

The optimal number of cycles of MOPP chemotherapy depends on the individual patient and the characteristics of his disease. Basically, patients should be treated until they have achieved a complete response of their disease and then two additional cycles of drug administered. It is vitally important to define the completeness of the response prior to discontinuation of therapy. This should be documented by reperforming all of the studies that were considered to be positive or abnormal at the initiation of treatment. This must include a repeat random iliac crest marrow biopsy and liver biopsy, if they were positive at the outset. It should include a repeat lymphogram, if that test was positive at the outset and there is not sufficient contrast material remaining in the nodes to characterize the status of intra-abdominal lymph nodes. A scout film of the abdomen will help you decide. In an occasional instance the scout film or repeat lymphogram is equivocal, and it may be necessary to resort to surgical biopsy and, in rare instances, to laparotomy to define the completeness of the response.

Under circumstances in which the patients have been carefully restaged to confirm the completeness of their response, therapy should stop. There is no data to support a survival advantage for patients receiving maintenance therapy. Because of the complications of prolonged combina-

TABLE 4. **Dosage Adjustments**

IF WBC COUNT BEFORE STARTING NEW COURSE WAS	THEN DOSAGE WAS ADJUSTED TO
>4000	100% of all drugs
3999–3000	100% of vincristine, 50% nitrogen mustard and procarbazine
2999–2000	100% of vincristine, 25% nitrogen mustard and procarbazine
1999–1000	50% vincristine, 25% nitrogen mustard and procarbazine
999–0	No drug

IF PLATELET COUNT BEFORE STARTING NEW COURSE WAS	THEN DOSAGE WAS ADJUSTED TO
>100,000	100% of all drugs
50,000–100,000	100% of vincristine, 25% nitrogen mustard and procarbazine
< 50,000	No drug

tion chemotherapy, maintenance therapy should be avoided in the management of advanced Hodgkin's disease.

Management of MOPP Failures

There is a major problem in Hodgkin's disease in that once patients have become refractory to MOPP chemotherapy their response to so-called noncross resistant combinations of chemotherapy has been less than optimal. It is important, however, to define the characteristics of patients who are considered to be resistant to MOPP chemotherapy. It is quite clear that patients who have their remission induced with MOPP for 6 to 10 cycles and relapse 1 to 3 years later in unmaintained remission probably have 60 per cent chance of responding to MOPP the second time with prolonged disease-free survival. On the other hand, patients who show progressive disease while receiving MOPP combination chemotherapy or who have an early recurrence of their disease within a year of achieving complete response, would be considered candidates for a number of three and four drug combinations that have been tested in this setting. ABVD (Figure 2) has produced significant numbers of complete responses in MOPP-resistant Hodgkin's disease patients. It combines doxorubicin (Adriamycin), bleomycin, vinblastine, and dacarbazine (DTIC). All four drugs are administered intravenously on days 1 and 14 and then restarted on day 29. A long-term follow-up on MOPP-resistant ABVD responders is not available at this time. Dose adjustments for the ABVD regimens are seen in Table 5.

Radiotherapy Plus Chemotherapy

The role of radiotherapy and adjuvant chemotherapy in the management of Hodgkin's disease remains experimental. Virtually all studies to

DAYS	1	2–14	15	28
Drugs (mg./m²)				
Adriamycin	25		25	No
Bleomycin*	10		10	Therapy
Vinblastine	6		6	
DTIC†	375		375	

*Units/m²
†Dimethyl-triazeno-imadazole-carboxamide.

Figure 2.   ABVD—single cycle.

date have failed to show a survival advantage for the combination although disease-free survival in each stage had been significantly prolonged. The administration of combination chemotherapy followed by low dose radiotherapy in advanced disease (IIIB, IV) has resulted in a high complete response rate and excellent disease-free survival with follow-up to 5 years.

Management of First Relapse Following Radiation Therapy

Patients with localized Hodgkin's disease who undergo radiotherapy are candidates for additional radiotherapy when the recurrence is localized and clearly outside a previous radiation therapy port. When the relapse is in a site marginal to prior radiotherapy ports, specific judgment needs to be made in coordination with the radiotherapist. MOPP combination chemotherapy is clearly indicated under circumstances in which the recurrence is within the previously irradiated field or where extensive extranodal sites are involved. The risk of complete response to MOPP combination chemotherapy is not reduced in patients who have received prior radiotherapy. The only important problem occurs when patients have residual compromise of bone marrow function from their previous radiotherapy, and under

TABLE 5.   **Dose Adjustments Recommended in Presence of Myelosuppression**

LEUKOCYTE COUNT BEFORE STARTING A NEW COURSE	PLATELET COUNT BEFORE STARTING A NEW COURSE	DOSAGE WHICH CAN BE ADMINISTERED
>4000	>130,000	100% of all drugs
3999–3000	129,000–90,000	100% of BLM, DTIC 50% of ADM, VLB
2999–2000	89,000–60,000	100% of BLM 50% of DTIC 25% of ADM
1999–1500	59,000–40,000	100% of BLM 25% of DTIC
<1500	<40,000	100% of BLM

HN₂: Nitrogen mustard; ADM: doxorubicin (Adriamycin); VLB: vinblastine; CCNU: chloroethyl-cyclohexyl-nitrosourea; PCZ: procarbazine; VCR: vincristine; DTIC: imidazole carboxamide; BLM: bleomycin; PRD: prednisone.

these circumstances careful management of their chemotherapy at attenuated doses is indicated.

Special Therapeutic Problems

Hodgkin's Disease in Children. The management of Hodgkin's disease in children is a considerably different problem than it is in adults. There are serious complications of an infectious nature that occur in children who undergo staging laparotomy and splenectomy. The indications for this procedure in that age group are even more stringent. Furthermore, the use of high dose radiotherapy in patients with localized disease has produced significant growth retardation. There are studies currently underway in which limited radiotherapy, in combination with chemotherapy, is under consideration for management of this group of patients.

Superior Vena Caval Syndrome. Occasionally, patients with localized disease and, less commonly, patients with advanced disease present with this problem. Radiotherapy is the treatment of choice in patients with localized disease and should be employed as an emergency procedure prior to complete definition of the extent of disease. In patients who have clinically advanced disease, nitrogen mustard alone, administered into a lower extremity or central venous line, is most effective in reducing this and avoiding the problem of extravasation of the drug associated with injection into a high pressure upper extremity vein.

Spinal Cord Compression. This is a relatively common emergency in the management of patients with Hodgkin's disease. It should be approached in a multidisciplinary fashion that includes immediate combined consultation with a medical oncologist, radiotherapist, and neurosurgeon. The treatment of choice in the management of this complication is immediate surgical laminectomy for decompression of the spinal cord. This should then be followed by localized radiotherapy. One should not be misled by what appears to be a slowly progressive onset of cord compression. The sudden appearance of paraplegia can occur at any time in this group of patients.

Pleural Effusion. The management of pleural effusion in patients with Hodgkin's disease is principally that of the proper management of the patient based on the stage of his disease. The pleural fluid should be examined for malignant cells and a pleural biopsy done to determine whether or not there is evidence of more advanced disease. More commonly, pleural effusion is related to mediastinal or abdominal lymph node involvement or both, and proper therapy directed to those areas can effectively control the pleural effu-sion. If the disease is of an advanced nature, systemic MOPP combination chemotherapy is the treatment of choice. Under extremely rare circumstances and only in patients with refractory disease should consideration be given to intrapleural administration of nitrogen mustard (12 mg. per square meter of body surface area in 30 ml. of saline) or bleomycin (30 to 40 units) following removal of as much pleural fluid as possible.

Ureteral Obstruction. Ureteral obstruction is a serious problem that requires careful evaluation of patients with advanced disease. Radiotherapy directed to the area of obstruction is the management of choice.

Hyperuricemia. Hyperuricemia and attendant precipitation of urate crystals in the renal tubules and collecting ducts is a highly preventable and very serious complication in the management of patients with lymphoma. This is much more common a problem in patients with non-Hodgkin's lymphoma than Hodgkin's disease. It can be avoided by the administration of allopurinol (Zyloprim), 100 to 200 mg., four times a day prior to the initiation of chemotherapy or radiotherapy or both. Once the tumor has been debulked, the allopurinol can be discontinued.

Long-term Complications. Development of nonlymphomatous second malignancies, particularly acute leukemia, is an acknowledged complication of the management of Hodgkin's disease. It is now an established fact that second malignancies in Hodgkin's disease are related to the intensity of the treatment. Acute leukemia has been identified as the most common second malignancy. These hematologic malignancies occur with increased frequency in patients still in complete remission of their Hodgkin's disease and among patients who receive intensive combination chemotherapy and radiotherapy. Data from Stanford as well as from the Southwest Oncology Group indicate that radiotherapy alone is not associated with increased risk of hematologic malignancy. Chemotherapy alone and chemotherapy in combination with radiotherapy clearly have oncogenic potential. Because of the risk of acute leukemia developing in patients treated for Hodgkin's disease, some of the survival advantage achieved by an aggressive approach to the management of patients may be cancelled by the development of acute leukemia in patients who have no evidence of Hodgkin's disease. Because of this problem, the unrestrained use of combined modality management of all patients with Hodgkin's disease is not indicated. An amount of chemotherapy or radiotherapy or both just sufficient to control the disease should be administered to each patient based on precise staging.

HODGKIN'S DISEASE: RADIATION THERAPY

method of
RALPH E. JOHNSON, M.D.
St. Petersburg, Florida

Clinical Presentation

Effective and potentially curative treatments have been developed for Hodgkin's disease, a malignancy almost inevitably fatal several decades ago. These therapeutic advances have stimulated an increased interest in the initial clinical presentation. Indeed, such factors as the physical findings and the presence of constitutional symptoms exert a major influence on not only the choice of diagnostic studies used for staging but also the ultimate treatment decision. However, the spectrum of presentations is so variable as potentially to confuse the physician who is concerned infrequently with the management of Hodgkin's disease. For this reason, it seems preferable that patients be referred immediately upon diagnosis to specialists with sufficient clinical experience to pursue an individualized diagnostic evaluation, thereby sparing patients from needless (or even hazardous) procedures, and to reach a correct treatment decision.

Staging of Disease

Certain highly specialized centers routinely undertake nearly every available diagnostic procedure in the staging of Hodgkin's disease in order to collect data on the relative merits of different tests. Such a comprehensive approach is not warranted in everyday practice. Only the utilization of those staging studies having a reasonable probability of influencing the selection of treatment is justified in the latter situation. At present, this policy is not always adhered to because of less than ideal communication between radiation oncologists and medical oncologists as to treatment philosophies and whether or not therapy might be altered by positive (or negative) results of staging tests. Close communication between these specialists is imperative, and a continuing dialogue must be maintained as the results of sequential diagnostic studies become available. It is not appropriate for the staging evaluation to be directed by a single physician with preconceived concepts that an unalterable series of tests is required for every patient, irrespective of the clinical presentation. In particular, one must be certain that the likelihood of detecting findings via invasive procedures such as staging laparotomy that will alter the treatment approach are at least several fold greater than the risk of serious morbidity to the patient.

TABLE 1. Staging for Hodgkin's Disease—Ann Arbor System

Stage I:	Involvement of a single lymph node region (I) or a single extralymphatic site (I_E).
Stage II:	Involvement of two or more lymph node regions on the same side of the diaphragm (II) or localized involvement of an extranodal site and one or more lymph node regions on the same side of the diaphragm (II_E).
Stage III:	Involvement of lymph node regions on both sides of the diaphragm (III), which may include the spleen (III_S), or localized extranodal involvement (III_E), or both (III_{SE}).
Stage IV:	Diffuse or disseminated involvement of one or more extranodal sites with or without lymph node involvement.

A and B subclasses indicate absence or presence of any of the following systemic symptoms: fever, sweats, or weight loss of 10 per cent of body weight.

CS and PS refer to clinical staging and pathologic (surgical) staging, respectively.

The Ann Arbor staging classification (Table 1) is accepted universally and takes into account those features of disease, except for histology, that have major prognostic importance, i.e., the anatomic extent of disease and presence versus absence of constitutional symptoms. The Ann Arbor conference also recommended a series of diagnostic studies to be routinely employed, as outlined in Table 2. Other studies were termed optional with a suggestion that they be utilized only when indicated by other circumstances and if having a reasonable chance of modifying the treatment decision. Thus, whole chest tomography finds its utility only in those patients with marked mediastinal or hilar adenopathy, as it is these selected patients who have a substantial risk of parenchymal involvement. Likewise, bone scans are likely to yield positive results only in patients with otherwise extensive disease (at least Stage III), an elevated serum alkaline phosphatase,

TABLE 2. Laboratory Investigation of Hodgkin's Disease

Required:
    CBC, platelets
    BUN, liver function studies, uric acid
    Chest x-ray
    Lymphangiogram
    Bone marrow aspirate and biopsy ("B" patients, stages III and IV A&B)

Optional:
    Sedimentation rate, serum copper
    Chest tomograms, IVP
    Liver-spleen scan, bone scan
    Laparotomy
    Immunologic testing
    Gallium scan
    CT scan
    Ultrasound

symptomatic bone pain, or bone tenderness on percussion.

A liver-spleen scan is considered of value in all patients with clinically limited disease for the purpose of assessing splenic size. Although it is recognized that splenomegaly does not necessarily imply actual involvement by Hodgkin's disease, the risk of involvement is clearly greater in those patients having an enlarged spleen. Consequently, an enlarged spleen on isotopic scan mandates a staging laparotomy as it is these particular patients who have a significant risk of hepatic involvement. Staging laparotomy also is routinely warranted in those patients with extensive retroperitoneal adenopathy detected by bipedal lymphography as they have a selectively high risk of otherwise undetectable involvement of lymph nodes outside the standard radiation therapy fields. Furthermore, bone marrow biopsy now has become optional in many centers since the rate of positivity is extremely low in patients otherwise considered at Stage I-II.

An "E" subclassification was introduced into staging at Ann Arbor to denote those patients with direct extension of nodal disease into contiguous nonlymphatic tissues. This type of contiguous spread does not appreciably alter prognosis as contrasted with noncontiguous spread (e.g., multiple nodules in the pulmonary parenchyma) although it may increase the complexity of treatment with irradiation. The Ann Arbor system also introduced the concept of "clinical" versus "surgical" staging. This innovation has produced some confusion with respect to comparing results between clinically and surgically staged series. Even more important is the question of how to extrapolate radiotherapy methods of proven efficacy for clinically staged patients to those patients having been surgically staged. For example, historical results with the radiotherapy of Clinical Stage III patients are not necessarily relevant to those Stage I-II patients (negative lymphogram and liver-spleen scan) who are upstaged to Surgical Stage III on the basis of minimal microscopic involvement of para-aortic nodes detected by laparotomy.

To illustrate this problem, we achieved a 95 per cent 10-year survival rate in Clinical Stage IIA Hodgkin's disease of the nodular sclerosis type prior to the advent of staging laparotomy by extending treatment beyond the mantle field to encompass the para-aortic lymph nodes and spleen because of suspected potential occult involvement. This demonstrated the high curability when prophylactic irradiation was employed, despite the fact that one third of these patients would have been upstaged to Surgical Stage III had a staging laparotomy been performed. Thus, it seems highly conjectural as to whether treatment decisions deserve to be changed in this situation because of *detecting what is already suspected.*

Contrarily, it must be appreciated that even staging laparotomy may be falsely negative. Current information indicates that fully 25 per cent of patients with negative laparotomy findings will relapse below the diaphragm because of undetected disease in the absence of prophylactic treatment. Therefore, we have concluded that the major role of staging laparotomy should be to investigate the presence of disease outside the usual radiotherapy fields in selected patients at high risk as described above, rather than serving as a reliable guide for withholding treatment.

Selection of Treatment

A multiplicity of therapeutic approaches has been investigated and proposed for all stages of Hodgkin's disease in recent years. This may present a perplexing dilemma for the community practitioner for whom the simple solution of randomizing patients to a protocol is not in effect. Under the best of circumstances, treatment decision making can be quite complex and any broad recommendations automatically suffer from oversimplification. Nonetheless, it seems acceptable to propose certain generalizations on the basis of currently available information.

In an attempt to avoid an excessively complicated approach, we have elected to identify patients with Hodgkin's disease as being at different risks of being cured by treatment with radiotherapy alone after completion of staging evaluation. The "good" risk patients are those with Stage I-II disease of the lymphocyte predominant and nodular sclerosis histologic types. These patients can be anticipated to have an 80 to 90 per cent survival rate following extended field irradiation. The latter includes, for those patients with presentations of disease above the diaphragm, the treatment of infradiaphragmatic lymphatics down to the level of the aortic bifurcation, the splenic pedicle, and the spleen (if intact). It also seems reasonable at present to include patients in the good risk category with the same histology who are Clinical Stage I-II and have occult disease detected by laparotomy and are reclassified as Surgical Stage III.

The "intermediate" group is comprised of patients with Clinical Stage III involvement but a favorable histology and in whom staging laparotomy fails to disclose hepatic involvement. An additional category within the intermediate group is Stage I-II patients with mixed cellularity or lymphocyte depletion histology. The intermediate group has an approximate control rate of 60 per cent when treated with total nodal irradiation. There is considerable current interest in the combined treatment using radiotherapy plus chemotherapy for such patients in an attempt to reduce the relapse rate and improve survival. While some indication of lower relapse rates have been forthcoming following combined treatment, definitive results must be awaited in terms of improved survival. Alternatively, about 50 per cent of patients who relapse following primary treatment with radiotherapy alone can be salvaged with modern combination chemotherapy. For the moment, it remains our preference to approach the intermediate group of patients in a conservative fashion and attempt the salvage of relapsers rather than subject all such patients to the toxicity of combined radiotherapy-chemotherapy at the onset and incur the risk of inducing acute myelocytic leukemia which may range as high as 5 to 10 per cent.

The "poor" risk category for primary treatment with radiotherapy alone obviously includes nearly all patients with Stage IV involvement as well as Stage III patients with unfavorable histologic types. Here, combination chemotherapy is viewed as having the primary role in initial treatment with radiotherapy serving as an adjunct. Several programs have documented that the addition of modest radiation doses (1500 to 2000 rads) to sites of initial bulky disease following the completion of chemotherapy has significantly reduced the relapse rate in patients with Stage III-IV disease.

It needs to be appreciated that situations are frequently encountered wherein patients are not easily assigned to any given category as defined earlier. Here the selection of primary treatment remains a matter of personal preference, and the choice cannot be dictated by current information. One can only plead for a spirit of cooperation between medical oncologists and radiation oncologists in such instances in the recognition that neither modality provides the ultimate answer. A willingness to modify what otherwise might be standard treatment is often called for because of experience that attempts to submit patients to unattenuated courses of both radiotherapy and chemotherapy imposes a serious risk of complications. Above all, specialists with divergent opinions must remain acutely aware of the need for judicious modification of standard regimens on a patient-by-patient basis.

Technique of Irradiation

A fundamental requirement in the radiotherapy of Hodgkin's disease is the administration of adequate doses to ensure local control (i.e., to reduce the probability of in-field recurrences to 5 per cent or less). A total dose of 3600 to 4000 rads, given at a daily rate of 180 to 200 rads using five fractions per week, will accomplish this aim in most patients. Treatment is preferably given with high energy x-rays (e.g., with a linear accelerator) rather than using cobalt 60 teletherapy because of the more sharply defined beam at the edge of the field. Optimal sparing of normal tissues has become ever the more critical, with many patients being cured and then being subjected to the late effects of treatment. In this respect, the minimizing of radiation exposure to the bone marrow via a well-collimated beam having little penumbra is essential to permit the delivery of adequate chemotherapy in those patients who relapse. In addition, there is no place for the use of multiple small fields in the modern radiotherapy of Hodgkin's disease because of the inherent danger of either underdosage or overdosage at the junction. It does not seem justified to refer patients to those facilities unprepared to treat the mantle field in continuity using individually designed blocks for shielding of the heart and lungs. The latter is not yet standard in all communities and demands that patients be assured of management at centers where the chance for cure is maximal and the risk of complications is minimal.

Our long experience with irradiation of large fields in Hodgkin's disease has shown that treatment is more readily tolerated by employing a so-called "split course" technique. Allowing a 2-week break in the treatment of a field not only attenuates the acute reactions, but the continued regression of tumor masses permits construction of more adequate shielding blocks and reduces the late complication rate. Likewise, boost doses above 4000 rads to nodes persisting at the completion of treatment has been found totally unnecessary. Resolution of disease may continue for months following irradiation, and we have not observed that persistent adenopathy immediately after treatment heralds the development of subsequent local recurrence.

Whereas some centers elect to treat the infradiaphragmatic area with a so-called inverted Y field, such a technique may result in severe hematologic depression after treatment of the mantle field, despite an intervening 4-week rest period. Our preference is to irradiate the upper abdominal area (para-aortic nodes, splenic pedicle, and spleen if intact) and pelvic-groin area sequentially. This will obviate the occasional need to interrupt treatment because of bone marrow toxicity and greatly reduces the gastrointestinal toxicity experienced by the patient.

Early and Late Consequences of Therapy

During and immediately following treatment, a variety of reactions may be observed, one of the most common being fatigue. Nearly all patients experience some degree of anorexia and nausea, especially when the upper abdominal area is being irradiated, and occasional emesis may occur. These gastrointestinal reactions are most intense during the several hours following each daily treatment and can be moderated by having patients abstain from eating during this interval, adhere to a bland diet, and use antiemetics if required.

Pharyngitis and esophagitis may be distressing during mantle field irradiation and result in considerable weight loss and dehydration and may occasionally necessitate temporary hospitalization. However, the split-course technique of irradiation virtually eliminates serious problems of this type. The loss of hair in the occipital region is unavoidable, but patients can be reassured that regrowth can be anticipated within several months after treatment.

The frequency of delayed complications is inversely proportional to the concern of the radiotherapist over their prevention. While total avoidance of iatrogenic complications is inconsistent with aggressive cancer therapy using any modality, the majority of serious late complications from irradiation will be sharply curtailed by proper attention to treatment details and a willingness to modify treatment when required rather than insisting on a "cookbook" prescription.

Radiation pneumonitis usually has its onset during the first two months of treatment in the form of dyspnea, a febrile course, and a dry, nonproductive cough. During the early phase, radiographic changes may be absent or minimal, but eventually a streak-like fibrosis develops that may progress to a dense confluency outlining the treatment field. A superimposed bacterial infection may occur and demands prompt institution of appropriate antibiotic therapy. In some patients, the acute phase resolves spontaneously without apparent residual effects. When the process is more extensive, some permanent respiratory disability can persist and predispose toward recurrent infections. Occasionally, the initial pneumonitis will extend from a localized area to well outside the field of treatment and cause acute respiratory decompensation. In such instances, oxygen is mandatory and corticosteroids can produce a dramatic improvement in both symptoms and arterial oxygen concentration. However, relapse of symptoms can occur when attempts are made to withdraw corticosteroids and there is no documentation that the degree of eventual fibrosis can be reduced by their use.

Pericarditis is a late complication noted most commonly when massive mediastinal adenopathy demanded that most if not all of the cardiac silhouette be encompassed within the treatment field. The initial manifestation can vary from the insidious development of a clinically asymptomatic effusion detected only radiographically to a picture resembling acute pericarditis. Tamponade can ensue and necessitate a pericardiectomy, the latter being preferable to a pericardial window so as to avoid subsequent constrictive fibrosis.

Whereas transient signs of spinal cord irritation (Lhermitte's sign) may be observed in one quarter of patients, a true progressive neurologic deficit is almost never observed in the absence of overlapping fields or predisposing conditions or both. The pathogenesis of radiation myelitis appears to involve radiation injury of the small blood vessels supplying the spinal cord and particular care should be exercised in the radiotherapy of patients with underlying small vessel disease (e.g., juvenile diabetes or hypertension).

One of the most common consequences of mantle-field irradiation is a relentless deterioration of the teeth, resulting from impaired salivary flow. Recent studies have demonstrated conclusively that decay problems can virtually be eliminated by the conscientious use of good dental hygiene, prompt restoration of caries, and the prophylactic use of fluoride treatments.

Some reduction in the sperm count can be expected when the male pelvis is irradiated, even when special testicular shields are employed. However, infertility is far less common among males than females, in whom amenorrhea occurs uniformly with pelvic irradiation unless the ovaries are repositioned surgically to the midline and shielded during treatment. Even under the latter circumstance, about one half of women cease to menstruate.

Another unavoidable consequence is retardation of bone growth and a reduction in the sitting height as well as shoulder girdle development following treatment of young children. The practitioner must also be alert to the possibility of hypothyroidism after cervical irradiation, especially in children where a perceptible slowing of the growth rate and other problems can result from thyroid deficiency. Fortunately, hypothyroidism is easily corrected by replacement therapy and does not pose a serious problem despite an incidence of 10 to 20 per cent. Finally, the development of a second malignancy is extremely uncommon (about 3 per cent) among patients treated only with radiotherapy. The exact risk remains to be defined for those patients treated with combined radiotherapy and chemotherapy, as insufficient time has elapsed for a reliable determination, but clearly the risk is much greater than after treatment with irradiation alone.

Conclusion

While many advances in the field of radiotherapy have contributed to a dramatic improvement in the outlook for patients with

Hodgkin's disease, this remains one of the most challenging tasks facing the radiation oncologist today. The highest level of expertise in both treatment planning and delivery are imperative if the gains are to be exploited. Precise daily reproduction of patient positioning, careful dosimetric calculations, meticulous construction of beam-shaping devices, and understanding of the need at times to modify treatment from a projected plan are all essential ingredients without which only disaster can be invited. When properly done, the management of these patients is extremely rewarding and even when cure is not achieved, a useful and significant prolongation of life is the rule rather than the exception.

ACUTE LEUKEMIA IN ADULTS*

method of
W. R. VOGLER, M.D.
Atlanta, Georgia

Objectives

At the present time there are two major objectives in treating acute leukemia. The first is to achieve a complete remission, currently defined as the return of bone marrow to normal cellularity with a normal differential cell distribution, restoration of normal blood counts and disappearance of all clinical evidence of leukemia. The second objective is to maintain the duration of remission for as long as possible. Not all patients with acute leukemia require immediate treatment. Only those with progressive disease should be promptly treated. Progressive disease is defined as a rising leukocyte count, thrombocytopenia, or severe anemia. In the elderly patient considerable caution should be exercised in assessing the necessity to treat with chemotherapeutic agents. In this instance the toxicity from the treatment may be more harmful than the disease.

Diagnosis of Leukemia

In order to make a diagnosis of leukemia the bone marrow is usually hypercellular and contains greater than 30 per cent leukemic blast cells. Maturing granulocytes, megakaryocytes, and erythroid precursors are reduced in numbers. The type of leukemia can be distinguished by morphologic criteria and more precisely by histochemical stains. Recent studies suggest that there is a subset of acute leukemia that cannot be distinguished by any of these criteria. Acute leukemia may be classified as lymphoblastic (T cell and non-T cell), myeloblastic, myelomonocytic, monocytic, erythroleukemia, and undifferentiated leukemia.

---

*Some agents mentioned in this article are considered investigational. Before using any of the drugs mentioned, the physician should be well aware of their actions and of the information in the manufacturer's official directives.

Principles of Treatment

At our current state of knowledge remission can be achieved only by treatment with drugs that are cytotoxic. With the exception of corticosteroids, most of the effective drugs are active against proliferating cells and have little if any effect on nonproliferating cells. Kinetic studies have indicated that mean cycle times of a leukemic cell population is usually longer than that of normal marrow cells. In a given treatment program drugs should be continued to allow the maximum number of leukemic cells to come into cycle, restricted only by the toxicity of the chemotherapy on other organ systems. This usually cannot be accomplished with less than 5 to 7 days of treatment. The objective is to obtain an hypoplastic marrow that, it is hoped, will repopulate with normal marrow cells. Obviously, extensive supportive care is mandatory if success is to be achieved.

Methods of Supportive Care and Treatment of Complications

In order to provide the best opportunity to enable the patient to obtain a remission, the nature of other diseases afflicting the patient should be thoroughly evaluated. Renal, hepatic, cardiovascular, and pulmonary functions should be assessed and appropriate therapeutic measures undertaken when possible.

Hypercalcemia is rarely a problem in acute leukemia but should be treated by appropriate measures with adequate hydration, mithramycin, or corticosteroids.

Hyperuricemia secondary to increased purine turnover in patients with high white blood counts can be worsened by therapy and result in renal damage by precipitation of uric acid crystals in the renal tubules. This may lead to acute renal failure. Methods to prevent this include adequate hydration and occasionally alkalinization of urine. Allopurinol, given in a dose of 300 mg. twice daily, will rapidly lower serum uric acid levels and should be used whenever hyperuricemia is present. Hyperuricemia is anticipated as a result of treatment in those situations in which the white count is high and preexisting renal disease or bulky disease (large lymph nodes, hepatomegaly, or splenomegaly) is present.

Leukostasis. Patients admitted with leukocyte counts in excess of 100,000 per microliter have a high risk of developing complications related to plugging of small vessels by the blast cells. This may produce central nervous system symptoms as well as pulmonary complications. The treatment for this condition requires rapid reduction in the circulating blasts. This can best be accomplished by leukapheresis using a cell separator. This should be followed by the prompt initiation of chemotherapy. If an anthracycline and cytosine arabinoside are used (see below), very rapid lysis of cells frequently occurs and the use of such agents as hydroxyurea is not necessary.

Anemia. Red cell transfusions should be given to maintain a hemoglobin concentration above 9 grams per dl. (100 ml.). Packed red cells should be used rather than whole blood.

Hemorrhagic Disorder. THROMBOCYTOPENIA. Platelet transfusions should be given to those patients with low platelet counts who are bleeding. Platelet concentrates collected from a minimum of eight random single donors should be given once or twice daily to control major bleeding and once daily or every other day to control minor bleeding. Patients who are not bleeding should receive prophylactic platelet transfusions to maintain platelet count above 20,000 to 30,000 per microliter. Patients refractory to random platelets (failing to show an increment in platelet count 1 hour post-transfusion) should be given platelets collected by means of a cell separator from a single donor with the best HL-A antigen match possible.

Disseminated Intravascular Coagulation. Patients presenting with ecchymoses or in whom promyelocytes are the predominant cell type in the marrow should be evaluated for disseminated intravascular clotting. Measurement of prothrombin time, partial thromboplastin time, fibrin degradation products, and fibrinogen should be obtained. Patients diagnosed as having disseminated intravascular clotting disorder should be treated with heparin in doses of 5 to 10 units per kg. per hour by continuous infusion. If there is progression of the bleeding disorder, the dose should be raised to 10 to 20 units per kg. per hour.

Infections. Fever appearing in the patient with acute leukemia must be promptly evaluated and antibiotic coverage initiated prior to obtaining the results of cultures. Broad-spectrum antibiotics which include carbenicillin, gentamicin, and cephalothin should be used. If an anaerobic infection is suspected, such as might occur with perirectal abscess, chloramphenicol should be added. If a fungal infection is suspected amphotericin B should be administered.

Granulocyte Transfusions. Several recent studies have demonstrated the efficacy of granulocyte transfusions in infected, neutropenic patients. This requires a compatible ABO blood group donor. Granulocytes should be transfused daily until marrow recovery occurs. The effectiveness of prophylactic granulocyte transfusions has not been established.

Protection Against Infection. Good hand washing techniques for personnel caring for patients should be encouraged. The number of visitors should be held to a minimum and private rooms used whenever possible. Prophylactic oral antibiotics have been shown to be of some help in preventing infectious complications. Nystatin (Mycostatin) oral suspension used as a mouth wash is helpful in reducing the frequency of oral moniliasis. Laxatives and stool softeners are helpful in preventing rectal and anal complications that may result from constipation.

Vaginal Care and Menstruation. Vaginal care should include povidone-iodine (Betadine) douches and the use of nystatin (Mycostatin) suppositories. Menstruating women with low platelet counts or in whom reduction of platelet counts is anticipated from the chemotherapy should have menses suppressed by progesterone-estrogen combination drugs.

CHEMOTHERAPY OF LEUKEMIA

Acute Myeloblastic Leukemia

Remission Induction. The two most effective drugs in treating acute myeloblastic leukemia are cytosine arabinoside and an antracycline (daunorubicin or doxorubicin [Adriamycin]). The best results have been reported with a schedule as follows:

Cytosine arabinoside, 100 mg. per square meter of body surface infused continuously for 24 hours daily for 7 days. Daunorubicin, 45 mg. per square meter daily by rapid (20 to 30 minutes) intravenous injection for 3 days. An alternative antracycline, doxorubicin (Adriamycin), can be given on the same schedule as daunorubicin, but at a dose of 30 mg. per square meter daily for 3 days.

One or two courses of this treatment at intervals of 21 days should result in remission in greater than 60 per cent of the patients. The majority of patients require extensive supportive care during this treatment.

Consolidation Phase. It is now generally considered that the number of leukemic cells that remain following remission induction is sizable, and efforts should be made to further reduce the leukemic population. "Consolidation" is a term that implies continuation of rather intensive chemotherapy for several cycles following the onset of remission. There have been numerous programs described. None have proved better than continuation of the same or similar drugs. One program involves a 5 day course of cytosine arabinoside, 100 mg. per square meter given by rapid intravenous injection, and 6-thioguanine, 100 mg. per square meter given by mouth every 12 hours, and daunorubicin, 10 mg. per square meter given intravenously every 24 hours. Courses are repeated every 28 days for 3 to 6 cycles. Approximately one third of patients will relapse during the consolidation program. Those completing three consolidation courses and remaining in remission are then considered for maintenance programs.

Maintenance Program. To date no completely satisfactory maintenance program has been established. In general, when no further treatment is given remissions last about 3 to 6 months. The use of methotrexate in doses of 30 mg. per square meter twice weekly has been demonstrated to prolong remissions in children. In adults one would expect a remission duration of about 6 months with methotrexate. More effective treatment for maintaining remission has employed the use of doxorubicin (Adriamycin) and cytosine arabinoside. This combination has maintained remissions for 12 months.

More recently, several reports have indicated that immunotherapy given in addition to chemotherapy will prolong the duration of remission. Immunotherapy programs have included bacille Calmette Guérin vaccine (BCG) given intradermally by the Tyne technique, Heaf gun or scarification, MER (methanol extractable residue of BCG), and allogeneic leukemic cells, untreated or treated with neuraminidase. The latter procedure changes the cell surface in the hope of making the cell more antigenic. Results of randomized studies comparing immunotherapy plus chemotherapy to chemotherapy alone have varied but tend to suggest that the addition of immunotherapy is advantageous, either in prolonging remission duration or increasing the chances of obtaining a second remission.

The duration of maintenance therapy required to prevent recurrence of leukemia is unknown. In one preliminary study patients in remission for 1 year or longer were given three courses of intensive chemotherapy. Of 19 patients so treated, five relapsed from 2 to 62 weeks after cessation of treatment and the remainder continued in remission. Time will tell which is the most effective program. Studies are underway in patients whose treatment is stopped after 1 to 2 years of maintenance therapy. Late relapses are known to occur, but whether more patients are being "cured" is uncertain.

Acute Lymphoblastic Leukemia

Remission Induction. Remissions can be induced rather promptly with prednisone, 350 mg. per square meter daily for 10 days followed by 70 mg. per square meter every other day until day 21; vincristine, 1.4 mg. per square meter weekly, and methotrexate, 2 mg. per square meter every 6 hours for four doses on days 1, 5, 9, 14, 17, and 21. A marrow examination should be done on day 21, and if leukemia persists, the course must be repeated. One would expect to obtain a remission in approximately 80 per cent of patients.

Remission Consolidation. Remissions may be consolidated by giving a 5 day course of cytosine arabinoside, 100 mg. per square meter every 12 hours intravenously, and thioguanine, 100 mg. per square meter every 12 hours by mouth. A week following this treatment a 5 day course of L-asparaginase in doses of 2000 units per square meter daily should be given.

Central Nervous System Prophylaxis. Evidence has been obtained that therapy directed to the central nervous system (CNS) significantly delays the appearance of CNS leukemia. Following consolidation the cerebral spinal fluid should be examined and if negative for leukemic cells the CNS prophylaxis program should be initiated. This consists of radiation therapy, 2400 rads to the whole brain given over a 2 to 3 week period, and methotrexate, 10 mg. per square meter given intrathecally in saline or Elliott's B solution every 4 days for 3 weeks. Subsequently, intrathecal methotrexate should be given every 2 months for 2 years.

Maintenance Therapy. Following consolidation and during central nervous system treatment, maintenance therapy should be initiated. This consists of methotrexate, 40 mg. per square meter, and cyclophosphamide, 50 mg. per square meter once weekly, and 6-mercaptopurine, 50 mg. per square meter daily. Doses are adjusted downward if hematologic toxicity occurs. Treatment should be continued for 2 years.

Every 2 months during maintenance therapy 14 day courses of prednisone, 100 mg. per square meter daily, and vincristine, 1.4 mg. per square meter weekly, for three doses should be given. The program should be continued for the 2 year period of maintenance.

The average remission duration on this program is approximately 14 months.

Relapsing Patients. Patients who relapse after remission induction may be reinduced with the same drugs in some instances, if they have not received large quantities of these drugs in the recent past. However, those failing to respond to this type of treatment may be tried on different drugs. An active agent in acute myeloblastic leukemia appears to be 5-azacytidine, given in doses of 150 mg. per square meter daily for 5 days by continuous infusion and repeating courses every 15 to 21 days. In acute lymphoblastic leukemia relapsing patients may sometimes be reinduced with L-asparaginase or with a treatment protocol such as used with acute myeloblastic leukemia (antracycline plus cytosine arabinoside).

Central Nervous System Leukemia

Patients diagnosed as having central nervous system (CNS) involvement should be treated with CNS radiation (3000 rads) to the brain and intrathecal methotrexate as described in the section on acute lymphoblastic leukemia. Cytosine arabinoside may be given intrathecally (this use of cytosine arabinoside is not listed in the manufacturer's official directive) if methotrexate is ineffective or causes severe side effects. The placement of an Ommaya reservoir in a lateral ventricle may facilitate drug administration.

CHILDHOOD ACUTE LEUKEMIA*

method of
ROBERT M. WEETMAN, M.D.,
and ROBERT L. BAEHNER, M.D.
Indianapolis, Indiana

Prognosis and survival of children with acute leukemia can be related to certain factors present at the time of diagnosis. The most important factor is the morphologic cell type. Acute lymphocytic leukemia (ALL) has a much better prognosis than acute myelocytic, acute monocytic, or acute myelomonocytic leukemia. Current induction therapy for acute lymphocytic leukemia employs vincristine, prednisone, and L-asparaginase and 90 to 95 per cent of children will obtain complete remission with this regimen. In contrast, multiple drug induction therapy for acute myeloid leukemia results in successful remission in less than 70 per cent of patients. More than half of the patients with ALL remain in continuous complete remission for five years, compared to a median duration of complete remission of 12 to 14 months in acute myeloid leukemia.

Other important prognostic factors predicting survival outcome in childhood leukemia include age at diagnosis and the initial level of white blood cell count (as a reflection of the total leukemic cell burden of the body). Children with normal initial white cell counts (less than 10,000 per cu. mm.) and between the ages of 3 and 7 years at diagnosis tend to have a much better prognosis with their mean disease-free survival ranging between 80 and 83 per cent at 48 months postdiagnosis. Children of any age with initial white cell counts greater than 50,000 per cu. mm. at diagnosis have mean disease-free survival of only 35 to 40 per cent at 48 months postdiagnosis. The good

and poor risk groups each account for approximately one third of the entire group. An intermediate risk group of children either less than 3 years of age or over 7 years of age with initial white blood cell counts of less than 10,000 per cu. mm. or children of any age with white cell counts between 10,000 and 50,000 per cu. mm. at diagnosis experience a 60 to 70 per cent mean disease-free survival 48 months after diagnosis. When these same general criteria are applied to children with acute myeloid leukemia, initial white cell counts less than 20,000 per cu. mm. are associated with a longer median survival than are initial white cell counts of greater than 20,000 per cu. mm. at diagnosis. In the Children's Cancer Study Group series, the median remission duration for children with less than 20,000 per cu. mm. initial white cell count was 16 months, in contrast to the group with greater than 20,000 per cu. mm. who had a 9 month median remission duration. Similarly, children in the age range of 5 to 10 years compared to the groups below age 5 and above age 10 appear to have an improved remission induction and duration. Children in the 5 to 10 year age range had a 90 per cent remission induction rate and a 30+ month median remission duration in contrast to 64 and 79 per cent remission induction rate and a 12.5 and 8.5 month median remission duration for children greater than 10 years or less than 5 years, respectively, at diagnosis ($p < 0.007$). In acute lymphocytic leukemia, these prognostic variables lose their significance after the patient has remained in remission for 2 years and are no longer of value in predicting the outcome of the disease. Other prognostic factors at the time of diagnosis that have been shown to have prognostic significance of one degree or another in childhood acute lymphoblastic leukemia include the sex of the patient (females tend to survive longer than males), central nervous system disease at the time of diagnosis, presence of a mediastinal mass, blast cell morphology (patients with the morphologically larger L-2 type blast tend to have a poorer survival than those with the smaller L-1 lymphoblastic morphology), lymphoblast cell markers (null cell leukemia has a better prognosis than T cell or B cell leukemia), and the occurrence of central nervous system or extramedullary relapse during remission. An in-depth discussion of these prognostic variables is beyond the scope of this article.

Other prognostic variables that may affect the outcome of acute myeloid leukemia in childhood include the increased incidence of bleeding and disseminated intravascular coagulopathy in acute promyelocytic leukemia, the increased incidence of central nervous system leukemia in children with acute monocytic or myelomonocytic leukemia, and the high risk of infection during

*Some agents mentioned in this article are considered investigational. Before using any of the drugs mentioned in this article, the physician should be well informed of their actions and of the information in the manufacturer's official directive.

induction therapy for all subgroups of nonlymphocytic leukemia.

The combination of multiagent chemotherapy and prophylactic central nervous system therapy has been the one factor responsible for the prolongation of complete remission in childhood acute lymphoblastic leukemia. Following successful induction therapy, the administration of 2400 rads to the craniospinal axis or cranial irradiation in combination with intrathecal methotrexate therapy has reduced central nervous system relapse rates from 50 to 60 per cent to 5 to 7 per cent. As central nervous system relapse regularly leads to bone marrow relapse, elimination of this complication in the majority of patients has resulted in increased disease-free survival for a much larger number of patients. Central nervous system relapse also occurs in acute myeloid leukemia, but to date, central nervous system prophylaxis has not led to an increase in the median duration of survival.

Therapy Designed to Restore Physiologic Balance

There are many important areas of management of the child with acute leukemia in addition to the chemotherapy of the disease.

Hyperuricemia. Hyperuricemia reflects the increased degradation of purines through the xanthine-xanthine oxidase pathway, either from an increased leukemic cell turnover and increased leukemic cell death occurring during the natural course of the disease or as a result of chemotherapy. Hyperuricemia in excess of 10 mg. per dl. (100 ml.) frequently results in precipitation of uric acid crystals in the acid environment of the renal tubules and subsequent renal failure. Although this complication may occur in any child with acute lymphocytic leukemia, it is most prevalent in those with high white blood counts and massive organomegaly and in those children with B cell leukemia or leukemic transformation of a non-Hodgkin's lymphoma. Consequently, all patients with acute leukemia and lymphomas must be screened for hyperuricemia and renal function abnormalities at the time of diagnosis. The patient should receive intravenous hydration with approximately 3000 ml. per square meter of appropriate intravenous fluid in order to assure a good urine flow. The urine should be alkalinized by administering 3 to 4 grams per square meter per 24 hours of sodium bicarbonate intravenously to the patient. Sodium bicarbonate dosage should be adjusted based upon the pH of the urine and monitored frequently to obtain a pH value in the 7.0 to 7.5 range as uric acid is more soluble in an alkaline urine. As purines are degraded by xanthine oxidase, the production of uric acid can be decreased markedly by administration of the xanthine oxidase inhibitor, allopurinol, in a dosage of 10 to 20 mg. per kg. per day (divided dosage of three or four times per day). In instances of oliguria or anuria due to hyperuricemia, diuresis may be induced by intravenous mannitol infusions. Diuretics, such as furosemide, produce an acid urine and thiazides increase serum urate levels and decrease urate excretion through competitive inhibition with uric acid for renal tubular secretion sites. In addition, salicylate therapy inhibits secretion of uric acid and raises serum urate levels. Uricosuric agents are also contraindicated since they transiently elevate urine uric acid levels while lowering serum urate levels and therefore can enhance precipitation of uric acid crystals in the kidney and worsen urate nephropathy. Obviously, all antileukemic agents should be withheld until the urate nephropathy problem is adequately controlled.

Anemia. Anemia results from the loss of normal erythroid progenitor cells in the bone marrow, owing to leukemic infiltration, and may be accentuated by bleeding. When the hemoglobin falls to less than 8 grams or the child becomes symptomatic, the anemia should be corrected. The use of frozen erythrocytes is more desirable than the use of fresh packed red cells, as the possibility of sensitization to HL-A and white cell antigens foreign to the child is reduced. Furthermore, sensitization may preclude a later bone marrow transplant if the patient has a refractory leukemia. For this same reason, relatives and immediate family members should not be used as erythrocyte or platelet donors.

Bleeding. In a newly diagnosed child with acute leukemia, thrombocytopenia and the threat of bleeding are usually present. Spontaneous hemorrhage from thrombocytopenia may occur as the platelet count falls to 20,000 per cu. mm. or below, necessitating platelet transfusion support in the child undergoing lumbar puncture or surgical procedures, or in the child with active sepsis or bleeding. Salicylates block platelet aggregation and formation of a hemostatic plug. Therefore, aspirin should be assiduously avoided and acetaminophen substituted for fever and pain control. In patients with acute promyelocytic leukemia, release of cytoplasmic granular contents may trigger both the coagulation and fibrinolytic pathways, initiating disseminated intravascular coagulopathy. Coagulation abnormalities have also resulted in some patients with acute myeloid leukemia from the release of an elastaselike protease from granules resulting in proteolysis and depletion of coagulation factors and a hemorrhagic diathesis. In each instance, the coagulation factors should be replaced with 10 to 15 ml. per kg. of fresh frozen plasma and platelets replaced with platelet transfusions, 1 unit per 13 lbs. (5.9 kg.) of body weight. When bleeding or disseminated intravascular coagulation (DIC) is present, platelet transfusions may be required more frequently than once or twice weekly. Ideally, HL-A identical or similar donors are selected to prevent or minimize the risk for development of platelet antibodies in the patient. When bone marrow transplantation is contemplated, then random unrelated donors are used. Heparin therapy has a therapeutic advantage in disseminated intravascular coagulation (DIC) associated with promyelocytic leukemia.

Metabolic Imbalance. Electrolyte abnormalities may occur during the course of acute leukemia. Initially, alkalinization of the urine with intravenous sodium bicarbonate may lead to hypocalcemia or hypokalemia. These situations are managed by appropriate replacement therapy and discontinuing the alkalinization until the deficiency is corrected. Hypocalcemia may also result from an increased phosphate load and calcium chelation following antileukemic therapy. Occasionally, clinical tetany may be observed. Rarely, hypercalcemia has been observed in patients with acute leukemia. Renal function may be disturbed similar to that in patients with hyperparathyroidism Hyponatremia due to inappropriate antidiuretic hormone secretion has been described in patients with malignancy and in patients following therapy with vincristine or cyclophosphamide. Inappropriate antidiuretic hormone (ADH) secretion is documented by observing a urine osmolarity greater than the serum osmolarity in the presence of oliguria. Treatment requires fluid restriction and discontinuance of drugs that may have caused the response.

Infection. Infection is the leading cause of death in children with acute leukemia. A number of factors are responsible for this enhanced susceptibility to infection. Neutropenia is usually present at the time of diagnosis, owing to depressed granulopoiesis by leukemic infiltration of the bone marrow, and often later in the course of the disease, owing to marrow suppression by chemotherapeutic agents. As many as 25 per cent of patients are infected at the time of presentation and approximately 50 per cent sustain a significant infection during the first few weeks of therapy. Patients with fever associated with an absolute neutrophil count below 1000 per cu. mm. (total white count × percentage of neutrophils) should be suspect for severe infection and should receive broad-spectrum antibiotic coverage intravenously following appropriate cultures. Often the usual clinical and radiologic signs of infection are absent in the leukemic patient. The majority of severe infections (i.e., sepsis, meningitis, pneumonia, cellulitis) occurring in children with leukemia are associated with absolute neutrophil counts of less than 200 per cu. mm. With documented sepsis, or an obvious site of infection, the granulocytopenic patients should receive white cell transfusions for a minimum of 5 days or until the granulocyte count begins to rise and the infection clears. In addition to *Staphylococcus aureus, Escherichia coli, Pseudomonas,* and *Candida albicans,* which can cause infection at any stage in the course of leukemia, many more common organisms are noted to cause sepsis in children at the time of diagnosis, including *Hemophilus influenzae, Diplococcus pneumoniae,* and the beta hemolytic streptococci. The sources of infection in the neutropenic patient include the skin, mucous membranes, and enteric and respiratory tracts. The blood, cerebrospinal fluid, perineal area, and gingiva are frequent sites of infection and must be frequently examined during periods of neutropenia.

Another factor increasing the susceptibility of patients with leukemia to infection is the transient suppression of the immune response induced by the disease itself or the chemotherapy and radiation therapy. Neutrophil bactericidal killing function is altered during and shortly after craniospinal irradiation. Intermittent suppression of both humoral and cellular immunity occurs during the early phases of therapy. Anatomic barriers may be broken down, a specific example being the gastrointestinal tract ulceration associated with methotrexate and other drug therapies allowing a portal of entry for both gram-negative and gram-positive organisms. Steroid therapy adds to the masking of signs of infection owing to its anti-inflammatory action. Suppression of cellular immunity reaches its nadir during the latter part of central nervous system prophylaxis and the early phases of maintenance therapy. Opportunistic and atypical infections often become a problem during this period. Interstitial and other pneumonias frequently occur and require open lung biopsy for diagnosis. Some of the more common organisms responsible for bilateral interstitial pneumonias in these patients include *Pneumocystis carinii,* cytomegalic inclusion virus, herpes viruses (varicella-zoster, simplex), adeno virus, and fungal organisms such as Candida, Histoplasma, and Aspergillus. Rarely, the picture of interstitial pneumonia can result from leukemic infiltration of the lungs or from a cyclophosphamide or methotrexate-induced chemical or hypersensitivity pneumonitis.

Certain prophylactic measures may be required to combat the high risk for life-threatening infection in the leukemic patient. The daily administration of trimethoprim-sulfamethoxazole has prevented the occurrence of Pneumocystis pneumonia at centers previously known to have high attack rates. Administration of zoster immune globulin (obtained for emergency use by contacting the ZIG distribution center, 617-732-3121) within 3 days after exposure to varicella will modify or prevent clinical varicella in the susceptible child receiving chemotherapy for leukemia. During the period of risk for development of varicella, chemotherapy, especially prednisone, should be tapered or discontinued.

Chemotherapy of Acute Lymphocytic Leukemia

Although we now recognize the low risk, average risk, and high risk groups of children with acute lymphocytic leukemia, we have not yet formulated ideal therapy for all groups. At present, investigative studies are in progress to determine whether more intensive therapy will be of benefit for the poorer risk groups. Following initial attempts to restore physiologic balance, children with acute leukemia should be referred to a cancer treatment center experienced in the management of childhood leukemia. The diagnosis of acute leukemia is confirmed by reviewing the bone marrow aspirate and biopsy. At the time of diagnosis, the child should be screened for prognostic indicators such as central nervous system disease, mediastinal mass, white cell count, age, sex, blast morphology, and immune markers on the lymphoblasts.

Remission induction is attempted with vincristine sulfate, 1.5 mg. per square meter per week intravenously (maximum = 2.0 mg.), prednisone, 40 mg. per square meter per day orally given in a divided three times daily dosage, and L-asparaginase, 6000 I.U. per square meter intramuscularly (Table 1). The vincristine is given on the first day of therapy and then every 7 days thereafter for a total of 5 doses. The prednisone is continued on the three divided doses daily dosage schedule for a total of 28 days and then is tapered over a period of 10 days. The L-asparaginase is begun on day 3 and continued every other day for a total of 9 doses. In addition, during the induction period, methotrexate is given intrathecally on the first day of therapy and again 2 weeks later. The intrathecal methotrexate dosage is based upon cerebrospinal fluid volume rather than body surface area in order to reduce toxicity. The dosage schedule is as follows:

Age	Intrathecal Methotrexate Dose
<1 year	6 mg.
1–2 years	8 mg.
2–3 years	10 mg.
≥3 years	12 mg.

On the twenty-eighth day of chemotherapy, a bone marrow aspiration is again performed to determine the state of remission. If the bone marrow reveals less than 5 per cent lymphoblasts, the marrow is considered to be in complete remission.

Following marrow remission, central nervous system prophylaxis is begun. Standard prophylactic central nervous system therapy includes 2400 rads of cranial irradiation utilizing a supervoltage source, i.e., cobalt 60 or 4 to 6 MeV source administered in a dose schedule of 200 rads per day for 5 days a week. In addition, intrathecal

TABLE 1. Chemotherapy of Acute Childhood Leukemia

ALL	AML
Induction:	*Induction:*
Vincristine: 1.5 mg./m.²/week I.V., Day 0, 7, 14, 21, & 28 (Maximum = 2.0 mg.)	Daunomycin: 30 mg./m.²/day I.V. × 3 doses (Maximum = 540 mg./m.²)
Prednisone: 40 mg./m.²/day p.o., Day 0 to 28 (divided T.I.D.)	5-Azacytidine: 50 mg./m.² I.V. B.I.D. × 8 doses
L-Asparaginase: 6000 I.U./m.² I.M., Day 3, 5, 7, 10, 12, 14, 17, 19, & 21	Cytosine arabinoside: 25 mg./m.² I.V. q8h × 12 doses
Methotrexate intrathecally (see text for dosage: Maximum = 12 mg./dose) Day 0, 14, & 28	Vincristine: 1.5 mg./m.²/dose I.V. × 1 dose (Maximum = 2.0 mg.) on first day of each course
	Prednisone: 40 mg./m.²/day p.o. (divided TID) × 4 days
Central Nervous System Prophylaxis:	*Repeat each course every 14 days*
Cranial irradiation: 2400 rads (200 rads/day, 5 days/week)	*Maximum = 6 courses*
Methotrexate intrathecally (see text for dosage: Maximum = 12 mg./dose) Day 28, 35, 42, & 56	
Prednisone: Taper over 10 days	*Maintenance:*
6-Mercaptopurine: 75 mg./m.²/day p.o.	5-Azacytidine: 100 mg./m.²/day I.V. × 4 days
	Cytosine arabinoside: 75 mg./m.²/day I.V. × 4 days
	Cyclophosphamide: 75 mg./m.²/day I.V. × 4 days
Maintenance:	Vincristine: 1.5 mg./m.²/dose I.V. on first day of each course (Maximum = 2.0 mg.)
6-Mercaptopurine: 75 mg./m.²/day p.o.	6-Thioguanine: 75 mg./m.²/day p.o. × 28 days
Methotrexate: 20 mg./m.²/week p.o.	*Repeat each course every 28 days*
Vincristine: 1.5 mg./m.²/dose I.V. every 28 days (Maximum = 2.0 mg.)	
Prednisone: 40 mg./m.²/day p.o. (divided T.I.D.) × 5 days, every 28 days	Methotrexate intrathecally (see text for dosage: Maximum = 12 mg./dose) every 28 days × 6 courses

methotrexate is continued once weekly for 4 additional dosages to a total of 6 doses using the same dosage schedule as above. During this period of time, 6-mercaptopurine, 75 mg. per square meter per day orally, is given for maintenance of the bone marrow remission. On day 56, or approximately 2 months since the beginning of chemotherapy (and one month following the beginning of cranial-spinal prophylaxis), bone marrow and spinal fluid surveillance are again repeated. If the bone marrow has remained in remission and the spinal fluid is clear of lymphoblastic involvement, maintenance therapy is begun.

Maintenance therapy consists of 6-mercaptopurine, 75 mg. per square meter per day orally, methotrexate, 20 mg. per square meter per week orally, and periodic doses of vincristine and prednisone, given monthly. Vincristine is given at a dosage of 1.5 mg. per square meter per dose (maximum = 2.0 mg.) and prednisone is given at a dosage of 40 mg. per square meter per day in divided (three times daily) dosage for a total of 5 days. Maintenance therapy is normally continued for 3 years. However, the optimal length of time for continuation of maintenance therapy is not known at the present time.

The physician responsible for the therapy of childhood acute lymphocytic leukemia should be familiar with the side effects and mechanism of action of the drugs administered and must have available supportive therapy in the form of white cell transfusions, platelet transfusions, and frozen red blood cell transfusions. The chemotherapy outlined here is probably optimal therapy for the child in the low risk category of acute lymphocytic leukemia. However, children in the moderate risk or high risk groups probably will require more potent or newer investigational forms of therapy available at a reputable cancer treatment center.

Extramedullary Leukemia. As with bone marrow relapse, relapse in the central nervous system or testicular area predicts a poor prognosis. Central nervous system relapse may be managed in one of several ways: (a) the cranium may be reirradiated and 6 additional courses of intrathecal methotrexate administered, (b) cranial-spinal irradiation, (c) injection of intrathecal methotrexate or injection of methotrexate, cytosine arabinoside, and hydrocortisone intrathecally. Testicular relapse usually presents as a unilateral painless testicular swelling. However, in most cases, both testes are involved and both should be biopsied to confirm the diagnosis. Testicular relapse is treated with 3000 rads of irradiation to the involved gonads. As bone marrow relapse frequently follows central nervous system or testicular relapse within a few months, most pediatric oncologists follow relapse treatment of these extramedullary areas with a reinduction program similar to that employed for the initial induction prior to continuing maintenance therapy.

Chemotherapy of Acute Nonlymphocytic Leukemia (Acute Myelocytic Leukemia, Acute Monomyelocytic Leukemia, Acute Monocytic Leukemia, Acute Histocytic Leukemia and Acute Erythrocytic Leukemia)

Perhaps to an even greater degree than with acute lymphocytic leukemia, physicians undertaking the therapy of acute nonlymphocytic leukemia must have available supportive therapy including white cell transfusions, platelet transfusions, and frozen red cells, and expertise in handling infection in the neutropenic patient. The diagnosis of acute nonlymphocytic leukemia is established by observing a predominance of blast cells of nonlymphoid origin in the bone marrow aspirate or biopsy. Peroxidase, sudan black, nonspecific esterase activities and Auer rods in the blast cells are helpful in some patients to establish the correct diagnosis. The Children's Cancer Study Group currently employs a 5 drug regimen for the treatment of acute nonlymphocytic leukemia. For remission induction, the following agents are employed in 4 day courses every 14 days for a minimum of 4 courses and a maximum of 6 courses: Daunomycin, 30 mg. per square meter per day intravenously for three doses, 5-azacytidine, 50 mg. per square meter intravenously twice daily for eight doses, cytosine arabinoside, 25 mg. per square meter intravenously every 8 hours for 12 doses, vincristine, 1.5 mg. per square meter per dose intravenously for one dose (maximum = 2.0 mg.), and prednisone, 40 mg. per square meter per day orally for 4 days (Table 1). Bone marrow aspirations are performed after each second course and the courses are repeated until remission is attained or until 6 courses have been given. Daunomycin is discontinued when a total dose of 540 mg. per square meter is reached in order to avoid cardiac toxicity. Upon attaining remission verified by bone marrow aspiration containing less than 15 per cent blast cells, maintenance therapy is begun with the following drugs given in 4 day courses every 28 days: cyclophosphamide, 75 mg. per square meter per day intravenously for 4 days, cytosine arabinoside, 75 mg. per square meter per day intravenously for 4 days, vincristine, 1.5 mg. per square meter per dose intravenously on the first day of each course, and 5-azacytidine, 100 mg. per square meter per day intravenously for 4 days. In addition, 6-thioguanine, 75 mg. per square meter per day

TABLE 2.   **Side Effects and Toxicities of Drugs Used in Therapy of Acute Childhood Leukemia**

DRUGS	SIDE EFFECTS AND TOXICITIES
Vincristine sulfate	Neurotoxicity (paresthesias, jaw pain, loss of deep tendon reflexes, constipation, obstipation, ileus, hoarseness, sensory loss, ptosis, muscle weakness, slapping gait); local reactions with injection site extravasation, alopecia, inappropriate ADH secretion, fever, rare seizures
Prednisone	Hypertension, increased appetite, weight gain, salt retention, Cushingoid appearance, personality changes, myopathy, osteoporosis, diabetes mellitus, pancreatitis, increased susceptibility to infection, immunosuppression, and gastrointestinal ulceration
L-Asparaginase	Hypersensitivity reactions (urticaria and anaphylaxis), hepatotoxicity, fever, coagulation abnormalities, azotemia, weight loss, anorexia, nausea, vomiting, transient hyperglycemia, diabetes mellitus, pancreatitis, EEG changes, encephalopathy and hyperammonemia
6-Mercaptopurine	Bone marrow suppression, hepatotoxicity, oral ulcerations, nausea and vomiting (toxicity accentuated by allopurinol administration)
Methotrexate	Bone marrow suppression, megaloblastosis, gastrointestinal tract ulcerations, renal toxicity, hepatotoxicity, osteoporosis, pneumonitis, necrotizing enteropathy, anorexia, nausea, vomiting, skin rash, immunosuppression, cerebrospinal fluid pleocytosis, meningismus, arachnoiditis, leukoencephalopathy
Cytosine arabinoside	Bone marrow suppression, megaloblastic marrow, oral ulcerations, anorexia, nausea, vomiting, fever, diarrhea and abdominal pain, hepatotoxicity, and alopecia
5-Azacytidine	Bone marrow suppression, nausea, vomiting, diarrhea, rash, fever, hepatotoxicity, phlebitis, and local reaction with injection site extravasation
Daunomycin	Bone marrow suppression, gastrointestinal tract ulcerations, anorexia, nausea, vomiting, fever, alopecia, cardiac toxicity, abdominal pain, phlebitis, local reactions with injection site extravasation, and dark urine
Cyclophosphamide	Bone marrow suppression, alopecia, anorexia, nausea, vomiting, hemorrhagic cystitis, bladder fibrosis, sterility, immunosuppression, inappropriate ADH secretion
6-Thioguanine	Bone marrow suppression, hepatotoxicity, gastrointestinal abnormalities

orally, is begun and continued throughout the 28 day cycle.

Lumbar punctures are performed at time of diagnosis and at the beginning of maintenance therapy for surveillance of central nervous system leukemia. Intrathecal methotrexate in the dosage described earlier for acute lymphocytic leukemia is given intrathecally every 28 days for 6 doses during the maintenance phase of therapy. Generally speaking, absolute granulocyte counts less than 1000 per cu. mm. and platelet counts less than 100,000 per cu. mm. require alterations in drug dosage for toxicity. A list of toxicities commonly seen with drugs used in the therapy of acute childhood leukemia can be found in Table 2.

Because of the disappointing long-term results in acute nonlymphocytic leukemia of childhood, currently selected patients with ABO, HL-A, and MLC compatible sibling bone marrow donors are being referred for bone marrow transplantation early in their first remission.

Psychosocial Management

One of the most important aspects in the management of the child with acute leukemia is the need for psychosocial support of the child and family created by the diagnosis. Confirmation of the diagnosis must be obtained by bone marrow aspiration or biopsy or both, following explanation of the procedure and obtaining consent from the child. After verification of the diagnosis, a frank but sympathetic discussion of the diagnosis, should be carried out with both parents. Depending on the specific hospital situation, in addition to the attending hematologist, the ward physician, nursing specialist, and social workers may take part in the initial conference. This conference should be held at a time and in a place where distractions and interruptions will be held to a minimum, allowing ample time for questions and discussion. During this conference an explanation of the diagnosis, as well as important aspects of supportive therapy and chemotherapy, should be outlined. Other topics requiring discussion in this conference include misconceptions about the disease, current knowledge about the cause of the disease, expectations for the child's well being during the next few months and years, and guidelines for the psychosocial management of the patient and siblings. The importance of restoring normal activities and discipline for the patient should be reinforced, and avoidance of over indulgence emphasized. Sibling reactions and anxieties to the diagnosis should be discussed. Options available for alleviating social and financial hardships should be revealed. The importance of open communication between the physician, parents, and child should be stressed and the parents encouraged to contact the physician whenever they consider it necessary. The willingness of the hospital staff and attending physician to answer questions as they arise should be stressed, and both office and home phone numbers given to the family at the time of initial interview. Attempts to alleviate parental guilt feelings should be made at the time of the first interview. The initial reaction of the family usually is one of shock, emotional turmoil, or denial, and repeated conferences are usually necessary to reinforce those points made during the initial conference.

The diagnosis should be discussed with the child at a level commensurate with his or her understanding and age. A great deal of emotional support and comfort may be engendered by active communication between physician and child. It is most important to develop and maintain an environment in which the child is able to ask questions and to feel confident that he or she will receive an honest answer. The child must be allowed to retain hope of recovery, but it must be remembered that inappropriate answers lead to increased fear and anxiety, decreased communication, and feelings of abandonment. It has been shown that there is a decreased incidence of withdrawal and depressive reactions among patients with whom the diagnosis has been honestly discussed. Establishment of a sound route of communication in this manner helps the child later to be able to discuss his fears and anxieties concerning impending death with both parents and physician, thus protecting him from the lonely death.

Green, a leader in the field of psychosocial management of the pediatric patient and his family, has enumerated the following guidelines for the care of the dying child which should be followed scrupulously: The physician must attend to the needs of the child and the family in a competent, conscientious manner and be available when needed. It is advantageous to the family to have a home as well as an office telephone number to increase availability and in the case of unavailability for whatever reason, competent, responsible physician coverage must be provided. Continuity of care with a single physician is desirable, with the ultimate development of more sensitive, personalized care. Prior preparation of the patient for forthcoming procedures, hospitalization, changes in therapy, or temporary absences of the physician should be the rule and help to decrease anxiety. The child should not be excluded entirely from discussions of his diagnosis and care; he or she should be involved to a level commensurate with age. The physician must exhibit a willingness to answer questions and be sensitive to the child's emotional needs in order to dispel anxieties, fears, anger, or guilt feelings. The physician must remain sympathetic, comforting, and supportive to the child and the family's needs. He must avoid loss of control of his own feelings; on the other hand, he must not become distant or impersonal and thus sacrifice his effectiveness as a physician.

In the instance in which all reasonable therapeutic measures have failed and the death of a child is imminent, a frank but sympathetic discussion concerning the impending death should be held with the family. Parents should be assured that the child will be made comfortable and all pain alleviated if medically possible. The decision to withdraw supportive care must be made by the physician caring for the child and then discussed with parents in terms of the necessity for not prolonging the child's suffering. Should the parents indicate a desire for prolongation of supportive care, the physician is obligated to continue supportive therapy. The parents should be given a chance to discuss their feelings engendered by the patient's impending death. The physician must make a special effort to remain sensitive to the dying child's needs, with maintenance of adequate care and attention. He must minimize his own tensions and anger, recognize and control his natural repulsion to death, and make a particular effort to not reinvest his energies elsewhere until after the patient dies. It is particularly important that the physician continue to comfort and support the child with his physical presence until death.

The physician should recognize that parents will progress through a mourning reaction, including sadness, anger, and finally reinvestment of energies into life and other activities that may require several months for completion. Parents of the deceased child should be encouraged to return in several months for an interview. This interview will not only allow discussion of autopsy findings, if appropriate, but will be therapeutic to the parents, allowing them to ask previously unanswered questions. It will allow discussion of the deceased child by the parents in an understanding setting, which may not be available elsewhere. It also provides the physician an opportunity to try to extinguish any lingering guilt feelings or anxieties that may remain with the parents.

THE CHRONIC LEUKEMIAS

method of
THOMAS C. HALL, M.D.
Pasadena, California

The treatment of neoplastic diseases has improved in recent years with increased knowledge of their pathogenesis and also their natural history. This is particularly true of the leukemias, for which we have now an improved understanding of pathogenesis as expanded clones of cells blocked at specific stages in their ontogeny. In the case of chronic myelogenous leukemia (CML), this has led us to understand that in 85 per cent of cases, there is malignant cellular transformation marked by a change in chromosomal structure shown by all normal marrow elements in the affected patient. Thus, the term "myelogenous" is more appropriate than "granulocytic." It can be assumed that at the earlier stages of CML, a stem cell is transformed but there is relatively normal maturation of "daughter" cells into erythrocytes, granulocytes and platelets, all bearing the Ph^1 chromosome. This results from the transfer of chromosomal material from number 22 to number 9. Initially, the effects on the host are due to proliferation of stem cells in marrow and spleen, with some secondary effects of the inhibition of normal marrow cell growth, and some tertiary effects such as hyperuricemia due to overproduction of short-lived granulocytes. At these stages, therapy has been traditionally directed at slowing down the replication rate of the abnormal clone by the use of agents, such as busulfan, that have very slightly stronger effects on the malignant than on normal marrow elements. Busulfan can be given in large initial doses if the disease seems to be moving steadily or started at very low doses if progression of disease is slow.

Recently, attempts have been made to eradicate the abnormal Ph^1 chromosomal cell population at an early stage, when the malignant clone was minimally expanded. This requires differential eradication of malignant marrow stem cells from among normal marrow elements, and to date no therapeutic methods have been developed that do this well. Patients desiring to participate in such therapeutic trials can be referred to one of the National Cancer Institute Treatment Centers engaged in such research.

About 10 per cent of CML patients lack the Ph^1 chromosome, and proliferation of such clones is characteristically more malignant. They usually have normal white cell alkaline phosphatase levels, the patient may be either juvenile or older than the midadult age common to patients with Ph^1 CML, and the process is harder to treat.

As CML progresses over 3 to 5 years, the malignant stem cells expand and the nature of the disease changes to one in which the rather mature circulating granulocytes are replaced by immature cells. These often have the surface properties and biochemical characteristics, such as terminal deoxynucleotide transferase ("tdt"), of highly primitive stem cells resembling those of acute stem-cell leukemia. We now expect that virtually all patients with chronic myelogenous leukemia will experience this "blast cell" transformation and plan to treat blasts that are tdt positive with intensive vincristine and prednisone. This has recently resulted, for the first time, in some remissions in this blastic phase.

Some understanding of the pathogenesis and history of chronic lymphocyte leukemia (CLL) has also occurred recently. We now understand that lymphomas and leukemias arise also by proliferation of immunocyte clones blocked at stages along their ontogenesis. Diffuse well-differentiated lymphoma and chronic lymphocytic leukemia both appear to be the consequence of slow proliferation of highly differentiated B lymphocytes similar to those found in the lymph nodes and peripheral blood. In contrast to CML, there is little evidence of transformation of a primitive lymphoid cell. Hence, there is great sensitivity to agents that are effective in lysing mature lymphocytes, such as alkylating agents, radiation, and corticoids. There is usually no late "blast cell" phase of the disease. The manifestations of disease are almost entirely due to the slow accumulation of masses of long-lived, almost normal, "B" lymphocytes with a single class of surface immune globulins, which are being produced at a slightly faster than normal rate. As myeloid cells in CML accumulate naturally in the marrow and later in the spleen, so these CML lymphocytes appear to accumulate first in nodes and spleen and only later in the marrow. The symptoms that arise are, hence, initially due to enlargement of nodes and spleen, later due to replacement of normal immunocyte function, often with hypogammaglobulinemia, and only much later due to decreases in red and white cells and platelets. Early therapeutic measures in CLL are directed toward decreasing the numbers of mature lymphocytes, both circulating and in lymphoid storage sites. This can be done by alkylating agents, titrated doses of ^{32}P or low dose radiation.

No rationale exists for early aggressive therapy directed at eradicatory "cure" of a CLL stem cell population. If, late in the disease, a rapidly dividing clone of blast cells appears, it is apt to resemble immature myelomonocytoid cells transformed by prior antileukemic therapy. Slow proliferation and long life span leads to gradual accumulation of cells and very slow presentation of symptoms; this "latent" period may last 5 to 10 years. Hence, there is nothing to be gained by therapy prior to the onset of mild symptoms, and thereafter, therapy is desirable with agents showing the greatest ratio of damage to tumor vs. damage to normal tissue. At the early stages, these include local low dose radiation to an enlarged spleen or lymph nodes, followed by intermittent courses with oral alkylating agents such as chlorambucil, a mild alkylating agent that does not cause alopecia or cystitis. Later, lysis of larger circulating or nodal CLL cell volumes or the correction of hemolytic anemia due to abnormal immunoglobulin production by the CLL cells may require more aggressive systemic therapy. A clinical staging classification has been initiated based upon extent of disease and effects upon the host. This may provide a reasonable guideline for sequential use of therapeutic measures in this disease.

"Hairy cell leukemia" or leukemic reticuloendotheliosis is a recently described clinical entity that results from the proliferation of clones of cells resembling both B lymphocytes and those histiocytic cells lining the medullary sinuses of lymph nodes. On smears there are irregular nuclei and cytoplasmic projections; histochemically, the cells are acid phosphatase positive and l-tartrate resistant. There is a characteristic involvement of the red pulp of the spleen and of the hepatic sinusoids; splenomegaly is always found. These are also slowly proliferating clones with little tendency to invade lymph nodes or bone marrow until late in the disease. Systemic effects such as anemia, neutropenia, and thrombocytopenia are common. At the later stage, therapy with alkylating agents alone is not as effective and corticoids may improve peripheral blood counts. Splenectomy decreases pancytopenia and may prolong survival.

We present here a summary of our treatment practices in a Clinical Stage-Related Treatment Program.*

A. Chronic lymphocytic leukemia:
Stage 0: lymphocytosis only; careful watching
Stage I: bulky lymphadenopathy; local radiation therapy
Stage II: Spleno-hepatomegaly; oral chlorambucil, 0.4 mg. per kg. body weight daily for 5 days each month
Stage III: anemia <11 grams; prednisone, 1.0 mg. per kg. daily orally for 1 week each month
Stage IV: neutropenia <1500, infection, thrombocytopenia <100,000; chlorambucil plus prednisone as above; splenectomy if hypersplenism or autoimmunity occurs

B. Chronic myelogenous leukemia:
Stage 0: granulocytosis >10,000; low alkaline phosphatase and Ph^1 chromosome; watchful waiting
Stage I: hyperuricemia/splenomegaly; localized splenic radiation therapy, busulfan, 2 mg. per day orally, increase by 2 mg. per day every other week, target: WBC <50,000
Stage II: Hgb <11 grams, platelets >1 million, WBC >150,000; busulfan, 0.1 mg. per kg. per day orally, reduce by 50 per cent when platelets or WBC have fallen by 50 per cent; discontinue when WBC ≤15,000 or platelets ≤150,000

Stage III: Special situations, e.g., CNS symptoms, busulfan, 2 mg. orally 6 times daily for 5 days; severe hyperuricemia, allopurinol, 0.3 gram per day orally; WBC rising on busulfan, 6-mercaptopurine, 0.4 mg. per kg. per day orally, or hydroxyurea, 20 mg. per kg. per day orally, also cyclophosphamide (Cytoxan) has been tried; pregnancy, fragile patient, drug resistant Stage II patient, leukapheresis until WBC <50,000
Stage IV: Blast crisis
  a. Lymphoid-looking cells, positive for tdt enzyme, intravenous vincristine, 1 mg. per week plus oral prednisone 1 mg. per kg. per day
  b. Nonlymphoid cells, negative for tdt, cytarabine, 0.5 mg. per kg. intravenously 6 times daily for 5 days, plus thioguanine, 0.5 mg. per kg. intravenously 6 times a day for 5 days, plus daunorubicin (investigational), 1 mg. per kg. intravenously on 1st day. Repeat in 2 to 3 weeks
  c. Experimental, total body radiation followed by cryopreserved pre-blast buffy coat or marrow, with or without splenectomy/chemotherapy.

NON-HODGKIN LYMPHOMA*

method of
RICHARD A. GAMS, M.D.
Birmingham, Alabama

Introduction

The non-Hodgkin lymphomas represent a heterogeneous group of lymphoid malignancies with diverse histologic appearance, prognosis, and response to therapy. Much of our current approach to these disorders remains experimental, and controversy exists in their diagnosis, staging, and management. In this discussion I will attempt to provide a rational and acceptable way to deal with the lymphomas which, while reflecting our current knowledge in the area, may differ substantially from the recommendations of others in the field.

---

*It is recommended that the administration of drugs listed here be under the supervision of a qualified physician experienced in their use. The manufacturer's official directive should be consulted for current dosage recommendations and other pertinent information before prescribing.

*Some of the agents or treatment methods mentioned in this article are investigational. Before using any of the drugs mentioned, the physician should be well informed of their actions and of the information in the manufacturer's official directive.

Pathology

Before the introduction of effective therapy for non-Hodgkin lymphoma the terms lymphosarcoma, reticulum cell sarcoma, and giant follicular lymphoma were widely used. It is now clear that these terms are of little practical benefit in predicting the behavior of these disorders. In 1956 Rappaport introduced the classification shown in Table 1, which remains the system with most clinical relevance. In general terms, lymphomas with a nodular pattern have a much better prognosis than those with a diffuse pattern, and lymphocytic proliferation has a better outlook than histiocytic. Unfortunately, current progress in our understanding of the immunobiology of lymphocytes has pointed out some serious pathophysiologic defects in this classification system. It is now recognized that nodular lymphomas in fact represent the proliferation of B lymphocytes originating in lymph node follicles. Furthermore, those cells previously classified as histiocytes in effect represent a stage in lymphocyte differentiation and many of them also are B lymphocytes. A number of new classification systems have been introduced based on this understanding, which employs surface markers and morphologic appearance to arrive at a more accurate pathophysiologic classification. Clinical relevance of these newer systems, however, remains to be determined, and for the present the system of Rappaport, notwithstanding the deficiencies noted, remains the most relevant.

Unfortunately, the use of any histologic classification continues to require the opinion of an experienced hematopathologist. Experience in the Southwest Oncology Group and the Southeastern Cancer Study Group has indicated a high frequency of disagreement in the classification of lymphomas between community and university pathologists and an experienced lymphoma review panel. Fortunately, these disagreements are largely in the subclassification of lymphocyte types and the recognition of nodular vs. diffuse lymphoma is generally understood. A final difficulty has been the recognition of more than one histologic type in the same patient and even in the same lymph node. It is my feeling that the presence of nodularity in any part of a lymph node carries with it a favorable prognosis although the final answer on this question is certainly not in.

As can be seen from Table 1, the marked difference in the behavior of nodular and diffuse lymphomas necessitates an adequate biopsy for initial diagnosis and the opinion of an experienced hematopathologist if any question exists. For the purposes of this discussion we will divide the lymphomas into favorable and unfavorable categories. Favorable categories include: all the nodular lymphomas except nodular histiocytic and in addition the diffuse lymphocytic, well-differentiated lymphoma. All the other histologic classifications are considered unfavorable histologic types.

Staging

The importance of accurate clinical staging in the non-Hodgkin lymphomas is uncertain. There has been an unfortunate tendency to utilize the Ann Arbor staging system, which is currently useful in Hodgkin's disease, for the non-Hodgkin lymphomas. In contrast to Hodgkin's disease, however, the non-Hodgkin lymphomas are most often disseminated, and the presence of extranodal involvement in bone marrow, liver, gastrointestinal tract, and so on does not necessarily carry with it an ominous prognosis. The only circumstance in which accurate staging appears to be important is in defining the very rare occurrence of truly localized disease. Such local disease occurs most frequently in the histiocytic lymphomas and there is some evidence that true Stage I disease may be curable by local radiation therapy. Such localized disease is often extranodal and frequently occurs in bone, gastrointestinal tract, or nasopharynx. One might argue that in such circumstances meticulous staging up to and including exploratory laparotomy might be indicated to define true Stage I disease. On the other hand, other than in diffuse histiocytic lymphoma, we shall see that systemic therapy offers little hope for

TABLE 1. The Non-Hodgkin Lymphomas*

| | NODULAR | | | | DIFFUSE | | |
Abbreviation	Relative Incidence	Median Survival	CELL TYPE	Abbreviation	Relative Incidence	Median Survival
—	—	—	Undifferentiated	DU	4%	0.6 yr.
NH	7%	3.0 yrs.	Histiocytic	DH	28%	1.1 yrs.
NM	19%	7.5 yrs.	Mixed histiocytic and lymphocytic	DM	10%	1.5 yrs.
NLPD	18%	7.5 yrs.	Lymphocytic, poorly differentiated	DLPD	10%	1.8 yrs.
NLWD	1%	>7.5 yrs.	Lymphocytic, well differentiated	DLWD	3%	>7.5 yrs.

*Adapted from Jones, S. E.: JAMA 284:683, 1975.

a cure. Even in the diffuse histiocytic histology there is little evidence that prompt and early therapy is beneficial. In consequence, I have taken the approach that meticulous staging in the non-Hodgkin lymphomas is probably important only for investigational purposes in order to obtain a true assessment of the influence of therapy in large groups of patients. Thus, unless a patient is to be included in a randomized prospective study evaluating various treatment programs, I would consider the following schema of staging adequate in most instances.

A complete history and physical examination will frequently reveal the presence of disseminated disease, as reflected by diffuse lymphadenopathy or splenomegaly or both. Because of the frequent occurrence of bone marrow involvement, particularly in the lymphocytic lymphomas, two needle biopsies of the bone marrow from opposite iliac crests are taken at the time of the initial visit and often reveal bone marrow involvement. In our own hands, gallium scanning and B mode ultrasonography have largely replaced lymphangiography and exploratory laparotomy to demonstrate abdominal lymph node enlargement. Finally, the new technique of whole body computerized tomography shows considerable promise in evaluating the presence of subdiaphragmatic involvement with lymphoma.

Since I am satisfied that anything other than truly localized lymphoma will require systemic therapy, it is clear that the demonstration of lymphoma in more than two sites would preclude the necessity for further staging evaluation. If there is apparent Stage I disease, I see no objection to treating that area with local radiation therapy and withholding systemic therapy until such time as systemic disease becomes manifest.

A final word needs to be said concerning systematic restaging of patients following completion of a course of therapy. Again, for the purposes of a randomized control trial evaluating various forms of management, it is clear that an accurate knowledge of the degree of response will be necessary for a final analysis of the results. It is my feeling, however, that for the routine management of patients with non-Hodgkin lymphoma there is little evidence that systematic restaging is required.

Although the measurement of immunologic parameters may be interesting from an experimental point of view, at the moment it has little impact on therapy and consequently is not recommended on a routine basis.

Therapy

The brilliant success of extended field radiation therapy in Hodgkin's disease has led to its intensive investigation as a treatment modality in the non-Hodgkin lymphomas. Current evidence would suggest, however, that radiation therapy has limited application in these disorders.

As mentioned earlier, there is some evidence that patients with truly localized disease are potentially curable utilizing involved field radiation treatment. As mentioned earlier, localized disease occurs infrequently and usually in histiocytic lymphomas. Furthermore, the ability to control localized disease with radiation is variable, some of the lymphomas being remarkably sensitive to even small doses of radiation and others being resistant even to extremely high doses. Nevertheless, an attempt should certainly be made to utilize intensive local irradiation in localized disease.

In patients with other than localized disease there has been interest in total nodal irradiation, total nodal irradiation plus total abdominal irradiation, and finally, total body irradiation. In my opinion, total nodal approaches have shown little benefit in the management of the disseminated non-Hodgkin lymphoma and are not indicated in routine practice. Total body irradiation utilizing low doses appears to be relatively nontoxic and may have some indication for palliation of patients resistant to chemotherapy. Nevertheless, my general opinion is that any form of radiation therapy for other than localized disease remains an experimental approach and should not be used in the primary management of these patients.

Management of Patients with Favorable Histologies (NM, NLPD, NLWD, DLWD)

The management of patients with favorable histology non-Hodgkin lymphoma remains controversial. Advocates of intensive combination chemotherapy or even combined modality therapy using various forms of irradiation with combinations of drugs claim higher remission rates and longer survivals for these modalities. Most workers in the field, however, agree that intensive therapy confers no survival benefit and may in fact shorten survival due to the adverse effects of the toxicity of the therapy. My personal approach to the management of these patients is to avoid therapy when possible. Many of these patients show little progression of their disease and may be considered in an indolent phase of a chronic disorder. Should therapy be required due to progression of disease, discomfort caused by enlarged lymph nodes or even perhaps extreme concern on the part of the patient, then minimal therapy is most often useful. My own approach is to use the alkylating agent, chlorambucil, in much the same way that one might treat chronic lymphatic leukemia. Although chlorambucil is usually administered as a daily oral dose, experience in our Cooperative Study Group has indicated that high dose intermittent chlorambucil may be preferable. After starting the patient on allopurinol, 300 mg. daily, to prevent urate nephropathy, the patient is treated with chlorambucil in a single dose of 20 mg. per square meter of body surface, repeated every 2 weeks. (This dosage is not listed in the manufacturer's official directive.) The minimal gastrointestinal toxicity associated with this single high dose can be avoided by asking the patient to take the tablets at night just before retiring. The dose is usually escalated on alternate courses in increments of approximately 4 mg. per square meter until dose limiting toxicity, usually myelosuppression, is reached. At such time as the white count falls below 4000 or the platelet count below 100,000, the dose should be reduced to a previously tolerable level. The proper duration for this therapy is uncertain; it is my practice to maintain patients for at least 2 years before discontinuing the medication. The allopurinol may be discontinued at such time as the disease has stabilized and no further shrinkage of the lymphadenopathy is occurring.

Some patients will prove resistant to this therapy or, after an initial period of response, may show progressive disease. At this time it is often recommended that a more intensive combination of drugs be used such as that outlined for the non-Hodgkin lymphomas with unfavorable histology. Although it is true that this may at times induce a response in patients with resistant or progressive disease, my own experience in this situation has been disappointing. It is under these circumstances that one might consider total body irradiation for palliation. Such treatment should be administered only by a radiation therapist with experience in this technique.

Management of Patients with Unfavorable Histologies (NH, DU, DH, DM, DLPD)

Patients with these histologic types have a much poorer prognosis than patients with favorable histologies and require more intensive management. There seems little question that survival in patients with unfavorable non-Hodgkin lymphoma is improved if there is a response to therapy. In only one histologic category however, DH, have unmaintained remissions been sufficiently long to suggest that some patients may be cured. In all other histologies, survival curves show a relentless decline, suggesting that cure has not been obtained despite the most vigorous therapy.

The uncertainty in the field is reflected by the proliferation of chemotherapeutic modalities including combinations with the exotic acronyms of COP, HOP, CHOP, BCOP, BACOP, COMA, etc., most of which are variations on the theme of combining alkylating agents, vinca alkaloids, nitrosoureas, antimetabolites, and adrenal steroids.

Although not an absolute certainty, it would seem that the traditional combination of cyclophosphamide (Cytoxan), vincristine, and prednisone (COP) is probably insufficient therapy in this unfavorable group of non-Hodgkin lymphomas. In choosing among the various potential combinations, current evidence would indicate that one including the anthracycline antibiotic doxorubicin hydrochloride (Adriamycin) may be the most beneficial to the largest number of patients with unfavorable histologic categories. Consequently, I will outline one regimen, CHOP, that should be acceptable for the management of most of these patients. Although the addition of bleomycin to this regimen enjoyed a recent vogue as in CHOP-Bleo or BACOP (bleomycin, doxorubicin [Adriamycin], cyclophosphamide [Cytoxan], vincristine, prednisone), my current feeling is that bleomycin adds considerable risk of pulmonary toxicity with little benefit of additional remission or survival.

As in the favorable category of lymphoma, a patient should be started on allopurinol, 300 mg. daily, to avoid urate nephropathy. My own formula for CHOP consists of cyclophosphamide (Cytoxan), 600 mg. per square meter, doxorubicin (Adriamycin), 60 mg. per square meter, and vincristine, 2 mg., all administered intravenously on the first day of therapy. The patient then starts prednisone, 100 mg. daily by mouth, for 5 days. The entire cycle is repeated every 21 days. It should be noted that an adequate bone marrow biopsy is an important part of the staging of these patients, as we have found severe bone marrow depression to occur if full doses of these drugs are used in the face of bone marrow involvement with lymphoma. Should bone marrow involvement be present we usually start with doses of cyclophosphamide (Cytoxan) and doxorubicin (Adriamycin) at a level of 50 per cent of those recommended above, with a gradual escalation of doses toward the 100 per cent level should bone marrow toxicity not occur. A complete blood count (CBC) should be done weekly after the first course of therapy to determine the nadirs of the white count and platelet counts. If the nadir of the absolute granulocyte count is less than 750 per cu. mm. or the platelets less than 75,000 per cu. mm. the doses of cyclophosphamide (Cytoxan) and doxorubicin (Adriamycin) should be reduced to 50 per cent at the next course of therapy. At the time the next course of therapy is due, should the absolute granulocyte count be less than 1500 per cu. mm. or platelets less than 100,000, per cu. mm., therapy should be delayed until bone marrow recovery occurs. If peripheral neuropathy such as severe constipation, foot drop, or disabling paresthesias occurs, vincristine should be eliminated. It might be wise to start all drugs at half dose in patients over the age of 65 because of reduced bone marrow reserve and increased sensitivity to vinca alkaloids in this age group. Additional toxicities that may be expected include alopecia, nausea and vomiting, and potential hemorrhagic cystitis from cyclophosphamide. The alopecia and gastrointestinal effects are, unfortunately, unavoidable. Hemorrhagic cystitis may be prevented by cautioning the patient to ingest large amounts of fluid for 24 hours after therapy.

The proper duration of therapy with these agents remains uncertain. Current practice is to treat patients at 3-weekly intervals for a total of 6 months or 8 cycles of therapy at which time treatment is discontinued but may be reinstituted at the first sign of relapse. It should be noted that the maximum permissible total dose of doxorubicin (Adriamycin) is probably 450 mg. per square meter when it is given in combination with cyclophosphamide (Cytoxan). Although this dose will not be exceeded if treatment is confined to a total of 6 months, the total dose should be recorded if further therapy is necessary. Irreversible cardiac toxicity has occurred at total doses of doxorubicin higher than 450 mg. per square meter when this agent has been used in conjunction with cyclophosphamide or following mediastinal irradiation.

These comments should be considered only in the context of non-Hodgkin lymphoma in adults. Children with these disorders have a high incidence of T cell lymphoma which has a more ominous prognosis, behaves differently, and might more suitably be treated in a manner similar to the treatment of acute lymphoblastic leukemia in childhood. As the disorder is uncommon in children, every effort should be made to refer these patients to an experienced pediatric oncologist or to a specialized treatment center.

The manner in which I have described my approach to non-Hodgkin lymphomas should indicate that I consider our understanding of the treatment of these disorders totally unsatisfactory. I cannot emphasize strongly enough that what I have outlined are only general considerations and that, if at all possible, consultation with a hematologist/oncologist experienced in the management of non-Hodgkin lymphoma would be useful in almost every instance.

Although the outlook for patients who respond to the various forms of management mentioned has improved, the situation is much less satisfactory for the majority of patients who are either refractory to treatment at the outset or relapse and show disease progression after an initial favorable response. It is hoped that our recommendations for management will become more definitive and more optimistic in future years.

MYCOSIS FUNGOIDES AND THE SEZARY SYNDROME

method of
PAUL A. BUNN, JR., M.D.,
and BETTY FISCHMANN, M.D.
Washington, District of Columbia

Mycosis fungoides (MF) and the Sezary syndrome comprise a spectrum of distinct malignant lymphomas for which the term "cutaneous T-cell lymphomas" has been proposed. These disorders are characterized by an atypical lymphocyte ("mycosis cell," "Sezary cell"), which has the light microscopic appearance of an atypical hyperchromatic lymphocyte with a convoluted nucleus. The nucleus has a distinctive cerebriform appearance under the electron microscope. These cells have the membrane characteristics of thymus-derived lymphocytes (T cells) and may exhibit functional properties of normal T cells, including production of migration inhibitory factor (MIF) and the ability to function as "helper" and "suppressor" lymphocytes. Originally, mycosis fungoides was divided into three skin stages: (1) premycotic or eczematoid stage, (2) plaque stage, and (3) tumor or ulcer stage. Later, an erythrodermic variant and a d'emblee tumor variant without antecedent plaque stage were recognized. The Sezary syndrome consists of the generalized erythrodermic form of MF with an abundance of atypical peripheral blood lymphocytes.

The clinical course of progression is frequently indolent, and signs of a chronic cutaneous disorder often have been present for many years. Early skin stages can be confused clinically and histologically with other chronic conditions. Thus, in the past, advanced stages of disease were often present by the time a diagnosis of mycosis fungoides was made. Consequently, therapy with corticosteroids, localized radiation, or topical drug administration, used for palliative purposes over the past several decades, had no effect on survival. Recent studies have suggested that more intensive therapy might prolong survival in some patients and lead to long-term disease-free survival in patients with early skin lesions. This had made early diagnosis increasingly important, and it is mandatory that the histologic material be reviewed by pathologists or dermatopathologists experienced with this problem. Since multimodality therapy is often required, the close collaboration of oncologists, hematologists, dermatologists and radiotherapists is necessary for optimal management. Because this disease is relatively uncommon and requires considerable collaborative efforts, several cooperative groups including the Mycosis Fungoides Cooperative Group and the National Cancer Institute are conducting clinical trials. Referral of patients to these trials will provide answers to questions of early diagnosis, staging, natural history, and therapy.

Staging

Histologic confirmation of disease must be obtained in all patients. This often requires multiple skin or lymph node biopsies. In patients with generalized erythroderma, classic "mycosis" cells may be identified more easily in peripheral blood smears and lymph node biopsies than in skin biopsies.

Age, absolute lymphocyte count, and extent of disease are proven prognostic variables. Functional immune status is under investigation. Extent of disease is the most important variable. Advanced skin stage, palpable lymphadenopathy and visceral involvement are associated with shortening in survival. Consequently, the routine staging procedures provided in Table 1 should be performed for determining prognosis and therapy.

Abnormal parameters should be repeated to determine response to therapy. Investigational procedures whose usefulness for prognostication has not been established are also included in the Table.

In difficult cases there are several useful diagnostic adjuncts, also included in Table 1. Electron micrographs demonstrating clusters of cells with the ultrastructural properties of "mycosis" cells in the skin, blood, or lymph nodes are highly suggestive of MF. Similarly, the demonstration that the atypical peripheral blood or lymph node cells have T cell surface markers is suggestive of MF. Histochemical staining with acid phosphatase (with or without tartrate) and β-glucuronidase may also demonstrate the T cell nature of these atypical lymphocytes. Cytogenetic studies of peripheral blood, lymph node, or bone marrow cells have revealed abnormalities in all patients studied to date, although there has been no single consistent abnormality.

There is no uniform staging classification such as the Ann Arbor Classification of Hodgkins Disease. A TNM system has been adopted by the Mycosis Fungoides Cooperative Group. A simple staging system used at the National Cancer Institute is shown in Table 2.

Therapy

Several forms of therapy, including radiation, topical chemotherapy, systemic chemotherapy, ultraviolet (UV) light, and immunotherapy, have been used or are investigational. The advantage and disadvantages of each will be discussed and followed by alternatives for each stage.

Topical Chemotherapy. 1. Topical nitrogen mustard (HN_2). A 10 mg. vial of nitrogen mustard is diluted into 50 to 60 ml. of tap water. (The topical use of nitrogen mustard is not mentioned in the manufacturer's official directive.) After a cleansing bath the patient applies the solution over the entire body surface using gloves to protect the hands from excessive exposure. Daily treatment is

TABLE 1. **Staging Procedures**

Routine

1. Complete history and physical examination (photographs)
2. CBC and platelet count. Detailed examination of peripheral blood smear for the presence of atypical lymphocytes
3. Liver and renal function tests, other serum chemistries
4. Chest x-ray
5. Liver spleen scan
6. Lymphangiogram

Biopsies

7. Skin (multiple if necessary)
8. Lymph node if palpable
9. Liver
10. Bone marrow

Investigational

11. Blind lymph node biopsy
12. Peritoneoscopy with directed liver biopsies
13. Staging laparotomy

Useful Adjuncts

A. Electron microscopy
B. Membrane markers of atypical lymphocytes
C. Histochemical stains
D. Cytogenetics

TABLE 2. **Staging System for Cutaneous T Cell Lymphomas**

Stage 1:	Premycotic lesions or plaques over less than 10 per cent of the body surface
Stage 2:	Plaques or erythroderma over more than 10 per cent of the body surface
Stage 3:	Cutaneous tumors or ulcers
Stage 4:	Lymphadenopathy and/or peripheral blood involvement with any skin stage
	A. Histologic appearance of dermatopathic lymphadenopathy on lymph node biopsy
	B. Histologic replacement of lymph nodes with mycosis cells
Stage 5:	Visceral involvement with any skin stage

continued until the skin is completely clear, which may take weeks to months. Therapy may be continued less frequently for at least 1 to 2 years if complete clearing occurs. The principal advantages of this therapy include the absence of systemic toxicity and the accessibility of this form of treatment to all patients. However, the therapy is inconvenient, and long periods of administration are required. In addition, more than a third of patients develop cutaneous delayed hypersensitivity reactions. In some patients this hypersensitivity may be overcome by patch testing with dilute solutions (10^{-2} to 10^{-8}) of HN_2 and continuing treatment with the highest tolerated drug concentration. Intravenous desensitization has not been uniformly successful.

2. Other topical therapies. Topical corticosteroid creams are often useful for relief of pruritus and are occasionally associated with objective tumor response. Topical 5-fluorouracil and carmustine (BCNU) frequently produce objective remissions but the duration is generally short and skin toxicity may limit the duration of therapy. (This use of these agents is not listed in the manufacturer's official directive.)

Radiation Therapy. 1. Kilovoltage (100 to 140 KeV) therapy to local lesions provides effective palliation for large tumors and ulcers in the majority of instances. However, only limited areas of the body can be treated because of the risks of systemic toxicity.

2. Electron beam radiation can be applied over the entire body surface with minimal systemic toxicity. To achieve a uniform dose distribution over the entire body surface, a 6-field or a rotating table technique is utilized. Total dose, fractionation schedules, and electron energy vary between centers. This therapy should be delivered by a center experienced with the technical difficulties involved to avoid under- or overtreatment and excessive cutaneous toxicity. We give 400 rads weekly using 3.2 MeV electrons and a rotating table dual field technique to a total dose of 2400 rads. Complete remissions can be achieved in at least 60 per cent of patients. Long-term disease-free survival has been reported in a significant minority of patients with early skin lesions. The advantages of this therapy are that it may lead to long-term disease-free remission, does not require maintenance therapy, and has limited systemic toxicity. The disadvantage is the expense, the radiation damage to the normal skin, and the limited number of centers capable of delivering this form of radiation.

Systemic Chemotherapy. Significant response rates are produced by a large number of chemotherapeutic agents, listed in Table 3. Unfortunately, with single agent chemotherapy there have been few complete responses, the duration of response has generally been short, and prolongation of survival has not been shown. The two most commonly used drugs are nitrogen mustard and methotrexate.

1. Nitrogen mustard can be given with conventional doses of 0.1 mg. per kg. intravenously for 4 days every 4 to 6 weeks or as a 2 mg. intravenous push or intravenous infusion daily for 14 days every 2 to 4 weeks.

2. Methotrexate can be given orally, intramuscularly, or intravenously. An intermittent weekly schedule of 30 mg. per square meter is as effective as other schedules. High dose methotrexate (240 to 2000 mg. per square meter) given intravenously over 6 hours and followed in 6 hours by leucovorin rescue (15 mg. per square meter every 6 hours for 3 days) and repeated at 5 day to 3 week intervals also gives high response rates. This therapy is experimental and should be given only in centers experienced with its use. It has not been proved superior to conventional doses.

Limited information on the effectiveness of combination chemotherapy is available (Table 3). High dose intermittent administration of combinations of cyclophosphamide, vincristine, and prednisone (COP) alone or with doxorubicin (Adriamycin) (CHOP) or bleomycin (COP-Bleo) have received the largest trials. Complete remissions appear to be more frequent with drug combinations than with single agents and the remission duration may be longer. Other drug combinations with lower doses given more frequently are under investigation and are also provided in Table 3.

Experimental Therapy. 1. PUVA (psoralen and long wave ultraviolet A Light). Oral 8-methoxypsoralen followed in 2 hours by graded longwave ultraviolet A light causes regression of skin lesions in many patients. The effect of this treatment on the natural history of MF is unknown and it should be given only on an experimental basis in centers studying its effectiveness.

2. Antithymocyte Globulin (ATG). Anecdotal reports of benefit in patients with the Sezary syndrome have been published. This form of therapy is also experimental and should be performed only in centers with experimental protocols. Multiple courses of ATG are limited by sensitization to animal protein.

3. Leukaphoresis. Leukaphoresis has provided temporary palliation in a few patients with high count Sezary syndrome. This process is still experimental and should be reserved for pa-

TABLE 3. **Systemic Therapy**

DRUG	DOSAGE AND ROUTE OF ADMINISTRATION	RESPONSE RATE (%)	RESPONSE DURATION
Single Agents			
HN_2	0.1 mg./kg. I.V. qd × 4 q 4–6 weeks	60–100	1–5 + months
	2 mg. I.V. qd × 14 q 2–4 weeks	60–100	1–12+ months
Methotrexate	30 mg./m.^{2} I.V. weekly	~80	4–20+ months
	240 mg./m.^{2} I.V. with CF q 5 days to q 3 weeks (4 cycles then maintenance)	100	6–30+ months
Cyclophosphamide	75 mg. p.o. daily	60–100	1–14+ months
	50 mg./m.^{2} I.V. q 3 weeks		
Chlorambucil	0.1–0.2 mg./kg. p.o. daily	25–70	—
Adriamycin	60 mg./m.^{2} I.V. q 3 weeks	85	3–10+ months
Bleomycin	15–20 units I.M. biweekly	50–60	1–8+ months
Vinblastine	5–10 mg. I.V. weekly	70	1–11+ months
Combination Chemotherapy			
COP or COP-Bleo			
Cyclophosphamide	200 mg./m.^{2} p.o. day 1–5		
Vincristine	1.4 mg./m.^{2} I.V. day 1		
Prednisone	60 mg./m.^{2} p.o. day 1–5	Repeated in 3 week cycles — 92	11 months
±Bleomycin	10 units/m.^{2} I.V. day 1		
CHOP			
Cyclophosphamide	500 mg./m.^{2} I.V. day 1		
Adriamycin	40 mg./m.^{2} I.V. day 1	Repeated in 3 week cycles — 91	11 months
Vincristine	1.4 mg./m.^{2} I.V. day 1		
Prednisone	60 mg./m.^{2} p.o. day 1–5		
CP*			
Chlorambucil	2–6 mg. p.o. daily	60	—
Prednisone	10–20 mg. p.o. daily		
VAB-CMP†			
Vinblastine	4 mg./m.^{2} I.V. weekly		
Adriamycin	10 mg./m.^{2} weekly		
Bleomycin	5 units/m.^{2} weekly		
Cyclophosphamide	50 mg./m.^{2} p.o. days 1–14	Repeated in 3 week cycles	
Methotrexate	10 mg./m.^{2} p.o. biweekly		
Prednisone	50 mg./m.^{2} p.o. days 1–7	—	—

*Used primarily with the Sezary syndrome
†Regimen VAB given for 9 weeks, alternating every 9 weeks with 3 week cycles of CMP.

tients with the Sezary syndrome with white blood counts of more than 20,000 cells per cu. mm.

Recommended therapeutic options for each stage are included below:

1. Stage I and II (Table 2): (a) electron beam irradiation, (b) topical HN_2, (c) electron beam plus topical HN_2, and (d) electron beam plus intravenous HN_2.

Many patients have long-term disease-free remissions after electron beam radiation alone. Patients may relapse because of the inability to treat uniformly all the cutaneous areas or because of extracutaneous disease. We have elected to combine 3 two-week courses of intravenous HN_2 with electron beam in an attempt to increase the frequency of long-term disease-free control. Topical HN_2 is used for patients who do not achieve complete remission or who relapse in cutaneous sites alone.

2. Stage III, IV, V (Table 2): (a) systemic chemotherapy alone, (b) topical HN_2 and systemic chemotherapy, and (c) electron beam and systemic chemotherapy.

Both topical HN_2 and electron beam allow for tumor reduction and symptomatic relief without systemic toxicity, and we feel they should be combined with systemic chemotherapy. We believe that simultaneous electron beam radiation and systemic combination chemotherapy is currently the optimal therapy for these stages. Our chemotherapy regimen (VAB-CMP) is provided in Table 3. The VAB combination is given simultaneously with electron beam radiation.

The pessimistic attitude that therapy for these disorders is only palliative has been replaced by an optimistic hope that thorough staging and restaging techniques with combined modality therapy may lead to long-term disease-free survival (? cure) in many patients and prolonged symptom-free survival in the remainder.

MULTIPLE MYELOMA

method of
ROBERT A. KYLE, M.D.
Rochester, Minnesota

If myeloma is suspected, the patient should have—in addition to a complete history and physical examination—determinations of hemoglobin or hematocrit; leukocyte, differential, and platelet counts; measurements of serum creatinine, calcium, phosphorus, alkaline phosphatase, and uric acid; roentgenographic survey of bones (bone scans with ^{99m}Tc are inferior to conventional x-rays), serum protein electrophoresis (including immunoelectrophoresis); quantitation of immunoglobulins and tests for cryoglobulins and viscosity; bone marrow aspiration and biopsy; routine urinalysis; and electrophoresis and immunoelectrophoresis of an adequately concentrated 24-hour urine specimen.

Minimal criteria for diagnosis include a bone marrow specimen that contains more than 10 per cent abnormal, immature, and atypical plasma cells and at least one of the following: monoclonal (M) protein in the serum, M protein in the urine, or osteolytic lesions. Because marrow involvement may be focal rather than diffuse, repeated bone marrow aspirations may be necessary. Connective tissue diseases, chronic infections, carcinoma, lymphoma, and leukemia should be excluded unless other features make the diagnosis of multiple myeloma clear. One must also exclude benign monoclonal gammopathy (monoclonal gammopathy of undetermined significance), which is characterized by an M serum protein less than 3 grams per dl. (100 ml.), normal serum albumin, fewer than 5 per cent marrow plasma cells, absence of anemia, osteolytic bone lesions, and absence or minimal amounts of M protein in the urine—and no change through at least 5 years of observation. It should be emphasized that all clinical and laboratory features must be considered before the diagnosis of multiple myeloma is made. Most patients who fulfill these diagnostic criteria have symptoms or findings that require therapy. Some, however, have low-grade or smoldering myeloma, and these should not be treated but must be reexamined at 3 to 6 month intervals. If clinical and laboratory examinations show no progression of the disease, continued observation with repeated evaluation is indicated.

Therapy of Special Problems

Hypercalcemia. Hypercalcemia occurs in one third of patients with myeloma and must be suspected in the presence of anorexia, nausea, vomiting, polyuria, increased constipation, weakness, confusion, stupor, or coma. Hypercalcemia often leads to renal insufficiency, so prompt treatment is essential. Because dehydration frequently accompanies hypercalcemia, the patient should be hydrated. Isotonic saline solution is the agent of choice, as sodium promotes renal excretion of calcium. The addition of furosemide (Lasix), 40 mg. every 4 to 8 hours, may be beneficial. During diuretic therapy the electrolytes must be monitored closely. With hydration, we recommend prednisone, in an initial dose of 100 mg. daily. This must be reduced after a few days and discontinued as quickly as possible. Hydrocortisone sodium succinate (Solu-Cortef) or methylprednisolone sodium succinate (Solu-Medrol) in equivalent doses may be used if the patient is comatose. Inorganic phosphate (Neutra-Phos) may be given with prednisone but must be avoided when hyperphosphatemia and renal insufficiency are present. I prescribe 150 ml. orally 4 times daily (2.0 grams of phosphorus).

If the patient is comatose, the inorganic phosphate solution can be given by a gastric tube or rectally. If the patient is comatose and critically ill, inorganic phosphate may be given intravenously, slowly and cautiously. If these measures fail, mithramycin should be given intravenously in a dose of 25 micrograms per kg. body weight. It produces its effect within 24 to 48 hours, but hypercalcemia often recurs after 2 to 3 days. (See manufacturer's official directive before using mithramycin.) Thrombocytopenia may follow, so depression of bone marrow function is a relative contraindication to the use of mithramycin. Prolonged bed rest often contributes to hypercalcemia, so patients with myeloma should be encouraged to be as active as possible.

Renal Insufficiency. More than 50 per cent of patients with myeloma eventually develop renal insufficiency, and it is one of the major causes of death. Hypercalcemia, protein casts in the proximal and distal tubules (myeloma kidney), hyperuricemia, deposition of amyloid, pyelonephritis, and infiltration of the kidney with plasma cells may have a part in causing the renal insufficiency. If hyperuricemia occurs, allopurinol, 300 mg. daily, provides effective therapy. If this cannot be given because of hypersensitization (allergy), alkalinization of the urine with sodium bicarbonate or an oral citrate mixture (Polycitra) is helpful. Intravenous pyelography can precipitate renal insufficiency, but it can be performed with little danger if dehydration is avoided. Dehydration should be avoided also in preparing the patient for a barium enema. Acute renal failure must be recognized and treated promptly. It it does not respond to conservative measures, peritoneal dialysis or hemodialysis should be tried. Many patients will recover adequate renal function. Long-term hemodialysis has been used successfully, but this is subject to availability and other local circumstances.

Infections. Bacterial infections are more common in myeloma than in the normal population. Their frequency is related to a deficiency of normal immunoglobulins, impairment of antibody response, reduction of delayed hypersensitivity, and, in some instances, depression of reticuloendothelial function and reduction of the numbers and activity of neutrophils. Significant fever is an indication for appropriate cultures, roentgenography, and consideration of antibiotic therapy. The selection of antibiotics can be made more specific once the results of the cultures are known. Injection of gamma globulin for prevention of infections has been of no value. Occasionally, in cases of recurrent, severe gram-positive bacterial infections, we have used penicillin prophylactically with good results. Employment of gentamicin in multiple myeloma must be carefully monitored because marked decrease of renal function may occur. Pneumococcal vaccine may be beneficial for preventing pneumococcal infection.

Anemia. Anemia occurs eventually in almost every case of myeloma and may be severe. The anemia of myeloma is due mainly to inadequate production of red cells by the bone marrow, but mild shortening of red-cell survival, iron deficiency, and extravascular loss of blood also may have significant influence. Increase of plasma volume from the osmotic effect of the monoclonal protein may produce hypervolemia and lower the hemoglobin or hematocrit concentration. Thus, significant anemia may be indicated by the hemoglobin value when the red cell mass is only slightly reduced. Transfusions with packed red cells remain the cornerstone of therapy, but successful treatment of the primary disease may restore erythropoiesis. A hemoglobin level of 8 to 10 grams per dl. is adequate unless there is significant coronary artery disease or cerebrovascular insufficiency. Androgens such as fluoxymesterone (Halotestin),* 10 mg. three times daily, or testosterone enanthate (Delatestryl),* 400 mg. intramuscularly every 4 weeks, or oxymetholone (Anadrol-50), 50 mg. three times daily, may be helpful.

Skeletal Lesions. These constitute a major problem. Although bone lesions are reported to heal with chemotherapy, we have been disappointed in this regard. Frequently, a brace or supporting garment is helpful, but avoidance of trauma is more important because even mild stress may result in multiple fractures. Nevertheless, the patient should be encouraged to be as active as possible because confinement to bed increases demineralization of the skeleton. Analgesics should be given to control pain so the patient can be ambulatory. Physical therapy may also be beneficial. Fixation of long-bone fractures with an intramedullary rod and methacrylate has given

very satisfactory results in our experience. The combination of sodium fluoride, 50 mg. twice daily with meals (investigational), and calcium carbonate, 1 gram four times daily 1 hour after meals, increases bone formation and appears to be a useful adjunct in treatment of myeloma bone disease.

Hyperviscosity Syndrome. The symptoms may include oronasal bleeding, decrease of visual acuity, neurologic symptoms, or congestive heart failure. Most patients have symptoms when the relative serum viscosity reaches 6 or 7, but the relation between serum viscosity and clinical manifestations is not precise. Although this syndrome occurs more commonly in macroglobulinemia, it may also be associated with either IgG or IgA myeloma, especially if the IgA monoclonal protein is polymerized. Plasmapheresis should be vigorous and can best be accomplished with a Haemonetics blood processor or an NCI-IBM continuous-flow blood cell separator, which can remove 6 liters of plasma daily. If these instruments are not available, removal of 2 units of plasma daily by phlebotomy for 7 to 10 days is also helpful. The results of plasmapheresis alone are usually transient, but concomitant treatment with alkylating agents contributes to long-term benefit.

Specific Therapy

Chemotherapy. Chemotherapy is the best initial treatment for generalized myeloma, unless there is disabling pain that is clearly the result of a well-defined focal process. If analgesics together with chemotherapy can control the pain, chemotherapy is preferred to repeated local irradiation because the bone marrow reserve of many patients is limited and irradiation does not benefit systemic disease.

The most effective chemotherapeutic agent is melphalan (L-phenylalanine mustard, L-sarcolysine [Alkeran]). We prefer to give it intermittently because such administration seems to achieve as much benefit as is obtained with daily use, and it requires fewer blood counts and patient visits for monitoring of its effects. We give 0.15 mg. per kg. orally each day for 7 days at 6 week intervals. The addition of prednisone in a dosage of 15 mg. four times daily for the same 7 day period increases the favorable response to approximately 70 per cent of cases. When prednisone is being given, the patient should follow a bland diet and take antacids. Leukocyte and platelet counts should be made at 3 week and 6 week intervals after the initial course of therapy. If the counts have not decreased, the daily dose of melphalan may be increased by 2 mg. daily for the next 7 day course; if the counts have decreased, the dose of melphalan should be lessened accordingly. In the presence of renal insufficiency the dosage of mel-

---

*This use of these agents is not mentioned in the manufacturer's official directive.

phalan should be modestly reduced (approximately 25 per cent). The dose of prednisone rarely needs to be reduced. In a few patients abrupt cessation of prednisone is associated with weakness, fatigue, and generalized aching, and in those cases we taper the prednisone dosage to zero over 3 to 4 days.

The major side effects of melphalan include leukopenia and thrombocytopenia. Nausea, vomiting, pruritus, and skin rash are seldom significant problems. Although acute leukemia has occurred in some patients treated with melphalan, the benefit of the drug outweighs this risk and does not constitute a contraindication to chemotherapy. At least three 7 day courses should be given before the melphalan and prednisone program is abandoned, unless therapy causes significant toxic reactions or the disease progresses rapidly despite clearly adequate therapy. Maximal improvement may not be achieved for several months.

Combinations of melphalan, cyclophosphamide (Cytoxan), carmustine (BiCNU), and prednisone have been reported to produce impressive results, but in a prospective randomized study we found this combination not superior to melphalan with prednisone except in patients with increased risk or high tumor-cell mass. Toxicity was greater in patients receiving the combination of alkylating agent drugs. Survival was essentially the same in both groups of patients.

How long to continue chemotherapy after response is controversial. Some recommend cessation of chemotherapy after 1 year if the patient has had a satisfactory response. We do not advise this, and I continue to treat patients for 5 years because most patients relapse and not all respond again to the chemotherapy.

If there is no response to melphalan, or if the patient becomes resistant after responding, one may give cyclophosphamide intravenously in a dose of 15 mg. per kg. every 4 weeks or in a daily oral dose of 2 mg. per kg. for long periods. The leukocyte and platelet counts should be performed every 2 weeks and the dosage should be modified in accordance with the results. Occasionally, hemorrhagic cystitis or alopecia develops in a patient who is taking cyclophosphamide, and long-term treatment with cyclophosphamide may produce interstitial fibrosis of the bladder or lung or damage to the ovaries or testes.

We have used the following combinations of drugs with some benefit for patients who have developed resistance to melphalan:

1. Doxorubicin (Adriamycin), 30 mg. per square meter of body surface and cyclophosphamide, 400 mg. per square meter, both given intravenously every 3 weeks, plus prednisone, 0.6 mg. per kg. daily for the first 7 days of each cycle.

2. Doxorubicin (Adriamycin), 30 mg. per square meter, and prednisone, 0.6 mg. per kg. daily, for 7 days every 3 weeks; plus carmustine (BiCNU), 75 mg. per square meter every 6 weeks.

Criteria for response to therapy include: (1) increase of hemoglobin by 2.0 grams per dl. from an initial value of <11.0 gram per dl.—without transfusion; (2) decrease of monoclonal serum protein by 50 per cent or more; (3) decrease of monoclonal urinary globulin by at least 50 per cent if initial value was 1.0 gram per 24 hours or more; (4) decrease of number of plasma cells in bone marrow by 50 per cent or more in repeated marrow specimens; (5) recalcification of skeletal lesions and absence of new osseous lesions. Response to therapy is not influenced significantly by the type of heavy or light polypeptide chain.

Irradiation. X-ray treatment is not effective as the only therapy, because multiple myeloma is a generalized disease. Irradiation should not be used unless pain is severe and localized. Palliative radiation in a dosage of 2,000 to 2,500 rads is usually effective. Although radiation therapy relieves pain in most instances, the patient frequently returns in a short time with pain at another site. Although irradiation may be repeated, it ultimately is limited by the development of leukopenia or thrombocytopenia, which in turn restricts the use of chemotherapy. If radiation therapy is given, it is advisable to complete the palliative therapy 3 weeks before starting chemotherapy. Leukocyte and platelet counts should be repeated before the start of chemotherapy, because the myelosuppressive effects of radiation therapy and chemotherapy are cumulative. Thus, irradiation in multiple myeloma is adjunctive and limited; and it should be used only for "focal lesions."

Treatment of Variant Forms of Myeloma

Solitary Plasmacytoma (Solitary Myeloma of Bone). Solitary plasmacytoma may remain solitary, but in most instances widespread multiple myeloma develops. The diagnosis depends upon histologic evidence of a plasma-cell tumor and the absence of other bone lesions; the bone marrow aspirate must contain no evidence of multiple myeloma; immunoelectrophoresis of serum and urine should show no monoclonal protein persisting after adequate radiation therapy; and no other abnormalities should develop during observation. Treatment for solitary plasmacytoma consists of irradiation in the range of 4000 to 5000 rads. There is no evidence that surgical removal of a plasmacytoma is superior to adequate irradiation.

Extramedullary Plasmacytomas. These are plasma cell tumors that occur outside the bone marrow. The upper respiratory tract—including the nasal cavity and sinuses, nasopharynx, and larynx—is the most frequent location of such lesions. Epistaxis, rhinorrhea, and nasal obstruction are the most common symptoms. Extramedullary plasmacytomas usually spread locally but may develop into widespread multiple myeloma. As in solitary plasmacytoma, a tumoricidal dose of 4000 rads is the most satisfactory treatment for localized disease.

For any patient with myeloma who states that his legs are weak or who has difficulty in voiding or defecating, the possibility of extradural myeloma and spinal cord compression must be considered. Neurosurgical consultation is urgently needed, and myelography is essential. Radiation therapy in a dosage of approximately 3000 rads is usually beneficial. If the neurologic deficit progresses during radiation, one must proceed with surgical decompression followed by radiation therapy.

Plasma Cell Leukemia. Increase of plasma cells in the peripheral blood (more than 20 per cent and more than 2,000 per cu. mm.) characterizes plasma cell leukemia, which should be considered a phase of multiple myeloma and not a separate entity. Treatment is usually unsatisfactory, but melphalan, cyclophosphamide, and prednisone have produced impressive temporary benefit.

Psychologic Factors

Any patient with a serious disease such as multiple myeloma has psychologic problems and needs substantial, continuing emotional support. The approach must be positive. The physician must have confidence in his ability to cope with the patient's problems, and the patient should be able to sense this confidence. Potential benefits of therapy should be emphasized. It reassures the patient to know that some persons survive for 5 or more years while receiving treatment. It is vital that the physicians caring for myeloma patients have the interest and capacity to deal with incurable disease over a span of months to years with assurance, sympathy, and resourcefulness.

POLYCYTHEMIA VERA*

method of
ALEKSANDER WEINFELD, M.D.
Göteborg, Sweden

Polycythemia vera is a chronic disease characterized by an abnormal proliferation of all hematopoietic bone marrow elements for which no cause is known. This uncontrolled panmyelosis causes an absolute increase of the red cell mass with increased blood viscosity in all patients and in most of them a variable degree of thrombocytosis and leukocytosis. Hematopoiesis is also reactivated in extramedullary sites such as liver and spleen. The polycythemic state is dominated by symptoms caused by plethora and to a lesser degree, thrombocytosis or splenomegaly or both. This erythrocytotic state may last for more than 20 years and, if properly managed, the survival of these patients does not differ much from that of the normal population. The disease progresses from the erythrocytotic state into a "spent phase" associated with myelofibrosis and myeloid metaplasia, and this evolution is independent of the therapeutic management of the disease. About 10 per cent of patients terminate with the picture of acute leukemia but this occurs almost exclusively in those patients who obtained myelosuppressive therapy.

Treatment of polycythemia vera is aimed at decreasing the circulating red cell volume to normal and, when indicated, to reduce the platelet and leukocyte count and the spleen size towards normal ranges. The normalization of the red cell volume can be accomplished by phlebotomies alone; the normalization of the remainder requires myelosuppressive treatment.

Treatment*

General Remarks. Before treatment is applied, the diagnosis of polycythemia vera must be assessed by rigid criteria and differentiated from pseudopolycythemia and secondary polycythemia according to the outlines given by the Polycythemia Vera Study Group (PVSG).

There is no treatment of choice applicable to all categories of patients. Phlebotomy, radiation, and alkylating agents all have their characteristic advantages and drawbacks and fit best for certain clinical situations. The optimal treatment of polycythemia vera must therefore be based on the individual characteristics of the disease and the patient as a whole.

Most of the complications, morbidity, and causes of deaths during the state of uncontrolled polycythemia vera are due to increased red cell volume, which causes vascular distention and increased viscosity, giving rise to complications such as hemorrhage, thrombosis with embolism, and most of the other symptoms associated with the plethora. It is therefore imperative to reduce the red cell volume and blood viscosity as soon as the diagnosis of absolute polycythemia is confirmed by red cell volume determination with the chromium-51 dilution technique. Phlebotomy is the only way by which blood viscosity can be reduced quickly. The need to lower the hematocrit

*Supported by grant from the Swedish Cancer Society (77:158)

*The use of certain drugs in this article is considered investigational in the United States. See manufacturer's official directive before use.

towards a normal level should be looked upon as a semiemergency measure. In some patients with symptoms of an imminent cerebrovascular catastrophe, phlebotomy is a real emergency. Consequently, the initial treatment of patients in all categories of polycythemia vera is repeated phlebotomy until a hematocrit level of 42 to 47 per cent is achieved. Thereafter, the patient should be controlled at 4 to 6 week intervals and the rate of the rise of the hematocrit observed. It is our policy to treat all new polycythemia vera patients during the first 6 to 12 months with phlebotomies alone, provided that no contraindications for such treatment are present.

Following the initial series of phlebotomies, the degree of the erythroid activity should be judged by the observation of the rate of the hematocrit rise and by the frequency of phlebotomies required in order to keep the hematocrit within normal limits. Other symptoms associated with a high platelet number or a massive enlargement of the spleen but not caused by increased viscosity might be assessed during this period of observation. The age and the particular characteristics of the polycythemia vera disease, as well as an acquaintance with the rest of the patient's symptomatology will be decisive for the choice of therapy to be applied in the individual patient.

It should be noted that the main symptoms of the erythrocytotic phase of polycythemia vera are circulatory in nature and that this disease, which is usually confined to older persons, is often accompanied by other diseases affecting circulation such as hypertension, heart disease, and general arteriosclerosis. Treatment of polycythemia vera must therefore embrace the whole of the patient and should preferably be controlled by a specialist in internal medicine with hematologic training.

Management with Phlebotomy

The primary goal of therapy is reduction of the increased red cell mass and maintenance of a venous hematocrit in a range of 42 to 47 per cent. This can be quickly accomplished by repeated phlebotomies of 300 to 500 ml., which can initially be performed every second or third day until the hematocrit has dropped below 47 per cent. In the elderly patient and in those with circulatory failure, who tolerate less well rapid hemodynamic changes, it is preferable to remove smaller amounts of blood (200 to 300 ml.) at intervals of 3 to 4 days. Usually there is no need to replace the removed blood by plasma or a plasma substitute in order to get an immediate decrease of the hematocrit level. It is, however, important to maintain an adequate fluid balance in patients undergoing frequent bloodletting and intake of fluids before and after the venesections must be encouraged to ensure expansion of plasma volume. In the majority of patients the series of initial phlebotomies is performed in the out-patient clinic. In elderly and disabled patients it is preferable to have them hospitalized.

In exceptional patients who have very severe plethora and an imminent risk of a vascular complication, normalization of the blood volume and blood viscosity might be an emergency problem. In such patients, depending on the initial hematocrit level, 1 to 2 liters of blood can be exchanged by the following technique. After an intravenous injection of 5000 units of heparin a venous tourniquet is applied and blood is taken from one arm. Plasma or dextran 70 (in isotonic saline or glucose solution) is given into the other arm in an amount corresponding to half the quantity of the blood removed. When necessary, the procedure may be repeated on following days. There is, however, seldom need for these drastic measures in polycythemia vera. This technique is the method of choice in the case of a surgical emergency in a patient with a high hematocrit.

Phlebotomies should be done by a skilled staff and is preferably performed at a blood bank unit. In patients with excessively high hematocrits the mechanics of withdrawing the blood may be difficult. Large bore needles are recommended, and attention should be paid to atraumatic venipunctures. In some instances it might be necessary to administer 5000 to 10,000 units of heparin intravenously in order to avoid coagulation. Because of the vascular distention and high blood viscosity, there is a risk for either prolonged bleeding or thrombophlebitis at the site of the venipuncture. These complications may be avoided by meticulous atraumatic management and perfect hemostasis with application of a pressure bandage. It is of prime importance to preserve the arm veins of the polycythemic patient, as it probably will be necessary to perform phlebotomies many times during the course of this chronic disease.

This initial phlebotomy program aimed at normalizing quickly the red cell volume and the hematocrit to the levels recommended for all patient categories, has been practiced by the PVSG in 500 patients with negligible occurrence of thromboembolic complications. A transient modest rise in the platelet count may occur but is without clinical significance.

Upon completion of the initial phlebotomies and with a stable hematocrit level below 47 per cent, the patient should be seen 4 to 6 weeks later for assessment of symptoms and blood values. After observation for some time, the rate of the hematocrit rise can be assessed and the physician will be able to order phlebotomies in advance and in this way avoid undesirable hematocrit peaks between the visits. Patients with active disease usually need a phlebotomy of 400 ml. every 4 to 6 weeks. The patient must be instructed to avoid medicines containing iron. In some instances it is necessary to forbid the intake of food with high iron content, such as liver. If a good contact is established between doctor and patient, and provided no symptoms from the cardiovascular system are present, 2 phlebotomies with appropriate intervals may be ordered in advance at the time of the visit. A new visit and laboratory control should be arranged 4 weeks after the last phlebotomy. I am accustomed to seeing the patient treated with phlebotomy every 2 or 3 months. In some patients with indolent disease when no more than 2 or 3 phlebotomies a year are required, the interval of the visits may be lengthened. At the time of the visit a complete physical examination should be done, with particular emphasis on assessment of the spleen and liver size. A venous hematocrit and a complete peripheral blood count are routine at every visit. Occasionally, serum uric acid, creatinine, and liver tests may be performed. It is of interest to measure the red cell mass again when the hematocrit is normal, but this is not necessary from the practical point of view. Patients with major splenomegaly often have an increased plasma volume and thereby may mask an increased red cell mass in spite of a normal venous hematocrit. In such patients the hematocrit level should be kept at a somewhat lower level.

Bone marrow histology with respect to cellularity and fibrosis should be assessed every 2 years and whenever indicated. It is also of interest to assess the size of the spleen by scintigraphy or flatplate x-ray at similar intervals.

Advantages and Drawbacks of Treatment with Phlebotomy Alone. Phlebotomy is the quickest way to reduce the red cell mass to normal and to alleviate all symptoms due to plethora and increased blood viscosity. Even hypermetabolic symptoms and the pruritus are most often ameliorated or relieved. The potential toxicity of radiation and alkylating agents is avoided, but the most important advantage of all is that the risks of transition into acute leukemia are small in phlebotomy-treated patients as compared with those treated with myelosuppression.

Phlebotomy, however, is useful only in treating the end product of erythroid proliferation. It has no suppressive effect on the proliferative process and the panmyelosis. Phlebotomy will not control thrombocytosis, leukocytosis, hyperuricemia, or progressive and painful splenomegaly. The principle of phlebotomy is based on the induction of iron deficiency. Hemoglobin production is curtailed, but red cell prolif-

eration continues with the resulting development of hypochromic microcytic polycythemia. The characteristic picture is that of a normal hematocrit with a red cell count of 6 to 8 million per cu. mm. and a hemoglobin level below normal. Some of these patients get symptoms of anorexia, weight loss, and asthenia, and in some patients, symptoms of impending senility and cerebral disorientation have been observed. These symptoms are said to be reversible by iron administration. Patients who do not require phlebotomies for a very long time and develop an anemia might erroneously be regarded as spent polycythemia. In fact, they might appear to have active polycythemia masked by iron deficiency and caused by decreased absorption of food iron. In some instances the polycythemia is unmasked first when parenteral iron is administered. Progressive splenomegaly and a painful spleen with hypermetabolic symptoms leading to cachexia is another important drawback that might occur after many years of successful therapy with phlebotomy alone. In such instances phlebotomy should be combined with temporary treatment with alkylating agents. The same is true if the patient has symptomatic thrombocytosis.

In summary, phlebotomy as a treatment modality is used initially in all patients; it is the only treatment available for emergency situations and may be used as the sole treatment in an appreciable number of patients during the entire course of the disease and when necessary can be combined with myelosuppressive treatment. The patient of choice for phlebotomy treatment alone will be discussed later.

Myelosuppressive Therapy

Myelosuppressive therapy provides efficient control of the panmyelosis in the bone marrow and of the hematopoietic proliferation at extramedullary sites. The objective of treatment is to maintain a normal blood volume and viscosity, a normal platelet count, and to achieve a shrinkage of hepatosplenomegaly when indicated.

Radiation or drugs are the two types of myelosuppressive treatment frequently used. The period of induction with either of these methods may extend over 1 to 3 months until the desired effect is achieved. During this time the hematocrit level should be controlled with phlebotomy. Because of the relative long life span of the red cell the myelosuppressive effect is noticed earlier in the peripheral blood by a fall of the leukocyte and platelet counts. It should be pointed out, however, that it is generally easier to achieve a suppression of the granulocytic and platelet precursors as compared to the erythrocytic series with either of the myelosuppressive methods used. There are patients with active polycythemia in whom suppression of erythropoietic activity can hardly be achieved with doses that are not severely toxic for the granulocytes and platelets. As the patient has usually undergone a series of phlebotomies before myelosuppressive therapy is given, it may be difficult to assess whether erythropoietic suppression has taken place or if the hematocrit level remains within the normal limits because of severe iron depletion. This should be tested by administration of iron salts and subsequent control of the venous hematocrit. Iron should not be administered earlier than 6 weeks after the start of myelosuppressive therapy, however, or at the time when the physician feels that suppression of erythropoiesis has taken place. Otherwise, there is a risk of a sudden rise of the hematocrit and of thrombohemorrhagic complications. If iron is administered, the patient should have a laboratory control with a 2 week interval. I have found it valuable to control the serum iron before and during the myelosuppressive therapy for the assessment of erythropoietic activity. The serum iron is usually extremely low after the initial phlebotomies and prior to therapy. A spontaneous rise of the serum iron during therapy indicates that erythropoiesis is suppressed.

The physician must clearly realize his objective in giving myelosuppressive agents; whether this is for erythrocytosis, a high platelet count, or an enlarged spleen. He should also delineate whether he aims to obtain complete normalization or whether amelioration of the status will be satisfactory. Finally, and no less important, he must determine whether or not he achieves the intended purpose. There is no justification for continued myelosuppressive therapy that does not give the desired result. Neither is there justification for giving more therapy than necessary if the objective delineated by the physician is fulfilled. Normalization of a platelet count might, for instance, require less therapy than the normalization of the red cell mass, which can be managed by phlebotomy. Less therapy might be necessary for lowering the platelet count below 1 million per cu. mm. if that is the objective, than for a complete normalization of the platelet count. This must be borne in mind with regard to the potential leukemogenic effects of myelosuppressive therapy.

There is no general agreement whether alkylating agents or radioactive phosphorus is the best treatment if myelosuppression is chosen as the mode of therapy. The preliminary data of the Polycythemia Vera Study Group favor radioactive phosphorus favor ^{32}P, and this is also my opinion if we consider an unselected sample of patients.

However, in the individual patient, and especially if myelosuppressive therapy is to be combined with phlebotomy, both alternatives may have advantages for a given situation.

Radiation. Radioactive phosphorus has been extensively used for more than 30 years and is the current choice for radiation myelosuppression. ^{32}P can be administered orally or intravenously. Because of variations in absorption, it is recommended that it be given intravenously. The dose recommended by the Polycythemia Vera Study Group for initial treatment is 2.3 millicuries (mCi) per square meter of body surface intravenously. The first dose should not exceed 5 mCi. If the oral route of administration is chosen, the dose should be increased by 25 to 50 per cent. The blood count is monitored at 4 week intervals. If no significant spontaneous fall of the hematocrit occurred after treatment, the suppression of erythropoietic activity should be assessed by an iron administration trial as delineated earlier, even though the hematocrit remained within normal limits. If a remission is not achieved after 3 months, the administration of ^{32}P is repeated with an increase of the dosage by 25 per cent. Should the patient be refractory, a third and fourth dose may be administered with a 25 per cent increment of the last dose, each with no less than 3 month intervals. No dose should exceed 7 mCi. If the patient does not respond to four doses of ^{32}P, no more ^{32}P should be given. It is preferable not to give more than 15 to 18 mCi and a maximum of 28 mCi during a 12 months treatment period. ^{32}P therapy should not be repeated whenever the white blood count (WBC) is less than 4000 per cu. mm. or the platelet count is less than 150,000 per cu. mm.

Radiophosphorus is easy to administer and gives good control of the disease with long-lasting remissions in about 80 per cent of patients. Bone marrow hypoplasia and dangerous leukopenia or thrombocytopenia are rarely produced. ^{32}P therapy is predictable and reliable and is at present the most convenient form of therapy because of the long intervals between treatments and fewer visits to the physician.

The drawback of radiation therapy is the development of acute leukemia, which occurs in 10 to 15 per cent of patients treated with ^{32}P. There is no consensus about whether there is a relationship between the total dosage of ^{32}P and the incidence of leukemia, but at least two large series of patients show such a relationship. Radiation therapy is therefore not advisable in younger patients and is contraindicated in women in the reproductive age group. When it has been decided to treat the erythrocytosis with myelosuppression alone, it is our preference to do it with ^{32}P because of its many advantages and patient convenience. The risk of developing acute leukemia is not lessened when the patient is maintained with alkylating agents. Patients with massive and huge spleens who respond less well to ^{32}P, patients with short lasting remissions (less than 6 months), and those who require very high doses of ^{32}P should be given an alternative therapy.

Drug Treatment. A number of alkylating agents have been used in the treatment of polycythemia vera. Busulfan, dibromomannitol, chlorambucil, melphalan, cyclophosphamide, and pipobroman all produce remissions and provide an efficient control of the symptoms and signs caused by panmyelosis. These drugs are particularly effective in bringing about shrinkage of a massively enlarged spleen. The most commonly used compounds are busulfan, chlorambucil, and melphalan. The Polycythemia Vera Study Group has used the latter two drugs. Cytotoxic drug therapy requires more frequent visits and blood counts than ^{32}P therapy and is impracticable in patients who cannot be relied upon to take the proper dose of the prescribed medication. The hope that treatment with alkylating agents will not be complicated by acute leukemia has not been fulfilled. A comparison of the leukemogenic affects of ^{32}P and alkylating agents has not as yet been possible, as the latter drugs were introduced much later than ^{32}P. The randomized study of the PVSG cannot, as yet, give a definite answer to this question. There are, however, more cases of acute leukemia in the chlorambucil group than in the ^{32}P group. Furthermore, the period from the start of chlorambucil therapy to the development of leukemia appears to be shorter than that previously reported for ^{32}P. This is in accordance with our experience. The advantage of alkylating agents over ^{32}P is that the dosage and length of therapy can be maneuvered at the deliberation of the physician. Chemotherapy might therefore be more suitable for short periods of treatment, for instance, to lower the platelet count below a dangerous level or to diminish a painful spleen. This flexibility makes drug therapy more convenient when it is used sporadically as an adjuvant to basic treatment with phlebotomy. The possibility of teratogenesis and the mutagenic properties of alkylating agents makes therapy with these compounds contraindicated in pregnancy and not advisable for young patients. The risks of infertility in males must also be considered.

Busulfan. Dependent on the initial white blood cell (WBC) and platelet count and the size of the patient, therapy is started with a daily dose of 4 to 6 mg. taken in the morning on an empty stomach. The blood count must be controlled weekly and the initial dose reduced by about 50 per cent when the WBC and platelet count de-

crease. The drug should be discontinued when the WBC falls to 3000 per cu. mm. (see manufacturer's official directive) and the platelet count to below 150,000 per cu. mm. When suppression of erythropoiesis is achieved, the drug is withdrawn and no maintenance given. Remissions induced with busulfan are gratifying because they may last for many months or for several years without maintenance therapy. Some patients may show an exaggerated sensitivity to the drug, however, and develop a long-standing leukopenia and thrombocytopenia. In rare patients marrow hypoplasia may take place.

Because of these untoward effects the use of busulfan has been relegated to a minor role by some physicians. It has also been suggested that myelofibrosis might develop with greater frequency in busulfan-treated patients. With careful management, however, busulfan has its place as a good therapeutic agent, mostly because of the long-lasting remissions it produces without the necessity of maintenance.

Chlorambucil. Treatment is initiated during the induction period with 10 mg. a day and administered in the fasting state. (This use of chlorambucil is not listed in the manufacturer's official directive.) The patient is initially seen at 3 week intervals and the dosage may be reduced by 2 to 4 mg. per day if the WBC is less than 5000 per cu. mm. or the platelet count is less than 150,000 per cu. mm. Therapy is discontinued if the WBC falls below 3000 per cu. mm., the platelet count below 100,000 per cu. mm. or the venous hematocrit falls below 42 per cent. Supplementary phlebotomy is performed if the hematocrit rises above 47 per cent. If suppression of erythropoiesis is not achieved after 6 weeks and toxicity is not present, the chlorambucil dose might be increased by 2 mg. Further increase in dose may be allowed in refractory cases after an additional 3 weeks. When the hematocrit is stable in the normal range for 8 weeks without supplementary phlebotomy, maintenance therapy is started with a dose of 5 to 10 mg. per day for 1 month, every other month. Some refractory patients may require continuous therapy. Sensitive patients, however, may get a long-lasting remission after short-term therapy. The suppression of erythropoiesis should be assessed by iron administration. A sudden drop in the blood counts during therapy may be caused by toxicity but may also herald the transformation into acute leukemia. This schedule has been extensively used by the PVSG. A hematocrit response was achieved in more than 90 per cent of patients and the median time until hematocrit response was 13 to 15 weeks. Although the observed toxicity was mild and reversible, it must be realized that such a regimen scheduled for both remission induction and maintenance in patients with long life expectancy will require a tremendous consumption of many kilograms of drug and too many visits to the physician. This regimen is, according to our experience, inferior to ^{32}P treatment. However, short periods of treatment with chlorambucil for thrombocytosis or a massive enlargement of the spleen, or both, in combination with phlebotomy is more realistic.

MELPHALAN.   This drug was extensively used by the PVSG and other workers. Treatment is initiated with 6 to 8 mg. per day in one fasting dose for 7 days and continued with 2 to 4 mg. daily until control of the hematocrit and platelet count is achieved. (This use of melphalan is not listed in the manufacturer's official directive.) An efficacy trial performed by the PVSG has shown that hematocrit response is obtained in 93 per cent of the patients and that the median for the time required to get this response is 8 to 9 weeks. Bone marrow toxicity is somewhat more frequent than with chlorambucil, but is reversible and without harm to the patient if adequately controlled. The difference in toxicity between the two drugs does not seem to have clinical significance. Melphalan reduces the platelet count quickly and is especially suitable for thrombocytotic patients. When the platelet count is brought down to a desired level, the drug may be withdrawn for some time or a maintenance dose of 2 to 6 mg. a week may be necessary. Patients with refractory disease that requires larger doses are encountered. I prefer melphalan over chlorambucil because of its faster action and comparable toxicity, which in practice means fewer days on the drug. Patients refractory to chlorambucil may respond to melphalan. Melphalan seems to be as good as chlorambucil to bring about a shrinkage of the spleen.

CYCLOPHOSPHAMIDE.   Cyclophosphamide, in daily doses of 75 to 100 mg. and administered intermittently for maintenance, can be effective and may particularly be used if the platelet count is rather low. (This use of cyclophosphamide is not listed in the manufacturer's official directive.) The side effects of alopecia and hemorrhagic cystitis, however, make the drug less acceptable for the management of polycythemia vera.

OTHER DRUGS (investigational).   There is an urgent need for an effective noncarcinogenic and nonmutagenic drug for treatment of polycythemia vera. The PVSG, which is currently looking for such potential drugs, has now started an efficacy protocol with hydroxyurea since several studies have failed to find evidence for carcinogenicity and mutagenicity. In my preliminary experience hydroxyurea, given in a dose of 1.0 gram twice a day for 1 week and thereafter 0.5 gram twice daily, will lower a platelet count of about 1 million or more towards normal within 2 to 3 weeks. The drug is also highly effective in bringing about a prompt shrinkage of the spleen. Without maintenance therapy the platelet count however tends to rise again very soon. For depression of erythropoiesis, a longer treatment will be required and the time of unmaintained remission seems to be shorter than for alkylating agents. The place of hydroxyurea in the treatment of polycythemia vera and the myeloproliferative syndrome requires further evaluation and we must await the results of the initiated PVSG study.

The Treatment "of Choice" for the Individual Patient

The guidelines given here are only my firm feelings based on the present incomplete knowledge of many aspects of the disease and on personal experience in treating polycythemia vera patients with phlebotomy alone, on one hand, and with myelosuppressive drugs for remission and maintenance, on the other. None of these forms of therapy is completely satisfactory. However, during the first 5 to 10 years of the erythrocytotic disease in the younger or middle-aged subject there is no great difference in terms of wellbeing whether he is treated with phlebotomy or myelosuppression. Even if some differences exist, they are not significant enough to motivate an early loading with myelosuppressive treatment. This is of particular importance nowadays, when patients with early asymptomatic disease come to our attention by medical monitoring. Some of these patients could live for 5 years or more without knowledge of their disease and I feel it is wrong to give to such patients myelosuppression of any kind. However, after many years of phlebotomy treatment, the disease may change character and the patient may urgently need and get benefit from myelosuppression. It is, therefore, my policy to postpone myelosuppressive treatment to a period when the patient will really need it.

The decision for the choice of therapy is dependent on the age, cooperability, distance from a medical center, and life expectancy with regard to associated diseases. Of the specific characteristics of the disease, the most important for the treatment decision are the presence of severe thrombocytosis (>1 million), thrombocytosis with symptoms of clinical significance, and symptomatic splenomegaly with hypermetabolic disturbances not alleviated by normalization of the red cell volume. The age limits given below are arbitrary; the biologic age of the patient is of more importance.

1. The Case for Phlebotomy Alone.   Indolent disease, unclassified erythrocytosis, patients below the age of 60 years with a good life expectancy and without the association of cardiovascular disease, provided symptomatic thrombocytosis, severe thrombocytosis (>1 million), or symptomatic splenomegaly is not present.

2. The Case for ^{32}P. Elderly patients and patients with cardiovascular insufficiency, patients with poor life expectancy, and patients who do not want to be treated with phlebotomies. Patients above 40 years of age living at a long distance from a medical center, provided they respond to ^{32}P treatment with prolonged remissions. Women in child-bearing age should be excluded from ^{32}P therapy. Patients with very huge spleens are better treated with myelosuppressive drugs.

3. The Case for Myelosuppressive Drug Therapy in Combination with Phlebotomy. Patients who, in spite of a good control of the red cell volume with phlebotomy, have symptoms caused by thrombocytosis. Patients with asymptomatic thrombocytosis but with an excessive high platelet count (above 1 million). Patients presenting initially with very huge spleens and those who during the course of phlebotomy treatment develop symptomatic splenomegaly. To all these categories of patients, temporary myelosuppressive drug treatment should be given for alleviation of symptoms, decrease of the platelet count below a dangerous level in asymptomatic patients, and for a decrease of the spleen to an acceptable size. The hematocrit level should be controlled basically by phlebotomy. In this way drug therapy can be reduced and given periodically when indicated.

Management of Complications

Thrombosis and Hemorrhage. Thromboembolic complications are managed with anticoagulants in the same way as in nonpolycythemic patients. Because of the increased danger of hemorrhage in patients with polycythemia vera, chronic treatment with coumarin anticoagulants should be used with caution and must be monitored carefully. In emergency bleeding situations fresh blood for transfusion should be used. According to laboratory tests, the platelets are functionally deficient in polycythemia vera and benefit has been reported from platelet transfusion. It should be reemphasized that for prevention of thrombohemorrhagic phenomena the control of the red cell volume and blood viscosity is most important.

SURGERY. Emergency surgery should, whenever possible, be preceded by a rapid reduction of the hematocrit towards normal with phlebotomy and exchange infusion of an appropriate amount of plasma or plasma substitute as described earlier. In nonemergency cases surgery should be performed when the patient's red cell volume has been under good control for a longer time. If marked thrombocytosis is present a course of myelosuppressive treatment should be given. Tests for disseminated intravascular coagulation should be taken before surgery and monitored postoperatively.

SYMPTOMS SPECIFIC FOR THROMBOCYTOSIS. 1. Pain in the fingertips, toes, pad, and margin of the foot may be severe and is often, but not always, associated with a ruddy discoloration of the affected area. This symptom occurs in patients with thrombocytosis and is not influenced by treatment with phlebotomy but disappears after reduction of the platelet count with the aid of myelosuppression. One dose of 0.3 to 0.5 gram of aspirin will bring about a prompt and complete relief of symptoms lasting for 2 to 5 days. It is probable that the symptom is caused by platelet aggregation and that the antiaggregating capacity of acetylsalicylic acid has a specific effect. This symptom should be distinguished from the paresthesias and erythromelalgia, which are ameliorated by reduction of the red cell volume with phlebotomy alone.

2. Painful subcutaneous, pea-sized infiltrations that dissolve after 1 to 2 days with a rainbow discoloration of the skin. This rather rare symptom occurs only in patients with thrombocytosis and is not relieved by phlebotomy treatment. It is not known whether aspirin has any effect, but with reduction of the platelet count these infiltrations disappear. It is possible that even here platelet aggregation with secondary extravasation is the primary cause.

Cutaneous Manifestations. The skin becomes red, warm, slightly swollen and tender. The involved area is of the size of a palm, but may embrace the whole lower extremity. In some cases the patient may be feverish. These manifestations are often misinterpreted as erysipelas, thrombophlebitis, thrombosis, or gouty arthritis when confined to the joint but usually disappear spontaneously after a few days. Rest and small doses of acetylsalicylic acid may be helpful. These manifestations occur in 10 to 15 per cent of our patients with longstanding disease and varies widely with respect to intensity and recurrency (once a year or every month). During myelosuppressive treatment this symptom is more rarely encountered.

Hyperuricemia. Allopurinol, 100 to 300 mg. per day, normalizes the serum uric acid level and is commonly given to patients with hyperuricemia for prevention of urate nephropathy. The indications for therapy in asymptomatic patients are cloudy, but side effects of allopurinol administration are very rare. After myelosuppressive treatment the serum uric acid becomes normal and allopurinol should be discontinued. Those patients who, after myelosuppression, have persistently elevated values of uric acid are either taking diuretics, have a renal insufficiency or a latent primary gout.

Pruritus. This symptom occurs with varying severity in about 40 per cent of patients and is most pronounced during the plethoric state. Reduction of the blood volume by phlebotomy alone results in amelioration or disappearance of symptoms in only a part of the patients. Patients maintained with myelosuppression have fewer symptoms. Treatment with a variety of antihistaminic drugs has given marginal results. Their effect seems to be more sedative than specific. Cyproheptadine (Periactin), 4 mg., two to four times per day, may be tried. It should be recognized also that factors other than polycythemia vera may be the cause of general itching.

Transition into Myelofibrosis with Myeloid Metaplasia (the Spent Phase). About 10 to 15 per cent of patients with polycythemia vera develop a clinical picture characterized by bone marrow failure with anemia and a massive enlargement of the spleen with myeloid metaplasia. The anemia may be associated with thrombocytopenia, thrombocytosis, leukocytosis, or leukopenia. The growing spleen may become space-encroaching and painful and is often associated with hypermetabolic symptoms, asthenia and cachexia.

ANEMIA. Iron, folate, and B_{12} deficiency must be excluded as a cause. The red cell volume should be assessed, since splenomegaly is associated with an increased plasma volume, which may mask a normal or even increased red cell volume. The anemia may be due to decreased production or increased destruction or both. If hemolysis and trapping of red cells in the enlarged spleen is the dominating cause of anemia, treatment with prednisone in combination with cautious administration of melphalan or busulfan may be indicated. Such treatment will also bring about a shrinkage of the spleen. Stimulation of erythropoiesis with moderate doses of androgens may be tried if necessary, provided that the continuous growth of the spleen can be balanced by simultaneous administration of small amounts of alkylating substances.

THROMBOCYTOPENIA. The cause should be assessed in the same way as for red cells. Thrombocytopenia in the spent phase is more often caused by a deviation of platelets to an increased exchangeable splenic platelet pool than to a decreased production. The huge spleen may conceal 80 to 90 per cent of body platelets. The destruction of platelets is also moderately increased. Treatment with alkylating agents to decrease the size of the spleen might be dangerous because of the concomitant decrease of platelet production. If the thrombocytopenia is moderate, a very cautious use of these agents together with prednisone may be tried by the experienced physician. Severe thrombocytopenia might be an indication for splenectomy. An evaluation of platelet production and the splenic platelet pool size should be done before a decision is made. Splenectomy may also be indicated if the large spleen is the major cause of anemia, especially if drug therapy is unsatisfactory or causes undesirable side effects. An eventual dangerous thrombocytosis that may develop after splenectomy must be balanced with myelosuppressive drugs. The decision for doing a splenectomy in patients with postpolycythemic myelofibrosis with myeloid metaplasia requires laboratory work-up and good hematologic and clinical judgment. When performed on good premises it is gratifying.

Acute Leukemia. Acute leukemia occurs in about 10 per cent of patients treated with myelosuppression. The treatment is the same as if the patient did not previously have polycythemia. Although the leukemia is myelomonocytic in type, complete remissions have been achieved in very few patients with the combination of vincristine-prednisone, according to a schedule used for lymphoblastic leukemia. If no result is obtained after the second injection of vincristine, no further treatment of this kind should be given. If aggressive antileukemic treatment is not desirable, moderate doses of prednisone may give some palliation and diminish the number of blood transfusions needed.

PORPHYRIA

method of
D. MONTGOMERY BISSELL, M.D.
San Francisco, California

As knowledge of the biochemistry of heme synthesis and porphyria has expanded during the past decade, so has therapy of this group of diseases. To an ever-increasing extent, management of porphyria is specific for each individual type. Thus, implicit in any discussion of therapy is the assumption that the patient's condition has been fully investigated with determination of the specific type of porphyria involved. The essentials of porphyria typing will be reviewed briefly here; several detailed reviews are available.

Porphyrins are derived from porphyrinogens, which are intermediates of heme synthesis (Table 1). Small amounts of these compounds normally appear in the circulation and undergo excretion into urine or bile. Defects in the heme pathway, localized to a specific enzyme, may partially block the flow of heme precursors, which then spill over into the circulation in abnormally large amounts. A pathologic increase in the excretion of heme precursors in urine or feces is termed *porphyria*. Clinically, the most important porphyrias are those due to the presence of a *hereditary* abnormality of the heme synthetic pathway. Several types of hereditary porphyria have been described: each represents a discrete enzymatic defect, and four involve predominantly the liver (AIP, PCT, HCP, and VP*). Erythrohepatic protoporphyria (EPP) appears to involve both liver and bone marrow. Finally, a type involving the bone marrow only, congenital erythropoietic porphyria, is extremely rare and will not be discussed here. The biochemical characteristics of the hereditary porphyrias are shown in Table 1. From this group, secondary (or acquired) porphyria must be differentiated. The latter involves variable elevation of delta-amino levulinic acid (ALA), uroporphyrin (URO), or coproporphyrin (COPRO), with normal porphobilinogen (PBG), and is seen in persons with heavy metal intoxication, liver disease, and occasionally other causes. The porphyrinuria per se rarely is associated with symptoms, and therapy should be directed at the underlying cause of porphyrin overproduction.

The symptom complexes associated with the hereditary porphyrias are listed in Table 2. Neurologic attacks are characteristic of the heme-deficient porphyrias (AIP, HCP, and VP),

comprising a spectrum of abnormalities from tachycardia and abdominal pain to psychosis and quadriplegia. Cutaneous photosensitivity is due directly to increased circulating porphyrins (but *not* porphyrin precursors), occurs on light-exposed skin, and is the only significant clinical problem associated with most cases of porphyria cutanea tarda (PCT) and erythrohepatic protoporphyria (EPP). Cutaneous findings are exhibited by 20 to 30 per cent of persons with hereditary coproporphyria (HCP) and 80 per cent with variegate porphyria (VP), although in these types the cutaneous manifestations are secondary in importance to the neurologic symptoms. Persons with acute intermittent porphyria (AIP), overproducing ALA and PBG only, do not exhibit cutaneous photosensitivity.

The pathogenesis of symptoms in the hereditary porphyrias is under investigation. In addition to the inherited enzyme defect in each type, environmental factors play a key role in precipitating clinical episodes. In AIP, HCP, and VP, drugs often are responsible for acute neurologic attacks (Table 3). Administration of these compounds stimulates cytochrome synthesis in the liver, thereby increasing the demand for heme. In normal persons, this demand is met by new heme synthesis. However, in these types of porphyria, the capacity for heme synthesis appears to be limited by the respective enzyme defect in each type, so that drug administration may result in a "heme-deficient" state. Consistent with this postulate is the fact that the biochemical abnormalities and, in many cases, the symptoms of these porphyrias can be reversed by administration of heme (see below).

*For abbreviations, see Table 1.

TABLE 1. **Biochemical Characterization of the Porphyrias[1]**

$$\text{glycine} + \text{succinyl CoA} \longrightarrow \text{ALA} \longrightarrow \text{PBG} \xrightarrow{(1)} \text{UROGEN} \xrightarrow{(2)} \text{COPROGEN} \xrightarrow{(3)} \text{PROTOGEN} \xrightarrow{(4)} \text{PROTO} \xrightarrow{(5)} \text{HEME}$$

UROGEN → URO ; COPROGEN → COPRO

TYPE OF PORPHYRIA	HEME PRECURSORS EXCRETED IN ABNORMAL AMOUNTS		ENZYME DEFECT	COMMENT
	Urine	*Feces*		
1. AIP	ALA<**PBG**≫URO	(normal)	UROgen-I synthetase (1)[2]	Heme-deficient type
2. PCT	**URO**≫COPRO	(normal)	UROgen decarboxylase (2)	Heme-compensated type
3. HCP	ALA<PBG<URO<COPRO	**COPRO**≫PROTO	COPROgen oxidase (3)	Heme-deficient type
4. VP	ALA<PBG<URO<COPRO	COPRO<**PROTO**	?PROTOgen oxidase (4)	Heme-deficient type
5. EPP	(normal)	COPRO≪**PROTO**	Ferrochelatase (5)	Erythrocyte **PROTO** elevated

[1]This is a simplified presentation, adequate for clinical diagnosis; detailed discussion of heme synthesis and the porphyrias is available elsewhere.

[2]The position of the enzyme in the heme-synthetic pathway above is indicated by the number in parenthesis.

Abbreviations: ALA, δ-aminolevulinic acid; PBG, porphobilinogen; URO, uroporphyrin; COPRO, coproporphyrin; PROTO, protoporphyrin; AIP, acute intermittent porphyria; PCT, porphyria cutanea tarda (symptomatic porphyria); HCP, hereditary coproporphyria; VP, variegate (South African) porphyria; EPP, erythrohepatic (erythropoietic) protoporphyria.

For each condition, the diagnostic abnormality is represented in bold type.

TABLE 2. **Symptoms in the Hereditary Porphyrias**

TYPE OF PORPHYRIA	NEUROLOGIC	CUTANEOUS	HEPATIC
Acute intermittent porphyria	+ +	0	0
Porphyria cutanea *tarda*	0	+ +	+*
Hereditary copro- porphyria	+	+	0
Variegate porphyria	+ +	+ +	0
Erythrohepatic protoporphyria	0	+	(+)†

*Hepatic dysfunction is clinically evident or biochemically detectable in most persons with PCT, although its severity varies widely

†Uncommonly, in persons with markedly elevated plasma protoporphyrin, cholestatic liver disease develops, progressing rapidly to cirrhosis and portal hypertension

In PCT, overproduction of porphyrins appears to require both a genetic defect and the presence of excess iron in the liver, these combining to produce a partial block in heme synthesis and porphyrin overproduction. The block is not of sufficient magnitude to cause a heme-deficient state, and persons with PCT exhibit no sensitivity to drugs that increase the demand for heme synthesis, as in AIP, HCP, or VP. However, drugs (in particular, ethanol and estrogens) that add to the inhibitory effect of iron on the heme synthetic pathway may be important in the pathogenesis of PCT.

Inheritance in all of the genetic porphyrias appears to be autosomal dominant, except for congenital erythropoietic porphyria, an autosomal recessive condition (not discussed here).

Acute Intermittent Porphyria (AIP)

Prophylaxis. In acute intermittent porphyria (AIP), as in the pathogenically related HCP and VP, prevention of acute attacks is of primary importance. Drugs that may precipitate attacks (Table 3) must be avoided; fasting, strenuous dieting, or fad diets also have been associated with acute

TABLE 3. **Drug Sensitivity in Porphyria**

TYPE OF PORPHYRIA	DRUGS IMPLICATED IN THE PATHOGENESIS OF SYMPTOMS
AIP	Barbiturates, griseofulvin, estrogens, phenytoin (and related compounds), sulfonamides, meprobamate, and ethanol
PCT	Ethanol, estrogens and possibly other drugs with a direct hepatotoxic effect
HPC	As in AIP
VP	As in AIP
EPP	None recognized

porphyric exacerbations. Weight loss may be undertaken in individual patients but should involve no more than modest caloric restriction. On the other hand, there is no evidence that a diet rich in carbohydrate prevents attacks. Seizures—apart from those associated with acute attacks (see below)—present a special problem, in that the routinely employed anticonvulsants are contraindicated in porphyrics. In these patients, bromides represent a possible therapeutic approach. A number of other drugs have been administered safely to persons with AIP (aspirin, penicillins, tetracyclines, aminoglycosides, chlorpromazine, meperidine, hydromorphone hydrochloride (Dilaudid), diazepam, glucocorticoids, nitrous oxide, ether, and others), so that adequate therapy of intercurrent illness is possible.

Genetic Counseling. The appropriate screening procedures for family members of a person with documented AIP are quantitative determination of urinary PBG and also assay of erythrocyte UROgen-I synthetase activity (Table 1). While urinary PBG may be normal in carriers that are asymptomatic (also in most prepubertal carriers), the erythrocyte UROgen-I synthetase assay will be abnormal, regardless of the age or clinical state of the patient.

Acute Attacks. If seizures occur with the acute presentation, they usually are transient and may be treated with intravenous diazepam. Abdominal pain in some patients responds to chlorpromazine; in others, meperidine is required. Severe hyponatremia develops in some patients and may be managed as is the syndrome of inappropriate antidiuretic hormone secretion. General supportive therapy includes the administration of oral or intravenous fluids, which should contain at least 300 grams of carbohydrate per day. Propranolol will control tachycardia in most patients; therapy, however, should be initiated conservatively, since some patients will react with marked hypotension to as little as 10 mg. of this compound.

Progressive neurologic symptoms, occurring in the face of the above measures, constitute a potentially life-threatening development and are an indication for hematin therapy. Hematin is prepared by dissolving recrystallized pyrogen-tested hemin in 1 per cent sodium carbonate. The solution is passed through a sintered glass filter, adjusted to pH = 8.0 and finally sterilized by membrane filtration (0.20μ pore size). The resulting preparation, containing 10 to 20 mg. heme per ml. is infused into a large vein over a period of 15 to 20 minutes. The maximal recommended dose is 4 mg. per kg. body weight per 12 hours, and smaller doses may be effective in many patients. Hematin is given at 12 hour intervals until a clinical and biochemical response occurs (usually within 72 hours). To date, no significant side effects of hematin infusions have appeared, provided that the recommended dose schedule is adhered to. Solutions should be prepared fresh and infused within 24 hours.

Porphyria Cutanea Tarda (PCT)

Cutaneous Symptoms. Chemicals implicated in this disease (ethanol, estrogens, or other) should be proscribed. While these measures alone may ameliorate PCT, phlebotomy is uniformly successful in producing a remission. This maneuver presumably mobilizes and eventually depletes the burden of iron in the liver, relieving the iron-mediated inhibition of heme synthesis. A unit is withdrawn once or twice monthly, provided that a satisfactory hemoglobin concentration is maintained. Phlebotomy is continued until a response occurs, which consists of uroporphyrin excretion <1000 micrograms per 24 hours and resolution of cutaneous photosensitivity or fragility. The time required for a response varies widely among patients from a few months to more than a year. With a clinical response, phlebotomy may be discontinued with the expectation that uroporphyrin excretion will decline still further, often reaching normal amounts (<50 micrograms per 24 hours). For patients unable to tolerate phlebotomy and seriously disabled by cutaneous symptoms, "low-dose" chloroquine phosphate (0.5 gram twice weekly) may be introduced. (This use of chloroquine is not listed in the manufacturer's official directive.) Persons taking chloroquine should be monitored for hepatotoxic reactions to the drug.

Genetic Counseling. In PCT, identification of carriers within a family generally is not pursued, as the disease is clinically benign and readily treated. Silent carriers may be detected by measurement of urinary porphyrins, in some cases. Assay of the enzyme defect in PCT (decreased URO decarboxylase activity) is not widely available at the present time.

Hereditary Coproporphyria (HCP)

Prophylaxis. See AIP (above). For cutaneous symptoms, avoidance of sunlight is indicated. Phlebotomy, chloroquine, topical sunscreens, and beta-carotene are of no apparent value.

Genetic Counseling. Carriers may be identified by their excretion of abnormal amounts of fecal coproporphyrin (Table 1). Assay of the enzyme defect in this disease (decreased COPRO oxidase activity) requires blood leucocytes or skin fibroblast cultures and is a research procedure at the present time.

Acute Attacks. See AIP (above).

Variegate Porphyria (VP)

Prophylaxis. See HCP (above).
Genetic Counseling. The appropriate test for carriers is quantitative determination of fecal protoporphyrin (Table 1).
Acute Attacks. See AIP (above).

Erythrohepatic Protoporphyria (EPP)

Prophylaxis. The acute effects of sunlight (burning, itching, edema) can be mitigated to a large extent by oral beta-carotene, the dosage being titered for the individual patient. Side effects of this treatment are minimal, consisting mainly of carotenodermia.

Hepatic Disease. All patients with EPP should have liver function studies, including sulfobromophthalein (Bromsulphalein) retention. Those with demonstrable abnormalities, as well as those with plasma PROTO in excess of 1000 micrograms per 100 ml. blood, should undergo liver biopsy to assess the possibility of liver damage secondary to PROTO deposition. Preliminary reports suggest that in patients with the hepatobiliary form of EPP, therapy with cholestyramine (investigational) or hematin infusion may be beneficial. Presumably, cholestyramine binds PROTO in the intestinal lumen, preventing its enterohepatic circulation, while hematin may suppress the hepatic component of excess PROTO production.

Genetic Counseling. The appropriate tests for identifying carriers are quantitative determination of erythrocyte and fecal PROTO. Both tests are necessary, because increased erythrocyte PROTO may occur also in iron-deficiency anemia or lead intoxication (in the absence of cutaneous symptoms). In EPP, the increase in erythrocyte PROTO is usually (but not invariably) accompanied by elevation of fecal PROTO. The enzyme defect in EPP (decreased ferrochelatase activity) has been measured in skin fibroblast cultures from affected persons.

THERAPEUTIC USE OF BLOOD COMPONENTS
method of
WILLIAM V. MILLER, M.D.
St. Louis, Missouri

Introduction

The principal indications for the transfusion of human blood components are hypovolemia and diminished oxygen carrying capacity. Patients are more sensitive to decreases in blood volume than to diminished red cell mass and require early and vigorous replacement of blood volume deficits. This difference in physiologic requirement is the basis of blood component therapy.

As the risks of blood transfusion are substantial, a transfusion of whole blood or blood components should be avoided whenever possible. The principal risks include the transmission of viral hepatitis, immediate and delayed transfusion reactions, circulatory overload, and alloimmunization to cellular and plasma constituents of blood. Careful choice of the appropriate blood product makes the other components of blood available for other transfusion requirements. The use of only necessary components leads to the efficient use of a complex tissue in short supply. Blood should not be given as a "tonic," as neither blood nor any of its components given for this purpose will shorten convalescence, heal wounds, or nonspecifically make patients feel better.

Treatment of Hypovolemia

As the blood volume becomes depleted, the pulse increases, and blood pressure falls. Peripheral vasoconstriction may lead to pallor and sweating. As cardiac output continues to fall, the patient lapses into deep shock and unconsciousness. As some of the changes may be irreversible, it is important to treat the hypovolemic patient as soon as possible, and to replace lost blood volume.

Crystalloid Solutions. Sterile, protein-free solutions such as lactated Ringer's and isotonic saline solution are used in the initial treatment of hypovolemia and are usually sufficient when blood volume losses are less than 1000 ml. Infusion should be rapid and in sufficient quantity to maintain pulse and blood pressure.

Colloid Solutions. Isotonic solutions of plasma protein in saline are better able to maintain oncotic pressure and provide long-term support of the hypovolemic patient. In colloid solutions, 5 per cent albumin and plasma protein fraction are prepared by biochemical fractionation of human blood and, because they are not lost to surrounding tissues, provide direct expansion of the intravascular space. Because they are nonantigenic and carry no risk of hepatitis, they are safe as well as effective. Unfortunately, they are expensive and must be derived from human plasma. As with crystalloid solutions, they are infused rapidly in sufficient quantity to maintain vital signs.

Single Donor Plasma (Human). Single Donor Plasma (Human) is separated from whole blood shortly after collection, and frozen to maintain vital clotting factors and assure sterility for long-term storage. In addition to providing volume expansion, fresh frozen plasma, as it is also called, provides stable and labile clotting factors for

hemostasis. Because plasma is antigenic and carries a risk of hepatitis equivalent to the transfusion of whole blood, its use is generally restricted to situations in which plasma clotting factors are required, as indicated by abnormal tests of hemostasis.

Whole Blood (Human) and Red Blood Cells (Human). Whole Blood (Human) should be used to treat only those patients with hypovolemia in whom there is significant decrease in red cell mass (generally greater than 1500 ml. whole blood loss). Because whole blood is stored at about 6°C. for up to three weeks, the concentration of labile clotting factors and viable platelets may be significantly diminished. The transfusion of the cellular portion of whole blood, of Red Blood Cells (Human), is important not only in maintaining oxygen carrying capacity but blood volume as well.

Treatment of Diminished Red Cell Mass

Patients are much more sensitive to diminished red cell mass when it occurs suddenly, as in major trauma, bleeding, or surgery, than when it occurs over a period of days or weeks, as it does in most forms of chronic anemia. Compensatory mechanisms permit the red cell to increase its oxygen delivery to the tissue, when the anemia is long-standing. In general, patients with long-standing anemia can function quite successfully with hematocrits as low as 20 to 25 per cent. In contrast, signs of difficulty with tissue oxygenation may occur at higher hematocrits when the red cell loss is sudden. Because the replacement of red cell mass requires the transfusion of products which carry a substantial risk of hepatitis, which are known to stimulate the formation of antibodies, and which are known to be associated with immediate and delayed transfusion reactions, the benefits of transfusion should be carefully weighed against the known risks. Each red cell preparation has different characteristics and specific indications for administration. Patients should usually be transfused with group and type specific red cells, but during relative blood shortages, it is perfectly acceptable to give crossmatched compatible group O red cells to patients of other blood types. Group AB patients can safely receive red cells from group A, group B, or group O donors. Whenever group nonspecific blood is administered, the plasma should be removed.

Red Blood Cells (Human). Red Blood Cells (Human), also known as packed red cell concentrates, are prepared by sedimenting whole blood and removing most of the supernatant plasma. The volume of the unit is 250 ml., and it has the same oxygen carrying capacity and the same amount of iron (250 mg.) as a unit of whole blood. Plasma removal reduces the risk of volume overload and citrate toxicity. If the plasma is removed immediately prior to transfusion, the quantity of transfused potassium, sodium, and ammonia will also be reduced, which may be important to patients with liver, heart, and renal disease. Because plasma removal may increase the viscosity of Red Blood Cells (Human), the infusion may flow slowly. The addition of 30 to 50 ml. of isotonic saline solution to the bag via a Y tubing is acceptable and will correct this problem.

Red Blood Cells (Human), Leukocyte-Poor. Leukocyte-poor red cells are prepared by differential centrifugation of freshly collected units and are of value in those patients requiring replacement of the red cell mass who have a history of frequent or severe febrile nonhemolytic transfusion reactions. These reactions are often due to patient antibodies directed against antigens on donor leukocytes, and removal of leukocytes from donor blood will usually prevent these reactions. Because up to 25 per cent of the red cells may also be lost during processing, chronically ill patients with no history of febrile reactions should not be given Red Blood Cells (Human) that are leukocyte-poor, as it will increase the transfusion requirement and associated risks.

Red Blood Cells (Human), Frozen, Deglycerolized. Freezing blood with a cryoprotective agent such as glycerol allows the storage time of blood to be extended for up to 3 years. Unfortunately, after thawing the blood must be repeatedly washed to remove the glycerol. The washing process removes plasma protein, white cells, and platelets, but introduces the risk of bacterial contamination and is expensive and time consuming. The cells must be used within 24 hours after thawing. Frozen red cell concentrates are most helpful in the therapy of patients with rare red cell types and permit storage of cells from rare donors to be stored for subsequent autologous or heterologous transfusion. Frozen red cells are thought to be associated with a lower risk of post-transfusion hepatitis, but there is little evidence to support widespread use in preventing this illness. Saline washed and frozen red blood cells are nearly free of all tissue antigens, but there is considerable controversy regarding the benefits of these products for potential transplant recipients.

Whole Blood (Human). There are no clinical situations that absolutely require the use of whole blood. Whole blood transfusions may be given to patients who are suffering from acute blood loss of sufficient magnitude to cause hypovolemic shock, where an increase in both the intravascular volume and oxygen carrying capacity is needed. Red cell concentrates and crystalloid or colloid solutions can also supply the patient's needs, however.

Whole blood is contraindicated in normovolemic patients with depleted red cell mass. Here, the plasma contained in whole blood increases the risk of transfusion and is of no additional benefit.

Blood Components for Hemostasis

A third major indication for the transfusion of blood components is the treatment of patients with disordered hemostasis. Briefly, hemostatic defects may be due to quantitative or qualitative platelet abnormalities, to congenital or acquired abnormalities of the clotting scheme, or to a combination of both. In any bleeding patient it is essential to maintain an adequate circulating volume and adequate oxygen carrying capacity. Appropriate blood components should be infused in sufficient quantity to support these vital functions. In the great majority of bleeding patients, evaluation of the history, sites, and nature of bleeding, and laboratory tests can provide much information about the cause of the bleeding and, inferentially, a choice of appropriate blood component. Prothrombin time, partial thromboplastin time, estimation of the fibrinogen level, and platelet enumeration, will generally provide sufficient data to allow most patients to be treated successfully.

Many clotting factor deficiencies are not associated with an increased risk of hemorrhage. In fact, clotting factors can be reduced to approximately 25 per cent of normal levels without increasing the bleeding potential. Platelet counts over 15,000 to 20,000 per cu. mm. are generally sufficient to prevent spontaneous hemorrhage, and counts over 50,000 per cu. mm. provide essentially normal hemostasis, even in major surgery or trauma. Abnormal laboratory values alone are not indications for therapy; the site, volume, and cause of bleeding must be assessed before replacement therapy can be intelligently selected.

Platelet Transfusions. Patients with severe thrombocytopenia, abnormal bleeding, and decreased platelet production may respond favorably to platelet transfusion. Patients who have received great quantities of blood rapidly (more than 12 units in a few hours) may develop abnormal bleeding, resulting in dilutional thrombocytopenia. Platelets may be efficacious in these patients if the blood loss can be controlled. In thrombocytopenic states in which there is rapid platelet destruction of the patient's own platelets, it is likely that transfused platelets would also be rapidly destroyed, and transfusion would be of little value.

Platelets are prepared by differential centrifugation of closed plastic collection sets, resulting in a concentrate that contains about 0.6×10^{11} platelets in a volume of 30 to 50 ml. of plasma. A small number of red cells is present, but rarely represents risk to an ABO incompatible recipient. Except for small children and women in their reproductive years who may be expected to bear children, platelet concentrates are given without regard to ABO or Rh type. Because the platelets from a single donor are relatively few, concentrates from 5 to 10 donors are usually pooled for a single therapeutic dose. In the absence of splenomegaly and alloimmunization by previous transfusion, donor platelets circulate normally and may be expected to provide an increment in the peripheral blood platelet count according to the following formula:

$$\text{Platelet Increment} = \text{pc } 2 - \text{pc } 1 \times \text{bsa} \div \text{c}$$

$$\text{where pc } 2 = \text{Post-transfusion platelet count}$$
$$\text{pc } 1 = \text{Pre-transfusion platelet count}$$
$$\text{bsa} = \text{Body surface area (M}^2\text{)}$$
$$\text{c} = \text{Number of concentrates given}$$

One platelet concentrate per 10 kg. body weight will increase the platelet count approximately 50,000 per cu. mm., so a pool of 8 platelet concentrates will ordinarily provide a significant increment and effective hemostasis in a 70 kg. man.

Because it is impossible to prevent sensitization to platelet antigens, and most recipients will ultimately develop antiplatelet antibodies, repeated platelet transfusions will lead to progressively smaller platelet increments and shorter platelet survival. For this reason, platelet transfusion should be accompanied by an immediate pretransfusion platelet count and by a platelet count 12 to 24 hours after transfusion. The effectiveness of each platelet transfusion should be monitored daily, and when post-transfusion increments are reduced, there is presumptive evidence of alloimmunization to platelet antigens. If the patient will continue to require platelet transfusion despite alloimmunization, platelets collected from HL-A matched single donors may be effective. There is, however, no evidence to suggest that the early use of HL-A matched platelets is of special benefit, and there are theoretical considerations suggesting that early exposure to HL-A matched products may lead to more difficult problems with refractoriness.

Replacement of Labile Clotting Factors. A congenital or acquired disorder of the clotting mechanism may lead to severe depletion of labile clotting factors, requiring replacement therapy. The differential diagnosis of these disorders is considered elsewhere in this book. Maintenance of blood volume and red blood cell mass is essential during any bleeding episode, and single donor plasma (human) is the mainstay of therapy in these conditions. This product contains normal levels of all the labile clotting factors and can be used to treat any of the hereditary clotting deficiencies. In addition, it is a therapeutic source of factor VIII and factor IX for hemophiliacs and is the least wasteful therapy available. However, the large volumes required to permit normal coagulation make other products more attractive. Plasma can be used for short-term hemostasis in some patients with diminished hepatic synthetic function, and for patients suffering from vitamin K deficiency. Vitamin K deficiency often can be treated by oral or parenteral vitamin K and transfusion is often not necessary. Patients receiving great quantities of stored blood are occasionally routinely given fresh frozen plasma to replace protein coagulation factors, but there is very little evidence that such practice is indicated in patients with normal hepatic function. Patients receiving more than 10 to 12 units of blood in a few hours should be examined closely for the development of abnormal or excessive bleeding or both. Thrombocytopenia is more likely to occur than labile clotting factor deficiencies. If the clinical and laboratory data suggest that abnormal bleeding has occurred because of clotting factor defects, then fresh frozen plasma may be administered, but other products may be more appropriate. Other hemorrhagic syndromes may develop in patients receiving great quantities of blood, and fresh frozen plasma is not routinely indicated in all situations. Where there is evidence of a clotting factor defect as shown by abnormalities of the prothrombin time or partial thromboplastin time or both, then 3 to 5 units of fresh frozen plasma may be required to restore labile clotting factors to the normal range.

The treatment of hemophilia A and hemophilia B are specialized problems requiring medical consultation. Classic hemophilia A is routinely treated with cryoprecipitated factor VIII or with antihemophilic factor VIII concentrates. Factor IX concentrates are used for the treatment of hemophilia B. Before either product is given, an accurate diagnosis must be made and the dose calculated on the basis of estimated clotting factor level, and the concentration of the product. Both factor VIII and factor IX concentrates carry a high risk of post-transfusion hepatitis.

Special Uses of Blood Components

Treatment of Infection. Recently, granulocyte concentrates have become available for the treatment of the severely granulocytopenic infected patient. Granulocyte concentrates are prepared from single donors by either differential centrifugation or nylon fiber filtration. Granulocytes are apparently useful in patients with granulocyte counts of less than 500 per cu. mm. and who have evidence of infection. The concentrate should consist of at least 1×10^{10} granulocytes, and should be administered each day while the patient is infected and profoundly leukopenic. Because many red cells contaminate granulocyte concentrates, the product should be ABO compatible and crossmatched for red cells. A granulocyte crossmatch is advisable, but routine HLA typing is not recommended. As granulocytes are distributed throughout the body, post-transfusion increments may be small, if detectable at all.

Protein Replacement.   Rarely, normovolemic patients with severe hypoproteinemia may require temporary elevation of serum protein levels. Twenty-five per cent albumin solution is available for this purpose, containing about 12.5 grams per bottle. It is well to remember that concentrated albumin solutions have considerable oncotic activity and will pull fluid into the intravascular space, temporarily increasing blood volume and providing some danger of cardiac overload. Usually no more than 2 or 3 bottles are administered per 24 hour period. Intravenous protein replacement has little value as a long-term therapeutic procedure.

Immunoglobulin Replacement.   Patients with immunoglobulin deficiency can be treated by transfusion of plasma or by injecting gamma globulin concentrates intramuscularly on a monthly basis. The first dose of gamma globulin should be 0.25 gram per kg. of body weight and further administration schedules determined to control symptoms and infections in the individual patient.

Infusion of Blood Components

Crystalloid and colloid solutions may be infused through a standard intravenous infusion set, but most blood components are best infused through a Y blood infusion set. In a Y set, isotonic saline solution is used to begin and terminate the transfusion, and a filter is imposed to remove particulate matter from the blood component. The same Y infusion set can be used for red cells, plasma, and platelets, but because of the large chamber size, significant doses of the platelet concentrate may be trapped in the filter, requiring rinsing at the end of the infusion to deliver the entire dose. Steps for the infusion of blood components are as follows:

1. Select the appropriate product and, if necessary, provide a tube of the patient's blood for compatibility testing and a signed requisition.

2. Prepare the infusion site, using a Y infusion set and isotonic saline solution. Lactated Ringer's, 5 per cent dextrose in water (D_5W), dextrose solutions and the like, should *not* be used to begin and end blood transfusions because of undesirable effects on citrated blood.

3. On receipt of the blood product, carefully check the type of product and numbers on the bag and the product identification tag against the patient's wrist band and patient record. More transfusion accidents result from failure to observe this precaution than any other.

4. After beginning the infusion, the patient should be observed carefully, especially during the first 15 to 30 minutes when reactions are most likely to occur. Vital signs should be recorded prior to transfusion and every 15 minutes during the transfusion. The patient should be urged to report all symptoms. Following transfusion, the effectiveness should be evaluated by appropriate clinical and laboratory observations. Should an adverse effect develop during or after transfusion, the transfusion service director should be notified immediately and appropriate therapeutic steps initiated.

UNTOWARD REACTIONS TO BLOOD TRANSFUSIONS

method of
HAROLD S. KAPLAN, M.D.
New York, New York

Even though blood transfusion is a relatively safe procedure, for every 100,000 transfusions given as many as 3000 adverse reactions may occur. The great majority of these are benign and without lasting significance. However, approximately 30 of these 3000 reactions may be acute hemolytic transfusion reactions and perhaps 5 of these will be fatal. At the current annual transfusion rate in the United States, this frequency would approximate one fatal hemolytic transfusion reaction per day.

This discussion will consider first the immediate reactions, that is, those occurring during or within several hours of transfusion, and then the delayed reactions, those occurring days, weeks, or months following transfusion.

IMMEDIATE REACTIONS

Acute Hemolytic Transfusion Reaction (AHTR)

It is ironic that this most dramatic and disastrous of transfusion complications is perhaps the most preventable. Acute hemolytic transfusion reactions are most often caused by errors simply related to ABO blood group incompatibility and not some arcane and subtle limitation of test methods. These are almost invariably clerical errors, often in patient identification, either in the collection and labeling of the original crossmatch blood sample or in the identification of the recipient at the time of transfusion. In this situation red cells are infused into patients already having potent, often hemolytic antibodies. The resultant immune destruction of red cells may lead to anaphylactic shock, disseminated intravascular coagulation, and renal failure.

Although symptomatology of AHTR may occur with transfusion of just a few milliliters of strongly incompatible blood, in general the greater the volume of incompatible blood transfused and the longer the delay in treatment, the greater the chance for severe and irreversible damage. This is one reason why no patient should be left unattended during a transfusion and why the initial 25 to 50 ml. should be given as slowly as possible. The patient should be carefully observed for any signs of an untoward reaction. There is no absolute pathognomonic sign or symptom for hemolytic transfusion reaction. *Any adverse change in the patient's status, even if only chills, fever or urticaria, or any other change or complaint, must be considered significant and be further evaluated.* When this occurs in anesthetized surgical patients, the only signs may be those of increased and unexpected bleeding or oozing from previously dry surgical areas and hypotension not responsive to further blood transfusions.

Whenever suspected reactions occur during transfusion, the transfusion must be discontinued immediately and the infusing line maintained patent with a slow drip of 0.9 per cent saline solution. Clerical rechecking is done to verify that the unit transfused was indeed the correct unit intended for that recipient, and the Blood Bank is notified of the reaction. The remainder of the blood unit, even if empty, is returned to the Blood Bank along with two blood samples, one in a clotted tube and the other in an anticoagulated (EDTA) tube. These samples should always be drawn away from the site of infusion and special care be taken to avoid artifactual hemolysis.

Careful monitoring of the urinary output is begun and an initial urine sample is examined for evidence of hemoglobinuria. It is important to remember that red cells in the urine are *not* an early sign of AHTR, and therefore a red urine should be centrifuged to establish whether the red color remains in the supernatant or is spun out as red cells with the sediment. Also, some hemolysis may be due to nonimmunologic causes such as extracorporeal circulation, improper storage of blood in a ward refrigerator, distilled water irrigation, and infusion of the blood along with potentially hemolytic agents including dextrose and water solutions.

The initial laboratory investigation is directed at the rapid establishment of whether significant immune red cell hemolysis has occurred. The anticoagulated sample is centrifuged and examined for visible evidence of hemolysis. Hemoglobin levels of approximately 30 mg. per dl. (100 ml.) will cause a faint but definite pink tinge to the supernatant plasma. A direct antiglobulin (Coombs') test is then performed on this EDTA sample.* If these initial screening tests are negative, it is unlikely that AHTR has occurred and therefore aggressive prophylactic and therapeutic intervention for AHTR will not likely be required. Further serologic testing is then done on the clotted sample.

The primary focus of therapy is, if possible, to *prevent* rather than to treat shock, renal tubular necrosis, and disseminated intravascular coagulation. Efforts are directed mainly at maintaining intravascular volume with crystalloid solutions, promoting diuresis and, when indicated, anticoagulation with heparin.

The salient point of therapy is to support intravascular volume and urinary output. The urinary output is an important index of renal function, and its response to hydration and diuretics a useful guide to management. The goal is to maintain urinary output of at least 60 ml. per hour. Vigorous fluid replacement may be necessary to ensure that hydration is not the limiting factor in diuretic response and to prevent excessive diuresis and reduction in blood volume. Central venous pressure or pulmonary wedge pressure measurements may provide important information to guide fluid replacement, especially in patients with compromised ability to handle a fluid load. Provision to obtain these measures should, however, not delay initiation of therapy.

The customary approach to therapy with mannitol as the primary diuretic agent has been questioned in recent years, and arguments have been made for furosemide or ethacrynic acid. This controversy is unlikely to be resolved in clinical experience and must await further experimental evidence. For the present, an empirical approach based on an assessment of the patient's clinical status appears to be reasonable.

In the hypovolemic patient, in whom maintenance of adequate intravascular volume is of concern, mannitol would tend to support volume and

---

*If either or both of these tests are positive, without other known cause, treatment for AHTR should be initiated without delay.

be advantageous. Furosemide, a very potent diuretic, would limit volume and be advantageous in patients with compromised cardiac function who would not tolerate well an acutely expanded blood volume.

In other patients, who have no significant or potential volume problems, the choice is less well-defined. Although mannitol has been in use longer than furosemide, experimental evidence for furosemide's ability to produce an increase in renal cortical blood flow and its powerful diuretic effect make it an attractive alternative.

Mannitol Regimen. 1. 100 ml. of 25 per cent mannitol solution given rapidly intravenously over a 5 to 10 minute period.

2. Over the first two hours, administer 1500 to 2000 ml. of isotonic saline solution with an added 45 mEq. of sodium bicarbonate.

3. Monitoring urinary output. If expected diuresis of 1 to 3 ml. per minute is achieved, maintain diuresis with a 5 per cent solution of mannitol and electrolyte solution to keep up with the urinary output. Up to 150 grams of mannitol may be administered in 24 hours in a patient who responds to the diuretic.

4. If no diuretic response is observed by two hours, further fluid and mannitol administration are unlikely to be effective and may be harmful, so restrict fluid intake and manage as for acute renal failure.

Furosemide (Lasix) Regimen. 1. Furosemide, 40 to 80 mg. intravenously in well-hydrated patient.

2. Monitor urine volume which should be 1 to 3 ml. per minute during the first hour, confirming diuretic response.

3. Maintain diuresis by either: intravenous infusion of 1500 ml. of isotonic saline solution with an added 45 mEq. of sodium bicarbonate, or two additional doses of 40 to 80 mg. furosemide every 6 hours. Prevent overdiuresis by careful monitoring of blood pressure and support of adequate hydration.

4. Monitor serum potassium levels, and estimate urinary losses since furosemide therapy may require potassium supplementation.

5. If urine volumes remain below target levels for 2 hours, further fluid and diuretic are unlikely to be effective and may be harmful. Restrict fluid intake and manage as for acute renal failure.

Anticoagulation. Because of the powerful thromboplastic effect of an acute hemolytic transfusion reaction (AHTR), anticoagulation with heparin has been suggested in order to prevent disseminated intravascular coagulation (DIC), but its use has not been widespread.

In the absence of a contraindication to anticoagulation, in a high risk patient, one with immune hemolysis following 200 ml. or more of whole blood or 100 ml. or more of packed cells, the use of heparin would appear warranted if there are other signs of a severe reaction or a strong incompatibility such as ABO or both.

Acute Nonhemolytic Immunologic Reactions

Febrile Nonhemolytic Reactions (FNHR). These reactions are characterized by chills or fever or both, sometimes accompanied by other signs and symptoms, but without immune hemolysis. They occur during or shortly after transfusion and are usually mild and self-limited. Their major significance is the overlap of these symptoms with those of AHTR. No presumption of a benign febrile reaction can be made. The transfusion must be stopped and AHTR ruled out.

Febrile nonhemolytic reactions (FNHR) are reactions to nonred cell antigens of the donor, typically due to donor leukocyte antigens and recipient antileukocyte antibodies (anti–HL-A) in a multiparous or multitransfused patient. Less often, antiplatelet and anti-immunoglobulin antibodies are the cause. The treatment of these reactions is symptomatic with an antipyretic such as acetaminophen, 650 mg.

Although ordinarily benign, FNHR can be of significance in the critically ill, and in patients requiring frequent transfusions. Fortunately, these reactions are often preventable. Since the severity of these reactions is related to the rate and amount of antigenic material tranfused, slow administration of leukocyte-poor blood (about 70 per cent depleted) is all that is required for prevention in the great majority of patients. This may be achieved by simple removal of the buffy coat in the Blood Bank prior to issue. If reactions persist, premedication with acetaminophen, 650 mg., just before transfusion of buffy-coat–poor blood is usually sufficient.

For the few still persistent or severe reactions, more thorough methods of white cell removal may be required. These include multiple centrifugation techniques, red cell washing, and the reconstitution of frozen red blood cells. The last product is as free of leukocytes as is currently technically feasible.

Pulmonary Hypersensitivity. This is a more severe form of reaction due to antileukocyte antibodies, which may be recipient or donor antibody reacting with foreign leukocytes. It usually presents as a febrile, nonhemolytic reaction with variably severe dyspnea, and hypoxemia. This noncardiac pulmonary edema shows a patchy infiltrate on chest x-rays with a normal-sized cardiac silhouette and normal central venous pressure or pulmonary wedge pressure.

TREATMENT. 1. Nasal oxygen.

2. Furosemide intravenously in sufficient dose to achieve and sustain diuresis (e.g., 40 mg.). Monitor potassium levels and central venous pressure. If excessive diuresis, replace fluid volume with salt-poor albumin.

3. There is some question of the effectiveness of steroid therapy. However, if not contraindicated, hydrocortisone, 200 mg. intravenously at 4-hour intervals over a 24-hour period, can be considered.

4. Prevention of such transfusion reactions in the future. Determine whether donor or patient antibody is responsible. If the donor is responsible, exclude plasma containing fractions in future donations. If the antibody is produced by the patient, premedicate and use reconstituted frozen red cells. If HL-A–containing blood components are required, use blood components from HL-A–compatible crossmatched donor, along with premedication. Transfuse slowly.

Allergic Reactions. URTICARIAL REACTIONS. The development of hives occurs fairly commonly. It usually appears shortly after starting the transfusion. It most probably represents an IgE response to an antigen in the donor's plasma. It is rarely serious and responds well to antihistamines such as diphenhydramine (Benadryl), 50 mg. orally or intramuscularly. As usual, the transfusion should be discontinued. The venous line is kept patent and the reaction evaluated to:

1. Rule out more serious reaction when this is first seen.

2. Document the pattern of allergic reaction in this patient.

3. Establish appropriate preventive therapy if further transfusion is required.

Occasionally, the urticaria is accompanied by wheezing. If mild, it may likewise respond to antihistamines. However, severe symptoms may require aqueous epinephrine 0.5 ml. of a 1:1000 solution subcutaneously.

If further transfusion is required:

1. Premedication with 50 mg. diphenhydramine either orally or intramuscularly about 15 minutes before initiating transfusion.

2. When plasma components are not required, use appropriate component, for example, packed cells. Patients with severe reactions in whom premedication is not effective may require washed or reconstituted frozen red cells.

ANAPHYLACTIC REACTIONS. These are the most severe of allergic reactions. They often occur shortly after the start of transfusion and may rapidly develop from flushing and wheezing into anaphylactic shock. They are due to IgG antibodies to donor IgA. These reactions occur most commonly in patients lacking IgA but may also be seen in some non-IgA deficient patients.

1. Immediately stop the transfusion and maintain a patent line. It is most important to prevent further transfusion of blood products until the cause has been defined. Crystalloid solution may be used to maintain an adequate intravascular volume.

2. Epinephrine, 0.5 ml. of a 1:1000 solution, may be administered subcutaneously or *slowly* intravenously.

3. Oxygen and other supportive therapy may be required, including hydrocortisone, 200 mg., intravenously repeated at 4 hour intervals for 24 hours.

Once the diagnosis is confirmed, further transfusions must be of IgA deficient material. A registry of IgA deficient donors is maintained by the American Association of Blood Banks and the Red Cross. Reconstituted frozen red cells have been successfully transfused in some patients with anti-IgA. But reactions have been reported even with these fully washed (deglycerolyzed) frozen cells.

Acute Nonhemolytic Nonimmunologic Reactions

Volume Overload. Volume overload is one of the most common adverse reactions to transfusion. It occurs typically in the very young or elderly. This hypervolemia may first become manifested as tachypnea during a transfusion and may ultimately result in congestive heart failure. Treatment is as for acute pulmonary edema, with elevation of the head of the bed (Fowler position), digitalization, diuretics, etc. In the majority of circumstances it is a preventable complication:

1. Red cell concentrates (packed red cells) should be used whenever transfusing to correct anemia. This is especially true in patients who are at risk of developing congestive heart failure, as in the severely anemic elderly patient.

2. The transfusion should be administered as slowly as possible, over several hours. To facilitate this, blood banks should divide these units in half volumes and issue only one portion at a time. The second half of the unit is refrigerated until the first half has been infused. This decreases the risk of sepsis (see below) and allays the anxiety of staff who might otherwise feel the need to hasten the infusion. In this way one unit may be conveniently transfused over 2 to 4 hours. Once hung at the bedside, the first half of the unit should be administered within 2 hours. While refrigerated the second half of the unit has a 24 hour expiry. For the very young, even smaller volume "quad" packs are available.

3. Monitoring of the central venous pressure and maintaining the patient in a sitting position further reduces the risk of volume overload reactions.

4. If necessary, a partial exchange can be

done to limit the expansion of the blood volume. This may be achieved by withdrawing one unit of the patient's own blood and replacing it with two units of packed red cell concentrates.

Septic Reactions. Septic reactions are rare. The limited number of organisms that may be introduced during blood collection does not ordinarily survive storage at 4°C. The advent of closed component preparation has further reduced the chance of contamination. However, the risk still exists. Cryophilic gram-negative organisms are capable of growing at refrigerator temperatures. Also, when blood is allowed to warm to room temperature, organisms remaining from the time of collection or introduced during subsequent manipulation may rapidly multiply. Contamination carries both the risk of infusing viable microorganisms and of producing endotoxic shock. Hyperpyrexia, hypotension, and other signs and symptoms indicative of gram-negative sepsis and shock require urgent therapy as outlined elsewhere in this book.

Diagnosis is made primarily by the clinical presentation. Confirmation by Gram staining of the stored blood may be technically difficult, and information derived from blood culture is necessarily delayed. Therapy may have to be started before confirmatory laboratory work-up is completed.

Prevention depends on rigorous attention to technique in blood collection and transfusion. Stored blood is a good culture medium and the time lapse between its issue and administration must be kept to a minimum. Once transfusion is initiated, it should be completed within 2 hours. If this is not possible, the unit should be divided in the Blood Bank and stored and issued as outlined above.

Other Immediate Reactions

Problems Associated with Massive Transfusion. Transfusion of massive amounts of blood, for example, the exchange of one blood volume or more in 24 hours, may have undesirable effects.

BLEEDING PROBLEMS. With rapid transfusion of large amounts of stored blood, a "washout" or dilutional coagulopathy may occur, but this is infrequent. Even with amounts equivalent to one blood volume, the platelet count in an otherwise healthy person remains above levels necessary for surgical hemostasis (approximately 50,000 per cu. mm.). However, in urgent large volume transfusions, it is not unreasonable to administer prophylactically approximately 4 to 6 units of platelets after the first 12 to 15 units of stored blood have been infused. Coagulation factors are even less likely to present a problem than platelets,

but selected circumstances may require a similar approach with 1 to 2 units of fresh frozen plasma. Optimally, coagulation studies should be initiated prior to replacement, to document deficiencies and provide a rational baseline for further therapy.

In instances of rapid blood loss, the effects of "washout" of any component may be minimized by rapid replacement of the full volume lost instead of just staying even with current volume losses. This phenomenon is a function of the exchange transfusion curve and is present even when the replacement medium is devoid of the component in question. Undue delay in replacing the full volume deficit may magnify the washout effect.

COLD BLOOD. The rapid infusion of large amounts of cold blood (at refrigerator temperature 4°C.) can cause cardiac arrhythmias and arrest. This can be prevented by warming the blood prior to infusion. The preferred method is infusion through a warming coil between the blood unit and the patient.

CITRATE AND POTASSIUM, AMMONIUM AND HYDROGEN IONS. The levels of plasma potassium, ammonium and hydrogen ions increase significantly with storage time. However, even with large transfused blood volumes this excess seldom leads to difficulty. In special circumstances, such as patients with acute renal failure, the transfused plasma potassium load can be minimized by administering blood less than 1 week old that has been resuspended and subsequently converted to red cell concentrate by centrifugation just prior to issue.

Although rapid infusion of large volumes of citrated blood (for example, 1 unit every 5 minutes) may produce hypocalcemia, the body's capacity to metabolize citrate is impressive, and overzealous replacement of calcium should be avoided. With very rapid rates of infusion the patient is monitored for electrocardiographic changes suggestive of hypocalcemia. The latter may be treated with 10 ml. of a 10 per cent calcium gluconate solution for every 1000 ml. of blood transfused.

MICROAGGREGATES. During blood storage, particulate material consisting primarily of degenerating platelets and granulocytes accumulates. These microaggregates are small enough to pass through the 170 micron filter used in routine blood administration. It has been suggested that with massive transfusion, significant amounts of this debris accumulates in the pulmonary capillaries and may impair ventilatory function. It is clear that other factors play a role in this postresuscitative respiratory complication, and the significance of the microaggregates is as yet unresolved. Regardless of this debate, cellular debris exist, and special filters with a pore size at 40 micron and below, effectively remove them from stored blood. Since filtration of blood is required in all transfusions, microaggregate filters would seem indicated in patients receiving approximately 5 units of blood or more, in infants, and in patients with preexisting pulmonary function impairment.

DELAYED REACTIONS

Delayed Hemolytic Reactions

This reaction occurs in patients previously sensitized to red cell antigens but with clinically undetectable circulating antibodies. Transfused blood may carry the corresponding antigen and serve as a "booster" dose with a resultant secondary response and concomitant rapid rise of antibody titer. This anamnestic response to the transfusion may result in a shortened red cell survival 4 to 14 days following the transfusion. These reactions are characteristically self-limited and often go undetected. The removal of red cells is predominantly extravascular and slow. During the reaction, there may be a slight elevation of temperature, some jaundice, and a gradual drop in hemoglobin levels. These changes are seldom correlated and rarely associated with a transfusion given within the prior week or two. Laboratory studies reveal not only a fall in hemoglobin and an elevation of bilirubin but spherocytes in the peripheral smear and a positive direct antiglobulin test (Coombs'). The diagnosis is confirmed by the positive direct antiglobulin test, in which there is a "mixed-field" pattern with a minor population of clumped donor cells detected in a field of uninvolved recipient cells. With large transfusion volumes, the positive direct antiglobulin test may not give the "mixed-field" picture and may resemble that of an autoimmune hemolytic anemia. In regard to the treatment of these reactions there is little concern because, in general, the vast majority of these are benign in nature and require no therapy. Only rarely has significant intravascular hemolysis occurred in delayed reactions, and in such circumstances treatment would be as for an acute hemolytic transfusion reaction. In general, however, the importance of these reactions is in recognizing that they do occur and that the patient be carefully monitored. Until the specificity of the antibody is resolved, further transfusion is withheld.

Post-transfusion Purpura

Post-transfusion purpura is a rare form of delayed immunologic reaction to blood transfusion. The patient becomes sensitized by transfusion not only to donor platelets but to his own platelets as well. This reaction is characterized by a severe thrombocytopenia, which may appear days or weeks following transfusion and may persist for several weeks. The thrombocytopenia in these reactions may be severe and even life-threatening. It is mostly unresponsive to steroids, but has been successfully treated with exchange transfusion.

Graft vs. Host Reaction

This unusual complication of transfusion therapy could occur when large numbers of donor leukocytes are transfused into an immunologically compromised patient. Examples of such cases are intrauterine blood transfusions and leukocyte transfusion to leukemic recipients. Clinical evidence for graft vs. host reactions following intrauterine transfusion is equivocal, and in the leukemic patient is difficult to assess. Irradiation of the donor blood units with 1500 rads has been utilized to prevent this potential complication.

Alloimmunization

Another delayed immunologic reaction to blood transfusion is the sensitization of the recipient to foreign antigens of plasma proteins or of formed elements of the blood. Recipients of appropriate ABO and Rh type specific blood become sensitized to other red cell antigens at a rate of about 1 per cent per unit transfused. Except in special circumstances of Rh immunization, there is no current method of preventing these sensitizations except by minimizing transfusion exposure.

In the Rh negative recipient (especially a young girl or a woman in her child-bearing years) who receives Rh positive platelet concentrates, Rh immune globulin may be administered to prevent sensitization to the Rh antigen. The standard single intramuscular dose may prevent sensitization to a dose of as many as 20 units of Rh positive platelet concentrates. It should be remembered, however, that this must be administered intramuscularly. In a patient with significant hemostatic compromise beyond simple thrombocytopenia such injections may carry the risk of a significant intramuscular bleed.

Transmission of Infectious Diseases

Although a number of infectious diseases may be transmitted by transfusion, by far the most significant is post-transfusion hepatitis (PTH). PTH remains a significant complication of transfusion therapy. However, with the advent of sensitive screening methods for Hb_sAg and decreased use of high-risk "commercial" donors, there has been a greater than 50 per cent reduction in disease incidence of PTH. Recent studies suggest that incidence of PTH is now approximately 5 cases per 1000 transfusions. Hepatitis B comprises less than 10 per cent of the PTH currently seen. Hepatitis A, as is the case with EB virus and cytomegalovirus, appears to be an insignificant cause of PTH. The term "non-A, non-B hepatitis" has been coined for the remaining cases of PTH, which may be due to one or more other agents. Like hepatitis B and unlike hepatitis A, non-A, non-B hepatitis may be complicated by chronic active or chronic persistent hepatitis.

Evidence has been presented in one report that the incidence of non-A, non-B PTH may be reduced by injection of standard gamma globulin preparations prior to transfusion. However, this single report is as yet unconfirmed and there is no current recommendation regarding routine gamma globulin use in blood transfusion recipients.

Hepatitis B immune globulin (HBIG) is not recommended for routine preexposure prophylaxis in current transfusion practice because of the decreased incidence of hepatitis B due to sensitive screening tests and increased volunteer donor use.

Rarely, a physician may be advised that his patient has received blood from a donor who has subsequently shown evidence of clinical hepatitis. If this is serologically demonstrated to be hepatitis B, the chances are considerable that the donor has been infective for at least one month. The recipient should be tested for both hepatitis B surface antigen and antibody. If the patient lacks antibody and is therefore susceptible, and the transfusion was received within the prior week, the patient should be given hepatitis B immune globulin (HBIG). The dose is approximately 5 ml. for adults. This dose should be repeated 28 to 30 days after exposure. If the donor in question is negative for hepatitis B surface antigen, one might consider the similar use of a standard immune globulin dose of about 10 ml. intramuscularly for adults.

Syphilis may be transmitted by blood transfusion but it apparently does not represent a significant hazard with nondirect transfusion, since there has been only one possible case report in the American literature. This is probably due less to routine serologic testing for syphilis than to the inability of the spirochete to survive storage at 4°C. for 72 hours. Post-transfusion syphilis appears as a secondary syphilis rash a week to several months post-transfusion. Specific treatment for syphilis will be found on pages 542 through 544.

The transmission of malaria by blood transfusion is less rare than that of syphilis but is still an uncommon event in this country. Specific therapy for malaria is found on pages 37 through 39.

Cytomegalovirus disease (CMV) may be transmitted by blood transfusion. CMV, however, does not appear to survive in stored blood at 4°C. for more than 2 days. The disease, however, is usually self-limited and requires no specific therapy.

The Digestive System

BLEEDING ESOPHAGEAL VARICES

method of
JOE U. LEVI, M.D.,
and EUGENE R. SCHIFF, M.D.
Miami, Florida

When the patient with a history of recent or active upper gastrointestinal bleeding arrives at the hospital, usually the emergency room, a series of rapid events should take place. These include: establishing an intravenous route as soon as possible with a large needle, preferably a 16 gauge venous catheter; obtaining a blood sample for type and cross matching of blood, as well as complete blood count, prothrombin time, partial thromboplastin time, platelet count, and a chemical profile, which includes standard liver chemistries and electrolytes; starting an infusion of Ringer's solution, pending the arrival of the blood for transfusion; and taking a history for ingestion of drugs, particularly salicylates, alcoholism, bleeding diathesis, previously established liver or pancreatic disease, and a past history of gastrointestinal bleeding. One wants to know, first, why is the patient bleeding and, second, if from varices, what is the basis of the varices, e.g., liver disease, portal vein thrombosis. The physical examination is directed towards signs of chronic liver disease, such as hepatosplenomegaly, spider angiomata, icterus, encephalopathy, ascites, and evidence of a bleeding diathesis, such as petechiae and ecchymoses.

A nasogastric tube is then placed and the stomach is lavaged with iced isotonic saline solution to ascertain whether or not there is active bleeding and to prepare the patient for endoscopy. Gastric lavage is facilitated by the use of a #18 French Levin tube with an air vent, which prevents the occlusion of the tip of the tube by mucosa sucked against it. If large clots are present, an Ewald tube is preferred. During gastric lavage an attempt is made to stabilize the vital signs with appropriate replacement of volume, preferably in the form of fresh whole blood. The patient is moved to an intensive care unit as soon as possible and will undoubtedly require the insertion of a central venous catheter and a Foley catheter for more accurate monitoring of central venous pressure and urinary output, respectively. If there are signs of congestive heart failure or any question as to the cardiovascular status of the patient, a Swan-Ganz catheter should be placed and appropriately monitored.

The management of a patient with bleeding esophageal varices requires a team approach. Both the internist, preferably a gastroenterologist, and the surgeon should evaluate the patient and jointly plan the tentative therapeutic approach. Endoscopy should be performed as soon as possible to establish the site of the gastrointestinal bleeding. Once it is clear that one is dealing with bleeding gastroesophageal varices, and sometimes earlier if conditions warrant it, peripheral vasopressin therapy is begun. The initial infusion of 20 units of vasopressin (Pitressin) in 100 ml. of D5W is infused over 20 minutes while the apparatus to institute continuous intravenous infusion is being set up. (This use of vasopressin is not listed in the manufacturer's official directive.) Four hundred units of vasopressin (Pitressin) is added to a solution of 500 ml. of D5W and is infused ideally through an infusion pump at a rate of 30 ml. per hour which will deliver 0.4 unit of vasopressin (Pitressin) per minute. Constant electrocardiographic (ECG) monitoring for cardiac complications is required at this infusion rate. If vasopressin infusion is successful in stopping the bleeding, the patient is weaned off the therapy gradually. After 24 hours of 0.4 unit per minute, the rate is reduced to 0.3 unit per minute for 12 hours, then 0.2 unit per minute for 8 hours, then 0.1 unit per minute over an additional 6 to 8 hours.

Lactulose in a dose of 30 ml. four times daily is given through the nasogastric tube to prevent or treat hepatic encephalopathy, and parenteral vitamin K should also be given to ensure adequate substrate for prothrombin synthesis. The nasogastric tube is attached to low continuous suction, which is stopped hourly for the instillation of antacids. If bleeding continues in spite of peripheral vasopressin therapy, however, a Sengstaken-Blakemore tube should be properly placed after it has been checked for proper function and for possible leaks. The gastric balloon is not inflated until the tube tip has been passed into the stomach and proper placement has been confirmed by monitoring over the epigastric area with a stethoscope while flushing air through the tube. Inflation of the balloon is then done slowly and stopped immediately if resistance to the inflation is felt or the patient complains of pain. A total of 300 ml. is instilled into the balloon which is then held against the gastroesophageal junction by traction. A properly equipped helmet for continuous traction in the range of 1 to 2 pounds of pressure is available (Preston Traction Unit, E.J.T. Industries, Inc., Chicago, Illinois). When the helmet is used, petrolatum gauze is placed on the forehead and chin, as well as foam padding, to avoid pressure injuries from the helmet. The straps on the helmet are adjusted to ensure a snug fit. All patients in whom the Sengstaken-Blakemore tube is used should be intubated with an endotracheal tube to prevent aspiration. Diazepam, in a dose of 2.5 mg. given slowly through an intravenous route, will help to sedate the patient for endotracheal as well as Sengstaken-Blakemore intubation. An additional nasogastric tube is inserted through the open naris to aspirate secretions above the gastric and esophageal balloons as they accumulate. If bleeding continues, the esophageal balloon is inflated and maintained at a pressure between 30 and 45 mm. Hg. The esophageal balloon is connected via a Y connector to a manometer, which is used to monitor the pressure on an hourly basis. The tube connected with the gastric balloon is clamped and taped to prevent leakage. A scissors should be available to cut across both balloon tubes if any signs of occlusion of the airway by the balloons develop. The gastric tube is attached to intermittent suction and lavaged every 30 minutes. If bleeding stops, the esophageal balloon should be kept inflated for 24 hours, but the esophageal balloon should be periodically deflated for a few minutes to prevent pressure necrosis. The esophageal balloon is then gradually deflated over one and a half hours and the patient monitored for evidence of recurrent bleeding. After 24 hours, if bleeding has not recurred, the gastric balloon is taken off the traction but left inflated to maintain the position for an additional 24 hours prior to being removed. An attempt should be made to maintain the hematocrit at about 30 per cent through the management of the gastrointestinal hemorrhage.

If bleeding is not controlled with the Sengstaken-Blakemore tube, the patient is sent to the radiology department, where arteriography is carried out. First celiac, then superior mesenteric arteriography is performed. Tolazoline (Priscoline), in a dose of 25 mg. in 10 ml. of saline, is injected into the superior mesenteric artery over a 30 second period before the arteriography. (This use of tolazoline is not listed in the manufacturer's official directive.) This will allow for better visualization of the venous phase depicting the portal vein and its collaterals. The arteriography is done for three reasons: first, to characterize the direction of blood flow through the portal vein, i.e., toward the liver (hepatopetal) or away from the liver (hepatofugal), in anticipation of surgery; second, to look for evidence of a hypervascular tumor, e.g., hepatocellular carcinoma in the liver; and third, to look for other possible sites of bleeding, e.g., a Mallory-Weiss lesion or previously undetected bleeding ulcer. A wedged hepatic venous pressure, as well as hepatic venography is done to determine if one is dealing with postsinusoidal portal hypertension, which is typical of cirrhosis, or a presinusoidal process, e.g., portal vein thrombosis, schistosomiasis. Hepatic venography will establish whether or not the portal vein is patent in the presence of hepatofugal flow. A portogram, utilizing a portal vein catheter passed percutaneously, is then attempted. Twelve to 15 passes through the liver may be necessary. The needle is directed toward the right horizontal branch of the portal vein, which was previously delineated on the venous phase of the arteriogram. Once the portal vein is entered, selective catheterization and embolization of the left gastric or coronary vein with a Gelfoam preparation is performed. Additional collaterals may have to be thrombosed to stop the bleeding. This technique requires a skilled radiologist but can be accomplished usually within 2 to 4 hours. If, in spite of all these measures, bleeding continues, an emergency shunt procedure is planned. At surgery, if bleeding is uncontrolled, the stomach is opened and the varices are oversewn; then preparations are made for a definitive shunt procedure.

Whether or not the shunt is done on an emergency basis or, as is more often the case, on an elective basis, the type of shunt is tailored to the portal hemodynamic and anatomic pattern, which has been characterized radiographically. When it is apparent that blood flow through the portal vein is primarily toward the liver, hepatopetal, a selective decompressive shunt (distal splenorenal shunt) is performed. Less commonly, the hemodynamic pattern is hepatofugal and under such circumstances a "central" shunt is performed, e.g., portacaval, mesocaval, mesorenal. Prior to the performance of an elective shunt, every attempt is made to maximize the patient's nutritional status, to mobilize ascites, to correct encephalopathy, and to treat active liver necrosis.

CHOLECYSTITIS AND CHOLELITHIASIS

method of
RONALD K. TOMPKINS, M.D.,
F.A.C.S.
Los Angeles, California

Operative treatment of gallstones and their complications is among the safest of major surgical procedures because of advances in pre- and post-operative care, earlier diagnosis, and the more widespread realization that asymptomatic gallstones should not be allowed to remain until they cause serious pain or complications. Indeed, elective operation for gallstones in experienced hands now carries a mortality risk of only 2 per 1000 operations and is 95 per cent curative. This article will attempt to detail current surgical therapy that should result in this favorable outcome.

Definitive Medical Treatment of Cholelithiasis

It is important to realize that, at this writing, experiments are being carried out with agents that have the potential for dissolving human gallstones in vivo. Two of these, lecithin and chenodeoxycholic acid, have been the subject of many reports. Lecithin, a phospholipid, has not been shown to dissolve preexisting stones in several patients who have taken up to 48 grams a day of a commercial product for two years. Bile from these patients, however, has been shown to be less saturated with cholesterol, thus raising hopes that lecithin might be a preventive agent in patients at high risk of forming gallstones. Lecithin has been found very safe when taken in large doses.

On the other hand, chenodeoxycholic acid, a primary bile acid, has been associated with the disappearance of gallstones in humans ingesting 0.75 to 1.0 gram daily for periods up to 2.5 years or more. In one series from Guy's Hospital in London, 50 per cent of patients treated for 1 year with chenodeoxycholic acid showed disappearance of their gallstones. Unfortunately, about 50 per cent of these patients had recurrence of gallstones 6 months to 1 year after stopping chenodeoxycholic acid ingestion. At this writing, there is a National Cooperative Gallstone Study underway in the United States to evaluate the safety and efficacy of chenodeoxycholic acid therapy. The results should be available within 2 to 3 years. Until the results are available, the drug remains strictly experimental and cannot be prescribed in the United States.

Chronic Cholecystitis and Cholelithiasis

Operative removal of the gallbladder and gallstones remains the only proven cure for this malady. We favor early elective operation in patients unless some medical problem such as hypertension, recent myocardial infarction (within 6 months), or other illness requiring medical control prevents surgery. In patients with frequent attacks, some of these contraindications become relatively less restrictive. Obesity has often been used as a reason to delay operation. In our experience, patients have not been successful in losing large amounts of weight and therefore we do not use obesity per se as a contraindication for elective operation. This is especially true if, when the patient lies supine on the examining table, the costal margins in the midclavicular line are visible. This finding indicates lax obesity, and these patients do not present unusual technical difficulties because of the thickness of their abdominal wall at the time of operation.

Patients with diabetes, whether requiring insulin or not, should be given the opportunity of early elective cholecystectomy since, as a group, they tend to have higher mortality and morbidity risks with the complications of acute cholecystitis, jaundice, or pancreatitis. Diagnosis of the gallstones is usually made by oral cholecystography. If nonvisualization occurs on double-dose cholecystography, we use ultrasound to examine the gallbladder and confirm the presence of stones. We have tended away from the use of intravenous cholangiography with the increasing effectiveness and reliability of grey-scale ultrasonography. One should consider surveying the upper and lower gastrointestinal tract with contrast as well as performing an intravenous pyelogram (IVP) before operation for demonstrated gallstones. There may often be concomitant gastrointestinal or renal pathology that may mimic cholecystitis and for which cholecystectomy would not provide relief.

Our patients are prepared for operation with povidone-iodine (Betadine) abdominal scrubs on the day prior to surgery. They are placed on a clear liquid diet the afternoon before operation and tap water or saline enemas are given the night before to evacuate the colon. Cathartics are usually not given, lest they cause abdominal cramping. Prophylactic antibiotics are not used in the elective cases since only 30 per cent of these patients will have bacteria in the gallbladder bile and the gallbladder is rarely entered during the operative procedure. We no longer routinely type and cross match these patients for blood since the frequency of giving blood during cholecystectomy has been nil. Instead, we type the patients and if transfusions are necessary during the operation, blood is cross-matched at that time.

On the day of operation, a solution of 5 per cent dextrose and Ringer's lactate given intravenously is started preoperatively unless the patient has some medical condition (such as cardiac insufficiency or hepatic disease or is on corticosteroids) that renders them susceptible to salt overloading. The patient is placed on an x-ray cassette table with the right arm at the side and positioned with the right side of the patient at the edge of the table. When anesthesia has been induced, the left shoulder is elevated on folded sheets to elevate the patient's left side 15°. This rotates the area of the ampulla of Vater to the right of the spinal column and facilitates visualization of the entire bile duct during cystic duct cholangiography. It is important to also elevate the left arm on towels so that brachial plexus stretch does not occur. If the anesthesiologist permits, the left arm can be placed at the patient's side as well. A rubber Levin tube is passed into the stomach by the anesthetist after the patient has been premedicated.

Although it takes a bit longer, we prefer a right subcostal incision for its superior exposure and lower incidence of postoperative muscle spasm and wound herniation. Thorough exploration of the abdomen is carried out and then the gallbladder is exposed by retracting the duodenum medially and the right colon inferiorly. If the area of the cystic duct–common duct junction (Triangle of Calot) is easily visualized, we begin by incising the anterior and posterior layers of parietal peritoneum there and encircle the cystic duct with two 2-0 silks. The cystic duct is traced into the ampulla of the gallbladder and the distal 2-0 silk is ligated at this junction only when the surgeon is convinced that it indeed is the cystic duct and not an aberrant duct. The 2-0 silk nearest the common duct is left untied and both silks are used as retraction devices while a transverse incision is made in the cystic duct between them. A malleable steel probe is passed down the cystic duct to dilate the spiral valves of Heister and an 18 gauge cholangiocatheter, or pediatric feeding tube, which has been filled with saline to eliminate all air bubbles, is passed into the cystic duct and secured in place with the proximal 2-0 silk. Aspiration of bile confirms the tube's position in the duct and cholangiograms are taken. Fifty ml. of 60 per cent meglumine diatrizoate (Renografin) is diluted into 100 ml. of isotonic saline solution to make a 20 per cent contrast solution and 7 ml. of

this solution is then injected into the cystic duct catheter and a film taken. A second film is taken after infusion of 15 to 20 ml. of dye while the surgeon's fingers compress the ampulla or distal common duct to allow visualization of the intrahepatic ducts. These films are reviewed in the operating room and the surgeon's impression is checked with a radiologist.

While x-rays are being developed and interpreted, the surgeon proceeds with identification and ligation of the cystic artery with 2-0 silk and subserosal dissection of the gallbladder from its bed in the liver. Prior to dissecting the gallbladder, we obtain a needle biopsy of the liver for permanent record of any coexistent intrahepatic disease and a sample of bile is aspirated into a syringe through a needle placed in the fundus of the gallbladder. The bile is cultured for aerobic and anaerobic bacteria, and a clamp is placed on the needle puncture site to prevent spillage of bile while the gallbladder is being dissected.

If the cystic duct cholangiogram is normal, the cystic duct stump is trimmed and ligated near the common duct with 2-0 silk. In addition, a medium hemostatic clip is applied to the cystic duct stump for radiologic identification in event of future problems related to the biliary system.

It is seldom necessary to divide the ligamentum teres in the subcostal approach. We do not use hemostatic clips for control of bleeding but rely on fine silk ties. The gallbladder bed is reperitonealized and a 1 inch Penrose drain is placed in the Foramen of Winslow, led out along the gallbladder bed through a stab wound in the right flank.

There is no question that removal of the gallbladder from the fundus downward (antegrade method) is a safer, although bloodier, procedure. We use this method frequently when the region of the cystic duct-common duct junction is not easily visualized. Removal of the gallbladder from the fundus downward allows more certain visualization of the cystic duct and cystic artery in difficult cases.

Serum amylase and venous hematocrit are determined the evening of operation. If the amylase is normal, the nasogastric tube is removed the first morning after operation and the patient is begun on clear liquids by mouth. The Penrose drain is removed 24 hours after operation if no bile staining is seen. Otherwise, it is left in place as long as indicated by any bile drainage. Patients are usually discharged between 5 and 7 days postoperatively.

Acute Cholecystitis

Approximately 6 per cent of all biliary tract operations in our experience are done for acute cholecystitis. All patients in whom the diagnosis of acute cholecystitis is strongly suspected are admitted to the hospital for treatment and observation, since the course of the disease is unpredictable. Initial diagnostic tests include liver function tests, amylase and creatinine in serum and urine for calculation of amylase-creatinine clearance ratios, and complete blood count with differential. Chest and abdominal x-rays and ultrasound examination of the liver, biliary tract and pancreas are obtained.

Initial treatment consists of stopping oral intake, inserting a nasogastric tube, beginning intravenous hydration with 5 per cent dextrose in Ringer's lactate and intravenous antibiotics, either ampicillin, 500 mg. every 6 hours, or a cephalosporin, 1 gram every 6 hours. Seventy-five to 100 mg. of meperidine every 3 to 4 hours is given for pain relief after physical examination has been performed. Morphine and morphinelike drugs are to be avoided, as they constrict the sphincter of Oddi and may raise intrabiliary pressure. If the patient is unable to tolerate meperidine, levorphanol tartrate (Levo-Dromoran) may be substituted. This synthetic narcotic does not constrict the sphincter of Oddi to any appreciable degree and is given in dosages of 2 mg. subcutaneously every 4 to 6 hours.

The patient is observed by repeated physical examination, white blood count, and vital signs at least every 4 hours. If a temperature of 102°F. (38.9°C.) or a pulse of 120 per minute occurs or persists after hydration; or a white blood count of 20,000 or above is noted; or hydrops of the gallbladder is detected, the patient is taken to the operating room as an emergency. A cholecystectomy and operative cholangiogram are performed, as about 12 per cent of these patients will have coexistent common duct stones. Approximately 70 per cent of acute cholecystitis patients will have bacteria recoverable from the bile at operation, hence we place all of these patients on antibiotics preoperatively.

In a series of more than 150 cases of acute cholecystitis, 60 per cent of patients responded to initial medical management and underwent elective cholecystectomy within 5 to 10 days of admission. Twenty per cent responded to initial medical management, but symptoms recurred with initiation of a diet, and these patients, plus an additional 20 per cent who did not respond at all to medical measures, underwent emergency operation. Thus, it was possible to convert more than half of all patients entering with acute cholecystitis to an elective operation with a mortality risk 14 times lower than the 2.8 per cent mortality observed in our emergency series.

We do cholecystostomy in those poor risk patients who require emergency biliary decompression under local anesthesia. When this procedure is done, we try to follow it in 4 to 6 weeks with cholecystectomy if the patient's condition permits. It is important to perform a cholangiogram at the time of cholecystostomy, since the failure to remove obstructing stones of the common duct will lead to the patient's continuing cholangitis and sepsis.

Acalculous Cholecystitis

This entity accounts for about 5 per cent of all acute cholecystitis and therefore represents only 0.3 per cent of all biliary tract surgical procedures done in most hospitals. In its acute stage, it is most often seen in the postoperative patient who frequently has undergone an operative procedure remote from the abdomen. The time of onset may vary from 2 to 14 days after such an operation and the abdominal pain may be misdiagnosed in such patients. Males and children have a higher incidence of acalculous acute cholecystitis. Gangrene and perforation tend to occur early in the course of the disease. Ultrasound often makes the diagnosis by showing a distended or edematous ("fuzzy walled") gallbladder. Mortality risks range from 36 per cent in the cholecystitis stage to 88 per cent if perforation occurs. The mortality risk is much higher in older patients. The cause of the disease is not known.

In its chronic stage, acalculous cholecystitis is seen in association with cholesterolosis ("strawberry gallbladder"), cholesterol polyps, and adenomyoma (either single or multiple). We recommend that patients with recurrent symptoms related to these lesions undergo elective cholecystectomy. Our experience has been that pain is relieved in almost all these patients by removal of the gallbladder.

Relatively Asymptomatic Gallstones

There is difficulty in decision making regarding proper treatment for patients with so-called "silent gallstones." Among the questions that arise is whether they really are silent or whether their symptoms are mild or atypical. Another problem is that there are no epidemiologic studies to determine the actual incidence of such stones. Data from Europe indicate that 25 per cent of males and 44 per cent of females autopsied between the ages of 10 and 99 years have gallstones, while only 4 per cent of males and 7 per cent of females have had previous cholecystectomy. Thus it may be that 85 per cent of gallstones in this population are "silent," i.e., did not require cholecystectomy. These are imperfect data, but no good prospective surveys of representative American population groups have been done.

Finally, there is a problem with our knowledge of the natural history of gallstone disease in a given patient. Again, from Europe there are longitudinal data on patients with cholelithiasis who had mild to severe symptoms which demonstrated that 51 per cent developed symptoms between 1 and 11 years after diagnosis. The incidence of emergency operation in this group of patients was 13 per cent within the first year with a mortality of 15 per cent. Emergency operations were needed in 18 per cent of the patients followed beyond 1 year with a similarly high mortality.

Our approach has been to recommend elective cholecystectomy, with its very low mortality risk and high cure rate, to patients with "silent gallstones" if they are satisfactory operative risks, have a life expectancy of several years, have an informed understanding of the risk to benefit ratio, and that no safe and effective nonsurgical therapy is available.

Common Duct Stones

Approximately 7 to 14 per cent of patients having cholecystectomy with and without common duct exploration will have recurrent or retained gallstones. Five per cent of these will be unsuspected at the time of cholecystectomy and can only be recognized by cystic duct cholangiography done routinely at cholecystectomy. The remainder are those stones that either are left behind or recur after common duct exploration.

Recently, a prospective, multicenter trial has demonstrated that the addition of operative choledochoscopy to the usual exploration of the common duct plus completion cholangiography after the T tube is in place will lower the incidence of unsuspected retained common duct stones to zero.

We utilize operative choledochoscopy and cholangiography in all patients in whom the common duct has been opened. In addition to the discovery of unsuspected retained stones, tumors of the bile ducts have been observed in a few patients by this endoscopic procedure.

CIRRHOSIS

method of
STEPHEN C. WRIGHT, M.D.,
and NORMAN D. GRACE, M.D.
Boston, Massachusetts

Introduction

Cirrhosis of the liver can be defined as a chronic progressive fibrotic reaction that follows a variety of hepatic injuries and is characterized by regenerative nodules that distort the normal lobular architecture. The therapeutic management of this disease, therefore, is twofold: (1) measures aimed at eliminating, where possible, the injurious agents responsible for the fibrogenesis and (2) measures aimed at managing the complications of cirrhosis once it is established.

Therapeutic Measures to Eliminate Progressive Hepatic Fibrosis

Chronic Active Hepatitis. As has been emphasized in several recent editorials, clear, universally accepted criteria for the diagnosis of chronic active hepatitis have been difficult to obtain, thus leading to confusion in the interpretation of the data dealing with treatment of this problem. Since it is not the purpose of this text to give a detailed analysis of the conflicting data, certain general assumptions can be made. Most investigators would accept as chronic active hepatitis a clinical course of at least 10 weeks with abnormal transaminases (or other tests of hepatocyte injury), increased gamma globulin, and histologic evidence of hepatitis with piecemeal necrosis and bridging. The additional features of bridging necrosis, multilobular necrosis, or cirrhosis may also be present. It is important to exclude other disorders that can produce a similar histologic picture such as drug induced chronic hepatitis (oxyphenisatin, methyldopa [Aldomet], aspirin, etc.), primary biliary cirrhosis, alcoholic liver disease, or Wilson's disease. Once the diagnosis is clearly established, patients tend to fall into three groups that need to be considered separately in determining the proper course of treatment. Since the accepted therapeutic agents, corticosteroids and immunosuppressive agents, have the potential for serious complications, the risk-benefit ratio must be kept clearly in mind.

GROUP I. Asymptomatic patients with chronic active hepatitis. Of three published controlled trials dealing with chronic active hepatitis, none have included asymptomatic patients with mild to moderate abnormalities of liver function tests. Since the natural history of this illness is variable, with the possibility that some of these patients may never progress beyond this initial stage, it is difficult to recommend treating them based on our current knowledge. A controlled trial in this group is clearly needed. At present, careful follow-up would seem to be the only reasonable course.

GROUP II. Symptomatic patients with chronic active hepatitis. In those patients with the histologic lesion limited to chronic active hepatitis, patients in the treatment groups have had a good response. However, very few patients with this lesion in the control groups have been shown to progress to cirrhosis. Therefore, the decision to treat needs to take into consideration the degree of biochemical abnormality and the potential risk of treatment to any coexisting disorders. Based on the results of the controlled trials, the preferred treatment schedule is a combination of prednisone, 10 mg., and azathioprine, 50 mg. per day. (This use of azathioprine is not listed in the manufacturer's official directive.) The prednisone is usually started at 30 to 40 mg. per day and then tapered over a few weeks to the maintenance dose. Treatment is continued until biochemical and histologic remission is achieved. Since there is a high relapse rate (up to 50 per cent in one study), treatment may need to be reinstituted. This course of therapy has been shown to be superior to azathioprine alone or alternate day steroids. Although the remission rate is similar to higher doses of steroids used alone, azathioprine in combination with steroids allows the use of a lower dose of steroids and thus fewer steroid complications.

GROUP III. Subacute hepatitis with bridging necrosis (SHB), subacute hepatitis with multilobular necrosis (SHMN), or chronic active hepatitis with cirrhosis. All three controlled trials have found steroids or combination therapy to be beneficial to this group of patients. The mortality was significantly less in the treated group, with corresponding improvement in biochemical and histologic features. Treatment failure was associated with the presence of hepatitis B surface antigen (HB$_s$Ag), a longer duration of symptoms, a more prolonged prothrombin time or higher serum glutamic oxaloacetic transaminase (SGOT) levels, and the presence of SHMN or cirrhosis. The treatment schedule for these patients is the same as outlined for Group II patients.

Wilson's Disease (Hepatolenticular Degeneration). Wilson's disease is an inherited autosomal recessive disorder characterized by cirrhosis of the liver, degeneration of the basal ganglia of the brain, and greenish-brown pigmented rings in the periphery of the cornea (Kayser-Fleischer rings). A defect in copper mobilization and transport leads to excessive accumulation of copper in the affected organs, resulting in tissue damage. Thus, treatment is aimed at depleting copper stores in affected patients and also asymptomatic heterozygous relatives. Penicillamine, a chelating agent that binds copper, is the treatment of choice. The usual dose is 250 mg. given orally 3 to 4 times a day, which can result in urinary excretion of as much as 3000 mg. of copper per day. In severe cases, the dose can be increased up to 2.0 grams per day. Once the copper stores are depleted, the patients should be maintained on 900 to 1200 mg. per day. Unfortunately, penicillamine has its complications, which include the nephrotic syndrome, skin rashes, leukopenia, and a lupus-like syndrome. Because of penicillamine's effect

on pyridoxine, it is advisable to give supplemental pyridoxine, 50 mg. orally twice per week. For patients who cannot tolerate penicillamine, other chelating agents such as BAL or triethylene tetramine dihydrochloride have been used but are not as effective. Finally, the physician should render genetic counseling to patients with this disorder.

Hemochromatosis (See also p. 280). Hemochromatosis is best defined as a pathologic entity characterized by cirrhosis or fibrosis of the liver with increased iron stores, primarily in the parenchymal cells of the liver, but also in other organs including the pancreas, heart, and pituitary gland. Iron may also be present in Kupffer cells. Diabetes mellitus and skin pigmentation are often present but are not essential for diagnosis. This definition would include the following entities: idiopathic (familial) hemochromatosis, cirrhosis of the liver with secondary iron overload (e.g., alcoholic liver disease), liver disease associated with certain anemias (e.g., thalassemia), liver disease associated with dietary iron overload (e.g., Bantu), and liver disease associated with transfusions.

Treatment of these entities is predicated on the assumption that increased iron stores are harmful to the hepatocyte. The evidence to support this concept is controversial. Despite numerous attempts over the years, an animal model in which increased iron, given either orally or parenterally, causes a pathologic entity similar to human hemochromatosis is lacking. There is some recent evidence on the cellular level that when the usual cellular mechanisms for handling iron are exceeded in the iron overload state, there is a rupture of lysosomal sacs with release of hydrolytic enzymes which cause cell destruction.

At the clinical level, the efficacy of the use of phlebotomy or chelating agents to remove excess iron stores needs to be considered separately for the entities listed above.

IDIOPATHIC (FAMILIAL) HEMOCHROMATOSIS (SEE ALSO P. 280). Based on a series of case reports starting in 1942 and a few recent retrospective studies, removal of excess iron stores via phlebotomy in both patients with hemochromatosis and relatives with increased iron stores in the latent or precirrhotic stage is thought to be beneficial. This is usually done by removing 1 to 2 units of blood per week until the patient develops evidence of iron deficiency anemia as reflected in the peripheral blood smear, red cell indices, reticulocytopenia, decreased (< 15 per cent) saturation of transferrin, and decreased serum ferritin levels. When this point is reached (usually when the hematocrit falls to around 80 per cent of the pretreatment level), deficient iron stores should be confirmed by bone marrow and liver biopsy. The patients should then be maintained in a mild iron deficient state by periodic phlebotomy. In one large study recently published, patients receiving this form of therapy showed improvement in survival as well as in liver function, decrease in liver size, and decrease in skin pigmentation. The effect on diabetes was variable, although there was no improvement in hypogonadism, arthropathy, or portal hypertension. Other studies have shown those patients with cardiac involvement to benefit. However, the most disturbing feature of recent studies is the failure of removal of excess iron to prevent the development of hepatoma in up to 25 to 30 per cent of patients.

THALASSEMIA MAJOR (SEE ALSO P. 255). In contrast to idiopathic hemochromatosis, a well controlled prospective study has been performed in children with β thalassemia major, in which the results indicated a marked reduction in hepatic iron accumulation that was associated with a significant retardation in the progression of hepatic fibrosis. Since these patients were anemic, they were treated with 500 mg. deferoxamine intramuscularly for 6 days per week to deplete excess iron stores. Chelating agents were also added to any blood transfusions they received. Larger quantities of iron may be removed by continuous intravenous infusion of deferoxamine. In addition to impeding hepatic fibrosis, patients receiving the chelating agents had a normal onset of puberty compared to the control group. There is no conclusive data yet on the effect of chelation therapy on survival.

LIVER DISEASE ASSOCIATED WITH SECONDARY IRON OVERLOAD. In contrast to the previously discussed conditions, both retrospective and prospective studies have shown that phlebotomy treatment of patients with alcoholic liver disease and secondary iron overload does not increase survival or decrease morbidity when compared to patients treated with standard medical therapy. There is no data in patients with nonalcoholic liver disease and secondary iron overload on which to base a therapeutic discussion.

Primary Biliary Cirrhosis. Primary biliary cirrhosis is a disease of unknown cause, but with significant immunologic associations, that largely affects middle-aged women. It is a disease of insidious cholestasis, often presenting with pruritus as the initial symptom, which slowly progresses to deep jaundice and ultimately liver failure. The disease may remain asymptomatic for many years. In the liver, small bile ducts are destroyed and surrounded by granuloma in the initial stage. The lesions then progress to a stage of ductular proliferation, scarring, and finally cirrhosis with paucity of bile ducts. Associated diseases include rheumatoid arthritis, arteritis, glomerulitis and the sicca syndrome. There is a familial clustering

of cases, with more than 90 per cent of patients demonstrating a positive antimitochondrial antibody in the serum.

At present, there is no validated treatment of the primary hepatic lesion. Steroids and immunosuppressive agents such as azathioprine have not been successful when subjected to controlled trials. The most promising agent is penicillamine, currently being studied by three groups in a prospective fashion. The basis for this treatment is the high copper levels that accumulate in patients with primary biliary cirrhosis, often equalling or exceeding the amounts found in Wilson's disease. The retention of the copper is probably due to decreased biliary excretion. Copper concentration correlates with the stage of primary biliary cirrhosis, suggesting that the continuous increase in copper concentration may be hepatotoxic. Support for copper acting as a hepatotoxin is found in experimental animals, acute poisoning, and Wilson's disease.

In the three current trials, the patients have received 1.0 to 1.2 grams of penicillamine per day. As expected, the initial data show a significant reduction in hepatic copper in the treatment groups. The data are too premature to assess the effect on hepatic histology or survival.

Since there is no specific treatment for primary biliary cirrhosis, treatment is aimed toward relief of symptoms and prevention of complications. One of the most annoying symptoms is pruritus secondary to retention of bile salts. This is usually effectively treated with cholestyramine, an anion exchange resin, which interrupts the enterohepatic circulation of bile salts by binding them in the gut. The usual dose is 4 grams orally three times daily, but the lowest effective dose is preferable, since cholestyramine may aggravate the steatorrhea that occurs in this disease. Because of the problems with fat absorption, supplemental vitamins A, D, and K are often needed, given either orally or parenterally as conditions warrant. Also, medium chain triglycerides have been successfully used as a dietary supplement for patients on a low-fat intake. Osteoporosis can be a debilitating complication, requiring calcium supplements in addition to vitamin D. Complications such as portal hypertension with esophageal hemorrhage or hepatic encephalopathy are treated in the usual fashion, discussed in the next section.

Alcoholic Hepatitis. In a patient with a history of excessive alcohol consumption, a liver biopsy showing hepatocyte necrosis with a leukocyte infiltrate associated with fat and alcoholic hyaline is defined as alcoholic hepatitis. This is a potentially reversible lesion and the patient should be advised to abstain from further alcohol consumption and to consume a well-balanced diet.

Folic acid supplements, 1.0 to 2.0 mg. per day, are often helpful, since these patients usually have an associated folic acid deficiency. A variety of agents have been examined in an attempt to prevent progression to cirrhosis. Of these, the most widely tested has been the use of corticosteroids with conflicting results in controlled trials. If useful, the group that seems to respond best are those patients with moderately severe lesion, often associated with hepatic encephalopathy. The accepted regimen is 40 mg. of prednisolone daily for 30 days, and then tapered over a 2 week period.

Cardiac Cirrhosis. Treatment of cardiac cirrhosis should be aimed at the underlying cause, minimizing the degree of hepatic congestion.

Therapeutic Measures to Control the Complications of Cirrhosis

Bleeding Esophagogastric Varices. See page 335.

Hepatorenal Syndrome. Hepatorenal syndrome is defined as functional renal failure in the setting of advanced liver disease. The physiologic defect appears to be one of maldistribution of renal blood flow with shunting of blood away from renal cortex with preferential perfusion of the renal medulla. It is usually associated with hyponatremia, oliguria (less than 300 ml. per 24 hours), very low urine sodium values (usually less than 10 mEq. per liter) and rapidly developing azotemia. This diagnosis can only be established by excluding all other reversible causes of renal failure, including sepsis, prerenal factors (such as volume depletion, low cardiac output) and postrenal factors (such as obstruction). This condition, once clearly established, almost always follows an inexorable downhill course and carries with it a high fatality rate.

Treatment of this entity is largely supportive once other causes of renal failure have been diligently sought and treated. Occasionally, volume expansion with salt-poor albumin may be associated with a transient increase in urine output, but response raises the question of volume depletion. Similarly, furosemide administration, in the presence of adequate circulating volume, may be associated with a transient improvement. Caution must be exercised, however, as the administration of diuretics often precedes the hepatorenal syndrome and, though not causally related to the syndrome, prerenal dehydration is easily induced in these patients.

Alternative support measures such as hemodialysis, peritoneal dialysis, and intra-arterial (renal) infusion of sympathomimetic amines have failed to improve renal function consistently. The hepatorenal syndrome continues to carry a grave prognosis.

Ascites. The accumulation of ascites is a common complication of cirrhosis, especially in its more advanced stages. The physiologic defects are multiple, but central to ascites formation is the inappropriate retention of sodium such that most ascitic cirrhotics will have elevated total body sodium, despite hyponatremia. Examination of the urine will usually reveal a sodium output that is less than the intake, and the cirrhotic will gain weight in the form of ascites. Ascitic fluid must be examined microscopically and bacteriologically to be certain it is of neither neoplastic nor inflammatory origin prior to initiation of therapy.

Recognizing the defect as one of inappropriate sodium (and water) retention, therapeutic measures are those aimed at (1) decreasing the oral intake of sodium and water, (2) enhancing the renal clearance of sodium, and (3) enhancing free water clearance. Dietary sodium restriction is usually essential to mobilize ascites and in some patients this will be all that is required. Diets with less than 1 gram of sodium are unpalatable and patient acceptance is poor. If urine sodium values are elevated while a patient is on a presumed salt-free diet and still gaining weight, one conclusion is that dietary sodium indiscretion is likely, and further dietary counseling will be necessary.

Diuretic administration is the next mainstay in the mobilization of ascitic fluid, though great caution must be exercised. The rate at which fluid may be mobilized from the ascitic compartment is limited, probably to about 900 ml. per day. Therefore, weight loss of greater than 2 pounds per day (purely from the abdomen) usually means the patient may be losing from his circulating volume as well, and prerenal dehydration becomes a concern. The first diuretic of choice is spironolactone, which can be administered as a single daily dose orally, beginning at 50 to 100 mg. and escalating dosage until the desired effect is achieved. If no response is noted after 200 to 300 mg. daily, then furosemide may be added, again with great caution. Serum potassium levels must be followed closely as a low sodium diet is an obligate high potassium diet and spironolactone interferes with the renal clearance of potassium. Rapidly developing hyperkalemia may complicate this program.

Hyponatremia is a common finding in the ascitic cirrhotic and usually requires no treatment. Many cirrhotics have serum sodiums in the 125 to 130 mEq. per liter range. Falling serum sodium values should be managed by restricting oral fluid intake (with careful attention to blood urea nitrogen and creatinine levels). Only in cases of severe hyponatremia with impending central nervous system (CNS) disturbances should parenteral hypertonic saline be given, as its intravascular retention will be very brief and it will ultimately only aggravate the ascites formation. Hyponatremia of a worsening degree often precedes the development of the hepatorenal syndrome.

Additional maneuvers include the intravenous administration of salt-poor albumin, but this effect is short-lived and costly. The removal of large volumes of fluid via paracentesis should be reserved only for those patients in whom ascites accumulation is massive enough to cause respiratory embarrassment. Finally, in severe medically-refractory ascites formation, the placement of a peritoneoatrial shunt (LeVeen) may be necessary.

Hepatic Encephalopathy. Hepatic encephalopathy can be defined as a spontaneously developing state of cerebral dysfunction in the setting of advanced hepatic insufficiency. The central nervous system (CNS) derangements are presumed secondary to the accumulation of toxic substances normally cleared from the circulation by the healthy liver. Clinically, the syndrome varies from mild symptoms to confusion, disinterest, and disorder of normal sleep rhythm, with asterixis present to deep coma and flaccid paralysis. Often patients may change levels of impairment depending on the presence and successful treatment of numerous "precipitating factors." These factors include gastrointestinal bleeding, injudicious sedative administration, fluid and electrolyte imbalance (especially hypokalemia and alkalosis), azotemia, sepsis, and even constipation. Hypoglycemia and CNS trauma, especially in the alcoholic, must be rigorously excluded before the diagnosis of hepatic encephalopathy can be established.

The primary treatment of hepatic encephalopathy therefore, is the elucidation of precipitating factors and, where possible, their elimination. In large studies of patients with this syndrome, offending agents or metabolic derangements can often be found. In addition, the oral administration of neomycin, 1 gram orally four times daily, or lactulose, 15 ml. orally three times daily (endpoint is the induction of 2 to 3 loose stools per day), has been associated with improvement. As the breakdown of dietary protein is thought to be a major contributor to the pathogenesis of this syndrome, dietary protein restriction to the level of 40 to 60 grams per day is also useful. Depending on the severity of the encephalopathy, some cirrhotics may require temporary total protein withdrawal from the diet. This maneuver can be a two-edged sword however, as cirrhotics, especially alcoholic cirrhotics, need optimal substrate of protein for hepatic repair and protein synthesis.

Spontaneous Bacterial Peritonitis. This complication of chronic cirrhosis with ascites is said to occur at a frequency of about 8 per cent. Clinically, the syndrome may be characterized by fever, abdominal pain, abdominal tenderness and hepatic encephalopathy, although all of these features may be absent. Early recognition of the peritonitis is critical, as infection is poorly tolerated in cirrhosis, attested to by a survival rate of 40 per cent. The mechanism by which the peritonitis becomes established is unclear. It has been speculated that the ascites becomes secondarily inoculated during transient bacteremias and the infection becomes established by this means. Asymptomatic bacterascites without apparent inflammatory response has been described. The organisms usually implicated are enteric organisms, often *Escherichia coli*, but frequency of the presence of other organisms mandates therapy with broad-spectrum antibiotics until the identity of the offending agent is established. Anaerobes have not been shown to be significant causative organisms.

Therapy of this complication begins with a high index of suspicion that spontaneous bacterial peritonitis (SBP) may be present. Paracentesis abdominis should be performed promptly and the fluid subjected to rigorous bacteriologic analysis, including Gram stain and culture. The fluid is usually exudative in quality (protein > 2.5 mg. per cent, specific gravity > 1.015). The clinical value of the white blood count (WBC) and percentage of polymorphonuclear leukocytes is somewhat controversial, though clearly WBC counts in excess of 500 per cu. mm. are highly suspect. Lower values have been associated with SBP and it would appear the safer approach to obtain all material for culture and then begin treatment with broad-spectrum parenteral antibiotics (ampicillin, gentamicin, and clindamycin) pending culture confirmation. The effectiveness of treatment is predicated on a drop in ascitic fluid WBC and negative cultures on repeat paracentesis. Of course, other noninfectious inflammatory disorders of the peritoneum and abdomen remain in the differential and must be excluded.

CONSTIPATION

method of
FRANZ GOLDSTEIN, M.D.
Philadelphia, Pennsylvania

Introductory Comments and Definitions

Although every physician and lay person would presume to know what constipation is, a precise definition of it is lacking. In general terms, constipation refers either to the passage of unusually hard stools or to the abnormally infrequent passage of stools. Any abnormality refers to a deviation from normal, but there is no agreement as to what constitutes normal bowel habits, and definitions differ depending upon cultural and regional standards, individual perceptions, or any changes from any individual's usual pattern. While it is not mandatory to have a single bowel movement every morning, such a pattern is an ideal to strive for, provided it does not produce an obsession. Constipation is but a symptom, and treatment generally should be directed at causes and not at symptoms. This is true to a point with regards to constipation, and if an underlying disease producing constipation can be found and treated, so much the better. Examples are hypothyroidism, where the constipation can be improved by the use of thyroid substitution therapy; Hirschsprung's disease, where specific surgical treatment is available; and a few other unusual illnesses. Neurologic illness can cause severe constipation, but specific treatment is usually lacking; this pertains to Parkinson's disease, spinal cord lesions, and a variety of other neurologic disorders. Carcinoma of the colon can present as constipation, and here it is clearly of utmost importance that the underlying disease be recognized and treated rather than offering symptomatic measures for relief of constipation. A number of proctologic conditions present with constipation, and frequently a vicious cycle is established of constipation producing fissures and hemorrhoids that in turn produce painful defecation and a fear of defecation, leading to further constipation, and so on. Local therapy of the hemorrhoids and fissures may be needed to cope with the problem. The remaining discussion will deal primarily with the approach to the symptomatic relief of constipation in adults, omitting the specialized problems of constipation in early childhood and infancy.

Classification

Constipation not related to any underlying organic illness, also referred to as functional constipation, can be broadly classified into two categories, a hypertonic or *spastic* type and a hypotonic or *atonic* type. Spastic constipation is usually part of the irritable bowel syndrome and is often associated with lower abdominal crampy pain and with frequent alterations in bowel habit fluctuating from constipation to diarrhea. The condition tends to start in late adolescence or early adult life, but occasionally starts in early childhood or in middle age, rarely later. In spastic constipation stools tend to be scybalous, i.e., pelletlike, or ribbony, and frequently tend to change in shape from day to day. The presence of scybalous stool is tantamount evidence of segmental contractions of the sigmoid colon, one of the major

pathophysiologic characteristics of the irritable bowel syndrome. The sigmoid colon is frequently palpable through the abdominal wall in such patients and in thin persons one can often feel stool particles as well. Mucus may be mixed with the stool, but the presence of blood should always suggest underlying organic disease and requires full investigation. On rectal digital examination the rectum tends to be empty, and on sigmoidoscopic examination, done without bowel preparation, the entire rectosigmoid colon tends to be empty or may contain a few particles of scybalous stool. The sigmoid lumen is usually contracted and may make it difficult to pass the instrument. If a barium enema is obtained, spastic constipation is often characterized by marked haustral indentations and hypercontraction of the colon on the postevacuation films, so-called colonic hypertonicity. Some observers have linked spastic constipation and the irritable bowel syndrome to emotional disturbances and have directed their attention to correction of suspected anxiety neurosis. The vast majority of patients with irritable colon–spastic constipation have no demonstrable neuroses and their condition is a physiologic, not a psychiatric, disturbance. However, severe emotional problems are found in a small percentage of patients with spastic constipation.

Hypotonic or atonic constipation tends to occur in older people but can be seen in youngsters as well. Infrequent large bowel movements with a tendency to impaction are the usual complaints expressed by affected patients. Low abdominal discomfort may be present but is more in the nature of distention and fullness rather than cramps. The condition is far more common in women. Faulty bowel habits, sometimes going back to faulty bowel training in infancy, based on a mother's misconceptions about what constitutes normal bowel habits, are other features of the history. Patients often tend to ignore the urge to defecate, eventually lose their normal reflexes, and resort to the use of harsher and harsher laxatives with diminishing effectiveness. Some patients resort to the frequent use of enemas, often containing irritants, to produce bowel movements, never allowing the colon to fill and to elicit the normal defecatory reflex. Faulty dieting, such as the recent craze for liquid protein diets, tends to produce atonic constipation. The ingestion of a variety of drugs, particularly anticholinergics and opiate analgesics, may lead to severe atonic constipation. On physical examination the abdomen is frequently distended, the rectum is usually filled with feces as noted on digital examination, and initial proctosigmoidoscopy done without bowel preparation usually can not be completed because of excess feces. It is nevertheless important to do these initial examinations without bowel preparation in order to ascertain whether the rectum is empty or filled and to check on the mucosal integrity without the disturbance produced by enemas or laxatives. When sigmoidoscopy is performed, after bowel preparation, the rectosigmoid is usually relaxed and the examination is easily carried out. On barium enema the colon tends to be equally relaxed, frequently distended, with haustral markings tending to be flattened, and the colon may be redundant. The most severe cases present with the picture of a megacolon.

Treatment

Despite their enormous frequency, functional disturbances of the colon have been subjected to few controlled studies, hence clinicians have had to depend upon their own empirical methods or on those evolved by others. However, recent studies have clearly shown the importance of fiber in the diet as a prerequisite for normal bowel function. In past generations, bran-containing foods provided the necessary dietary fiber; constipation is said not to have been a problem among our forefathers and is not a problem now in peoples of the developing countries. The diet of present-day Americans and western Europeans is clearly deficient in fiber, the producer of fecal bulk. In our experience, the introduction of bulking materials into the diet is a necessary prerequisite for any bowel regimen to succeed. This is true for both spastic and atonic constipation.

In dealing with patients suffering from spastic constipation, we provide the patient with a sheet of written instructions that includes a brief and admittedly over-simplified explanation of the mechanisms of spastic constipation, followed by a list of therapeutic suggestions:

1. Patients are advised to avoid excessive amounts of spicy foods because they are believed to increase spasm. Patients with milk intolerance are advised to abstain from eating lactose-containing foods.

2. Patients are advised to eat a balanced diet, including a "normal" amount of fruits and vegetables. Patients are encouraged to eat bran-containing foods, such as bran cereals and whole wheat or whole rye bread, in reasonable quantities.

3. Patients are advised to take additionally a daily dose of a bulking agent such as psyllium hydrophylic muciloid (Konsyl, Metamucil, L.A. Formula). Konsyl is a brand of pure psyllium hydrophylic muciloid, whereas Metamucil and L.A. Formula are premixed with equal amounts of dextrose. Hence, twice the amount of the latter products has to be taken to get the equivalent effect of taking Konsyl. Patients are instructed to take a heaping teaspoon of Konsyl or equivalent every day, preferably at bedtime, and they are advised in advance that it takes days to weeks to get any appreciable effects and that it may take months to obtain optimal effects. Most patients should continue indefinitely with the use of these agents once the need for their use has been established.

4. Patients are advised to try having a bowel movement every morning after breakfast and to take extra time to accomplish this important task.

5. Patients who tend to be tense and anxious are offered the use of mild tranquilizers. Anticholinergic drugs are usually not prescribed. They may be helpful in patients who have diarrhea as the outstanding manifestation, but they tend to aggravate constipation.

In the United Kingdom the use of bran has become popular for the treatment of spastic constipation. There is not enough bran in the usual bran foods to provide patients with sufficient bulk, unless 10 to 15 servings of bran cereals or about a pound of pumpernickel bread are ingested daily, clearly unacceptable quantities. The use of pure bran can be substituted, in amounts of approximately 2 tablespoons three times a day. This will usually relieve spastic constipation, but will produce frequently unacceptable gaseousness and distention. Bran is a relatively inefficient bulking agent in terms of its water-holding capacity, the measuring stick of bulking activity. Psyllium muciloid has a far greater capacity to hold water and is approximately 10 times more efficient than bran, hence much smaller quantities of these substances are required for proper action. Approximately 90 per cent of patients seen in our offices will respond to the previously listed measures and will usually require no more than 1 to 2 visits to have their bowel function normalized. If results are not satisfactory, we frequently add a stool softener and a peristaltic stimulant to the regimen prescribed, or increase the amount of bulking agent, or use various combinations of the above.

The treatment of atonic constipation also requires the use of a bulking agent, with a preference also for psyllium hydrophylic muciloid. However, patients with atonic constipation tend to require additional measures already alluded to. As a rule, we prefer three agents to be used for patients with atonic constipation. These are (1) a bulking agent, usually in somewhat larger amounts than used for spastic constipation, e.g., a heaping teaspoon of Konsyl three times a day; (2) a peristaltic stimulant, and our preference is for standardized senna concentrate (Senokot) tablets or granules. The dose has to be adjusted individually and may vary from half a tablet a day to two tablets three times a day or corresponding amounts of the granules up to 1 teaspoon three times a day; (3) a stool softener, either dioctyl calcium sulfosuccinate (Surfak), 240 mg. daily, or dioctyl sodium sulfosuccinate (Colace), 100 mg. one to three times per day. For proper results, all three agents should be taken daily, with individual adjustment in dosage depending upon the results produced. Although some theoretical objections to the long-term use of stool softeners have been expressed and some changes in the structure of mucosal cells have been shown, no clearly demonstrable clinical side effects have been reported and we have not observed any adverse effects in our patients on this regimen used for many years. If patients are impacted when first seen, the impaction has to be manually extracted, and at times softening agents must be used from below and above. Oil enemas and stool softeners taken by mouth are frequently needed to clean out the impaction. Patients who have had prolonged atonic constipation and had been using harsh laxatives for long periods of time may be difficult or impossible to bring under control and some may have to continue using enemas. We prefer isotonic saline solution or water enemas to harsher mixtures and advise patients not to use soapsuds enemas or other irritants.

Among chronically constipated patients will be encountered some severely depressed patients who present with the somatic complaint of constipation. In such patients the underlying psychotic depression may require treatment before any improvement in the constipation can be expected, and such patients are best referred to psychiatrists.

DYSPHAGIA AND ESOPHAGEAL OBSTRUCTION

method of
H. JUERGEN NORD, M.D.,
and H. WORTH BOYCE, JR., M.D.
Tampa, Florida

Dysphagia is one of the most important symptoms of esophageal disorders. It indicates obstruction to a bolus either as a result of a motility disorder or mechanical obstruction. Dysphagia typically is a late symptom of esophageal stricture and usually indicates at least 50 per cent narrowing of the lumen. This symptom regularly occurs when the maximum lumen diameter is reduced to 13 mm. Intermittent dysphagia may occur with lesser degrees of narrowing when the patient inadvertently swallows a large bolus. Dysphagia should therefore never be regarded as trivial or functional and all patients with this complaint require thorough evaluation.

A detailed history and physical examination provide sufficient clues to make a correct presumptive diagnosis in most patients. A standard barium meal may not detect the area of stenosis and a bolus challenge (marshmallow, barium tablet) is necessary for complete evaluation. Esophagoscopy, with biopsy and cytology in cases of mechanical obstruction, is necessary in the evaluation of most patients. By utilizing cineradiography and manometry, the nature of the dysphagia should be clearly identified in those patients not adequately evaluated by the aforementioned radiographic and endoscopic methods.

The main goal of therapy is to establish and maintain a patent esophagus at the lowest cost and risk to the patient. Peroral bougienage with various dilators is safe and effective and best suited for this purpose. Surgical treatment rarely is necessary for benign esophageal strictures.

Instruments for Dilation

Metal olives (Eder-Puestow) sizes Fr. 21 to 45 (1 French unit = 0.3 mm.) attached to a flexible metal rod and passed over a guide wire with flexible Fr. 7 spring tip are most commonly used for initial therapy of tight or tortuous strictures.

Mercury-filled rubber dilators with rounded tip (Hurst) or tapered tip (Maloney) are supplied from Fr. 12 to Fr. 60, each being 2 Fr. wider than the preceding. Dilators of less than Fr. 36 are so flexible that little effective pressure from above may be applied and consequently, tight stenoses are not reliably dilated by these sizes. Metal olives are more effective in these cases. Because of the tapered tip, Maloney dilators are preferred for most of our stricture work when rubber bougies are used.

The Rider-Moeller (Eder) pneumatic cardia dilator is used for treatment of achalasia. It is supplied in three balloon sizes. The balloon has a "dumbbell" shape that allows easy seating of its waist in the lower esophageal sphincter to ensure proper fixation for optimum dilation.

Patient Preparation

1. The patient should be fully evaluated, applying all appropriate diagnostic means (see above).

2. Full patient information and education about technique, results, and possible dangers is mandatory. Any instrumentation within the esophagus bears the risk for complications. In experienced hands, dilation is remarkably safe and effective.

3. Local anesthesia of the hypopharynx is unnecessary in most patients. If desired, a gargle with diluted lidocaine (Xylocaine Viscous) is sufficient. Sedation, analgesia, or anesthesia is not required and is undesirable, since patient response should be monitored. The value of at-

ropine sulfate as premedication is unproved but often helpful in patients bothered by sialorrhea.

4. Patients are usually kept on clear liquids for 12 to 24 hours before initial dilation to ensure a clean esophagus. In the case of complete obstruction or achalasia, emptying of the esophagus with a Fr. 34 Ewald tube may be necessary prior to dilation. Suction equipment for oropharyngeal aspiration should be readily available.

5. We perform all dilations under fluoroscopic control. This is mandatory for patients with tight or tortuous strictures, diverticula secondary to strictures or diverticula in other parts of the esophagus, and all malignant strictures. An uncomplicated benign stricture after the initial dilation may be managed in the office without x-ray control if the operator is certain that no angulations or diverticula are present in which the dilator tip could become trapped.

General Technique of Dilation

1. *Position.* Dilation may be performed with the patient in the sitting or standing position. In general, our patients are lying on the fluoroscopy table with the head of the table elevated 15 to 30°.

2. *Cleaning.* All dilators are thoroughly washed with povidone-iodine (Betadine) prior to use to prevent instrument-induced infection and bacteremia.

3. *Eder-Puestow Dilator Set.* The Eder-Puestow guide wire is passed under fluoroscopic control until the spring tip has passed the gastroesophageal junction and is positioned in the proximal stomach. The tip usually points towards the greater curvature. If the wire cannot be readily passed because of a tight or irregular stricture, it may be passed under direct vision through the operating channel of a standard fiberoptic panendoscope. The shaft with the proper olive attached and lightly lubricated is passed over the guide wire until it has passed the stricture. This is easily felt by the experienced operator. The assistant assures with fluoroscopic control that the spring tip remains in proper position. This is particularly important during withdrawal of the shaft. After a maximum of three dilations has been completed, the spring tip is pulled against the dilator shaft and the entire apparatus is withdrawn.

4. *Hurst and Maloney* dilators are lightly lubricated at the distal end and passed gently into the hypopharynx much like a flexible endoscope. At this point the patient is asked to swallow to relax the cricopharyngeus, allowing easy advance into the esophagus. After the maximum width of the instrument has passed the stenosis, it is rapidly withdrawn.

5. *Dilations per Sitting.* As a rule no more than 3 successive size dilators are passed per visit.

This number appears safe for most strictures and is well tolerated by patients. However, each stricture is different and requires an individually tailored approach. For very tight, far advanced, or long segmental strictures, only 1 or 2 dilators may be passed initially.

6. *Frequency of Dilations.* Initially, dilations are performed every 2 to 4 days. At these visits the last dilator used in the previous session is usually passed first. Later dilations every other day appear safe until the desired lumen size has been achieved. After patients have been treated successfully, the follow-up interval must be determined individually but should not exceed 3 to 6 months after completion of the initial dilation series. Annual evaluation should be the longest follow-up interval between evaluations once lumen patency is assured.

7. *Endpoint of Dilation.* In an uncomplicated short distal stricture due to reflux a maximal lumen size of Fr. 52 to 56 can usually be reached. In long-standing or chronic cicatricial strictures one may have to be satisfied with maximal passage of a smaller bougie (perhaps Fr. 46). Patients dilated to this size are able to eat a regular diet, provided they chew their food well and take plenty of liquids with their meals. Patients with strictures dilated to less than 13 mm. (Fr. 39) maximal diameter can be expected to experience solid food dysphagia at least intermittently. Therefore, the optimal lumen size to keep patients asymptomatic will be about Fr. 46.

Specific Treatment Regimens

Distal Esophageal Stricture. This is usually a short segmental stricture secondary to gastroesophageal reflux and depending on its size should be treated initially with metal olives if tight (<30 Fr.), then followed by rubber dilators as outlined above.

Long Segmental Strictures. They are usually secondary to ingestion of corrosive agents or long-standing nasogastric intubation with reflux. The same regimen as for distal esophageal strictures applies except that a more cautious approach is taken. Fewer dilators are passed per session and larger time intervals allowed between visits (see Frequency of Dilations.)

Acute Corrosive Esophagitis. Daily esophageal dilation should be initiated as soon as esophagoscopy has determined degree and extent of injury. This practice should be maintained for the period of hospitalization. Less frequent dilations are necessary for up to one year and periodic passage of bougies is usually required for lifetime. It should be emphasized that prevention of a stricture by this method is far easier than treating an established lesion.

Other methods (systemic steroids and broad-spectrum antibiotics) may be applied to suppress the inflammation and infection that are regularly present. The value of steroid therapy for acute esophageal injury by corrosive agents is unproven in adults.

Scleroderma.   The distal esophageal stricture that develops with scleroderma of the esophagus is treated like any other distal stricture (see above). Problems may arise with skin changes in face and neck that make introduction of instruments extremely difficult. Nevertheless every effort should be made to treat these patients using flexible rubber dilators.

Rings and Webs.   Lower esophageal rings should not be taken as a ready explanation for dysphagia, and other causes should be eliminated by the diagnostic studies. Should therapy be necessary, this is easily achieved by dilation with Hurst or Maloney dilators in a manner similar to benign strictures.

Webs are easily treated. Frequently they are ruptured by passage of the endoscope; the same can be achieved by passage of rubber dilators of adequate size. Only rarely will it be necessary to remove sections of a tough web with the endoscopic biopsy forceps in order to produce symptom relief.

Food Impaction.   A large food bolus (usually meat) may impact in the distal esophagus if hastily eaten without proper mastication or may become lodged above a stricture.

A nasogastric tube should be passed to clear the esophagus of retained secretions above the obstruction and then contrast studies carried out to determine exact size and location of the bolus. Occasionally, a piece of meat may pass spontaneously within 24 hours, particularly if the obstruction is in the area of the ampulla.

Usually one should take one of two steps:

1. Removal with forceps through an endoscope. Occasionally rigid esophagoscopy has to be applied because of the larger forceps size. Never should a bolus be pushed forward.

2. Dissolution: The enzyme papain is capable of dissolving lean meat. Commercially available meat tenderizer containing papain (preferably nonspiced variety) is commonly used for this purpose. A rounded teaspoon of meat tenderizer dissolved in 4 ounces of water is instilled through a Levin tube every 30 to 60 minutes following removal of the previous dose. The patient senses relief easily which usually occurs after 4 doses. When there is suspicion or evidence of a piece of bone or other foreign body it probably is wise not to use papain or similar enzymes for this purpose.

Esophageal disease should be ruled out in all patients following relief of the impaction by radiography and esophagoscopy. Also, dentures should be checked for proper fit and function.

Motility Disorders

Globus Hystericus.   This is not a true motor disorder. It is usually caused by anxiety or a conversion reaction. No specific therapy is indicated. Reassurance after a complete work-up will usually convince the patient that this is a functional disorder.

Achalasia of the Cricopharyngeus Muscle.   The inability of the upper esophageal sphincter to open after a bolus arrives in the hypopharynx can cause serious problems of aspiration. Usually there is underlying disease of the pharyngeal musculature or disordered function of cranial nerves IX and X, or both.

Initially, dilation with a large rubber bougie is preferable over surgery which may further compound the problems. The prognosis is usually guarded because of the underlying disorder, which is often focal damage to the central nervous system.

Hypertrophic Cricopharyngeus Muscle.   This disorder is best diagnosed by cineradiography, which will usually indicate poor coordination of the pharyngeal musculature. Periodic dilations with a large rubber dilator may give some relief. Surgical myotomy has been used in some cases.

Diffuse Esophageal Spasm.   This is best diagnosed by cineradiography or manometry, or both. The troublesome retrosternal pain may be relieved for periods of time by intermittent passage of a large (Fr. 58) Hurst bougie. Nitroglycerin or a long-acting nitrate, isosorbide dinitrate (Isordil), may be helpful, especially in those persons who do not have gastroesophageal reflux as an associated problem. Should pain be incapacitating or weight loss occur in spite of these regimens, surgery (long esophagomyotomy) may be the only other alternative. The response to surgery is unpredictable.

Achalasia.   Pneumatic dilation is simple and inexpensive and gives results comparable to surgery (Heller myotomy), making it the preferred initial treatment. It should be carried out only by an experienced operator under fluoroscopic control. After the diagnosis is firmly established and the esophagus has been emptied of retained fluid, a large Hurst bougie (Fr. 56) is passed into the stomach to assure patency of the cardia, since balloon dilation of a stricture or carcinoma would be disastrous. In recent years we have abandoned our previous experience with the Starck dilator in favor of the pneumatic dilator. The well-lubricated, collapsed pneumatic dilator is passed and the waist of the "dumbbell" shaped balloon is positioned in the cardia. Prior passage of a guide wire (provided with the Rider-Moeller dilator) enhances easy passage through a markedly dilated esophagus with sigmoid distal segment. The balloon is inflated to 300 mm. Hg and held in position for 3 minutes, then deflated and rapidly removed. Patients usually complain of marked retrosternal pressure pain during the procedure. We do not use analgesia but on rare occasion in select patients have used mild sedation. Streaks of blood on the bag indicate adequate stretching. Should achalasia recur, a second pneumatic dilation may be tried before a Heller procedure is recommended. Patients should be alerted that relief of the obstruction does not relieve all dysphagia, since the lack of primary peristalsis in the body of the esophagus persists. All patients require surveillance for carcinoma of the esophagus that reportedly occurs with increased frequency after many years with achalasia.

Neoplasms

Benign mucosal tumors can be removed via the esophagoscope with polypectomy snares. The operator must be certain he is not dealing with a vascular lesion or a submucosal neoplasm since these lesions should be removed only by surgery.

Squamous cell carcinoma is initially best treated by radiation therapy. Most lesions are far advanced when diagnosed and show significant obstruction at the time of diagnosis or re-stenose after radiotherapy. Only a patent esophagus can assure adequate nutrition and prevent aspiration. Peroral dilation with metal olives or rubber bougies under fluoroscopic control (see above) should be started as soon as the diagnosis of esophageal obstruction is made and as needed may be carried out simultaneously with radiotherapy. Due to the great variation in extent of tumor and growth rate no standard program can be recommended. Dilation of carcinoma by proper technique is safe.

Should a malignant obstruction become too firm for further dilation or when a satisfactory lumen size cannot be maintained without frequent dilations, a permanent peroral polyvinyl prosthesis can be inserted.

The prosthesis also may be used to block a tracheoesophageal fistula, a serious complication of esophageal carcinoma.

Adenocarcinoma of the cardia involving the esophagus may be more amenable to surgical resection in some patients but otherwise should be treated in a similar fashion. Unfortunately, these tumors are less sensitive to radiation therapy and represent difficult problems to dilation since the stomach is involved as well. Nevertheless, dilations under fluoroscopic control with or without a guide wire should be used for palliation in these patients.

DIVERTICULA OF THE ALIMENTARY CANAL

method of
GRANT V. RODKEY, M.D.
Boston, Massachusetts

Esophagus

Esophageal diverticula are relatively common among patients of older age groups, and may occur in the upper, mid, or lower segments of that structure. Pharyngoesophageal and epiphrenic diverticula are of the pulsion type, whereas those of the midesophagus are usually secondary to adhesions and traction from previously inflamed adjacent lymph nodes.

Symptoms are largely limited to those diverticula which are of the pulsion type, and are chiefly dysphagia, regurgitation, and substernal pain. Rarely local perforation may occur or hemorrhage may complicate the disease.

Treatment of these lesions is essentially surgical. Pharyngoesophageal diverticula are now believed to develop chiefly as a secondary manifestation to spasm of the cricopharyngeal sphincter. Thus small diverticula may be managed by extramucosal posterior myotomy of the cricopharyngeus muscle through a left cervical approach. Larger diverticula should be excised with layer closure of the esophagus, carefully avoiding stenosis, and combined with posterior myotomy. Complications may include infection, esophagocutaneous fistula, and unilateral cord palsy secondary to injury of the recurrent laryngeal nerve. However, with modern surgical techniques the incidence of such complications should be minimal, and all patients with symptomatic pharyngoesophageal diverticula should be advised to have surgical repair.

Epiphrenic diverticula may be associated with neuromuscular dysfunction of the lower esophagus, hiatus hernia, or stricture. If symptoms are significant, transthoracic excision of the diverticulum with concomitant repair of associated defects of the esophagus, cardia, or diaphragmatic hiatus is indicated.

For all practical purposes, traction diverticula of the midesophagus do not produce symptoms and do not require specific treatment.

Stomach

Diverticula of the stomach are uncommon, but not rare. They usually occur at a point near the cardia on the posterior wall of the stomach, but in a small proportion of cases may be found in the prepyloric area. When they occur, they are usually solitary lesions.

Symptoms from gastric diverticula are ill defined, in part because of the frequency of concomitant structural or functional disorders of the upper digestive tract. The diverticula have been thought to be capable of causing epigastric or retrosternal pain, and they are occasionally the site of ulceration and hemorrhage. If the severity of symptoms requires treatment and other diseases have been excluded by careful study, including endoscopy, surgical excision of the diverticulum is the only effective therapy. However, the experienced surgeon will exercise extreme caution to be sure that he does not overlook some accompanying occult lesion which has been the real cause of the symptoms.

Duodenum

In contrast to those of the stomach, duodenal diverticula are frequently present and are often multiple, although it is rare for more than three or four to be present in a single patient. They usually arise on the mesenteric (pancreatic) side of the duodenal loop, and are intimately attached to pancreas lying on the posterior surface of that organ or protruding into the head of the gland. They are usually to be found in the second and third portions of the duodenum and commonly occur near the papilla of Vater. Pseudodiverticula may occur in the first portion of the duodenum as a sequel to peptic ulceration or scarring, or to previous surgery (e.g., pyloroplasty). Duodenal diverticula are usually discovered during x-ray examinations of the gastrointestinal tract with contrast medium, and are easily overlooked at the time of surgical exploration unless their presence has been noted previously.

Symptoms from duodenal diverticula undoubtedly do occur occasionally, but their precise definition is difficult unless there is hemorrhage or local inflammation with perforation—both extremely rare occurrences.

From a practical point of view, one should usually regard duodenal diverticula as an incidental finding not responsible for dyspeptic symptoms. However, it is of extreme importance to the surgeon doing surgery on the biliary tract to be wary of diverticula near or at the lower termination of the common bile duct, lest unrecognized perforation of the thin-walled portion of the duodenum occur.

If symptoms are clearly attributable to diverticula of the duodenum, the only therapy to be recommended is surgical excision. This is not a simple problem, and operation may be followed by acute pancreatitis or by duodenal leakage, peritonitis, and fistula. The operation should be undertaken thoughtfully and only by experienced surgeons.

Small Intestine

Diverticula extending into the mesentery of the small bowel, contained by a covering of serosa, submucosa, and mucosa, and analogous in structure to duodenal diverticula are occasionally encountered. Their frequency is considerably less than that of duodenal diverticula, and when they are present they are more often found in upper jejunum than in lower segments of the intestine. Diverticula of the small bowel are usually multiple, and they may involve long segments of the bowel or its entirety. Diagnosis is usually made on the basis of a barium meal followed through the intestine by means of serial films.

Symptoms caused by small bowel diverticula of this type are vague. Acute inflammation, perforation, hemorrhage, and obstruction rarely occur but are clearcut indications for surgical intervention. More frequently, symptoms of intestinal dysfunction—flatulence, abdominal pain, bloating, weight loss, megaloblastic anemia, or steatorrhea—may occur. Even these are rare, and when present they may represent a variant of the so-called "blind loop syndrome." Relief of symptoms may be obtained by intermittent short courses of antibiotic therapy (i.e., tetracycline, 250 mg. four times daily for 2 to 3 days), or by varying the diet pattern. Parenteral vitamin supplements may infrequently be required.

If significant symptoms are present from diverticulosis of the small bowel, surgical treatment may have to be considered. The only effective way to deal with these lesions is resection of a segment of the bowel; but if a large proportion of the small bowel is affected (as it usually is if symptoms are severe), this therapy is inappropriate.

Meckel's diverticulum of the ileum is a congenital remnant of the omphalomesenteric duct which may be manifested in a variety of ways. These include a blind pouch projecting from the antemesenteric border of the ileum (usually within 2 or 3 feet of the ileocecal valve) or a mucus-lined tract extending from ileum to umbilicus or to adjacent small bowel mesentery.

Symptoms caused by Meckel's diverticulum fall mainly into three categories: (1) those consequent to the present of heterotopic tissue—mainly gastric mucosa—in the diverticulum; (2) those resulting from mechanical factors set up by the presence of the diverticulum; and (3) those secondary to acute inflammation of the diverticulum. Rarely, Meckel's diverticulum may be the site of origin for tumors, either benign or malignant.

Symptoms relevant to the presence of heterotopic tissue in the diverticulum are chiefly those of gastrointestinal hemorrhage, often massive and secondary to acid-peptic digestion of mucosa adjacent to the base of the diverticulum. Most of these cases occur in children. The blood presenting in the stool in these patients usually varies from dark to light red, depending upon the rate of hemorrhage.

Mechanical effects of Meckel's diverticulum which cause symptoms are those of small bowel obstruction or, infrequently, intussusception.

Inflammation of Meckel's diverticulum is the third most frequent manifestation of its presence, and the signs and symptoms are those of appendicitis. Perforation and peritonitis may occur if diagnosis is delayed.

Finally, occult neoplasms of Meckel's diverticulum may become manifest by hemorrhage, obstruction, or metastases, or may be discovered incidentally in the course of laparotomy for another illness.

The treatment of all complications of Meckel's diverticulum is surgical excision. Indeed, such a diverticulum should be removed whenever it is discovered during the course of operation of another cause, the patient's condition permitting.

Appendix

It is not generally appreciated that the appendix may be the site of diverticulosis. The condition is rare, and its clinical significance, if any, is obscure. Diagnosis is always an incidental finding at laparotomy, and it seems reasonable to advise incidental appendectomy in such instances. If diverticulitis of the appendix occurs, the symptoms and pathologic findings are indistinguishable from those of acute appendicitis and the treatment is identical.

Colon

Diverticula of the colon should be classified as congenital or acquired. Congenital diverticula occur in the region of the cecum; are composed of serosa, muscularis, submucosa, and mucosa; and occur with comparable frequency among all population groups. They may be discovered as incidental findings on barium enema or may become manifest because of complications of acute inflammation or (rarely) hemorrhage. The symptoms of diverticulitis of the cecum mimic those of appendicitis, although progression of symptoms may be more leisurely, and nausea occurs less frequently than with appendicitis. Treatment is limited to patients with acute diverticulitis, and consists of operation with excision of the lesion. This may be accomplished by local excision if the pathology is recognized. Sometimes it is not possible to exclude the diagnosis of cancer of the cecum at operation, and in such cases a right colectomy should be performed. In a few instances, inflammation may involve only the poste-

rior wall of the cecum and may be difficult to discover unless the cecum is detached from its peritoneal fixation and rolled forward for inspection. Excision of the diverticulum and performance of cecostomy at the site is an alternative method of managing some of these lesions. Diverticula of the cecum discovered incidentally during laparotomy for another illness should be treated by excision or by simple inversion.

Colonic diverticula of acquired origin rarely occur among Orientals, but are common among Western populations. They are composed of serosa, submucosa, and mucosa only; arise first in the sigmoid region and tend to proliferate proximally from this point; and seem to represent intermuscular or perivascular herniations as an expression of increased intraluminal tension arising from neuromuscular dysfunction and altered patterns of peristalsis. Although they may appear earlier, they do not commonly occur before age 40. They become progressively more frequent with advancing age. These diverticula have narrow mouths and tend to collect inspissated feces. Mechanical irritation and bacterial digestion may frequently induce pathologic changes in the diverticula which may be manifested by symptoms of local inflammation or perforation, local or general peritonitis, hemorrhage varying from microscopic to massive, small or large bowel obstruction, cystitis, pelvic abscess, or fistula formation. Because of the comparable age groups involved, differentiation between diverticulitis and carcinoma of the colon may be difficult.

Despite the potential hazards of diverticulosis of the colon, most patients with this disease may be managed without surgical intervention. Medical therapy consists of a diet of normal or high fiber residue (except during attacks of acute diverticulitis), supplemented by 1 to 2 teaspoonfuls of powdered psyllium seed husk (Metamucil) per day. Anticholinergics and mild sedation should also be a part of the regimen.

During attacks of acute diverticulitis, the bowel should be put to rest by giving intravenous fluids, restriction of oral intake, and use of nasogastric suction as required. Systemic antibiotics (cephalothin [Keflin], 6.0 grams per day, or other broad-spectrum agent) should be given parenterally until the acute phase of the inflammation subsides and gastrointestinal function returns.

For less severe attacks of diverticulitis, manifested by left lower quadrant tenderness but without systemic illness, the patient may be managed with a liquid or very low residue diet, antibiotics or phthalylsulfathiazole (Sulfathalidine), 2.0 grams every 6 hours by mouth (this use of phthalylsulfathiazole is not listed in the manufacturer's official directive), and physical rest. Interestingly, many of these patients may gain relief of symptoms of diverticulitis following a barium enema, perhaps because of filling of the diverticula by the barium.

The complications of diverticulitis that may require surgical intervention include persistent or recurrent local inflammation, abscess formation, free perforation with peritonitis, obstruction, fistula formation, and hemorrhage. In the case of hemorrhage, it has been established that bleeding may often originate in the right colon even though diverticulosis is chiefly left-sided. Also, massive hemorrhage may occur because of so-called "angiodysplasia" (arteriovenous malformations), which may occur in the right colon with or without associated colonic diverticulosis. If facilities for selective mesenteric angiography are available, all patients with massive lower gastrointestinal hemorrhage should be studied by this method as early as possible. Intra-arterial or systemic infusion of vasopressin will control acute hemorrhage in a significant proportion of these patients after the bleeding source has been identified. If bleeding persists despite vasopressin infusion, surgical resection of the appropriate segment of bowel is indicated.

If angiographic studies are not available, massive lower intestinal bleeding associated with diverticulosis should be treated by subtotal colectomy and ileosigmoidostomy, as accurate localization of the bleeding point during operation is usually not possible.

The aim of surgical treatment for the remaining complications of diverticulitis is the extirpation of the diseased segment and restoration of intestinal continuity. However, the complicating factors may make a primary resection unwise, and in such circumstances staged resections (preliminary transverse colostomy, resection, and final colostomy closure; or sigmoid resection, end colostomy, and rectal turn-in with delayed reanastomosis) have been found to contribute to lowered mortality. Appropriate parenteral nutrition and antibiotic therapy should be adjuncts to operation. Technical problems involved in the surgical treatment are too complex for consideration here, but they tax the skill of the most expert surgeons and should never be considered lightly.

Simultaneous occurrence of diverticulitis and carcinoma of the colon may cause confusion in diagnosis, especially in those patients in whom a partial obstruction is seen on barium enema examination. These patients should be carefully studied, and early operation should be recommended unless carcinoma can be clearly excluded.

With a view to reducing the morbidity required by staged resections for complications of diverticulitis, serious consideration should be given to elective operation in patients with the following manifestations:

1. Recurrent attacks of diverticulitis, especially in patients under 50 years of age.

2. Marked narrowing or deformity of the colon by x-ray with stasis of the proximal bowel.

3. Persistent palpable mass.

4. Dysuria, frequency, or pneumaturia.

5. Repeated serious episodes of hemorrhage.

Fortunately, diverticulitis does not affect the extraperitoneal rectum, and it should be possible to restore continuity of the bowel in those cases not complicated by a low-lying carcinoma.

Hazardous complications, prolonged morbidity, and serious economic losses may be averted by judicious selection of patients in the categories described for elective primary colonic resections. Clinical judgment in such patients is enhanced by close cooperation between internist and surgeon.

CROHN'S DISEASE

method of
ROBERT W. SUMMERS, M.D.
Iowa City, Iowa

Principles of Therapy

Before initiating treatment of a chronic disease, one should perform adequate studies to eliminate potentially curable disorders such as tuberculosis or amebiasis. The cause of Crohn's disease remains unknown and management based on specific therapy is not presently possible. The principle aims in therapy are to (1) maintain adequate nutrition, (2) alleviate symptoms such as emotional disorders, diarrhea, or pain, (3) attempt to control or suppress the disease through the use of anti-inflammatory drugs, (4) attend to extraintestinal manifestations of the disease, and (5) be alert to situations in which surgical intervention will be helpful.

Nutritional Therapy

Basic Diet. Most patients should be advised to eat a well-balanced, high-protein, high-caloric, and unrestricted diet. There is seldom one type of food that causes problems in all patients; therefore, we advise common sense in the choice of foods and advise patients to eliminate only foods which they recognize to cause problems. For some patients fresh fruits and vegetables produce cramps or diarrhea; for others highly spiced foods cause symptoms. A food-symptom diary is sometimes helpful to identify poorly tolerated foods or areas of gross nutrient neglect.

Problems Requiring Specific Restrictions. Specific dietary restrictions apply to some patients; however, problems should be well documented before recommending severe alteration in diet.

MILK INTOLERANCE. A few patients with excessive flatus and diarrhea are intolerant of milk on the basis of lactase deficiency, but the incidence is no higher than in the general population. The problem should be well documented by a specific test such as the lactose tolerance test and a trial of a lactose-free diet may be in order. If no clear-cut benefit results, there is no reason to restrict milk.

PARTIAL INTESTINAL OBSTRUCTION. Low-grade obstruction can be aggravated by certain high-fiber foods. If there is a suggestive clinical picture of postprandial cramping, abdominal pain, loud borborygmi, abdominal distention, and radiographic intestinal stricture, restriction of indigestible food residues should be advised.

Steatorrhea. Significant steatorrhea should be managed with a low-fat diet (40 to 75 grams or less). Unabsorbed fatty acids are hydroxylated in the colon and aggravate diarrhea. A low-fat diet should be initiated if steatorrhea is documented by fecal fat analysis. Reducing fat will significantly reduce caloric intake, and these calories should be replaced with appropriate protein and carbohydrate and the addition of medium chain triglycerides (MCT). A diet manual or dietitian should be consulted to aid in the use of MCT in cooking or Portagen, a commercial formula using MCT oil. Excessive MCT, over 100 grams per day, in the diet can aggravate diarrhea because of high osmolality.

HYPEROXALURIA. Increased colonic absorption of oxalate leads to increased urinary oxalate excretion and calcium oxalate renal stones. Normally, dietary calcium combines with oxalate, forming insoluble precipitates which are unavailable for absorption. With steatorrhea, calcium combines with fatty acids to form calcium soaps and increased oxalate is available for colonic absorption. Unabsorbed bile acids from ileal disease or resection increase colonic permeability to oxalate and also increase its rate of absorption. The increased absorption can be decreased by the restriction of high-oxalate foods and drinks such as nuts, spinach, rhubarb, tea, colas, or grapefruit juice, as well as restriction of dietary fat, which allows calcium to complex with oxalate instead of the formation of fatty acid soaps. These measures along with the encouragement of a large fluid intake may be enough to reduce the lithogenic potential of the urine; however, further reduction

can be accomplished through the use of aluminum or calcium antacids to bind oxalate in patients with steatorrhea, cholestyramine (Questran) to bind excessive colonic bile salts and reduce oxalate absorption or thiazide diuretics which decrease urinary calcium excretion.

Dietary Supplements. Severe diarrhea or steatorrhea can result in excessive loss and depletion of sodium, potassium, bicarbonate, magnesium, or calcium ions, all of which must be replaced if serum measurements indicate depletion. Fat-soluble vitamins A, D, E, and K can be poorly absorbed when steatorrhea is significant and result in deficiency. Vitamin B and C stores are sometimes low because of anorexia or a low-fiber diet. A variety of vitamin supplements will be necessary, depending on which vitamins are depleted. Because of frequent blood loss, poor iron utilization, and possible interference of iron absorption with sulfasalazine, iron deficiency anemia is a common problem and iron sulfate or gluconate, 300 mg. three time daily, must be given when serum iron saturation or bone-marrow iron stores are low. Vitamin B_{12} deficiency is another common cause of anemia. It occurs as a result of extensive ileal resection or ileal disease and is aggravated in some patients by intestinal stasis and bacterial overgrowth. If serum levels or a Schilling's test indicate that B_{12} malabsorption is responsible, 30 micrograms of hydroxocobalamin (Neo-Betalin) should be given per month. Folic acid deficiency is another cause of anemia because of poor intake, increased utilization from inflammation, and rapid cell turnover and decreased absorption aggravated by sulfasalazine. If low serum or red blood cell folic acid levels are found, 5 mg. per day should be given.

Special Formulas. For some patients, food intake is difficult or impossible. Such patients include those with an enteric fistula, stricture with partial or complete obstruction, short bowel syndrome, abscess, or extensive inflammatory disease. The so-called elemental or chemically-defined diets are useful to improve caloric intake and reduce indigestible residue. These diets include Vivonex HN, Precision High Nitrogen, Warren Teed-Low Residue, and Flexical. When prepared, each contains 1 calorie per ml., which often produces diarrhea initially, especially when flavored, because of high osmolality. This can be minimized by choosing diets with no flavoring, beginning with at least half-strength solutions, and slowing the rate of administration. Over several days the concentration and infusion rates are increased. We have found that a small pediatric feeding tube and an infusion pump help to control the rate of administration.

Central Venous Nutrition. The intestinal tract

should be the route of nutrition whenever possible but in patients in whom the digestive tract cannot be used, parenteral alimentation provides the potential to restore nitrogen balance, supplies totally adequate nutrition, allows time for severely ill patients to respond to intensive medical therapy, or corrects malnutrition prior to surgical therapy. A central venous catheter is placed into the superior vena cava under strict sterile conditions and concentrated glucose, nitrogen, as protein hydrolysates or pure L-amino acids, and sometimes lipids are infused. These solutions contain all required vitamins and trace minerals. Extreme care must be utilized to prevent infectious and thrombotic complications. Other complications include extreme hyperglycemia, hypoglycemia, osmotic dehydration, essential fatty acid deficiency, trace metal deficiencies, and hypophosphatemia.

Symptomatic Therapy

Psychologic Aspects. The disease is not caused by psychologic stress but produces psychiatric disturbances by the nature of the symptoms and their chronicity. The symptoms often produce personal and marital concerns such as anxiety, irritability, or sexual dysfunction or economic problems because of chronic fatigue or frequent absence from work. Therapy is aimed at providing solid information about the disease process, supportive psychotherapy, and a sense of concern on the part of the physician about the relief of disabling symptoms. We find pamphlets from the National Foundation for Ileitis and Colitis to be especially helpful for patient information. Routine use of psychotropics or psychiatric referral is not indicated; however, minor tranquilizers, antidepressants, sedatives and hypnotic agents can be useful as adjuncts in patients with excessive anxiety, depression, and insomnia.

Diarrhea. There are several causes of diarrhea requiring several approaches to therapy. For patients with active disease the most important factor in control of diarrhea is control of the inflammatory process through the use of sulfasalazine or corticosteroids (see below).

For many patients diarrhea improves simply through the use of a bulk hydrophilic agent such as psyllium mucilloid (Metamucil or Effersyllium), 1 to 2 teaspoonfuls 2 or 3 times per day with fruit juice or water. We rarely use antidiarrheal agents but temporary relief may be obtained with diphenoxylate hydrochloride, 2.5 to 5 mg., with atropine sulfate (Lomotil), 3 or 4 times daily, loperimide (Imodium), two 4 mg. tablets initially, followed by one with each loose stool, to a maximum of 8 tablets per day, or deodorized tincture of opium, 6 to 10 drops 3 to 6 times per day as needed. We urge caution regarding possible habituation, and never use these agents in the fulminant stage of the disease. With severe diarrhea these agents are frequently ineffective and they may contribute to toxic dilatation when the colon is involved. Anticholinergic agents, 15 mg. of propantheline (Pro-Banthine) or 0.4 mg. of atropine sulfate, given before meals relieves diarrhea in patients with a prominent gastrocolic reflex.

Bile salt diarrhea results from interruption of the enterohepatic circulation and occurs when extensive (10 to 100 cm.) ileal disease is present or after ileal resection. Impaired absorption results in increased amounts of bile salts entering the colon. Here they are deconjugated and interfere with salt and water absorption to produce watery diarrhea. The diarrhea will be controlled in many such patients with cholestyramine (Questran) or cholestipol (Colestid), bile salt-binding resins, 2 to 5 grams in water or juice before each meal. As stated earlier, fat malabsorption aggravates diarrhea, which improves through reduction of fat in the diet. Steatorrhea should be suspected when active ileal disease or ileal resection or both exceeds 100 cm.

Pain. The pains of ureteral obstruction, perinephric, pelvic or perianal abscess or partial bowel obstruction have differing clinical characteristics, but the cause of the pain must be discovered, usually through radiologic studies, in order to plan specific therapy. Many of these problems will respond to control of the disease process with anti-inflammatory therapy, others will require surgical intervention. The routine use of narcotics is to be discouraged because of the chronic nature of the problems and the fact that pain usually implies some complication of the disease requiring specific therapy.

Control of Disease Activity

Sulfasalazine. Sulfasalazine (Azulfidine, Rorasul) has recently been shown to be effective in active disease in the National Cooperative Crohn's Disease Study. The drug was nearly as effective as prednisone in inducing a remission of active disease. The drug was effective in patients with ileocolitis and colitis but ineffective when only the ileum was involved. In distinction to the prophylactic effect in ulcerative colitis, there was no benefit in the maintenance of a remission in patients with inactive disease or with recent resection. Therefore, we find the drug most useful in treating active disease whenever it involves the colon. It is given in a dosage range of from 2 to 6 grams per day in divided doses. We discontinue the drug when a complete remission is achieved.

The drug is made up of two molecules, 5-amino salicylate and sulfapyridine, joined by a diazo bond. It passes unchanged through the small intestine, unless there is bacterial overgrowth, to the colon, where it is split. A significant amount of sulfapyridine but very little 5-amino salicylate is absorbed from the colon. The 5-amino salicylate is probably responsible for the beneficial effects of the drug in Crohn's disease as it is in ulcerative colitis. The mechanism of action is unknown but the drug may be anti-inflammatory or interfere with prostaglandin metabolism. The antibacterial activity of sulfapyridine probably is not responsible since there is no significant change in bowel flora. Sulfapyridine is responsible for most of the dose related side effects of headaches, nausea, anorexia, dyspepsia and vomiting. Reducing the dose or the use of enteric-coated tablets lessens side effects. Agranulocytosis, Heinz-body or glucose-6-phosphate dehydrogenase-deficient hemolytic anemia, sulf- and methemoglobinemia, and pancreatitis are serious but fortunately uncommon toxic complications. A variable drug eruption is a more common and limiting problem.

Corticosteroids. Corticosteroids appear to suppress the disease activity through an anti-inflammatory mechanism but are not curative. In the National Cooperative Crohn's Disease Study, prednisone was effective in induction of a remission of active disease, but lower doses were ineffective in prevention of relapse in inactive disease. The drug was beneficial in patients with isolated ileal disease or ileocolitis, but not effective in patients with only colonic involvement. We use doses of 40 to 60 mg. per day in severely ill patients, 20 to 40 mg. per day in moderately ill patients and attempt to taper the dosage and discontinue the drug in patients with mild or inactive disease. Some patients experience a relapse whenever the drug is withdrawn and require long-term therapy. Severity is judged by the degree of fever, abdominal pain, diarrhea, amount of blood loss, weight loss, and radiologic and endoscopic changes. Careful evaluation is important in order to differentiate severe inflammatory disease requiring intensive medical therapy from an intraperitoneal abscess requiring surgical intervention. Patients with either problem can have fever, right lower quadrant pain, severe diarrhea, a tender inflammatory mass, signs of low grade obstruction, and leukocytosis. Therapy should be initiated while diagnostic studies are being done. Supine and upright abdominal radiographs can show signs of obstruction or extra-intestinal gas and a barium enema or B-mode ultra-sound examinations sometimes demonstrate an extra-intestinal mass. Definitive demonstration of an abscess or septicemia are indications for surgical intervention. Equivocal or absent signs justify expectant medical therapy consisting of nothing by mouth, nasogastric suction when the patient has signs of obstruction, central venous nutrition if oral intake is inadequate for more than several days, 10 to 15 mg. of prednisone orally 4 times daily or equivalent parenteral steroids, appropriate fluids and electrolytes, and systemic antibiotics. Clindamycin, 1 to 3 grams per day in 6 hour intervals, and gentamicin, 3 to 5 mg. per kg. per day in 8 hour intervals, or chloramphenicol, 4 grams per day in 6 hour intervals, are appropriate choices. Worsening diarrhea could indicate a complicating pseudomembranous enterocolitis in patients receiving clindamycin. Patients must be observed carefully for several days; improvement will allow gradual reduction in the steroid dosage and resumption of oral intake, while deterioration or failure to improve will usually require surgical therapy.

Extraintestinal Manifestations

Most extraintestinal manifestations of the disease have a relationship to the activity of the bowel disease; i.e., successful treatment of the enterocolitis also reduces the activity of the extraintestinal disorders. Some require specific therapy, but some are unresponsive to treatment.

Mucocutaneous Disease. Pyoderma gangrenosum and erythema nodosum usually accompany active disease and respond to systemic corticosteroids, or resection of diseased bowel. Some authorities advocate dapsone (Avlosulfon), 100 mg. daily initially with gradual increase to 400 to 600 mg., watching carefully for methemoglobinemia. (This use of dapsone is not listed in the manufacturer's official directive.) Aphthous stomatitis may improve with zinc sulfate in a few patients with zinc deficiency.

Liver Disease. The spectrum of liver disease in Crohn's disease is very broad, including hepatic granulomata "pericholangitis" (portal triaditis), chronic active hepatitis, postnecrotic cirrhosis, fatty metamorphosis, sclerosing cholangitis and amyloidosis. There is poor correlation between biochemical and histologic abnormalities. The cause is unknown and the course is extremely variable as it is in ulcerative colitis. Very little is known regarding therapy and the response to corticosteroids or surgical resection is equivocal.

Arthritis. The joint manifestations tend to parallel the activity of the disease, especially colitis. The arthritis is usually minor and nondeforming, involves the larger joints, and responds to aspirin or other nonsteroidal anti-inflammatory agents. Sacroileitis and ankylosing spondylitis pursue a more independent course.

Renal Disease. The urinary tract is affected by a wide variety of complications, including amyloidosis, perinephric abscess, nephrolithiasis, fistulas to the renal pelvis, ureter, or bladder, or ureteral obstruction and hydronephrosis secondary to involvement of the ureter in an inflammatory mass. Perinephric abscess requires a surgical drainage and antibiotics. Symptomatic stones, fistulas, and ureteral obstruction also require surgical intervention. Management of recurrent calcium oxalate stones was discussed earlier.

Ophthalmic Disease. Uveitis and iritis usually parallel the disease activity but local corticosteroids are always indicated. The disease process in the eye should be managed by an ophthalmologist. Posterior subcapsular cataracts sometimes are a complication of long-term steroid therapy.

Surgical Therapy

The disease is constantly changing and the physician must be alert to conditions in which surgical therapy is indicated. However, because of the high rate of recurrence, especially at the anastomotic sites, resection is indicated only when medical therapy fails to control the problem. The indications include: free perforation; massive uncontrolled hemorrhage; total or near-total bowel obstruction; blind-loop syndrome; a fluctuant, tender mass suggestive of abscess; persistent fistulae to skin, genitourinary tract, or other loops of bowel; growth retardation; toxic dilatation of the colon; severe extraintestinal manifestations not controlled with medical therapy, ureteral obstruction, or intractable symptoms. For most of these problems resection of involved bowel is indicated with end-to-end anastomosis rather than bypass of the involved segment. Unfortunately postoperative therapy with anti-inflammatory agents does not appear to reduce the incidence of recurrence.

HEMORRHOIDS, ANAL FISSURE, AND ANAL FISTULA

method of
GUY L. KRATZER, M.D.
Allentown, Pennsylvania

Hemorrhoids

Hemorrhoids develop from normal structures, tiny veins present at birth. These veins swell slightly when the person is standing or straining and in this manner aid the pursestring muscles of the anus to control gas and stool. Hemorrhoids are the most common cause of bleeding from the rectum. These veins may enlarge or become varicose. Although the reason for it is unknown, they occasionally become inflamed, and thrombosis and phlebitis occur. Superficial gangrene of the internal ones may even occur.

Practically everyone has occasional attacks of "piles" or hemorrhoids. An attack may be triggered by trauma such as straining at stool or childbirth and does not constitute an emergency.

Over a period of years these veins may become enlarged and varicose to the extent that they protrude and have to be replaced after each bowel movement. Sometimes they do not stay in, and the constant or chronic protrusion causes a "wet" anus.

Hemorrhoids can be graded according to their severity and size. Internal and external hemorrhoids should be graded separately because their anatomy and symptoms differ. Internal hemorrhoids are covered by mucosa, which is not sensitive to pain. External hemorrhoids are covered by skin and can be very painful when thrombotic or inflamed.

Management. Modern local anesthesia has made it possible to avoid hospitalization in the treatment of most anorectal diseases; however, in actual practice more and more complete hemorrhoidectomies are performed in the hospital, as nervous tension on the part of the patient and medicolegal considerations are becoming factors of great importance. Fortunately, the vast majority of patients suffering from hemorrhoids may be treated by simple office procedures.

The approach to problems of anorectal disease has undergone many changes in recent years, with preventive measures certainly representing the most reasonable approach, as they do to other phases of medicine.

Once in several hundred cases, a patient with normal hematologic studies (including coagulation profile), will bleed profusely from hemorrhoids. Sometimes transfusions are required. Usually such hemorrhoids are of the spongy or "arterial" type. Surgery in the hospital is required in such cases.

With few exceptions, the complications need not occur if the formation of dry, firm stools is prevented. Diet should include bulk. The anus should be cleaned thoroughly with tissue followed by cotton soaked in witch hazel after each bowel movement. Soothing ointments or lotions such as hydrocortisone acetate and pramoxine hydrochloride (Proctofoam-HC) are sometimes indicated.

Hemorrhoids are treated only when they are symptomatic. If they are small, do not protrude and the internal ones are bleeding, sclerosing therapy with 5 per cent phenol in almond oil may suffice. The purpose is not to inject the solution in the veins but to inject it submucosally, with the expectation that the resulting inflammatory reaction will create fibrous tissue and "shrink" the hemorrhoid. Larger protruding internal hemorrhoids are treated by the rubber band method, except in obese women with short anal canals. In such patients, it is difficult to maintain reduction.

A rubber band can be placed around the hemorrhoid with the aid of an ingenious instrument invented by Barron. Anesthesia is not necessary. The internal hemorrhoid is choked off and falls away with the rubber band in a few days. Because hemorrhage from slough is a possibility that requires coagulation as an emergency procedure, some of the larger hemorrhoids are treated two or more times rather than choking off too much tissue at one time. One hemorrhoid is treated relatively painlessly every 3 weeks until all of them have been removed. Usually there are 3 internal ones to be treated. Often after such treatment, the external ones cease to be a problem. If not, they can be treated by simple excision in the office under local anesthesia.

Acute Hemorrhoidal Disease. Acute hemorrhoidal disease, characterized by acute prolapse of the anal canal with thrombophlebitis of all hemorrhoids and, occasionally, necrosis or gangrene, is usually best treated conservatively with hot or cold compresses and mineral oil by mouth to ensure easy bowel movements. The condition will eventually resolve itself. When it is seen within the first 24 to 48 hours, injection of a local anesthetic with hyaluronidase (Wydase) will occasionally cause the edema to disappear and make immediate hemorrhoidectomy possible. This is seldom necessary, however, since it is far safer to use conservative measures until the acute inflammatory process has subsided. By this time, the patient feels so much better that surgery becomes optional.

Thrombotic Hemorrhoid. Perhaps the most frequent anorectal surgical condition encountered in the office is a thrombotic hemorrhoid. After introducing a small amount of anesthetic solution beneath and around the thrombosis, it can be removed with a simple elliptical incision. Often the wound margins fall together after the clot is removed. Usually nothing is needed to control bleeding, and primary union follows. If bleeding occurs, it can be controlled by fulguration, or the vessel, usually a small vein, can be ligated with ooo chromic catgut. A small pressure dressing can be used to prevent development of another thrombus. If in doubt, the skin wounds may be easily closed with ooo chromic catgut.

Management in the Hospital. The indications for hospital surgery are huge hemorrhoids associated with severe protrusion where the lowermost portion of the rectal lining is "turned inside out," and the association of hemorrhoids with other extensive rectal problems such as deep fistulas.

Usually there are 3 and sometimes more groups of hemorrhoids and radial incisions are required to remove them. It is wise to save as much "normal" tissue between the groups as possible. Primary closure with interrupted or running ooo chromic catgut is preferred when this can be done without tension. Sometimes it is necessary to remove the subcutaneous plexus of veins from underneath the preserved anoderm before proceeding with the primary closure. However, one must treat each case individually, and when in doubt, it is good practice to leave the external wound open and free of real or potential tags.

Since open wounds, particularly in the midline posteriorly may be slow healing, there is a trend to avoid them if possible. The posterior sliding skin graft is a simple, effective way of avoiding this annoying complication.

Partial lateral sphincterotomy, when indicated in patients with a contracted anal canal due to fibrous tissue that is usually due to chronic use of laxatives, is another way to relieve the patient's symptoms and encourage primary healing. This should not be used in the very elderly or in a patient suffering from diarrhea.

Idiopathic Pruritus. Persistent itching at the anal area known as idiopathic pruritus ani is probably a functional problem. It is not due to hemorrhoids and seldom is a fungus involved. Surgery will only make the condition worse and compound the problem. Dermatologic and systemic treatment is indicated.

Cryotherapy. Extirpation of hemorrhoids by cryotherapy is also available but will not be discussed here, as it is too early to assess its true value.

Fissure

The treatment of fissure depends upon the cause, and relationship to the general condition of the patient. It may be possible to prevent fissures by proper anal hygiene, high residue diet to encourage regular normal stools, and control of nervous tensions.

Acute Fissure. Acute fissures or abrasions that are a consequence of trauma from too firm a stool are easily recognized for what they are, slitlike superficial linear ulcers. Many heal spontaneously with good anal hygiene—thorough cleansing after each bowel movement with cotton and witch hazel.

A topical 1 per cent hydrocortisone foam preparation (Proctofoam-HC) applied to the folds of the anal verge several times a day helps relieve symptoms and aids the healing process. If pain is severe, 1 per cent benzocaine and 5 per cent sulfathiazole in ointment base can be introduced freely and frequently with the finger, utilizing finger cots.

The acute type of fissure is often found in children. Surgery is necessary so seldom that it is practically contraindicated. Especially in children, the general condition and home environment must be considered.

Application of silver nitrate in treating acute fissures or persistent abrasions will not help and may do harm by converting an acute condition to a chronic one.

Some acute fissures progress to chronic fissures or ulcers because of repeated trauma of hard or too frequent stools and associated infection in the crypts. They are usually located in the posterior portion of the anal canal below the anorectal line and overlying the lowermost portion of the internal sphincter muscle. They usually have a clean, punched-out appearance associated with an enlarged papilla, skin tag, and narrow, spastic anal canal. They are usually small, oblong ulcers, seldom larger than 0.5 cm. A fissure produces pain disproportionate to its size.

Chronic Fissure. The chronic fissure is easily recognized because of its classic features. It is important to rule out the shaggy, large, indolent ulcers associated with Crohn's disease, leukemia, tuberculosis, or even cancer. General study, including proctosigmoidoscopy, barium enema, and colonoscopy, as well as biopsy, may help in diagnosis. Surgery, except for incision and drainage of abscesses in these conditions is contraindicated because the wounds will not heal and there is danger of sepsis and fecal incontinence.

The chronic fissure requires surgery for cure. The patients usually have taken mineral oil or laxatives for years, and, therefore, the anal canal has lost its ability to accommodate a normal stool with resultant fibrous contraction.

Some surgeons would advise simple anal dilatation or sphincterotomy. These "simple" procedures are associated with a high rate of permanent incontinence as well as recurrence.

The "old fashioned way" is to denude the appropriate quadrant, utilizing local anesthesia. The fissure, along with the skin tag, papilla, internal and external hemorrhoids and crypts immediately adjacent to it, is dissected free from the underlying muscle. Usually the respective anal quadrant is left completely denuded. The cut edge of the mucosa is closed with ooo chromic catgut. If the cut edge of the mucosa is too wide for closure, it can be anchored to the muscle at the anorectal line.

Sometimes a band of scar tissue (pecten band) at the lower border of the internal sphincter is encountered and this is divided in one of the lateral quadrants.

The lateral partial internal sphincterotomy has added a new dimension to surgical management of fissures. The obvious reason for this procedure is to reduce to a minimum the necessary associated surgery. A large papilla or tag or associated large hemorrhoids should be removed. I have not performed enough of these "limited" procedures to fully endorse them.

It is here that the posterior midline sliding skin graft has proven itself. Most fissures occur here and since this method constitutes a primary closure, it should be considered a modern procedure.

Postoperative Care. A suitable daily regimen begun the day after operation is as follows: a full diet; sitz baths, meperidine (Demerol) 50 mg. administered by mouth, 1 tablet every 4 hours or as required; milk of magnesia and mineral oil, 1 oz. (30 ml.) of each. These laxatives provide comfortable bowel movements until a regular bowel habit is established. Usually the patient can be discharged from the hospital on the second or third day after operation. After the twelfth postoperative day, the patient is encouraged to have firm, well-formed stools to prevent contracture of the anal canal. At any time after the twelfth day the patient may resume his customary work. He is told to report to the physician's office to determine the condition of the wound. This method of postoperative care is applicable to all anorectal operations.

Fistula

Most fistulas originate as infections in the anal crypts or ducts, and from these sources of infection they burrow outward, through, between, or superficial to the anal sphincter muscles. After they have passed beyond these muscles, they involve the loose areolar ischioanal tissues and become localized there in the form of abscesses. Occasionally, they may "point" internally to the pectinate (anorectal) line and discharge through an opening higher in the rectal wall. Sometimes they may proceed superficially and point into the perianal skin, or they may rupture through the surface of the buttocks.

The diagnosis can be made by palpation or digital examination of the rectal outlet and adjacent structures. If necessary, anesthesia should be used.

Treatment. Abscesses which point externally (in the perianal area) may be incised and drained as an office procedure, providing that suitable anesthesia (local) is available.

Subsequently, after a lapse of time determined by the extent of involvement, definitive surgery may be performed. The procedure usually requires hospitalization. Local anesthesia has proved satisfactory. If possible, the entire fistulous tract, including the involved crypt, should be removed. It may be laid open as a fistulotomy if conservatism is desirable.

Rarely, patients with supralevator and pelvirectal abscesses may be encountered. In such patients hospitalization and regional or general anesthesia are required. The abscesses should be incised and drained intrarectally. Often the communication between the abscess and its crypt of origin can be discovered when the abscess is opened, but if this is not possible, it must be sought when the curative operation is performed.

Tuberculous Anorectal Abscess. Tuberculous anorectal abscess and fistulas can be treated in the same manner as other fistulas, with the exception that attention should be devoted to concomitant treatment of the pulmonary and systemic manifestations of the disease.

Complications. A survey indicates that at least 5 per cent of anorectal surgery is followed by various degrees of incontinence and other sequelae. Conservatism is the modern approach to advising and conducting treatment.

GASTRITIS

method of
ARTHUR B. FRENCH, M.D.
Ann Arbor, Michigan

Management of gastritis really is management of *symptomatic* gastritis. It is difficult to convince students, either medical students or mature postgraduate audiences, that while the majority of patients are completely asymptomatic, a minority will have severe and very troublesome symptoms. Bleeding or hypoalbuminemia may be late manifestations of previously asymptomatic gastritis. On the other hand, severe nausea, vomiting, and abdominal pain may be the result of either acute or chronic gastritis, which does not appear severe to the gastroscopist or histopathologist.

Our understanding of the cause of gastritis is limited in large part to the various agents that can contribute to its causation and to a sequence of histopathologic and immunologic events, which constitute a description of the course of some forms of gastritis without giving an understanding why some patients are symptomatic and others are not. Management of gastritis will be discussed in terms of (1) noxious agents that should be avoided or withdrawn, (2) substances the abnormal mucosa fails to secrete when it should or allows to pass its injured barrier when it should not, and (3) treatment of symptoms in general. Except for variation in the nature of the injury produced by a noxious agent, a traditional detailed classification of the types of gastritis does not help in its management.

Noxious agents have often done their damage before they can be detected and withdrawn. Others have beneficial medicinal effects and are deliberately given until symptoms occur. The most common noxious agents are infectious. *Infectious gastroenteritis* is self-limited in most cases. It is most commonly found in epidemics of food- or food handler-transmitted food poisoning. Agents vary from the Staphylococcus with its toxin to a wide variety of Salmonellae and, by inference, to viruses, the traditional but virologically elusive "gastrointestinal flu."

Symptoms vary from minimal to severe nausea, vomiting, and cramps. In addition to the gastric component, there is often an intestinal component with diarrhea. Treatment is usually limited to rehydration, either by mouth, if tolerated, or intravenously, if not. Intravenous replacement should include not only isotonic saline solution with or without dextrose but also 20 to 40 mEq. of potassium as KCl per liter of fluid. Vomiting may also require an antiemetic, such as prochlorperazine (Compazine), 5 or 10 mg. intramuscularly every 3 to 4 hours, not to exceed 40 mg. daily and followed by 10 mg. as Spansules by mouth every 12 hours. Even with antibiotic-sensitive organisms such as Salmonellae, antibiotic therapy has little effect on intraluminal infection and is useful only if there is systemic invasion. In the acute phase, diarrhea should probably not be stopped with powerful drugs like diphenoxylate (Lomotil), or loperamide (Imodium). It is generally believed that diarrhea speeds elimination of toxins and organisms.

Although salicylate, and particularly alcohol, may cause the acute gastric symptoms of nausea, vomiting and epigastric pain, or more chronic cyclic epigastric pain alone, they may also produce an acute erosive hemorrhagic gastritis with severe hematemesis or melena with or without antecedent pain. Fortunately, this bleeding almost always stops when the agent is withdrawn, blood lost is replaced as necessary, the general measures as listed at the end of this article are taken, and surgery is avoided. Replacement of blood is not needed at all in most patients and should be used only for (1) *shock*-tachycardia and fall in blood pressure, (2) *persistent* tachycardia and fall in blood pressure on standing, (3) *substantial* fall in hematocrit, or (4) failure to bring the hematocrit substantially back toward normal after *many* days.

Surgery should be avoided in all forms of gastritis, particularly in patients with more chronic disease, since postoperative complications and postgastrectomy symptoms are much more frequent than in patients after surgery for peptic ulcers.

Other noxious agents usually cause a milder, often chronic gastritis with pain, which may be severe. Nausea and vomiting are usually less prominent than in patients with infectious gastritis. Bleeding or protein loss are minimal and usually asymptomatic. It is difficult to distinguish between chronic gastritis and pharmacologic effects on the motor activity of esophagus, stomach, and duodenum as a cause of the same discomfort. Many agents can have either or both of these effects. Some are also ulcerogenic. Conveniently, simple withdrawal of the drug is usually all that is required in either case. Beyond alcohol and salicylates, the list of drugs is large. Phenylbutazone, indomethacin, and the corticosteroids are considered *primarily* ulcerogenic and may cause gastrointestinal bleeding on that basis. Antimetabolites such as 5-fluorouracil, 6-mercaptopurine, and nitrogen mustard may also cause either bleeding or protein loss. Reserpine, caffeine, sulfonamides, ferrous sulfate, ammonium chloride, iodides, bromides, mycin antibiotics and fluphenazines are not uncommonly involved.

In addition to gastritis known to be drug induced, there is a large group of patients in whom no reason for gastritis can be determined. However, management at this time fortunately does not depend on type of inflammation (infiltrative, eosinophilic or granulomatous), on extent (antral or diffuse) or on etiology.

When gastric mucosal damage is diffuse and severe: (1) The stomach fails to secrete acid, or else the one way permeability of the membrane, which permits secretion but not back diffusion of hydrogen ion, is damaged, resulting in achlorhydria by gastric analysis. This back diffusion of hydrogen ion may be responsible for initiating tissue damage through the mechanism of histamine release. We certainly do not replace acid with our therapy. (2) Intrinsic factor is not secreted or may be inactivated by antibodies. Since vitamin B_{12} cannot be absorbed from the ileum unless it is coupled to intrinsic factor, monthly injection of vitamin B_{12} (100 micrograms) should be given to patients who have an abnormal Schilling test without intrinsic factor. (3) The same damage to the permeability of the gastric mucosa, which permits back diffusion of hydrogen ion, permits serum proteins to ooze into the lumen, leading to hypoalbuminemia. When hypoalbuminemia is present, a high protein diet is needed to encourage increased albumin synthesis.

In addition to measures directed at circumventing specific gastric mucosal defects, a series of arbitrary intuitive measures seems to be helpful. They are directed at reducing the acid-peptic injury, resting the stomach, and preventing mucosal injury from regurgitated, then deconjugated bile salts.

1. The usual method of therapy to prevent acid-peptic injury is antacid therapy. It seems to help even when gastric analysis shows achlorhydria. Relief of pain by antacids may be partly due to a little understood but clearly demonstrated effect on gastrointestinal motor activity. In any case, antacid-peptic injury is antacid therapy. It seems to two hours, not uncommonly every hour, to give relief. With most nonabsorbable antacids, these doses are cathartic. Enough aluminum hydroxide (Amphojel) must be included to avoid catharsis and give a normal bowel habit. If constipation occurs with use of a magnesium-aluminum formulation (Maalox, Gelusil) or magaldrate (Riopan), or others, milk of magnesia is an effective cathartic and antacid. Cimetidine (Tagamet), 300 mg. four times daily, provides the opportunity to suppress rather than neutralize gastric acid secretion. Most reported studies deal with peptic ulcer, but it logically can be expected to be helpful in gastritis and is widely used. We look forward to reports of scientifically meaningful studies, which may provide a scientific basis for its use or, less likely, relegate it to oblivion. Safety of long-term use (more than 8 weeks) is not established.

2. If acid neutralization or suppression is justifiable only on an intuitive basis, what can one say about stomach rest? In the vomiting patient, one has no choice. In other cases, opinions differ widely. Most recommend the avoidance of spices, but there agreement ends. We permit nonspicy foods as long as they do not seem to aggravate symptoms. Alcohol, tobacco, and coffee are, however, avoided. We would use the word forbidden if the number of patients who follow our advice was larger. We do not believe that food allergies contribute significantly to symptoms in this group of patients, and we do our best to discourage a patient's belief in individual food idiosyncrasies.

3. Bile regurgitation may well contribute significantly to gastric mucosal damage when regurgitated bile salts are deconjugated by bacteria growing in the achlorhydric stomach. Deconjugated bile salts can be rendered harmless to the mucosa by the resin cholestyramine. However, the amount and frequency of administration become prohibitive for this expensive drug. Aluminum hydroxide gel (Amphojel), but not other antacids, binds bile salt as effectively as cholestyramine. Magnesium hydroxide or trisilicate are much less effective binders of bile salts. Therefore, in a frequent antacid program, as much Amphojel as tolerated should be used.

The reader will be impressed that this therapeutic program is almost entirely intuitive and without scientific proof. We can only say that its use results in satisfaction for many patients who come in for consultation after the failure of other programs. It must be given with enthusiasm and it is apparent that strong supportive psychotherapy is an important part of the program.

GASEOUSNESS

method of
JOHN H. BOND, M.D.
Minneapolis, Minnesota

Introduction

Complaints of gaseousness or "too much gas" are frequently encountered in every type of medical practice. Until recently, little reliable scientific information was available defining the true role of gas in the pathophysiology of these symptoms. For this reason, it has been difficult for the practicing physician to deal rationally with these problems and an extensive folklore of misbeliefs and unproved remedies related to intestinal gas has evolved. This article briefly outlines current concepts of the relation of gas to several clinical problems and defines a rational approach to the patient with gas symptoms.

Volume and Composition of Intestinal Gas. The intestinal tract of healthy adults normally contains less than 200 ml. of gas. Five gases, N_2, O_2, H_2, CO_2, and CH_4 (methane), make up greater than 99 per cent of this volume. Of these gases, N_2 is usually present in greatest concentration, and O_2, which is rapidly utilized by the intestinal bacteria, is present in very small amounts. The remaining three gases are found in differing quantities depending on several factors described below. The volume of gas passed per rectum is highly variable, ranging from 200 to 2000 ml. per day with a mean of about 600 ml. per day.

Source of Intestinal Gas. Although it has been traditionally thought that swallowed air is the main source of intestinal gas, recent data indicates that gas production within the gut lumen may frequently be substantial. O_2 and N_2 enter the esophagus and stomach in swallowed air; however, it appears that normally most of this gas is eructated and little passes on into the duodenum. Eructation is easiest in the upright position. When a person is supine, air becomes trapped below fluid overlying the gastroesophageal junction, and more gas passes into the small bowel. This effect of body position may explain the rapid gaseous distention of the small bowel that frequently occurs during surgical or radiologic procedures performed with the patient in the supine position. In addition to swallowed air, N_2 and O_2 also enter the gut lumen by diffusing from the blood. H_2, CH_4, and CO_2 are present in negligible concentrations in the atmosphere, and therefore, must be produced in the gut. These three gases often account for more than 50 per cent of bowel gas, and hence it is apparent that swallowed air is not always the major source of intestinal gas.

CO_2 is produced in large quantities in the upper intestinal tract when gastric hydrochloric acid or dietary fatty acids are neutralized by bicarbonate. Rapid distention of the upper bowel by this gas may account for some of the symptoms of postprandial pain and bloating suffered by many patients with "functional" bowel disease. Most of this CO_2 is rapidly absorbed as it passes down the bowel and never appears in flatus. Flatus, however, may contain as much as 50 per cent CO_2, most of which is derived from colonic bacterial metabolism.

H_2 and CH_4 are produced solely by the intestinal bacteria, and more than 99 per cent of this production occurs in the colon. The bacteria produce appreciable quantities of H_2 only in the presence of dietary fermentable substrate, primarily unabsorbed carbohydrate. The excessive gas commonly observed by patients with malabsorption presumably results from failure to absorb normally ingested carbohydrate, which then passes down to the colonic bacteria. In healthy persons, excessive H_2 production may result from ingestion of vegetables, fruit, and whole grains containing carbohydrate that cannot be digested and absorbed by the normal small intestine and hence serve as substrates for H_2 production in the colon. The effect of eating beans on flatus excretion is a well-known example.

Unlike, H_2, CH_4 production is not related to carbohydrate malabsorption, and the substrate for CH_4 production is not known. CH_4 production also differs from that of H_2 in that only about one third of the normal population appears to have the colonic bacteria capable of producing CH_4 (almost everyone's flora can produce H_2). The tendency to harbor CH_4-producing bacteria appears to be a familial trait determined by early environmental factors.

Since each of the five major components of intestinal gas are nonodorous, it is obvious that other gases must be present in flatus. Odoriferous gases such as NH_3, hydrogen sulfide, indole, skatole, volatile amines, and short chain fatty acids comprise less than 1 per cent of flatus. However, these gases are readily sensed by the nose, which can detect noxious gases in minute concentrations.

Clinical Problems Related to Intestinal Gas

There are four clinical problems in which gastrointestinal gas is thought to be responsible for symptoms—repetitive eructation, functional abdominal pain and bloating, excessive passage of flatus, and explosion during electrosurgery in the colon.

Repetitive Eructation.　A small amount of air enters the stomach with each swallow of food or liquid. In addition, some foods contain appreciable gas as part of their structure (about 20 per cent of an apple's volume is air) or is added in processing (whipped foods, breads, carbonated beverages). The occasional "normal" belch that follows a meal represents the expulsion of part of this ingested gas. Although it is commonly believed that certain "abnormal" forms of swallowing that may occur with rapidly gulping food or drink, chewing gum, sucking on candy, drinking through a straw, having loose dentures, or smoking increases air swallowing, no studies have ever proved these relationships.

Persons who complain of chronic repetitive belching have been shown to take air into the esophagus prior to each belch. Most of this air is noisely regurgitated and does not reach the stomach. Repetitive belching is thus a nervous habit, often exacerbated by emotional stress, or sometimes appears to be precipitated by other symptoms of organic disease in the abdomen or thorax. A vicious cycle of aerophagia and belching may develop in which unconscious air swallowing distends the esophagus and stomach, producing mild discomfort, which is then relieved by belching. In order to have a good belch, however, additional air is swallowed which again produces the discomfort. The patient, unaware he is swallowing air, believes there is an abnormality of his digestive system causing excessive gas production, and this concern increases his anxiety and further aggravates his symptoms.

Patients complaining of chronic belching first require appropriate x-ray and laboratory tests to rule out the presence of organic disease of the thorax or abdomen. The mainstay of treatment is then thorough reassurance that no serious disease is responsible for their belching, that each belch simply represents the expulsion of air which has just been taken into the esophagus. The physician should then demonstrate, using a mirror and palpation of the neck, that each of the patient's eructations is preceded by an elevation of the larynx corresponding to aspiration of air into the esophagus. If the physician himself can belch at will, a personal demonstration of this process will often convincingly persuade the patient of the aerophagia-eructation sequence. Minor tranquilizers may occasionally be needed in the presence of severe emotional upsets, but their long-term use should be avoided. Even when patients continue to belch following this simple therapeutic program, they usually cease complaining or worrying about this symptom once they are convinced of its functional origin.

Functional Abdominal Pain and Bloating.　Abdominal pain and bloating, often worse after meals, are the most common gastrointestinal complaints attributed to gas. Based on little or no scientific data, both patients and their physicians commonly attribute such symptoms to abnormally increased volumes of intestinal gas. However, a recent study in which intestinal gas volumes were carefully measured using a wash-out technique failed to demonstrate increased gas in such patients either in the fasting state or following a large meal. The patients did, however, have an abnormality of intestinal motility resulting in the disordered passage of gas through the bowel with a painful response to the presence of gas volumes well tolerated by normal subjects. Symptoms resulting from this abnormal motility and pain response to distention seem to be interpreted by the patient as a feeling of excessive gas, when, actually, the total intestinal gas volume is normal. The observation by such patients that certain foods "turn to gas" may represent the tendency of these foods to stimulate abnormal motility rather than their tendency to gasify in the gut.

Patients with functional abdominal pain and bloating first require thorough laboratory and x-ray evaluation to ensure they do not have organic disease. Initial treatment then consists of strong reassurance that no serious organic pathology exists. This approach frequently increases substantially the patient's tolerance of abdominal sensations, even though they may continue to exist. Relief of apprehension about the origin of these symptoms may also favorably influence the motor function of the gut and thereby decrease the frequency and severity of abdominal pain.

Whether drugs that alter intestinal motility might be useful in patients with functional abdominal pain and bloating is not known. Claims have been made for anticholinergic agents in this situation; however, well-controlled studies have not yet shown clear-cut benefits from such medications in these patients. A trial course of one of the several available anticholinergic agents might be tried in a given patient who continues to have severe symptoms, but the drug should be discontinued if no improvement occurs within a few weeks.

Although these patients do not have excessive

gas, it appears they have painful responses to volumes of gas which are normally well tolerated. Thus, it may be beneficial to attempt to reduce the volume of gas that accumulates in the bowel as a result of both air swallowing and intestinal gas production. The patient should be cautioned to avoid repeated belching, since a portion of the aspirated air may enter the stomach, and should avoid reclining immediately after meals. Postprandial production of CO_2 in the duodenum may be decreased by a low fat diet and by giving the patient a hydroxide-containing antacid 30 minutes after each meal. Since H_2 and CO_2 production by the colonic bacteria require fermentable substrate, the patient should be counseled to decrease ingestion of vegetables and fruits (e.g., beans, cabbage, apples) that contain nonabsorbable carbohydrates. In addition, since the sugar in milk, lactose, is not completely absorbed even by subjects without obvious lactase deficiency, a lactose-free diet may be helpful.

Excessive Flatus. The passage of large volumes of gas per rectum is another common gas-related complaint. This symptom may simply be an annoying source of social embarrassment to the patient or it may cause him to believe something is seriously wrong with his digestive tract.

Normal subjects on a standard diet rarely excrete more than 100 ml. of flatus per hour. When a group of healthy volunteers was fed a diet containing 50 per cent of its calories as baked beans, flatus elimination increased from a basal level of 15 ml. per hour to 176 ml. per hour. The number of passages of gas per rectum is quite variable, and, in one study of 7 healthy adult males, averaged 13.6 ± 6 (1 SD) per day over a 7 day period.

Conventional blood, x-ray, or endoscopic studies are of little value in the evaluation of the patient with excessive flatus. A more rational approach is to first document the presence of increased gas excretion by inserting a rectal tube attached to a syringe, and measuring gas excretion. Although it is less precise, the frequency of gas passage also may be used to document the problem.

If available, gas-chromatographic analysis of a sample of rectal gas will quickly determine whether excessive flatus excretion is due to air swallowing or to intraluminal gas production. When making this determination, the rectal tube and syringe must first be completely cleared of gas by flushing with water, and care must then be taken to prevent contamination of the sample with room air during collection and analysis. If swallowing air is the source of the excessive flatus, rectal gas will contain high concentrations of N_2. Since excessive air swallowing is of psychogenic origin, simple counseling is the treatment of choice.

If rectal gas contains high concentrations of H_2 and CO_2, which are largely derived from fermentation of unabsorbed carbohydrate in the colon, the patient should be evaluated for a malabsorptive problem. Carbohydrate malabsorption may be due to a generalized malabsorptive disorder (e.g., sprue, pancreatic insufficiency) or more commonly may result from an isolated abnormality such as lactase deficiency. If carbohydrate malabsorption is not found, excessive colonic production of H_2 and CO_2 may be due to ingestion of fruits or vegetables containing large amounts of nonabsorbable carbohydrates. A low carbohydrate diet, including reduction or elimination of milk, will usually reduce flatus volume.

Most patients with documented excessive flatus excrete mainly H_2 and CO_2. Therefore, if rectal gas analysis is not feasible, the first approach should be to search for malabsorption of carbohydrate and reduce dietary carbohydrate.

Gas Explosion in the Colon. Both CH_4 and H_2 are combustible gases and in the proper mixtures with room air may be explosive. There have been many reports of life-threatening explosions and colonic perforations resulting from ignition of these gases by an electrocautery device used to resect or fulgurate rectal lesions through the rigid proctosigmoidoscope. In spite of the current widespread use of electrosurgical snare resection of colonic polyps using the fiberoptic colonoscope, no such explosions have been reported during colonoscopy. Presumably the extensive bowel cleansing required for colonoscopy lowers the concentration of both H_2 and CH_4 by mechanically removing bacteria responsible for their production.

In patients undergoing proctosigmoidoscopy who are not prepared in this extensive manner, the risk of explosions during electrosurgical procedures may be reduced by first aspirating gas from the lumen and then perfusing the operative site with an inert gas such as CO_2 or N_2 prior to coagulation.

ACUTE AND CHRONIC VIRAL HEPATITIS
method of
WILLIAM A. KNIGHT, JR., M.D.,
and ALA E. IMAM, M.D.
St. Louis, Missouri

Viral hepatitis remains a major worldwide public health problem. The number of cases of viral hepatitis reported annually in the United States has reached

70,000, which represents an incidence of 33 cases per 100,000 population.

Viral hepatitis type A and type B have been implicated as the main causative agents in this systemic infection. Occasional cases may be attributed to non-A, non-B types, also referred to as hepatitis C or D. Hepatic involvement is also a feature of infections by the Epstein-Barr virus, cytomegalovirus, herpes simplex virus and other viruses.

Hepatitis A Virus

Hepatitis A virus has been identified by immune electron microscopy in fecal specimens from volunteers during the early incubation period. The virus is 27 nm. in diameter, exhibits cubic symmetry, and stains as an RNA virus of the enterovirus family. The virus survives at 56°C. for 30 minutes but is inactivated by a 1 minute exposure at 98°C.

Hepatitis B Virus

Electron microscopic studies have revealed the presence of three distinct morphologic forms in serum obtained from patients with hepatitis B virus infection.

1. Hepatitis B surface antigen (HB_sAg) appears as a spherical particle 22 nm. in diameter and as a tubular filamentous form of the same diameter but over 200 nm. in length. This surface antigen has no nucleic acid, contains eight to nine polypeptides and three phospholipids, and resides on the surface of the virion.

Four subtypes of this surface antigen have been identified; all share the same *a* antigen and are referred to as *adw, adr, ayw,* and *ayr.* HB_sAg is synthesized in the cytoplasm of infected hepatocytes.

2. Dane particles are spherical, measuring 42 to 45 nm. in diameter. The outer surface containing HB_sAg surrounds a 27 nm. inner core. The Dane particle is probably the complete hepatitis B virion. The concentration of Dane particles in the blood is usually low in the carrier state but high in the presence of active liver disease. No correlation is found between concentration of Dane particles and HB_sAg concentration. Infectivity correlates better with Dane particle concentration than with HB_sAg concentration.

3. Hepatitis B core antigen (HB_cAg) is demonstrable in the serum only after the Dane particles are disrupted by treatment with detergent. HB_cAg is 27 nm. in size and contains DNA polymerase activity, DNA template, and circular double stranded DNA. This inner core is synthesized in the nucleus of infected hepatocytes.

Immunologic Pattern of Hepatitis B Infection.

1. DNA polymerase activity and Dane particles appear in the serum late in the incubation period and decline before the maximum rise in transaminase activity.

2. HB_sAg appears in the serum several weeks after exposure, before the onset of clinical illness and may remain as long as the infection is clinically apparent.

3. Hepatitis B core antibody (HB_cAb) in the serum often coincides with the onset of clinical illness, falls gradually, and may become undetectable 2 to 3 years after the infection. A high titer is observed in those persons who become chronic carriers, particularly those with chronic active liver disease. Thus this antibody may

be a sensitive indicator of viral replication and the presence of hepatitis B virus infection.

4. Hepatitis B surface antibody (HB_sAb) seroconversion usually occurs during convalescence, after HB_sAg has disappeared. The demonstration of this antibody indicates that the person has previously had type B hepatitis and is immune to reinfection by all of its subtypes (all share the same *a* antigen).

5. The *e* antigen (e-Ag) is another antigen that is associated only with hepatitis B infection. It is immunologically distinct from both HB_sAg and HB_cAg. It is not known whether e-Ag originates in the virus or in the host. It is a mucopolysaccharide with a molecular weight of 300,000. The presence of this e-Ag in sera positive for HB_sAg is associated with the presence of chronic hepatitis, high titers of HB_sAg and Dane particles in the serum, and high infectivity. The presence of *e* antibody (e-Ab) is associated with normal liver histology, low titers of HB_sAg and Dane particles in the serum, and low infectivity.

Prevention and Prophylaxis

Until vaccines are available, prevention and control of hepatitis A and B must be directed toward interrupting the route of transmission.

Hepatitis A. Strict sanitation methods are necessary to prevent fecal-oral contamination. The patient and his close contacts should not be permitted to prepare food or water for others. Strict personal hygiene, washing of hands, wearing of gloves, proper handling and disposal of feces and urine, the use of 0.5 per cent sodium hypochlorite (1:10 Clorox) as disinfectant, and the use of disposable plates and eating utensils are essential in preventing the spread of hepatitis A during the acute phase of the illness and for several weeks thereafter. Only disposable needles, syringes and lancets should be used. The patient's clothes and linen should be laundered separately.

Immune serum globulin (ISG) prepared from large pools of normal adult plasma confers passive protection against hepatitis A in 80 to 90 per cent of exposed persons if given within the first 4 to 6 weeks after exposure. ISG, 0.02 to 0.04 ml. per kg. intramuscularly, will prevent symptoms and jaundice, although subclinical infection may occur. ISG is recommended for close contacts or for common source exposure. To interrupt epidemics in institutions or camps and to protect persons at high risk, ISG, 0.06 to 0.10 ml. per kg. intramuscularly, every 4 to 6 months is recommended. ISG has no proven value after the onset of clinical hepatitis.

Hepatitis B. Education concerning hepatitis B transmission and continuous surveillance for hepatitis B cases are necessary for those in the high-risk group. Whenever practical, disposable needles and syringes are recommended and instruments should be autoclaved, boiled, or gas sterilized. Clorox 1:10 destroys HB_sAg in material having a low concentration of protein and can be used in special situations, such as cleaning fiberoptic endoscopic instruments. The wearing of gloves and protective clothing is encouraged to avoid contamination with blood and other infective fluids.

To reduce the risk of post-transfusion hepatitis, persons who have had hepatitis are currently not accepted as blood donors; however, blood containing detectable HB_s antibody carries no increased risk of transmitting hepatitis B. Since commercial whole blood or blood from first-time donors carries a higher risk, transfusion from these sources should be avoided. The use of frozen red blood cells is preferable. Pooled plasma should be made from no more than five donors and each should be tested for HB_sAg. A sensitive method such as radioimmune assay should be used for detecting HB_sAg.

Hyperimmune serum globulin (HISG) contains a very high titer of hepatitis B surface antibody (HB_sAb). HISG has been shown to be effective in preventing hepatitis in persons exposed to hepatitis B via needle stick, in hemodialysis units or in close contact with patients who have hepatitis B. It is necessary to administer 5 to 10 ml. of HISG immediately after known contact. However, HISG fails to provide long-term immunity and should be administered every 3 to 4 months. Standard immune serum globulin (ISG) containing HB_sAb has demonstrated some benefit in preventing clinical hepatitis in nonparenteral transmission of hepatitis B infection. Unlike HISG, ISG permits passive active immunization with long-term immunity and may be used for prophylaxis among contacts of hepatitis B patients or carriers.

Highly purified formalin-treated and heated HB_sAg has been used as a vaccine against hepatitis B infection. The antigen prepared by this method lost its infectivity but maintained its antigenicity. The vaccine has been tested in chimpanzees and a limited number of humans. It appears safe, produces active anti-HB_s response and protects against hepatitis B infection upon challenge with hepatitis B virus. This vaccine, when available, may be used to protect those at high risk and those who live in endemic areas of hepatitis B virus infection.

Non-A, Non-B Hepatitis. The incidence of non-A, non-B viral hepatitis may be reduced by the use of volunteer rather than commercial blood donors. Information suggests that standard ISG administered at the time of transfusion lowers the risk of non-A, non-B hepatitis and significantly reduces the number of cases that progress from non-A, non-B hepatitis to chronic hepatitis. Actual identification of these viruses will aid the development of means to prevent the disease and its complications.

Therapy for Acute Hepatitis

Typical Acute Hepatitis. There is no specific therapy for typical acute viral hepatitis. Hospitalization may be required for correct diagnosis and clinically severe illness with persistent anorexia, nausea, and vomiting. Patients with minimal symptoms and good appetite with an adequate caloric oral intake may be managed at home.

REST. Complete bed rest is not required. The patient may ambulate but should not become exhausted or fatigued. The patient's clinical course should be followed daily while in the hospital and hepatic function studies repeated twice weekly, more often if necessary. When the patient's oral caloric intake is adequate and there is significant clinical improvement as manifested by symptoms and laboratory studies, the patient at home may gradually return to normal activity and the hospitalized patient may be discharged, to be followed at home. Minor abnormalities in liver chemistry do not preclude gradual resumption of normal activities.

DIET. Acutely ill patients with nausea and vomiting may not be able to ingest adequate fluids and calories by mouth and should be given 5 to 10 per cent glucose solutions intravenously. Oral intake should be encouraged, and a diet that provides adequate protein, carbohydrate, and fat is prescribed. The dietitian should calculate the daily food and caloric intake and this record will provide a valuable index of the patient's clinical course. Alcohol consumption is prohibited during the acute illness and excessive alcoholic intake should be avoided for 6 to 12 months.

DRUGS. Steroids are not indicated in the treatment of typical acute viral hepatitis and should be avoided. Cholestyramine, 8 to 12 grams per day in divided doses, with meals, may be used if significant pruritus is present. Nausea and vomiting usually subside in a few days, but if medication is needed, phenothiazines may be of value. Chlordiazepoxide hydrochloride in small doses is used for anxiety. All drugs, especially those with hepatic toxicity, are avoided unless absolutely essential.

Following discharge the patient should be re-evaluated in two weeks, then monthly until complete recovery.

Fulminant Hepatitis. The aim of therapy in fulminant hepatitis is to prolong survival in order to permit the liver to recover. The complications that usually contribute to mortality are hepatic encephalopathy, cerebral edema, fluid and electrolyte abnormalities, hypoglycemia, bleeding and hemorrhage, respiratory failure, cardiovascular collapse, and renal failure. Frequent, astute observation for the early signs of these complications and prompt therapy may enhance survival. This therapy may include maintaining an open airway with or without endotracheal tube or positive or assisted ventilation, and maintaining fluid and electrolyte balance, intravascular volume, and urine output by intravenous fluids, glucose, and electrolytes. A nasogastric tube may be used for decompressing the stomach or the administration of drugs. Cimetidine, 300 mg. every 6 hours intravenously, may reduce the risk of gastrointestinal bleeding. (This use of cimetidine is not listed in the manufacturer's official directive.) If the patient is tolerating some oral feedings and signs of encephalopathy develop, the protein intake should be limited to 30 grams or less per 24 hours and lactulose, 30 to 50 ml. every 4 to 6 hours, tetracycline, 0.25 to 0.5 gram, or neomycin, 1 gram with sorbitol every 4 to 6 hours, may be given orally or by nasogastric tube. Saline enemas with or without neomycin may be given. Coagulation abnormalities can be corrected temporarily by using fresh frozen plasma. Levodopa, 250 mg. every 4 to 6 hours orally or by nasogastric tube, may induce a temporary improvement in the level of consciousness and in the changes in the electroencephalogram. (This use of levodopa is not listed in the manufacturer's official directive.) The therapeutic value of this latter drug is still uncertain. Similarly, insulin and glucagon combined have been shown to decrease the mortality rate in experimental animals. Its value in human fulminant hepatitis is unproved.

Heroic procedures, e.g., exchange transfusion, cross circulation and total body wash-out, do not enhance the survival rate. The use of corticosteroids in patients with severe hepatitis is still controversial and may be detrimental.

Bridging Hepatic Necrosis. The effectiveness of corticosteroids in reversing this form of severe hepatitis has not been established and may be hazardous in some patients.

Therapy for Chronic Hepatitis

Chronic Persistent Hepatitis. Chronic persistent hepatitis is a nonprogressive disease and requires no treatment except reassurance, observation, repeat liver function studies, and liver biopsy, primarily for the purpose of confirming the initial diagnosis.

Chronic Active Hepatitis. Piecemeal necrosis alone without any evidence of cirrhosis or bridging hepatic necrosis in the asymptomatic patient can be observed for 3 to 6 months with repeat liver function studies and liver biopsy. If there is no evidence of progression, the patient can be observed without treatment. If the patient is symptomatic and there is evidence of progression, early treatment may prevent progression of the disease process and possibly cirrhosis.

Bridging hepatic necrosis with or without piecemeal necrosis and all patients who have chronic active hepatitis with cirrhosis should be treated after establishing the histologic diagnosis.

Prednisone is the drug of choice. The initial treatment should be 40 to 60 mg. a day and tapered over a period of 4 to 6 weeks to a maintenance dose of 15 to 20 mg. a day. This therapy should be continued until remission is established based on clinical and histologic criteria. After remission, treatment should continue for 4 to 6 months and then be slowly stopped over a 6 to 8 week period. Relapse after discontinuing treatment occurs in 50 per cent of patients and is usually evident in the first 6 months. If relapse occurs, the course of prednisone should be repeated.

Azathioprine, 50 to 100 mg. a day, can be used in addition to prednisone in those patients who cannot tolerate high doses of steroids, if there is a contraindication to steroid therapy, and in those patients who are not responding to steroids. (This use of azathioprine is not listed in the manufacturer's official directive.) With azathioprine, the maintenance dose of prednisone may be as low as 5 to 10 mg. per day.

THE MALABSORPTION SYNDROME

method of
IRWIN H. ROSENBERG, M.D.,
and JAMES M. RABB, M.D.
Chicago, Illinois

In planning therapy, we view the malabsorption syndrome in two ways: (1) as the primary manifestation of a specific disease process, e.g., celiac disease, whose identification and treatment will improve or restore normal absorption, or (2) as a complication of a large number of conditions, e.g., Crohn's disease, short gut, or postgastrectomy states, where we may be unable to correct the underlying situation, but must evaluate and treat malabsorption as an important part of the general therapy.

Recognition of the Malabsorption Syndrome

The symptoms most common in patients with malabsorption syndrome are nonspecific: weight loss, weakness, and lethargy. Intestinal abnormalities are suggested by diarrhea, borborygmi, abdominal bloating, anorexia, light colored, greasy, oily, foul smelling stools, or passage of

TABLE 1.　**Pathophysiologic Basis for Symptoms and Signs in Malabsorptive Disorders**

CLINICAL FEATURES	PATHOPHYSIOLOGY
Generalized malnutrition as manifested by weight loss, muscle wasting and growth retardation	Malabsorption of fat, carbohydrate, and protein → loss of calories
Diarrhea, abdominal distention, flatulence	Impaired absorption of sodium and water; osmotic effects of unabsorbed carbohydrate; ? "irritant" effect of unabsorbed fatty acids, bile salts
Weakness	Anemia; electrolyte depletion; malnutrition
Anemia	Impaired absorption of iron, vitamin B_{12}, and/or folic acid
Glossitis, cheilosis	Deficiency of iron and B vitamins
Peripheral neuritis	Deficiency of vitamin B_{12} and/or other B vitamins
Edema	Impaired absorption of amino acids → protein depletion → hypoproteinemia
Amenorrhea	Protein depletion → secondary hypopituitarism
Bone pains	a. Protein depletion → impaired bone formation → osteoporosis b. Vitamin D and calcium malabsorption demineralization of bone → osteomalacia
Tetany, paresthesias	Calcium malabsorption → hypocalcemia; magnesium malabsorption → hypomagnesemia
Hemorrhagic phenomena	Vitamin K malabsorption → hypoprothrombinemia

TABLE 2.　**Tests in the Diagnosis of Malabsorption States**

I. *Initial Screening Tests*
  A. Stool exam
    1. Microscopic fat
       Neutral fat
       Fatty acids
    2. Undigested muscle fibers
    3. Fecal leukocytes
  B. Blood tests
    1. Hgb, Hct
    2. Serum albumin, Ca, Mg, Fe
    3. Serum prothrombin—response to Vitamin K
    4. Serum folate
    5. Vitamin A, carotene (serum)
    6. Serum cholesterol
    7. Serum 25-OH-Vitamin D
II. *Documentation and Workup of Malabsorption*
  A. Fecal fat (72 hours, quantitative)
  B. Carbohydrate absorption tests
    1. Xylose tolerance test
    2. Lactose breath test
    3. Lactose tolerance blood test
  C. Peroral intestinal biopsy
  D. Gastrointestinal x-ray
  E. Vitamin absorption tests
    1. Schilling test (B_{12}) + I.F.
    2. Folate absorption
  F. Pancreatic function tests
    1. Secretory tests (secretin, pancreozymin)
    2. Stool enzymes (trypsin)
  G. ^{14}C Bile acid breath test

undigested food. Protein, vitamin, and mineral deficiencies may present as edema, muscle wasting, ecchymoses, bleeding, paresthesias, numbness, stomatitis, glossitis, cheilosis, pallor, dermatitis, alopecia, bone pain, and tetany. Table 1 illustrates the correlation between the clinical presentation and the corresponding nutrient deficiencies. Table 2 enumerates the laboratory tests employed to document, quantify, and identify the cause of malabsorption.

Principles of Treatment

1. Treat the underlying disease to the extent possible.
2. Manage the manifestations of malabsorption.

Treatment of Specific Causes of Malabsorption

Pancreatic Insufficiency. 1. Low fat diet. Begin at 50 grams and liberalize fat intake as tolerated.

2. Divide daily dietary intake into six rather than the usual three feedings.

3. Pancreatic enzyme replacement: Preparations with the highest trypsin and lipase are Ilozyme, Ku-Zyme HP, Cotazym, and Viokase. Begin with 2 or 3 capsules or tablets with each feeding. Titrate the severity of diarrhea or fat response by increasing the enzyme replacement.

4. If the response to pancreatic replacement is unsatisfactory, consider acid neutralization to enhance the action of pancreatic supplements by preventing enzyme digestion in the stomach. Use sodium bicarbonate, 500 mg., 2 to 6 tablets with each meal, or cimetidine, 300 mg. 1 hour prior to each meal.

Celiac Disease. 1. Gluten-free diet (for all diets in this chapter refer to William, S. R.: *Essentials of Nutrition and Diet Therapy*, C. V. Mosby Co., 1974).

2. For refractory cases:

a. Be sure patient is adhering strictly to the gluten-free diet.

b. If response to strict diet is unsatisfactory, add corticosteroids, e.g., prednisone, 40 to 60 mg. per day, and taper according to the patient's response.

Tropical Sprue/Tropical Enteropathy. 1. Broad-spectrum antibiotics: Tetracycline, 250 mg. four times daily or sulfasoxazole 500 mg. four times daily for 2 weeks to 6 months, depending on the patient's response. (This specific use of sulfasoxazole is not listed in the manufacturer's official directive).

2. Folic acid, 1 to 5 mg. intramuscularly, acutely for folate deficient megaloblastic anemia then 1 mg. daily orally; vitamin B_{12}, 1000 micrograms intramuscularly in a single dose.

Whipple's Disease. 1. Antibiotics: procaine penicillin, 1.2 million units intramuscularly daily until there is a good clinical response. Then phenoxymethyl penicillin, 250 mg. four times daily for 4 to 6 months or until the biopsy returns to normal.

2. Relapses and drug resistance are to be expected. Treat relapse with the agent initially employed. If the patient does not respond, switch to an alternate antibiotic. Alternate regimens: tetracycline, 250 mg. four times daily, or ampicillin, 250 mg. four times daily for 4 to 6 months as above.

Ileal Resection, Disease, or Damage With Disorders Such as Crohn's Disease and Radiation Enteritis. 1. *Less than 100 cm. resection or involvement.* Diarrhea caused by bile salt action on the colon: give cholestyramine, 4 grams with each meal. Cholestyramine itself can induce malabsorption of some drugs and fat-soluble and some water-soluble vitamins. Check the prothrombin time, vitamin A, and vitamin D levels periodically and adjust drug and vitamin dosages accordingly (see below).

2. *Greater than 100 cm. resection.* Diarrhea secondary to bile salt deficit and steatorrhea. Use a low fat diet. Supplement with vitamins and minerals.

3. *Vitamin B_{12}.* In both (1) and (2) above where vitamin B_{12} malabsorption is documented or expected, treatment is initiated with a 1000 micrograms loading dose (often given with the Schilling test). Maintenance treatment is 100 micrograms per month intramuscularly or 1000 micrograms intramuscularly every 6 months.

4. *Intestinal hyperoxaluria and oxalate nephrolithiasis*

a. Patients comply poorly with a low oxalate diet because of its unpalatability. However, chocolate, cola beverages, tea, potatoes, spinach, rhubarb, and nuts, as well as "mega" doses of vitamin C, should be avoided. This form of diet therapy should be combined with the other modifications listed below.

b. Lessen steatorrhea by lowering fat intake, often to 50 to 60 grams.

c. Calcium supplementation: begin at 1 gram per day of elemental calcium (Titralac, 420 mg. tablets, 6 tablets, or Titralac liquid, 12.5 ml. [1 gram per 5 ml.]) given in divided doses throughout the day.

Increase the calcium in weekly increments of 1 gram per day until the urine oxalate excretion falls into the normal range.

Protein-losing Enteropathy. This disorder may be caused by lymphatic obstruction, inflammatory disease, or congenital lymphangiectasia.

1. Treat underlying disease medically or surgically if possible.

2. Low fat, high protein diet (less than 50 grams of fat per day).
To replace calories lost through fat restriction, utilize diets or commercial formulas in which calories from carbohydrate or medium chain triglycerides replace those derived from long chain fatty acids.

Eosinophilic Gastroenteritis. 1. Omit the offending dietary agent if known.

2. Corticosteroids: Prednisone, 30 mg. per day for 7 to 10 days; then taper to levels which maintain freedom from symptoms.

Bacterial Overgrowth, "Blind Loop" Syndrome. 1. When possible, surgically repair strictures, fistulas, and poorly emptying loops causing the overgrowth.

2. Antibiotics: Tetracycline, 250 to 500 mg. four times daily, erythromycin, 250 to 500 mg. four times daily, phenoxymethyl penicillin, 500 mg. four times daily, or clindamycin, 150 to 300 mg. four times daily. After improvement give antibiotics 2 weeks out of each month or 4 days per week. Drug resistance may necessitate changing the antibiotic.

Cholestasis (Primary Biliary Cirrhosis, Sclerosing Cholangitis, etc.). 1. Low fat diet.

2. Supplementation of fat soluble vitamins:

a. *Vitamin A,* 25,000 units per day is usually required to maintain normal serum levels.

b. *Vitamin D,* the optimal replacement dose is uncertain. 100,000 units of ergocalciferol (vitamin D_2) per month intramuscularly is often used. Oral 25-hydroxyvitamin D, 100 to 200 mg. daily (approval by the FDA pending). Follow replacement therapy by serum calcium, phosphate, alkaline phosphatase, and, when possible, serum 25-hydroxyvitamin D levels.

c. *Vitamin K,* 5 to 25 mg. of phytonadione (AquaMephyton) intramuscularly as necessary to normalize the prothrombin time, then vitamin K, (Mephyton), 5 to 10 mg. by mouth per day, as needed to maintain this state.

Disaccharidase Deficiency. 1. *Lactase deficiency, lactose intolerance.* Low lactose diet. It is usually sufficient to remove full glasses of milk, ice cream, and creamed cottage cheese. Rigid removal of all milk products is unnecessary.

2. *Glucose-galactose malabsorption.* Give glucose, galactose-free formulae such as Galactomin

and Cho-Free for infants. For older children and adults give foods low in starch, glucose, and lactose.

3. *Sucrase deficiency.* Low sucrose diet.

Management of Malabsorption in General

Resuscitation for Acute Nutritional/Metabolic Depletion. Patients with severe diarrhea and malabsorption may present acutely ill with dehydration, hypotension, mineral and electrolyte abnormalities, and florid signs of malnutrition. The physician's strategy should be to attend emergently to the patient's vital functions and to correct potentially lethal metabolic aberrations.

1. Immediately replete intravascular volume to support adequate blood pressure and then more gradually correct the total volume deficit, i.e., 50 per cent over the next 8 to 12 hours. Avoid excessively rapid fluid shifts.

2. Transfuse as necessary.

3. Albumin infusions, 25 to 50 grams per 24 hours, are necessary when the patient's hypoalbuminemia might contribute to pulmonary edema or severely threaten his recovery, for example, from poorly healing decubiti, wounds, or fistulas.

4. Hemorrhagic phenomena: Treat acute hemorrhage due to vitamin K deficiency with 10 to 50 mg. of vitamin K intravenously and fresh frozen plasma infusion, the latter repeated until the prothrombin time has normalized.

5. Electrolyte imbalance: Correct electrolyte balance gradually, 50 per cent correction over 8 to 12 hours. The electrolyte disorders most likely to occur in the malabsorption syndrome are hypokalemia, hypocalcemia, and hypomagnesemia.

a. Hypokalemia. A serum potassium of 3 mEq. per liter at normal pH represents approximately a 100 mEq. deficit and a serum potassium of 1.5 mEq. per liter represents approximately a 600 mEq. deficit. Alkalosis lowers and acidosis raises the serum potassium. Corrections can usually be made with KCl, up to 40 mEq. per liter in the intravenous fluids.

b. Hypocalcemia. Symptomatic hypocalcemia with stridor or tetany must be reversed emergently. Give 20 to 30 ml. of 10 per cent calcium gluconate intravenously over 15 minutes, then titrate the serum calcium to the required level with a slower infusion. Be sure to correct hypomagnesemia.

c. Hypomagnesemia. For a magnesium of less than 0.8 mEq. per liter give 2 mEq. of magnesium per kg. body weight over 4 hours.

6. Severe vitamin deficiencies. Therapy for florid hypovitaminosis is best begun parenterally. See below for dose guidelines.

Management of Chronic Malabsorption. FAT MALABSORPTION. Fat malabsorption (steator-

rhea) induces diarrhea and contributes to deficiency of calories and fat-soluble vitamins.

Treatment with a low fat diet alone will frequently remedy these abnormalities. The degree of fat restriction should correspond to the patient's symptomatic response but reduction to a 50 to 60 gram fat intake is often most helpful.

Replenish the calories lost by fat restriction with increased dietary carbohydrate and, if preferred, medium chain triglyceride oil.

Repletion of fat-soluble vitamins (see below).

PROTEIN/CALORIE DEFICIENCIES. Significant protein and calorie deficits lead to weight loss, muscle wasting, decrements in serum proteins such as albumin and transferrin, and immune depression as manifested by a low lymphocyte count and loss of delayed hypersensitivity to skin antigens. To supply the required protein and calories:

Increase the protein and calorie content of the diet until the patient responds with weight gain and evidence of improved protein status such as increased serum albumin, serum transferrin, lymphocyte count, positive tests of delayed hypersensitivity, 24 hour urine creatinine, and arm muscle area.

If the patient cannot tolerate the increased dietary intake try liquid formula supplements:

Modular feedings. There are available a vast array of protein and calorie sources, alone or in combination, which can be added to the patient's diet. Products which we frequently use are: *protein,* Pro-Mix, Liquid Protein Formula, EMF; *calories:* carbohydrate, Polycose, Hycal; lipid, MCT Oil; *combination,* Citrotein.

Elemental feedings (Vivonex, Vivonex HN, Precision, Precision HN, Portagen). Patients with severe short-gut syndrome, extensive Crohn's disease, or radiation enteritis, for example, may tolerate little or no dietary intake. For them, elemental diets may be ideal. Protein and calorie sources in these commercially available liquid feedings need little or no digestion, so assimilation is considerably more efficient than that from the normal diet. Along with each 1800 calories of an elemental feeding is included the recommended dietary allowance for all vitamins and minerals. For most preparations, 30 ml. of safflower oil per day must be added to purify essential fatty acids. If any of the aforementioned products except Portagen are to serve as the patient's sole dietary source, 30 grams of safflower oil or 50 grams of corn oil should be added daily to supply essential fats. With the additions described, a patient can derive 100 per cent of his nutritional requirements from an elemental diet. Many of these products are administered in hypertonic form which can induce cramps and diarrhea. Therefore, begin feedings with 1 liter of solution diluted to isotonicity and increase to full concentration in 2 to 3 steps as tolerated. Then increase the volume until protein and calorie requirements are met. If necessary and not contraindicated, employ antidiarrheal agents such as paregoric, diphenoxylate (Lomotil), or loperamide.

Parenteral nutrition. Within the past several years it has become possible to satisfy nutritional needs entirely through intravenous feedings. The practitioner should reserve total parenteral nutrition for the following situations: (1) the critically malnourished patient in whom enteral nutrition of any kind would be inadequate or harmful, and (2) the patient with short gut syndrome whose malabsorption or electrolyte losses through diarrhea are so severe that oral alimentation would not sustain life. Because the remaining small bowel hypertrophies somewhat, many patients are ultimately able to make a gradual transition from parenteral to formula alimentation and then to a diet consisting of normal foods. However, some may still require permanent parenteral support. The details of the technique of parenteral nutrition are beyond the scope of this article. The reader is referred to Fischer, J. E. (ed.): *Total Parenteral Nutrition,* Little, Brown & Co., 1976.

VITAMIN DEFICIENCIES. Fat-soluble vitamins: Vitamin A. When vitamin A deficiency is clinically apparent as night blindness, xerophthalmia, and keratomalacia, 100,000 to 300,000 I.U. of vitamin A per day should be temporarily employed. Thereafter for maintenance, mild dark adaptation changes or low serum vitamin A levels, 25,000 I.U. per day are usually needed.

Vitamin D. 2500 to 12,500 I.U. per day of vitamin D (ergocalciferol, cholecalciferol) is adequate for most malabsorptive disorders except cholestasis (see above).

Vitamin K. For chronic replacement vitamin K_1 (Mephyton), 5 to 10 mg. per day by mouth or phytonadione (AquaMephyton), 10 to 25 mg. intramuscularly, intermittently according to the prothrombin time.

Water-soluble vitamins: B complex, vitamin C. The use of a multivitamin preparation that supplies up to five times the recommended daily allowance is probably sufficient on a daily basis. If oral consumption is not possible, then vitamins B and C may be administered, intravenously or intramuscularly.

Dose guidelines for these vitamins include: vitamin C, 50 to 250 mg.; thiamine, 5 to 25 mg.; riboflavin, 5 to 25 mg.; niacin, 25 to 50 mg.; pyridoxine, 2 to 10 mg.; pantothenic acid, 10 to 25 mg.; and biotin, 150 to 300 mcg. (Deficiency state in man is not well defined for pantothenic acid and biotin. Therapy is therefore optional.)

In general, for treatment of manifest vitamin deficiency these doses should be given three times per day orally or once parenterally. A single daily oral dose is then adequate for maintenance.

Folic acid. Initial treatment for deficiency, 1 to 5 mg. intramuscularly. Maintenance therapy, 1 mg. orally per day.

Vitamin B_{12}. Initial treatment 1000 micrograms intramuscularly, thereafter 100 micrograms per month, or 1000 micrograms intramuscularly every 6 months.

MINERALS AND TRACE ELEMENTS. *Calcium.* Calcium supplementation is required for treatment of metabolic bone disorders resulting from calcium and vitamin D malabsorption and for treatment of intestinal hyperoxaluria as already described. For this former situation give 2 grams of elemental calcium per day as Titralac, 420 mg. tablet, 12 tablets per day, or Titralac liquid (1 gram per 5 ml.) per day.

Magnesium. For chronic requirements give magnesium sulfate, 1 to 6 grams per day by mouth. Diarrhea, a troublesome complication of oral therapy, sometimes necessitates intermittent intramuscular magnesium injections of 8 to 16 mEq. of magnesium sulfate per day, every other day, or weekly.

Iron. Ferrous sulfate, 300 mg., or ferrous gluconate, 650 mg., 4 times per day until the serum iron is restored to normal, then as often as necessary to maintain the serum iron, usually 1 to 2 times per day.

Other trace elements. Includes zinc, copper, manganese, cobalt and chromium. The doses, safety, and indications for therapy are under study. For zinc, zinc sulfate, 66 to 400 mg. orally per day, is recommended.

INTESTINAL OBSTRUCTION

method of
PHILIP C. JOLLY, M.D.,
and LON S. ANNEST, M.D.
Seattle, Washington

Obstruction of the alimentary tract produces a life-threatening illness that usually requires operative intervention. Early diagnosis and treatment are critical if strangulation, gangrene, perforation, and sepsis are to be avoided.

Recognition of bowel obstruction is facilitated by the following:

1. A history of vomiting, obstipation, and episodic abdominal pain is usually elicited. Continuous abdomi-

nal pain suggests strangulation or an inflammatory process producing an ileus. Vomiting usually occurs early in small bowel obstruction but may not develop for several days in large bowel obstruction. A history of previous abdominal surgery, malignancy, or abdominal irradiation should be sought.

2. A careful abdominal examination should include a search for laparotomy scars and evaluation of degree of distention. Localized abdominal tenderness, tachycardia, elevated temperature, and postural hypotension suggest compromised bowel. A groin mass may indicate an incarcerated hernia or metastatic tumor.

3. Supine and upright abdominal x-rays usually show dilated small bowel with air fluid levels but are diagnostic in only 60 per cent of patients. If the colon is dilated and contains a large amount of gas with an abrupt cut-off, a large bowel obstruction can be diagnosed. In this latter instance diagnosis may be safely confirmed by proctoscopy and barium enema. A small amount of air in the colon and a history of intermittent passage of flatus suggest partial obstruction. Occasionally, a closed loop obstruction (a segment of bowel obstructed at both ends) will not show any roentgenographic evidence of gas in the small bowel. Barium by mouth can be of assistance in the diagnosis of small bowel obstruction, but should not be given to patients suspected of having compromised bowel or large bowel obstruction.

4. Leukocyte count above 15,000 per cu. mm. suggests compromised bowel or an inflammatory process with associated ileus. Very high counts above 25,000 per cu. mm. are found in patients with mesenteric vascular occlusion and infarction. An elevated hematocrit may mean significant third space sequestration of fluid and electrolytes, often found when bowel is compromised. A low hematocrit initially may indicate blood loss from a carcinoma. Electrolyte determinations before operation are mandatory. Low serum potassium, phosphorus, or magnesium levels may cause a paralytic ileus, which masquerades as mechanical obstruction. Blood gas determinations are important in guiding replacement therapy and in assessing pulmonary status. Serum amylase values two to three times normal may occur with bowel obstruction and do not necessarily mean pancreatitis.

Initial Management

When a diagnosis is made within 24 hours of the onset of symptoms early operation is usually needed. Alternately, in the absence of "grave signs" (localized tenderness, fever, tachycardia, and leukocytosis), a period of cautious observation may be planned since an occasional adhesive bowel obstruction will be relieved by nonoperative means. During this period initial resuscitation consists of the following:

1. Nasogastric intubation with intermittent or sump tube suction is mandatory. Long tubes are ineffective and only cause delays in resuscitation. General anesthesia is not safe without first decompressing the stomach.

2. Intravenous fluid replacement is started usually with isotonic saline in 5 per cent dextrose. Rate of administration depends on external and internal losses and on cardiac status. Generally, fluid replacement is begun at 200 to 1000 ml. per hour.

3. An indwelling urinary catheter is used in most patients to monitor urinary output. Urine volumes of 40 to 60 ml. per hour indicate adequate fluid replacement and satisfactory intravascular volume.

4. Analgesics are needed for control of pain.

5. Antibiotics should be administered before operation if nonviable bowel is suspected.

Laparotomy after a minimum of delay for the indicated resuscitation is necessary in most patients. The urgency for operation is increased if any of the "grave signs" are present. These signs suggest compromised circulation to bowel. Prolonging resuscitation when one or more "grave signs" are present will not succeed in improving the patient's risk for operation and may result in gangrene of bowel. Immediate surgical resolution of the obstruction will be of much greater benefit to the patient.

When the diagnosis of intestinal obstruction is made more than 24 hours after the onset of symptoms the following should be added to the above steps:

6. Intravenous antibiotics should be administered before operation. Cephalosporin, 1.0 gram, or a combination of clindamycin and gentamicin are satisfactory.

7. Central venous pressure or pulmonary artery wedge pressure should be monitored.

8. Additional time may be taken for fluid and electrolyte replacement, since compromised circulation to the bowel is less likely in a patient who has been sick for several days. Potassium replacement, 100 to 200 mEq., may be necessary in order to restore the serum to a safe level of at least 3.3 mEq. per liter.

9. Intravenous hyperalimentation for a period of 3 to 7 days before operation may benefit patients with severe protein caloric malnutrition caused by a long-standing partial bowel obstruction. With the exception of these patients who require hyperalimentation, resuscitation should not necessitate a delay in laparotomy of more than 24 hours. This period must be shortened if the patient shows instability of blood volume or other "grave signs" of bowel compromise.

The Surgical Procedure

Access to the peritoneal cavity is best obtained through midabdominal midline or paramedian incisions. A generous incision is needed so that the entire small bowel can be examined. The obstructing point will be below the transverse colon and may reside in the pelvis. The entire small bowel is examined proceeding from the cecum to the ligament of Treitz. After the obstructing adhesion is released and the mesentery untwisted, the bowel is examined for viability (peristalsis, arterial pulsations, and return of normal color are important). Enterotomy for decompression is avoided, as the incidence of septic complications is markedly increased if the bowel is opened. Gas and fluid in the dilated small bowel are best removed by stripping the contents gently toward the stomach. Here they are removed by the anesthesiologist via the nasogastric tube. If a nonviable bowel must be removed or enterotomy must be done to remove a gallstone or bezoar, direct decompression can be carried out using a large Foley catheter or abdominal suction tube.

Recurrent Small Bowel Obstruction

Tube jejunostomy with a Baker tube (9-foot balloon-tipped tube) inserted one foot distal to the ligament of Treitz and threaded down the entire length of the small bowel is justified in an effort to prevent additional episodes of adhesive bowel obstruction. All existing adhesions must be lysed and the bowel is reduced into the abdomen in gentle folds. The tube exits through a Witzel tunnel, which is fixed to the parietal peritoneum and is left in place for two weeks. The Baker tube has the advantage of intraoperative decompression and restoration of a smooth intraperitoneal course, which allows formation of natural adhesions without the presence of an intraperitoneal foreign body. It is superior to serosal and mesenteric plication procedures.

Nonoperative Treatment of Small Bowel Obstruction

In the following situations prolonged gastric decompression and intravenous hyperalimentation may be sufficient treatment of mechanical bowel obstruction:

1. Early obstruction after surgery (within the first two weeks) caused by fibrinous adhesions.

2. Inflammatory bowel disease (Crohn's disease).

3. Irradiation enteritis or proctitis. Intravenous steroids, 300 mg. of hydrocortisone daily tapering to 50 mg. daily, are used. When oral alimentation is possible prednisone, 5 to 15 mg., is continued and sulfasalazine (Azulfidine) is added. Operation with intestinal bypass or resection may be required.

4. Peritoneal carcinomatosis.

Large Bowel Obstruction

Colonic obstruction is usually due to carcinoma and less frequently to diverticulitis or sigmoid volvulus. The latter can usually be treated nonoperatively by proctoscopy. Resection of the redundant sigmoid may be required later. The following principles are useful in managing colonic obstruction:

1. Resection of right colon cancer with primary anastomosis is usually feasible. If there is marked dilatation of the small bowel temporary ileostomy may be safer.

2. For obstructing cancers of the transverse and left colon, a Hartmann's resection is preferred with end colostomy and closure of the distal colon or rectum. Reconstruction of bowel continuity is performed in approximately 3 months. Primary anastomosis of the distended, unprepared colon is never indicated. Alternately, if the patient cannot tolerate a resection, a proximal loop colostomy may be constructed followed by a primary resection after preparation in about two weeks.

ACUTE PANCREATITIS

method of
W. CREUTZFELDT, M.D.,
and P. G. LANKISCH, M.D.
Göttingen, Federal Republic of Germany

Acute pancreatitis may present itself as a mild disease with upper abdominal pain and amylase elevation in serum and urine due to edema of the pancreas and a favorable outcome or with severe pain, shock, pulmonary and renal insufficiency, electrolyte and metabolic derangements due to hemorrhagic necrosis of the gland, and high mortality. Diagnosis must often be made on clinical grounds only, as there are no biochemical findings specifically indicating acute pancreatitis. Raised amylase and lipase values are also found in diseases other than pancreatitis, and levels may be normal or borderline in severe pancreatitis. Lowering of serum calcium levels is indicative of a severe form of the disease. The presence of methemalbumin in acute pancreatitis indicates the hemorrhagic form and thus a grave prognosis, but methemalbumin is also found in intravascular hemolysis and in a few abdominal disorders such as ileus and ruptured ectopic pregnancy. Therefore, surgical exploration may still be necessary in selected patients in whom perforated ulcer, gangrenous gallbladder, and infarcted bowel cannot be ruled out.

Assessment of Severity and Complications

Therapy must be tailored to the severity of the disease. As complications of acute pancreatitis may develop at any time, patients (except those with very mild forms) are best put in an intensive care unit for assessment and frequent reassessment of severity and complications for the first 48 hours at least. Obtain *hourly:* blood pressure and pulse and urine output; *every 6 to 12 hours:* temperature, hematocrit, blood glucose, electrolytes, arterial blood gas analysis, and fluid balance; *twice daily:* physical examination, including observation for abdominal distension, ascites, abdominal (Cullen's sign) and flank ecchymoses (Grey-Turner's sign), epigastric mass, and tetany; *daily:* serum amylase, white blood count, thrombocytes, albumin, total protein, creatinine, serum calcium, methemalbumin, Quick's test and fibrin-monomer-complexes. At the beginning obtain an x-ray of the chest and abdomen; this may have to be repeated in the later course. In addition, ultrasound examination may be indicated when epigastric masses develop.

Basic Therapy

The therapy of acute pancreatitis is largely empirical, as the effectiveness of many aspects of treatment has not been demonstrated by controlled trials. For the time being, the following methods are recommended.

Splinting of the Pancreas. A patient with acute pancreatitis should be given nothing by mouth. Until further confirmation of a recent report that nasogastric suction is unnecessary in mild or moderate pancreatitis, suction should be applied to relieve gastric distention and small bowel ileus as well as to prevent secretin release caused by hydrochloric acid entering the duodenum. In mild cases, nasogastric suction may be replaced by ingestion of antacids or cimetidine. Pharmacologic splinting of the pancreas has been tried with atropine or propantheline bromide (Pro-Banthine) and acetazolamide (Diamox). A beneficial effect of both drugs has never been proved, and both may have serious side effects: enhancement of paralytic ileus, tachycardia, psychosis (atropine or propantheline bromide) and hypokalaemia (acetazolamide). We are not using them anymore. For hormonal inhibition of pancreatic secretion, glucagon, calcitonin, and somatostatin have been recommended. Several controlled studies failed to show a beneficial effect of glucagon or calcitonin on the lethality of acute pancreatitis. Somatostatin therapy has not been tested in man, but in animal experiments it had no effect on the fatal outcome of the disease.

Pain Relief. Pain is relieved with 50 to 100 mg. meperidine hydrochloride (Demerol) intramuscularly every 4 to 6 hours as needed. Its effect can be potentiated by promethazine (Phenergan), 12.5 to 25.0 mg. Morphine is contraindicated because it may cause spasm of the sphincter of Oddi.

Fluid and Electrolyte Substitution. Fluid and electrolyte losses may be critically high because of vomiting, ascites, or ileus and retroperitoneal edema and have to be carefully replaced intravenously. Central venous pressure is kept at approximately 10 cm. H_2O and urine output at 40 to 60 ml. per hour at least. Potassium is given according to the serum level. Ten per cent calcium gluconate infusions should correct a drop in serum calcium below 8 mg. per dl. (100 ml.). Minimum caloric need can be supplied in the form of glucose infusion. Parenteral hyperalimentation may be helpful if the course of pancreatitis is prolonged.

Enzyme Inhibitors. A few years ago a controlled study seemed to indicate that extremely high doses of aprotinin (Trasylol) lower the lethality of acute pancreatitis. This study has been criticized for statistical reasons and three further controlled studies with equally high doses of aprotinin had a negative result. We avoid this very expensive form of treatment.

Prevention and Treatment of Complications

Shock. Irreversible shock with anuria is the main cause of death in acute pancreatitis. Shock and anuria seem to be due to hypovolemia and, to some extent, also to toxic protein breakdown products. To counteract hypovolemia in addition to intravenous fluid substitution, 40 to 60 grams of albumin or other colloids should be infused daily. Blood transfusion may be indicated. When hypotension persists, dopamine has to be given.

Anuria. When anuria occurs, mannitol (250 ml. of a 20 per cent solution intravenously in 30 minutes under control of central venous pressure) is indicated. This is followed by peritoneal dialysis with or without surgical drainage of the lesser sac when anuria persists. Though the effectiveness of peritoneal dialysis has been proved only in animals and in man shown only in uncontrolled studies, this method is recommended for shock therapy and electrolyte balance in severe acute pancreatitis when ascites is present, even before anuria occurs.

Respiratory Insufficiency. Acute respiratory insufficiency occurs frequently in severe acute pancreatitis, even in the absence of obvious clinical or radiographic pulmonary signs. Arterial blood gas measurements revealed that a drop of Po_2 is a severe prognostic sign. Close monitoring is required and humidified oxygen has to be applied when Po$_2$ is lowered below 70 mm. Hg. If it drops further in spite of this therapy controlled ventilation with positive end-expiratory pressure has to be started without further delay. Though enhancing diabetes, steroids might be given in pharmacologic doses as in other forms of shock lung.

Septic Infections. Several studies have demonstrated that prophylactic use of antibiotics has no effect on the course of pancreatitis. However, antibiotics should be given in severe pancreatitis because of the difficulty in differentiating signs and symptoms of infection from those of severe pancreatitis.

Hyperglycemia. Insulin administration is indicated when blood glucose levels increase above 250 mg. per dl.

Disseminated Intravascular Coagulation. Heparin is given when signs of intravascular coagulation occur. Its application to improve microcirculation of the pancreas is still in the experimental phase.

Surgical Therapy

Recently, in severe acute pancreatitis several surgical methods have been recommended varying from resection of necrotic tissue to total pancreatectomy. Until now no convincing evidence has been presented that such invasive therapy is beneficial.

Pseudocysts and abscesses of the pancreas (continuing elevation of amylase, fever) require surgery. However, watchful waiting may be wiser than early surgical intervention. The decision depends on the clinical course. Clinical evidence of empyema of the gallbladder should lead to cholecystectomy or common duct drainage.

Length of Treatment and Prevention of Relapses

Total fasting, nasogastric suction, and parenteral fluid substitution have to be continued until marked clinical improvement (disappearance of pain, fever, distention, and hyperamylasemia). Oral treatment must be started slowly (low-fat and low-protein diet). Caffeine-containing and alcoholic beverages should be avoided.

Diagnostic evaluation to ascertain the cause of pancreatitis can now be done. Absolute cessation of alcohol intake is essential to prevent recurrences. Biliary tract diseases should be corrected surgically. Careful investigation for hyperparathyroidism and hyperlipoproteinemia and appropriate treatment if these conditions are present is mandatory. Avoidance of thiazide diuretics and glucocorticoids is advised if pancreatitis occurs in the course of such treatment.

CHRONIC PANCREATITIS*

method of
I. N. MARKS, B.Sc., M.B., F.R.C.P., Ed., F.A.C.G.,
and P. C. BORNMAN, M.B., M.MED. (SURG.), F.R.C.S., Ed.
Cape Town, South Africa

Alcohol is the major cause of chronic pancreatitis in most western countries and accounts for some 90 per cent of calcific pancreatitis in these areas. Gallstones, allegedly responsible for up to 30 per cent of chronic pancreatitis in some countries, are seldom causative in calcific pancreatitis. The dominant clinical presentation in calcific pancreatitis is pain. This accounts for almost half the patients and may take the form of severe attacks, mild attacks, or persistent pain. About a third present with diabetes, steatorrhea, or both, and the picture in the remainder is dominated by persistent jaundice, gastrointestinal bleeding, an abdominal mass, or pyloroduodenal obstruction. Thus, the treatment of chronic pancreatitis is usually directed against pain, pancreatic insufficiency or other complications and includes, in addition, stern advice regarding alcohol withdrawal.

Medical Approach

Pain. RELAPSING ATTACKS. Although acute fulminating attacks are rare in chronic pancreatitis, patients not uncommonly present with severe attacks necessitating hospitalization and the urgent management of acute pancreatitis. The majority suffer relatively milder attacks. Some attacks are associated with slight pyrexia, subclinical jaundice or an elevated alkaline phosphatase, while others may be unaccompanied by constitutional effects or even an elevated serum amylase level. The intensity of treatment varies according to the severity of the attack, and most attacks subside within 3 to 7 days with bed rest, analgesics (e.g., avoforten [not available in the U.S.A.]; pethidine [meperidine]), oral fluids or a bland diet, and perhaps antibiotics.

PREVENTION OF FURTHER ATTACKS. An attempt should be made to establish the cause in patients suffering recurrent attacks unassociated with alcohol abuse. In this connection, it should be noted that recurrent clinically-acute attacks in patients enjoying a moderate intake of alcohol may

---

*The authors acknowledge M.R.C. support.

occasionally be due to gallstones rather than alcohol-induced pancreatitis. Conventional investigations such as barium meal, cholecystogram and intravenous cholangiography (IVC), serum lipids, and serum calcium should always be carried out. Despite this, there is a hard core of patients in whom the cause cannot be established.

The importance of complete alcohol withdrawal in alcohol-induced chronic pancreatitis cannot be overemphasized, and considerable time should be spent with the patient, stressing the need for complete abstinence and the hazards of continued drinking. All therapeutic measures, medical or surgical, are virtually doomed to failure if alcohol is not abandoned. Further attacks are nearly always precipitated by a recurrence of drinking, although pork and other fatty foods are sometimes incriminated. Recurrent attacks developing despite alcohol withdrawal or in patients with idiopathic pancreatitis clearly require a detailed pancreatic work-up to exclude a cyst, significant duct obstruction, or other surgically treatable condition.

PERSISTENT PAIN. Persistent or virtually persistent pain may occur after a severe attack or develop gradually during the course of the disease. In the absence of continuing alcohol it often presents a diagnostic and therapeutic dilemma. The main causes are: (a) an unsuspected cyst; (b) hyperplastic fibrosis, tumefaction, and abscess formation, usually in the head of the pancreas; (c) major duct obstruction e.g., due to calculi; (d) common bile duct stones secondary to stasis; (e) development of pancreatic carcinoma; (f) associated disease; or (g) no obvious cause. Again, conventional investigations, a sonogram, endoscopic retrograde cholangiopancreatography (ERCP), and possibly even angiography may be necessary to help define the problem and assess pancreatic duct status. Failure of the usual measures to control pain warrants surgery.

Complications. CYST FORMATION. The natural history of chronic pancreatitis is complicated by cyst formation in at least 30 per cent of patients. Once diagnosed, it is our policy to observe the patient for a few weeks in the unlikely event of spontaneous resorption, a broad-spectrum antibiotic being given to patients with a leukocytosis or a markedly raised sedimentation rate. The majority, however, will remain static or enlarge and in these one of the internal drainage procedures is recommended. Hemorrhage into a cyst is a rare but potentially lethal complication, particularly after cystanastomosis.

JAUNDICE. Persistent or progressive jaundice is usually due to compression of the distal common bile duct by a swollen pancreas, hyperplastic fibrosis or cyst, or to the development of common bile duct stones secondary to biliary stasis. Associated alcoholic hepatitis, complicating carcinoma of the pancreas, or biliary cirrhosis following long-standing cholangitis are other rare causes. Common bile duct obstruction not infrequently presents as cholangitis with a high fever, chills, and jaundice. This requires urgent treatment with a broad-spectrum antibiotic such as a cephalosporin or chloramphenicol. The jaundice in these and in other patients with common bile duct compression may settle on conservative measures, but the majority require appropriate surgery.

GASTROINTESTINAL BLEEDING. Chronic pancreatitis is complicated by hematemesis and melena of variable severity in about 9 per cent of patients. Bleeding associated with attacks are usually due to extrahepatic portal hypertension caused by splenic vein compression by an enlarged pancreas, acute gastric erosions secondary to contiguous pancreatitis or local venous compression, a Mallory-Weiss tear due to retching, alcoholic gastritis, or salicylate-induced erosions. Bleeding during the intervals between attacks of pancreatitis is usually due to peptic ulceration or to varices associated with cirrhosis.

PANCREATIC ASCITES. The development of ascites with a high amylase content in chronic pancreatitis is almost always due to rupture of a cyst or a pancreatic duct into the peritoneal cavity. The ascites frequently follows an attack of variable severity but may be insidious in development. Pancreatic ascites may settle on conservative treatment, comprising bed rest, anticholinergics, diuretics, hyperalimentation, and repeated paracenteses. Radiotherapy is occasionally of value. However, the majority will persist until internal drainage or resection of the offending area is carried out, after confirmation of the pancreatic leak by preoperative or operative pancreatography. *Pleural effusions,* usually left-sided, may occasionally follow an attack of pancreatitis. The high amylase content is diagnostic, and treatment is medical unless a communication with the pancreatic duct system can be shown on endoscopic retrograde cholangiopancreatography.

METASTATIC FAT NECROSIS. Subcutaneous fat necrosis, intramedullary fat necrosis, calcified medullary lesions of the long bones, and arthritis are rare complications that usually settle on little more than bed rest and analgesics.

OTHER COMPLICATIONS. Pulmonary tuberculosis, peripheral neuropathy, cirrhosis of the liver, and peptic ulcer may complicate or be associated with chronic pancreatitis and require specific therapy.

Pancreatic Insufficiency. Weight loss is almost universal in calcific pancreatitis. Overt diabetes occurs in about 70 per cent of such patients and eventual steatorrhea in 30 per cent, and there is a particular liability to tuberculosis and infection.

DIABETES. The treatment of pancreatic diabetes is influenced to some extent, by the rarity of ketosis and angiopathy and the hazard of insulin-induced hypoglycemia. These factors underline the importance of controlling diabetic symptoms and promoting weight gain rather than maintaining a glycosuria-free state. However, treatment should never be undertaken without knowledge of the blood sugar level because of the occasional occurrence of marked hyperglycemia of the order of 1000 mg. per dl. (100 ml.) unassociated with ketosis or severe symptoms. With this proviso, asymptomatic diabetes or patients with mild symptoms should be treated with diet and oral hypoglycemic agents. These measures may also be tried in patients with symptomatic diabetes, although the majority of these will be found to require insulin. The dose varies widely from patient to patient and, indeed, from time to time in the same patient. Careful follow-up is mandatory because of fluctuations in the diabetic state. The great danger in patients who continue drinking is insulin-induced hypoglycemia, and perfect diabetic control should be attempted only in reliable patients. Ketosis is almost invariably due to a further attack, infection, tuberculosis, or poor patient management. With regard to diet, most patients with pancreatic diabetes require at least 2000 or 2500 calories a day. Patients on insulin should be on an unlimited protein and moderate to high carbohydrate intake.

STEATORRHEA. Many highly effective preparations of pancreatic enzyme (pancreatin triple BP, Viokase, Cotazym, Nutrizyme) are available for replacement therapy. The choice of preparation and the dose should be titrated according to the patient's requirements. One to 5 tablets with meals and teas may suffice, but patients with gross steatorrhea may require an hourly dosage schedule. Pancreatic replacement therapy usually improves the nature and frequency of the stools but seldom restores fecal fat entirely to normal levels. Long-term replacement therapy is necessary in some patients, while others display spontaneous improvement in steatorrhea that makes continued therapy unnecessary. It is questionable whether the tedium of replacement therapy is warranted in patients with nontroublesome or occult steatorrhea on the grounds of improving absorption and nutrition.

Graduated dietary fat restriction is of undoubted benefit, but it is seldom necessary to reduce the fat intake to less than 70 grams a day in patients on replacement therapy. Sodium bicarbonate and, more recently, cimetidine have been advocated to prevent acid inactivation of the oral pancreatic enzymes, and medium chain triglycerides have been used with variable success in reducing steatorrhea. More important, perhaps, are protein supplements and anabolic steroids in patients with low serum albumin levels, attention to diet, and constipating agents such as codeine phosphate or diphenoxylate. Long-term antibiotics are probably justified in patients with steatorrhea associated with evidence of infection or a smouldering cholangitis. Surgery may be indicated in patients with gross steatorrhea unassociated with diabetes if proximal pancreatic duct obstruction or a cyst can be demonstrated on endoscopic retrograde cholangiopancreatography.

Surgical Strategy

The management of chronic pancreatitis requires patience and flexibility, with close teamwork between the physician and surgeon, their relative roles varying according to the severity and persistence of the pain and the type of complications. The indications for *emergency surgery* in chronic pancreatitis are limited to the occasional laparotomy in patients with clinically acute attacks in whom there is any doubt about the diagnosis and to the infrequent operation for uncontrollable gastrointestinal bleeding. For the rest, the surgery of chronic pancreatitis is usually an elective affair. *Complications* such as cyst, pseudocyst, and abscess formation, persistent jaundice due to common bile duct obstruction with or without secondary choledochal stones, duodenal obstruction, and pancreatic ascites obviously invite surgical correction. Timing of surgery in patients with cysts or jaundice, especially when these develop in the wake of a clinically acute attack, may pose a problem in clinical judgment.

Relapsing attacks or persistent pain despite alcohol withdrawal is, perhaps, the major indication for surgery in chronic pancreatitis. In general, the surgical procedure should be governed by the findings of sonography, ERCP, angiography, and operative pancreatography on the one hand, and by knowledge of the preoperative functional status of the pancreas on the other. The findings of a previously undiagnosed *cyst* at laparotomy offers the best chance of a surgical cure, and *sphincteroplasty* may be of value in the occasional patient with true sphincteric stenosis. *Pancreaticojejunostomy* with distal resection of variable extent may be carried out for single or multiple areas of duct stenosis, but pancreaticojejunostomy without distal resection is preferred in patients with a single stricture in whom pancreatic function is still adequate. Obstruction of both the pancreatic and biliary duct systems warrants treatment by one of the elegant *combined internal drain-*

age procedures described by Cattell or Mercadier. Rarely, *pancreaticoduodenectomy* may have to be considered in patients with relentless pain with gross abnormality confined to the head of the pancreas, particularly if there is any question about malignancy, and *95 per cent pancreatectomy*, reserved as a last resort in patients with intractable pain and gross pancreatic insufficiency. At all times, the possible advantages of pancreatic ablative procedures and, in particular, near total pancreatectomy should be weighed very carefully against the risk of further deterioration in diabetes and steatorrhea. Definitive surgery has little to offer if the pancreatic duct is normal, especially if pancreatic function is reasonably good. Such patients should be treated with benign neglect, the judicious use of analgesics being clearly preferable to unwarranted ablative procedures that only add to the existing problem.

Unfortunately, the results of surgery in chronic pancreatitis do not necessarily parallel the logic of the procedure. Operative pancreatography and ERCP are the current barometers of surgical thinking, but it is possible that factors other than duct narrowing or stenosis may be strategic in the cause of symptoms in some patients. In any event, many will continue to suffer further attacks after a tailored procedure because of a resumption of drinking. Others subjected to an illogical procedure may remain free of pain because of progressive impairment of pancreatic function and continued avoidance of alcohol. In surgery, as in the other arts, good things may fail and bad things impress.

Opinions differ as to the advisability and extent of surgery in patients who are unable to stop abusing alcohol and in whom medical measures are ineffective. It is our policy to consider surgery in such patients only in the event of a complication or persistent, unyielding pain with ERCP evidence of significant duct narrowing. If not, we are inclined to treat the pain with heavy analgesics and reinforce the importance of alcohol withdrawal.

PEPTIC ULCER

method of
WILLIAM J. GRIFFITHS, M.D.,
and JACK D. WELSH, M.D.
Oklahoma City, Oklahoma

Since the release of the H₂ receptor antagonist, cimetidine, there has been a renewed interest in the medical therapy of peptic ulcer disease. As a consequence, a few better controlled double-blind trials of therapy have been reported. It is hoped this trend will continue. Other aspects of therapy will probably never be adequately appraised to everyone's satisfaction. The effects of diet are harder to assess than drug therapy, and there is no financial impetus for good controlled trials of diets. The importance of the physician's personality and the patient-physician relationship have not been weighed. Also, how much patient education influences adherence to therapy and improves results is not known. Underlying difficulties in appraising specific therapeutic modalities are the lack of concordance among symptoms, healing, and recurrence. Other problems in evaluating therapeutic results also relate to our lack of understanding of the factors that influence exacerbations or remissions of the disease.

The goals of therapy remain unchanged: relief of symptoms, complete healing of the ulcer, and prevention of complications and recurrence.

Patient Education

In typical chronic duodenal ulcer disease the patient's first attack is usually not the last. At least 80 to 90 per cent will have a recurrence or relapse. Also, approximately half the patients with gastric ulcers may have a recurrence. Although it is of no proven benefit, we feel each patient should be informed that disappearance of symptoms does not mean the ulcer has healed, as well as the fact that they have a disease that may recur. Endoscopic studies have revealed that many duodenal ulcers do not heal for 6 weeks and that gastric ulcers may not heal for as long as 3 months. The need for continued therapy for these periods of time is emphasized, and the patient is told that after healing of the ulcer if there is a recurrence of symptoms he should return to his physician.

Antacids

Action and Rationale. The rationale for the use of antacids is based on the concept that if the acid and pepsin are reduced, the ulcer should heal. Recent studies have confirmed, at least in part, that antacids taken in adequate amounts will heal peptic ulcers. However, some data suggest that antacids do not relieve ulcer pain more than a placebo. Different preparations vary in their effectiveness and duration of antacid action. Sodium bicarbonate almost immediately reacts with hydrochloric acid in the stomach but is emptied rapidly, so its duration of antacid effect is short-lived. Any excess is absorbed in the small intestine. When calcium carbonate is given, the calcium chloride formed with the acid is soluble; however, the majority of it is converted to in-

TABLE 1. **Antacid Potencies—The Number of mEq. in 10 ml. of Antacid Titrated to pH 3.0 with 0.1 N HCl, 60 RPM, 37° C.**

ANTACID	CONTENTS	0 TIME mEq.	%*	120 MIN.† mEq.
Ducon	Al and Mg hydroxides, Ca carbonate	20.2	29	70.4
Mylanta II	Mg and Al hydroxides, simethicone	4.3	10	41.4
Titralac	Glycine, Ca carbonate	32.9	85	38.7
Camalox	Al and Mg hydroxides, Ca carbonate	12.7	49	35.9
Aludrox	Al hydroxide gel, Mg hydroxide	6.4	23	28.1
Maalox	Mg and Al hydroxide gel	5.5	21	25.8
Creamalin	Hexitol stabilized Al hydroxide gel, Mg hydroxide	11.1	43	25.7
Di-Gel	Al and Mg hydroxides, simethicone	5.6	23	24.5
Mylanta	Mg and Al hydroxides, simethicone	4.1	17	23.8
Silain-Gel	Mg and Al hydroxides, simethicone	3.3	14	23.1
Marblen	Mg and Ca carbonates, Al hydroxide, Mg phosphate, Mg trisilicate	17.2	75	22.8
WinGel	Al and Mg hydroxides, hexitol stabilized	8.4	37	22.5
Gelusil M	Mg trisilicate, Al hydroxide, Mg hydroxide	11.1	49	22.3
Riopan	Mg and Al hydroxides	3.5	16	22.1
Amphojel	Al hydroxide gel	3.9	20	19.3
A-M-T	Mg trisilicate, Al hydroxide gel	6.5	36	17.9
Kolantyl Gel	Bentyl, Al hydroxide, Mg hydroxide, methylcellulose	5.7	34	16.9
Trisogel	Mg trisilicate, Al hydroxide gel	7.2	43	16.5
Gelusil	Mg trisilicate, Al hydroxide	4.1	31	13.3
Robalate	Dihydroxyaluminum aminoacetate	3.4	30	11.3
Phosphaljel	Al phosphate gel	2.5	59	4.2

*Percentage of total buffer capacity at 120 minutes. Indicates the rapidity of onset of action.

†The value in this column is a measure of buffer capacity of the antacid in milliequivalents per 10 ml. after 120 minutes. (Modified from Sleisenger, M. H., and Fordtran, J. S. [eds.]: Gastrointestinal Disease. Philadelphia, W. B. Saunders Co., 1973, p. 726.)

soluble calcium salts in the small intestine. It is emptied at a somewhat slower rate from the stomach than sodium bicarbonate. Aluminum hydroxide reacts with gastric acid to form aluminum chloride. Magnesium hydroxide reacts rapidly with hydrochloric acid but has a slow emptying rate, so it has a more prolonged action. In the fasting subject, liquid antacids have only a transient intragastric buffering effect of 20 to 40 minutes because of their being emptied by the stomach. Since gastric emptying is slowed by food, the optimal buffering appears to occur when the effective dose is given 1 and 3 hours after each meal. Potency varies widely among commercially available antacids (Table 1).

Dosage. To achieve optimum neutralization, hypersecretors may require 80 to 160 mEq. of buffer, while hyposecretors may take 40 to 80 mEq. of buffer. Specifically, the patient with a duodenal ulcer should receive a dosage equivalent to 80 mEq. of buffer per dose each hour until pain-free for 7 to 10 days. This usually amounts to at least 30 ml. per dose of the more potent antacids. After this period the patient should take equivalent amounts 1 and 3 hours after each meal and at bed time for at least a total of 6 weeks. Similar amounts of antacids are usually given to patients with gastric ulcers for at least 3 months. The evidence supporting this program is not too good, and patient compliance is poor for this

length of time, in our experience. Although more convenient to carry, antacid tablets are not as effective as the liquid forms. The new nonbreakable bottles make it easier for the patient to carry liquid antacid with him at all times.

Side Effects. The adverse effects from antacids must always be taken into consideration. Calcium carbonate is effective, but the calcium can be absorbed and produce increased gastric acid secretion, hypercalcemia, and impaired renal function. Aluminum hydroxide gels produce constipation and hypophosphatemia. It may be beneficial

TABLE 2. **Sodium Content of Some Antacids per 10 ml. Dose**

ANTACID	SODIUM CONTENT (MEQ.)
Ducon	0.64
Mylanta II	0.74
Titralac	1.10
Camalox	0.22
Aludrox	0.43
Maalox	0.22
Creamalin	0.26
WinGel	0.31
Gelusil M	0.62
Riopan	0.06
Amphojel	0.46
A-M-T	0.84
Kolantyl Gel	0.53
Gelusil	0.59

to alternate magnesium antacids with aluminum hydroxide gel to achieve the best balance in stool frequency. Sodium content varies and in some patients needs to be taken into account when selecting an antacid (Table 2).

H₂ Receptor Antagonist

Action and Rationale. Cimetidine blocks the effects of histamine on gastric acid secretion. It has been demonstrated to inhibit basal and nocturnal acid secretion and acid secretion to all stimulants, such as food, insulin, pentagastrin, and caffeine. The kidney is the major route of excretion of cimetidine. Cimetidine, 300 mg., given orally to a patient with a duodenal ulcer decreases basal acid by 85 per cent for at least 5 hours, and at bed time inhibits nocturnal acid over 80 per cent and maintains nocturnal pH above 4 for about 6 hours.

Dosage. Cimetidine should be given in doses of 300 mg. four times daily with meals and at bed time for 6 weeks to patients with duodenal ulcers. The majority of the drug is excreted in the urine, so the dosage should be modified to 300 mg. each 12 hours for patients with severe renal insufficiency. Cimetidine has not been shown to be superior to intensive antacid therapy in the healing of duodenal ulcers. No acid rebound has been demonstrated on stopping cimetidine. Although at present it does not have Food and Drug Administration approval, chronic administration of cimetidine twice a day or at bed time may prevent recurrence. Cimetidine has not been demonstrated to be superior to a placebo in the outpatient or inpatient treatment of gastric ulcers in this country; however, the use of antacids has confused these studies.

Adverse Effects. Mild increases in the serum glutamic oxaloacetic transaminase (SGOT) and creatinine may occur but return to normal when the drug is discontinued. Headache, mental confusion, diarrhea, muscular pain, dizziness, fever, and rashes have been reported. Gynecomastia may occur when the drug is given for prolonged periods for hypersecretory states, such as the Zollinger-Ellison syndrome.

Anticholinergics

Action and Rationale. The drugs inhibit the action of acetylcholine on structures innervated by postganglionic cholinergic nerves and the smooth muscle responses to acetylcholine. Their clinical usefulness is limited by the generalized parasympathetic blockade produced. In spite of many papers on the influence of anticholinergics on gastric secretion and their consequence in patients with peptic ulcer, their clinical effectiveness, particularly as the single therapeutic agent, is controversial.

Dosage. It is the opinion of physicians with the most experience with these agents that they should be titrated to an individualized dose for each patient. The aim is to achieve the dosage that is just at or below the dose producing mild symptoms. Their use may be confined, along with antacids or cimetidine, to patients with persistent pain or nocturnal pain.

Side Effects. Urinary hesitancy, constipation, headache, insomnia or dizziness, and gastric retention are common side effects. These difficulties can usually be controlled by reduction of the anticholinergic, or if not, the drug should be discontinued. Anticholinergics should not be given if the patient has glaucoma, gastric retention, achalasia, or reflux esophagitis. Anticholinergics should be used cautiously in older patients.

Diet

Many patients and their physicians are convinced that certain foods contribute to exacerbation of their peptic ulcer disease and vigorously champion specific diets. At least two problems exist in evaluating such claims. First, symptoms following ingestion of food may represent intolerance and not exacerbation of an ulcer. Patients with and without ulcers have similar food intolerances. Second, many physicians are so personally assured of the necessity of special diets that their personality and conviction influence the patient, possibly more than the diet. If one examines the available evidence, special diets (bland, peptic ulcer diets, etc.) are not more effective in promoting healing than a regular diet. Since they have *not* been shown to be *better* and do take more time to prepare and serve, we see no need for their use. Other restrictions and allowances are also of questionable value. Decaffeinated coffee stimulates gastric acidity as much as regular coffee. If one feels that coffee should be restricted, then decaffeinated coffee should be restricted. Frequent feedings have also not been demonstrated superior to three regular meals. The usually prescribed night time feeding only stimulates nocturnal acid secretion. Hourly milk has little proved value and should be deleted from diet recommendations. If the patient is convinced that certain foods repeatedly cause symptoms, then they should be eliminated.

Hospitalization

Early data suggested that hospitalization improved the healing of duodenal and gastric ulcers. Present data do not support this supposition. With increasing costs of medical care, this assumes more importance. Worry about the bill may be far more detrimental than any benefit from hospitalization. This, like the other aspects of the treatment of peptic ulcer, must be individualized. Most patients with uncomplicated duodenal or gastric ulcers can be treated as out-patients. It must be emphasized in those with gastric ulcers that certain healing criteria should be met, and if not, they may have to be hospitalized. For patients who appear to be refractory to therapy, or find their home or business situation intolerable, a period of hospitalization may be warranted.

Smoking and Medications

Early studies demonstrated that gastric ulcers healed better in nonsmokers than in smokers. Newer data suggest that duodenal ulcers heal as well in smokers as nonsmokers, when the patient is receiving antacids or cimetidine therapy. Aspirin and alcohol should be restricted or eliminated during acute attacks of peptic ulcer disease.

Therapy

Now, with more options available, what should the physician prescribe and recommend for his patient? The acute duodenal ulcer patient can be treated as an out-patient with three regular meals a day. Excessive coffee, alcohol, pepper, and foods that the patient feels repeatedly produce symptoms should be eliminated from the diet. Heavy smokers should probably be advised to decrease their smoking. Large doses (at least 210 ml. or more a day) of a potent antacid or cimetidine have equal healing effects over a 6 week period, and the costs in our area are similar, so initial therapy may begin with either. In our practice, patient acceptance of cimetidine seems to be better than the large doses of antacids required. If adverse effects are prohibitive with the first agent used, or the patient will not take it, then another agent should be used. Anticholinergics should not be prescribed as the only agent, unless for some reason antacids or cimetidine are contraindicated or have produced too many side effects. However, in particularly refractory cases anticholinergics, especially at bed time, may potentiate the effect of the antacid or cimetidine. Therapy should be continued for at least 6 to 8 weeks. In patients with uncomplicated duodenal ulcers we do not feel that the added expense of a followup x-ray or endoscopy is beneficial to determine when therapy should be discontinued unless the patient's response is unusual. Although not approved now for duodenal ulcer patients, some maintenance program of cimetidine at least at bed time may prevent relapse or recurrence.

In the patient with an uncomplicated gastric ulcer, assurance that the lesion is benign should be established by radiographic and endoscopic criteria and followed to healing. The majority of patients can be treated as out-patients on a regular diet. If they have an antral ulcer or a channel ulcer with nausea and vomiting secondary to obstruction, they should be hospitalized, at least initially. In all cases the physician should make clear to the patient how the healing of the ulcer will be followed and the criteria for an adequate therapeutic response. At the moment antacids would appear to be somewhat more effective than other agents.

Previously accepted therapy is now being questioned, and a number of studies are underway that should further clarify the role of cimetidine and other therapeutic agents. Newer agents are being used in other parts of the world. It is hoped that the experience gained in the evaluation of cimetidine will be beneficial when these agents become available in this country.

TUMORS OF THE STOMACH

method of
EDWARD WEINSHELBAUM, M.D.
Gainesville, Florida

Carcinoma

The most common malignant tumors of the stomach are carcinomas. These have been classified in several ways based on gross and microscopic characteristics and include a variety of types designated in older terminology as simple, papillary, colloid, medullary, and scirrhous. Bormann's classification divides gastric carcinomas into four categories based on the degree of cellular differentiation found within the tumors. Although these classifications have some prognostic significance, all gastric carcinomas are treated similarly, that is, by extensive gastric resection unless extraperitoneal metastases are evident or the tumor is so far advanced that resection is obviously not feasible.

Preoperative Preparation. If weight loss has been severe and an extensive operation is planned, hyperalimentation by the intravenous route according to the method developed by Dudrick is begun several days prior to operation and continued in the postoperative period. The patient is usually provided 3000 to 4000 calories per day. Obstruction, if present, is treated by decompression via a nasogastric tube. Anemia is corrected so that the preoperative hematocrit is 30 per cent or greater.

Operation. For carcinomas of the distal stomach or midstomach a high subtotal gastric resection is performed that includes the gastrocolic ligament, the greater omentum, the hepatogastric ligament, and a cuff of the first portion of the duodenum. When the tumor is situated proximally and lies along the greater curvature, the spleen is included in the resection. Gastrointestinal continuity may be restored by antecolic or retrocolic gastrojejunostomy or by gastroduodenostomy. Our preference has been to use antecolic gastrojejunostomy because of its simplicity and because this places the anastomosis away from some of the sites where tumor recurrence is likely.

For carcinomas of the fundus or esophagogastric junction or for those tumors situated so high on the lesser curvature that they extend to within a few centimeters of the esophagus, proximal esophagogastrectomy with esophagogastrostomy is done, usually with splenectomy. Our preference has been to approach these tumors through the left chest using a peripheral diaphragmatic incision. This approach gives excellent exposure of the left upper abdomen and, in contrast to radial incisions, preserves diaphragmatic innervation. The exposure obtained by this approach is such that a thoracoabdominal extension or a separate abdominal incision is unnecessary. Even though the resection results in vagotomy, a pyloroplasty or other gastric drainage procedure is usually not needed in these patients. (Total gastrectomy with esophagojejunostomy may also be done by this approach. In these patients a small laparotomy may be necessary to complete the closure of the duodenal stump.)

Because of the complexity of the lymphatic drainage of the stomach a variety of resections more extensive than the ones described have been used. These have included routine total gastrectomy and extended subtotal gastrectomy with wide node dissection, splenectomy, and, in some procedures, routine removal of the body and tail of the pancreas. Although total gastrectomy is indicated in order to encompass a bulky tumor, it is generally agreed that routine removal of the entire stomach in an effort to improve long term survival is not warranted.

Palliative Resection and Bypass. It is often found at the time of operation that a carcinoma is more extensive than was anticipated. In particular, involvement of the celiac axis by direct extension or by tumor bearing lymph nodes may preclude resection for cure. When curative resection is not possible, palliative resection is done unless the peritoneal cavity is widely seeded with metastases or the tumor is fixed to retroperitoneal or other adjacent organs. Unresectable tumors are bypassed when possible, but the results of bypass alone are disappointing in that the patient often remains unable to eat.

Disseminated or Recurrent Carcinoma. Little other than supportive care can be offered to patients with disseminated or recurrent gastric carcinoma. Radiation therapy is usually not effective. Chemotherapeutic regimens that use a combination of agents have been reported to achieve an objective response in 40 per cent of patients but the regimens are toxic and the improvement in survival is small. In one study using a combination of 5-fluorouracil and BCNU, 50 per cent of patients undergoing treatment died within 7 months of the time of diagnosis and 85 per cent did not survive beyond one year.

Prognosis. Of all patients in whom the diagnosis of gastric carcinoma is made, approximately 85 per cent will be suitable for operation. Resection that apparently removes all gross tumor will be possible in 45 per cent. Forty per cent of all patients undergoing operation will not have tumor in the regional lymph nodes. The 5 year survival of this more fortunate group is 50 per cent, but these patients represent only one third of all patients in whom the diagnosis is made. When tumor is present in the regional nodes, the 5 year survival rate drops to 20 per cent.

After palliative resection, 35 per cent of patients may be expected to survive at least 1 year and 20 per cent more than 2 years. Although very few patients survive more than 3 years, an occasional patient will have a surprising and gratifying longevity. The results of bypass alone are poorer, mean survival being 3 months. The overall 5 year survival for all patients in whom the diagnosis of gastric carcinoma is made is approximately 10 per cent. Once a patient has survived 5 years, the prognosis for that individual patient is good in that there is little difference between 5 and 10 year survival rates.

Lymphoma

Lymphomas are the second most common malignant tumors of the stomach and account for 1 to 2 per cent of all malignant gastric lesions. They may arise as primary gastric tumors or the stomach may be involved secondarily in disseminated disease. Primary lymphomas are treated by resection as described for carcinoma. In addition, a course of intensive postoperative radiation therapy is given. The overall 5 year survival of patients with primary gastric lymphoma treated by resection and radiation is 50 per cent. For those patients in whom all tumor appears to be encompassed by resection, the 5 year survival rate is 65 per cent. Although removal by operation followed by radiation is the usual method for treating primary gastric lymphoma, some studies have reported sufficiently good results with radiation alone, so that this modality may be considered when a tumor is so bulky that total gastrectomy would be required for resection. When the stomach is involved in disseminated lymphoma, treatment is by a combination of radiotherapy and chemotherapy appropriate to the cell type and degree of dissemination.

Pseudolymphoma. In this entity there is extensive proliferation of normal appearing lymphocytes and lymphocytic follicles associated with ulceration of the gastric mucosa. It is not known whether this represents an inflammatory reaction to chronic gastric ulceration, hyperplasia, or very well differentiated neoplasm. In general, pseudolymphoma is considered to be a benign condition and is usually diagnosed after resection of an indeterminate gastric mass. Once the diagnosis is confirmed, no additional treatment is necessary.

Leiomyosarcoma

Leiomyosarcomas are friable bulky tumors that vary histologically from very well to poorly differentiated. They account for 1 per cent or less of all gastric cancers. Most are over 3 cm. in size at the time of diagnosis. Smooth muscle tumors smaller than 3 cm. are likely to be benign. Leiomyosarcomas are treated by resections similar to those done for gastric carcinoma. The prognosis is considerably better however in that the overall 5 year survival rate is 40 to 50 per cent compared to the 10 per cent survival rate in carcinoma.

Indeterminate Gastric Ulcer

The combination of radiologic and endoscopic evaluation of ulcerating gastric lesions is reasonably accurate in that the number of malignant lesions misdiagnosed preoperatively as benign is approximately 3 per cent (false negative rate). When undertaking resection of an ulcer which has been diagnosed as benign preoperatively there is little problem when the lesion can be encompassed by a distal gastrectomy. On rare occasion, however, an ulcer may be situated so far proximally that an esophagogastrectomy would be appropriate if the lesion were known to be malignant. In these cases a wedge of stomach encompassing the ulcer is excised and submitted to the pathologist. If no cancer is found, the gastric wall is closed and the operation concluded.

Gastric Polyps

The majority of gastric polyps are small proliferations of well-differentiated epithelium composed of glands lined by normal-appearing mucus secreting cells. An inflammatory component is often present in the lamina propria. Polyps of this type have been called hyperplastic, regenerative, or differentiated. In addition to these, less well-differentiated polyps are seen. These include types classified as adenomatous or dedifferentiated polyps and villous tumors. The overall incidence of carcinoma in or associated with polypoid lesions of the stomach has been variously reported from 7 to 35 per cent. The incidence in lesions less than 2 cm. in size is 5 per cent or less. The incidence reported in lesions larger than 2 cm. ranges from 25 to 55 per cent. In general, polyps larger than 2 cm. or those which have been shown to be dedifferentiated or villous by endoscopic biopsy should be removed in toto. The indications for polypectomy are less clear in the case of small hyperplastic lesions.

When a decision has been made for removal, the polyp with a margin of normal mucosa is excised through a gastrotomy and suture ligature is used to close the mucosa and control bleeding at the base. The specimen is submitted to the pathologist for examination by frozen section and, if invasive carcinoma is found, gastrectomy appropriate to the site is performed. A more limited gastrectomy may also be done as an expeditious way to remove multiple benign polyps confined to one area of the stomach. As more experience is gained it may prove feasible to remove the majority of gastric polyps by use of endoscopically controlled cautery snare.

Other Benign Gastric Tumors

There are a variety of benign gastric tumors in addition to hyperplastic and adenomatous polyps. Those of epithelial origin include carcinoid, heterotopic pancreas, and mucosal cyst. Leiomyoma is the most common tumor of mesenchymal origin. Other benign mesenchymal tumors are fibroma, neurofibroma, lipoma, and angioma. Many benign gastric tumors persist through life asymptomatic and undiscovered. Others give rise to bleeding or to pain similar to that of peptic ulcer disease. A number are discovered incidentally. In general, benign-appearing lesions that are symptomatic are removed. The decision as to whether or not operation should be undertaken to remove asymptomatic lesions that appear to be benign on radiologic and endoscopic evaluation is a difficult one and is individualized according to the degree of suspicion of malignancy and the age and condition of the patient.

At the time of operation, small tumors or tumors near the cardia are removed by full thickness excision of the involved portion of the stomach and submitted for histologic examination. If the benign nature of the tumor is confirmed, nothing other than closure of the gastric wall is necessary. Large benign tumors situated distally are removed by distal gastrectomy. In these patients our preference is to use gastroduodenostomy to restore continuity.

TUMORS OF THE COLON AND RECTUM

method of
ROBERT S. NELSON, M.D.
Houston, Texas

Tumors of the colon and rectum, the majority of which are polypoid, occur in 5 to 10 per cent of all persons. Many are entirely undetected during life and found only at routine postmortem examination. The greatest proportion of such tumors are also benign, but may often be associated with cancer of the large bowel, which makes their detection and histologic examination important. As they occur and grow initially in an asymptomatic manner, early detection is difficult. Screening measures are expensive and even more difficult to impose on the general population. Nevertheless, such methods, consisting of stool testing for occult blood, routine proctosigmoidoscopic examination, and in some cases barium enema and colonoscopy, are being tried in a limited measure with varied degrees of success. Routine studies on selected persons may also be quite productive.

Until the last 10 years, our knowledge of unresected tumors above the level of the sigmoidoscope was limited to radiologic studies, and judgment as to whether the individual lesion should be removed depended on its appearance and size as shown on the x-ray film. The advent of colonoscopy has changed the approach. Tumors may now be visualized, mobilized with a biopsy instrument, biopsied, and even resected in toto (the most complete biopsy) by a relatively noninvasive procedure. When used as part of a screening study, colonoscopy ideally complements radiology and adds another dimension to the detection and treatment of colorectal tumors. Further use and development will be necessary to determine the impact of this increased capability on the mortality of colorectal cancer, but some gains have been made. Tumors found on radiologic examination in poor-risk patients are now subject to objective scrutiny that truly assesses the risk and allows the best possible judgment. Routine colonoscopy sometimes also reveals polyps or early carcinomas not shown on radiologic examination. When in doubt, both x-ray and endoscopic studies should be done.

Benign Tumors

These come under the general headings of (1) hamartomas (juvenile polyps, Peutz-Jeghers polyps, endometriosis), (2) inflammatory polyps (specific infectious granulomas, such as amebiasis, schistosomiasis, and others, pseudopolyps as in chronic ulcerative colitis or reactive granulomas), (3) hyperplastic polyps, and (4) neoplasms (simple adenomas, villous adenomas, villoglandular tumors and hereditary polyposis), as well as a variety of other tumors, extraepithelial in type (lymphoid, lipomas, carcinoids, leiomyomas).

Although those tumors listed as neoplasms are in the main entirely benign, there is evidence that a small number (1 to 2 per cent) of adenomas may undergo malignant degeneration. In addition, villous or villoglandular tumors may become malignant with considerably greater frequency (estimated at 25 to 50 per cent). Patients with hereditary polyposis and Gardner's and Turcot's syndromes develop colon cancer with extreme frequency. Although essentially "benign," chronic ulcerative colitis persisting over 10 years in a person, particularly with chronic intestinal changes such as pseudopolyps, is also associated with an increasing risk of cancer.

Carcinoma can occasionally develop in an originally benign polyp, but more frequently the development of polyps in any colon or rectum may be associated with carcinoma, even when there is little evidence that the tumor is the result of carcinomatous degeneration in a benign polyp. The aim, therefore, is to find and obtain proper histologic identification of all polypoid and other tumors of the colon and rectum. The combination of air contrast barium enema, proctosigmoidoscopy, and colonoscopy will make this identification in all but a few patients. Diagnosis may be made by adequate biopsy specimens, or removal of the whole lesion. In most patients, polyps, even multiple, can be removed by proctosigmoidoscopy or colonoscopy, depending on their level of origin. When the polyp has an unusually broad base, and cannot be removed entirely, the burden of proof is with the physician if he chooses to rely on biopsies alone. This is especially hazardous in the case of villous adenomas or mixed villoglandular tumors, in chronic ulcerative colitis with marked mucosal distortion, or in hereditary polyposis. Removal of multiple polyps in the polyposis syndromes is no protection against cancer. Hamartomas, inflammatory lesions, and hyperplastic polyps are usually easily diagnosed and proper treatment or follow-up instituted.

Emphasis must be particularly placed on the complete removal of all villous or villoglandular tumors. When these occur in the rectum, it is sometimes possible to remove them completely with the operating sigmoidoscope, but they should be widely excised and the base carefully examined. Many harbor carcinoma in some area of the tumor that may be inaccessible to previous biopsy. It is doubtful that removal of such tumors can be accomplished above the level of the sigmoidoscope through colonoscopy, although attempts are sometimes advocated. Our procedure is surgical resection of all such broad-based lesions above the level of the rectosigmoid. Those in the latter area will frequently be so large as to require extensive resection. Although some of these tumors are reported to produce watery diarrhea and hypokalemia, they are extremely rare in our experience, and the malignant potential should be the main focus of attention.

Malignant Tumors

Adenocarcinoma is by far the most common malignant colorectal tumor, comprising 97 to 98 per cent of all such lesions. It is currently the second most common malignancy in males and third most common in females in the United States. The remaining malignant tumors are squamous cell, cloacogenic carcinoma, carcinoid tumors, sarcoma, lymphoma, or melanoblastoma. These latter are seldom seen, require special considerations as to treatment, and will not be dealt with in detail.

Diagnosis. All the malignant tumors must be diagnosed histologically, and this can be performed with a high degree of accuracy by the use of proctosigmoidoscopy, x-ray, and colonoscopy, as already described.

However, the symptoms that bring the patient to the doctor may be vague and inconsistent, so that the opportunity for diagnosis is delayed. Right-sided cancers are particularly insidious in this regard. The liquid stool delivered from the small intestine at this level does not obstruct, even in the largest tumors, which may grow massively until a severe, slowly-developing anemia or palpable mass prompts radiologic examination. Tumors of the transverse and descending or sigmoid colon are much more likely to produce crampy pain and eventually true obstruction. Grossly diagnostic blood with or between stools is seldom seen. Changes in bowel habit may or may not be significant features.

Because of these inconsistent and often disregarded symptoms, screening tests to determine occult blood in the stools have been advocated in all persons over 50 years of age. Studies have been carried out in a limited manner, employing Hemocult stool testing on 3 successive days following a high-residue meat-free diet. A positive test for blood on any specimen is the signal for further evaluation to consist of sigmoidoscopy, barium enema, and, in suitable instances, colonoscopy. In at least one study, the latter test has been done routinely. Varying results have been reported, although without question a certain number of asymptomatic early colorectal cancers have been discovered and removed. Many questions need to be settled concerning such routine testing and costs are considerable. Any patients with persistent, even though vague, symptoms should, however, be thoroughly evaluated, particularly in the older age group.

If the physician is reasonably aware of the possibility of colorectal cancer, the diagnosis should be made prior to the necessity for emergency surgery because of obstruction or perforation. A fair number of tumors are nevertheless first discovered at surgery for these complications. Needless to say, this is not the optimum time for treatment. When a preoperative diagnosis has been made, careful search for metastases should be carried out to include, if necessary, liver scan and bone survey. A preoperative carcino-embryonic antigen (CEA) test may be valuable in follow-up if elevated, and should be done if available. A finding of metastatic disease does not preclude surgery, and removal of the primary tumor must be carried out wherever possible.

Treatment. Surgery remains the only method of cure, and should be attempted only by an experienced surgeon who can perform adequate removal. Proper histologic identification of metastatic disease in the abdomen (nodes, mesentery, ovaries, and other organs) is extremely helpful in later management and should be metic-

ulous. In particular, biopsy of suspected liver tumor, or even routine needle biopsy of the liver when metastases are suspected may be worthwhile. Rectal lesions must be adequately resected, and attempts to spare the patient the discomfort of a colostomy are risky with a high rate of recurrence. Occasional very old or poor risk patients and those with massive metastases may be managed by fulguration but should be strictly selected. When colostomy is necessary, the patient must be thoroughly oriented and instructed in its care. A team of from 1 to 3 "ostomy" nurses are invaluable for this purpose and should be available in all cancer institutions or hospitals where colorectal cancer is treated.

Radiation has been used both pre- and post-operatively. Preoperative doses of 2500 to 5000 rads have been shown to reduce the number and size of lymph node metastases and effect some shrinkage of the primary in rectal cancer, but there is an appreciable increase in postoperative complications from radiation effect, and overall improvement in outcome has not been shown. Postoperative radiation, up to 6000 or more rads, has been used to ablate residual tumor. Experimental studies are still progressing, but side effects, such as severe radiation proctitis and sphincter incompetence, are common, and long-term improvement in results has yet to be shown. Radiation for localized bone or pelvic lesions can give excellent palliation in disseminated disease, and is superior to chemotherapy for this purpose.

Chemotherapy has been used extensively for all types of colorectal carcinoma, especially since 5-fluorouracil (5-FU) became available 18 years ago. As a single drug, this agent is capable of producing some type of remission (not all objective) in 20 to 25 per cent of patients. No other single drug has approached these figures, and many combinations are now being tested, particularly those containing 5-FU, one of the nitrosoureas, such as methyl CCNU, and vincristine. Remissions have been reported with these combinations in as many as 43 per cent, although the majority of results are closer to 35 per cent. With the reports of increased remissions in disseminated disease, studies have been initiated using combinations of agents as adjunctive therapy in Duke's B and C colorectal cancers. As there are no clear parameters to measure in these patients, results must be assessed in terms of survival of at least 5 years, and anything less must be rated as premature and possibly misleading. A number of authorities have cautioned against the use of adjuvant therapy in colorectal cancer other than in carefully controlled series, and this has been our practice. Nevertheless, we see many patients who have been started on adjuvant chemotherapy without being included in a controlled group. Most of the drug combinations, especially those containing nitrosourea, are extremely toxic, and severe reactions may be life-threatening as well as lowering life quality. Until their usefulness is definitely demonstrated experimentally, they have no place in treatment. Thus far, no patient with colorectal cancer has been cured of disease with chemotherapy. This fact should be thoroughly impressed on each patient prior to drug treatment.

A considerable number of patients with colorectal cancer can be shown to be immunosuppressed when first evaluated. Attempts are now underway to determine effectiveness of nonspecific immunostimulants such as BCG (bacille Calmette Guérin) and the methanol extraction residue of BCG (MER). Preliminary results are not encouraging, and some researchers have temporarily abandoned attempts to include immunostimulants in therapy until better agents and methods are found. The majority of evidence would seem to support this stand.

Follow-up. Regardless of the classification of colorectal cancer at initial evaluation or surgery, long-term follow-up is essential. After surgery, a control air contrast study of the colon should be done for future comparison, routine chest x-ray, liver function, and blood tests. If a CEA value was elevated prior to surgery, a repeat determination should be performed during convalescence and at intervals thereafter. If the tumor was originally in the rectosigmoid region and resected anteriorly, proctosigmoidoscopy should be added routinely to the follow-up. Patients with evidence of metastases, particularly to the lungs and liver, should be initially followed at intervals of 3 to 4 months, to determine progress of disease; this is mandatory if chemotherapy is used. Duke's A and B patients should be seen every 4 months for 1 year, then every 6 months for a total of at least 3 years, when checks may be advanced to a yearly basis if no evidence of tumor is found. One of the more important elements of follow-up in colon cancers is air contrast colon x-rays and colonoscopy, which are alternated every 6 months during the first 3 years. New lesions do appear in colons that have produced one cancer, and we have so far uncovered four such cancers in as many patients. These were early and probably curable lesions at resection. Patients who form polyps and those with a strong family history of colon cancer should have particularly meticulous evaluation of the colon at regular intervals.

Many approaches are being evaluated for the diagnosis and treatment of colorectal cancer. At present, the best results will be obtained with maximum efforts at early diagnosis, particularly in those groups especially susceptible to carcinomatous degeneration of the colon or rectum, and the earliest possible resection by a competent surgeon. Treatment of disseminated disease is still in its early stages.

ACUTE VIRAL AND BACTERIAL DYSENTERIES

method of
ARVEY I. ROGERS, M.D.
Miami, Florida

Acute diarrhea is among the most common symptoms affecting man. Global in distribution and of pandemic proportions, infectious diarrheas, both viral and bacterial, account for the majority of causes of disease. Though usually self-limiting, these acute dysenteries can have devastating consequences, both morbid and mortal, in the malnourished and underdeveloped populations of the world, and in infants, the elderly, and the debilitated anywhere. The health worker, whether physician or nonphysician, who deals with acute diarrheal disorders, should think in terms of cause, clinical recognition, comprehensive management, and cure.

Cause

Organisms that invade mucosa or stimulate it to secrete fluid and electrolytes or do both are responsible for acute, infectious diarrheal states. *Salmonella* species (most often *typhimurium* subtype), *Shigella* species (usually *sonnei*), *Escherichia coli*, both toxigenic and nontoxigenic strains, and viruses of the orbi- and reovirus groups are capable of producing diarrhea by one of the above mechanisms. The toxigenic prototype is *Vibrio cholerae*; other bacteria with similar properties include *Vibrio parahemolyticus*, *E. coli*, *Staphylococcus aureus*, *Clostridium perfringens*, and *Pseudomonas aeruginosa*, organisms that may all be capable of stimulating gut wall–associated levels of cyclic AMP, a mediator of fluid secretion. Once past the gastric acid barrier, the small intestine, colon, or both may be the target organ for bacterial pathophysiology. *Shigella* prefers the colon, while *Salmonella* stimulates secretion proximally and invades the ileum and colon distally. The inoculum size and sites of proliferation are determinants of clinical disease and mechanisms responsible. Invasiveness is responsible for infectious manifestations of fever, malaise, and generalized illness not attributable to volume depletion.

Comprehensive Management

Therapeutic objectives include rehydration and prevention of further dehydration, replacement of electrolyte losses, shortening the course of the illness, and symptomatic therapy.

Hospitalization should be undertaken for patients with moderate to severe dehydration or concomitant illnesses, such as congestive heart failure, chronic renal disease, or diabetes, which will complicate replacement efforts. As soon as it is determined that an infant is unable to tolerate oral replacement sufficient to maintain urine flow, hospitalization should be planned. Oral therapy should be allowed in patients who are not vomiting or in whom vomiting can be satisfactorily controlled. Balanced, isotonic glucose-electrolyte or sucrose-electrolyte solutions are superior to many commercial preparations such as Pedialyte, Lytren, or Gatorade, which are low in electrolytes or contain extremes of glucose concentrations. Sodium chloride, 3.5 grams; sodium bicarbonate, 2.5 grams; potassium chloride, 1.5 gram; and glucose or sucrose, 20.0 grams per liter (quart) of boiled tap water should yield close to an ideal solution containing (mEq. per liter): Na^+, 90; K^+, 20; HCO_3^+, 30; Cl^-, 80; and glucose, 111.

Another preparation includes 1 teaspoon of table salt, 1 heaping teaspoon of baking soda, and 4 tablespoons of table sugar in a quart of boiled tap water. This also produces near balance and isotonicity. The finding of reducing substances in the stool of an infant should alert the observer to reduce glucose content in oral solutions, consider sucrose substitution or hospitalization for parenteral therapy. Clear soups, apple juice, carbonated beverages, Karo syrup, and water may all be allowed in addition to the administration of a mixed glucose-electrolyte solution orally at a rate and volume sufficient to maintain an adequate urine output and volume status.

The prevention of further losses is accomplished by the administration of antiemetics or cessation of oral intake and by the judicious application of motility suppressants for the control of diarrhea. There is a small body of data suggesting that the carrier state for *Shigella* may be prolonged and that noninvasive organisms may become converted to invasive forms when severe suppression of motility prevents elimination of organisms via the rectum. *Salmonella* infections locally have been converted to septicemic forms with the use of motility suppressants. These occurrences may be coincidental to drug use but do raise the caution sign, nonetheless. If used, they should not be overused. Diphenoxylate (Lomotil), one 2.5 mg. tablet every 4 to 6 hours, codeine, 15 to 20 mg. every 6 hours, or paregoric, 4 to 8 ml. every 4 hours, are reasonable dosage schedules with a built-in need to consider whether or not renewal is necessary after 24 hours. Kaolin and pectin may also be utilized to provide some bulk.

Cure

Generally, it should be recalled that *Shigella* and *Salmonella* infections are usually self-limited and do not require antibiotic therapy. They do not usually shorten mild to moderate illness and may prolonged carrier state and encourage development of communitywide resistant strains. If a septic form of salmonellosis is suspected or the patient with shigellosis is very ill, antibiotics should be utilized. Ampicillin, trimethoprim-sulfamethoxazole (this use of this agent is not listed in the manufacturer's official directive), or chloramphenicol can be used for salmonellosis and should be selected based on antibiotic sensitivity testing or antibiotic susceptibility patterns for salmonella strains isolated in the community. Because of widespread resistance to sulfa and tetracycline preparations, shigella requiring antibiotics should be treated with ampicillin, 500 mg. every 6 hours in adults and 50 mg. per kg. per 24 hours in children.

Comment

Prophylaxis should be considered for individuals traveling to areas in which "traveler's diarrhea" outbreaks are prevalent, especially Mexico. A combination of neomycin and sulfa or tetracycline alone may be adequate in preventing the development of such an occurrence taken the day before traveling and for several days following arrival. *Isolation* of patients ill with acute bacillary dysentery should be attempted but is usually unsuccessful, and spread of illness to others in a close environment should be anticipated. *Giardiasis* should be considered as a nonbacterial, nonviral cause of an acute, nonbloody diarrhea, occurring in isolated or epidemic form, often 7 to 10 days following "exposure"; outbreaks have been described in Aspen, Colorado, Mexico, and Leningrad, U.S.S.R. Diagnosis can be made by careful stool examination for trophozoite forms (loose stools) or cyst forms (formed stools) in up to 50 per cent of cases; duodenal aspirate with small bowel biopsy stained for *Giardia lamblia* with Giemsa or iron-hematoxylin usually confirms the diagnosis. A therapeutic trial with metronidazole (Flagyl) or quinacrine (Atabrine) can provide dramatic results in strongly suspected cases. (This use of metronidazole and quinacrine is not listed in the manufacturer's official directive.)

INTESTINAL PARASITES*

method of
LEE S. MONROE, M.D.
La Jolla, California

Ever-expanding travel and population shifts have introduced exotic parasitic infections into the United States and have required that, on occasion, the physician be acquainted with the treatment of a wide spectrum of parasitosis. Help can be obtained in unusual cases from the Parasitic Disease Division, Center for Disease Control, Atlanta, Georgia, 30333 (telephone 404-633-3311). When supplied with adequate information by the inquiring physician, this Division provides consultation and unapproved drugs.

Pregnancy

Careful consideration must be given the treatment of a parasitosis in association with pregnancy. The hazards of parasitic infection must be weighed against potential damage to the fetus and mother by drugs that are often toxic. Inasmuch as many intestinal parasites produce few problems, a knowledge of their potential is indispensable in arriving at a therapeutic decision. Unfortunately, the literature contains little information on the safety of antiparasitic drugs in pregnancy.

Intestinal Protozoa

Amebiasis. See section on amebiasis for *Entamoeba histolytica.*

Dientomoeba Fragilis. This protozoan, seldom recognized, can produce a noninvasive colitis. See Table 1 for drugs used in treatment.

Nonpathogenic Ameba. Although infections with *Entamoeba coli, Iodamoeba bütschlii,* and *Endolimax nana* are not associated with symptoms and do not mandate treatment, it should be remembered that the finding of these forms indicates ingestion by the patient of fecally contaminated material. For this reason when such forms are encountered, the clinician should call for additional studies to rule out pathogens and, when in doubt, institute prophylactic treatment. When small race *Entamoeba histolytica (Entamoeba hartmanni)* is found, treatment as for *E. histolytica* should be instituted. The overlap in size between *E. histolytica* and *E. hartmanni* precludes an accurate differentiation by the average laboratory.

---

*Some drugs mentioned in this article may be considered investigational. See manufacturers' official directives before using.

Intestinal Flagellates. GIARDIA LAMBLIA. Giardiasis is cosmopolitan in its distribution and can exist either as a commensal or as an infection capable of producing a diarrheal state, tissue invasion, and malabsorption. Infection is frequently attributed to a contaminated water supply. In addition to the usual stool studies, diagnosis may require aspiration of the duodenal fluid with microscopy of duodenal mucus or the performance of a string test. The infection is not uncommonly seen in association with dysgammaglobulinemias. See Table 1 for the drugs used in treatment.

Nonpathogenic flagellates (*Chilomastix mesnili, Trichomonas hominis, Retortamonas intestinalis,* and *Enteromonas hominis*) do not require treatment, but their presence in stool examination raises the question of the ingestion of contaminated material and suggests the need for additional studies to ensure that pathogens are not present.

Ciliates. *Balantidium coli* is a ciliate commonly infecting primates, rats, and swine. Less commonly, humans, usually living in close contact with pigs, become infected. The organism in humans can exist as a commensal or as a life-threatening infection. See Table 1 for the drugs used in treatment.

ISOSPORA. Nearly every species of animal is known to harbor, on occasion, its species-specific coccidium. *Isospora belli* and *hominis* in man can produce a self-limited diarrhea or in rare instances be associated with a malabsorption syndrome. If coccidial forms are recognized in the stool or biopsy of the small intestine, a nitrofurantoin or a pyrimethamine-sulfadiazine combination can be tried, although treatment has not been standardized.

Intestinal Helminths

Nematodes. ASCARIS LUMBRICOIDES. The drugs used in the treatment of ascariasis are detailed in Table 2 and eradicate the parasite in greater than 90 per cent of the patients. Because of the potential problems occasioned by asymptomatic infections, all patients deserve therapy. Massive infection with the production of intestinal obstruction is a medical emergency and requires fluid and electrolyte replacement, intestinal decompression by intubation and suction, and the instillation of an anthelmintic via intestinal tube. Surgery is reserved for persisting ileus and carries a high mortality. Rarely, migration of ascarids into the biliary or pancreatic ductal system will require surgery if repeated medical therapy is unsuccessful.

ENTEROBIUS VERMICULARIS. The treatment of pinworm infection many times requires the administration of drugs (which are 90 per cent effective) to an entire family as cross-infection is the rule. Despite attempts to prevent the transmission

TABLE 1. Drug Therapy of Protozoal Infections

ORGANISM	DRUG	AVERAGE ADULT DOSE*	DAYS DURATION	INDICATIONS	ADVERSE DRUG EFFECTS
Entamoeba histolytica	See section on amebiasis				
Dientamoeba fragilis	1. Diiodohydroxyquin U.S.P.	0.65 gram t.i.d.	10	Commensal state or symptomatic intestinal	*Occasional:* Diarrhea, cramps, rash, thyroid enlargement. *Rare:* Optic atrophy
	2. Tetracycline	0.25 gram q.i.d.	7	Commensal state or symptomatic intestinal	*Common:* Nausea, vomiting, diarrhea, staining of teeth in children and neonates when given to pregnant women. *Occasional:* Liver damage infrequent. *Rare:* Allergy, blood dyscrasias
Giardia lamblia	1. Quinicrine hydrochloride	0.1 gram t.i.d.	5	Commensal state or symptomatic intestinal	*Common:* Headache, nausea, tinnitus. *Occasional:* Blood dyscrasias, arrhythmias
	2. Metronidazole	0.25 gram t.i.d.	5	Commensal state or symptomatic intestinal	*Common:* Antebuse-like reaction with ethanol, nausea, headache. *Occasional:* Dizziness, vomiting, diarrhea, rash, paresthesias. *Rare:* Ataxia
Balantidium coli	1. Tetracycline	0.5 gram q.i.d.	10	Commensal state or symptomatic intestinal	See above.
Isospora	1. Nitrofurantoin			Standard treatment for isosporiasis (coccidiosis) in humans has not been established.	*Occasional:* Nausea, emesis, diarrhea. *Rare:* Hepatitis, hypersensitivity lung disease
	2. Pyrimethamine-sulfadiazine				*Occasional:* Folic acid deficiencies, blood dyscrasias, rash. *Rare:* Convulsions, shock

*When prescribing in infants or children, the drug packaging information and/or the Parasitic Disease Division should be consulted.

of eggs from the environment, even heroic efforts towards personal hygiene and household cleanliness are usually futile. It is important to educate the family to the benign nature of enterobiasis and to emphasize that therapy is chiefly important for symptom relief. See Table 2 for the drugs currently used in therapy.

HOOKWORM (NECATOR AMERICANUS AND ANCYLOSTOMA DUODENALE). Light infections with hookworm sp. may be asymptomatic and unaccompanied by evidences of anemia or iron deficiency. Nevertheless, as a public health measure, treatment is recommended in all patients. Fortunately, the primary drugs of choice, pyrantel pamoate and mebendazole, have few side effects. Oral iron replacement should be added to the therapeutic program when anemia with iron deficiency is present. A follow-up stool examination should be done within 4 weeks to evaluate the residual worm burden; and retreatment given if evidences of infection persist. Repeated treatments produce a cure rate in the neighborhood of 90 per cent.

TRICHOSTRONGYLIASIS. The drug of choice is thiabendazole with pyrantel pamoate as an alternate. Bephenium hydroxynaphthoate (Alcopara) is a nonapproved drug that is probably effective in a dose of 5 grams. Most human infections are light and do not lead to symptoms, but a heavy infection with hundreds of worms can lead to duodenitis and jejunitis.

TRICHURIASIS. The intestinal roundworm, *Trichuris trichuria* is markedly resistant to therapy. Of the drugs currently available for treatment mebendazole is the drug of choice; it has a high therapeutic index with cure rates of 65 per cent or

TABLE 2. **Drug Therapy of the Common Helminth Infections**

ORGANISM	DRUG	AVERAGE ADULT DOSE*	DAYS	ADVERSE DRUG EFFECTS
NEMATODES				
Ascaris lumbricoides	1. Pyrantel pamoate (Antiminth)	11 mg./kg. (max. 1 gram)	1	*Occasional:* nausea, vomiting, headache, fever, rash
	2. Mebendazole (Vermox)	0.1 gram b.i.d.	3	*Occasional:* abdominal discomfort, diarrhea
	3. Piperazine citrate (Antepar)	0.075 gram/kg. (max. 3.5 grams)	2	*Occasional:* nausea, vomiting, dizziness, urticaria *Rare:* visual disturbance, ataxia, exacerbation of epilepsy
Enterobius vermicularis	1. Mebendazole (Vermox)	0.100 gram	1 repeat in 2 weeks	See above
	2. Pyrantel pamoate (Antiminth)	Single dose per Ascariasis	Repeat in 2 weeks	See above
	3. Piperazine citrate (Antepar)	6 mg./kg. (max. 2.5 grams daily)	7 repeat in 2 weeks	See above
	4. Pyrvinium pamoate (Povan)	5 mg./kg. (max. 0.250 gram)	1-repeat in 2 weeks	*Common:* red stools *Occasional:* nausea, vomiting, diarrhea *Rare:* photosensitivity
Hookworm sp. (*Necator americanus, Ancylostoma duodenale*)	1. Pyrantel pamoate (Antiminth)	See under Ascariasis	1	See above
	2. Mebendazole (Vermox)	See under Ascariasis	3	See above
	3. Bephenium (Alcopara)	5.0 grams b.i.d.	3	*Occasional:* nausea, vomiting, diarrhea
Trichostrongylus sp.	1. Thiabendazole (Mintezol)	0.025 gram/kg. b.i.d.	2	See under Trichuris
	2. Pyrantel pamoate (Antiminth)	See under ascariasis	1	See above
Trichuris trichuria	1. Mebendazole (Vermox)	0.100 gram b.i.d.	3	See above
	2. Thiabendazole (Mintezol)	0.025 gram/kg. b.i.d.	2	*Common:* dizziness, nausea, vomiting *Occasional:* Hallucinations, leukopenia, rash *Rare:* tinnitus, Stevens-Johnson syndrome, shock
Strongyloides stercoralis	1. Thiabendazole (Mintezol)	See under Trichuris	2	See above
Trichinella spiralis	1. Corticosteroids— for acute symptoms	20 to 40 mg./day (prednisone) with gradual reduction	Not established	
	2. Thiabendazole (Mintezol)	See under Trichuris	5	See above
CESTODES				
Taenia saginata *Taenia solium* *Diphyllobothrium latum*	1. Niclosamide (Yomesan)	2.0 grams in a single dose	1	*Occasional:* abdominal discomfort, nausea
	2. Paromomycin (Humatin)	1 gram every 15 min. for 4 doses	1	*Common:* nausea, abdominal discomfort *Rare:* 8th nerve, renal toxicity
Hymenolepis nana *Hymenolepis diminuta*	1. Niclosamide (Yomesan)	2.00 grams	5–7	See above
	2. Paromomycin	45 mg./kg. daily	5–7	See above
Dipylidium canium	1. Niclosamide (Yomesan)	As for *T. saginata* (reports scarce)	1	See above

*When prescribing for infants or children, the drug packaging information and/or the Parasitic Disease Division should be consulted.

TABLE 2. **Drug Therapy of the Common Helminth Infections** (*Continued*)

ORGANISM	DRUG	AVERAGE ADULT DOSE*	DAYS	ADVERSE DRUG EFFECTS
TREMATODES				
Clonorchis sinensis	1. Chloroquine (Aralen)	0.250 gram t.i.d.	42	*Occasional:* headache, confusion, pruritus, nausea, vomiting, corneal opacities, retinitis, ocular palsies, alopecia *Rare:* blood dyscrasias, 8th nerve damage, discoloration of nails and mucous membrane
Fasciolia hepatica	1. Bithionol	0.030 to 0.050 gram/kg. daily × 10 to 15 doses		*Common:* urticaria, nausea, vomiting, diarrhea, photosensitivity, skin eruptions
Schistosomes 　*S. haematobium*	1. Niridazole (Ambilhar)	0.025 gram/kg. (max. 1.5 grams)	5–7	*Common:* nausea, vomiting, dizziness, headache *Occasional:* paresthesias, rash, EKG changes, diarrhea *Rare:* hemolytic anemia in G6PD-deficient persons, psychosis, convulsions
	2. Antimony sodium dimercaptosuccinate (Stibocaptate)	8 mg./kg. I.M. 1 to 2 times per week for 5 doses		*Common:* pruritus, rash— same effects but to lesser degree than potassium antimony tartrate—see below
S. japonicum	1. Antimony potassium tartrate U.S.P.	0.5% sol. intravenously, 8, 12, 16, 20, 24 ml. on alternate days then 28 ml. on alternate days for 10 additional doses		*Common:* coughing and vomiting with rapid injection, muscle and joint pains, bradycardia, pain on I.V. extravasation *Occasional:* rash, pruritus, myocardial damage, diarrhea *Rare:* shock with sudden death; hepatocellular and renal damage; hemolytic anemia
S. mansoni	1. Niridazole (Ambilhar)	As for *S. haematobium*		See above
	2. Antimony sodium dimercaptosuccinate (Stibocaptate)	As for *S. haematobium*		See above
	3. Stibophen (Fuadin)	1.5 ml. intramuscularly followed by 3.5 ml. intramuscularly 2 days later, followed by 5 ml. intramuscularly daily, for total dosage of 100 ml.		*Occasional:* myocardial damage, rash, pruritus *Rare:* sudden death, shock, encephalopathy, sulfhemoglobinemia. Same effects, but to a lesser degree than antimony potassium tartrate

greater and a low incidence of side effects. If more than an occasional egg is found in the follow-up stool examination in 4 weeks, the course can be repeated.

STRONGYLOIDIASIS. The treatment of *Strongyloides stercoralis* is important, as autoinfection can progressively increase parasitic burden. Thiabendazole (see Table 2) has proven to be a therapeutic advance. Pyrvinium pamoate, 5 mg. per kg. repeated for 5 to 7 days, also apparently has significant activity. Inasmuch as it is important to eradicate this infection thoroughly, careful follow-up stool studies in 4 weeks are mandatory. Further assurance of cure can be obtained by duodenal drainage with search for ova and rhabditiform larvae.

TRICHINOSIS. Patients with myocarditis, cerebral edema, or pneumonia are candidates for suppressive treatment with ACTH or oral corticosteroids during the inflammatory stages of larval invasion. It is probable that treatment with thiabendazole (see Table 2) is of value early in the course, before massive invasion and encystation have occurred. Thiabendazole may also be of value as a prophylactic measure when it is determined that the patient has recently ingested infected meat.

Cestodes

The large tapeworms (*Taenia saginata, Taenia solium* and *Diphyllobothrium latum*) can be effectively treated with niclosamide (Yomesan) (see Table 2). It has been postulated that, in the case of *T. solium*, degenerating proglottids resulting from therapy might lead to cysticercosis. Experience, however, has not justified this theory. Paromomycin (Humatin) is an effective alternative to niclosamide but is not currently approved for this usage in the United States of America by the Food and Drug Administration.

Cysticercosis, produced by tissue invasion of the intermediate stage of *T. solium*, most often manifests itself as a central nervous system problem, and treatment is usually surgical. If the condition is recognized, mebendazole may be effective in killing the larval stage. Drug therapy is limited in value, however, as the larvae may be degenerating when first symptoms appear.

Hymenolepis nana and *Hymenolepis diminuta* infections are responsive to the same drugs as the large cestodes. Treatment should be prolonged from 5 to 7 days (see Table 2).

Infection with *Diphylidium caninum* is uncommon so that reports of therapeutic efficacy are scarce. The infection is harmless, but treatment with niclosamide, as for large tapeworms, appears to be effective.

Trematodes

Clonorchiasis. Infection with *Clonorchis (Opisthorchis) sinesis* responds rather poorly to treatment, particularly in advanced cases. Chloroquine (see Table 2) is the drug most effective and, in rare cases, cures have been reported. Therapy usually suppresses egg production without killing the adult. In patients with advanced cases, on rare occasion, surgical intervention for bile duct strictures and abscesses is warranted. Hetol (chloxyle), a drug not approved in the United States, gives significant cure rates but has proved toxic in laboratory animals.

Fascioliasis (hepatica and gigantica). Bithionol (Table 2) is the drug of choice and can be obtained from the Parasitic Disease Division of the Center for Disease Control in Atlanta, Georgia. Clinical reports documenting this therapy in fascioliasis are scarce, but the therapeutic index in paragonimiasis, from a related fluke, is high.

Schistosomiasis (*Schistosoma haematobium, S. mansoni* and *S. japonicum*). This constitutes one of the most important and dangerous of the parasitic infections. Unfortunately, the drugs used in treatment are toxic and the clinician must weigh the severity of the infection against risk of treatment. In light infections and when there are nonviable ova recovered from biopsy material or stool, withholding treatment is the procedure advocated.

Niridazole (Ambilhar), an orally administered drug, is available from the Parasitic Disease Drug service and is useful in both *S. haematobium* and *S. mansoni* infections; however, side effects are frequent. When given to patients with liver disease, niridazole may produce cerebral symptoms and, in such cases, stibophen should be used. Antimony sodium dimercaptosuccinate (Stibocaptate) is an alternate drug for these infections and can be given intramuscularly. *S. japonicum* is most resistant to treatment and the drug of choice is the toxic antimony potassium tartrate (tartar emetic). This compound should be given slowly intravenously. Rapid intravenous administration can produce a cough, vomiting, and even a fatal reaction. Antimony preparations are contraindicated in patients with concurrent infections or in the presence of liver or heart disease. The results of treatment should be assayed at intervals of 2 months for a total of 6 months after therapy to ensure that the patient is cured. It should be remembered that nonviable ova are often passed for years after successful treatment and that viability is determined by observing motility of the flame cell, or the miracidium, and also by observing hatching of the miracidium.

ULCERATIVE COLITIS

method of
BURTON I. KORELITZ, M.D.
New York, New York

Ulcerative colitis is a distinct, usually chronic, inflammatory disease of the colon that was first described in its classic form in England during the second half of the nineteenth century. Now, more than 100 years later, its cause remains unknown. During the past decade the intensity of research has been accelerated and the results suggest that the immunologic surveillance or defense of the colonic mucosa is somehow compromised, permitting either invasion or perpetuation of damage by an invader from the lumen of the colon. The invader may yet prove to be viral, bacterial, or a material as yet not even considered. There may be a genetic, an environmental or even an emotional predisposition to the compromise of the immunologic integrity.

Although the pathology of ulcerative colitis is reasonably diagnostic, the number of ways in which the colon can respond with inflammation are limited. Therefore, differential diagnosis from other forms of colitis is frequently necessary. These forms include amebic, bacillary, ischemic, and antibiotic, most of which can be excluded by historical evidence and fortunately often appear different as well. Another form of colitis that often requires distinction from ulcerative colitis is Crohn's disease when it is limited or almost limited to the colon. These two diseases, grouped under the terminology *inflammatory bowel disease,* must be separated in order to administer proper therapy for each.

Treatment

Consideration must be given to the severity of illness. Whereas mild disease may be treated on an ambulatory basis, severe disease warrants hospitalization and close observation. Ulcerative colitis is a disease process that can rapidly become worse and be complicated by hemorrhage, toxic megacolon, or perforation.

General Supervision

The patient must be seen frequently by the managing physician when the disease is active. Symptoms or lack of them can be misleading. As the rectal segment is always involved, sigmoidoscopy is indicated at almost every office visit for accurate determination of disease activity. The management of ulcerative colitis requires a great deal of personal attention. More than in other conditions, the emphasis must be on the care of the patient rather than on the specific disease process. The physician who is both knowledgeable about the course of ulcerative colitis and actively caters to the patient's needs is clearly more successful in management than the physician who is guided by symptoms alone.

The managing physician must be aware of complications of the disease and of the drugs being used in treatment. In the very ill patient, a plain film of the abdomen will occasionally outline the ulcerated colon so that sigmoidoscopy can be temporarily postponed. After sigmoidoscopy a barium enema is performed to determine severity, extent, and perhaps differentiation from other forms of colitis. Usually this procedure is reasonably well tolerated, but it should be postponed in the very sick patient until there is some clinical improvement. Sometimes this examination provokes the development of toxic megacolon. If there is no clinical improvement and no dilatation of the colon, barium enema should no longer be delayed. The abdomen must be examined for tenderness, masses, peristalsis, and signs of free air. The general evaluation should include consideration of anemia, dehydration, and depression, as well as side actions of the specific drugs being used.

Supportive Measures

Diet. Specific food restriction has little place in the treatment of ulcerative colitis and this concept is well supported by vast experience. Good nutrition is important in this disease, and the patient's appetite should be used in any way necessary to achieve this. Although some fruits and vegetables might increase gaseousness, they do not intensify the disease process and often seem to increase the patient's morale as well as his nutrition. If a specific food is consistently poorly tolerated it should be avoided on that basis only. In an occasional patient milk and milk products will aggravate symptoms. Usually a lactase insufficiency is then demonstrated, which is similar to that in patients who have lactase insufficiency but who do not have ulcerative colitis. Even in very sick patients there is no advantage to keeping the patient on nothing by mouth unless a toxic megacolon or impending toxic megacolon is demonstrated. If the intake is limited, multivitamin supplements may be used. If the oral intake is poor, intravenous feedings with vitamins should be added.

Minerals. With chronic disease and prolonged diarrhea, hypopotassemia and anemia due to blood loss often follow. In many patients oral potassium and iron preparations are poorly tolerated and if foods high in potassium and iron content do not suffice, parenteral supplements should be used. These include 20 to 40 mEq. KCl per liter of intravenous fluids and 2 ml. of iron dextran (Imferon) intramuscularly daily.

Antidiarrheal Agents and Medications for Pain. The use of these drugs must be based on the recognition that symptoms are due to the persistence of active disease. Therefore, these agents should have only a temporary and supplemental role in management. Their use should be monitored carefully, particularly those containing narcotics, as they predispose to toxic megacolon.

The most effective of the antidiarrheal agents is deodorized tincture of opium. The usual dose is 10 drops following every other diarrheal stool, to a maximum of 30 drops daily. For some patients a lesser dose is satisfactory. Paregoric, in doses of 5 ml., might have an equivalent effect. Codeine sulfate, 30 to 60 mg. every 4 to 6 hours, might be preferable when abdominal pain rather than diarrhea dominates the picture. Acetaminophen (Tylenol) or propoxyphene hydrochloride (Darvon) or combinations are preferable if they are effective. Aspirin compounds should be avoided.

Sedatives. Phenobarbital, chlordiazepoxide (Librium), diazepam (Valium), or equivalent drugs may be used when indicated for the specific patient. Valium is sometimes responsible for a superimposed lethargy or an accentuation of depression. Chlorpromazine (Thorazine) is of value in the treatment of toxic psychosis, which may complicate steroid therapy.

Anticholinergics. This group of drugs should be avoided in managing ulcerative colitis. Although they might relieve cramps temporarily, they often cause atony of the bowel and contribute to the complication of toxic megacolon.

Antibiotics. This group of drugs has no specific action against ulcerative colitis. They should be reserved for the treatment of complicating infections and for use in postoperative periods. There is a definite role for parenteral antibiotics (ampicilin, cefazolin sodium [Ancef], gentamicin) as part of the program in the management of toxic megacolon and impending perforation.

Blood Transfusions. If the patient is both anemic and actively ill, blood transfusions should be used. In the very ill patient with ulcerative colitis the transfusion often leads to a degree of improvement above and beyond that expected from blood replacement alone and permits steroid therapy to be more effective. If the serum albumin is under 3 grams per dl. (100 ml.), the infusion of salt-poor albumin may be considered as well.

Hyperalimentation. The indications for this form of treatment are limited in ulcerative colitis, as opposed to Crohn's disease. When the patient may not eat, as is the case in managing toxic megacolon, hyperalimentation may be favored over peripheral intravenous nutrition. This is particularly true when the state of nutrition was poor to begin with or when surgical intervention seems imminent.

Small Bowel Tube. In the event of toxic megacolon or impending megacolon, a small bowel tube should be passed immediately and connected to a constant suction apparatus.

Specific Drug Therapy

Sulfasalazine. Sulfasalazine is the mainstay of drug therapy. Its action is more specific for ulcerative colitis than that of other sulfonamides. The drug has a di-azo linkage between acetylsalicylic acid and sulfapyridine that is broken down in the colon. The therapeutic benefit from the drug seems to correlate with the blood level of free sulfapyridine, although this does not mean the good result is dependent on this cleavage. Side actions such as nausea and headache are common. Generalized skin eruptions of the type caused by sulfonamides also occur frequently. These reactions occur more often in patients in whom the free sulfapyridine is slowly acetylated by the liver than in those in whom the acetylation is rapid. Seemingly, however, patients prone to these reactions are also those who have the best therapeutic results. Therefore, it is appropriate to start the drug slowly, such as 1 tablet (0.5 gram) daily, and increase the dose by 1 tablet daily until a maintenance level of 8 tablets (4 grams) daily is reached. If nausea or headache intervene, the increase should be stopped and the dose maintained at that level. It may then be slowly increased at a later date. The onset of a rash in most instances requires stopping the drug. Severe rashes might be modified by coincident steroid therapy or steroids might be appropriately introduced at that time. After the rash subsides, desensitization with sulfasalazine should be seriously considerd, as there are few drugs available for the treatment of ulcerative colitis and in general sulfasalazine is still probably the least toxic. Desensitization might be started with a quarter of a tablet daily and increased at various rates over long periods of time. About 80 per cent of patients will respond to this plan and eventually tolerate the drug. Leukopenia is common during treatment with sulfasalazine but usually the white blood count remains between 4000 and 5000 per cu. mm., despite continuation of the drug. If the white count falls below 4000 per cu. mm. the drug should be stopped. It might be tried again at a later date. Agranulocytosis is the greatest concern when attempting desensitization but occurs rarely. Anemias have also occurred in the course of sulfasalazine therapy. One type results from the interference with folic acid absorption and in many cases can be counteracted by intramuscular followed by oral folate.

Corticosteroids. Steroid therapy usually results in dramatic remissions of ulcerative colitis. Whereas sulfasalazine has been proven to be effective for maintenance against recurrences and will often be effective in the mild attack, the sicker patient usually does not respond, and his symptoms might be aggravated by the side actions of the drug. On the other hand, steroids have little role in maintenance but will reduce the inflammation of the disease to permit the introduction of the sulfasalazine.

If the patient with ulcerative colitis is sick enough to be hospitalized and requires intravenous fluids, the choice form of steroid therapy is ACTH in crystalline form added to the intravenous fluid. The preferable initial dose is 40 units per 1000 ml., which will total 120 units when 3000 ml. are given over a 24-hour period. If clinical improvement is forthcoming with increase in sense of well being, increase in appetite, decrease in number of stools, and increase in consistency of stools, the intravenous ACTH may be stopped or reduced in dose after a few days. At that point intramuscular ACTH (crystalline or gel) may be substituted for the interim, or oral prednisone may be introduced, starting at 60 mg. daily, or both may be used at once. The dose of prednisone is gradually reduced in proportion to the rate of clinical response. The average rate of reduction is 5 mg. per week but may be faster. At some point in the reduction, such as at the level of 15 to 20 mg. of prednisone per day, sulfasalazine should be introduced for maintenance.

In some hospitalized patients and others managed on an ambulatory basis, steroid therapy may be initiated in the form of prednisone. Ideally, the dose should not be less than 60 mg. daily if this drug is to be started at all. This dose can then be reduced fairly rapidly. If the initial dose level chosen is too low, raising the dose later does not always accomplish the same results as when a 60 mg. dose is used initially, and the clinical advantage is lost.

6-Mercaptopurine and Azathioprine (Imuran). Immunosuppressives are considered experimental in the treatment of ulcerative colitis, as double blind studies have not as yet proved their efficacy. In some patients clear-cut improvement has occurred coincident with their use. In many instances these agents have been used in young adults and children in whom sulfasalazine had failed and reintroduction of steroids had been required many times. In most of these patients long periods of well-being have resulted, and growth and development have occurred coincidentally. The average dose is 50 to 100 mg. daily. Weekly complete blood counts, including platelet counts, are required near the beginning. Later, once monthly is satisfactory for most. Patients for whom this form of therapy is being considered should be both intelligent and conscientious. Ideally, the responsibility for dosage and blood tests should be in the hands of a hematologist who should manage the case in close cooperation with the primary physician.

Goals of Therapy. If sulfasalazine is successful in the treatment of ulcerative colitis and does not cause any serious complications in itself (these always occur within the first few weeks), the drug should be continued indefinitely. The dose may be reduced either to lessen nausea or headaches, or for psychologic purposes, from 4 grams daily to 3 or 2 grams daily. Even 0.5 gram is sufficient to maintain remission in some patients, although dosage should not be reduced to this level unless necessary. Sulfasalazine should be considered primarily a chronic phase drug. On the other hand, steroids should be introduced at the time of severe exacerbation (or onset of the disease) to effect a reversal; therefore, they should be considered acute phase drugs. Once their role has been accomplished, the steroid dosage should be gradually reduced and then stopped. Low-grade maintenance treatment of ulcerative colitis with steroids permits smoldering disease and potentially irreversible complications. If the reintroduction of steroid therapy is required frequently, then treatment with immunosuppressives should be considered. These drugs have none of the side actions of steroids; neither are they followed by a dramatic response. They behave more like sulfasalazine and should be considered chronic phase drugs. The therapeutic effect might not be seen for as long as 4 to 6 months, although it usually occurs sooner. The toxic complications of these drugs, like those of sulfasalazine, occur early. The leukopenia, which occurs in almost all patients at some time, is reversible by either reducing the dose or temporarily stopping the drug. The therapeutic benefit varies, but immunosuppressives provide a steroid sparing effect if not a complete remission.

Surgery

Perforation of the colon and massive hemorrhage are absolute indications for surgical intervention. Impending perforation and toxic megacolon are relative indications increasing with lack of response to appropriate medical management. When toxic megacolon is recognized, oral feedings should be stopped immediately. This condition is frequently reversed by using small bowel tube decompression, by the use of blood transfusions and albumin infusions, and by increasing the steroid dose when inadequate or starting steroids (intravenous crystalline ACTH) in high dose. Antibiotics are appropriate in these circumstances. The cautious use of a rectal tube is also of help. With early recognition of toxic megacolon and attentive enthusiastic management, the condition can be reversed in more than half the patients. Elective surgery is indicated for carcinoma, for dysplasia accompanying universal disease, and for retarded growth and development in children with narrowed and shortened colons. Chronic disease and failure to thrive are indications for surgery only when all appropriate forms of medical therapy have failed. The operation of choice is ileostomy with total proctocolectomy; in some patients with toxic megacolon preliminary surgical decompression is indicated. Subtotal colectomy with ileorectal anastomosis is no longer encouraged because of persistent diarrhea, possible addiction to opiates, and the enduring risk of carcinoma of the rectum. Fortunately, ulcerative colitis may be cured by resection of the diseased colon and rectum. When the surgery is performed electively the patient may choose a newer procedure, the Kock or continent ileostomy, in which an ileal pouch is constructed posterior to the rectus muscle and, as there is no stoma to protrude from the abdominal wall, no appliance is required.

Treatment of Common Complications

Systemic or Extraintestinal Manifestations of Ulcerative Colitis. Arthritis, erythema nodosum, and uveitis usually respond effectively to steroid therapy. When the uveitis or arthritis is active while the primary bowel disease is quiescent, local steroid infiltration or antiarthritic medications may be preferable. Pyoderma gangrenosum also usually responds to large dose steroid therapy although not as dramatically as do other complications.

Retarded Growth and Development. Usually other complications than retarded growth and development dictate proper management. If retarded growth and development are present while the disease is otherwise quiescent, this complication deserves total proctocolectomy for its own sake, particularly if the epiphyses are not yet closed. Before puberty a trial of hyperalimentation and supplementary elemental feedings should be tried to effect a growth spurt.

Strictures and Carcinomas of the Rectum and Colon. Carcinoma occurs in approximately 10 per cent of patients with universal or almost universal ulcerative colitis after a 20-year history of the disease. The incidence increases more rapidly after 10 years. A carcinoma diagnosed by x-ray or by x-ray and biopsy warrants immediate total proctocolectomy. Barium enemas should be performed at least once yearly after the diagnosis of ulcerative colitis is made, even if the patient is asymptomatic.

A stricture occurring in the course of ulcerative colitis is more likely to be benign than malignant, but since radiologic signs are lacking to aid in the differential diagnosis, all strictures should be considered malignant until proven otherwise. Colonoscopy with biopsies should be performed when strictures are discovered by rectal examination, sigmoidoscopy or at the annual barium enema x-ray examination.

Dysplasia. Ulcerative colitis is a premalignant lesion. Premalignant histologic changes in the form of dysplasia may be found on mucosal biopsies and, if persistent, warrant total proctocolectomy. Rectal biopsies should be performed at least once yearly after the diagnosis of ulcerative colitis is made. After 10 years of disease, colonoscopy with multiple biopsies should be performed annually, and rectal biopsies should be performed twice a year. Exfoliative cytology should be done during colonoscopy when a competent cytologist is available.

Management During Pregnancy

The influence of pregnancy on the course of ulcerative colitis varies with the state of activity at the time of conception. If the disease is quiescent, the ulcerative colitis usually remains inactive. If the disease is active, the risk is high that it will worsen. This is particularly true if the pregnancy is unwanted. Worsening is most likely to take place in the first trimester of pregnancy. If the patient is already receiving steroids, the dose should be raised, and if not, steroids should be started. If the condition continues to worsen, therapeutic abortion should be considered, and if it is to be done, the decision should be made as early in the first trimester as possible. After the first trimester every effort should be made to maintain the pregnancy, even if high dose steroid therapy is required thereafter. Therapeutic abortion is usually but not always followed by remission. If the pregnancy is continued for a full term, there appears to be little risk to the fetus from the disease or steroid treatment. If indications for surgery in the patient with ulcerative colitis arise, it must be performed any time during the course of pregnancy, even though the child is unlikely to survive. Ulcerative colitis has a particularly ominous prognosis when it has its onset during pregnancy.

If the patient is established and symptom free on sulfasalazine at the time when pregnancy is recognized, this drug should be continued. Theoretically, the drug should be stopped during the ninth month as it might compete with bilirubin for binding sites on the plasma proteins and result in kernicterus after birth.

Patients on immunosuppressives should not become pregnant, because of the risk of genetic damage to the fetus. If pregnancy does occur, a therapeutic abortion is advisable.

Ulcerative Colitis in the Aged

Whether the patient has onset of the disease after age 60 or has had continued or intermittent disease since childhood, the course in the older patient is more likely to be complicated by drug reactions and the presence of coincident diseases.

These patients should be followed particularly closely, and signs of activity should warrant enthusiastic treatment. Rectal bleeding in the aged is often considered due to hemorrhoids or diverticulosis so that proper diagnosis and treatment, unfortunately, are postponed.

Ulcerative Proctitis

Patients with ulcerative colitis limited in extent to the rectal segment fall into two therapeutic groups: those who respond best to local steroid therapy and those who respond best to sulfasalazine. Of the two local forms of steroid applications, the *steroid enemas* (100 mg. of hydrocortisone in 60 ml. of isotonic saline solution) are more effective in patients in whom the entire rectum and rectosigmoid are involved as the liquid spreads more extensively and covers the entire area. Sometimes the use of a steroid enema is appropriate for patients with disease extending more proximal (proctosigmoiditis). The frequency with which hydrocortisone enemas are given varies but the therapy is usually initiated on a program of 2 enemas daily, then with improvement is reduced to 1 daily, then further reduced to one enema 2 of 3 days, then one enema every other day, etc. The hydrocortisone acetate (Cortifoam) aerosol, when available, is better suited to those patients with ulcerative proctitis limited to the rectal ampulla or just beyond. This form of treatment is better tolerated, as it does not provoke the tenesmus or urgency which often accompanies a fluid enema. The initial dose is usually one application twice daily and is then reduced according to a formula similar to that for the steroid enemas. The suppository forms of steroid have little place in the treatment of left-sided or universal ulcerative colitis. Occasional local applications may facilitate reduction of the oral dose when the rectal segment is the one most markedly involved.

Prognosis

In most patients who withstand the first few years of ulcerative colitis without requiring colectomy, the primary bowel symptoms decrease in severity. Management is then dominated by considerations of the later complication of carcinoma. Some gastroenterologists have recommended elective total proctocolectomy and ileostomy after 10 years of ulcerative colitis (involving all or most of the colon), even if the patient is then symptom free. Even if statistically valid, this advice is usually refused by the young patient, who has already tolerated the early years of disease and currently is doing well. Therefore, the close periodic follow-up of patients after the first 10 years becomes essential—with annual or more frequent sigmoidoscopy, barium enema, colonoscopy, and biopsies. With these techniques the risk of late mortality from ulcerative colitis is markedly diminished.

The National Foundation for Ileitis and Colitis, Inc. (NFIC)

This group was founded 11 years ago by patients with ulcerative colitis or Crohn's disease, by their families, and physicians for purposes of fund raising to support research and for education. The efforts of NFIC have benefited many physicians and their patients by disseminating knowledge as to the natural course and optimum management, based on current knowledge. There are now 26 chapters of NFIC throughout the country and others are being organized. Physicians who would like more information for their patients or themselves concerning purpose, functions, nearest chapter, informative brochures, or research, should contact the National Foundation for Ileitis and Colitis, Inc., 295 Madison Avenue, New York, N.Y. 10017.

Metabolic Disorders

BERIBERI

(Thiamine [Vitamin B₁] Deficiency)

method of
RICHARD W. VILTER, M.D.
Cincinnati, Ohio

Classic beriberi is rare in the United States except in the chronic alcoholic. It may occur occasionally, however, in persons with diseases predisposing to increased nutritional requirements such as hyperthyroidism, pregnancy, lactation, malignant diseases, or malabsorption syndromes. In the Orient it occurs in adults who are dependent for calories on vitamin-poor polished rice. An infantile form presenting as acute cardiac failure, aphonia, pseudomeningitis, or vomiting, constipation, and failure to thrive also occurs in infants of thiamine-deficient mothers. Since thiamine is involved in carbohydrate metabolism, mainly as a codecarboxylase of alpha keto acids such as pyruvic acid and to a lesser extent as a cotransketolase in the pentose phosphate pathway, long use of unsupplemented intravenous glucose solutions may precipitate a thiamine deficiency state. Psychoneurotic symptoms, peripheral neuritis, edema, heart failure (usually of the high output type), and Wernicke's encephalopathy (ophthalmoplegia, nystagmus, ataxia, and global confusion) are the classic manifestations of thiamine deficiency.

Prevention

A diet rich in meat, cereals, vegetables, and dairy products will prevent beriberi, even in the chronic alcoholic. Ingestion of bread or rice enriched with the vitamins of the B complex will afford a large measure of protection. In pregnant women or in persons with systemic diseases that limit the appetite or interfere with proper absorption of vitamins from the gastrointestinal tract, 2 to 5 mg. of thiamine a day, usually prescribed in capsule form or as an intramuscular injection with other members of the vitamin B complex, will prevent the deficiency state. The dietary allowance of thiamine recommended by the Food and Nutrition Board of the National Research Council is approximately 0.5 mg. for each 1000 calories; when the caloric intake of adults is less than 2000, the thiamine intake should not fall below 1.0 mg. per day. Pregnant and lactating women should receive an additional allocation of 0.3 mg. per day over that of nonpregnant women.

Treatment

Patients with peripheral neuritis due to thiamine lack should abstain from alcohol and should be given a diet rich in meat, vegetables, cereals, dairy products, and fruit, as well as thiamine 5 mg. four times daily by mouth or parenterally. In addition, a multiple vitamin capsule should be taken several times a day, because it is almost certain that a patient deficient in one of the B complex vitamins will be deficient in all of them. Very occasionally, an anaphylactic reaction occurs when thiamine is given intravenously.

Analgesics often may be necessary to relieve the painful burning of the feet and legs. Acetylsalicylic acid and codeine are usually sufficient, but occasionally meperidine (Demerol) may be necessary. Hyperesthetic feet and legs, the usual sites of the most severe neuropathy, should be protected from the bedclothes by a cradle; when foot drop develops, the feet should be supported by a footboard at the end of the bed or by light splints to avoid contractures.

As soon as pain will allow, physiotherapy should be started; it should be passive at first, then active, as muscles begin to function. Convalescence is prolonged, particularly in the chronic alcoholic, and may take 6 months or longer. Damaged nerves regain function slowly. Dead nerves never recover.

Patients with beriberi heart disease should be kept at absolute bed rest, since mild activity may bring about sudden death. A diet low in salt and residue and rich in protein and B complex vitamins is important. If patients cannot eat such a diet, tube feedings may be necessary until the most acute stage of the disease has passed. It is customary to give the initial dose of 25 to 50 mg. of thiamine intravenously followed by an oral dose of 5 mg. four times daily. Administration should be continued parenterally if the patient cannot take medication orally. Larger doses, especially when administered parenterally, are rapidly excreted in the urine. The other vitamins of the B complex should be administered as described for peripheral neuritis. Congestive heart failure is managed in the usual fashion, with diuretics and digitalis, which may be helpful after the thiamine deficiency has been alleviated. Occasionally, thiamine therapy alone may be sufficient to induce massive diuresis. Convalescence may be prolonged, but usually, if the patient recovers and remains on an adequate diet thereafter, there will be no noticeable residuals of cardiac damage. Alcoholic cardiomyopathy (low output failure) is a frequent complication and interferes with a dramatic response to thiamine and with eventual recovery.

Wernicke's encephalopathy may be treated in the same way as beriberi heart disease. Ophthalmoplegia disappears rapidly, and nystagmus and ataxia usually do also, but psychosis and neuritis may persist for months or may gradually merge into Korsakoff's psychosis, which is usually but not invariably irreversible. Improvement in mental capabilities may occur over 6 to 12 months with good medical management.

Patients with delirium tremens should receive 25 mg. of thiamine parenterally to prevent the development of the manifestations of acute beriberi, particularly if glucose solution is to be given intravenously. For infantile beriberi 10 mg. of thiamine should be given parenterally at once, followed by 5 mg. twice a day for a week. In patients who are treated early in the course of the disease, improvement may be dramatic. Those who have been ill for several days may not recover. Nutritional repletion of the nursing mother of the infant is important.

HYPO- AND HYPERVITAMINOSIS A

method of
DARWIN KARYADI, M.D., Ph.D.,
and A. SOMMER, M.D.
Bogor, Indonesia

Hypovitaminosis A

The usually recommended dietary allowances provide ample amounts of vitamin A so that deficiency may be avoided and optimum nutrition may ensue. Once a deficiency is manifest, the most effective therapy consists of (1) prescribing large doses of vitamin concentrates, (2) removing or

curing any condition that interferes with efficient utilization of food, and (3) correcting the diet so that vitamin intake again becomes normal.

The treatment of night blindness, conjunctival xerosis, and Bitot spots should consist of 200,000 I.U. of vitamin A by mouth on two successive days. Corneal xerosis should be treated by the intramuscular injection of 100,000 I.U. of a water-miscible preparation and 200,000 I.U. vitamin A by mouth the following day (if no water-miscible vitamin A is available use oral schedule above). In addition, a local eye ointment (gentamicin and bacitracin) applied five times a day until the cornea is clear is recommended.

Corneal ulceration, corneal destruction, or keratomalacia should be managed basically with the same vitamin A dosage and local eye ointment treatment as for corneal xerosis. However, in addition, systemic antibiotic therapy (gentamicin and penicillinase-resistant penicillin) appropriate for weight and age is required. All patients with malnutrition, in particular, protein energy malnutrition, respiratory tract infection, diarrhea, and other disorders, should receive appropriate therapy.

Hypervitaminosis A

Acute vitamin A toxicity in man is characterized by drowsiness, headache and vomiting and is associated with a transitory increase in intracranial pressure. Other signs one may detect are bone and joint pain, anorexia, weight loss, vertigo, hyperesthesia, and alopecia.

The prolonged ingestion of very large amounts of vitamin A, at least 7500 times the amount of vitamin A required for normal nutritional needs, is considered toxic. The management of hypervitaminosis A consists in (1) early diagnosis from the signs and symptoms, including especially the art of taking a careful medical history to reveal the consumption of large doses of vitamin A, and (2) the discontinuance of the consumption of high potency preparations of vitamin A. This should eliminate the signs and symptoms of vitamin A toxicity within days to weeks.

DIABETES MELLITUS SYNDROME IN THE ADULT

method of
JOSEPH C. SHIPP, M.D.
Omaha, Nebraska

Each physician knows that diabetes mellitus is a common, chronic disorder manifest by:

1. Generalized disturbance of metabolism (more than a sugar problem) affecting carbohydrate, lipid, and protein metabolism. The intensity of the metabolic disorder presents a full spectrum ranging, from impaired glucose tolerance, with normal fasting glycemia, to the other extreme of diabetic ketoacidosis. The catabolic nature of the diabetes syndrome is best shown by the profound weight loss in those with diabetes of moderate or severe intensity.

2. Nonmetabolic features, which are represented by altered response to infections, neuropathy, and vascular disease (microangiopathy of a characteristic type, clinically manifest by retinopathy and nephropathy; and large vessel disease). Whether and to what extent these manifestations relate to the metabolic disturbance remains a controversy.

In the usual clinical situation treatment is directed at the metabolic component, usually viewed or assessed in terms of hyperglycemia and glycosuria. Intervention aimed at restoring a more normal metabolic state is done because the physician believes that this will help the patient. Because of the continuing controversies related to the incomplete understanding of the syndrome, the physician is often ambivalent about his recommendations. However, the practicing physician (1) knows what diabetes is, (2) detects diabetes commonly, (3) initiates and carries out some type of treatment plan, and (4) he and the patient become frustrated and discouraged because the treatment plan often does not work.

The following *points of view* will be addressed to specific questions focused on the treatment of adults with diabetes mellitus in the office setting.

Why Treat?

1. Patients will feel better and be able to pursue activities at work and at home more fully.

2. Prevent infections.

3. Prevent coma (diabetic ketoacidotic and hyperglycemic nonketotic).

4. Prevent or retard the development of neuropathy and microangiopathy. This remains controversial. It is established that the diabetic state (in man as well as in experimental animals) produces neuropathy and microangiopathy. Furthermore, treatment that ameliorates the diabetic state prevents and, under certain conditions, reverses the microangiopathic changes.

Who Should Be Treated?

Should everyone with glucose intolerance be treated? I think not. Physicians caring for adults know that diabetes mellitus is often one of 5 to 10 problems of a given patient. The only manifestation of diabetes mellitus may be impaired glucose tolerance. This may be of much less clinical significance than problems of other organ systems. Thus, in the older or the very sick patient with multiple problems, the hyperglycemic state of modest degree does not merit treatment in the same manner as does the patient with more severe or symptomatic diabetes mellitus.

Treatment: Office Setting

The following suggestions (see Fig. 1) are applicable to the "typical adult patient." He is age 50, a college graduate, married and a successful businessman with income in the upper middle class. He smokes one and a half packs of cigarettes daily and rarely exercises. He is 5 feet 10 inches tall and weights 230 pounds. Blood pressure is 160/100. Glycosuria, fasting plasma glucose concentration of 230 mg. per dl. (100 ml.) (repeated twice), and plasma triglycerides of 360 mg. per dl. were demonstrated during a periodic medical examination.

Physician Attitude. The physician's attitude is crucial from the moment that the diagnosis is communicated. If, as often happens, the busy physician says, "Yes, you have diabetes. Your sugar is a little high. It's no problem. All you need is diet," the results will be predictable. The patient is not reassured and will usually see another physician.

In contrast, if the physician takes the necessary time to indicate what the diagnosis of diabetes means for this particular patient, he can, over

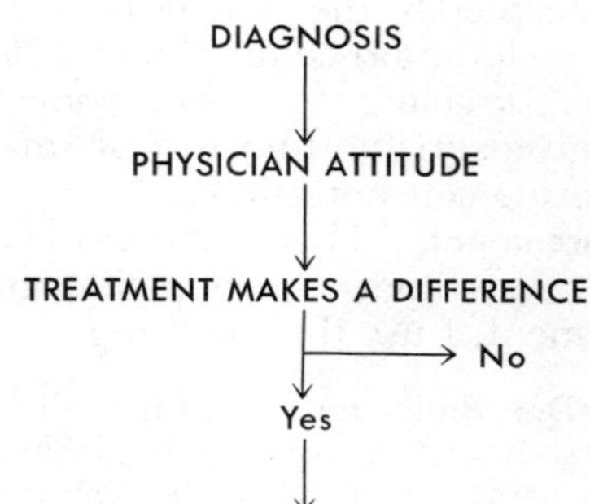

Figure 1. Anatomy of treatment plan.

weeks or months, carry out a successful treatment plan. The patient needs to know that treatment is desirable, that it can be done effectively and safely, and that there is no emergency.

Education/Understanding/Practice. These are three distinct phases. The initial educational program needs to be individualized and specific. The areas of information include: (a) general, (b) diet, (c) urine testing, (d) insulin, (e) hypoglycemia, (f) coma, (g) foot care, and (h) others (for example, sick day rules).

Thus, initially the patient presented needs (a), (b), and (c) only.

How To Provide Information. *Book-form.* Choose one and use it. I like The Good Life with Diabetes by T. G. Duncan. (Published by Garfield Duncan Research Foundation, 829 Spruce St., Philadelphia, PA 19107).

Video cassettes. I like the series compiled by the Medfact Patient Education System (Medfact, Inc., Box 458, Massillon, Ohio).

Individualized time with physician: Time is best used to set objectives and assess progress. Discussion with nurse and dietitian: They are more effective in providing information and in listening to the patient, which permits individualization of treatment.

Practice is the translation of information into a new daily life style and is objectively assessed by the diabetic record, which should indicate weight and results of urine testing.

Specific Objectives. These must be understood and accepted by the patient. For our patient this should include: (a) commitment to learn, (b) diet and exercise change to approach ideal weight, and (c) no glycosuria and normal plasma glucose and triglyceride concentrations.

The Agreement. This is the *moment of truth* and should be a written, signed (patient and physician) agreement. I use the following:

"I, John Doe, understand that I have diabetes mellitus. I understand that treatment is important and that it is my responsibility. I agree to the objectives, which include:
  A. Commitment to learning.
  B. Specific diet, plus regular exercise, to achieve ideal body weight.
  C. No glycosuria and normal blood glucose and triglyceride (blood fats) concentrations.
  D. I agree to maintain a diabetic record. I will bring it with me at the time of each office visit.

Furthermore, I understand that insulin will be required now or later, if diet is not effective."

Patient: ________________

Physician: ________________

The Diabetic Record. PATIENT'S HOME RECORD. Use the Clinilog (Ames Co.). It is compact, check-book size, has space for 1 year, and is low in cost. He should bring this at the time of each office visit.

OFFICE RECORD. This should be a flow sheet with recordings done by a nurse (or appropriate office assistant) prior to the physician-patient review.

Figure 2 shows my office Flow Record. I have found this to be especially useful for the office care of the adult with diabetes and associated problems such as obesity, hypertension, hyperuricemia, and renal disease. The data presented are for the patient presented. It selectively shows initial successful regulation with diet and the progressive nature of diabetes to an insulin-requiring stage.

How Will We Know? We can look at the objectives and the diabetic record. It is quite specific:

What is the weight? Are there glycosuria and hyperglycemia? What are plasma triglycerides?

URINE TESTING. The patient must know how to test urine for glucose and ketones. I use the Clinitest Two Drop Method (quantitative) for glucose and Ketostix (Ames Co.) for ketones. The glucose oxidase strip tests (such as Testape) may be convenient to use when the aglycosuric state is reached.

Individualized Diet. Most diets are not followed. Reasons for this, among others, include failure to communicate the importance of the diet and failure to individualize the diet. Both features take time. However, unless done it is preferable not to proceed.

Options for the patient presented include:

1. Diet profile. Have the patient record the type and amount of food for one week. From this, negotiate where he will reduce calories.

2. Arbitrary diet of 1500 calories.

3. Fast for 1 week followed by 800 calorie diet.

Each approach can work. For this patient I would start with the first choice. If there is no success in 6 months I would move to the third option.

The patient will quickly grasp that all calories count, 1 pound (0.45 kg.) is equal to 3500 calories, and exercise helps.

The combination of reduced calories plus caloric equivalent of exercise will be reflected by weight on flow sheet.

Numbers: Assume 2500 calories are required to maintain ideal body weight. If he eats 1500 calories daily and walks 1 hour (500 calories), he will use 1500 calories from tissues (fat) and lose almost 0.5 pound (0.23 kg.) daily.

Compare the caloric game to the money game. There is so much and no more. Excessive caloric intake is like overspending, with an inevitable debt to pay.

The patient may discover that the recommended diet can be gourmet in quality.

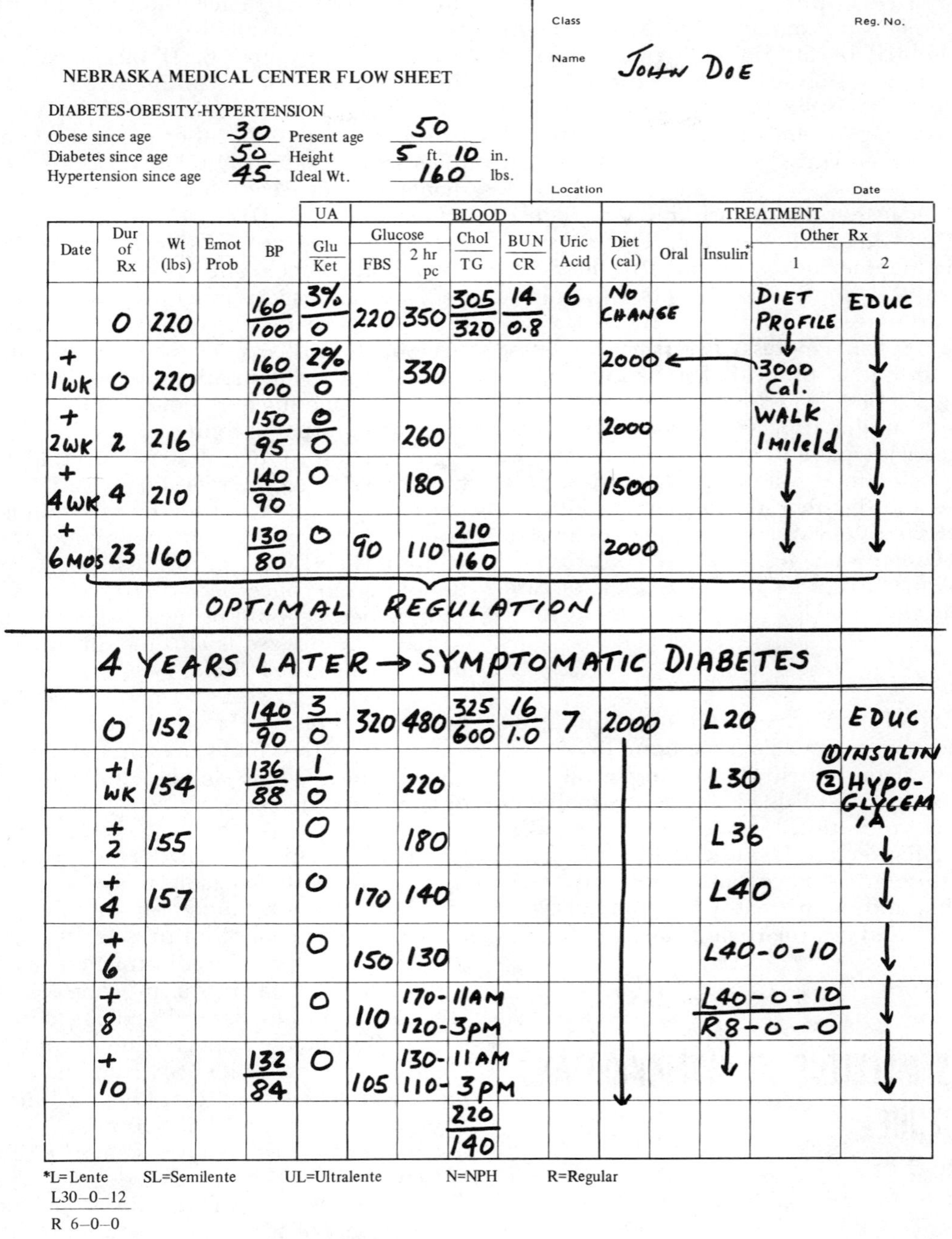

NEBRASKA MEDICAL CENTER FLOW SHEET

DIABETES-OBESITY-HYPERTENSION

Obese since age **30** Present age **50**
Diabetes since age **50** Height **5** ft. **10** in.
Hypertension since age **45** Ideal Wt. **160** lbs.

Date	Dur of Rx	Wt (lbs)	Emot Prob	BP	UA Glu/Ket	FBS	2 hr pc	Chol/TG	BUN/CR	Uric Acid	Diet (cal)	Oral	Insulin*	Other Rx 1	Other Rx 2
	0	220		160/100	3%/0	220	350	305/320	14/0.8	6	No Change			Diet Profile	Educ
+1 wk	0	220		160/100	2%/0		330				2000 ←			3000 Cal.	↓
+2 wk	2	216		150/95	0/0		260				2000			Walk 1 mile/d	↓
+4 wk	4	210		140/90	0		180				1500			↓	↓
+6 mos	23	160		130/80	0	90	110	210/160			2000			↓	↓

OPTIMAL REGULATION

4 YEARS LATER → SYMPTOMATIC DIABETES

Date	Dur of Rx	Wt (lbs)	Emot Prob	BP	UA Glu/Ket	FBS	2 hr pc	Chol/TG	BUN/CR	Uric Acid	Diet (cal)	Oral	Insulin*	Other Rx 1	Other Rx 2
	0	152		140/90	3/0	320	480	325/600	16/1.0	7	2000		L20		Educ
+1 wk		154		136/88	1/0		220						L30		① Insulin ② Hypo-glycemia
+2		155			0		180						L36		↓
+4		157			0	170	140						L40		↓
+6					0	150	130						L40-0-10		↓
+8					0	110	170-11AM / 120-3PM						L40-0-10 / R8-0-0		↓
+10				132/84	0	105	130-11AM / 110-3PM / 220/140						↓		↓

*L=Lente   SL=Semilente   UL=Ultralente   N=NPH   R=Regular
L30—0—12
R 6—0—0
May 1975 J C.S

Figure 2. Flow chart for treatment of diabetes mellitus in the adult.

The diet formulation is and should be presented as a prescription. It is beyond the scope of this presentation to detail the variations on diabetic diets. These are widely available to physicians and are less effective than the individualized diet.

I recommend, in addition to the appropriate calorie level, high carbohydrate (60 per cent calories) and low fat (20 per cent calories), low cholesterol (eliminate eggs), and low salt.

Insulin. Insulin is indicated for ketosis and persistent hyperglycemia.

When indicated: Tell the patient insulin is indicated and will be needed twice daily.

Personally assist with first injection (conveys the importance directly to the patient).

Use only U-100 Lente and regular insulin.

Begin with 20 units of Lente each morning and adjust.

Add presupper Lente if fasting hyperglycemia is present after maximal morning dose (as judged by afternoon hypoglycemia) is reached. Most insulin-dependent diabetics require twice daily insulin for optimal regulation.

Add regular insulin to morning injection if hyperglycemia and/or glycosuria remain in late morning.

Make clear that diet is basic and that regular frequent food intake is essential. This must include three regular meals and midafternoon and bedtime snacks. Snacks should not be omitted based on urine tests.

Office Visits: Progress Assessment. These should be frequent (biweekly for 3 months); patient brings Clinilog; patient tests urine for glucose and ketones, under supervision of nurse; review Flow Sheet with patient; physician time can be spared by telephone follow-ups and office visits with nurse and dietitian, if available.

Health Care Maintenance. Cigarettes must be stopped! Unlike diabetes, it is not controversial that smoking produces cardiovascular disease. The physician should take a clear and strong stand on this.

When to Refer

For initial patient education if time and interest do not permit this to be done by you.

For regulation during unstable periods; the ultimate expression of this is the brittle diabetic.

For complications such as retinopathy (photocoagulation may be indicated for proliferative changes), severe and symptomatic neuropathy, and nephropathy with renal failure (some are candidates for renal transplantation).

DIABETES MELLITUS IN CHILDHOOD AND ADOLESCENCE

method of
MARK A. SPERLING, M.D.
Cincinnati, Ohio

Introduction

Diabetes mellitus in children and adolescents is usually of the insulin dependent (juvenile) type, in which the ability to secrete insulin is totally or near totally lost. The disease appears to have a prevalence of approximately 1 in 800 children. Recent evidence suggests that affected children have a genetic predisposition to an autoimmune destruction of their pancreatic islets as well as possibly other endocrine target tissues conferred through, and associated with, the inheritance of certain histocompatibility loci (HL-A) located on chromosome number 6. Among these HL-A loci, the inheritance of the antigens B8 or BW15 increases the relative risk of developing diabetes two-fold, whereas the inheritance of B8 and BW15 together increases the relative risk of developing diabetes some seven-fold; the presence of still other antigens (DW3, CW3) confers an even higher relative risk of developing diabetes. Although still in the realm of research, these findings provide new insights into understanding the cause of the underlying disease process. In susceptible persons this process may be triggered by viral infections and is commonly associated with the presence of circulating antibodies not directed against insulin but rather at components of the islets, leading ultimately to their destruction. It is the loss of the ability to secrete insulin in response to the physiologic stimulus of food intake that is the cardinal factor in the pathophysiology of the symptoms and signs of this disease. Accordingly, the physician concerned with the care of children with diabetes should be aware that:

1. The disease is chronic, in the sense that insulin deficiency is lifelong, except for a relatively short period of weeks to months, the so called honeymoon phase, that occurs frequently but not always after the initial presentation. Oral hypoglycemic agents have no place in the management of childhood diabetes.

2. Relative psychologic disturbances occur frequently, as in other chronic diseases.

3. Currently available modes of therapy do not restore the fine moment-to-moment control of intermediary metabolism present in normal persons. Thus, even careful adjustment of insulin, diet, and exercise results in varying degrees of imperfect control rather than physiologic control.

4. Despite the imperfection of control, an increasing mass of evidence from clinical experimental and biochemical studies in humans and animal models links the development of complications that affect the microvasculature of the eye, kidney, and nerves to the degree of control. Hence, the fostering of appropriate attitudes is an integral part of treating diabetes in children.

5. Therapy must always be tailored to suit the best needs of each patient.

The management of children with diabetes can be conveniently divided into

1. The treatment of acute disturbances such as diabetic ketoacidosis of hypoglycemia.

2. Daily management of diabetes including type, dose and frequency of administered insulin, diet, and exercise.

3. Special situations such as surgery.

4. Psychologic counseling and support.

Diabetic Ketoacidosis

Definition. Diabetic ketoacidosis is said to exist when deficiency of insulin causes severe hyperglycemia, accumulation of ketoacids such that arterial blood pH is 7.25 or less and serum bicarbonate 15 mEq. per liter or less, and polyuria resulting in dehydration and electrolyte losses. This condition must be distinguished from:

1. Nonketotic hyperosmolar coma, in which plasma osmolality is greater than 300 mOs. per liter but few ketones are present.

2. Salicylate intoxication, in which acidosis is marked but ketosis and hyperglycemia is minimal.

3. Uremic coma with grossly elevated BUN (blood urea nitrogen) and acidosis, but not ketosis.

4. Vomiting in a child with renal glycosuria (Fanconi's syndrome). Glycosuria and ketonuria are present but blood glucose is normal.

Pathophysiology. Insulin deficiency is the primary defect, but the rate of development of all features depends on the presence of excessive amounts of other hormones, particularly epinephrine, glucagon, cortisol, and growth hormone. In concert, these hormonal changes result in:

1. Hyperglycemia due to increased glycogenolysis and gluconeogenesis, and decreased peripheral glucose utilization. In turn hyperglycemia results in glycosuria, osmotic polyuria, and dehydration with significant losses of electrolytes, in particular sodium, chloride, potassium, and phosphate.

2. Increased lipolysis in fat tissue with a resultant rise in circulating free fatty acids (FFA).

3. The conversion of these FFA to ketone bodies, namely acetoacetic acid and β-hydroxybutyric acid, the formation of which exceeds the capacity for tissue utilization, resulting in ketonemia, ketonuria, and acidosis. Nonenzymatic conversion of acetoacetate to acetone is responsible for the characteristic fruity odor of the breath.

Clinical Presentation. These mechanisms are responsible for the clinical picture of polydipsia, polyuria, dehydration, weight loss, metabolic acidosis with attempts at respiratory compensation through expiration of CO_2, i.e., deep rapid respirations of Kussmaul, fruity odor on the breath, and progressive obtundation of consciousness leading ultimately to coma. In addition, diabetic ketoacidosis is often associated with abdominal pain that mimics, to some extent, the features of an acute abdomen, particularly appendicitis, and the presence of elevated serum amylase levels that do not necessarily indicate the existence of pancreatitis. It is important to be aware that diabetic ketoacidosis develops over a period of hours to days and even weeks, in contradistinction to hypoglycemia, which develops suddenly or over a period of minutes.

Management of Acute Diabetic Ketoacidosis. 1. Establish the diagnosis through the clinical picture and confirm by rapid screening tests *on blood* for hyperglycemia and ketonemia (Dextrostix provides a semiquantitative measure of blood glucose, Acetest tablets measure acetoacetate). Also, there should be glucosuria and ketonuria. However, urinary tests are notoriously misleading and cannot be relied upon to initiate treatment. For example, a child with renal tubular glycosuria (Fanconi's syndrome), vomiting, dehydration, and mild ketonuria will have normal blood glucose. Hence, the blood tests provide the clue that insulin therapy is not warranted lest iatrogenic hypoglycemia be precipitated. Similarly, when a child with Kussmaul respiration has only mild ketonuria in undiluted plasma, acidosis due to salicylate intoxication should be suspected. Finally, with marked hyperglycemia in the absence of commensurate ketonemia, nonketotic hyperosmolar coma should be suspected. Although less common in children than adults, it is important to recognize it and to minimize the use of insulin while placing more reliance on fluids alone, because these highly insulin-sensitive patients may rapidly develop hypoglycemia.

2. Draw blood for determination of the concentration of the serum electrolytes, sodium, potassium, chloride and phosphate, blood urea nitrogen (BUN), blood glucose, pH, and bicarbonate concentration.

3. If physical examination suggests the possibility that an infection has precipitated the episode, obtain a complete blood count, blood culture, and microscopic examination of a clean catch urine. Use condom or bag drainage collection of urine. Avoid catheterization of the bladder unless urine flow is in doubt.

4. Perform an electrocardiogram (ECG), since it will indicate the presence of hyperkalemia (high peaked T waves) and results are available more quickly than from the serum determination.

5. Assume the patient is 10 per cent dehydrated with losses as outlined in Table 1. Also, hyperosmolality is invariably present to some extent since osmolality can be expressed by the formula

$$[Na^+ (mEq./L.) + K^+ (mEq./L.)] \times 2$$

$$+ \frac{glucose\ (mg.\ per\ dl.)}{18}$$

For example with a blood glucose of 720 mg. per dl. (100 ml.) and normal serum concentrations of Na^+ and K^+, the normal osmolality of approximately 300 mOsm. per liter is increased to 340 mOsm. per liter.

TABLE 1. **Fluid and Electrolyte Maintenance in Diabetic Ketoacidosis**

	MAINTENANCE REQUIREMENTS*	LOSSES†
Water	1500 ml./m.²	100 ml./kg. (Range 60–100 ml./kg.)
Sodium	45 mEq./m.²	6 mEq./kg. (Range 5–13 mEq./kg.)
Potassium	35 mEq./m.²	5 mEq./kg. (Range 4–6 mEq./kg.)
Chloride	30 mEq./m.²	4 mEq./kg. (Range 3–9 mEq./kg.)
Phosphate	10 mEq./m.²	3 mEq./kg. (Range 2–5 mEq./kg.)

*Maintenance is expressed in surface area to permit uniformity because fluid requirements change as weight increases.

†Losses are expressed per unit of body weight since the losses remain relatively constant as a function of total body weight.

When diabetic ketoacidosis is strongly suspected, therapy can be initiated before the laboratory results are reported. As therapy is initiated, a flow chart that permits recording of the following should be established: fluid input and output; clinical status of the patient including pulse and blood pressure; serum electrolyte and acid-base status; and insulin dosage and time of administration.

Aims of Therapy. Correct fluid and electrolyte disturbances; provide adequate insulin to restore and maintain near normal intermediary metabolism; treat the precipitating event, e.g., an acute infection; also, educate the patient and the family in the management of diabetes so as to avoid a recurrence of ketoacidosis.

Fluid and Electrolyte Therapy. The initial fluid therapy should consist of isotonic (0.9 per cent) or 0.5 isotonic saline solution, because this fluid is still hypotonic relative to the patient's osmolality, and because a gradual decline in osmolality is desirable to prevent cerebral edema. Too rapid a decline in plasma glucose and therefore in plasma osmolality may be responsible for cerebral edema. Therefore, only half the total deficits should be corrected in the first 8 hours and thereafter treatment should proceed more slowly. In addition, blood glucose should not be allowed to fall below 250 to 300 mg. per dl. in the initial 24 to 36 hours of therapy. Subsequent therapy can proceed as outlined in Table 2, which illustrates the volume, composition, and rate of fluid administration in a child weighing 30 kg. Important points to be stressed include:

The initial therapy of 500 ml. of isotonic saline solution contains no potassium, provides approximately 15 to 20 ml. per kg., and is designed to expand circulating volume. This can be ongoing while the results of initial laboratory tests are pending.

TABLE 2. **Fluid and Electrolyte Losses and Replacement in a 30 Kg. Child with Diabetic Ketoacidosis**

LOSSES	LOSS IN 10% DEHYDRATION	REQUIRED FOR MAINTENANCE	TOTAL	WORKING TOTAL
Water (ml.)	3000	1700	4700	5000
Sodium (mEq.)	180	50	230	250
Potassium (mEq.)	150	40	190	200
Chloride (mEq.)	120	30	150	150
Phosphate (mEq.)	90	10	100	100

Replacement Procedures*	Sodium	Chloride	Potassium	Phosphate
A. 500 ml. isotonic saline solution	75	75		
B. 500 ml. 0.5 isotonic saline solution with 20 mEq. KCl	35	55	20	
C. 1000 ml. 0.5 isotonic saline solution with 40 mEq. (KH₂PO₄ + K₂HPO₄)	75	75	40	40
D. 1000 ml. 0.5 isotonic saline solution with 40 mEq. (KH₂PO₄ + K₂HPO₄)	75	75	40	40
E. 2000 ml. 5% dextrose with 40 mEq. of potassium per liter as KCl or the phosphate		40	80	40
Totals	260	320	180	120

*Steps in fluid and electrolyte replacement:
A. 1 hour
B–D. 6–8 hours (if blood glucose has fallen to 300 mg./dl., then the 0.5 isotonic saline solution is made up with 5 per cent dextrose).
E. 20–30 hours

Start K^+ early, because total body K^+ is always depleted, although acidosis, by causing K^+ to move from the intra to extracellular space, may maintain normal or elevated serum K^+. In providing insulin, glucose and relieving acidosis, therapy results in a shift of K^+ back into the cells, so that hypokalemic complications are more frequent than hyperkalemia. Monitor the patient with frequent ECGs or serum K^+ determination or both.

Provision of excess chloride is almost inevitable (see Table 2); minimize it by administering phosphate, which is frequently depleted in ketoacidosis. Phosphate deficiency can cause a number of clinical and biochemical problems, including a deficiency of 2,3-DPG, which governs the dissociation of oxygen from hemoglobin. With deficiency of 2,3-DPG less oxygen is available to tissues, thereby promoting lactic acidosis and aggravating tissue acidosis. Provision of phosphate ameliorates all of these potential problems.

Proceed slowly with fluid and electrolyte replacement. Only half the total deficit is given over the first 6 to 8 hours and the remainder is given over the ensuing 18 to 20 hours.

If the pH is 7.2 or less one ampule of bicarbonate (40 mEq.) added to the infusate may be given over 1 to 2 hours. If the pH is 7.1 or less, two ampules of bicarbonate may be given. Do not administer bicarbonate by intravenous push because this may trigger cardiac arrhythmias. Concern regarding the use of excessive bicarbonate relates to two major factors. First, bicarbonate may aggravate cerebral acidosis while plasma pH is rising toward normal. This is because the HCO_3^- combines with H^+ and dissociates to H_2O and CO_2. Bicarbonate cannot pass the blood brain barrier, whereas CO_2 freely diffuses, thereby exacerbating cerebral acidosis. Second, repleting bicarbonate according to the calculated base deficit may overcorrect the acidosis and result in alkalosis.

Start glucose as a 5 per cent solution as soon as blood levels approach 300 mg. per dl., since rapid reduction of blood glucose may lead to cerebral edema.

Plasma levels or urinary persistence of ketones are poor indices of therapeutic progress, and their measurement is less valuable during therapy than in establishing the initial diagnosis. This is because the standard test for ketones measures acetoacetate but not β-hydroxybutyrate. Since the ratio of β-hydroxybutyrate to acetoacetate in diabetic ketoacidosis is commonly 7:1 and may be as high as 30:1 compared to the normal 3:1, and since β-hydroxybutyrate dissociates to acetoacetate with correction of acidosis, the persistence of ketones merely reflects that a greater fraction of existing ketoacids is now being measured.

Insulin Therapy During Ketoacidosis. Two approaches are commonly used. The first, or traditional approach, employs doses and routes of administration as follows. If blood glucose is above 900 mg. per dl., 2 units per kg. are given, half by intravenous route and half by intramuscular injection; if blood glucose is 600 to 900 mg. per dl., 1 unit per kg. is given in equally divided intravenous and intramuscular injections; and if blood glucose is 300 to 600 mg. per dl., 0.5 unit per kg. is given again divided equally for intravenous and intramuscular injection. Blood glucose and serum electrolytes are determined every 2 hours to judge initial progress.

After blood glucose has fallen below 300 mg. per dl., subsequent insulin therapy (0.25 unit per kg.) is given every 6 to 8 hours, while maintaining an infusion of 5 per cent glucose solution until the patient can fully tolerate a diet. During this period sips of clear liquid, progressing to carbonated beverage and orange juice rich in K^+, may be given. Once the patient can fully tolerate a diet, the previous day's regular insulin is summed, and one half to two thirds given as an intermediate acting form (NPH or Lente), with further coverage by regular insulin according to the pattern of glucose excretion in urine.

The second form of insulin administration, named constant low-dose infusion, has gained wide acceptance. A priming dose of 0.1 unit per kg. of insulin is given intravenously followed by constant infusion at a rate of 0.1 unit per kg. per hour. For example, in a 30 kg. child, 3 units would be given as an intravenous priming dose followed by 3 units per hour. To achieve this, add 25 units to 500 ml. of 0.5 isotonic saline solution and infuse at 60 ml. per hour. The infusion can be given via a pediatric intravenous set without a controlled infusion apparatus. However, we prefer to infuse into a separate vein from the one used for fluid and electrolyte replacement. The advantages of this method are its simplicity, effectiveness, and physiologic appeal. The rate of decline in blood glucose is virtually linear for each individual patient, although the actual rate (slope) varies from patient to patient. Thus, a reasonable prediction can be made when the blood glucose will reach approximately 300 mg. per dl. so that glucose can be added to the infusate. Moreover, hypoglycemia can be avoided since there will be no residual intramuscular or subcutaneous insulin depots when the intravenous infusion is stopped. Concern that a large portion of the insulin will stick to the glass and tubing has proved unfounded. Despite this simplicity and effectiveness, each patient must be carefully monitored and failure of response, i.e., true insulin resistance, recognized and treated by large doses of insulin. Once the blood glucose has fallen to 300 mg. per dl., and 5 per cent glucose is begun, the insulin infusion may be discontinued and insulin therapy given subcutaneously as outlined earlier. Alternatively, the insulin infusion may be continued but at one half the previous rate, i.e., 0.05 unit per kg. per hour until the patient can fully tolerate a diet.

Hypoglycemia

In contrast to diabetic ketoacidosis, which develops over hours and days, hypoglycemia occurs suddenly or over minutes. Symptoms and signs are those due to an outpouring of catecholamines, including shaking, sweating, tachycardia, apprehension, and hunger, and those due to cerebral glucopenia including drowsiness, mental confusion, seizure, and coma.

The occurrence of hypoglycemia in a diabetic indicates inappropriate insulin therapy for that patient's energy intake and expenditure. Common causes include an error in insulin dosage, missing meals, and exercise in the absence of reducing the insulin dose or taking extra calories.

Treatment of Hypoglycemia. All patients must be educated to be familiar with the symptoms and signs. Acutely, a carbohydrate-containing snack, drinks such as orange juice, or candy each containing 5 to 10 grams of glucose should be taken. Patients, parents, and teachers should also be instructed in the use of glucagon; 0.5 to 1.0 mg. given intramuscularly is particularly useful when the patient is losing consciousness or vomiting. If exercise has been the precipitating factor, the patient should be instructed to reduce the morning insulin dose by 10 per cent and to take additional calories prior to exercise. Recent studies indicate that hypoglycemia following exercise in diabetics is due to increased blood flow and resultant increased absorption of insulin from the injection site. Therefore, a diabetic whose exercise involves mostly the lower limbs should inject insulin into an upper limb on the morning of exercise or vice versa. When both upper and lower limbs are exercised, the abdominal wall should be the preferred injection site.

Long-Term Management of Diabetes in Children and Adolescents

Therapy is based on the assumption that endogenous insulin secretion is totally absent, although some residual insulin secreting ability may persist. This is particularly common following initial presentation when residual insulin-secreting ability is adequate to maintain almost normal metabolism. The insulin dose should be gradually reduced to avoid precipitating hypoglycemia. Our own policy is not to completely discontinue insulin injections even if daily doses are small (less than 5 units daily) because this "honeymoon" period is, with few exceptions, transient, lasting weeks to months, during which the patient and family should not believe that the disease is "cured." However, the physician may decide to completely discontinue insulin treatment if this is in the patient's best interest. The principles of management that we follow include:

Education. The family and patient should be repeatedly taught the principles of the disease, appropriate technique and site of insulin injection, and its modification according to need, recognition of symptoms of hypoglycemia, and monitoring of urine for the degree of glucose and acetone spill.

Insulin. An approximate working rule is 0.5 to 1 unit per kg. daily. In the belief that we obtain smoother control with fewer wide fluctuations in blood glucose, we encourage the use of "splitting" the dose for morning and evening injection prior to meals. Thus, two thirds of the total daily dose is given in the morning before breakfast and one third in the evening before dinner. With each injection we recommend a ratio of intermediate to short acting insulin of 2 to 3:1. In the example of the 30 kg. child, the daily dose would be 30 units divided as follows: morning, 14 units of NPH plus 6 units of regular; evening, 6 units of NPH plus 4 units of regular. With encouragement and explanation, our experience of patient compliance with this regimen has been good. If patients resist twice daily injections, we accept single daily injections before breakfast.

Special Problems with Insulin. 1. Patients should be taught to adjust their insulin dose according to the prevailing degree of control. Thus, if urinary glucose is repeatedly 2 per cent (4+) for two consecutive days, increase daily insulin by approximately 10 per cent. If episodes of hypoglycemia are recurrent and cannot be explained by an error in insulin, missed meals or exercise, reduce the daily insulin dose by approximately 10 per cent.

2. Patients with infection should take additional insulin; 10 to 20 per cent of total daily insulin should be given as the regular (short-acting form) before meals if urine glucose remains 4+ so that the development of ketoacidosis is aborted.

3. Patients who are vomiting should nevertheless take some insulin; approximately 50 per cent of daily dose is a general rule. If vomiting continues and the patient cannot tolerate clear liquids, admission to the hospital for intravenous therapy may be warranted.

4. *Major surgery in the diabetic.* If surgery is elective, admit the patient 24 hours prior to surgery and provide usual diet and insulin. On the evening prior to surgery, begin an infusion of 5 per cent glucose in 0.45 per cent saline solution plus 20 mEq. of KCl per liter adding 1 unit of insulin to the infusate for each 2 to

4 grams of administered glucose. This regimen may be continued during the operative period and discontinued when the patient is awake and capable of maintaining oral food and fluid intake, at which time the regimen used prior to surgery can be reinitiated. An alternative and equally effective approach is to begin the infusion at 7 A.M. on the morning of surgery, omit the intravenous insulin, and provide approximately one half to two thirds of the usual morning dose of intermediate acting insulin. Following recovery from anesthesia, subcutaneous regular insulin is given at approximately 0.25 unit per kg., and the dose is repeated, decreased or increased at 6-hourly intervals, depending on the level of hyperglycemia, until the patient can tolerate his usual diet, at which time the insulin regimen used prior to surgery can be reinitiated. If emergency surgery needs to be undertaken, an intravenous line that provides 5 to 10 per cent glucose in 0.45 per cent saline solution plus 20 mEq. of KCl per liter is begun and insulin added to the infusate so as to provide 1 unit for each 2 to 4 grams of glucose infused. Following surgery, the regimens described above can be instituted. The major risk to the patient is unrecognized hypoglycemia while under anesthesia; hence, our cautious use of insulin and provision of glucose during the operative period.

5. *Injection site lipodystrophy.* Atrophy or hypertrophy at injection sites appears to be far less common now that the highly purified single peak insulins are routinely available. Indeed, injection of these purified insulins directly into the dystrophic area has been recommended as a form of therapy. Patients should be taught to rotate their injection sites regularly, using the upper arms, the outer portion of the anterior aspect of the thigh, upper outer quadrant of the buttocks, and lower quadrant of the abdomen. Injections should be given into the subcutaneous tissue at right angles to the plane of any of the above sites.

Diet. It should be clearly understood that there is no such thing as a diabetes diet. The principles are to provide adequate calories for growth and development including consideration of daily exercise; meals should be balanced and represent approximately 45 to 50 per cent carbohydrate, 35 to 40 per cent fat, and approximately 15 per cent protein, and calories should be evenly distributed throughout the day. Our recommended approach is to involve a dietitian and to take into account the dietary habits of the ethnic and cultural background of the patient and family. Total calories are based on the formula 100 cal. per kg. for the first 10 kg.; 1000 cal. plus 50 cal. per kg. in the weight range 10 to 20 kg., and 1500 cal. plus 20 cal. per kg. in the weight range 20 to 70 kg. Of these total daily calories, 2/10 should be taken at break-

fast, 2/10 at lunch, and 3/10 at dinner, leaving 1/10 each for midmorning, midafternoon, and evening snacks. Consistency in the eating pattern should be encouraged, since this is one of the most important factors in maintaining good control and preventing wide swings in blood glucose; once insulin has been injected, caloric intake must balance the available insulin or hypoglycemia must inevitably result. In our clinic we encourage the use of diet exchange lists, as these are flexible and permit a wide choice of equivalent portions that endow the diet with variety and enhance compliance. A large pictorial representation of diet exchanges in each of the classes carbohydrate, protein, and fat is available (The Diabetes Unit, Poster 304, National Health Systems, P.O. Box 1501, Ann Arbor, Michigan, 48106); it occupies the side of a refrigerator door, the number of exchanges of each class for each meal is indicated and is subject to easy modification. We also encourage the use of polyunsaturated fats, substituting margarine for butter and corn oil for animal fat, and encourage the use of lean meats, poultry, and fish. Occasional excesses in the form of cake or ice cream are tolerable, but in general the carbohydrate should be in the form of complex starch rather than rapidly absorbed glucose as in nondietetic carbonated beverages. Flexibility rather than rigidity is encouraged, and feelings of guilt because of noncompliance with diet are to be avoided.

Exercise. Exercise is an important aspect of childhood and adolescence. No form of exercise, including competitive sports, is forbidden to diabetics; indeed, it should be encouraged. Precautions regarding reduction in insulin dose, additional calories, and the use of an appropriate injection site depending on the predominant limbs to be exercised have been mentioned in the section on hypoglycemia.

Monitoring the Patient's Control. Patients should be taught to check their urine for glucose and acetone spill using Clinitest and Acetest tablets or the Ketodiastix strips. Urine checks should ideally be performed four times daily, before breakfast, lunch, dinner, and bedtime, using "second void" specimens of urine. Practically, school age children find it difficult to perform the Clinitest measurement at school, hence omission of the lunch time check is common. When using Clinitest tablets, we teach the 2 drop method, i.e., 2 drops of urine plus 10 drops of water. Ketodiastix have proved highly acceptable to patients, because of their simplicity and ability to dip them directly into the urinary stream during voiding. A carefully maintained record of the pattern of urinary glucose spill is helpful in managing the patient and making adjustments in insulin dosage. However, our experience has been that these urinary records are notoriously unreliable. Consequently, to assess more accurately the urinary loss of glucose, we ask the patient to provide a 24-hour urine specimen in three separate containers for the time periods 7 A.M. to 2 P.M., 2 P.M. to 10 P.M. and 10 P.M. to 7 A.M. After recording the total volume in each specimen, a quantitative assessment of glucose concentration is made. If most of the glucose is spilt in the first morning period, the dose of regular fast-acting insulin in the morning is increased; if glucose spill is greatest in the afternoon period, the morning intermediate-acting insulin is increased; and if the predominant glucose spill is during the night, the evening intermediate acting insulin dose is increased. Increases in insulin dose should be gradual and on the order of 10 per cent. Glucose spill in the urine should not exceed 5 per cent of daily caloric intake. For example, if total caloric intake is 2000 cal., the total glucose in the urine should not exceed 100 cal., i.e., 25 grams. It should be appreciated that this magnitude of urinary glucose loss is considered acceptable but is clearly not good control.

Somogyi Phenomenon

Hypoglycemic episodes, which may be mild, may manifest as early morning headache, sweating, or night terrors or may be asymptomatic, alternating rapidly (as quickly as 4 to 6 hours) with ketosis, hyperglycemia, ketonuria, and severe glycosuria, should arouse suspicion of the Somogyi phenomenon. This syndrome has been aptly described as "hypoglycemia begetting hyperglycemia" and is believed to be due to excessive insulin and counterregulation of its hypoglycemic effects by hyperglycemic hormones. The coexistence of this brittle form of diabetes with daily insulin doses of more than 2 units per kg. suggests that the phenomenon is present and that insulin should be gradually reduced.

Special Forms of Diabetes in Childhood

Asymptomatic carbohydrate intolerance occasionally occurs in children. Two major types are seen.

1. Abnormal carbohydrate tolerance in obese children in whom there remains adequate insulin secretion. In these children, as in their adult counterparts, weight reduction is indicated.

2. Abnormal carbohydrate tolerance with a strong family history of maturity (insulin independent) onset diabetes that affects multiple family members in a pattern suggestive of dominant inheritance. These patients have been termed MODY (Maturity Onset Diabetes of the Young). If symptomatic they should be treated with insulin as above.

Psychologic Support

Diabetes in a child affects the lifestyle and interpersonal relationships of the entire family unit. Feelings of anxiety and guilt are common in parents; similar feelings coupled with denial and rejection are equally common in children, particularly during the "rebellious" teenage years. These feelings take form as nonadherence to instructions regarding diet and insulin therapy and noncompliance with self-monitoring. Deliberate overdosage of insulin resulting in hypoglycemia, and omission of insulin or excesses in diet resulting in ketoacidosis are pleas for psychologic help, manipulative events to escape family surroundings perceived as undesirable, and occasionally manifestations of suicidal intent. Overprotection on the part of parents is frequent. Misinformation abounds regarding the risk of developing diabetes in siblings or offspring or the risk of pregnancy in young diabetic women. In turn, this misinformation fosters further anxiety. Many but not all of these problems can be averted through an attitude of knowledge, understanding, patience, counseling based on correct information, and the fostering of attitudes that do not perceive the patient as a cripple, but rather call for a productive and reproductive life. In some circumstances referral for expert psychologic help or for specialist advice is clearly indicated. In managing diabetes in children and adolescents, the pediatrician or family physician should be aware of his pivotal role as counselor and advisor as well as physician and of the recourse to expert advice when necessary.

GOUT

method of
EDWARD W. HOLMES, JR., M.D.
Durham, North Carolina

Introduction

Gout is a disorder of diverse causes characterized by the common biochemical feature of hyperuricemia. Hyperuricemia may be defined either on the basis of epidemiologic studies or on the physicochemical properties of urate. The physicochemical definition, which will be assumed in this discussion, states that serum is supersaturated with respect to urate when the concentration of urate is greater than 6.4 mg. per dl. (100 ml.) This value is based upon the determination of urate by the uricase or enzymatic methods, and it should be increased by 0.5 to 1.0 mg. per dl. if urate is determined by autoanalyzer techniques employed in most clinical laboratories.

Hyperuricemia may arise from a decrease in the renal clearance of uric acid, an increase in the rate of uric acid production, or a combination of these two mechanisms. Either of these pathogenic processes may be the consequence of an inherited abnormality or they may be the result of an acquired problem such as obesity, excessive ethanol ingestion or diuretic therapy. As will be discussed later, it is important to consider the pathogenesis of hyperuricemia when selecting a hypouricemic agent for the individual patient.

As mentioned, the biochemical feature common to all patients with gout is hyperuricemia. One consequence of hyperuricemia is the development of gouty arthritis, which presents as acute self-limited episodes of monarticular or polyarticular synovitis. If uncontrolled, gout may progress to a deforming arthritis characterized by chronic synovitis with destruction of the joint and surrounding bone. In addition to arthritis, hyperuricemia may lead to subcutaneous deposits of urate, or tophi. Although tophi are usually painless, they may erode through tendons and ulcerate with chronic drainage. Patients with hyperuricemia also deposit monosodium urate in the interstitium of the kidney, leading to chronic and progressive renal dysfunction. In addition, patients with hyperuricemia are prone to develop renal calculi, especially those individuals who excrete excessive amounts of uric acid in the urine. Rarely, patients with hyperuricemia may develop acute renal failure due to the deposition of uric acid crystals in the collecting tubules when uric acid excretion is markedly increased. In this discussion therapy for the attacks of acute gouty arthritis will be reviewed, as well as therapy for reducing the serum urate concentration to prevent the development of recurrent attacks of gouty arthritis, tophi, and urate nephropathy. Therapy for renal calculi will also be discussed.

Before initiating therapy, the diagnosis of gouty arthritis should be firmly established. As most patients placed on therapy for gout will take medication that is costly and potentially toxic for the remainder of their lives, the diagnosis of gout should be based on definite criteria. Any one of the following three criteria will usually suffice to firmly establish the diagnosis of gouty arthritis: (1) demonstration of monosodium urate crystals in synovial fluid leukocytes, (2) demonstration of monosodium urate crystals in tophaceous deposits, or (3) a classical clinical history, i.e., monarticular arthritis that completely resolves with a free intercritical period, hyperuricemia, and the demonstration of a classic response to oral or intravenous colchicine. The first two methods are unequivocal in establishing the diagnosis; the third is usually reliable in differentiating between gouty arthritis and other types of acute synovitis.

Management of Acute Gouty Arthritis

When the patient presents with acute gouty arthritis, the first step is to establish the diagnosis. The criteria for diagnosing gout are outlined above. If the patient already has crystal-proved gouty arthritis, any of a number of agents may be used in treating the acute attack. However, if the diagnosis has not been confirmed by the demonstration of crystals, colchicine may be employed as a diagnostic as well as therapeutic agent.

Colchicine. Colchicine may be administered either orally or intravenously. If used orally, one 0.6 mg. tablet is administered every hour until one of the following develops: (1) the patient responds with resolution of the acute arthritis, (2) gastrointestinal toxicity develops in the form of nausea, vomiting, abdominal cramps, or diarrhea, or (3) a total dose of 10 mg. has been administered. Oral colchicine is the safest route for administration since the patient usually develops gastrointestinal toxicity before systemic toxicity. If colchicine is to be administered intravenously, the usual dosage is 1 to 2 mg. infused over 1 to 2 minutes. The ampule of colchicine should be diluted to 10 or 20 ml. with isotonic saline solution and the intravenous line should be functioning well. These precautions are necessary, as colchicine is very caustic to the subcutaneous tissue if it extravasates. The intravenous route has the advantage of producing a quicker response than the oral route, but it has the disadvantage of not producing gastrointestinal toxicity before systemic toxicity develops. Consequently, the patient should be screened for significant renal, hepatic, or hematologic disease before administering colchicine intravenously.

Leukopenia is a potential complication of intravenous colchicine in patients with hepatic or renal disease and in subjects on long-term prophylactic therapy. If the patient does not respond to the first intravenous dosage, it may be repeated at 6 hours and again at 6 to 12 hours. Although a rapid response to colchicine is very suggestive of gouty arthritis, this response is not absolutely specific, since patients with other types of acute arthritis will respond to this agent on rare occasions. In addition, failure to respond to colchicine does not exclude the diagnosis of gouty arthritis. Often patients with an acute attack that has lasted more than 48 hours will not respond to colchicine.

Indomethacin and Phenylbutazone. If one is dealing with a patient in whom the diagnosis of gouty arthritis is well established, an agent other than colchicine may be preferable because of better patient acceptance and ease of administration. Indomethacin is used in a dosage of 50 mg. three times daily for a period of 2 days, or until the patient's attack begins to subside. At this time the dosage is reduced to 25 mg. three times daily and continued for another 2 to 3 days. The major toxicities associated with indomethacin are gastrointestinal intolerance and central nervous system disturbances, such as headache. Phenylbutazone is administered in an initial dose of 200 mg. followed by 100 mg. every 6 hours for the first

2 days, or until the patient begins to respond. At this time the dose is reduced to 100 mg. three times daily for the next 2 days. Phenylbutazone produces gastrointestinal discomfort and fluid accumulation, and occasionally it leads to toxicity of the bone marrow. Phenylbutazone, but not indomethacin, is uricosuric, and this may lead to confusion in the subsequent evaluation of the patient. Both of these agents are remarkably well tolerated when used for short periods to treat the acute attack of gouty arthritis, and they are not usually associated with serious toxicity during these brief periods of treatment.

The drug used to treat the acute attack can be tailored to the patient's and the physician's personal preference and should be limited to the period of the acute attack. Long-term administration of any of the agents is not warranted and may lead to toxicity. For subsequent attacks, it is advisable to instruct the patient to begin therapy with one of the above agents at the first signs of an acute attack. Most patients will respond more rapidly if therapy is instituted at the first signs of an attack, rather than waiting for a full-blown episode to develop.

In addition to the drug prescribed for the acute attack, it is our practice to initiate prophylactic therapy with 0.6 mg. of colchicine, once or twice daily, during therapy for the acute episode. This is useful in preventing a flare at the time of tapering of the anti-inflammatory drug and at the time of initiation of hypouricemic therapy. We do not recommend instituting hypouricemic therapy until the acute attack has completely resolved.

Occasionally, a patient is encountered who is intolerant of or unable to take oral medications and is not a candidate for intravenous colchicine therapy. In these patients intra-articular steroids may be of benefit. Triamcinolone hexacetonide, 5 to 20 mg., depending on the size of the joint, injected intra-articularly will reduce inflammation within 6 to 12 hours.

Management of Hyperuricemia

After the attack of acute gouty arthritis has subsided and the patient is on prophylactic colchicine, hypouricemic therapy may be started. It is recommended that hypouricemic therapy be initiated while the patient is on prophylactic colchicine because a sudden decrease in serum urate concentration with allopurinol or a uricosuric drug may precipitate an attack of gouty arthritis. Irrespective of the agent selected, the goal of hypouricemic therapy is to reduce the serum urate concentration below the supersaturation limit. When uric acid is determined by the uricase method, this value is 6.4 mg. per dl.; in the case of autoanalyzer determinations, a value which is 0.5 to 1 mg. per dl. higher is acceptable. The dose of hypouricemic agent required is the amount needed to lower the serum urate concentration to this level.

A useful method for selecting a hypouricemic agent for a given patient is the quantification of urinary uric acid excretion. At the time the patient is seen for the acute attack, he is instructed to collect a 24 hour urine sample while on an unrestricted diet. At the first return visit, a serum sample is obtained for urate and creatinine. The 24 hour urine is quantified for uric acid and creatinine excretion. With these simple tests it is possible to identify those patients who produce excessive quantities of uric acid, i.e., excretion of more than 1000 mg. per day, and to assess baseline renal function.

Patients who produce excessive amounts of uric acid should be treated with an agent that inhibits uric acid synthesis. At the present time, allopurinol is the only drug available in the United States that blocks uric acid synthesis and is approved for use in gouty patients. In patients who excrete less than 1000 mg. of uric acid per day, either a uricosuric drug or allopurinol may be used. However, there are several important exceptions to this: (1) patients with extensive tophaceous disease, even though they excrete normal amounts of uric acid, should be treated with allopurinol in preference to a uricosuric drug; (2) patients with a history of renal calculi, especially if they are known to be uric acid stones, should be treated with allopurinol, since a uricosuric drug may exacerbate renal stone disease; (3) patients with significant renal disease, creatinine clearance less than 30 ml. per minute, are unlikely to respond to a uricosuric drug and therapy should be initiated with allopurinol.

Allopurinol. If allopurinol is selected as a hypouricemic agent, therapy is usually begun with 300 mg. administered as one tablet. Since the half-life of oxipurinol, the major metabolite of allopurinol, is greater than 20 hours, there is no benefit to administering the drug in divided doses. In patients with significant renal impairment oxipurinol excretion is reduced. Consequently therapy may be initiated with a dosage of 100 mg. per day. The serum urate concentration begins to fall in 1 or 2 days and reaches its nadir at 1 to 2 weeks. Thus, if the patient has not attained normouricemia after 2 weeks on a given regimen, the dosage may be increased. Patients with extensive tophaceous deposits and the rare patient who markedly overproduces urate may require relatively high doses of allopurinol, 600 to 1000 mg. per day.

The major side effects of allopurinol are skin rash, hepatotoxicity and bone marrow toxicity. In some patients the skin involvement may be severe, i.e., vasculitic lesions develop, exfoliative dermatitis ensues or toxic epidermal necrolysis occurs. Rarely, clinically significant liver disease may develop. A few patients have been reported to develop a combination of skin rash, abnormal liver function tests, and progressive renal failure. The occurrence of this constellation of findings appears to be seen more often in patients concomitantly receiving thiazide diuretics. Allopurinol in combination with ampicillin is reported to lead to a higher incidence of skin reactions. In addition, allopurinol interferes with the catabolism of azathioprine and 6-mercaptopurine, thereby potentiating the toxicity of these drugs. Xanthine stones are rare in patients receiving allopurinol—the only documented occurrences being in Lesch-Nyhan patients or patients undergoing cytotoxic therapy for tumors.

Uricosurics. Of the uricosuric agents available, two drugs are commonly employed in the United States, probenecid and sulfinpyrazone. With either of these agents therapy is initiated with a small dose of the drug, such as 250 mg. twice daily of probenecid or 100 mg. twice daily of sulfinpyrazone. In addition, during the initial phases of therapy the patient is encouraged to drink large volumes of water to ensure a urine output of greater than 1 liter per day. If the urine is persistently acid, an alkalinizing agent is added. These precautions will retard the development of a renal calculus, which might result from the transient increase in uric acid excretion. The dose of probenecid or sulfinpyrazone is increased over the next 2 to 4 weeks until the patient is receiving a dosage sufficient to reduce the serum urate concentration to 6.4 mg. per dl. In the case of probenecid this is usually achieved with 1 to 3 grams per day given in divided doses; in the case of sulfinpyrazone, the usual maintenance dosage is 400 to 800 mg. per day. Once the patient is normouricemic, the alkalinizing agent may be discontinued and fluid intake reduced.

The major side effects of the uricosuric drugs are gastrointestinal intolerance, skin eruptions, and hypersensitivity. Another effect of sulfinpyrazone, which may or may not be beneficial, is on platelet function. Patients receiving sulfinpyrazone have lengthened platelet survival and decreased platelet turnover.

Patients being treated with either of these uricosuric agents should be cautioned against the use of salicylates in any form, as salicylates abolish the uricosuric action of both drugs.

After the patient has been stabilized on hypouricemic therapy and has been symptom-free for several months, prophylactic colchicine may be discontinued. However, in patients with extensive tophaceous deposits it may be helpful to continue prophylactic therapy with colchicine until the tophi have resolved. Continued therapy with prophylactic colchicine may also benefit patients who are erratic in taking their hypouricemic therapy, since wide swings in serum urate concentration may precipitate acute attacks.

Management of Associated Conditions

A significant proportion of patients with gouty arthritis are obese and many consume excessive amounts of ethanol. Weight reduction results in an increase in urate clearance and a decrease in the rate of uric acid production. Consequently, weight-reducing diets may be of benefit in some patients with hyperuricemia and may obviate the need for hypouricemic drugs. In addition, abstinence or moderation in ethanol intake may lead to a decrease in serum urate concentration, lessening the requirement for drug therapy. Other dietary measures, such as low purine diets, are not necessary in most patients and are usually reserved for patients with severe renal failure in whom there is no mechanism for eliminating preformed urate except through the gastrointestinal tract.

A commonly associated finding in patients with gouty arthritis is hypertension. All too often, the hypertension in gouty patients is not adequately controlled for fear of exacerbating hyperuricemia. Although the administration of diuretics may lead to renal urate retention and may even precipitate attacks of gouty arthritis on occasion, the effects of uncontrolled hypertension upon the kidney and cardiovascular tree are more damaging than those of hyperuricemia. Consequently, we recommend that hypertension be aggressively managed in all patients with gout. If the hypertensive medication leads to an increase in serum urate concentration, this can be reversed by either a uricosuric agent or allopurinol. In the near future a new class of drugs will be available and they may prove to be of benefit in treating persons with hypertension and hyperuricemia. These agents are uricosuric as well as natriuretic.

HYPERLIPOPROTEINEMIA

method of
J. DAVID SCHNATZ, M.D.
Hartford, Connecticut

Background

Composition and Separation of Lipoproteins. Lipids are insoluble in aqueous media, but are solubilized in vivo by association with proteins called apoproteins. The combination of an apoprotein with cholesterol, triglyceride and phospholipid is referred to as a lipoprotein. In terms of a clinical approach, the significant serum lipids are cholesterol and triglyceride, although phospholipids clearly have a role in the metabolism and modeling of the lipoprotein molecule. Elevations of cholesterol or triglyceride or both, along with their corresponding apoprotein, are referred to by the term hyperlipoproteinemia.

Several methods are commonly used for separating and characterizing lipoproteins. Ultracentrifugal separation utilizes the density of the lipoprotein molecule to effect separation. Chylomicrons (CHYLOS) have a density less than 0.96 gram per ml., and very low density lipoproteins (VLDL) have a density between 0.96 and 1.006 gram per ml. These fractions are not usually separated in the ultracentrifuge since the density of serum is 1.006. Each contains primarily triglyceride and small amounts of cholesterol. Because of their size, these lipoproteins produce opalescent or milky plasma when sufficiently increased. Intermediate density lipoproteins (IDL) have a density of 1.006 to 1.019, and contain roughly equal amounts of cholesterol and triglyceride. The triglyceride content imparts characteristic flotation properties to the molecule. Low density lipoproteins (LDL) have a density of 1.019 to 1.063 gram per ml., contain primarily cholesterol, and are associated with clear plasma. The high density lipoproteins (HDL) have a density greater than 1.063 gram per ml. The predominant lipid is phospholipid, with lesser amounts of cholesterol.

Electrophoresis utilizes the electric charge of the lipoprotein molecule as another means of separation. This method has been used commonly for clinical evaluation. After electrophoresis of fasting plasma, the stained lipoproteins produce a pattern of visible bands (Figure 1). Normal plasma has a faintly stained alpha band near the anode (+) and a more intensely stained beta lipoprotein band closer to the origin. Abnormal plasma may contain additional bands at the origin or in the prebeta lipoprotein region. The lipoproteins of the latter class may trail from the prebeta region toward the origin, particularly if electrophoresis is conducted on paper strips. These bands contain primarily triglyceride, whereas the beta lipoprotein band contains primarily cholesterol. The intermediate density lipoprotein migrates as a broad beta band (Type III) and contains roughly equal amounts of cholesterol and triglyceride, reflecting its intermediate status between VLDL and LDL.

The apoprotein moiety of the lipoprotein has been more difficult to study because of the tendency to denaturation during delipidation. Some understanding, however, has been achieved, leading to the awareness of three major apoproteins; A, B and C, varying in size from 57 to 245 amino acids. These apoproteins are incorporated into the various lipoproteins: chylomicrons and VLDL contain primarily B and C apoproteins, LDL contains primarily apoprotein B, and HDL primarily apoprotein A. An arginine-rich apoprotein E, contained in the IDL, is important in classifying disorders in which IDL predominate.

Metabolism of Lipoproteins. Recent data indicate that the lipoproteins do not exist in a static state in vivo. Rather, VLDL is synthesized in the liver as a combination of cholesterol, triglyceride, phospholipids, and apoproteins. It is secreted into the plasma where this molecule is converted, via an intricate series of transformations, to IDL and then to LDL. In initiating this sequence, it is probable that some VLDL also originates from CHYLOS. LDL is removed by peripheral tissues and in the normal state regulates the peripheral synthesis of cholesterol via an intricate mechanism termed the LDL pathway. Tissue receptors for LDL are necessary to the proper function of this pathway, and a deficiency in these receptors leads to abnormal states of cholesterol metabolism.

While the other lipoproteins transport lipids from the intestines or liver to peripheral tissues, HDL may be important in the transport of cholesterol from peripheral tissues to the liver. Thus, high levels of HDL are considered to give a protection against atherosclerosis and low levels a tendency toward this disorder. More information is necessary, but clearly this appears to be a potentially important area for classification and therapeutic intervention.

Thus, in the normal state, cholesterol circulates primarily as LDL (beta lipoprotein), and triglycerides circulate primarily as either CHYLOS (nonmigrating lipoproteins), VLDL (prebeta lipoproteins), or both. The presence of appreciable amounts of triglycerides in two distinct lipoprotein classes is significant. The former (CHYLOS) result from intestinal absorption of dietary lipids and are referred to as exogenous triglycerides. The latter (VLDL) result primarily from hepatic synthesis and are referred to as endogenous triglycerides.

Triglycerides are removed from the circulation for energy or storage through the action of lipoprotein lipase (LPL), an enzyme present in heart, fat, and possibly other tissues. Familial deficiencies in LPL occur, but more commonly acquired deficiencies appear, particularly in diabetes mellitus. Although the source of circulating cholesterol is similar to that of triglycerides, i.e., intestinal absorption and hepatic synthesis, distinction between these two sources cannot be made by electrophoresis or centrifugation. Cholesterol is not used

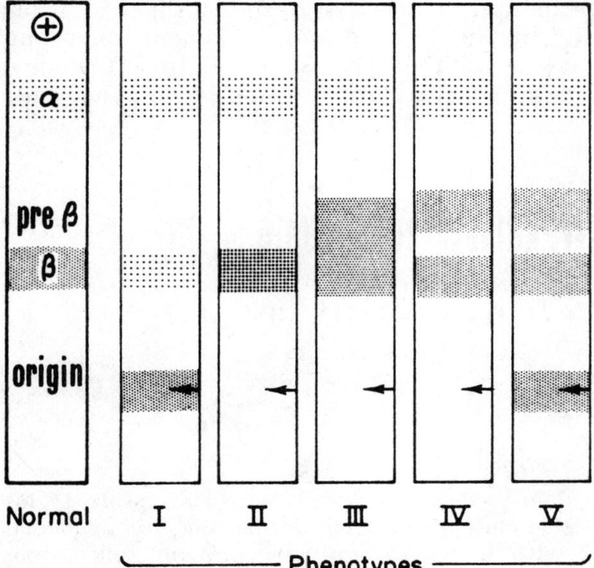

Figure 1. Classification of familial hyperlipoproteinemia by phenotyping.

for energy purposes, as is triglyceride, but instead is an important structural and functional component of tissue membranes. It is synthesized by many tissues, regulated by feedback control through the LDL pathway, and is excreted in the feces as bile acids and neutral sterols. Feedback regulation of hepatic cholesterol synthesis completes an enterohepatic circulation of cholesterol.

Evaluation and Classfication

Normal Values. Serum lipids should be measured after a 12 to 14 hour period without caloric intake. A definition of normal serum lipid values is difficult to achieve since sex, age, specific population group, and antecedent diet all influence the results. In dealing with a specific population, the distribution of values is unimodal and skewed to the right, presenting the problem of deciding where the normal values end and the abnormal begin. In approaching the problem from an investigational standpoint, some authors use the 90th or 95th percentile as the upper limit of normal. In clinical practice, however, this is probably too high and may not apply to the patient's specific population. Commonly used figures for normal can be obtained by reference to a standard table (Ann. Intern. Med., 77:267, 1972). Taking all of the preceding into account, the following generalization can be developed: adult values are normal, if cholesterol is less than 250 mg. per dl. (100 ml.) and triglyceride less than 150 mg. per dl. Levels are generally abnormal, if cholesterol is greater than 300 mg. per dl. and triglyceride greater than 200 mg. per dl. Intermediary values are questionable. Certain exceptions exist; children tend to have lower values, and recently some populations have been shown to have higher triglyceride values in apparently normal persons.

Approach to the Patient. For practical purposes the hyperlipoproteinemias can be classified as primary and secondary. The history, physical examination, and general laboratory evaluation should detect medical conditions that might produce a secondary elevation of serum lipids. Among these are diabetes mellitus, obesity, alcohol consumption, oral contraceptives, and estrogen deficiency as well as thyroid, renal, hepatic, and pancreatic disease.

Primary hyperlipoproteinemias can be characterized by family analysis, history of premature coronary vascular disease, xanthomas, or previous lipid abnormalities, and current lipid determinations on family members. Such screening can help to determine if the abnormality displays characteristics of monogenic or polygenic inheritance or if it appears to be sporadic. Monogenic inheritance is caused by a single gene, either dominant or recessive. An autosomal dominant trait is inherited vertically in the pedigree and manifested in approximately 50 per cent of first degree relatives, thus forming a bimodal pattern of values when frequency is plotted against the lipid level. A recessive trait will affect one of four siblings, often detected by an abnormal level of the gene product such as an enzyme. Clinical expression, however, is variable, depending upon the presence in the pedigree of heterozygotes versus homozygotes. Polygenic inheritance is influenced by more than one gene and is manifested by a unimodal distribution when

frequency is plotted against the lipid level. Near relatives are more likely to be affected than distant. If no inheritance pattern is apparent, the trait is termed sporadic, and inheritance appears to play no role.

When the patient has no diseases that produce secondary elevation in serum lipids and the family screening is positive for lipid abnormalities, primary familial hyperlipoproteinemia is present. When the patient has a medical illness that produces elevated serum lipids and family screening is negative, the hyperlipoproteinemia is classified as secondary. When both patient and family screening are positive, the medical condition may be familial, causing a secondary increase in lipids, or the patient may have a primary familial hyperlipoproteinemia. When all screening tests are negative, the lipid abnormality may be sporadic or an underlying medical condition is occult.

Classification of Familial Hyperlipoproteinemias by Phenotyping. Beginning in the mid-1960s it became accepted practice to do lipoprotein electrophoresis for phenotyping of the familial hyperlipoproteinemias (Circulation, 31:321, 1965) (Figure 1). By this method, Type I is characterized by nonmigrating lipoproteins (CHYLOS) associated with high levels of triglyceride, eruptive xanthomas, hepatosplenomegaly, and abdominal pain. The disorder is expressed in childhood and is due to a genetic deficiency of lipoprotein lipase or its plasma activator, apoprotein C-II. Type IIa is characterized by an intensely staining beta lipoprotein band associated with hypercholesterolemia, premature coronary vascular disease, and tendon xanthomas. Type IIb has characteristics similiar to IIa, but with mild elevations of triglyceride. Type II hyperlipoproteinemias, particularly the homozygous form, occur in childhood. Type III is characterized by a broad beta lipoprotein band, which floats in the ultracentrifuge. Both cholesterol and triglyceride are elevated. Characteristic features of Type III are aggravation of the hyperlipoproteinemia by ingestion of carbohydrate, a tendency to glucose intolerance, hyperuricemia, tuberous as well as palmar xanthomas, and vascular disease, both peripheral and coronary. Type IV is an endogenous hypertriglyceridemia characterized by an increase in the pre-beta lipoprotein band (VLDL) and aggravation of these abnormalities by ingestion of excessive amounts of carbohydrate. Patients with this disorder tend to be overweight, have carbohydrate intolerance and an increased incidence of vascular disease. Finally, Type V is a combination of exogenous and endogenous hypertriglyceridemia, manifested by nonmigrating and prebeta lipoproteins on electrophoresis. Patients display the following characteristics: glucose intolerance, hyperuricemia, pancreatitis, and xanthomas but a relative freedom from vascular disease.

Ten years after initiation of lipoprotein phenotyping, it became apparent that phenotyping had fallen short of expectations (Circulation, 51:209, 1975). First, quantitation is not possible, and Type III needs specific measurement of the cholesterol/triglyceride ratio in the separated lipoproteins in order to establish the diagnosis. A VLDL cholesterol/plasma triglyceride ratio greater than 0.3 can be considered diagnostic. Recently, immunologic measurement of apoprotein E has been used to identify the characteristic IDL. Second, phenotyping has proved of little value genetically, since phenotypic heterogeneity occurs commonly within a specific familial disorder. That is, relatives may have a variety of phenotypes; IIa, IIb, IV, V, and a given individual may display different phenotypes at different times. This has been particularly true of an entity described in the early 1970s, familial combined hyperlipoproteinemia. In this disorder, triglyceride and cholesterol levels are both elevated, while at other times one or the other may be increased. The mechanism of the disorder is uncertain and there are no biochemical tests to distinguish it as a specific entity. Familial studies are helpful in making the diagnosis.

Classification of Familial Hyperlipoproteinemia by Lipid Analysis and Family Study. Although lipoprotein phenotyping may be useful, the majority of patients with primary hyperlipoproteinemia can be separated into three groups, based on whether they have elevations of cholesterol, triglyceride, or both (Table 1). Cholesterol elevation alone is the familial, IIa, hyperlipoproteinemia with an increase in the beta lipoprotein. This condition is inherited as a monogenic, autosomal dominant, or polygenic trait. Homozygous forms of the monogenic hypercholesterolemia are manifested in childhood and have cholesterol levels greater than 600 mg. per dl. while heterozygous forms are apparent later in life and have cholesterol levels ranging between 300 and 500 mg. per dl. Though not available for clinical classification, measurement of LDL receptors in peripheral tissues will permit subdivision of this entity into those with no LDL receptors and those with defective LDL receptors.

Triglyceride elevations can be exogenous (Type I), endogenous (Type IV), or a combination of exogenous and endogenous (Type V). A rough differentiation between exogenous and endogenous hypertriglyceridemias can be achieved by placing plasma in the refrigerator over night. Exogenous particles will rise and form a layer on the top of the plasma, while endogenous particles remain homogeneously distributed. Other means of differentiating the two, if necessary, are by dietary trial or by electrophoretic separation of CHYLOS (nonmigrating) and VLDL (prebeta). Type I is a rare recessive disorder, usually detected in children. The other two types are rarely seen in children and are autosomal dominant.

Cholesterol and triglyceride elevations can occur as IIb, III, or the combined entity, which can be manifested by a variety of phenotypes. Type IIb has an increase in LDL and a mild increase in VLDL. Type III has an increase in the IDL and requires chemical analysis of the separated lipoprotein, or immunoassay for apoprotein E. Circulating cholesterol and triglyceride levels are roughly equal. The combined variety may have a combination of lipoprotein elevations, and family analysis is important for classification, inheritance being autosomal dominant. While IIb may appear in childhood, the other two rarely occur except in adults.

The foregoing discussion and deemphasis of lipoprotein phenotyping does not imply that I am against the most accurate classification possible. Indeed, the more accurate the classification, the better our chances of applying a rational therapy. Further work is necessary to arrive at a specific biochemical classification that will have the most meaning in terms of therapy. At the present time we are still dealing with a heterogenous group of patients at best, and there are serious limitations to the electrophoretic phenotyping when used alone.

Treatment

Reasons for Therapy. Therapy of primary hyperlipoproteinemia consists of two aspects: diet and drugs. It is generally based on the unproved assumption that lowering serum lipids will favorably influence existing or potential atherosclerosis and associated coronary vascular disease. Although the lipid hypothesis has not yet been proved in humans, there are data that suggest that the phenomenon observed in animals will ultimately be shown to exist in man. That is, an increase in serum lipids produces atherosclerosis, and a decrease in serum lipids leads to regression of the atherosclerosis. Thus, it is standard practice to advise a prudent attention to diet or drug therapy or both with the goal of lowering serum lipids, realizing that ultimate proof of the relationship between serum lipids and atherosclerosis is still lacking. A significant problem in this regard is patient education and acceptance of potential long-term benefits. To accomplish this the physician must take an active role.

Other reasons for considering therapy of hyperlipoproteinemias are to effect regression of bothersome or unsightly xanthomas, or relief of abdominal pain secondary to pancreatitis or both. Although some xanthomas may respond rapidly (eruptive xanthomas secondary to exogenous hypertriglyceridemia), others may respond poorly, if

TABLE 1. **Classification of Familial Hyperlipoproteinemia by Lipid Analysis and Family Study**

LIPID ELEVATION	LIPOPROTEIN PHENOTYPE	MODES OF INHERITANCE	OCCURS IN CHILDREN
Cholesterol	IIa	Autosomal dominant or polygenic	Yes
Triglyceride	I	Autosomal recessive	Yes
	IV	Autosomal dominant	Rare
	V	Autosomal dominant	Rare
Cholesterol & Triglyceride	IIb	Autosomal dominant or polygenic	Yes
	III	Autosomal dominant	Rare
	IIa, IIb, IV, or V	Autosomal dominant	Rare

at all (tendon xanthomas). The most remarkable results may come from control of massive triglyceride elevations, leading to relief of abdominal pain as well as regression of eruptive xanthomas.

General Therapy. Excessive body weight is frequently associated with increased synthesis of triglyceride-rich lipoproteins. Thus, caloric restriction should be a matter of primary attention for any overweight patient. The degree of obesity can be determined by use of the Body Mass Index, by measurement of fat folds with calipers, or by reference to standard tables such as the report of the Food and Nutrition Board published by the National Academy of Science, 1968.

A prescribed program of graduated exercise may be beneficial to caloric control and weight reduction, provided there is no medical contraindication. Furthermore, exercise may increase the circulating HDL levels, which are thought to provide a protective effect against atherosclerosis.

A number of the hyperlipoproteinemias seen in clinical practice will be secondary to some other disease such as diabetes mellitus, which when treated may eliminate the hyperlipoproteinemia. Diabetes mellitus may have both an exogenous and endogenous form of hypertriglyceridemia. The former is caused by a reduction in lipoprotein lipase activity as a result of insulin deficiency, and will respond to insulin therapy. The latter is due to increased synthesis of lipoproteins and at times to decreased clearance of endogenously synthesized lipoproteins. It may not respond completely to control of the diabetes unless other measures for managing endogenous hypertriglyceridemia (caloric and carbohydrate restriction) are followed. In certain cases it may be difficult to decide whether an abnormal glucose tolerance is part of a familial hyperlipoproteinemia (Types III, IV, or V) or whether the hyperlipoproteinemia is secondary to the glucose intolerance. Nevertheless, the principles of therapy to be stated subsequently remain the same.

Two of the more common factors that will produce hyperlipoproteinemia (primarily hypertriglyceridemia) are the use of oral contraceptives and alcohol. Discontinuance of oral contraceptives and moderation or abstinence from alcohol may reverse the abnormality.

Familial Hyperlipoproteinemias. For specific familial disorders, treatment may be prescribed according to the phenotypes described in the preceding discussion, and one may designate a specific therapy for each type of familial hyperlipoproteinemia (Table 2). However, recognizing the problems with classification and a basic heterogeneity that persists with all present classifications, I prefer to initiate treatment according to the classification in Table 1. This therapy is outlined in Table 3.

If cholesterol elevation is primary, mild elevations may respond to diet alone.* For significant hypercholesterolemia, I use a combination of diet and drug therapy from the outset, since these abnormalities are notoriously the most difficult to treat. Although disagreement still exists as to the effectiveness of cholesterol restriction, I recommend that the patient attempt to reduce cholesterol intake to less than 300 mg. daily. Polyunsaturated fatty acids appear to aid in lowering serum cholesterol by decreasing its absorption. Thus, reduction of saturated fatty acids and substitution of polyunsaturated fatty acids is advisable. The simultaneous restriction of cholesterol and saturated fatty acids is aided by the fact that they occur together in many foods.

Some of the foods to be avoided in restricting cholesterol are cream, butter, whole or 2 per cent milk, cheese, coffee whiteners, dessert toppings, sauces and gravies that are not made with allowed fat or oil, commercially fried foods, creamed foods, frozen or packaged dinners, olives, avocado, chocolate candies made with butter, cream, or coconut, fudge, commercial popcorn, foods containing egg yolks, sausages, cold cuts, weiners, organ meats, and shellfish. Meat should be lean and limited in amount to no more than 3 ounces three times per week. Poultry and fish, each without the skin, may supply the remainder of the protein needs. The use of skim milk should be encouraged to provide a balanced caloric, calcium, and protein intake.

The polyunsaturated to saturated fatty acid ratio of the diet (P/S) should be greater than 2:1. To increase the polyunsaturated fatty acids one should use liquid oils such as corn, safflower, sunflower seed, cotten seed, sesame seed, or soybean oil. Peanut and olive oil are not recommended, as they are low in polyunsaturated fats. The patient should be cautioned to read labels carefully; margarines to be acceptable should contain at least 25 per cent linoleic acid and not more than an equal amount of saturated fatty acids. The American Heart Association has made available a booklet entitled "Planning Fat-Controlled Meals," which can be obtained from local heart associations or the American Heart Association, 44 East 23rd Street, New York, New York, 10010. Recipes detailing the use of polyunsaturated fats are also available. These prepared diets are of considerable value in reviewing dietary prescriptions with a patient. Of course, the assistance of a therapeutic dietitian is invaluable.

A number of lipid-lowering drugs are currently available to aid with regulation of serum cholesterol. Their effectiveness in lowering lipids

---

*For young persons the mild elevation (225 to 275 mg. per. dl.) may be significant and warrant drug therapy as well as diet.

TABLE 2. **Treatment of Familial Hyperlipoproteinemia***

PHENOTYPE AND ELECTROPHORETIC CHARACTERISTIC	DIET†	DRUGS
I Exogenous hypertriglyceridemia, nonmigrating lipoproteins	Low fat and/or medium chain triglycerides	None
II Hypercholesterolemia, elevated beta-lipoprotein	Low cholesterol (less than 300 mg.) High polyunsaturated fatty acids P/S: 2/1	Cholestyramine or colestipol Nicotinic acid Clofibrate Sitosterol Consider ileal bypass
III Mixed hyperlipidemia, unusual beta-lipoprotein	Low cholesterol (less than 300 mg.) High polyunsaturated fatty acids P/S: 2/1	Clofibrate Nicotinic acid
IV Primarily endogenous hypertriglyceridemia, pre-beta-lipoprotein	Caloric restriction Restriction of alcohol and carbohydrates (less than 125 grams daily)	Clofibrate Nicotinic acid
V Exogenous and endogenous hypertriglyceridemia, nonmigrating and pre-beta-lipoproteins	Combination of regimens used for Types I and IV	Clofibrate Nicotinic acid

*Classified by electrophoretic phenotypes described by Fredrickson et al.: New Engl. J. Med., *276*:32, 1967. Classification implies that other diseases are ruled out and that the disorder has been shown to be familial.

†Booklets entitled "The Dietary Management of Hyperlipoproteinemia" by Donald S. Fredrickson, M.D., and Robert I. Levy, M.D. are available to the physician by writing the Office of Heart Information, National Heart and Lung Institute, Bethesda, Maryland, 20014.

and increasing life expectancy is currently debatable, although I believe it is prudent to act as if there is a relation. None of the drugs are ideal and all have side effects. Because of the incidence of side effects and the less than optimal results in many patients, we can expect that new lipid-lowering drugs will continue to be introduced. Among the drugs that may be useful in lowering serum cholesterol are cholestyramine, nicotinic acid, and clofibrate.

For marked forms of hypercholesterolemia, combinations of drugs may be necessary such as cholestyramine and nicotinic acid, or cholestyramine and clofibrate. In persistently resistant hypercholesterolemia with levels over 350 mg. per dl. and a strong familial history of hypercholesterolemia, coupled with premature coronary vascular disease, I consider using the ileal bypass procedure to effect cholesterol lowering (Circulation 49, Suppl., *1*:1, 1974). For homozygous forms of hypercholesterolemia, portocaval shunt has been used (Lancet *2*:449, 1974). This procedure is investigational, and any patient with the rare, extremely lethal, homozygous form of hypercholesterolemia, should be referred to the National Cooperative Study, if this procedure is contemplated.

If endogenous triglycerides are elevated, it is advisable to recommend caloric or carbohydrate restriction or both, and restriction of alcohol. In some instances it may be helpful to recommend reduction of refined sugars. Finally, substitution of polyunsaturated fats for saturated fats may make a difference in lowering endogenous triglyceride levels. Most patients with endogenous hypertriglyceridemia will respond effectively to an appropriate diet, but if dietary control is incomplete, clofibrate may provide additional lipid lowering. Although clofibrate is the drug of choice, nicotinic acid may be beneficial in this condition.

If the hypertriglyceridemia is exogenous, dietary fat restriction should be instituted, sometimes to as little as 5 grams daily. Such severe dietary fat restriction of necessity results in a high carbohydrate diet that will, in turn, aggravate any component of endogenous hyperlipidemia that may be present. In addition, such a low fat diet is unpalatable and difficult to follow. An alternate approach is to substitute medium chain triglycerides (MCT) for the usual dietary fat, and reduce the fat content of the diet to roughly 20 grams. MCT are effective in lowering circulating exogenous triglycerides because they are transported from the intestine via the portal vein rather than the lymphatics, and thus they by-pass the lipoprotein lipase clearing mechanism. MCT are available as a special nutrient formula, Portagen. Alternatively, MCT oil can be employed in a number of

TABLE 3. **Treatment of Familial Hyperlipoproteinemia***

LIPID ELEVATION	DIET	DRUGS
Cholesterol		
Mild (225–275 mg./dl.)	Low cholesterol (less than 300 mg.) High polyunsaturated fatty acids P/S: 2/1	
Moderate (275–350 mg./dl.)	Same as above	Cholestyramine or colestipol Nicotinic acid Clofibrate Combinations
Severe (Over 350 mg./dl.)	Same as above	Same as above Consider ileal bypass, if drugs fail
Triglyceride		
Endogenous	Caloric and/or carbohydrate restriction Restriction of alcohol	Clofibrate Nicotinic acid
Exogenous	Low fat and/or medium chain triglycerides	
Cholesterol and triglycerides	Caloric restriction, if overweight Low cholesterol, high polyunsaturated fatty acids	Clofibrate Nicotinic acid

*Classified by lipid analysis and family study (Table 1).

recipes as outlined in a recipe book available from Mead-Johnson. A simple and palatable method is to add MCT oil to skim milk.

Regardless of the type of hyperlipoproteinemias, our current state of knowledge is such that combined elevations of cholesterol and triglyceride are basically treated the same. They require a combination of the above noted therapies. Weight control and modification of the fat content of the diet may be all that is necessary, but reduction of carbohydrates and refined sugars as well as restriction of alcohol may be necessary to obtain optimal lowering of serum lipids by diet. Clofibrate is the drug of choice, but nicotinic acid may be beneficial as well. Cholestyramine is not recommended, as it may increase triglyceride, particularly if VLDL are elevated or IDL is present.

Specific Drugs

Cholestyramine (Questran). Cholestyramine is the chloride salt of a basic anion exchange resin. It is given in doses of 4 to 8 grams three to four times daily. The initial dose for adults is 12 to 16 grams and the maximal dose is 32 grams. Although patients may mind the taste when mixed with water, it can be made more palatable by mixing with juices or crushed fruit.

Cholestyramine is extremely effective in lowering LDL cholesterol and is the drug of choice in patients with Type II hyperlipoproteinemia. Reduction of serum cholesterol levels by cholestyramine in Type IIa familial hyperlipoproteinemia has been reported to be as much as 20 to 25 per cent, the mechanism generally being considered to be due to binding of bile acids in the small intestine and alteration of the enterohepatic recirculation. However, such reduction in enterohepatic recirculation will result in increased hepatic cholesterol synthesis. Thus, the decrease in cholesterol may be related to an increased fractional catabolic rate of the LDL apoprotein as brought about by cholestyramine. If the hypercholesterolemia is due to elevations of VLDL or IDL, a situation in which the triglyceride would be elevated also, cholestyramine may lead to increased levels of cholesterol as well as triglyceride, presumably due to stimulation of VLDL synthesis.

Patients receiving cholestyramine have frequent gastrointestinal complaints, particularly constipation and less frequently abdominal discomfort, flatulence, anorexia, nausea, vomiting, diarrhea, and rarely steatorrhea.

As an anion exchange resin, cholestyramine may have strong affinity for acidic drugs. In this regard, certain drugs should be taken at least one hour prior to cholestyramine administration. Among these drugs are digitalis, thyroid, chlorothiazide, warfarin, phenylbutazone, and phenobarbital. If the cholestyramine can be taken only 3 times daily and maintain effective action, the other drugs might be given at bedtime. Of further note is the fact that a patient on cholestyramine and one of these other drugs may have potentiation of the other drug if cholestyramine is discontinued. Finally, due to its effect on fat absorption, cholestyramine may affect fat-soluble vitamins. Vitamin K deficiency may result and lead to hypoprothrombinemia and an increased bleeding tendency. Deficiencies of vitamins A and D, though less common, may also occur.

The safety of cholestyramine in pregnancy has not been established, and the doses in children are currently under investigation, but the drug has been shown to be effective in children at reduced levels.

Nicotinic Acid. Nicotinic acid, a component of the coenzymes NAD and NADP, has been shown effective in lowering serum lipids when given in large doses. To avoid uncomfortable side effects, the initial dose is low, 100 mg. three times daily or 500 mg. twice daily. This is gradually increased over 2 to 4 weeks to a dose of 3 to 6 grams daily. If given with meals, the tendency to gastritis will be diminished.

Presumably, the decrease in serum lipids occurs through its suppression of free fatty acid release from peripheral adipose tissue stores with subsequent decreases in hepatic VLDL synthesis and secretion, and a decrease in circulating triglyceride levels within 4 to 6 hours. In turn, this leads to a decrease in IDL and LDL with a concomitant decrease in cholesterol over several days. Nicotinic acid has been shown to produce reduction in cholesterol between 15 and 30 per cent whereas reductions of triglyceride have been noted to be as much as 60 per cent. When combined with cholestyramine in treating familial Type II hyperlipoproteinemia, a significant additional effect may be shown.

The most frequent and uncomfortable side effect is that of cutaneous flushing and itching. In most patients this generally disappears after the first few weeks of therapy, but may be avoided if the initial dose is small and the subsequent doses increased slowly. Carbohydrate intolerance may be precipitated or diabetes mellitus aggravated. Hepatotoxicity and hyperuricemia may occur but will disappear after discontinuation of the drug. Thus, use of nicotinic acid should be avoided in patients with diabetes mellitus, liver disease, or gout. Hyperpigmentation and acanthosis nigricans may occur with prolonged therapy.

Clofibrate (Atromid-S). Clofibrate is a branched chain fatty acid ester that significantly reduces VLDL but has a variable effect on LDL when given in usual doses of 1 gram, twice daily. Serum triglycerides may be lowered by as much as 40 per cent with cholesterol no more than 20 per cent, and frequently less. Thus, it is the optimal drug for treatment of hypertriglyceridemia, but has considerably lesser effects on hypercholesterolemia. On the other hand, when used in conjunction with cholestyramine, it may produce a significant additional lowering of serum cholesterol levels.

Serum cholesterol is probably lowered via a number of mechanisms, among which may be decreased synthesis of cholesterol and increased sterol excretion. In lowering serum triglyceride, its major use, it appears to decrease free fatty acid release from peripheral tissues and to decrease hepatic triglyceride synthesis. Recent reports indicate that VLDL and IDL clearance may be increased by clofibrate, and that this may be the primary mechanism of the serum triglyceride lowering.

Among the most important side effects are its potentiation of coumarin anticoagulants and occasional elevation of circulating hepatic enzymes. Rarer side effects include cardiac arrhythmias, gastrointestinal disturbance, skin rash, myositis, dizziness, and alopecia. The syndrome of inappropriate ADH secretion has been noted and may

be more common than recognized. In fact, almost all organ systems can be involved in a variety of side effects that are rare.

Other Drugs. Colestipol and probucol have been introduced recently. Colestipol is a resin that presumably works like cholestyramine and could be substituted for cholestyramine in the treatment of familial, Type II, hyperlipoproteinemia. Some patients will find this more palatable than cholestyramine and may not develop constipation which is so common with cholestyramine. Probucol is a bis-phenol that works by unknown mechanisms, lowering cholesterol but not triglyceride. As a newly introduced drug, long-term experience is limited.

D-Thyroxine, an analogue of the metabolically active L-thyroxine, is still recommended by some authors, but I generally do not use it. The most important side effect is increased metabolic rate, and it is not advisable in the presence of organic heart disease or hypertension. In fact, it was discontinued from the Coronary Drug Project because of an excess of myocardial ischemia in those receiving the medication.

Estrogens have been used in the past, but were discontinued from the Coronary Drug Project due to adverse effects: an excess of nonfatal myocardial infarctions, pulmonary embolism, and thrombophlebitis. Previously, one might have considered using estrogen for the postmenopausal female to lower cholesterol. However, with the recent awareness of an increased incidence of uterine adenocarcinoma secondary to estrogen therapy, one must balance this risk against the risks of hypercholesterolemia, and one generally comes out against the use of estrogens.

Beta sitosterol (Cytellin), a plant sterol, interferes with cholesterol absorption and produces small decreases in cholesterol. It is safe and free of side effects.

Conclusion

Treatment of hyperlipoproteinemias depends upon characterization; primary versus secondary, type of lipid elevation, and, if possible, whether the source is endogenous or exogenous. Therapy is evolving continuously. It will improve as classification becomes more refined and as new forms of drug therapy are introduced. At present, a given therapy should be tried based on the foregoing description, but modified as soon as it is apparent that optimal results have not been obtained.

In following a patient under therapy for hyperlipoproteinemia, one should check serum lipids at intervals of 1 to 2 weeks, initially, and 1 to 2 months later on. If a given regimen is not effective in lowering serum lipids by 15 to 20 per cent within 1 to 2 months, adherence to diet and compliance with drug therapy should be verified. If the regimen is being followed but is unsuccessful, another drug should be added to or substitued for the one being used. If satisfactory control is achieved, maintenance follow-up should be at 4 to 6 month intervals.

REACTIVE HYPOGLYCEMIA

method of
JAMES W. ANDERSON, M.D.
Lexington, Kentucky

Reactive hypoglycemia is characterized by postprandial hypoglycemia and symptoms related to glucopenia. This combination of chemical hypoglycemia attended by symptoms is uncommon in adults, although nonspecific symptoms consistent with hypoglycemia are experienced with moderate frequency by many persons. The symptoms induced by hypoglycemia result from either stimulation of the sympathetic nervous system or neuroglucopenia. The release of catecholamines produces sweating, weakness, hunger, tachycardia, anxiety, numbness, and tingling. Under other circumstances, especially when the hypoglycemia develops slowly, symptoms of irritability, headaches, mental confusion, slurred speech, or convulsions may result from neuroglucopenia. Reactive hypoglycemia is usually self-limited and associated with only mild to moderate symptoms related to catecholamine release; however, some persons may develop seizures or transient neurologic defects associated with severe reactive hypoglycemia.

The diagnosis of reactive hypoglycemia is based on the presence of all of these criteria:

1. Recurring symptoms after meals that are consistent with hypoglycemia.

2. A plasma glucose value below 45 mg. per dl. (100 ml.) between 90 and 270 minutes after ingestion of a meal or oral glucose.

3. Symptoms of hypoglycemia that coincide temporally with the chemical hypoglycemia.

The most useful diagnostic procedure is a 5-hour glucose tolerance test. Plasma glucose values should be measured before and every 30 minutes after administration of the glucose load; plasma or serum insulin measurements should be made every 30 minutes for 3 hours. The plasma glucose concentration documents the presence of meaningful hypoglycemia, while the timing of the hypoglycemia and the insulin peak aid in the differential diagnosis. The nadir of the plasma glucose may not be observed if measurements are made less frequently than every 30 minutes.

Reactive hypoglycemia results from either an unusually rapid absorption of glucose (the alimentary type) or a delay in insulin secretion (the diabetic type). Other types of reactive hypoglycemia that can be related to hormone deficiencies (e.g., growth hormone), enzyme deficiencies (e.g., fructose-1,6-diphosphatase), or other genetic derangements (e.g., hereditary fructose intolerance) are rare. Idiopathic reactive hypoglycemia is unusual in my experience because, with appropriate diagnostic procedures, most patients can be classified into the alimentary or diabetic types. Nutritional management is the mainstay of treatment of all types of reactive hypoglycemia and drug therapy is reserved for those persons who do not respond to appropriate dietary therapy.

Alimentary Type of Reactive Hypoglycemia

Hypoglycemia results from the accelerated absorption of carbohydrate from the small intestine, coupled with an exaggerated secretion of insulin. Both the rapid absorption of simple sugars and the excessive secretion of insulinogenic gut hormones appear to produce the postprandial hyperinsulinemia. This sequence of events may occur after gastric surgery (e.g., subtotal gastrectomy) or in persons who have had no previous gastric surgery. The principal aim of therapy is to prevent postprandial hyperinsulinemia by regulating the intake and absorption of simple carbohydrates (monosaccharides and disaccharides).

Dietary Management. Restriction of the intake of monosaccharides (especially glucose) and disaccharides (sucrose, maltose and lactose) is the first step in nutritional therapy. A generous intake of complex carbohydrates and plant fibers is beneficial. Those persons who have had a partial gastrectomy usually benefit from a food plan consisting of three meals of moderate size and snacks between meals and at bedtime. Restricting total carbohydrate and encouraging increased protein intake is usually not required. A prototypical diet for treatment of alimentary hypoglycemia is outlined below:

Breakfast
Whole wheat muffin, 50 grams (one medium)
Oatmeal, 50 grams (½ cup, dry)
Skim milk, 100 grams (3½ oz.)
Peaches, water packed, 75 grams (¾ cup)
"Diabetic" jelly, 5 grams (1 teaspoon)
Margarine, 5 grams (1 teaspoon)

Morning snack
Rye crisp wafers, 36 grams (6 crackers)
"Diabetic" jelly, 5 grams (1 teaspoon)
Margarine, 5 grams (1 teaspoon)

Noon meal
Lean ham, 40 grams (1½ oz.)
White beans, 100 grams (½ cup, cooked)
Cornbread, 50 grams (1 medium muffin)
Kale, 150 grams (¾ cup)
Margarine, 5 grams (1 teaspoon)

Afternoon snack
Whole wheat muffin, 50 grams (one medium)
Orange, 95 grams (one small)
"Diabetic" jelly, 5 grams (1 teaspoon)
Margarine, 5 grams (1 teaspoon)

Evening meal
Baked chicken, 50 grams (~2 oz.)
White potatoes, 150 grams (¾ cup, raw)
Peas, 100 grams (½ cup)
Corn, 150 grams (¾ cup)
Lettuce, 50 grams (1 cup)
Tomato, 30 grams (¼ small)
French dressing, 40 grams (1½ oz.)

Evening snack
Turkey (light), 30 grams (1 oz.)
Mayonnaise, 20 grams (4 teaspoons)
Whole wheat bread, 46 grams (2 slices)

This 1850 calorie diet provides: protein, 94 grams; total carbohydrate, 229 grams; complex carbohydrate, 179 grams; simple carbohydrate, 50 grams; fat, 66 grams; and plant fiber, 50 grams. Approximately 50 per cent of the energy comes from carbohydrate but less than one fifth of the carbohydrate is of the simple type. Eating the simple carbohydrates in the form of whole fruits or with plant fibers slows their absorption and decreases the insulin response.

Drug Therapy. Most patients respond favorably to a restriction of simple carbohydrate intake and the other dietary modifications outlined above. No pharmacologic agents are available that specifically reverse the pathophysiology of this disorder and available drugs offer palliation only. Thus the health care team should work intensively to help patients modify their food habits before considering the introduction of drug therapy. The following agents have been reported effective in selected patients.

Anticholinergic agents inhibit gastric emptying and may be effective in some patients, especially those who have not had a subtotal gastrectomy. Propantheline, 7.5 to 15 mg., may be taken orally three times daily.

Sulfonylureas may attenuate insulin secretion by unknown mechanisms and prevent hypoglycemia and symptoms. Either tolbutamide, 250 mg. orally before each meal, or chlorpropamide, 250 mg. every morning, may be used. (This use of these agents is not listed in the manufacturer's official directives.)

Beta-adrenergic blocking agents inhibit insulin secretion and may reduce the hyperinsulinemia that induces the subsequent hypoglycemia. These agents should be used judiciously, since they also mask the catecholamine-induced symptoms of hypoglycemia. Propranolol, 5 to 10 mg., may be given orally before each meal. (This use of this agent is not listed in the manufacturer's official directive.)

Diabetic Type of Reactive Hypoglycemia

Before symptomatic diabetes develops, reactive hypoglycemia may occur in either the latent or chemical stages. During the glucose tolerance test abnormal hyperglycemia may not be observed at 60 to 180 minutes after glucose ingestion, but chemical hypoglycemia may be documented between 180 and 270 minutes. Usually, the plasma insulin response is delayed, with peak values occurring at 90 to 150 minutes instead of the normal peak at 30 to 60 minutes. The therapeutic aims are to improve insulin secretion by weight reduction, nutritional management, or, finally, by drug therapy.

Dietary Management. Increasing the intake of starch and decreasing the intake of fat leads to improved glucose metabolism and may alleviate symptomatic hypoglycemia. Furthermore, restricting simple carbohydrates and increasing plant fiber intake may reduce the likelihood of hypoglycemia. Weight reduction is important if the patient is obese. For lean persons we use a weight-maintaining diet, which provides 55 per cent of calories as carbohydrates (less than one fourth of this as simple carbohydrates), 15 to 20 per cent protein, and 25 to 30 per cent fat with at least 40 grams of plant fiber. This diet is similar to the one outlined earlier except it provides slightly more carbohydrate. Food can be taken in three main meals and an evening snack is optional.

Drug Therapy. Most patients respond to vigorous dietary management and pharmacologic agents are reserved for those patients who have persistent symptoms despite good dietary compliance. Treatment with the sulfonylurea agents may facilitate early insulin secretion and prevent the reactive hypoglycemia. Tolbutamide, 250 mg. given orally three times daily, or chlorpropamide, 100 to 250 mg. each morning, has been effective for some patients. (This use of these agents is not listed in the manufacturer's official directives.)

Other Types of Reactive Hypoglycemia

Rarely, a deficiency of growth hormone or of a gluconeogenic enzyme (fructose- 1,6-diphosphatase) may be associated with reactive hypoglycemia. When reactive hypoglycemia cannot be classified it is termed idiopathic reactive hypoglycemia. The dietary measures outlined earlier can be used to provide symptomatic relief for these patients. No specific pharmacologic agents are available to treat these disorders. Diazoxide is useful in treating *fasting* hypoglycemia associated with islet cell tumors but has no role in treatment of the reactive types of hypoglycemia.

OBESITY

method of
GEORGE V. MANN, M.D.
Nashville, Tennessee

The clinician confronts two practical questions in the management of obesity in his patients. The first is whom to treat—the second is how to treat. Neither problem has an entirely satisfactory solution, but for those who face them, here are the best available answers.

Whom to Treat

This issue immediately involves a measurement classification of obesity. There is no feasible clinical way to measure body fat directly, although that is the measurement we need. On the average, adult well-nourished women have about 25 per cent of their body weight as fat, and adult men have about 15 per cent. Women need to be reminded that there is no method for redistributing fat or for locally reducing, the raucous massage and shaking industry notwithstanding. Relative weight is presently the best index of obesity. It relates actual weight for a given height and sex to a reference population of insured persons who had the best health performances (see Table 1). Quetelet's index (W/H^2) may be a little more precise mathematically, but it lacks the ease of interpretation of relative weight.

The critical issue is how far individuals can deviate from relative weight 1.00 before health is impaired in either the short or long term. The best information comes from the insurance data now supplemented by the great prospective studies of selected populations at Framingham and Tecumseh. Health risks in those experiences increased when relative weight was less than 0.9 or more than 1.25. Lesser degrees of leanness and fatness are not importantly related to health, although they do often have great cosmetic and therefore social significance, especially for women.

Coronary heart disease is only weakly related to obesity. Weight reduction has not been shown to be an effective preventive or treatment. High blood pressure is related to obesity and there is some evidence for a lowering of blood pressure with weight loss, but such a treatment is not as effective as modern drug regimens. It seems reasonable that arthritis would be aggravated by obesity, but this has not been rigorously proven. In my experience, even minimal rheumatoid arthritis is worsened by exercise. This is one of the rare contraindications to a fitness program.

The fact that three fourths of all adult-onset diabetics are obese and that 80 per cent of such diabetics would heal their diabetes if they regained

TABLE 1. **Fogarty International Center Conference on Obesity Recommended Weight in Relation to Height***

HEIGHT		MEN		WOMEN	
Feet	*Inches*	*Average*	*Range*	*Average*	*Range*
4	10	. . .	. . .	102	92–119
4	11	. . .	. . .	104	94–122
5	0	. . .	. . .	107	96–125
5	1	. . .	. . .	110	99–128
5	2	123	112–141	113	102–131
5	3	127	115–144	116	105–134
5	4	130	118–148	120	108–138
5	5	133	121–152	123	111–142
5	6	136	124–156	128	114–146
5	7	140	128–161	132	118–150
5	8	145	132–166	136	122–154
5	9	149	136–170	140	126–158
5	10	153	140–174	144	130–163
5	11	158	144–179	148	134–168
6	0	162	148–184	152	138–173
6	1	166	152–189	. . .	. . .
6	2	171	156–194	. . .	. . .
6	3	176	160–199	. . .	. . .
6	4	181	164–204	. . .	. . .

*Height without shoes, weight without clothes. Adapted from the table of the Metropolitan Life Insurance Company.

normal weight ought to be a powerful tool for the physician in motivating obese patients. The emphasis in treatment and prevention of diabetes ought to be on fitness, since there is no real justification for the traditional diabetic diet. The old-fashioned practice of sending fat folks to a dietician for a preposterous 800 or 1200 kcal. diet is foolishness. The hub-bub raised over cyclamates and saccharin comes down to two simple facts— artificial sweeteners have no established efficacy for either diabetes or obesity, and they may be carcinogenic. Their promotion arises from the billion-dollar soft drink industry, which has no alternative sweeteners.

How to Treat

There is no effective dietary treatment of obesity. The perennial and profitable dietary regimens are promotional devices, usually for publishers and authors. Many of these regimens are harmful, because all starvation regimens will set in motion a train of physiologic adaptations, which are both uncomfortable and sometimes dangerous for the subject (see Table 2). This series of events occurs irrespective of the dietary mixture used in the starvation regimen. It is the body's response to the emergency of starvation. Many of the adaptations are energy-conserving and so tend to defeat the goal of the regimen. Only the most highly motivated persons can master the discomforts and persist. A research proposal suggested that a high protein/low energy diet (protein-modified fast) would allow the body to burn stored fat while minimizing some of these side effects, especially the negative nitrogen balance. The proposal is not yet thoroughly investigated, but even so, the protein-modified fast is the basis for the current ill-founded "last chance diet" and the scourge of overpriced protein supplements.

The most effective stimulus for preserving body nitrogen and minimizing the side effects of calorie deprivation while burning body fat is exercise. This is the strategy that coaches and horse trainers use in bringing athletes to high levels of fitness with extreme leanness. This strategy has the additional merit of developing fitness, which has other subjective and health advantages.

The physician confronted with an overweight patient, whether presenting as a cosmetic or a real health threat, must recognize that the first few weeks of treatment will require a great deal of professional support. Since many physicians cannot supply this, they are well-advised to send their obese patients to some paramedical organization in the community, such as TOPS or Weight Watchers. The physician's responsibility is that of evaluating the patient's suitability for exercise and dieting by making exercise cardiographs, ventilometry, and evaluating any disorders of bone and joint. The physician can also effectively motivate the patient by pointing out the health hazards of obesity and the advantages of fitness.

Amphetamines have now been essentially removed as a drug treatment of obesity for lack of efficacy. Ileal bypass remains a research procedure for the most desperate problems (relative weight greater than 3). It can be properly and safely done by only a few research centers. Such a device as jaw-wiring is hardly deserving of consideration.

In Summary

1. Determine the patient's relative weight (Table 1) and make a decision about the patient's motivation to lose weight.

2. Explain the relative risks of obesity to the patient.

3. Evaluate the patient's suitability for exercise by measuring heart, lung, and skeletal competency.

4. Refer the patient to a paramedical weight management program.

5. Ask the patient to return at 3-month intervals for measurement of his progress.

TABLE 2. **Adaptive Responses to Starvation**

1. Preoccupied with food
2. Social disorder
3. Escape—Migration
4. Lethargy
5. Depression (not suicidal)
6. Pigmentation
7. Loss of secondary sexual characteristics
8. Polyuria—edema
9. Bradycardia
10. Anemia
11. Cannibalism
12. Residual "gefangenitis"

PELLAGRA

method of
WILLIAM B. BEAN, M.D.
Galveston, Texas

Pellagra, first described by Casal in Spain, nearly 250 years ago, with a few elements resembling kwashiorkor, is likely to slip by most alert physicians and medical teams in this country today. Certainly the doctor in his office misses it because he has never seen it and has not been taught about it. The name "pellagra," *pelle agra*, means rough skin. It has nothing to do with photosensitivity. No photochemical reaction is required, although exposure to sunlight is the most common cause of nonspecific damage which determines its cutaneous localization. Most people who suffer from nicotinic acid deficiency have suffered a long time from a reduction of calories and protein of good biologic value. They develop pellagra as but one of a cluster of deficiencies. Absolutely pure nicotinic acid deficiency exists only among bacteria or in laboratory animals.

Pellagra has been a characteristic deficiency where maize, corn, has been the staple energy food. One of the mysteries which developed after it was known that nicotinic acid would correct black tongue in dogs and correct or prevent the manifestations of pellagra was that there was no sharp relationship—sometimes not a close one—between the level of reduction of nicotinic acid in the diet and the probability of getting pellagra. It turned out that tryptophan could be converted into nicotinic acid, although the reverse process does not occur in nature. Because nicotinic acid is a component of two coenzymes, NAD^+ and $NADP^+$, which are concerned with tissue respiration, fat synthesis, and glycolysis, it is not surprising that the energy output is connected with the development of clinical manifestations. We do not know whether North and South American Indians, who used much maize, had pellagra. Where maize was the only or main source of calories, they must have had pellagra.

In many cases, vitamin deficiency diseases are related to that recurring combination of poverty and ignorance. In most practice in the United States, pellagra is secondary to some disease, or process, which reduces the intake and assimilation of a balanced diet or greatly increases need. A diet dependent upon corn for energy not only lacks nicotinic acid but is not rich in tryptophan, which by way of kynurenine and hydroxyanthranilic acid becomes nicotinic acid, although it is not a simple relationship. About 60 mg. of tryptophan may be needed to make 1 mg. of nicotinic acid.

Pellagra used to be recognized by the four D's: dermatitis, diarrhea, dementia, and death. This brings back memories of days when brain tumors were diagnosed by convulsions, hemiplegia, and advanced destruction of the nervous system, not by the early manifestations. Today, in the United States, wheat and corn flour have had restored a modicum of the things milled out, and this flour or meal is referred to as "enriched." It does, indeed, contain added niacin, thiamine, riboflavin, and some minerals. Few persons on reducing diets develop pellagra, despite their poor choice of what they may eat. Others have malabsorption and do not get value returned for what they take in through the mouth. The person who drinks alcohol to excess may get the rest of his calories from salted crackers, potato chips, pretzels, and other naked calories.

If one looks sharply for the bright red tongue, the strange behavior of the alimentary canal, and mental aberration in hospitals where people with diseases of the alimentary canal, cancer, or other chronic ills of the ailing are, pellagra may be recognized. In old persons, the combination of aging, inertia, and neglect by children and friends leads to depression, which is likely to result in eating habits which almost selectively neglect food of good biologic value, especially meats and protein-rich foods.

Specific Treatment

One does not treat a disease, except accidentally, if it is not recognized. Once the notion that pellagra might exist gets into the mind of a physician, he will immediately do what is necessary. Pellagra occurring in hospital patients or in people who have not been exposed to sunlight is often associated with dermatitis from pressure or irritation. This is often overlooked. Diagnosis by exclusion is the resort of those destitute of ideas, but it is still important to remember that if there is a suspicion of vitamin deficiency, no harm will be done by using what is suspected of being the missing vitamin. Unfortunately with pellagra the sore tongue may make it impossible or difficult to ingest food or pills. Thus it may be necessary to start an attack on identified pellagra by giving a significant amount of parenteral nicotinic acid. Within a few hours the red and irritated tongue may resume its normal color. Its edema disappears. The alimentary canal becomes quiet, although it may not return to normal completely. Usually the mental aberrations are corrected rapidly. Most pellagra seen in hospitals is *secondary*, resulting from disease which increases metabolism, reduces absorption, or diminishes appetite and what is eaten. Thus it is likely to be but part of the manifestation of multiple nutritional deficiency states.

Once niacin has been given, the pellagrous patient may rapidly regain appetite, partly because the painful lesions of the mouth and tongue have begun to heal and partly because of a brighter mental outlook. There is also a surge in a sense of well-being, real but hard to measure.

Therapy for patients with less severe or complicated cases should begin with nicotinamide in doses of 100 to 150 mg. twice a day. Sequential release capsules are supposed to maintain a fairly constant level, but this is quite different from the natural three-meals-a-day sequence and advantages are not clearly known. In addition to specific therapy with nicotinamide, a good, balanced, nutritious diet selected from items a patient can and will eat should be prepared. A search should be made for other vitamin, protein, and mineral deficiencies and these corrected if found. Most patients with pellagra suffer from calorie shortage as well as protein deprivation, and these deficiencies should be corrected.

Supportive Therapy

When the patient has made his initial response, we begin a program of complete correction of dietary inadequacies and the employment of a truly balanced diet with approximately 1 gram of protein for each kilogram of body weight to help build up the deficiency in those chronically malnourished. Energy material should be provided to keep dietary protein from being used as fuel. For a 70 kg. person, 70 grams of protein will provide just over 11 grams of nitrogen. About 2250 kilogram calories are needed every day. Most routine hospital diets, if eaten completely, provide at least this much. There may be reason to give supplements between meals or to give a large number of small feedings for a while. Supplementary vitamin capsules containing the recommended daily allowances may be useful, but the sheet anchor of therapy is a judiciously chosen, ample, and balanced diet.

Prevention

Although the restoration to flour of portions of the vitamins and minerals milled out has been called "enrichment," this term suggests wishful and wistful thinking rather than careful evaluation. Its effect has been probably more important in reducing beriberi among chronic alcohol addicts, for most of them will eat at least a sandwich a day with some thiamine in white bread. We know that with intervening disease, poverty, and food fads with outrageously unbalanced diets, many forms of malnutrition will continue. Pellagra, although unusual, can be treated and corrected specifically. This may be lifesaving, and it invariably produces a welcome return or increase in the sense of well-being and a restoration of good health.

RICKETS AND OSTEOMALACIA

method of
BOY FRAME, M.D.,
and MICHAEL KLEEREKOPER, M.D.
Detroit, Michigan

Rickets and osteomalacia result from impaired mineralization of bone matrix. Rickets is a defect in enchondral bone formation and occurs before closure of the cartilaginous growth plates, whereas osteomalacia is an abnormality of appositional bone formation and occurs after the growth plates are fused. Pathogenesis and therapy of the two conditions are similar and can conveniently be considered together. The underlying metabolic derangement can often be pinpointed, and the response to adequate treatment is usually most gratifying in terms of alleviating the skeletal disability.

Recent major advances in our knowledge of vitamin D (ergocalciferol) metabolism have led to the realization that this compound is the precursor of a well-regulated hormonal system. Via a series of successive hydroxylation reactions, more active metabolites of the parent vitamin are formed in the liver and kidney (Figure 1). The terminology used in this chapter will reflect the hormonal nature of the vitamin D system (Table 1).

Ergocalciferol (Calciferol) remains the only compound in this system that is readily available and therefore is still the mainstay of current therapy for rickets and osteomalacia. However, several of the newly discovered metabolites are undergoing extensive clinical trial and should become more readily available in the near future. Where appropriate, we shall indicate the form and dosage of these newer compounds that have been successfully used in treatment. These metabolites offer several advantages over conventional ergocalciferol therapy: lower and more physiologic doses, more rapid onset of action, shorter half-life, which

TABLE 1.   **Nomenclature of Vitamin D and Metabolites**

AS A VITAMIN	AS A HORMONE
Vitamin D_2	Ergocalciferol
Vitamin D_3	Cholecalciferol
25 Hydroxyvitamin D_3(25OH D_3)	25 Hydroxycholecalciferol (25HCC)
1-25 Dihydroxyvitamin D_3 (1-25$(OH)_2D_3$)	1-25 Dihydroxycholecalciferol (1-25DHCC)
24-25 Dihydroxyvitamin D_3 (24-25$(OH)_2D_3$)	24-25 Dihydroxycholecalciferol (24-25DHCC)

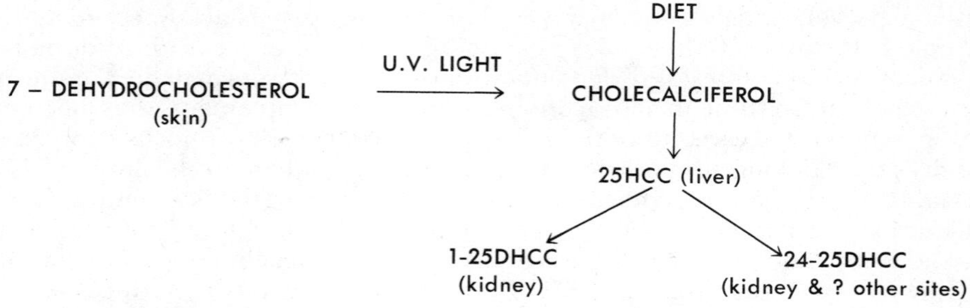

Figure 1. Schematic representation of the metabolism of vitamin D.

becomes important if hypercalcemia develops during treatment, and greater specificity for certain rachitic or osteomalacic states.

Since ergocalciferol and its metabolites are available in pure chemical form, units of weight rather than the older terminology of international units will be used. Forty thousand (40,000) International Units (I.U.) of ergocalciferol are equal to 1 mg. and 400 I.U. are equal to 10 micrograms.

Ergocalciferol Deficiency

The widespread use of vitamin supplements and fortification of foods has largely eliminated the occurrence of ergocalciferol deficiency rickets and osteomalacia in the western world. Their occurrence now is usually the result of poverty, ignorance, and unusual dietary habits within small segments of the population. Dark-skinned populations with little exposure to sunlight are particularly susceptible, because under these circumstances the synthesis of ergocalciferol that normally takes place in the skin is reduced. Rickets is most apt to occur in premature infants and infants receiving unenriched cow's milk.

Prophylaxis. The prophylactic dose of ergocalciferol required to prevent rickets in children is generally agreed to be 10 micrograms per day, whereas in adults 2.5 micrograms per day is considered adequate to prevent osteomalacia. Some enthusiastic mothers may give additional ergocalciferol supplements to infants who are already receiving the minimal daily requirement of the vitamin in fortified milk and other foodstuffs. This is to be discouraged, as some infants are unduly sensitive to the effects of ergocalciferol and may develop hypercalcemia with its attendant risks.

Treatment. Although smaller doses may occasionally be effective, it is advisable to administer at least 100 micrograms of ergocalciferol (Calciferol) daily for children and 50 to 100 micrograms daily for adults until a response is obtained. This is measured by a return of the serum calcium and phosphorus levels to near normal in 7 to 10 days and roentgenologic improvement of rachitic

changes or pseudofractures in 4 to 6 weeks. It may be several months, however, before the elevated alkaline phosphatase level returns to normal.

Not infrequently, symptomatic hypocalcemia may be present either before or immediately after initiation of treatment with ergocalciferol, especially in infants. Under these circumstances intravenous calcium gluconate should be given initially, to be followed by oral calcium supplements until normal serum calcium levels are attained.

Vitamin D Dependent Rickets (Pseudo-Calciferol Deficiency Rickets)

This form of hereditary rickets clinically resembles ergocalciferol deficiency rickets, with the exception that it requires lifelong pharmacologic doses (0.5 to 1.5 mg. per day) of ergocalciferol for correction of the mineral and skeletal defect.

Recent studies have demonstrated that patients with this disease appear to have defective synthesis of 1-25 dihydroxycholecalciferol in the renal cortex. Biochemical and skeletal response occurs with as little as 1 to 2 micrograms of 1-25DHCC and 1-αhydroxycholecalciferol given daily.

Intestinal Malabsorption

Both rickets and osteomalacia, resulting from impaired absorption of ergocalciferol, may occur in association with intestinal malabsorption from different causes.

If the underlying cause of the intestinal malabsorption can be successfully treated, a smaller initial dose or a reduction in the established dose of ergocalciferol may be required to prevent intoxication with the vitamin. Osteomalacia after gastric surgery can usually be treated by the oral administration of 100 to 200 micrograms daily. In gluten enteropathy, complete cure of rickets and osteomalacia is possible with a gluten-free diet alone. If more rapid treatment of the bone disease is required, 1 to 2 mg. of ergocalciferol may be administered daily until radiologic improvement is noted and the elevated alkaline phosphatase level returns to normal. Osteoporosis frequently accompanies the osteomalacia in malabsorption states and does not respond to this treatment. In those malabsorption states that do not respond to treatment of the primary intestinal disorder, lifelong administration of as much as 1 to 10 mg. of ergocalciferol daily, along with calcium supplements, may be necessary. Parental administration of ergocalciferol might normally be recommended in treatment of rickets or osteomalacia due to intestinal malabsorption, except that a reliable preparation for parental use is not readily available. Magnesium supplements may also be required before symptomatic hypocalcemia is corrected in some instances of intestinal malabsorption.

Primary Hypophosphatemia, Rickets, and Osteomalacia

Since the pathogenesis of this disorder has not been completely defined, treatment cannot be based on the rational correction of a specific metabolic error. Proper therapy requires a long-term close cooperation between the patient, his family, and the physician. There is a difference of opinion as to whether initiation of treatment in early infancy will result in normal growth and prevention of deformities.

In most cases the disorder is first recognized in a child who is just learning to walk. Therapy with 1 to 2 mg. of ergocalciferol daily is initiated, and 0.25 to 0.50 mg. increments in the dose are considered every 3 to 4 months. Only rarely are more than 3 to 4 mg. of ergocalciferol required daily. The ideal dose of ergocalciferol to initiate and maintain healing, but yet to deter vitamin toxicity, is often most difficult to achieve. Improvement is gauged by radiologic signs of healing and prevention of deformities, and toxicity is measured by the appearance of hypercalcemia with its attendant risks, mainly renal insufficiency. The levels of serum phosphorus may remain low and the alkaline phosphatase elevated, even in the presence of radiologic healing. Corrective osteotomics are best delayed, if possible, until after cessation of growth. The dose of ergocalciferol should be discontinued or markedly curtailed during the period of bed rest and casting before and several months after corrective surgery. If this is not done, the added factor of immobilization may be sufficient to cause hypercalcemia.

After closure of growth cartilages the dose of ergocalciferol can often be reduced to 0.5 to 1.0 mg. daily, but lifelong treatment is recommended to prevent reactivation of the disease which may occur during middle life.

There are theoretical reasons why additional measures to increase the serum phosphorus levels in resistant rickets are warranted. Since even optimal doses of ergocalciferol do not return phosphorus levels to normal, the administration of oral phosphate supplements has been used for this purpose. That phosphorus supplements alone do not initiate adequate healing in childhood resistant rickets is well documented. However, the administration of 1 to 2 grams of elemental phosphorus given each day, with the onset of diarrhea as the limiting factor, reduces the daily requirement of ergocalciferol by 0.5 to 1 mg., thus reducing the chance of vitamin toxicity. Frequent small doses of the oral phosphate supplements with a bedtime dose are better tolerated, and a more persistent elevation of the serum phosphorus is attained. Another maneuver that is occasionally helpful in increasing the tolerance of large amounts of supplemental phosphorus is the use of powdered forms of phosphorus in the cooking of stew, hamburgers, and so on. At the onset of therapy, 0.5 to 1.0 gram of extraelemental calcium per day is beneficial, but after optimal healing is attained the calcium present in a fully nutritious diet is adequate.

Rarely, sporadic and vitamin D-resistant hypophosphatemic osteomalacia occurs for the first time during adolescence or in adulthood. The biochemical findings are similar to the sex-linked form of vitamin D resistant rickets but are different, in that severe skeletal pain and muscle weakness are invariably present. The principles of calciferol administration are similar in both instances but phosphate supplements are more efficacious in the adult-onset variety. In fact, a number of such adult patients have shown improvement in both muscle weakness and osteomalacia with 2 to 3 grams of oral phosphate supplements as the only form of therapy. Excessive phosphate may lead to hypocalcemia and secondary hyperparathyroidism with its deleterious effect on the skeleton.

An acquired form of sporadic hypophosphatemic osteomalacia has been reported in association with certain vascular and giant cell tumors. This form of the disease will respond to phosphate supplements and ergocalciferol therapy. However, if the tumor is resectable, the osteomalacia is usually cured or greatly improved once the tumor is removed.

The general principles of therapy for primary hypophosphatemic rickets and osteomalacia also apply when there are associated findings of renal glycosuria and aminoaciduria, as in some of the complex renal tubular disorders.

Hyperchloremic Acidosis

Hyperchloremic acidosis occurring as a result of renal tubular acidosis and after ureterosigmoidostomy may be associated with clinical rickets or osteomalacia. The defect in mineralization may, in part, be related to the metabolic acidosis itself, but concomitant factors such as renal phosphate wasting and hypophosphatemia are also factors to consider. Since the skeletal disability is often incapacitating, it is desirable to initiate therapy with both ergocalciferol and alkali therapy. Usually 1 to 2 mg. of ergocalciferol given daily over a period of 6 to 8 months is sufficient to restore normal mineralization of the skeleton. In addition, sufficient alkali in the form of sodium bicarbonate or sodium citrate is given to correct the systemic acidosis as measured by normal or near normal levels of serum chloride and bicarbonate. Ten to 15 grams of sodium bicarbonate may be required each day, which might present a problem if cardiac decompensation is present. After healing of the bone disease, alkali therapy alone will prevent recurrence of the skeletal disturbance. When phosphate depletion is present, additional oral phosphate supplements will help initiate healing more rapidly.

Renal Osteodystrophy

Progressive renal glomerular insufficiency leads to a complex metabolic bone disorder that includes osteomalacia (or rickets), osteitis fibrosa, osteoporosis, and osteosclerosis. While the course of the bone disease is quite variable, biochemical evidence of secondary hyperparathyroidism can be demonstrated when the creatinine clearance falls below 70 ml. per minute. Osteomalacia, on the other hand, is not common before the creatinine clearance falls below 30 ml. per minute. In patients who are susceptible to osteomalacia from other causes (e.g., concomitant use of phenytoin [Dilantin or phenobarbital]) significant osteomalacia may occur earlier in the disease.

Since a combination of skeletal diseases is more usual in renal osteodystrophy than pure osteomalacia or osteitis fibrosa alone, one cannot discuss the treatment of one without some reference to treatment of the other.

Adequate attention to diet is probably more directly important in the treatment of renal osteodystrophy than in any other skeletal disease except nutritional osteomalacia. Dietary phosphate intake must be reduced as renal function declines, since phosphate retention promotes secondary hyperparathyroidism and soft tissue calcification, as well as contributing to the hypocalcemia. Impaired synthesis of 1-25DHCC in uremia is most directly reflected in decreased intestinal absorption of calcium. The dietary intake of calcium should be maintained at 1000 mg. per day and is best achieved by supplementing the diet with calcium carbonate. This form of calcium supplement has an advantage over calcium lactate or gluconate since it has significant phosphate binding effects in the intestine and thereby helps maintain a more normal serum phosphate. (Calcium carbonate is not as effective a phosphate binding agent as aluminum hydroxide and most patients will require aluminum hydroxide therapy in addition to dietary phosphate restriction and calcium carbonate).

Ergocalciferol in large doses (usually 2.5 mg. per day or higher) will cause significant healing of osteomalacia in most uremic patients. It is usual to start with 0.5 mg. daily and increase the dose until symptomatic improvement occurs. Biochemically there will be a progressive increase in the serum calcium as the ergocalciferol begins to take effect. The alkaline phosphatase usually rises as bone healing occurs (alkaline phosphatase flare), and this enzyme should be monitored as well as the serum calcium. As the phosphatase returns towards normal, one should start decreasing the dose of ergocalciferol to avoid hypercalcemia. Crystalline dihydrotachysterol (DHT) (investigational) has some theoretical advantages over ergocalciferol because it does not require 1-hydroxylation in the kidney to be effective. DHT has added practical advantages over ergocalciferol. Its onset of action is quicker and if hypercalcemia does complicate therapy, the serum calcium will return to normal more quickly after stopping the DHT. The usual dosage is 0.25 to 0.75 mg. of DHT daily.

The newer metabolites of calciferol, 25 hydroxycholecalciferol, 1,25 dihydroxycholecalciferol and 1-αhydroxycholecalciferol have been somewhat disappointing in clinical trials with respect to treatment of the osteomalacic component of renal osteodystrophy. They have, however, been shown to be of great benefit in reducing secondary hyperparathyroidism. The daily doses that have been used in these trials are 50 to 100 micrograms of 25HCC and 1 to 2 micrograms of 1,25DHCC or 1-αhydroxycholecalciferol.

The best treatment for renal osteodystrophy is unquestionably renal transplantation and restoration of normal renal function. However, there are certain skeleton complications peculiar to the post-transplant state. In the immediate post-transplant period there is a rise in the serum calcium, occasionally to hypercalcemic levels. This is usually a transient phenomenon and spontaneous return to normocalcemia usually occurs over a period of a few weeks to a few months. If hypercalcemia persists, subtotal parathyroidectomy may be indicated. A more frequent complication is aseptic necrosis of the femoral head (occasionally also the humeral head). The use of glucocorticoids for immunosuppression has been implicated in the pathogenesis. This cannot be the only factor, since it is occasionally seen in patients prior to transplantation and treatment with steroids. An occasional skeletal complication after renal transplantation is the development of hypophosphatemic osteomalacia. This is consequent to tubular dysfunction leading to a renal phosphate leak in the transplanted kidney. This lesion usually responds well to supplemental phosphate therapy.

SCURVY

(Vitamin C Deficiency)

method of
VICTOR HERBERT, M.D.
Brooklyn, New York

Vitamin C

Chemistry. Ascorbic acid is the physiologically active form of vitamin C. Iron and copper salts, alkaline pH, heat, and light facilitate the oxidation of ascorbic acid to dehydroascorbic acid, which remains active as a vitamin. Further oxidation renders the vitamin irreversibly inactive.

Sources. Ascorbic acid is widely distributed, chiefly in plant products, especially vegetables and fruits, whereas grains and cereals contain little. More than 100 mg. per 100 grams is found in broccoli greens, Brussels sprouts, collards, black currants, guava, horseradish, kale, turnip greens, parsley, and sweet peppers. About 50 to 99 mg. per 100 grams occurs in cabbage, cauliflower, chives, kohlrabi, orange pulp, lemon pulp, mustard greens, beet greens, papaya, spinach, strawberries, and watercress. About 30 to 49 mg. per 100 grams is found in asparagus, lima beans, Swiss chard, gooseberries, currants, grapefruit, limes, loganberries, melons (cantaloupe), okra, tangerines, potatoes, and turnips. Potatoes and cabbage may be consumed in large quantities by low-economic groups, and can provide rather large intakes of ascorbic acid.

Absorption. Intestinal absorption of ascorbic acid depends on the amount that is ingested, up to certain limits. If these limits are exceeded, there will be excessive loss of the vitamin in the gastrointestinal tract, with the corresponding osmotic attraction of water and production of diarrhea. Absorbed ascorbic acid is used for metabolic functions and saturation of tissue stores, and excess is largely excreted by the kidneys.

Metabolic Functions. (1) Metabolism of some amino acids. (2) Metabolism of iron and keeping folic acid in the reduced state. (3) Catecholamine metabolism. (4) Connective tissue metabolism via hydroxylation of proline and collagen crosslinking (wound healing). (5) Tooth and bone metabolism. (6) Blood coagulation. (7) Immune response. (8) Electron transport chain. (9) Possibly cholesterol metabolism.

Tissue Stores. Ascorbic acid has been found in large amounts in adrenals, pituitary gland, thymus, and corpus luteum. The saturated body pool of ascorbic acid has been estimated to be 1500 mg., with a daily utilization of 3 per cent (45 mg.). Signs and symptoms of ascorbic acid deficiency appear when tissue stores have been reduced over 80 per cent (body pool below 300 mg.).

Urinary Excretion. Ascorbic acid in excess of metabolic requirements and tissue storage capacity is excreted in the urine. The handling of ascorbic acid is similar to that of glucose. The renal threshold is approximately 1.4 mg. per dl. (100 ml.). When larger doses of ascorbic acid are present, the organism adapts by increasing the glomerular filtration rate and catabolism of the vitamin, with urinary excretion of its metabolites. Among these metabolites, one of the best characterized is oxalic acid. The further catabolism of this metabolite differs among individuals, with some persons more susceptible to oxaluria than others after the ingestion of large amounts (above 1 gram) of ascorbic acid.

Requirements

Because a saturated body pool of ascorbic acid is maintained in healthy men by 45 mg. per day, and because 10 mg. or slightly less per day will prevent and even cure clinical scurvy, the National Academy of Sciences recommends a daily dietary allowance (RDA: Recommended Dietary Allowance) of 35 mg. for infants, 40 mg. for children up to age 11 years, 45 mg. for adults, 60 mg. for pregnant women, and 80 mg. for lactating women. These recommendations meet (and actually exceed) the known nutritional needs of essentially all healthy persons. Needs for ascorbic acid may be slightly increased in situations of increased metabolism (e.g., hyperthyroidism), infections, inflammation, drug therapy (estrogens, antacids), smoking, and growth. However, no studies suggest that this increase would exceed the RDA, and alleged "antistress" actions of ascorbic acid have not been confirmed in man. Premature infants seem to do well with 50 mg. per day.

Treatment of Deficiency

Ascorbic acid deficiency is characterized by follicular hyperkeratotic lesions containing fragmented or coiled hairs, perifollicular petechiae, ecchymoses, spongy bleeding gums, poor wound healing, fatigue, swollen joints, muscular aches, and sometimes edema. There may be Sjögren's sicca syndrome or the "neurotic triad" of hysteria, depression, and hypochondriasis.

The only absolute indication for treatment with vitamin C is scurvy. Although as little as 10 mg. per day is enough to treat scurvy, oral doses of 100 mg. three times daily are recommended, and will replenish the body pools within about 5 days. If the patient's mouth is sore, swallowing is difficult, or intestinal absorption is impaired, parenteral administration of 250 to 500 mg. of vitamin C in an isotonic saline solution can be used. With these doses improvement is rapid, and after 1 week the doses should be gradually reduced until the patient is able to achieve a dietary intake of 45 mg. per day. Because malnutrition usually includes deficiencies of other vitamins, the patient should receive, in addition to vitamin C, one multivitamin capsule each day and, as soon as possible, a well-balanced diet. It is safe to continue vitamin supplements for up to 1 month. Doses greater than 100 mg. per day may induce increased catabolism of the vitamin, which continues after the doses have been reduced, and the increased catabolism can produce "rebound scurvy" if doses of 1 gram or more daily are stopped abruptly rather than tapered by about 10 to 20 per cent a day.

Toxic Effects

Although none of the published clinical trials have reported any significant toxicity of ascorbic acid in doses as high as 3 to 6 grams per day for a limited number of days, such large doses should be avoided because of these potential toxic effects: oxalic aciduria and renal stones, uric aciduria, increased urinary calcium, decreased urinary sodium, and hemolytic anemia in patients with glucose-6-phosphate dehydrogenase (G-6-PD) deficiency or sickle cell disease. A case has been reported of acute renal failure and death in a 68 year old man with G-6-PD deficiency who received 80 grams of ascorbic acid intravenously for 2 consecutive days. Large intakes of the vitamin have also been shown to interfere with certain tests for urine or serum vitamin B_{12}, glucose, uric acid, and iron, thus rendering these tests dangerously inaccurate. Destruction of food vitamin B_{12} by megadoses of ascorbate has been reported, but is disputed; vitamin B_{12} absorption may be reduced.

Allegations continue to be made that vitamin C is useful for the prevention and treatment of the common cold. A weak antihistamine effect is alleged. The available evidence, although implying that some slight effects may occur, suggests that any benefit is minimal and that there is no greater value of doses in excess of 200 mg. per day than is achieved by 200 mg. The alleged effects of the vitamin in treatment of cancer are compatible with placebo effect.

VITAMIN K DEFICIENCY

method of
RUTH ANDREA SEELER, M.D.
Chicago, Illinois

The physiologic requirement for the fat-soluble vitamin K is normally met from diet (K_1) or de novo bacterial synthesis (K_2) in the large bowel accompanied by normal gastrointestinal absorption. Vitamin K is not stored in the body and thus a constant supply is required for the synthesis of coagulation factors II, VII, IX, and X. Any pathologic process that affects fat absorption, gastrointestinal mobility, or bacterial flora may have significant effects on the coagulation status. The usual dietary source of vitamin K is from green leafy vegetables. The pharmacologic need is extremely small, approximately 4 to 6 micrograms per day for an infant, and 50 to 100 micrograms per day for an adult, compared to the conventional therapeutic dose, which is measured in milligrams (1000 micrograms).

Vitamin K is needed only for the addition of the calcium binding site, a gamma carboxyl amino acid, to the inactive precursor coagulation molecules. Precursor synthesis is not limited in the absence of vitamin K and thus correction of the hemorrhagic phenomenon is extremely rapid when vitamin K is administered parenterally (intravenously or intramuscularly). The hemorrhagic symptoms abate 1 to 1½ hours after parenteral vitamin K administration, and the prolonged prothrombin time and partial thromboplastin time will revert to normal in 4 to 12 hours after therapy. In fact, there is no faster way to correct a vitamin K deficient coagulation disturbance than parenteral administration of vitamin K. By the time one is able to get type specific fresh frozen plasma thawed and transfused into the patient, the same patient would synthesize sufficient amounts of the active coagulation factors II, VII, IX, and X to achieve hemostasis. Vitamin K_1 will not be as therapeutically dramatic in the face of vitamin K antagonist overdose. If a bleeding patient does not respond to vitamin K, there is no benefit to be derived from repeating the dose.

Vitamin K should be given either intramuscularly or subcutaneously whenever possible. There have been extremely rare anaphylactic type reactions following rapid intravenous administration. If intravenous administration is required, vitamin K should not be given faster than 1 mg. per minute.

Neonate

The normal neonate synthesizes factors II, VII, IX, and X after transplacental passage of vitamin K. In the fetus or in the newborn there is hepatic immaturity, which results in lower levels of factors II, VII, IX, and X than found in the adult but adequate to assure hemostasis. The circulating half-lives of these coagulation factors are measured in hours, and thus one would expect a decline if there is no further synthesis. Initially, after birth the baby must rely on exogenous dietary sources of vitamin K as the gastrointestinal tract is sterile. Artificial formulas are now all fortified with vitamin K_1. Thus, if the infant feeds well, it will be no problem. Breast-fed infants are still at considerable jeopardy, as colostrum contains even less vitamin K than human milk, which has only 1.5 micrograms per liter. In addition, there is delayed colonization of the large bowel and the flora are different from those of artificially fed infants. Thus, the breast-fed infant has a lower endogenous bacterial production of vitamin K_2 plus low dietary intake. To prevent hemorrhagic disease of the newborn, it is prudent to give all infants 1 mg. of vitamin K_1 (AquaMephyton, Konakion). Although the physiologic requirement is approximately 4 to 6 micrograms, the traditional dose is 1 mg. (1,000 micrograms) This dose has proven safe in prospective studies including glucose 6-phosphate dehydrogenase deficient infants.

Infants under 6 months of age who are exclusively breast-fed should probably receive an injection of 1 mg. of vitamin K_1 should they be scheduled for elective surgery. As mentioned, their vitamin K status is precarious.

Maternal Use of Anticonvulsants

A special subgroup of full-term infants with severe hemorrhagic disease due to vitamin K deficiency are those infants born to mothers with epilepsy taking hydantoins or barbiturate anticonvulsants. In contrast to the usual hemorrhagic disease of the newborn seen on the second or third day of life, the hemorrhage in these infants may be present at birth or within hours and is unusually severe, including a number of fatalities due to intracranial hemorrhage. The mothers of these infants uniformly have normal coagulation values.

The mechanism has been studied for phenytoin (diphenylhydantoin)). The drug crosses the placenta and exhibits a competitive inhibition with vitamin K similar to that of warfarin. In the fetus, phenytoin is metabolized very slowly and thus becomes concentrated in the liver. The depressed liver enzymatic activity characteristic of the perinate makes the drug more toxic to the perinate than to the mother.

Such women should receive 10 mg. of vitamin K_1 intramuscularly during early labor, and the infant should receive vitamin K_1 immediately after birth. If the infant has clinical hemorrhage, the child should be treated with 10 ml. per kg. of fresh frozen plasma. In the face of severe hemorrhage, one should not rely on vitamin K alone because the presence of the hydantoin will continue to provide competitive inhibition. Ideally, one does not wish to use the prothrombin complex concentrates (Konyne or Proplex) unless the hemorrhage is life-threatening because of the hepatitis risk and the fact that young infants frequently become chronic carriers of the hepatitis antigen. In extreme cases, an exchange transfusion with fresh whole blood should be considered.

Hepatitis

In acute viral hepatitis or toxic hepatitis there is decreased synthesis of the vitamin K–dependent coagulation factors due to hepatic cellular dysfunction, which is further compromised by low vitamin K levels resulting from fat malabsorption secondary to the decreased bile in the gastrointestinal tract. Thus, the prolonged prothrombin time in hepatitis frequently can be improved by intramuscular vitamin K_1. Patients with fulminate hepatitic necrosis will not respond to vitamin K and require infusion of fresh frozen plasma to supply the vitamin K–dependent coagulation factors and factor V and fibrinogen, which are also liver made but not vitamin K–dependent. The prothrombin complex concentrates (Konyne and Proplex) are contraindicated in this clinical setting. Normally, the liver inactivates the activated coagulation factors and the activated fibrinolytic system. These functions are also compromised in acute hepatic necrosis and sudden death caused by pulmonary emboli has resulted from the infusion of the prothrombin concentrates in such patients. Therapy should include 10 ml. per kg. of type specific fresh frozen plasma. Intensive plasmapheresis with the infusion of fresh frozen plasma will also restore the coagulation status to normal and should be considered in those patients with advanced hepatic failure and massive hemorrhage.

Malabsorption Syndromes

Patients with chronic malabsorption of any cause (ulcerative colitis, regional enteritis, short bowel syndrome, pancreatic cancer, biliary atresia, idiopathic cholestasis, cystic fibrosis, gluten enteropathy, sprue) are prone to develop vitamin K deficiency. Other pathologic processes that shorten the transit time in the large bowel also produce vitamin K deficiency secondary to failure to absorb vitamin K. Such patients should receive oral prophylactic water-soluble vitamin K_3, either as the sodium disulphate or sodium diphosphate salt (Hykinone, Synkayvite). An adequate prophylactic dose is 5 mg. by mouth once a day of either form of K_3. If the patient with a chronic malabsorption condition develops hemorrhagic symptoms, the therapy would be intramuscular vitamin K_1, 1 to 2 mg. for an infant, or 5 to 10 mg. for an adult.

Infantile Diarrhea Illness

Infants less than 6 months of age not infrequently develop severe coagulation abnormalities with acute diarrheal disease of bacterial or viral cause. This is probably the result of low vitamin K absorption during the diarrheal illness secondary to the hypermobility. The suppression of bacterial flora by antibiotic therapy may further decrease endogenous vitamin K_2 synthesis. Ordinarily, as the diarrhea subsides, the coagulation disturbance spontaneously corrects. Administration of vitamin K is not usually required so long as the diarrhea is not prolonged. In diarrhea lasting more than 7 days, hemorrhagic symptoms may be developed. Prompt correction of the coagulation disorder can be obtained by the administration of 1 mg. of vitamin K_1. This should be repeated at intervals of 4 to 7 days as long as the diarrhea persists. The hemorrhagic problems noted earlier are much less common now that the special formulas for infants with diarrheal illness are all fortified with vitamin K. However, normal vitamin K status requires normal fat absorption as well as sufficient time for absorption.

Infants on intravenous alimentation (hyperalimentation) will develop hemorrhagic disease due to vitamin K deficiency if they do not receive the vitamin K_1 supplementation. One mg. of vitamin K_1 every 7 days is usually adequate.

OSTEOPOROSIS

method of
C. CONRAD JOHNSTON, JR., M.D.
Indianapolis, Indiana

Osteoporosis may be defined as a condition characterized by a decrease in the amount of bone present in the skeleton and by fracture associated with minimal trauma. The bone present in patients with osteoporosis is thought to be normal qualitatively but reduced in quantity. This disorder remains asymptomatic until pain associated with fracture occurs. Microfractures may develop and be the cause of pain; however, microfracture is an unusual manifestation of the disease. The most common sites of fracture in patients with this disorder are the thoracic and lumbar vertebrae, the neck of the femur, and the distal radius. Vertebral collapse fracture is the hallmark of osteoporosis; however, fractures of these parts of the skeleton are often asymptomatic. The major morbidity and mortality associated with this disease is due to fractures of other locations. Postmenopausal women are the most common victims of this disease, but osteoporosis may also occur in elderly males and rarely in young adults of either sex.

The diagnosis may be made by finding a decreased quantity of bone in a patient presenting with fracture when other causes of low bone mass have been excluded. Standard radiographs are usually used to estimate the quantity of bone present, but it should be stressed that this method is both imprecise and insensitive. The standard x-ray does not provide a quantitative estimate of bone mass and only very large changes can be detected. More precise techniques for quantitatively measuring bone mass in the appendicular skeleton are available and include radiogrammetry (i.e., measuring cortical thickness of a phalanx) and photon absorptiometry. These methods are useful for following patients to determine if therapeutic intervention produces a change in bone mass, but neither technique is particularly useful for establishing a diagnosis, since neither separates osteoporosis from other diseases associated with low bone mass. In addition, the finding of abnormally low mass in an otherwise asymptomatic person does not indicate that the bones of that person will subsequently fracture.

Osteoporosis may occur as a secondary feature of another underlying disease. It occurs commonly in Cushing's disease and as a consequence of exogenous corticosteroid therapy. Bone loss occurs in hyperthyroidism and, although the mechanism of loss is different here, the clinical syndrome is indistinguishable from osteoporosis. Apathetic hyperthyroidism occurs more commonly among the older population, where osteoporosis is a major clinical problem and thus a high index of suspicion must be maintained to establish this diagnosis. Osteoporosis probably occurs more commonly in patients with diabetes mellitus and in alcoholics.

The principle differential diagnosis of the patient with low bone mass includes osteomalacia, hyperparathyroidism, and some malignancies. It is, of course, important to make the correct diagnosis, since the treatment is quite different for these disorders. Osteomalacia must be suspected, especially in the presence of gastrointestinal disorders associated with malabsorption (e.g., gluten enteropathy, sprue, postgastrectomy, small bowel surgery) and in patients with renal tubular disorders (e.g., renal tubular acidosis and Fanconi syndrome). In these disorders, patients may present with symptoms of osteomalacia. Some elderly patients may receive little or no sunlight and have very poor nutrition. Such patients may develop osteomalacia in association with osteoporosis. Most patients with osteomalacia will have hypophosphatemia or hypocalcemia or both and elevated serum alkaline phosphatase activity; however, histomorphometric evaluation of an undecalcified bone biopsy specimen may be necessary to establish the diagnosis. Hyperparathyroidism may also be associated with a decrease in bone mass and fractures. The serum calcium is most frequently continuously elevated, is occasionally only minimally or intermittently elevated, or is rarely within the normal range. Another cause of decreased bone mass is multiple myeloma, which can present with generalized skeletal demineralization and fractures rather than the more common finding, localized osteolytic lesions. Serum protein electrophoresis usually points toward this diagnosis.

Treatment

Loss of bone occurs with age in all persons after the fourth decade. There is an accelerated rate of bone loss in women from the late fifth decade through the middle of the eighth decade. Thereafter, the rate of bone loss slows. Since it is felt that fractures in osteoporosis are in part due to low bone mass, prevention of this age-related loss of bone should provide protection from the development of this disease. Unfortunately, it is currently impossible to predict accurately which person or group of persons at skeletal maturity is likely to develop later low bone mass and fracture. Thus, those at greatest risk of fracture cannot be identified for administration of preventive therapy. Current methods for preventing bone loss probably carry sufficient risk so that the treatment of the entire population is not warranted.

It is known that therapeutic oophorectomy in the premenopausal woman leads to accelerated bone loss and that this loss can be prevented by administration of estrogens. Thus, it seems quite reasonable to replace estrogens in all premenopausal women who have had an oophorectomy when administration of this drug is not otherwise contraindicated. It has also been shown in several small groups of postmenopausal women that bone loss can be slowed or prevented at least for several years if estrogen is administered. Whether this effect will persist for longer periods of time and be effective in reducing the incidence of fracture is unknown. Great caution should be exercised in the use of estrogen in postmenopausal women because of the suggested increased incidence of carcinoma of the uterus in this population. Should estrogen be prescribed, it should be used in low dose (0.625 mg. of conjugated estrogen or its equivalent), and it should be given cyclically. Some physicians also suggest that a progestational agent be added with every third or fourth cycle to assure endometrial shedding.

Administration of calcium to postmenopausal women has been shown to slow the rate of bone loss for at least several years. It is necessary to give approximately 1.5 grams of calcium to achieve a positive calcium balance in most postmenopausal women. Although any form of calcium supplement probably can be used, calcium carbonate provides the highest quantity of calcium per gram of drug administered and thus may somewhat more conveniently be taken by most patients. Since a few patients may be gastrointestinal hyperabsorbers of calcium and thus develop hypercalciuria, the urinary calcium should be checked especially in patients with a history of renal stones. The long-term effect of administration of calcium supplements has not been determined.

Most patients seek medical assistance only after a large quantity of bone has been lost and acute fracture has developed. Many of these patients require management by standard orthopedic measures. Acute vertebral collapse fractures are treated initially with bed rest and analgesics. When pain has subsided, a series of mild back and abdominal muscle-strengthening exercises should be undertaken. In addition, a program to slow subsequent bone loss should be planned. Calcium supplementation in a dose to provide an intake of approximately 1.5 grams of calcium should be given, if not contraindicated by development of hypercalciuria. Although there may be risk from estrogen substitution therapy, the gain achieved in slowing bone loss probably warrants its use, especially in those women who are within one decade of the menopause when symptomatic osteoporosis develops. Estrogen therapy should be given cyclically at low dose, and these patients must be observed very closely for evidence of uterine carcinoma. Androgens have also been shown to slow the loss of calcium from the skeleton, but these drugs have significant side effects and their place in the therapeutic armamentarium is as yet to be demonstrated.

Sodium fluoride, alone or in combination with calcium and vitamin D, has been suggested as a treatment for osteoporosis. Although it is known that this form of therapy increases bone mass, it is not known whether the newly formed bone is qualitatively normal. More importantly, it has not been demonstrated that there is a reduction in incidence of fracture in patients treated with sodium fluoride. Since sodium fluoride is potentially quite toxic, it should be only used in the investigational setting until the certainty of its efficacy and toxicity is established. Similarly, treatment of osteoporosis with calcitonin, or with one of the new phosphonate drugs, or with vitamin D or its metabolites, should be pursued only in the experimental setting.

PARENTERAL NUTRITION IN ADULTS

method of
MANUEL MARTINEZ-MALDONADO,
M.D.,
and LUIZ NASCIMENTO, M.D.
San Juan, Puerto Rico

Parenteral nutrition requires a team approach for effectiveness and safety. Thorough knowledge of the indications and potential complications of this form of therapy is essential. Moreover, the hospital setting must provide the facilities necessary to undertake this exacting procedure.

Clinical Assessment of Nutritional Deficit

Consider the patient as a whole, since no single value can be used to identify nutritional deficit. The following are clues to its presence:

1. History of dietary habits.

2. If there has been a loss of more than 25 per cent of ideal weight, malnutrition is most likely present.

3. If possible, determine subcutaneous fat by skin fold calipers or roentgenographically, but this is usually unnecessary. Estimation of skin folds in the triceps or subscapular area between one's fingers usually suffices. If the estimate is below 85 per cent of normal skin folds, malnutrition is present.

4. A serum albumin below 3.2 grams per dl. (100 ml.).

5. A total lymphocyte count below 1200 per cu. mm. but not due to the primary disease. (WBC × percentage of lymphocytes in differential = total lymphocyte count).

6. If 4 and 5 are not present, it is extremely unlikely that parenteral nutrition is required.

Indications

I. Impaired digestive function
1. Enteric or enterocutanous fistulas
2. Bowel inflammation or obstruction
3. Intractable diarrhea
4. Malabsorption syndrome
5. Ulcerative colitis
6. Short bowel syndrome
7. Mouth and throat carcinoma
8. Pancreatitis
9. Peritonitis
10. Chronic vomiting (e.g., hyperemesis gravidarum)

II. Obtunded sensorium (neurologic or metabolic)

III. Iatrogenic disturbances of nutrition
1. Radiotherapy
2. Chemotherapy
3. Corticosteroid therapy

IV. Hypercatabolic states
1. Trauma
2. Postsurgery
3. Severe burns
4. Acute renal failure

V. Malnutrition secondary to
1. Anorexia
2. Cancer
3. Alcoholism

Principles and Practice of Total Parenteral Nutrition (TPN)

A patient in a basal metabolic state will expend about 600 calories per day. An infusion of 3 liters of 5 per cent dextrose solution daily will meet this need; however, this regimen is clearly inadequate for most disease states in which the patient requires intravenous hyperalimentation. On an average, a healthy ambulatory person has a functional basal requirement of between 1600 and 1800 calories daily. Patients in need of total parenteral nutrition usually have energy requirements that exceed those of normal subjects. Frequently, these patients have a hypercatabolic state (infections, burns, trauma, etc.). It is impossible to deliver such high caloric infusions through a peripheral access; thus, the need to use a central vein. The subclavian route is the most commonly used. Placement of the catheter should be done with scrupulous adherence to aseptic technique. Under local anesthesia, the catheter is inserted and the tip advanced into the superior vena cava above the right atrium. After x-ray confirmation of position, the catheter end is sutured to the skin and connected to standard tubing. The wound care should consist of changing dressings three times a week. The use of millipore membrane filters in the infusion line is strongly advised; it has been shown to decrease significantly the incidence of infection. The TPN line should not be used as a means of administering drugs or transfusions or manipulated for measurement of central venous pressure (CVP) or for other reasons.

It is recommended that total parenteral nutrition in adults be started with 1 liter of infusion on the first day, 2 liters the second day, and reaching a total of 2.5 to 3.5 liters the third day. A constant rate of infusion is suggested to avoid some complications. Patients on total parenteral nutrition should have the following monitored: (1) electrolyte balance; (2) serum albumin; (3) transferrin levels; serum transferrin = (total iron-binding capacity × 0.8) − 43; normal levels, 170 to 250 mg. per dl. (100 ml.); and (4) daily weight. A patient undergoing successful total parenteral nutrition should gain one half pound per week. Table 1 summarizes the tests to be monitored and their frequency while the patient is undergoing TPN.

TABLE 1.   Monitoring a Patient on Total Parenteral Nutrition

I. To be evaluated daily:
1. Body weight
2. Vital signs
3. Intake and output
4. Blood measurements: blood sugar, osmolality, BUN and electrolytes (during the initial phase of therapy)

II. To be evaluated two or three times a week:
1. Calcium, phosphate and magnesium
2. Bilirubin and liver enzymes
3. Complete blood count
4. Blood NH_3

III. Urine measurements:
Glucose, acetone and osmolality should be evaluated four to six times daily during initial phase and at least twice a day throughout the therapy.

IV. Screening for infection:
1. Close medical observation
2. Temperature readings
3. WBC and differential as indicated
4. Cultures: blood, urine, infusate and filters as indicated

TABLE 2.   Composition of Typical Parenteral Nutritional Solution (Daily Intake)

Glucose	600–900 grams
Nitrogen (amino acid preparations)	10–20 grams
Water	2500–3500 ml.
Sodium	60–120 mEq.
Potassium	100–140 mEq.
Calcium	3–7 mEq.
Magnesium	20–30 mEq.
Phosphate	20–30 mEq.
Vitamins	
Ascorbic acid	80–120 mg.
Thiamine	3–9 mg.
Riboflavin	3–5 mg.
Niacin	30–45 mg.
B_6	3–5 mg.
B_{12}	4–6 mg.
Pantothenic acid	10–20 mg.
A	1500–3500 I.U.
D	100–300 I.U.
E	3–10 I.U.

It is of fundamental importance that total parenteral nutrition provide adequate calories, nitrogen, electrolytes, and water.

Calories.   The infusion of fat emulsion (1 gram can provide 9 calories) is potentially the most efficacious intravenous energy source. A solution (Intralipid 10 per cent) is available and is very useful; when a large central vein is not accessible this solution can be infused through a peripheral vein. Its composition is soybean oil, 10 per cent (54 per cent linoleic, 26 per cent oleic, 9 per cent palmitic, 8 per cent linoleic acids); egg yolk phospholipids, 1.2 per cent; glycerin, 2.2 per cent; and the pH adjusted to 5.5 to 9.0 with NaOH. The osmolarity of the solution is 280 mOsm. per liter. Peripheral thrombophlebitis can occur, and there is always a potential hazard of sepsis (excellent growth medium). Recently, solutions have been administered through a polytetrafluoroethylene arteriovenous conduit in nonuremic subjects. This technique promises a decrease in the incidence of phlebitis and infection at the infusion site. Carbohydrates, usually in the form of dextrose or fructose, are the major source of calories in any intravenous regimen. Dextrose, the most readily available parenteral substrate, can provide 4 calories per gram. An infusion of high concentrations of carbohydrates per day results in sparing of the protein breakdown that follows fasting states. The requirement for dietary nitrogen is therefore lowered. An outline of the composition of a typical solution used in total parenteral nutrition is shown in Table 2.

Nitrogen.   Approximately 80 to 120 grams of protein equivalent (crystalline amino acids, protein hydrolysate) infused in the solution is necessary to produce a positive nitrogen balance. The nitrogen intake through the infusate, 10 to 20 grams, plus the nitrogen-sparing effect of glucose administration usually combine to achieve a state of anabolism. In conditions in which renal or hepatic failure is present, the nitrogen intake may be severely restricted.

Electrolytes.   It has been shown that during long-term parenteral nutrition the requirements are usually increased; thus, a need for close monitoring and supply of electrolytes, phosphate, calcium, and magnesium (Table 2).

Water.   An adult requires approximately 35 ml. per kg. of body weight of water intake daily. Usually the parenteral nutrition involves the infusion of 2.5 to 3.5 liters per day. Special care should be taken regarding water intake in patients with renal, hepatic, and cardiac disease.

Contraindications for Parenteral Nutrition

1. A moribund or unsalvageable patient.
2. Good nutritional status or a short length of time needed for parenteral nutrition.
3. Oral nutrition feasible.
4. Uncorrected cardiac or metabolic derangements.

Complications

Sepsis.   With meticulous attention to aseptic technique, the infection rate can be reduced to between 2 to 4 per cent (based on 1000 patient-days with an average of 10 days per patient). Thorough knowledge of the special techniques required for the care of the catheters and lines is essential. The use of millipore membrane filters in the infusion line helps reduce the incidence of infection. Should sepsis supervene, discontinue parenteral nutrition and implement adequate diagnostic and therapeutic measures.

Fluid Administration. Correct blood volume adequately prior to starting feeding and assess renal function. This will make it easier to control the patient and avoid unnecessary manipulation of intravenous lines and the patient in general. Infuse the nutritional fluid at no more than 100 to 125 ml. per hour by gravity or, better yet, by pump. Do not exceed 1 liter the first day; one may go to 2 liters the second day and 3 the third day, after which constant daily infusion should be maintained. This will prevent overloading and its two possible consequences: hypertension and vascular congestion. Should these supervene, the rate of infusion must be reduced to that tolerated by the patient.

Electrolyte Disturbances and Hyperosmolality. Carefully monitor serum electrolytes so that any changes can be corrected early and promptly, lest they become clinically significant. Rises in serum sodium and chloride may be early indications of *hypertonicity* and will require solute-free water administration. Should sodium and chloride values fall, the amount of water being administered must be reduced. *Hypokalemia* and *hyperkalemia* may result. Hypokalemia is caused by inadequate intake, particularly in the protein anabolic phase of the procedure. Hyperkalemia results from administration of excess potassium or, if metabolic acidosis develops, even the amounts replaced as the daily requirements may result in hyperkalemia (see later). If calcium administration is inadequate, *hypocalcemia* may occur. In addition, if in attempts to replenish phosphate, calcium is not administered simultaneously, *hypocalcemia* may result. Excessive calcium administration will lead to *hypercalcemia*. *Hypomagnesemia* can result from inadequate administration relative to protein anabolism.

Glucose Metabolism Abnormalities. Excessive glucose administration or too rapid a rate of infusion may lead to *hyperglycemia*. If endogenous insulin production is normal, the problem may be of small clinical importance, but in patients with diabetes mellitus, hyperosmolar, nonketotic dehydration, and coma may result. Blood sugar must be monitored and insulin given to maintain blood sugar between 200 and 300 mg. per dl. If a nonketotic hyperosmolar situation occurs, insulin and hypotonic saline solution should be administered and the intravenous administration reduced or discontinued, at least temporarily. In diabetics in whom insulin therapy is inadequate, ketoacidosis and diabetic coma may supervene. On the other hand, in normal subjects persistence of endogenous insulin production as a result of prolonged stimulation of islet cells by high carbohydrate in-

take, may lead to *hypoglycemia* when the infusion is stopped.

Abnormalities in Phosphate Metabolism. *Hypophosphatemia* may result if exogenous phosphate administration is inadequate and the total parenteral nutrition period is more than 7 to 10 days. In addition, phosphate may be redistributed into muscle and red cells. Consequently, 2,3-diphosphoglycerate depletion may occur, increasing the affinity of hemoglobin for oxygen. Muscle weakness and exhaustion may also occur, particularly if the serum phosphate is less than 1 mg. per dl., and respiratory arrest may ensue. Follow-up of changes in serum phosphate and administration of this ion when needed will prevent this complication. *Hyperphosphatemia* because of diminished renal function or as a result of hydrolysation of casein may occur, leading in some patients to paresthesias and tetany. This can be corrected by giving synthetic aminoacids or 10 per cent Intralipid intravenously. Knowledge of renal function will also permit prevention.

Metabolic Acidosis. Preparations containing synthetic amino acids may cause hyperchloremic acidosis because of the presence of hydrochloric acid. In the presence of renal function impairment the tendency to metabolic acidosis will be greater. Follow-up of serum bicarbonate concentration and administration of protein hydrolysates will help prevent this situation.

Hyperammonemia. Subjects with liver disease may be unable to convert ammonia to urea. The ammonia comes from the protein hydrolysates or from deficiency of arginine, ornithine, and aspartic acid or glutamic acid or both.

Mechanical Complications. Insertion of the catheter or its manipulation during bottle changes might lead to a pneumothorax or, if the subclavian vein is punctured, a hemothorax may occur. Development of arteriovenous fistula, injury to the brachial plexus, cardiac tamponade, cavitating pulmonary infarction from catheter embolus, and thrombosis of the subclavian vein or superior vena cava or both can also take place. Catheter migration into other vessels (jugular vein) has also been observed.

Miscellaneous. Anemia as a result of deficiency of iron, folic acid, B_{12}, copper, and zinc has been described. Bleeding, which can in turn result from vitamin K deficiency, can also lead to anemia. Hepatic enzyme elevation (SGOT, SGPT, alkaline phosphatase) can also occur as a result of excessive glycogen or fat deposition in the liver. Proper replacement of hematopoietically necessary substances and reduction in the rate of parenteral nutrition will prevent these complications. Linoleic acid deficiency leading to dermatitis, poor healing, or thrombocytopenia may be corrected by 10 per cent Intralipid intravenously.

PARENTERAL FLUID THERAPY IN CHILDREN

method of
ROBERT C. KELSCH, M.D.,
WILLIAM J. OLIVER, M.D.,
and STEVE T. KOEFF, M.D.
Ann Arbor, Michigan

It is expedient to consider water and electrolyte needs in terms of maintenance requirements and deficit replacement. The theoretic basis will be reviewed briefly, but physicians caring for children should have a firm knowledge of the background.

MAINTENANCE REQUIREMENTS

Water

The metabolic rate determines the magnitude of maintenance requirements of water. These obligatory losses occur through the skin, lungs, and kidney and, to a minor extent, from the gastrointestinal tract. Since the metabolic rate of children is large in proportion to their size, their basal water needs appear large compared with adults. We have elected to use weight and age as the physical measurements which correlate with the metabolic rate.

1. Insensible water loss, not sweat, occurs through the skin and expired air as water vapor. Insensible water losses in the usual hospital circumstances approximate 30 ml. per kg. per day for infants, 20 ml. per kg. per day for children, and 12 ml. per kg. per day for adults.

2. Urinary losses of water are conditioned primarily by the quantity of wastes (solute load) and the concentrating ability of the kidneys. The solute load during usual parenteral fluid therapy in infants and children requires approximately 50 ml. of water per kg. per day when the urine specific gravity equals that of plasma (1.010).

3. Stool losses of water in the absence of diarrhea are small (10 ml. per kg. per day).

To summarize, maintenance water requirements may be illustrated for an infant in a resting state, who has no deficits or sources of excess water loss:

	ml. per kg. per day
Insensible loss	30
Urine requirement	50
Stool loss (no diarrhea)	10
Total fluid	90 ml. per kg. per day

The maintenance parenteral fluid requirements for varying ages are summarized in Table 1. Only the calculated total volumes are given, but the

TABLE 1. **Daily Maintenance Requirements of Water**

AGE	ML./KG.
Newborn	60
1 week–1 year	80–100
1 year–2 years	70
2 years–5 years	60
5 years–10 years	50
10+ years	40

distribution of water needs is similar to that of the infant.

The estimation of maintenance water requirements is essentially a balance problem. The amount of water given parenterally should equal the amount of water lost through all routes during the period of fluid administration. Daily weighing of the patients will confirm the accuracy of the total fluid given. It is apparent that the maintenance requirements for water will vary significantly, depending upon environmental factors and disease states.

Factors Increasing Maintenance Requirements

1. Fever.
2. Hyperpnea.
3. Sweating.
4. Defective renal water conservation (renal disease and pituitary disease).
5. Increased renal solute load (diabetes mellitus, increased tissue breakdown, inappropriate electrolyte administration).
6. Unusual intestinal losses (vomiting, gastric suction, diarrhea).

Each of the aforementioned factors increases water needs to a variable extent, and several may occur simultaneously. Some can be readily measured (i.e., urine, gastric suction); others can be only estimated. For example, insensible water loss is increased by 7 ml. per kg. per day per degree Fahrenheit of fever. Instances in which hyperpnea or sweating has increased water needs by 100 per cent are recorded. These losses can rarely be measured, but some concept of their magnitude is necessary. If any of the listed factors need to be considered in calculating maintenance fluids, an increase of 25 to 50 per cent above the usual parenteral fluid requirements listed in Table 1 usually will satisfy these needs. Rarely, an increase of 100 per cent in the minimal parenteral water requirements will be necessary.

Factors Decreasing Maintenance Requirements

Few factors decrease water needs. However, use of a cold steam tent (Croupette) may reduce insensible water requirements by as much as 30 per cent. In some patients a persistent decrease in the effective plasma volume (congestive heart failure, cirrhosis, and nephrotic syndrome) or inappropriate antidiuretic hormone (ADH) secretion (purulent meningitis) may result in urine of specific gravity above the 1.010 postulated in estimating water requirements. In those patients significantly less water for urinary requirements may be needed.

Electrolytes and Glucose

Sodium. Infants and children conserve sodium as avidly as adults, but also require several days to attain maximal sodium conservation. Thus sodium should be included in maintenance fluids (Table 2) except in anuria. Any excess is usually excreted.

Potassium. Potassium conservation is similar to that of sodium, but less effective. Therefore potassium should be included in the maintenance requirements (Table 2).

Bicarbonate. Bicarbonate is a product of metabolism. There are no maintenance requirements.

Chloride. Maintenance needs for chloride ion are adequately supplied if sodium is given in the form of NaCl. For this reason, we do not make a separate calculation of chloride needs.

Glucose. Sufficient glucose should be given to spare protein catabolism (Table 2.)

Example of Calculation of Maintenance Needs. Most hospitals have stock solutions containing 5 per cent glucose to which standard quantities of sodium chloride have been added. Common solutions are as follows:

0.9% NaCl in 5% glucose	(150 mEq. Na$^+$/liter or 0.15 mEq./ml.)
0.6% NaCl in 5% glucose	(100 mEq. Na$^+$/liter or 0.10 mEq./ml.)
0.45% NaCl in 5% glucose	(75 mEq. Na$^+$/liter or 0.075 mEq./ml.)
0.33% NaCl in 5% glucose	(57 mEq. Na$^+$/liter or 0.057 mEq./ml.)
0.2% NaCl in 5% glucose	(34 mEq. Na$^+$/liter or 0.034 mEq./ml.)

For simplicity, we use these solutions.

EXAMPLE.   Infant with weight of 8 kg.

Total fluid 80 ml. × 8 kg. = 640 ml.
Sodium   2 mEq. × 8 kg. = 16 mEq. Na$^+$
Potassium 2 mEq. × 8 kg. = 16 mEq. K$^+$
Glucose   3 grams × 8 kg. = 24 grams glucose

Examination of these solutions shows that 640 ml. of the 0.2 per cent NaCl in 5 per cent glucose supplies 21 mEq. of Na$^+$, which is only 5 mEq. more than the calculated requirement. The quantity of glucose (32 grams) is sufficient to minimize protein catabolism. Potassium chloride (16 mEq. K$^+$) must be added to the solution.

TABLE 2. Daily Maintenance Requirements of Electrolytes and Glucose

	NA$^+$	K$^+$	GLUCOSE
Infants (< 2 years of age)	2 mEq./kg.	2–3 mEq./kg.	3 grams/kg.
Children (> 2 years of age)	1 mEq./kg.	1 mEq./kg.	2 grams/kg.

Similar calculations hold throughout childhood. Therefore we find that a maintenance solution containing 0.2 per cent NaCl with added potassium to a volume determined by basal fluid requirements (Table 1) meets usual maintenance requirements. The adequacy of this therapy should be monitored by daily body weights and serial plasma electrolyte measurements.

DEFICIT THERAPY

Water

The magnitude of water deficit is *independent* of the route of water loss. Therefore the quantity required for replacement can be estimated without reference to the primary disease. Acute losses of body water are generally equivalent to acute losses of body weight. These losses may be associated with the classic signs of dehydration (poor skin turgor, sunken eyes, and so forth). Thus replacement requirements for water (Table 3) can usually be estimated by physical examination. During the first 6 months of life, severe dehydration is associated with a 12 to 15 per cent acute loss of body weight. This extreme loss is possible because of the large extracellular space of small infants. Note that for deficits calculated on a kilogram basis, per cent of deficit need be only multiplied by weight in kilograms to obtain the volume of fluids for repair. Since these estimates involve considerable error, no more than 50 to 70 per cent of the deficit determined in this manner should be given in the first 24 hours to severely dehydrated patients. One is always able to give more fluid, but it is difficult to remove an excess.

TABLE 3. Relationship Between Degree of Dehydration, Acute Weight Loss (Water Loss), and Water for Repair

DEGREE OF DEHYDRATION	ACUTE WEIGHT LOSS (%)	WATER FOR REPAIR (ML./KG. OF BODY WEIGHT)*
Severe	8–10	80–100
Moderate	5–8	50–80
Minimal	3–5	30–50

*In theory, these calculations should be based on preillness weight. In practice, we have found the patient's weight upon admission to be satisfactory for these calculations.

TABLE 4. **Deficits of Sodium and Water in Severe Dehydration**

	WATER DEFICIT (ml./kg.)	SODIUM DEFICIT (mEq./kg.)
Fasting and thirsting	100	5
Diarrhea (plasma sodium)		
Isotonic (130–155mEq./liter)	100	8–10
Hypertonic (>155 mEq./liter)	100	2–4
Hypotonic (<130 mEq./liter)	100	10–12

Electrolytes

Sodium. In *dehydration*, the sodium deficit has been usefully related to plasma sodium concentration. Table 4 describes these relationships and may be utilized for estimating sodium deficit.

Potassium. Potassium deficit may be large, but safe repair requires that no more than 3 mEq. per kg. per day be given unless significant hypokalemia is demonstrated (K^+ less than 3 mEq. per liter). Potassium should not be added to parenteral fluids until after the patient has urinated.

Bicarbonate. In *metabolic acidosis*, plasma bicarbonate concentration falls below the normal level of 23 to 25 mEq. per liter. Mild acidosis (HCO_3^- above 15 mEq. per liter) cannot be recognized clinically. Given appropriate fluids and electrolytes and adequate renal function, correction of mild acidosis will occur without alkali therapy. Intravenous bicarbonate will effectively lower the hydrogen ion concentration, and correct severe metabolic acidosis (HCO_3^- less than 10 mEq. per liter). For estimation of the bicarbonate requirements for correcting acidosis, an acute distribution space of 30 per cent body weight is utilized:

Dose of $NaHCO_3$ mEq. = Normal HCO_3^- 25 mEq. − Measured patient $HCO_3^- \times 0.3$ wt. in kg.

When serum bicarbonate analysis is not immediately available and the patient has hyperpnea, the following equation estimates the bicarbonate requirements:

Dose of HCO_3^- in mEq. = $(25-15) \times (0.3$ wt. in kg.$)$

Use of the acute distribution space of bicarbonate will not completely correct metabolic acidosis. Furthermore, complete correction is not desirable, because such correction may aggravate central nervous system acidosis. We therefore do not recommend the use of bicarbonate if plasma HCO_3^- is above 10 mEq. per liter.

Example of Calculation of Total Fluid and Electrolyte Requirements (Maintenance plus Deficit)

An infant with severe isotonic dehydration; admission weight is 10 kg. The infant is hyperpneic; plasma bicarbonate is 10 mEq. per liter.

Estimated deficits of water and sodium:
Water   1000 ml.   from Table 4
Na^+ 80 mEq. from Table 4
Estimated deficits of bicarbonate:
$(25 - 10) \times (0.3 \times 10$ kg.$) = 45$ mEq.
Calculated needs:

	Water	Na^+
Deficit	700 ml.*	56 mEq.*
Maintenance	800 ml.	16 mEq.
Total	1500 ml.	72 mEq.

These needs are best met by using 0.2 per cent NaCl in 5 per cent glucose. Add 45 mEq. of $NaHCO_3$ and 30 mEq. of potassium to this solution.

In practice, we have found that in the treatment of dehydration associated with diarrhea, there is a simple practical approach. It requires measurement only of serum sodium, and is useful when laboratory support is minimal:

1. Calculate water for maintenance and deficit needs.

2. For isotonic dehydration, give the above-calculated volume as 0.33 per cent NaCl in 5 per cent glucose. After the patient has voided, add K^+, 3 mEq. per kg. per day, to the intravenous fluids.

3. For hypotonic dehydration, give the above-calculated volume as 0.45 per cent NaCl in 5 per cent glucose. After the patient has voided, add K^+, 3 mEq. per kg. per day, to the intravenous fluids.

4. For hypertonic dehydration give the above-calculated volume as 0.2 per cent NaCl and 5 per cent glucose. After the patient has voided, add K^+, 3 mEq. per kg. per day, to the intravenous fluids. It is important that the fluid deficit in hypertonic dehydration be given over 48 hours or longer if convulsions occurring during the rehydration stage are to be avoided. This slow administration of intravenous fluids appears to be a critical factor in preventing intracerebral edema.

5. In each instance above if severe metabolic acidosis is present, calculate the required bicarbonate and give over the first 3 hours. This should be subtracted from the total sodium therapy.

In severe dehydration with impending or actual shock, intravenous fluids should be given rapidly to expand plasma volume. Usually 20 ml. per kg. lactated Ringer's solution is adequate.

Correction of deficits should always be by the intravenous route; subcutaneous fluids may be poorly absorbed and actually reduce circulating volume.

---

*Recall that only 70 per cent of water and electrolyte deficits should be replaced in the first 24 hours.

SPECIAL PROBLEMS

Metabolic Alkalosis

Pyloric stenosis and the use of diuretics are the major causes of metabolic alkalosis in childhood. The deficits involve sodium, chloride, potassium, and hydrogen ion. Effective therapy requires correction of the extracellular volume contraction with chloride-containing solutions and repair of the potassium deficit. Solutions containing 0.6 per cent sodium chloride in 5 per cent glucose with added potassium chloride will adequately correct the problem.

Diabetes Mellitus

In addition to the requirement for correction of deficits of water, Na^+, and Cl^-, an occult potassium deficit is present prior to the onset of therapy in diabetes mellitus. Correction of the metabolic acidosis unmasks the deficit in the early hours of treatment. Prevention of severe hypokalemia requires the addition of potassium to the intravenous fluids within the first 6 hours at a concentration of 40 mEq. per liter. In certain instances larger quantities of potassium may be required. The potassium may be given as half chloride and half phosphate salts.

Gastric Suction

Gastrointestinal losses by suction should be measured, and the volume should be used as an estimate of replacement needs. More precise information can be gained by laboratory analysis of the aspirate. If analyses cannot be made, intestinal fluids may be considered isotonic, and isotonic replacement solutions used. For periods of 1 to 2 days, 0.9 per cent NaCl is an adequate replacement solution. If longer periods of nasogastric aspiration are indicated, solutions producing potential hydrogen ion should be given and careful laboratory monitoring of the patient is required. Commercially available solutions are Electrolyte No. 3 [Baxter] and Ionsol-G Solution [Abbott]. Replace volume for volume.

Gastric replacement solution:

Cation	mEq. liter	Anion
NH_4^+ 70		Cl^- 150
Na^+ 63		
K^+ 17		

Salicylate Intoxication

Alkalinization of the urine promotes renal excretion of salicylate. We have found the Whitten et al. program of alkalinization (Am. J. Dis. Child. *101*:178, 1961) to be simple and effective.

1. Start an infusion of 0.33 per cent NaCl in 5 per cent glucose to which maintenance amounts of potassium have been added. The rate of infusion should be 1 to 3 ml. per minute, dependent upon the state of hydration.

2. Add 2 mEq. of $NaHCO_3$ per kg. of weight every 30 minutes until urine is alkaline (pH greater than 6.5).

3. Check urine pH every 15 minutes. Add additional $NaHCO_3$ to maintain an alkaline urine.

4. Improvement can be judged clinically or by measurements of plasma salicylate concentration.

Acute Renal Failure

1. Water is required for insensible loss (skin and lungs) and measured urine output. Fortunately, gastrointestinal losses are generally low or absent in children with anuria or oliguria. Estimate the fluid for insensible loss (30 ml. per kg. in infants, 20 ml. per kg. for children), subtract metabolic and preformed water (5 to 10 ml. per kg.), and add urine volume. For correct balance a daily weight loss of 1 to 2 per cent of body weight should occur. Gain of weight or a constant weight is an indication to reduce the fluid intake.

2. Electrolytes are not required in acute renal failure unless unusual losses are present.

3. Glucose will minimize protein catabolism. Give at least 3 grams of glucose per kg. per day for infants and 2 grams per kg. per day for children. If possible, give orally. For intravenous administration, hypertonic solutions may be used, but increase the frequency of venous thrombosis.

4. Life-threatening elevations of plasma potassium are more frequent in the presence of tissue breakdown (hemolysis or massive soft tissue injury). These may be prevented or treated by ion exchange resins. We use sodium polystyrene sulfonate (Kayexalate), 1 gram per kg. per day orally or rectally. Resins may require 12 to 24 hours to effectively reduce the potassium, so other measures are required in emergent circumstances. If plasma potassium is greater than 7 mEq. per liter give (a) Ca gluconate, 0.5 ml. per kg. of 10 per cent solution intravenously; (b) $NaHCO_3$, 2.5 mEq. per kg. intravenously; and (c) glucose 50 per cent, 1 ml. per kg. intravenously. This should be followed promptly by peritoneal or hemodialysis.

Postoperative State

Use minimal maintenance requirements (Table 1); give as 0.2 per cent NaCl in 5 per cent glucose. Recall that these figures assume a urine concentration of 300 mOsm. per liter (specific gravity 1.010). Less water can be given if the patient can concentrate his urine and if the surgical condition requires that a patient be kept "dry." After the patient has voided, add KCl, 2 to 3 mEq. per kg. per day for infants and 1 mEq. per kg. per day for children. If a mist tent is used, the water requirements may be reduced by 25 per cent and the electrolytes supplied by 0.2 per cent NaCl will still be adequate.

Comment

There are no rules or shortcuts that can substitute for experience and judgment in determining parenteral fluid requirements. The methods described provide a background for planning parenteral fluid treatment, but repeated observations of the state of hydration, change in weight, urine output, increase or decrease in gastrointestinal losses, and overall response to treatment should all be used in assessing the accuracy of the calculated needs. In seriously ill infants these observations usually must be made more frequently than once a day. For the additional clinical situations not discussed, the principles underlying maintenance needs combined with a common sense estimate of deficits incurred should provide sufficient information to permit valid estimates of parenteral fluid needs.

The Endocrine System

ACROMEGALY

method of
BERNARD KLIMAN, M.D.,
and RAYMOND N. KJELLBERG, M.D.
Boston, Massachusetts

Definition

Acromegaly is an illness produced by excessive and inappropriate secretion of growth hormone, almost always of pituitary tumor origin except in rare cases of secretion by a neoplasm such as a carcinoid lung tumor. Functional excess of growth hormone has been suggested in the past due to appearance of the disease before detectable enlargement of the sella turcica. More recent evidence, based on surgical exploration of such patients, indicates that this initial stage is related to a microadenoma, a less than 10 mm. diameter tumor, within the sella. In most instances, eosinophilic cells are identified in the tumor; however, the proportion of nonstaining cells may be in the majority or compose the entire tumor. Clinical signs of tissue growth or other changes were used as indices of active disease until growth hormone measurements by radioimmunoassay became available and demonstrated that inactivity of the disease or so-called "burned out acromegaly" was rare and usually associated with spontaneous infarction of the tumor. Active acromegaly is an evolution of progressive changes, both physical and metabolic, which lead to morbidity or mortality related to arthritis, diabetes mellitus, cardiovascular disease, or visual complications due to growth of the pituitary tumor. The purpose of treatment is to prevent complications and to reverse the metabolic effects of excess growth hormone.

Treatment Objectives

The preferred approach to treatment of acromegaly is to inhibit the growth and endocrine secretion of the pituitary tumor with the intention of avoiding future complications. Improvement of existing changes and preservation of normal anterior pituitary functions are desirable objectives. The removal of tumor tissue is essential, if possible, when damage has been caused by tumor expansion, particularly recent visual loss by chiasmal compression. Cessation of tumor growth and prevention of future recurrence are important in the choice of available therapeutic measures. At any time during the course of this disease the major and minor objectives may change due to existing circumstances or the effects of previous therapy. The physician must also consider the potential benefits and known risks of therapy for an individual patient. In general, treatment is preferred to observation, since disease changes are unpredictable in onset and may fail to reverse despite reduction of growth hormone levels. Exceptional patients include the very elderly or persons with other major diseases that limit the prospects for treatment. The physician has a choice of several modalities of treatment listed in Table 1. It is the responsibility of the attending physician to become familiar with the characteristics of each therapy and to obtain informed consent of the patient when one or more choices is recommended. When sufficient information is not available, consultation with physicians experienced in those techniques should be requested.

Preparatory Studies

The evaluation of each patient is intended to provide information needed to formulate therapy choices and to evaluate the status of acromegaly and any related or pertinent medical disorders. These studies should include assessment of the

TABLE 1. **Treatment of Acromegaly**

A. Therapy directed at the pituitary tumor:
Surgery
1. Transfrontal craniotomy
2. Transsphenoidal surgery:
    Sub-labial approach with microsurgery
    Cryosurgery
    Radiofrequency thermocoagulation
    Ultrasonic destruction
Radiation
1. Conventional radiation:
    High voltage x-ray
    ^{60}Co
    Linear accelerator
2. Intrasellar implantation:
    Yttrium-90 isotope
    Gold-198 isotope
3. Heavy particle
    Alpha particles
    Proton beam, Bragg peak
B. Therapy directed at growth hormone excess:
Reduction of growth hormone secretion
1. Bromocriptine
2. Chlorpromazine
3. Medroxy-progesterone
Antagonism of growth hormone action
1. Estrogens
C. Multiple forms of therapy:
Surgery by more than one approach
Surgery followed by radiation
Radiation followed by surgery
Radiation combined with chemotherapy
Surgery and radiation followed by chemo-
    therapy

degree of growth hormone excess with confirmation of current activity and baseline values for future reference. Fasting samples for serum growth hormone and glucose are drawn after overnight rest in a hospital location, avoiding ambulation, which may elevate the growth hormone level. Additional samples are drawn during 3 hours after 100 grams of glucose by mouth, with growth hormone samples at 1 and 2 hours, and glucose samples at ½, 1, 1½, 2, and 3 hours. In equivocal cases, further samples may be obtained during sleep or at frequent intervals. Radioimmunoassay of serum somatomedin levels may become useful in such patients as a means of detecting early acromegaly.

The status of other anterior pituitary functions is determined by screening laboratory tests and reserve tests as indicated. Basic studies can be obtained entirely by blood tests for follicle-stimulating hormone (FSH), luteinizing hormone (LH), 8 A.M. cortisol, testosterone in adult males, thyroxine, free thyroxine or free thyroxine index, thyroid stimulating hormone (TSH), and prolactin. In suspected deficiency states, TSH reserve is measured by thyrotropin releasing hormone (TRH) infusion and multiple sampling during 120 minutes, ACTH reserve is evaluated by plasma cortisol levels during an insulin tolerance test, and

FSH, LH reserves are measured in serum drawn after injection of LH-RH. When insulin-induced hypoglycemia is inadvisable or fails because of relative insulin resistance caused by acromegaly, a metyrapone test with plasma 11-deoxycortisol or urinary 17-hydroxysteroid response is obtained. The presence of menstrual function or the finding of elevated gonadotropin levels, FSH, and LH in women of menopausal age is adequate evidence of gonadotropin function and does not require LH-RH testing or serum estradiol assay. In our own laboratory, unbound plasma testosterone has proved more reliable in men with borderline or slightly low testosterone levels. It is rare to find impairment of posterior pituitary function unless intracranial surgery has been performed. In such patients, serum and urine electrolytes and osmolarity are obtained after at least 16 hours of fluid restriction.

Additional possibilities of multiple endocrine neoplasm syndrome are considered. All patients are screened for primary hyperparathyroidism with serum calcium, phosphorus, and alkaline phosphatase. A normal serum phosphorus may be considered suspect, since elevation is frequently related to the growth hormone effect on renal tubular resorption of phosphorus. If there is a history of renal calculi, or unexpected osteoporosis, or a finding of hypercalcemia, the plasma parathyroid hormone is measured and compared to a simultaneous serum calcium value. If hypertension is present, screening tests are obtained for pheochromocytoma and primary aldosteronism. If fasting hypoglycemia is noted, serum insulin is measured in the fasting state to screen for pancreatic islet cell tumor; however, acromegaly is associated with elevated insulin levels and further diagnosis may first require successful relief of acromegaly. In patients with a history of peptic ulcer, serum gastrin is measured to screen for gastrinoma. Medullary carcinoma of the thyroid gland and acromegaly have not been associated in our experience, although thyroid nodules are frequently observed. Iodine-131 thyroid scan and a serum calcitonin level are obtained in such patients.

The anatomic extent of the pituitary tumor is routinely determined to choose appropriate therapy and to search for complications due to the mass lesion. Initial skull x-rays with an inclined posteroanterior, true lateral, and coned view of the sella may reveal a gross enlargement or distortion of the sella. When possible, the DiChiro formula (length × width × depth ÷ 2) should be applied to provide a reference value for sella volume. Visual field examination by perimetry is essential and may indicate the presence of significant suprasellar extension. If visual impairment is noted, computerized tomography (CT scan) with intravenous contrast medium is obtained for early diagnosis of a suprasellar mass and to plan for prompt surgical intervention in order to relieve chiasmal compression. Tonometry is also advised as part of the visual examination, since a 10 per cent incidence of glaucoma has been reported in association with acromegaly. More detailed measurements of tumor location and extent are obtained in preparation for therapy. The patient is admitted to the hospital and on successive days has a cavernous sinogram and pneumoencephalogram. The sinogram demonstrates the lateral extent of pituitary tissues on both sides of the sella and may show extension beyond the bone of the sella floor or intrusion into one or both cavernous sinuses. Similar information can be obtained by carotid angiography, which is more subject to complications including stroke. The venous infusion used for the sinogram avoids that possibility, and we have only used arterial studies when the cavernous sinuses were occluded by tumor or scar tissue formation. The finding of "encasement" narrowing of the carotid artery is ominous, since it indicates extrasellar invasion, which is difficult to treat. Unless a decision has already been made in favor of surgery, the pneumoencephalogram is essential to provide localized irradiation to the tumor. Suprasellar extension of more than 1 or 2 mm. above the level of the clinoid processes interferes with effective heavy particle therapy with the proton beam since dosage above the clinoids is held to a minimum and may not be adequate for tumor in that area. When the major mass of tumor is below the clinoids, this may be a less important factor. Since some patients require both surgery and radiation, the pneumoencephalogram may show a partially empty sella with a tumor remnant that does not conform directly to the sella contours. It has proved to be extremely useful to obtain hypocycloidal polytomes of the sella and contiguous areas while air is present over the sella in the brow-up position. This provides a three-dimensional assessment of tumor location and leads to more effective use of treatment. If this procedure is not performed, detailed polytomes in lateral and anteroposterior positions at 2 mm. intervals are advised for localization of extensions into the sphenoid sinuses not always evident on routine films for sella volume. The computation of volume and normal ranges vary for the type of examination and should only be compared by similar technique during serial evaluations.

Radiation Therapy

The early experience with conventional high voltage x-ray therapy was obtained prior to the availability of growth hormone measurements, which have since indicated active acromegaly in most patients observed at major treatment centers. Proponents of this technique have noted successful results when patients with milder disease were treated and observed for up to 6 years for final results. This has not been favored, owing to the long observation period and uncertainty of response. Intrasellar implantation of radioactive yttrium (^{90}Y) or gold (^{198}Au) has been useful but subject to hazards of surgical implantation and proximity to adjacent structures with risks of cerebrospinal fluid leak or optic nerve or oculomotor nerve injuries, which are more frequent than with open surgery alone.

Extensive series of patients have been treated by heavy particle therapy at two cyclotron facilities in the United States. Lawrence and his associates at the Donner Laboratories, University of California, Berkeley, introduced this form of therapy with alpha particles. Initial dosages of 6000 rads were employed with limited success, whereas 9000 rads was found to be highly effective. This method does not use the Bragg peak and requires three or more sittings for completion.

A more rapid method has been developed by Kjellberg and colleagues, based on stereotactic fixation and use of the Bragg peak of the proton beam generated at the Harvard Cyclotron. This allows maximal concentration of radiation within the sella, up to 12,000 rads during a single 90 minute treatment period. The optic chiasm is exposed to no more than 1000 rads, and the skin dose is in the range of 600 rads so that no depilation is produced. Treated patients return home within 24 hours after therapy and can resume their usual activities immediately thereafter. The effectiveness of this method appears to be comparable to other methods, with 85 per cent either in clinical remission with fasting growth hormone levels 10 nanograms per ml. or less or improved to the extent that additional treatment is not desired. These results are achieved in the first 2 years of observation and longer term follow-up reveals that the improved patients have further decreases in growth hormone level. Factors that rule against using proton beam Bragg peak therapy are (1) significant degree of suprasellar extension (2) fasting growth hormone level over 200 nanograms per ml. and (3) exposure to 4000 rads or more of x-ray within the past 2 years. With these exceptions, we have favored this form of localized radiation to the sella for initial treatment, having a zero mortality experience and only an 11 per cent incidence of complete anterior pituitary insufficiency. The rate of recurrence has been very low, three cases in the first 450 treated to date. Patients not suitable for proton beam therapy are advised to have transsphenoidal microsurgery, also available at this medical center. Significant elevation of growth hormone after surgery or during follow-up is next treated with proton beam therapy unless extrasellar tumor is confirmed. Patients who fail to achieve satisfactory results with both of these treatments are then considered for palliative x-ray therapy to limit tumor growth or for bromergocriptine therapy to reduce the excessive growth hormone secretion. We have designated our approach as a "system of therapy," in which the mainstay of treatment is the proton beam, and other therapies are utilized as indicated when proton beam therapy is not appropriate for the specific problem or has not achieved optimum results after a 2 year interval of observation with pituitary function surveys at 6, 12, and 24 months.

Surgery

The role of craniotomy in the treatment of acromegaly has lessened in recent years due to improved techniques of transsphenoidal surgery. The inconvenience and hazards of intracranial surgery include prolonged hospitalization and convalescence, risk of seizure disorder, need for high-dose steroid therapy to prevent cerebral edema, risk of diabetes insipidus, risk of optic nerve damage, and a high frequency of anterior pituitary deficiency. This method is currently reserved for tumors with extensive suprasellar mass and severe visual impairment that are, fortunately, late manifestations and remain uncommon. Earlier recognition of acromegaly and the use of CT scans to detect suprasellar tumor should further reduce the need for craniotomy in the management of acromegaly.

The microsurgical methods introduced by Guiot of Suresnes, France, and Hardy of Montreal, Canada, have become available in many treatment centers around the world. The advantages of this technique include a rapid outcome of treatment, 1 week or less of postoperative care in the hospital, limited use of steroid support, no seizures, usually a transient diabetes insipidus that resolves in 1 or 2 days, and preservation of anterior pituitary function in the majority of patients. The mortality is estimated at about 1 per cent, based on hazards of general anesthesia, potential hemorrhage, or postoperative complications. The problems encountered during the operation are unpredictable findings of vascular tumors with bleeding, cavernous sinus invasion, or difficulty in finding a division between tumor and normal pituitary tissue. If a dissection plane cannot be developed between the tumor and diaphragma sellae, cerebrospinal fluid leakage may occur. In some patients the tumor is adherent to adjacent structures and its removal is incomplete. Favorable appearance at surgery is sometimes followed by unexpected residual activity or eventual recurrence. Consequently, postoperative follow-up and lifetime observation are important. There is no difficulty in applying proton beam therapy to such patients, provided that a suprasellar mass has not developed. It is also possible to attempt repeat transsphenoidal surgery if the location of tumor remnants can be demonstrated by radiographic methods. Disadvantages of this approach include a 1 month interval at home advised for adequate healing of the internal operative site, and nasal irritation or numbness of the upper lip that is variable in duration.

Chemotherapy

There has been a strong interest in new methods for treatment of acromegaly by chemotherapeutic means. Despite the apparent autonomy of the tumors with respect to glucose suppression, growth hormone levels have been responsive to a variety of agents. The first agent with beneficial results was diethylstilbestrol, a synthetic estrogen, used in high dosage of 5 to 25 mg. daily. Serum phosphorus usually decreases, soft tissue recession may occur, further acral growth is prevented, and glucose tolerance may improve. Hypertension is not improved and may worsen. Endometrial hyperplasia with bleeding is a side effect in women, and gynecomastia is a major limitation to its use in men. Tumor growth is not affected, and we have seen extrasellar extension develop in a patient treated elsewhere without provision of radiation therapy. The side effects of estrogen therapy have rendered this method obsolete, but it is important to note that growth hormone levels are not lowered, and the treatment appears to interfere with the action of growth hormone on peripheral tissues. A therapy of this type would be suitable if accomplished by a better tolerated drug.

Agents that have appeared successful due to initial lowering of growth hormone have included medroxy-progesterone, 10 mg. by mouth four times daily, or chlorpromazine, 25 mg. by mouth three times daily. Subsequent experience is that escape from the effects of these drugs takes place and the acromegaly becomes active again.

Successful treatment of growth hormone excess has been reported with the use of an ergot alkaloid, bromocriptine, in doses of 2.5 to 5.0 mg. four times daily. The apparent side effects are nausea, particularly in cortisone-dependent patients, and instances of Raynaud's phenomenon. Failure to respond initially or in the long term is also a problem in some patients. Evidence is not yet available as to whether inhibition of tumor growth can be achieved. Approval for use in the United States has not yet been obtained. Drug treatment while awaiting a response to heavy particle therapy would appear to be an indication for this form of therapy. It may also have application as a diagnostic test to determine whether a patient with residual but minor elevation of growth hormone may benefit by further treatment for acromegaly.

Choice of Treatment

Since more than one type of treatment can be shown to be effective, there is no "treatment of choice" and we prefer to consider "choice of treatment" for each patient and the particular problems involved. In some instances, the choice may depend on the preference of the patient. The degree of current symptoms, presence or absence of complications, and the time available for observation of response are examples of choice factors. Some patients fear surgery and others fear exposure to radiation, even when well informed. A need for prompt relief of acromegaly tends to support a choice of surgery. The presence of a larger tumor that may not be completely accessible to surgery tends to support a choice of heavy particle therapy. The greater speed of surgery is associated with more uncertainty as to future recurrence. When chemotherapy becomes more widely available, the differences in time to achieve remission may be eliminated. At present, each technique has applicability and either surgery or radiation may serve as the second form of therapy in the event of incomplete response to the first chosen therapy. As mentioned, heavy particle therapy has major advantages of convenience that have led to its extensive use in this country and to its initiation in one other country with similar facilities.

Associated Endocrine Disorders

When multiple endocrine neoplasm syndrome (MEN, type I) is present, consideration must be given to priority for treatment of the more threatening clinical problem. In most patients acromegaly is slowly progressive and can be treated at a later date. Pheochromocytoma merits treatment before acromegaly. Islet cell tumor is likewise a serious problem and may produce more severe hypoglycemia if the growth hormone level were to be reduced first. Hyperparathyroidism can usually await treatment of acromegaly unless marked hypercalcemia, over 11.5 mg. per dl. (100 ml.), is present.

Treatment of Anterior Pituitary Failure

The presence of defects in normal pituitary function should be defined and treated in the first evaluation of patients with acromegaly. When possible, hypothyroid patients should achieve full replacement for at least three weeks before major surgery. A covering dose of 40 mg. of methyl-prednisolone (Solu-Medrol) or 4 mg. of dex-amethasone is ordered for intramuscular injection on call to pneumoencephalography for all patients in order to be certain that the typical signs of nausea, fever, and headache are not due to adrenal insufficiency and to prevent hypotension in the event that ACTH reserve is inadequate for stress. In many patients, symptoms of gonadal deficiency may not attract attention in the presence of more urgent problems of acromegaly. Evaluation of such disorders and correction by available replacement therapy may result in other improvements such as muscle strength in the hypogonadal male who is given testosterone.

It is important to survey all patients who have received proton beam therapy at regular intervals and institute hormonal replacement as needed. The slow evolution of symptoms may not be recognized until function tests have demonstrated a change from pretreatment findings. Annual examination and screening tests are a part of the follow-up program recommended to the attending physician.

After transsphenoidal surgery, steroid therapy is tapered rapidly and 8 A.M. cortisol levels are measured on the sixth postoperative day. Low levels are measured again on the following day. Return of cortisol to the preoperative level is considered satisfactory. If ACTH function was deficient before surgery it will usually fail to improve and previous replacement is continued. Patients with uncertain results are studied in more detail with reserve tests. Patients with normal basal function but deficient reserve to hypoglycemia or metyrapone are not given daily replacement therapy but are instructed to take steroids for significant physical stress such as fever, infections, trauma, and surgical procedures. Thyroid replacement is not started on a trial basis but awaits results of hormone tests drawn 3 weeks after surgery since the majority do not become hypothyroid. Equivocal results are evaluated further with a thyrotropin-releasing hormone (TRH) test. Gonadal function in males can be measured while still in the hospital since plasma testosterone will fall rapidly if gonadotropin function is lost. A fasting growth hormone sample is also drawn prior to discharge, and the result is available at the time of the first follow-up visit in order to plan for future evaluations.

Problems in the Management of Acromegaly

The major hindrance to effective therapy of acromegaly is the delay in diagnosis of active disease. The first recognition of acromegaly is often made by a physician who has not seen the patient before. Carpal tunnel syndrome, prognathism, osteoarthritis, hypertension, and diabetes mellitus are clues to the presence of acromegaly that are often ignored. Negative results of serum phosphorus, serum growth hormone, or standard skull x-rays may delay the diagnosis despite the presence of obvious physical changes. An appreciation of the rarity of inactive disease in an untreated patient and the variable clinical and laboratory manifestations in a patient with early disease is necessary to confirm a suspicion of active acromegaly. Stability of acral overgrowth should not be taken as sufficient evidence of disease arrest. The patient who has had successful surgery should not be dismissed from follow-up since delayed recurrence may develop and evade notice in the initial stages when further treatment is most beneficial.

There remains a conservative group of physicians who prefer to await definite complications before making a decision for therapy. During such observation periods, unrestricted growth of the pituitary tumor may cause treatment failure or require more extensive therapy.

The unfounded belief that radiation treatment will interfere with subsequent surgery has limited the choice of therapy and should be discarded. A preference for initial surgery exists in some centers and should not be applied to all patients since unfavorable size or location of the pituitary tumor or presence of risk factors such as cardiac disease can influence the outcome. Some patients have not been informed that, because of the benign nature of the tumor, it does not require total removal by surgical means. The one case of malignant tumor we have reported was in a patient who was treated with estrogens for several years without radiation therapy and required craniotomy when first referred to be treated for the tumor.

Future Developments

The treatment of acromegaly can be improved. More convenient radiographic localization is desirable and should be possible by development of high resolution multidimensional CT scan equipment. A method for metrizamide liquid contrast encephalography has been proposed to the Food and Drug Administration and would provide a better-tolerated study than the pneumoencephalogram. Evaluation of a new radioimmunoassay method for the measurement of somatomedin, the growth factor derived from the action of growth hormone, is underway and has promise of earlier detection and more reliable evaluation of the effects of growth hormone on body tissues and functions. More versatile use of the proton beam has been introduced at the Harvard Cyclotron. Irregular tumors are being treated with different types of beams, including a hemi-beam, double beams applied successively to the outer and inner portions of large tumors, and wedges introduced in the beam path to change the shape of the Bragg peak, which thereby conforms to intrasphenoidal projection of tumor. The number of patients to be accommodated will be increased by additional stereotactic equipment so that as many as five patients can be treated during a simple daytime therapy session. These developments will allow wider availability of treatment and a reduced waiting interval for urgent cases. Ultimate general approval of medical suppressive therapy, presumably with bromocriptine, will allow inclusion of patients who need immediate relief of acromegaly while awaiting the response to heavy particle therapy. The advances of diagnostic tests, preparative radiography, chemotherapy, and new precision techniques in proton beam therapy combined with a general availability of microsurgery will provide effective management and more favorable results in the future treatment of patients with active acromegaly.

ADRENOCORTICAL INSUFFICIENCY

method of
J. C. LAIDLAW, M.D.
Hamilton, Ontario, Canada

Adrenal cortical insufficiency may be primary due to bilateral destruction of the adrenal cortex (Addison's disease). In this type there is a deficient production of all groups of adrenal steroids: glucocorticoids (principally cortisol), androgens, and mineralocorticoids (principally aldosterone). Secondary adrenal cortical insufficiency results from ACTH deficiency due either to pituitary disease or to the suppression of the hypothalamic-pituitary axis by corticosteroids used for the treatment of nonendocrine disorders. In this type there is a deficient production of cortisol and androgens but rarely of aldosterone.

Chronic Adrenocortical Insufficiency

When such insufficiency is primary, the glucocorticoid deficiency may be treated by the oral administration of 25 to 37.5 mg. of cortisone, 20 to 30 mg. of cortisol, or 5 to 7.5 mg. of prednisone daily. Ordinarily one half to two thirds of the dose is taken before breakfast and the remainder at dinner time. Administration of the second dose later in the evening may lead to insomnia. Mineralocorticoid deficiency is treated with 9α-

fluorocortisol (fludrocortisone) by mouth with the dose ranging from 50 micrograms every other day to 100 micrograms daily. One must be careful to avoid mineralocorticoid overtreatment, which is manifested by hypertension and edema due to sodium and water retention and weakness due to potassium loss.

When chronic adrenocortical insufficiency is secondary to pituitary disease, it is only necessary to give glucocorticoid in the manner described for primary insufficiency.

With onset of an acute illness or the occurrence of trauma, surgical or otherwise, glucocorticoid dosage must be increased to prevent adrenal crisis. This applies not only to patients with chronic adrenocortical insufficiency but also to those who are receiving pharmacologic doses of glucocorticoid for the treatment of nonendocrine disorders. With a mild illness such as an upper respiratory infection, an extra tablet of glucocorticoid is sufficient. With an illness complicated by vomiting of more than 12 hours duration, e.g., acute gastroenteritis, the glucocorticoid may not be retained and cortisol succinate, 50 to 100 mg. daily in two divided doses by intramuscular injection, will be required. For a severe acute medical illness, treatment as described below for a major operation should be instituted.

It is not ordinarily necessary to alter steroid dosage during pregnancy in a patient with Addison's disease. However, if edema should occur during the third trimester, mineralocorticoid dosage should be reduced. With the onset of labor, 100 mg. of cortisol succinate (hydrocortisone sodium succinate) should be given every 8 hours by intramuscular injection until delivery has been achieved. Following this, the previous maintenance therapy may be resumed.

With a minor surgical procedure such as dilatation and curettage in patients with treated chronic adrenal insufficiency or in those receiving pharmacologic doses of glucocorticoid, it is necessary merely to give 100 mg. of cortisol succinate intramuscularly or intravenously 1 hour before the procedure and repeat the dose every 6 to 8 hours during the operative day. Over the next 4 to 5 days the glucocorticoid dose is gradually tapered to oral maintenance levels, at which time mineralocorticoid treatment, if it has been part of the maintenance regimen, is resumed.

Every patient with chronic adrenocortical deficiency, as well as those patients on pharmacologic doses of glucocorticoid, should record this information on a card in his wallet and on an identification disc or bracelet. The need for additional glucocorticoid in the event of severe trauma, acute illness, or surgical procedure should also be recorded.

Acute Adrenocortical Insufficiency

The manner in which acute insufficiency can be prevented when acute illness or trauma occurs in patients with treated chronic adrenocortical insufficiency or in those on pharmacologic doses of glucocorticoid has just been described. Acute insufficiency can, of course, also develop when a patient with *untreated* chronic adrenocortical insufficiency falls prey to acute illness or trauma.

Serious suspicion of the presence of acute primary adrenocortical insufficiency requires that replacement therapy be administered forthwith. One hundred mg. of cortisol succinate are given intravenously immediately. Thereafter 100 mg. of this preparation are infused every 6 to 8 hours in 500 to 1000 ml. of 5 per cent glucose in isotonic saline solution depending on the degree of dehydration and salt deficiency. When severe salt depletion is present, as much as 4 liters of isotonic saline solution may be required on the first day of therapy. It is to be emphasized, however, that in the absence of appreciable salt deficiency, the excessive infusion of saline may induce cardiac failure in the addisonian patient. When clinical improvement is noted, gradual tapering of the cortisol dose is begun. Maintenance levels of glucocorticoid by mouth can be reached in 3 to 4 days, provided that the precipitating illness, e.g., an infection, has been brought under control. Large doses of cortisol given intravenously possess considerable mineralocorticoid activity; hence, maintenance 9α-fluorocortisol need not be instituted until the cortisol dose has been tapered to less than 100 mg. per day.

In acute secondary adrenocortical deficiency, treatment with cortisol is identical to that in acute primary adrenocortical deficiency. Replacement of fluid and salt, however, is much less critical in this form of adrenal insufficiency because there is little impairment of aldosterone secretion.

CUSHING'S SYNDROME

method of
LOUIS N. PANGARO, M.D.,
and JOHN J. CANARY, M.D.
Washington, District of Columbia

The treatment of Cushing's syndrome varies, depending on the cause, and thus hinges entirely on accurate diagnosis. The most frequent cause today is *iatrogenic exogenous corticosteroid* utilized in the therapy of nonendocrine disorders. The majority of patients with "endogenous Cushing's syndrome" will be found to have *bilateral adrenocortical hyperplasia* with at least minimally inappropriately elevated plasma levels of ACTH. In the majority of these patients a pituitary or parapituitary tumor cannot be demonstrated by current radiographic techniques. In a small number, ophthalmologic and radiographic techniques, including tomography, may demonstrate an abnormality in the pituitary area. Another variety of hyperplasia is also recognized, associated with low levels of plasma ACTH; this is bilateral *primary nodular hyperplasia* of the adrenal cortex. Finally, bilateral hyperplasia of the cortex with Cushing's syndrome may occur in the presence of neoplasm, usually malignant, but occasionally benign, most commonly of lung or pancreas. These extra-adrenal neoplasms secrete an *ectopic ACTH* leading to bilateral adrenocortical hyperplasia and reduction of the unusual hypothalamic-pituitary control. Cushing's syndrome also results from primary neoplasms of the adrenal cortex, usually *benign adenoma*, occasionally *carcinoma*. Rarely, Cushing's syndrome results from physiologic replacement with normal doses of corticosteroids or from treatment with small therapeutic doses. In patients with myxedema or primary liver dysfunction there may be decreased conjugation or excretion and thus prolonged physiologic effects.

In any case, this syndrome is directly related to the tissue exposure to excessive levels of cortisol. In the endogenous varieties of Cushing's syndrome this results from excessive secretion of this material by the adrenal glands. Diagnostically, the most accurate techniques are the quantitation of urinary free cortisol excretion or its metabolites and demonstration of excessive and non-suppressible secretion rates by the adrenal cortex. Loss of normal diurnal rhythmicity of plasma or urinary cortisol is a helpful diagnostic clue. In the case of hyperplastic adrenal conditions, lack of functional suppressibility by small doses of dexamethasone are useful. Also helpful is the response of 17-hydroxy metabolites to the administration of metyrapone; the excessive endogenous ACTH provoked by this drug will cause an excessive adrenocortical response in hyperplastic states but no stimulation or perhaps a decline in benign adenoma. Cancerous adrenal lesions almost uniformly show no response to these tests. The extra-adrenal neoplastic variety of Cushing's syndrome with ectopic ACTH is characterized by a rapid clinical course, very high levels of cortisol production, and hypokalemic alkalosis, the latter an uncommon manifestation of the other types of cortisol excess.

Preoperative scanning with iodocholesterol compounds has proved very helpful: persistent unilateral uptake (while on dexamethasone for suppression) favors a benign adenoma on the side with uptake; bilaterally persistent uptake favors simple hyperplasia or nodular hyperplasia. No persistent uptake on scan despite very high unsuppressible steroid values favors adrenal carcinoma.

Adrenocortical Neoplasm

After this diagnosis is made, surgical treatment should be carried out. Persistent unilateral uptake on iodocholesterol scanning gives preoperative localization of a *benign adenoma;* this can usually be removed without great difficulty. We recommend removal of the tumor with its attendant tissue. The contralateral gland should be exposed and biopsied to confirm the presence of atrophy of this cortex. With regard to *malignant lesions* of the adrenal cortex, we believe that these should be approached surgically and as much of the tumor as possible should be removed, all if possible. If carcinoma is found, and when the patient is stabilized after the immediate postoperative period, maintenance doses of corticosteroid should be given, such as dexamethasone. These carcinomas usually produce significant amounts of 17-ketosteroids and other metabolites, and since the remaining normal adrenal tissue will continue to be suppressed by the dexamethasone, plasma and urinary steroid levels can be used as a guide to a local recurrence or to increasing metastatic tumor burden.

If palliative therapy is to be utilized, *ortho-para'-DDD*, mitotane (Lysodren), may be given. Regression of primary tumor or metastases may be achieved in about 30 per cent of patients. The dosage is substantial, varying from 6 to 20 grams per day and treatment should be started in the hospital. A large number of patients will demonstrate nausea, vomiting, somnolence, vertigo, or other central nervous system (CNS) symptoms. We recommend the use of this drug for as long as possible and would try to control the symptoms with other medications. Maintenance doses of steroids should, as noted before, be given concomitantly. Some patients may require mineralocorticoids as well. *Aminoglutethimide* (Elipten, Cytadrene) effectively inhibits adrenocortical function by blocking production of pregnenolone from cholesterol. Thus it does not destroy tumor cells but decreases steroid production. At the usual dose of 250 to 500 mg. four times a day it may induce goiter, hypothyroidism, dermatitis, and lethargy. It remains investigational. If used in conjunction with mitotane, its occasional discontinuation to evaluate the mitotane effect is suggested. This compound may be useful preoperatively to reduce the nitrogen wasting of severe Cushing's, particularly with adenoma. It can be given in combination with moderate doses of dexamethasone for some weeks to restore tissues to a more normal quality preoperatively.

Some reduction in cortisol production can be achieved by the use of *metyrapone* (Metopirone) in doses of 500 to 750 mg. four times a day. The drug reduces cortisol production. It does this by inhibiting 11-beta hydroxylase activity in the adrenal cortex; however, increased production of desoxycorticosterone may cause hypertension and hypokalemia. There is no effect on tumor growth.

Bilateral Adrenocortical Hyperplasia

Cushing's Syndrome With Pituitary Tumor. The management of this problem depends upon the degree of severity of Cushing's syndrome. If there is marked evidence of protein wasting and features of severe cortisol excess, adrenalectomy should be carried out as the first therapeutic step. The pituitary tumor can then be treated, depending upon the neurosurgical indications by transsphenoidal resection (wherever possible), by other neurosurgical approaches, or by radiation. Radiation generally requires between 4000 to 5000 rads from a standard source or with higher doses concentrated at the pituitary by means of proton beams.

When the Cushing's syndrome is not severe enough to require immediate bilateral adrenalectomy, a trial with aminoglutethimide may decrease cortisol overproduction while waiting for therapies directed at the pituitary to be effective.

Cushing's Syndrome Without Demonstrable Tumor. Bilateral *total adrenalectomy* is recommended for the adult. It is always effective and is the treatment of choice for patients with severe Cushing's syndrome. When a milder syndrome is present, therapy may be directed at ablating excess ACTH production at the level of the pituitary. Further studies with exploratory *transsphenoidal surgery* may reveal that microadenomas of the pituitary, too small for preoperative detection, are present in many of these patients, despite hypothalamic suppressibility by high dose dexamethasone. This surgical approach may be considered in centers experienced in this technique since the low incidence of panhypopituitarism and immediate effectiveness may outweigh the uncertainty. Otherwise, cobalt or proton *irradiation* may be used.

Medical therapy with cyproheptadine (Periactin) is still investigational in Cushing's syndrome with excess ACTH of pituitary source. Presumably by its antiserotonin effect, this drug inhibits the releasing factor for ACTH and thus medically ameliorates the bilateral adrenal hyperplasia. Half to two thirds of patients may respond at a dose of 8 mg. three times a day. The drug produces no lasting effects and must be maintained indefinitely or until more definitive therapy is applied.

In patients previously treated with subtotal adrenalectomy or maximal pituitary radiation who have relapsed, cyproheptadine or transsphenoidal surgery should be considered before proceeding with second adrenalectomy.

Bilateral Nodular Hyperplasia. In this condition without ACTH dependence, bilateral adrenalectomy should be undertaken.

Bilateral Hyperplasia With an Extra-adrenal Neoplasm. When the *ectopic ACTH* syndrome is diagnosed, therapy is directed, if possible, at the primary tumor, particularly when a localized primary tumor—bronchial carcinoid, seminoma, parotid tumor, pheochromocytoma—is producing the syndrome. Surgical extirpation may completely relieve the syndrome. More commonly, the syndrome is from bronchogenic oat-cell carcinoma, often inoperable. Ectopic ACTH production may respond to irradiation or chemotherapy of the primary tumor or metastases. Orthopara'-DDD with aminoglutethimide may be used to palliate severe hypercortisolism. Thus far, aminoglutethimide is an investigational agent. If the underlying tumor has a relatively good prognosis and the Cushing's syndrome is severe, bilateral adrenalectomy might be considered as a part of the total therapy.

Management of Patients Undergoing Adrenal Surgery

For the purpose of the discussion it will be assumed that complications, e.g., infection, diabetes mellitus, and congestive heart failure, will be managed in the usual manner. In certain of these patients significant psychiatric problems, including frank psychosis, are present. Hypokalemia must be treated preoperatively. At the time of surgery the patient should be supported with full replacement doses of corticosteroids.

When unilateral adrenalectomy is done for a benign adenoma, a period of hypoadrenocorticism will occur postoperatively, since the remaining adrenal cortex will be atrophic. This atrophy is caused by inhibition of the pituitary mechanism by excessive and autonomous cortisol production by the tumor.

We have utilized the following schedule effectively: 100 mg. of cortisone acetate intramuscularly at midnight prior to surgery; 100 mg. of hydrocortisone by intravenous bolus immediately prior to surgery; a drip infusion with 100 mg. of hydrocortisone per 12 hour period is then begun for the day of surgery and the first postoperative day. Thereafter, as soon as the patient can take medication by mouth, dosage is decreased progressively in 50 mg. per day steps. By the seventh to tenth postoperative day a dosage range of 15 to 25 mg. of hydrocortisone is given orally every 6 to 8 hours. After the eighth to tenth day gradual tapering of the oral cortisol with daily decrements of 5 to 10 mg. for 2 to 3 days is recommended. Patients who have bilateral total adrenalectomy will usually require the addition of some salt-retaining steroids such as fluorinated hydrocortisone (Florinef) in a dose ranging from 0.2 mg. per day to 0.1 mg. three times a week. During this period of time, episodes of steroid withdrawal syndrome may be seen following reductions in steroid dosage. This syndrome comprises hypotension, lethargy, weakness, fever, myalgia, nausea, vomiting, or diarrhea. Intensive search for infection, particularly at the incision site, and other causes must be sought. In the absence of other causes, the presence of more than mild symptoms should be treated with an increase in steroid dosage sufficient to control the symptoms. Then, gradual reduction should again be resumed.

When a benign adrenocortical adenoma is removed, the remaining adrenal cortex is atrophic and may require 4 to 12 or more months to recover function. Since pituitary secretion of ACTH may itself require several months to recover from suppression, such patients may be treated with long-acting ACTH in doses of 80 units intramuscularly 3 or 4 times a week for the first few weeks, then 3 times a week for 2 months, and then in progressively decreased doses. When the patient's symptoms are minimal or when endogenous ACTH secretion returns, determined by rising radioimmunoassay levels, or when essentially normal plasma and urinary steroid values are found some days following the last ACTH injection, exogenous administration is no longer needed.

It is equally true that certain patients with adenomas and mild Cushing's syndrome may not require more than a few weeks of low dose steroid maintenance following surgery and then do well without further treatment.

Long-term Problems

Patients who have undergone bilateral adrenalectomy or who have glucocorticoid deficiency after pituitary ablation require intensive education in the problem of living without full adrenal capacity. Basically, this consists of being aware that more hydrocortisone is required with significant stress such as febrile illness, more than trivial injury or dental extraction. These patients should carry with them at all times the information that they are taking corticosteroids after an adrenalectomy. They should have available in their homes one of the readily injectable forms of glucocorticoid, so that if an episode preventing oral therapy occurs it will be available.

The physician should also be aware that after bilateral adrenalectomy about 15 per cent of patients develop *Nelson's syndrome,* characterized by a progressive intense pigmentation signaling the expression of a pituitary neoplasm producing excessive ACTH. All patients with this variety of Cushing's syndrome should have had careful tomography of the pituitary fossa prior to initial therapy. Skull x-rays and serial measurements of plasma ACTH should be followed, especially if there are pigmentary changes or elevated ACTH levels despite adequate replacement with glucocorticoids. Pituitary irradiation at the time of adrenalectomy has not been shown to prevent this syndrome. Treatment is with the use of surgical, radiation, or cyproheptadine therapies described earlier.

Iatrogenic Cushing's Syndrome

Prevention is the best form of treatment for this serious problem. Use of every-other-day administration and giving the pharmacologic dose at noon to reduce its effect on the hypothalamic-pituitary axis is, when possible, effective, providing that the steroid does not have a prolonged disappearance time.

When this syndrome is encountered, serious consideration should be given to the possibility of withdrawing the patient from the medication. With some patients this can be done; with others it cannot. When it can, it is best done by gradual reduction in dosage over weeks to months with careful evaluation of the response of the underlying disorder; periodic increases in steroid dosage may be required. When the underlying disease allows, giving a larger dose but on alternate days, at noon, also facilitates pituitary recovery.

In general, following successful withdrawal from long-term corticosteroid therapy, we recommend that extra attention to the risks to which such patients may be exposed in terms of their ability to respond to stress, in particular, to emergency or elective surgical stress, for up to 12 months. If significant stress is encountered during that period and stress response capacity is unknown, treatment should be given as if the patient were adrenally insufficient. For minor stress, such as mild febrile illness, an increase in cortisol from maintenance dosage (25 to 30 mg. per day) to 60 to 75 mg. per day for the few days of stress is sufficient. The patients must also be educated not to overtreat themselves.

The patient recovering from Cushing's syndrome caused by exogenous steroids is similar to one recovering after removal of an adenoma. In both cases it is worthwhile to test the recovery of the patient's pituitary adrenal axis. Specifically, adrenal response to exogenous ACTH can be tested simply with plasma cortisol levels before and at 30 or 60 minutes following an intravenous ACTH bolus, and if a response occurs, the higher levels of control can be tested in the usual fashion with metyrapone. This should not be done prematurely but only some time after discontinuation of steroid. If the responses are normal, exogenous steroid support for the stress should not be needed.

DIABETES INSIPIDUS

method of
MARGARET BIA, M.D.
New Haven, Connecticut

Diabetes insipidus is a disease characterized by polyuria and polydipsia that results from a failure of the kidneys to conserve water despite an increased plasma osmolality. The cause of this disorder can be central in origin owing to lack of the antidiuretic hormone, arginine vasopressin (central diabetes insipidus), or it can be caused by an inability of the renal tubule to respond to vasopressin (nephrogenic diabetes insipidus).

The hallmark of the derangement is a urine that is inappropriately dilute relative to plasma tonicity. In establishing the diagnosis, it is first essential to exclude other causes of polyuria such as diabetes mellitus, post obstructive states and certain kinds of chronic renal failure. In these conditions, the excessive urine output results primarily from a loss of solute (such as glucose in diabetes mellitus) that secondarily inhibits fluid reabsorption in the kidney, creating a solute diuresis. This results in a large volume of urine which is usually isotonic with plasma. In contrast, the typical patient with diabetes insipidus experiences polyuria due to excessive water losses and will have a urine that is relatively dilute (UOsm less than 200 mOsm. per kg. water or specific gravity less than 1.005). The diagnosis of diabetes insipidus is usually established following a fluid deprivation study designed to increase plasma osmolality and thus provide a strong stimulus for ADH secretion. Patients with complete central or nephrogenic diabetes insipidus will fail to concentrate their urine above plasma osmolality unless severe dehydration ensues. If exogenous vasopressin is administered after the period of fluid deprivation, the person with central diabetes insipidus will respond with a significant rise in urine osmolality. The patient with nephrogenic diabetes insipidus will respond neither to fluid deprivation nor to exogenous vasopressin. The patient with partial central diabetes insipidus may concentrate the urine above plasma osmolality following dehydration, but urine osmolality will still be less than that found in normal subjects under similar conditions.

In central diabetes insipidus, the lack of antidiuretic hormone can be either partial or complete, and the defect can be either temporary or permanent. Approximately 50 per cent of all cases are idiopathic while the remaining cases result from damage to the hypothalamic-pituitary tract from head trauma, pituitary surgery, or tumor. A thorough evaluation of the hypothalamic-pituitary tract in search of possible causes of secondary diabetes insipidus is therefore essential once the diagnosis of central diabetes insipidus has been established. The patient with uncomplicated diabetes insipidus rarely suffers serious water depletion since with an intact thirst mechanism and with free access to water, he will drink large amounts of fluid to prevent dehydration and plasma hyperosmolality. However, the marked polydipsia and polyuria is quite disturbing and interrupts sleep; therefore, replacement therapy is justified. In the unconscious patient who is unable to drink, replacement therapy is critical. Despite many new modes of treatment available in recent years, administration of some form of vasopressin remains the cornerstone of treatment of central diabetes insipidus.

Nephrogenic or vasopressin-resistant diabetes insipidus can occur as a familial defect, can result from a variety of metabolic disorders such as hypokalemia or hypercalcemia, or can be caused by a variety of drugs, most notably demeclocycline and lithium. The polyuria is usually not as marked in these patients as in patients with central diabetes insipidus. Treatment of this disorder should first be directed at correction of the underlying cause, if possible (also see thiazide diuretics).

Central Diabetes Insipidus

Once the diagnosis is established and a careful search for potentially remediable causes has been made, chronic treatment can be instituted. The development of new vasopressin analogues with less pressor activity and a longer duration of action has revolutionized the treatment of diabetes insipidus and will probably make the future use of nonhormonal drugs less essential. However, even with the availability of newer analogues it is likely that for any given patient, treatment will have to be individualized using one of several possible drugs.

1. *Aqueous vasopressin (Pitressin)* is a water-soluble posterior pituitary mixture containing a variable amount of lysine and arginine vasopressin. It is available in 1 ml. vials containing 20 units per ml. and is used mainly for diagnostic purposes and for management of the unconscious patient with acute central diabetes insipidus. It should not be used as a form of chronic treatment in patients with uncomplicated diabetes insipidus. When the usual dose of 5 to 10 units is given subcutaneously or intramuscularly, the onset of action occurs within 30 to 60 minutes and lasts approximately 4 to 6 hours. When used intravenously, in doses of 1 to 5 milliunits per minute, the onset of action is immediate and lasts 30 to 60 minutes. Intravenous usage should be reserved for investigational purposes only. Adverse reactions are similar to those listed under vasopressin tannate in oil.

2. *Vasopressin (Pitressin) tannate in oil* is a long-

acting preparation containing a mixture of lysine and arginine vasopressin. It is available in 1 ml. ampules containing 5 units per ml. When administered in the usual dose of 2 to 5 units subcutaneously or intramuscularly, the onset of action occurs within 2 to 4 hours and the antidiuresis lasts for 24 to 72 hours. Before injection of the preparation, care must be taken to shake vigorously and warm the vials in order to ensure that the brown precipitate, which can be seen at the bottom of the ampule before agitation, is properly suspended in the oil. This precipitate contains the active hormone, and failure to distribute it evenly in the emulsion is the most common cause for treatment failure with this regimen.

Adverse reactions with vasopressin include abdominal cramps, nausea, and menstrual cramps in females, owing to stimulation of intestinal and uterine contractility. Since vasopressin is a potent vasoconstrictor, patients with coronary artery disease should be treated with caution at the onset of therapy although blood pressure elevation and coronary insufficiency are uncommon at the recommended doses. Rarely, allergic reactions may occur and are treated by desensitization. Local abscesses at the site of injection have also been reported to occur after long-term usage. Perhaps the most common adverse reaction is dilutional hyponatremia secondary to excessive water retention that can result from too frequent use of the preparation. This complication can be prevented easily by training the patient to repeat the next dose of vasopressin only after polyuria recurs. In general, complications with vasopressin usage are uncommon, and it is a safe and effective form of therapy for many patients with diabetes insipidus.

3. *Synthetic lysine vasopressin (Diapid)* is a nonirritating saline solution (50 units per ml.) that is sprayed deeply into the nasal passages, 1 to 2 sprays in each nostril. It is administered every 4 to 6 hours with an additional dose before bedtime. Its major limitation is its short duration of action, but it has been useful as an adjunct to parenteral therapy during travel or at bedtime. In addition, it has obviated the need for injections in some patients, which is especially important in treating children.

4. *Desmopressin (DDAVP)* is a synthetic analogue of vasopressin with greater antidiuretic potency and greatly diminished pressor activity, so that the compound is more specifically a "water hormone" than is the parent substance. It is currently available in 2.5 ml. vials containing 0.1 mg. per ml. of solution. A small calibrated catheter comes with each ampule so that exact amounts can be measured and inhaled intranasally. When the usual dose of 5 to 20 micrograms is employed, the onset of action occurs within 1 hour and the antidiuresis lasts for 8 to 20 hours. Most patients can be maintained on 10 to 20 micrograms once or twice daily. Extensive investigations in Europe and in the United States in both adults and in children have confirmed the superiority of DDAVP over other available preparations of vasopressin. Unlike lysine vasopressin, it has a longer duration of action so that patients can be maintained on 1 or 2 daily doses. Unlike vasopressin tannate in oil, no agitation is required before administration. In addition, painful and unpleasant injections, which can be especially noxious to children, and local reactions are avoided. All studies to date indicate that patients receiving DDAVP clearly prefer this form of therapy over other hormonal and nonhormonal treatment regimens. DDAVP appears destined to become the drug of choice for this disease.

Adverse reactions have not yet been reported although it is expected that excessive water retention with resultant hyponatremia could occur if the doses were not adjusted to be given only when onset of symptoms recur.

5. *Nonhormonal therapy* includes the use of agents such as thiazide diuretics, chlorpropamide, clofibrate, and carbamazepine. It should be emphasized that the use of these agents in the treatment of diabetes insipidus is not listed in the manufacturer's official directive. These drugs, used alone or in combination with each other or as an adjunct to hormone therapy, have been efficacious in some patients. They are most effective in the treatment of patients with residual amounts of vasopressin and may even be used alone in patients with partial central diabetes insipidus. However, with the availability of new vasopressin analogues, these drugs may eventually be useful only in patients with sensitivity or refractoriness to exogenous vasopressin.

The *thiazide* diuretics are useful in reducing urine volume in patients with both central and nephrogenic diabetes insipidus. The conventional doses employed, 50 to 100 mg. of hydrochlorothiazide* or 500 to 1000 mg. of chlorothiazide* daily, are effective in decreasing polyuria in patients with both central and nephrogenic diabetes insipidus. Their mode of action depends on creating a state of negative salt balance with volume contraction. This reduces glomerular filtration rate (GFR) and increases fluid reabsorption in the renal tubule, thus decreasing total urine volume. Their effectiveness can therefore be abolished by a high salt intake. Side effects, mainly hypokalemia, are uncommon at the recommended doses except in cases of lithium induced diabetes insipidus where large potassium losses can occur.

---

*This use of this agent is not listed in the manufacturer's official directive.

*Chlorpropamide (Diabinese)** is an oral sulfonylurea hypoglycemic agent that is successful in reducing polyuria in about 50 per cent of patients with central diabetes insipidus. When given orally as a single dose of 250 mg., onset of action occurs in approximately 24 hours with peak antidiuresis occurring in 2 to 3 days. Dosage may be increased in a stepwise fashion up to 750 mg. daily, although the incidence of side effects is more common when larger doses are used. The drug is ineffective in patients with nephrogenic diabetes insipidus or patients with complete central diabetes insipidus, for its major mode of action appears to be a potentiation of the action of vasopressin on water reabsorption by the distal nephron. A good response to chlorpropamide can be predicted from the initial fluid deprivation study, since there is a positive correlation between patients' ability to concentrate the urine during dehydration and subsequent responsiveness to chlorpropamide. An increased antidiuresis can be expected when chlorpropamide is used in combination with thiazide diuretics or clofibrate. The major side effect is hypoglycemia, which occurs in up to 10 per cent of patients in some series. Children and patients with anterior hypopituitarism are most susceptible to this adverse effect. Other complications include a disulfiram (Antabuse)-like reaction with alcohol as well as dilutional hyponatremia. The latter is usually related to excessive ingestion of the drug. In addition, it is possible that, with prolonged usage, an increased incidence of cardiovascular abnormalities may occur, as has been suggested by the University Group Diabetes Program (UGDP) study with the use of tolbutamide.

*Clofibrate (Atromid-S)** is an oral hypolipidemic agent that is effective in patients with partial central diabetes insipidus but ineffective in nephrogenic or complete central diabetes insipidus. When given orally at doses of 500 mg. every 6 to 12 hours, its peak effectiveness does not occur for 48 to 72 hours. Its action depends on the presence of some residual vasopressin and when used in combination with chlorpropamide or thiazide diuretics, but not with vasopressin, its antidiuretic potential can be enhanced. Although its mechanism of action has not been well defined, it is thought to exert its effect through release of residual amounts of vasopressin. Although some physicians prefer clofibrate over chlorpropamide as therapy for diabetes insipidus because it avoids the danger of hypoglycemia, it has the disadvantage of having to be administered more frequently. In addition, gastrointestinal side effects, myositis, and liver function abnormalities have been reported.

*Carbamazepine (Tegretol)** is an oral agent used as an anticonvulsant and in the treatment of tic douloureux. It is similar to clofibrate in that, when given orally at doses of 200 mg. 2 to 4 times daily, peak effectiveness is achieved in 2 to 3 days. In addition, it is effective only in the presence of some residual amount of vasopressin and therefore cannot be used in the treatment of complete central diabetes insipidus. Lastly, its antidiuretic potential can be enhanced by concomitant use with chlorpropamide and thiazide diuretics, but not with vasopressin. Since its mode of action is similar to that of clofibrate and since it can induce the rare but serious side effect of aplastic anemia, its use in the routine treatment of diabetes insipidus is not recommended at this time.

Nephrogenic Diabetes Insipidus

In patients with nephrogenic diabetes insipidus, therapy should first be directed at correction of the underlying cause such as a metabolic defect or drug. If the cause is not correctable or if the defect is familial, treatment should then be focused on reducing the polyuria with the use of diuretics as discussed earlier. In addition, dietary restriction of protein and salt is quite effective. Such restriction limits the solute load to be excreted thereby reducing obligatory water losses and hence urine volume.

Two final points concerning the treatment of diabetes insipidus deserve emphasis. First, in patients with diabetes insipidus secondary to causes frequently reported to be temporary, such as head trauma, fluid deprivation studies of therapy should be performed periodically to assess the need for continued treatment and therefore avoid a lifetime of unnecessary therapy. Finally, in patients with uncomplicated diabetes insipidus, it is important to emphasize to the patient that he can never come to serious acute harm, treated or untreated, if he religiously follows the maxim "drink whenever, but only whenever, you are thirsty."

SIMPLE GOITER

method of
MARTIN I. SURKS, M.D.
Bronx, New York

Simple goiter represents a large category of thyroid diseases with diverse diagnostic, therapeutic, and prognostic implications. The criteria for inclusion in this group of disorders, also called nontoxic goiter, include

---

*This use of this agent is not listed in the manufacturer's official directive.

thyroidal enlargement and normal thyroid function based on clinical evaluation and normal concentration of serum thyroid hormones. Once a diagnosis of simple goiter is made, an attempt should be made to determine the cause of the disorder so that the most appropriate therapy will be employed. Specific diagnostic tests are generally directed at determination of the metabolic status with measurements of serum thyroxine (T_4), triiodothyronine (T_3), plasma hormone binding (T_3-resin uptake), and thyrotropin (TSH). Thyroid size and function are usually assessed with a radionuclide scan.

Simple goiters can be divided into two general types based on whether the enlargement is diffuse or nodular. Diffuse goiter includes patients with chronic thyroiditis, those with documented or presumed abnormalities of enzymes critical to hormonogenesis and iodine conservation, and patients with goiters induced by pharmacologic doses of iodides or by lithium therapy. These disorders may be associated with hypothyroidism as defined clinically by typical symptoms and signs and chemically by an elevation in serum TSH and a decrease in serum T_4 and T_3. Some patients may appear euthyroid clinically with serum T_4 and T_3 concentrations in the normal range but have an elevation in serum TSH and this probably represents the earliest stage of thyroidal failure. A specific diagnosis is important for appropriate treatment. Thus, for iodide- or lithium-induced goiters, with or without clinical hypothyroidism, removal of the offending agent alone will lead to a return to normal thyroid function and diminution in thyroid size. In chronic thyroiditis with elevated antithyroid antibody titers or thyroidal enzyme abnormalities, thyroid hormone production is or will be permanently reduced. Patients in these groups should receive lifelong hormonal replacement. L-thyroxine (levothyroxine) is the preferred agent for hormonal replacement since the pattern of plasma T_4 and T_3 concentration following drug ingestion closely mimics that seen in normal euthyroid subjects throughout the 24 hour period. Ingestion of hormone preparations that contain T_3 such as T_3 itself, combinations of T_4 and T_3, and desiccated thyroid results in wide fluctuations in T_3 concentrations. A daily dose of L-thyroxine between 0.1 and 0.2 mg. is sufficient to return most patients to the euthyroid state clinically, and this should be accompanied by normalization of the serum T_4 and TSH concentrations. The potential cardiovascular complications of hormonal replacement in patients with underlying heart disease should always be considered. In this group, the initial dose of L-thyroxine (T_4) should be small (0.025 mg. per day or less) and the dose incremented at about monthly intervals.

When diffuse goiter occurs in a euthyroid patient, the thyroidal enlargement is generally presumed due to exposure to increased concentrations of TSH over a long period of time. Although a significant increase in serum TSH or in the TSH response to thyrotropin releasing hormone (TRH) has not been demonstrated in such patients, an essential role for TSH in the pathogenesis of these thyroidal enlargements is still likely. This is because TSH is a potent stimulus for thyroid growth and because TSH secretion may be augmented even by a very small decrease in plasma thyroid hormone concentrations. Since the quantitative characteristics of the thyroid growth response to TSH are not well known, it is possible that a very small increase in TSH concentration that would be undetectable using available TSH assays could, over a long period of time, induce goiter formation. Another possibility is that increased TSH secretion, which is responsible for thyroidal enlargement, occurs at night rather than during the waking day when most clinical measurements are made. In this regard, it is now established in normal subjects that the main TSH release occurs during the several hours prior to sleep. Thus, the 24 hour pattern of plasma TSH concentration in goitrous subjects might reveal such an elevation.

The likelihood that TSH is responsible for these thyroidal enlargements makes suppression of TSH secretion by administered thyroid hormone the treatment of choice. The guidelines for TSH suppression therapy for these patients are roughly similar as those for hormonal replacement. Since only a minimal increase in serum T_4 and T_3 concentration suppresses TSH secretion, the range of L-thyroxine doses required for TSH suppression, 0.1 to 0.2 mg. per day for 90 per cent of patients, is similar to that for hormonal replacement. Different, however, are the criteria for determining when adequate TSH suppression has been achieved. A decrease in serum TSH concentration to the undetectable assay range is not adequate due to the insensitivity of the TSH radioimmunoassays available in most laboratories. Thus, some normal subjects may have undetectable TSH values. Some patients with undetectable TSH in samples obtained during the day still may release TSH prior to sleep or after TRH administration, indicating that they still have the ability to secrete TSH under appropriate physiologic or pharmacologic stimuli. My clinic relies heavily on the thyrotropin releasing hormone (TRH) stimulation test in conjunction with measurement of serum T_4 to determine whether the dose of L-thyroxine is sufficient to achieve adequate TSH suppression. The dose of L-thyroxine is adjusted until the serum T_4 concentration is similar to or 1 to 2 micrograms per dl. (100 ml.) greater than before therapy was instituted. Thyrotropin releasing hormone (protirelin), 500 micrograms intravenously, is then administered and a blood sample is obtained after 10 to 20 minutes for TSH measurement. Absence of a TSH response to TRH indicates that TSH secretion is adequately suppressed. If plasma TSH is measureable after TRH, the dose of L-thyroxine is increased by 0.025 to 0.05 micrograms per day and the testing procedure outlined above is repeated after 1 to 2 months.

Although TSH suppression therapy results in diminution in thyroid size in the majority of patients with diffuse goiters, diminution in size occurs in no more than one half of patients with nodular goiters. Benign nodular disease presumably arises after sequential hyperplasia and involution of the thyroid that is chronically exposed to increased TSH. Although most nodules are benign, the occurrence of nodules raises the possibilities of adenoma or carcinoma. If the thyroid scan shows that a single nodule is nonfunctioning or cold or that there is a significant cold area in a multinodular gland, the incidence of carcinoma is increased and surgical excision is usually recommended. There is also a higher index of suspicion of carcinoma when nodules occur in children, in men, or in patients who have a history of irradiation to the anterior neck for enlargement of the tonsils, thymus, adenoids, or for treatment of acne. Medical management of benign nodular disease is generally directed at the presumed causative factor, TSH. TSH suppression therapy is instituted as described here and the criteria employed for adequate TSH suppression are also used for patients with nodular goiters. Diminution in thyroid size occurs in about one half the patients with no change notable in the remainder. If thyroid size is decreased, long-term TSH suppression therapy with L-thyroxine is indicated. However, if the thyroid size is unchanged with adequate TSH suppression therapy, the indications for continued treatment are less clear. Some workers would discontinue TSH suppression therapy, whereas others suggest that continued TSH suppression may at least prevent further thyroidal enlargement or development of new nodules.

As indicated, surgical excision is carried out to exclude carcinoma in a number of patients with either single or multiple nonfunctioning nodules. Other indications for surgery may occasionally be symptoms of dysphagia or tracheal compression or continued growth of nodules during adequate TSH suppression therapy. If surgery proves benign disease, long-term TSH suppression therapy with L-thyroxine is usually instituted. The ra-

tionale for this management is to prevent the emergence of new nodules in predisposed patients.

HYPER- AND HYPOPARATHYROIDISM

method of
FREDERICK R. SINGER, M.D.
Los Angeles, California

Primary Hyperparathyroidism

Primary hyperparathyroidism is second to malignancies as a cause of hypercalcemia. The development of sensitive radioimmunoassays for the measurement of parathyroid hormone has greatly improved the clinician's ability to diagnose this condition. The use of routine screening tests of serum chemistries has altered the clinical presentation of the disease. In the past patients primarily presented with symptoms of hypercalcemia, bone disease, and renal stones. More recently a significant number of patients have been discovered with asymptomatic hypercalcemia. The definitive treatment of the disease remains surgical; but in view of the necessity of at least partially correcting severe hypercalcemia prior to operation, the medical treatment of symptomatic hypercalcemia will be discussed first.

Medical Management of Hyperparathyroidism.
DIET. Since excessive gastrointestinal absorption of calcium may contribute to the hypercalcemia, a low calcium diet (restriction of dairy products) is indicated.

HYDRATION AND DIURESIS. Vomiting, anorexia, and polyuria all may contribute to the development of dehydration. The intravenous administration of 0.9 per cent sodium chloride serves two purposes: it corrects dehydration and induces renal calcium diuresis by inhibiting renal tubular reabsorption of calcium. From 4 to 10 liters per day may be required. After rehydration and establishment of vigorous urinary output, furosemide, 40 to 80 mg., or ethacrynic acid, 50 mg., may be administered intermittently to further increase urinary calcium excretion. It is preferable to carry out this therapeutic regimen within an intensive care unit, as careful monitoring of central venous pressure and urinary output and electrolytes are necessary to minimize the possibility of the patient's developing congestive heart failure, hypokalemia, and hypomagnesemia. Full replacement of the potassium and magnesium losses should be accomplished. If adequate diuresis is achieved, serum calcium concentrations near normal usually can be attained within 24 to 72 hours. Other modes of treatment should then be considered, as this regimen is expensive, requires considerable physician time, and is fatiguing to the patient. Contraindications to its use are the presence of congestive heart failure and anuria.

ORAL AND INTRAVENOUS PHOSPHATE. In patients with low or low-normal serum phosphate concentration, phosphate treatment is highly effective in controlling hypercalcemia. Oral treatment should be instituted with 250 mg. of elemental phosphorus administered four times a day. It is important to administer the last dose at bedtime to avoid a prolonged period between doses. The dose may be increased by 500 mg. increments per day if the desired effects are not attained after 2 or 3 days on a given dose. The maximum tolerated dose is usually 3 grams daily. The serum phosphate concentration should be monitored daily to avoid hyperphosphatemia. Diarrhea may occur at higher doses and usually subsides after reducing the dose. Available commercial preparations are listed in Table 1.

Patients who cannot tolerate oral medication may receive intravenous phosphate as either a sodium or potassium salt in a dosage of 1 gram daily. This should be administered over at least a 6 to 8 hour period to avoid hyperphosphatemia. This regimen has proved safe, but if higher doses are administered over shorter periods of time, a patient may develop hypocalcemia and hypotension and expire.

Phosphate may be used for years in patients who refuse surgery or who have had unsuccessful surgery. The serum calcium will be suppressed in most patients, but there is no evidence to indicate that this treatment prevents the continuing deleterious effects of parathyroid hormone on the skeleton.

The use of phosphate is contraindicated in the presence of hyperphosphatemia. If renal function is impaired, the starting dose should be reduced. Potassium phosphate can be used in patients who are in congestive heart failure.

MITHRAMYCIN. Mithramycin is a cytotoxic antibiotic which has been used in the management of certain malignancies such as embryonal cell carcinoma of the testes. It is a potent hypocalcemic agent through its inhibitory effect on bone resorption. It is administered intravenously over a 10 minute period or longer in a dose of 25 to 50 micrograms per kg. The hypocalcemic effect is usually observed within hours, but the maximal effect is often noted after several days. This drug has considerable toxicity. Platelet depression leading to hemorrhage is the most dangerous complication. Impaired renal function and transient rises in hepatic enzymes may also develop. Nausea and vomiting are common side effects which may require treatment. It is preferable to use this drug only if other measures fail. Close monitoring of the toxic effects should be carried out. Repeat injections should be kept to a minimum and should not be administered without knowledge of the platelet count and renal function.

ESTROGENS. Primary hyperparathyroidism is most commonly diagnosed in postmenopausal females. If physiologic doses of estrogens are given to such patients, a decrease in serum calcium concentration of up to 1 mg. per dl. (100 ml.) may result. Ethinyl estradiol, 50 micrograms daily, or conjugated estrogens, 0.3 to 1.25 mg. daily, for 3 of every 4 weeks have proved effective doses. The effects on serum calcium concentration may persist more than 1 year on treatment.

CALCITONIN. Calcitonin is a peptide hormone which has been successfully used in the treatment of Paget's disease of bone. It is a natural antagonist of parathyroid hormone and should be an ideal agent in the management of primary hyperparathyroidism. It does acutely lower serum calcium concentration, but this effect is usually not sustained on repeated treatment. Salmon calcitonin is the form available for use, but it has not been approved for this purpose by the Food and Drug Administration. A dose of 50 to 100 MRC units given parenterally will induce a transient hypocalcemic response.

DIALYSIS. In an occasional patient in whom certain drugs are contraindicated or have proved ineffective, peritoneal dialysis or hemodialysis utilizing a calcium-free dialysate may be required to temporarily manage hypercalcemia. Such a patient may have associated complications such as chronic renal failure or congestive heart failure.

The aforementioned treatments may also be useful in managing other diseases which result in hypercalcemia. It should be kept in mind that adrenal corticosteroids are quite ineffective in patients with primary hyperparathyroidism but very

TABLE 1.   **Some Commercial Preparations of Phosphate**

PREPARATION	1 GRAM OF ELEMENTAL PHOSPHORUS IN:
Oral	
pHos-pHaid	8 tablets, 0.5 gram each
Phospho-Soda	1½ teaspoons
Hyper-Phos K	6 tablets
K-Phos	8 tablets
Intravenous	
Potassium phosphate	30 ml., 1.1 M solution

efficacious in managing the hypercalcemia of sarcoidosis and various malignancies.

Surgical Management of Hyperparathyroidism. The definitive treatment of primary hyperparathyroidism is surgical. In more than 80 per cent of patients this involves the removal of a single parathyroid adenoma. Because approximately 15 per cent of patients have hyperplasia of all four glands and because abnormal glands may be located in unusual sites such as the mediastinum, it is important that the surgery be undertaken by a surgeon experienced in parathyroidectomy. The following principles should be kept in mind:

PREOPERATIVE PREPARATION.   Severe hypercalcemia may lead to dehydration, hypokalemia, and hypomagnesemia. These abnormalities should be corrected prior to surgery.

SELECTIVE VENOUS CATHETERIZATION. In patients who have had previous unsuccessful parathyroid surgery or when a nonparathyroid neoplasm is suspected to be secreting parathyroid hormone, blood samples can be obtained from veins draining the parathyroid glands and other sites. Assay of the samples for parathyroid hormone will frequently point to the most likely site of the excessive hormone secretion. This information can greatly aid the surgeon but is probably unnecessary as a routine procedure owing to its expense and the likelihood that an experienced surgeon has an excellent success rate in previously unoperated patients.

SURGICAL STRATEGY.   The decision to operate on a patient with primary hyperparathyroidism should be based on the presence of symptoms, the detection of complications, the age of the patient, and the presence of other disorders which might influence the operative risk. The elderly asymptomatic patient can be followed with or without medical treatment and may never require surgical intervention. Younger patients who are asymptomatic may also be followed; but if the serum calcium concentration is consistently above 12 mg. per dl., surgery is probably advisable. The symptomatic patient, at any age, should be strongly considered as a surgical candidate.

Knowledge of the pathology of primary hyperparathyroidism is important in the surgical management. If on initial exploration of one side of the neck an enlarged gland is found, this should be removed and sent to the pathology laboratory for frozen sections to be made. Further exploration should be carried out to find the other gland on that side. The second gland should be biopsied or even removed for pathologic evaluation. If the large gland is consistent with a parathyroid adenoma histologically and the second gland is

normal, the exploration can be terminated, because the incidence of multiple adenomas is very small. If both glands are abnormal, the presence of hyperplasia is likely and the opposite side of the neck should be dissected until the other two glands are found. If hyperplasia is present in all the glands, a subtotal parathyroidectomy, including three glands and a fraction of the fourth gland, should be done. An estimated 100 mg. of parathyroid tissue should remain. A metal clip can be placed as a marker to allow future surgery should hypercalcemia recur because of further enlargement of the remaining gland. The presence of hyperplasia should be suspected in any patient with associated endocrine neoplasia or with a family history of endocrine neoplasia. Should no abnormal glands be found in the neck, the surgeon frequently can explore the superior mediastinum through the neck incision and locate a mediastinal tumor. If none is found, the incision should be closed. Mediastinal exploration through a sternal split should be done at a later time. Selective venous catheterization can be done prior to this procedure.

POSTOPERATIVE MANAGEMENT.   Serum calcium concentration begins to decrease within hours after successful surgery. In most patients the concentration will return to normal or slightly below normal levels. In patients with significant bone disease as manifested by increased serum alkaline phosphatase concentration and abnormal x-rays, the "hungry bone syndrome" may develop. Hypocalcemia occurs within several days after surgery and may persist for months if untreated. This state can be distinguished from iatrogenic hypoparathyroidism by measurement of the serum parathyroid hormone concentration. Postoperative magnesium deficiency may also cause hypocalcemia and can usually be diagnosed by measurement of the serum magnesium concentration. If magnesium deficiency is ruled out, the treatment should be a high calcium and phosphate intake, 1 to 2 quarts of milk daily, and pharmacologic doses of vitamin D_2 or dihydrotachysterol. The dose of these agents should be adjusted to maintain serum calcium concentration in the low normal range. A dose of 50,000 units of vitamin D_2 or 0.2 mg. or more of dihydrotachysterol daily may be necessary. As the serum alkaline phosphatase concentration falls with healing of the bone, the dose can be reduced.

Secondary Hyperparathyroidism

Secondary hyperparathyroidism develops as a physiologic response to a state of resistance to the effects of parathyroid hormone. Severe hyperplasia of the parathyroid glands develops most commonly in patients with chronic renal failure and hypocalcemia. Other disorders commonly associated with parathyroid hyperplasia are osteomalacia, rickets, and pseudohypoparathyroidism. The key to treatment is to increase the serum calcium concentration with the judicious use of vitamin D or an analogue and calcium supplementation. A prolonged state of normocalcemia will decrease parathyroid hormone secretion and thereby protect the skeleton against the deleterious effects of the hormone. In patients with chronic renal failure particular care must be taken to normalize the serum phosphate concentration to avoid metastatic calcification. This can be achieved by the use of aluminum hydroxide, 2 tablespoons given four times daily. Large doses of vitamin D_2, 50,000 units or more daily, or dihydrotachysterol, 0.2 mg. or more daily, with 1 to 2 grams of elemental calcium (calcium lactate, 7.7 to 15.4 grams, or calcium carbonate, 2.5 to 5 grams) are often required to correct hypocalcemia. Frequent monitoring of blood chemistries is absolutely imperative in these patients. In patients who are resistant to this treatment, symptomatic bone disease or severe pruritus may be an indication for subtotal parathyroidectomy. This may now be successfully accomplished by removing all parathyroid tissue from the neck and autotransplanting 100 mg. of parathyroid tissue in a forearm muscle. If continuing parathyroid hyperplasia occurs, reoperation can be done under local anesthesia.

Hypoparathyroidism

Hypoparathyroidism may arise as a complication of thyroid surgery, as a rare idiopathic disorder associated with other endocrine deficiencies such as Addison's disease and hypothyroidism, and, not uncommonly, as a reversible complication of severe magnesium deficiency. Tetany may be manifested early in the course of hypocalcemia and can be treated with a short infusion of 10 ml. of 10 per cent calcium gluconate. All patients found to be hypocalcemic should have a serum magnesium concentration determined. If magnesium deficiency is suspected because of alcoholism, malabsorption, or long-term parenteral therapy, magnesium sulfate, 4 ml. of a 50 per cent solution, can be administered parenterally while awaiting the result. If hypomagnesemia is found, treatment should be continued for at least 5 days with 12 ml. of 50 per cent magnesium sulfate to obtain a maximal increase in serum calcium concentration. The drug is best tolerated by intravenous infusion over 12 to 24 hours. Vitamin D or calcium supplementation is not necessary.

The management of chronic hypocalcemia caused by iatrogenic or idiopathic hypoparathyroidism is most easily achieved by the use of high doses of vitamin D_2, average dose 50,000 units daily, or dihydrotachysterol, average dose 0.2 mg. daily, and 1 gram of elemental calcium. The calcium may be obtained from a quart of milk daily, but in some patients persistent hyperphosphatemia will force discontinuation of the milk. In these patients calcium carbonate, 2.5 grams, or calcium lactate, 7.7 grams, will provide 1 gram of elemental calcium. The dose of these agents should be adjusted to maintain the serum calcium concentration at no greater than 9 mg. per dl. in order to avoid hypercalciuria. After changing the dose of vitamin D_2, a change in serum calcium concentration will not occur until at least 2 weeks have passed. Careful monitoring of this test is necessary to avoid hypercalcemia. If hypercalcemia does occur, rapid reversal of this complication can be achieved by inducing a diuresis with intravenous isotonic saline solution and by instituting adrenal corticosteroids in high doses (prednisone, 30 mg. daily).

HYPOPITUITARISM*

method of
JOHANNES D. VELDHUIS, M.D.,
and RICHARD J. SANTEN, M.D.
Hershey, Pennsylvania

Hypopituitarism embraces a spectrum of hormonal deficits ranging from isolated or monotropic deficiencies to panhypopituitarism. The causative process is often progressive and deficiency of additional hormones may be acquired over time in any sequence. Children with idiopathic selective growth hormone deficiency may also develop pluritropic deficits such as adrenocorticotropin hormone (ACTH) and thyroid stimulating hormone (TSH) deficiency in the absence of an identifiable pathologic process.

Prior to treatment, clarification of cause is imperative, since morbidity and mortality may derive from local mass lesion effects (visual field loss, extraocular nerve palsies, hypothalamic syndrome) or from progression of an underlying, more generalized disease manifested first by its effects upon the hypothalamus or pituitary (e.g.,

*This work was supported in part by an NIH Contract No. 1-CB-53851, and a Specialized Cancer Research Grant No. 1 P30 CA18450-01, both awarded by the National Cancer Institute, DHEW.

metastatic carcinoma to the sella turcica, vasculitis, histiocytosis). Precise and persuasive demonstration of hormonal deficits is required. Thereafter, replacement therapy may be organized according to a scheme that considers each of the anterior and posterior lobe hormones individually. Finally, patients must be monitored periodically to ascertain whether additional hormonal replacement becomes necessary as the primary disease process evolves.

In general, patients with hypopituitarism may be treated by providing the hormonal product of the respective target glands or by direct administration of the trophic polypeptide hormones when available. Hypothalamic releasing peptides are not yet approved for clinical replacement therapy, although GnRH (gonadotropin-releasing hormone, a synthetic decapeptide) has been used to provide selective replacement of isolated hypothalamic GnRH deficiency (Kallmann's syndrome) with administration by long-term intranasal instillation to avoid repetitive parenteral injection.

ACTH Deficiency

Patient Instructions. All patients should receive an identification card, bracelet or pendant (Medic-Alert or Life Guard, Maurer Metal Specialties, Box 2493, Springfield, Illinois 62705), and injectable glucocorticoid for emergency use. Preassembled syringes of dexamethasone, 4 mg. per ml., or 100 mg. hydrocortisone phosphate or hemisuccinate (Solu-Cortef Mix-O-Vial) are available. Hypoadrenal patients should be instructed in self-injection technique for use acutely after major trauma or if vomiting prevents oral intake and advised to seek medical assistance promptly. For minor illnesses (e.g., upper-respiratory infection), the daily maintenance dose of glucocorticoid is doubled until symptoms resolve for 48 hours. Bacteremia, stroke, myocardial infarction, or other major illnesses require prompt hospitalization with an increase in daily hydrocortisone equivalent to 100 to 200 mg. per day.

Maintenance Replacement. Symptoms and signs of cortisol deficiency appear within 12 to 36 hours of acute hormone deprivation, although low basal levels may support life in the absence of superimposed infection, surgery, or trauma. Glucocorticoids (rather than ACTH) constitute preferred replacement therapy. The daily maintenance dose of oral cortisone acetate in adult patients is approximately 25 mg. each morning and 12.5 mg. each evening, or of hydrocortisone, 7.5 to 10 mg. every 8 hours. A hydrocortisone schedule of three doses per day is suggested because of the relatively short biologic half-life of this steroid. In children, hydrocortisone administration should approximate the secretion rate of 12 (±

3) mg. per square meter per day, also in distributed doses, recognizing that patients may require twice this dose to account for incomplete oral absorption. Excessive glucocorticoid replacement should be avoided to assure normal height progression in growing children. While synthetic steroids such as dexamethasone, prednisone, and prednisolone have been commonly used as maintenance therapy, the metabolism of these compounds (but not of cortisone acetate or hydrocortisone) may be altered as much as four-fold by other drugs administered concurrently (e.g., phenobarbital). Consequently, the dosages of such synthetic steroids required may vary markedly in individual patients or in the same patient. For this reason we prefer using hydrocortisone or cortisone acetate.

Adrenal Crisis. Acute adrenal insufficiency requires immediate intravenous soluble glucocorticoid injection: hydrocortisone hemisuccinate (Solu-Cortef), 100 mg. bolus, and intravascular volume restoration with dextrose in isotonic saline solution to replace saline deficits and to avert hypoglycemia. Vigorous attention should be directed toward defining and treating any precipitating event (e.g., lobar pneumonia, pyelonephritis, perforated duodenal ulcer, myocardial infarction). Intravenous hydrocortisone infusion is continued at doses of 50 to 100 mg. every 6 hours until resolution of the underlying illness, and then reduced by 50 per cent every 24 to 48 hours to oral maintenance levels. Intramuscular cortisone acetate is not recommended as sole therapy under these circumstances because it may be absorbed slowly. Patients with panhypopituitarism require no additional mineralocorticoid replacement since aldosterone synthesis and release mechanisms are relatively intact. Furthermore, a dose of 300 to 400 mg. per day of hydrocortisone or cortisone acetate provides significant mineralocorticoid activity. As the use of saline and large amounts of hydrocortisone may cause hypokalemia through renal sodium-potassium exchange in the distal tubule, electrolytes should be monitored closely.

Elective Surgery. For general anesthesia or major surgery, administer 100 mg. cortisone acetate intramuscularly (a long-acting preparation) the evening before surgery and 100 mg. of hydrocortisone hemisuccinate (Solu-Cortef) intravenously immediately preoperatively. Postoperatively, 50 mg. intravenous infusions (or bolus injections) of hydrocortisone hemisuccinate should be continued at 6 hour intervals. This dose may be reduced by 50 per cent the next day and again every 24 to 48 hours by a similar amount. Maintenance therapy is resumed when the patient is eating and afebrile. Persistence of low-grade fever should prompt evaluation for infection or thrombophlebitis and continuation of approximately 80 mg. of hydrocortisone per day. If major postoperative complications arise or reoperation is necessary, resumption of larger amounts of glucocorticoid are required with the dosage decided on an individual basis.

Thyroid Stimulating Hormone (TSH) Deficiency

In patients with thyrotropin deficiency, a careful evaluation for coexistent glucocorticoid (ACTH) deficiency is necessary before initiating thyroid replacement. Augmentation of metabolic demands could otherwise precipitate adrenal crisis. This is of particular significance practically, since isolated TSH deficiency is rare (reported sporadically and in association with pseudohypoparathyroidism).

A single daily dose of levothyroxine provides sustained, uniform and predictable replacement. Adults require 2 micrograms per kg. per day or 0.1 to 0.15 mg. (range: 0.075 to 0.25 mg.) daily. In children, 3 to 5 micrograms per kg. per day of L-thyroxine approximates requirement confirmed by age-adjusted norms for serum T_4 and the clinical examination. Unlike the situation in primary hypothyroidism, suppression of TSH levels cannot be employed to ascertain adequacy of replacement, but serum thyroxine (T_4) determinations usually will be in the normal range in patients receiving adequate L-thyroxine replacement. Similarly, triiodothyronine (T_3) levels by radioimmunoassay should also approximate the normal range during replacement with L-thyroxine alone, since the preponderance of endogenous T_3 derives from extrathyroidal conversion of T_4 to T_3 (by 5'-monodeiodination) rather than from direct glandular secretion. Rare patients manifest a T_4-to-T_3 conversion defect (the T_3 level is inappropriately low with a normal T_4) and may be replaced preferably with triiodothyronine to achieve euthyroidism. Triiodothyronine (Cytomel) exhibits a shorter half-life than L-thyroxine and, therefore, usually requires administration in divided doses: 25 micrograms orally three times daily in adults (range: 50 to 100 micrograms per day or 1 microgram per kg. per day in children). Serum T_3, rather than T_4, must be determined by radioimmunoassay to assess replacement adequacy.

Dessicated thyroid preparations are less desirable because of variable biopotency (inconstant T_4-T_3 ratios); if employed, doses are 1 to 2 grains (60 to 120 mg.) per day. It should be stressed that tests of circulating thyroid hormone levels must be correlated with clinical parameters, and the physician should not rely solely on the laboratory as a final arbiter of appropriate dosage. In addition, therapy should be started slowly in older patients, particularly those with known or suspected ischemic or arrhythmic heart disease. In these instances, one eighth the usual replacement dosage is initiated and gradual increments made over a 3 month period, e.g., start with 25 micrograms L-thyroxine per day and increase by 25 micrograms every three-to-four weeks.

Although the tripeptide TSH-releasing hormone is available for diagnostic studies it has no practical utility in selective replacement of hypothalamic hypothyroidism.

Gonadotropin Deficiency

Monotropic Deficiency. Isolated FSH deficiency is exceedingly rare and purified human follicle stimulating hormone (FSH) for selective replacement is not generally available. Monotropic LH deficiency may occur within the spectrum of hypogonadotrophic hypogonadism as the "fertile eunuch" syndrome. Because of availability, human chorionic gonadotropin (hCG) is utilized as replacement therapy rather than human luteinizing hormone (LH). Both hormones stimulate Leydig cell production of testosterone with equal efficacy in males. However, because of considerations of cost and frequency of administration, direct replacement of testosterone (see below) can be accomplished more practically than hCG administration.

Bihormonal Gonadotropin Deficiency. Gonadotropin deficiency may arise in the setting of panhypopituitarism from a variety of causes or in Kallmann's syndrome, diagnosed when isolated hypogonadotrophic hypogonadism occurs in males or females with anosmia, hyposmia, a family history of hypogonadism, or midline facial defects. Both sex-steroid deficiency and fertility are therapeutic considerations in any of these conditions.

Treatment of testosterone deficiency may be accomplished by an injectable repository ester of this steroid such as testosterone enanthate or testosterone cypionate in doses of 200 mg. intramuscularly every 2 to 4 weeks. Initially, serum testosterone levels should be monitored just prior to a subsequent dose to determine the frequency of administration necessary to maintain the levels of this hormone within the adult normal male range.

The peripubertal boy should receive correspondingly lower doses initially in amounts of 50 to 75 mg. intramuscularly each month in order to stimulate pubertal progression and minimize premature epiphyseal closure. Alternately, in the absence of associated testicular disease, exogenous hCG in doses of 2000 to 4000 U.S.P. units three times per week intramuscularly will induce testosterone production and progressive male secondary sexual development. Clinical indices of androgenization and testosterone levels should be monitored at 3-monthly intervals to assess endogenous steroid production. The decision when to treat boys with delayed puberty is beyond the scope of this chapter and should include appropriate endocrine consultation.

Undesired effects may occur during testosterone replacement, including gynecomastia, extracellular fluid retention, acne, and rarely prostatic hypertrophic obstruction (particularly in elderly men). In such instances, a short-acting oral preparation such as fluoxymesterone (5 to 10 mg. per day) is appropriate for the first month of replacement. However, in other circumstances, available oral preparations may not provide clinical effects of full androgenic replacement.

When fertility is the therapeutic goal, replacement with pituitary hormones or their equivalent is necessary. Treatment is usually initiated with 2000 to 4000 U.S.P. units of hCG three times per week intramuscularly. In patients with only a relative deficiency of FSH, seminiferous tubular maturation and fertility can ensue after hCG alone. However, if FSH is undetectable, a preparation containing both FSH and LH (Pergonal, menotropins) is required to provide concordant Leydig cell and seminiferous tubular stimulation. The usual approach is to treat with hCG alone for 6 to 12 months, after which FSH is added. Such therapy is usually administered by an experienced endocrinologist.

In females, cyclic administration of sex steroids will induce withdrawal menses. Fewer adverse effects occur with lower doses of estrogens in the range of 20 to 30 micrograms ethinyl estradiol per day. A combination oral contraceptive may be employed. Alternately, daily oral conjugated estrogens, 0.625 to 1.25 mg. (e.g., Premarin), or ethinyl estradiol 20 or 50 microgram tablets, for days 1 through 25 of each cycle may be used with the addition of 5 to 10 mg. of medroxyprogesterone acetate on days 21 through 25. In peripubertal girls, initial replacement should include estrogen alone for 6 to 12 months to stimulate uterine and secondary sexual maturation (e.g., 0.625 mg. of conjugated estrogens or 20 micrograms ethinyl estradiol on a continuous daily regimen). Thereafter, cyclic hormonal replacement is appropriate.

During long-term replacement, periodic endometrial biopsies should be considered as a means of monitoring endometrial hyperplasia, which can arise as a result of excessive estrogen doses. This precaution may be particularly warranted in light of recent evidence linking estrogen replacement therapy to endometrial carcinoma.

Pregnancy may be accomplished in bihormonal hypogonadotropism or in panhypopituitarism. Human FSH and LH purified from postmenopausal urine are available as 75 I.U. of FSH and 75 I.U. of LH per ampoule, menotropins (Pergonal), for intramuscular administration. One major side effect of this therapy is ovarian hyperstimulation, which is associated with painful ovarian enlargement, ascites, pleural effusion, or ruptured ovarian cysts. Multifetation develops in approximately 20 per cent of patients and has resulted in live births of quintuplets and sextuplets. During ovulation induction, current practice requires measurement of estrogens and physical examination of ovarian size daily. The laboratory support necessary for this monitoring limits use of ovulation induction to centers experienced in the administration of these medications.

As typical therapy, 1 to 3 ampoules of Pergonal (75 I.U. of FSH, 75 I.U. LH per ampoule) are injected daily until follicular maturation is indicated by serum estradiol levels exceeding 500 picograms per ml. (or total urinary estrogens exceeding 10 micrograms daily) or until 12 doses have been administered in the absence of clinical ovarian hyperstimulation. Five thousand U.S.P. units of hCG are then injected intramuscularly to induce ovulation. The latter event should be assessed by serum progesterone or urinary pregnanediol determinations, by basal body temperature measurements and by clinical evaluation of vaginal cytology and cervical mucus. Coitus is recommended on alternate days in proximity to anticipated ovulation.

Human-Growth-Hormone Deficiency (HGH)

Human growth hormone obtained from cadaver sources is available through the National Pituitary Agency for authorized research protocols or commercially (Calbio or Kaby Pharmaceuticals). Unambiguous human-growth-hormone deficiency must be documented by two or more provocative tests. Adults do not require HGH replacement, but in children principal indications are hypoglycemia, which is related to diminished gluconeogenetic substrate mobilization, and statural deficit prior to epiphyseal closure (bone age 15 or 16 years). Human growth hormone (HGH) is usually administered as 1 to 2 units intramuscularly three times each week. Precise height measurements at 3 month intervals permit assessment of response, which may initially exhibit a "catch-up" increment exceeding growth velocity norms adjusted for corresponding bone age. Subsequent height velocity approximates that of normal patients of equivalent bone age. Resistance to currently available human growth hormone is rare. Although antibody development does occur commonly, neutralization of HGH bioactivity is infrequent. Thus, if response to therapy is poor, other causes should be sought including intercurrent hypothyroidism (which rarely may develop during HGH therapy and resolve with cessation of treatment); excessive cortisol replacement; premature epiphyseal closure sometimes related to overzealous sex-steroid replacement; or nonendocrinologic systemic disease (e.g., sprue, renal disease).

Optimal preservation of the pubertal growth spurt requires continuation of HGH treatment during sexual maturation, whether spontaneous or induced.

Prolactin Deficiency

Rare families with asymptomatic isolated prolactin deficiency have been reported (e.g., in pseudohypoparathyroidism), but in most other cases pluritrophic hypopituitarism is present. Exogenous human prolactin is not available for administration nor are specific physiologic indications defined for its replacement.

Beta-Lipotropin

β-MSH appears to represent a cleaved fragment of the native peptide β-lipotropin. β-lipotropin may constitute a central nervous system (CNS) precursor for met- and leuencephalins, recently recognized endogenous opiate-like neurotransmitter substances. Isolated deficiency of β-lipotropin has not been reported. No replacement therapy is available or suggested.

Antidiuretic (ADH) Deficiency

Deficiency of antidiuretic hormone (ADH) most often implies a lesion in the supraoptic and periventricular nuclei or the medium eminence of the hypothalamus, the site of neuronal synthesis of ADH. Disease confined to the sella or posterior lobe frequently permits continued ADH secretion by residual axons of the neurohypophyseal tract.

HYPERTHYROIDISM

method of
J. M. MCKENZIE, M.D.
Montreal, Quebec, Canada

Introduction

If the rare varieties are included, the list of causes of hyperthyroidism is lengthy and includes thyrotoxicosis factitia, functioning thyroid carcinoma, thyrotropin-secreting pituitary tumor, and several other entities. However, the great majority of hyperthyroid subjects suffer from one of only two conditions, Graves' disease or toxic adenoma of the thyroid. There are those who would proffer a third common diagnosis, toxic multinodular goiter, but probably all patients so labeled either have Graves' disease with incidental thyroid nodularity or have multiple adenomata of the thyroid gland. The relative incidence of Graves' disease and thyroid adenoma varies from country to country, perhaps related to the prevalence of endemic goiter; in North America, Graves' disease is currently much the more common. Similarly, the total prevalence of hyperthyroidism probably varies from one geographic area to another, having been reported as 0.23 per 1000 females in a review of hospital patients in Minnesota and 2 to 3 per 1000 females in a population survey in the north of England.

Causative factors in Graves' disease encompass the genetic, perhaps environmental, and probably emotional, all with certain implications regarding therapy. The familial incidence is well-recognized and recently reported analyses identify HL-A antigens (B 8 in Caucasians) as occurring with undue frequency in affected persons. As with other similar associations of specific HL-A antigens and particular disease entities, the correlation is far from absolute and it is probable that this reflects, whatever else, the comparatively undeveloped state of HL-A–typing. When the antigens on the gene-locus, perhaps specifically in the D-locus, are further defined, more complete correlation with Graves' disease may result; as it stands, there is some indication that the caucasian patient with the B 8 antigen is more likely to require ablative therapy for hyperthyroidism than is one who is B 8-negative.

Regarding environmental influences, the amount of iodide ingested, be it inadvertently in food or deliberately as medication or a nutritional supplement, appears to be important. Iodide lack may prevent the development of hyperthyroidism, and a relative increase or excess may precipitate the disease or be associated with a higher relapse rate, particularly after antithyroid drug therapy. However, it is not clear that deliberate reduction of iodide-containing foods has a significant effect on the outcome of therapy.

That emotional factors are important in "triggering" or maintaining the disease is still debated, but it now seems likely that they are indeed significant in some patients, although perhaps not through an influence on thyroid function per se but rather by modifying the activity of the immune system. Again, this concept has implications for therapy in that it reinforces and emphasizes the time-honored practice of prescribing rest and often some means of sedation for patients with Graves' disease.

Pathogenesis. Graves' disease is now accepted as one of the autoimmune syndromes. The cause of the hyperthyroidism is the existence in the blood of a thyroid-stimulating antibody (TSAb) that has been identified in greater than 90 per cent of a group of over 200 patients. Evidence is rapidly accumulating that the persistence of TSAb in the blood of a patient during treatment with antithyroid drugs indicates that clinical relapse will follow rapidly on discontinuation of the medication. It may be that the titer of TSAb measured at the time of initial diagnosis will turn out to be an efficient index of the type of clinical course to be expected; i.e., the higher the titer, the more likely will ablative therapy be required, or, the lower the titer, the more likely will the patient enter remission on therapy with antithyroid drugs. One must emphasize, however, that these interpretations and extrapolations are from the results of on-going research into the significance of TSAb. Even if this forecast of the prognostic significance and usefulness of the measurement of TSAb is borne out by additional studies, the general applicability of the information will have to await the development of an assay method more reproducible and with fewer logistic problems (e.g., one type of assay requires fresh human thyroid tissue as test material) than those currently in use.

Choice of Therapy

Toxic Adenoma.   Distinction between Graves' disease and toxic adenoma (or adenomata) as the basis for a patient's hyperthyroidism is of obvious importance in the choice of therapy, since the latter condition, being a reflection of benign neoplasia, requires ablation of the autonomous tissue for cure to be effected. Clinical features such as a diffuse goiter and the association of ophthalmopathy, with or without pretibial myxedema, may identify Graves' disease. Difficulty arises, more commonly in the older patient, if there is a nodular goiter and no ophthalmopathy. The presence of circulating antibodies to either thyroglobulin or to the thyroid microsomal antigen provides circumstantial evidence for Graves' disease as the diagnosis, but more precise data may be obtained by evaluating the thyroid "scan" obtained after the administration of radioiodine. If radioactivity is confined to the area of one or more nodules in the thyroid, indirect confirmation of the diagnosis of adenomatous disease may be obtained by the intramuscular injection of thyrotropin (10 units once or daily for 3 consecutive days) before repeating the scan. Appearance of radioactivity in paranodular tissue that was previously "cold" indicates that those areas were functionless because of suppression of pituitary thyrotropin by the hormone-output of the autonomous thyroid tissue; thus, the condition is not Graves' disease, in which all functional (in terms of concentrating radioiodine) tissue is stimulated by TSAb, at the time of the initial scan.

Ablative therapy for a thyroid adenomatous condition means either a surgical approach or the use of ^{131}I; the choice is based on considerations that are different from those arising in managing the patient with Graves' disease. Either form of ablation of adenomatous tissue ought not to lead to hypothyroidism and relapse of hyperthyroidism is not to be expected following initially effective treatment. Therefore, the two forms of therapy may be accepted as approximately equal in effectiveness and a choice ought to be made on more specific, individual considerations. Before adulthood, radiation to the thyroid may have a carcinogenic effect that is more significant than appears to occur in later years, so that ^{131}I therapy is, in general, inappropriate for patients of either sex under the age of 18 to 20 years. The theoretical mutagenic effect on gonadal tissue similarly weighs against ^{131}I use in women of child-bearing age, especially since "one-shot" effective therapy usually entails a higher dose of ^{131}I, e.g. 25 mCi., than would be contemplated in the treatment of hyperthyroidism of Graves' disease. On the other hand, the most essential factor in the choice of surgical therapy is the availability of the appropriate operative prowess; without this, the theoretical risks of radiotherapy pale into insignificance against the postoperative morbidity associated with inexperienced surgical technique.

Graves' Disease.   The choice of treatment for hyperthyroidism of Graves' disease is greater, and more difficult, than it is for toxic adenoma, for the reasons that the whole gland is involved and that a significant proportion of patients may go into remission with nonablative therapy. Thus, decision must be made primarily amongst treatment with thionamides (antithyroid drugs) and partial ablation surgically or by use of ^{131}I. (Recently reported experience with the use of ^{125}I indicates it offers no significant advantage to ^{131}I). Few patients are treated solely with iodide or propranolol, two agents that are used rather as adjuvants to the main forms of therapy.

Use of Thionamides

In North America the two drugs commonly used are propylthiouracil (in the United States, 50 mg. tablets; in Canada, 50 and 100 mg. tablets) and methimazole (in the United States, 5 and 10 mg. tablets; in Canada, 5 mg. tablets) whereas in western Europe methylthiouracil and carbimazole are more routinely prescribed. It has been stressed for decades that these drugs must be given in divided dosage, e.g., 6- or 8-hourly, to be effective, but recently it has been shown that a single daily dose is adequate in many patients. Consequently treatment schedules may now be offered as alternatives: propylthiouracil, 100 mg. every 8 hours or 300 mg. once daily; methimazole, 10 mg. every 8 hours or 30 mg. once daily.

The single daily dose, that is probably better tried with methimazole because of a somewhat more prolonged effect, is convenient and more readily followed. Prescribing multiple doses throughout the day often leads to erratic administration of the drug for nonhospitalized patients with the midday doses too frequently being forgotten. However, there are patients who require multiple doses for control of their hyperthyroidism and the more severely ill subject ought to be started on an 8-hourly or even more frequent regimen; a 6-hourly schedule ought to be avoided, since a continuous period of 8 or more hours sleep, if possible, is important in itself for the hyperthyroid subject.

Propylthiouracil has a property not shared by methimazole in that it impairs peripheral conversion of thyroxine to triiodothyronine, and this may be an important early effect in the extremely hyperthyroid subject. Otherwise, and for long-term medication, there is probably little to choose between these two thionamides, since they are both effective in blocking the synthesis of thyroid hormones and they have a similar low incidence of side effects. The most common adverse reaction is skin rash that can often be adequately cared for by a switch to the alternate drug and the administration of an antihistamine, such as chlorpheniramine or chlortripolon, 4 mg. twice daily, for a few days. Leukopenia or granulocytosis may occur, although rarely, with either drug; immediate cessation of the treatment is essential when the diagnosis is made and usually leads to a satisfactory outcome. Because of the rapidity of development of this complication there is no point in the routine measurement of blood leukocytes. Rather, it is mandatory that the patient be fully alerted to the possible significance of the occurrence of a sore throat, at which time she or he should be examined physically and by enumeration of leukocytes. It has become customary to maintain administration of a thionamide for periods ranging from 9 months to 2 or more years, with the implicit belief that some such length of treatment facilitates remission of the disease. However, there are no objective data to support any particular duration of therapy as being more effective than another, and recent studies indicate that, on average, a shorter period of 3 to 6 months is as likely to lead to remission as the longer courses. Therefore, our current practice is to maintain patients on a thionamide for 6 months and then stop the drug. Usually a euthyroid state is achieved within 3 to 8 weeks and then continued observation, on the same dose of thionamide, is indicated in order to identify hypothyroidism if it develops. An enlarging goiter is an early physical sign of this event, but the measurement of serum thyrotropin is the most sensitive laboratory index. If the clinical features or laboratory data indicate that the therapy has reduced thyroid hormone formation to an excessive degree (and many patients are maintained for 6 months on the initial dose of thionamide without this occurring) the dosage may be reduced by half; a simpler procedure, however, is to continue with the same dose of thionamide and, in addition, prescribe L-thyroxine, 0.1 mg. tablet daily.

Current research indicates that if TSAb is still present in blood after 6 months of thionamide therapy, relapse will occur shortly (usually within 2 months) of stopping the drug. When measurement of TSAb becomes routinely available, this index ought to rationalize the duration of antithyroid drug therapy.

Radioactive Iodine Therapy

Three objections are commonly raised to the use of radioiodine in treatment of hyperthyroidism of Graves' disease:

1. It may be carcinogenic, either to the thyroid or to other tissues, especially bone marrow. In fact, the evidence supporting this concern is extremely weak. Thyroid carcinoma may indeed be unduly common following head and neck external irradiation in childhood, but the incidence of carcinoma after ^{131}I therapy for Graves' disease is not clearly greater than the spontaneous rate of occurrence. Acute leukemia apparently develops with excess frequency after ^{131}I treatment (dosage commonly greater than 100 mCi.) of thyroid carcinoma but does not appear to be related to the quantity of ^{131}I usually given for hyperthyroidism (< 10 mCi.). On the basis of these rather tangential pieces of information it is reasonable to restrict ^{131}I therapy to the adult population without fear of a carcinogenic effect.

2. It may induce genetic mutation. Again, this is a theoretical hazard where the concern ought to be directly related to the dose of ^{131}I; with the conventional dosage of ^{131}I used to treat hyperthyroidism, the human gonads are not irradiated to a significantly greater extent than occurs in various routine radiologic procedures. This fact, of course, ought to reemphasize the advisability of restricting radiation, especially of younger sub-

jects, to the minimum but also it puts the theoretical risk of ^{131}I-induced genetic mutation into perspective. Nonetheless, since the magnitude of the hazard is not known, and mutations indeed may become overt only in succeeding generations, it is rational not to give ^{131}I as therapy to potentially fertile subjects unless there are positive contraindications to alternative forms of treatment.

3. Hypothyroidism will ensue. This is the most clear-cut and important restriction to the use of ^{131}I as therapy. It is now clear that the majority, probably all, of those so treated will become hypothyroid if they live long enough. Published experience varies but in general 10 to 40 per cent of ^{131}I-treated patients become hypothyroid within 2 years and, of the remainder, 2 to 3 per cent become hypothyroid each year. The consequences of this realization are two-fold. First, the younger the patient, the more reluctant one ought to be to give ^{131}I therapy. Second, any patient to be treated with ^{131}I should have the apparent inevitability of eventual hypothyroidism clearly explained. The danger to health, it should be emphasized, is not the hypothyroidism itself but unrecognized and untreated thyroid failure. Therefore, the ^{131}I-treated patient, after a euthyroid state is established, has to be seen routinely and regularly, preferably yearly, for life.

The dose of ^{131}I, presumably calculated by the specialist in nuclear medicine, is based on the 24 hour uptake of ^{131}I, the estimated size of the thyroid, and the desired quantity of radiation that is quoted as "rads," (the absorbed dose of radiation). Formerly, 6000 to 8000 rads were routinely prescribed for therapy, but we now prefer 3000 to 4000 rads, especially for the younger patient. This dose of ^{131}I produces a euthyroid state more slowly than does the larger (and often necessitates temporary medication with thionamide, starting 48 hours after administration of ^{131}I and lasting 2 to 3 months) but also seems to lead more slowly to the eventual state of hypothyroidism.

Surgical Therapy

The usual procedure is a subtotal thyroidectomy and in the hands of a competent surgeon, this is very effective treatment of hyperthyroidism. The major or most commonly occurring hazard is the same as with the use of [131]I: the development of hypothyroidism. Of those patients who become euthyroid after operation (and a significant proportion either relapse or become hypothyroid within the first 1 to 2 years, with the ratio of these two outcomes varying with the aggressiveness of the surgery) 1 to 2 per cent are expected to become hypothyroid every year. As with the late occurrence of post ^{131}I hypothyroidism, it appears that the annual incidence of this complication is maintained indefinitely. Therefore, the decision to choose a sur-

TABLE 1.   **Features that Influence the Choice of Therapy of Hyperthyroidism of Graves' Disease**

THERAPY	PRO	CONTRA
Thionamides	Preadult age group First episode, age less than 40 years Patient's preference Pregnancy Thyroid storm Short-term after ^{131}I treatment Short-term preoperative	Known allergy to thionamides Age greater than 40 years Previous relapse Large goiter Pressure symptoms from goiter (High concentration TSAb)*
[131]I	Age greater than 40 years Patient's preference Relapse after previous therapy Known allergy to thionamides Surgical risk high Small goiter (High concentration TSAb)*	Pregnancy Preadult group First episode, age less than 40 years Patient's fear of radiation Pressure symptoms from goiter Very large goiter
Surgery	Pressure symptoms from goiter Large goiter Patient's preference Relapse after thionamide therapy in preadult age group (High concentration TSAb, especially if age less than 40 years)	Surgical prowess not available Surgical risk high Relapse after previous surgical therapy Patient's fear of operation Pregnancy

*The evaluation of the significance of a high concentration of thyroid-stimulating antibody (TSAb) in the patient's blood is an area of active research, with initial indications permitting these categorizations. Most of the features listed are of relative importance in the choice of therapy; pregnancy is an absolute contraindication to treatment with [131]I.

gical approach to the therapy rather than ^{131}I becomes largely individual and is influenced by factors such as the availability of an experienced surgical team and the patient's personal preference. These and other aspects of the bases for electing a particular choice of treatment of hyperthyroidism are listed in Table 1.

The patient should be brought to a euthyroid status before operation; it must be rare that circumstances dictate the necessity of a subtotal thyroidectomy being carried out without this preparation. The usual routine is the administration of a thionamide drug for 4 to 8 weeks with the addition of iodide to the prescription for the last 1 to 2 weeks; the latter drug can be given conveniently as saturated solution of potassium iodide (SSKI), twice daily 2 drops on a scrap of bread that is swallowed without chewing (to avoid the bitter taste of iodide). The duration of each therapy ought to be dictated by the patient's response, and not by any prior decision regarding operation schedules. In the postoperative period, no medication usually is required.

As preparation for operation, propranolol (30 to 80 mg. per day in divided doses) has been recommended by some, but is probably best used only in the rare circumstances of surgery being required before thionamide and iodide therapy can be completely effective.

Special Problems of Therapy

Hyperthyroidism in Pregnancy. Because ^{131}I freely crosses the placenta and, therefore, would be harmful to fetal tissues in general and to the thyroid in particular (after the fourteenth week of gestation, the human fetal thyroid is capable of concentrating iodide from the bloodstream), this form of therapy is not to be considered for the pregnant woman. While subtotal thyroidectomy may be entirely successful (and is usually restricted to the second trimester), there seems little point in subjecting the pregnant woman to this degree of stress. Rather, the optimal therapy is the well-controlled use of a thionamide drug.

The concerns here are related to the control of the mother's hyperthyroidism, the avoidance of goiter with hypothyroidism in the fetus, and the identification and treatment of neonatal hyperthyroidism if it should occur. It is accepted that the risk associated with undertreatment, and the resultant mild hyperthyroidism, is greater than the consequences of maternal hypothyroidism. Therefore, antithyroid drug should be given as described but with care to keep the free thyroxine index (the mathematical product of the value for serum thyroxine concentration and a measure, such as resin uptake of ^{131}I-triiodothyronine, of the degree of saturation of thyroxine-binding globulin) in the upper half of the range of normal. This often means reducing the dose of thionamide to half within the second month of treatment. There is no advantage—indeed only positive disadvantage—in adding thyroxine to the treatment regimen, as may be done with the nonpregnant patient. The aim is to give the minimal required dose of thionamide, so that the fetus is not exposed to more of the drug than necessary. To continue a relatively large dose of thionamide and keep the mother euthyroid by giving thyroxine, in addition, obviously maintains an unnecessarily high concentration of the thionamide for transplacental passage. Prescribing only the minimal required dose of antithyroid drug (e.g., initially 300 mg. propylthiouracil daily and then 150 mg. as a maintenance dose) ought not to be associated with hypothyroidism or even goiter in the fetus.

Much less under the control of the physician is the possibility of hyperthyroidism, i.e., Graves' disease, in the neonate. This complication seems to be directly related to the concentration of TSAb in the maternal circulation. If TSAb is in high titer, neonatal hyperthyroidism must be expected and, if confirmed, treated expeditiously with thionamide and, in most cases, iodide as well; the doses are, for propylthiouracil, 5 to 10 mg. per kg. body weight per day, and for SSKI, 1 drop every 8 hours. In the usual instance of this syndrome treatment can be discontinued after 2 to 3 months without fear of relapse.

Thyroid Storm. Thyroid storm may be defined as an acute threat to life by severe hyperthyroidism; in this way the definition includes those patients who may, for instance, have cardiac or renal failure with acute decompensation being precipitated by the episode of hyperthyroidism. Whether this is the situation, or the rarer true "thyroid crisis" wherein the threat to life lies only in the severity of the thyroid disease, the emphasis must be on rapid and effective control of the overactive thyroid gland together with, simultaneously, amelioration of the consequences of the excess circulating hormone.

For this condition propylthiouracil is probably superior to methimazole because of its capacity to reduce the rate of peripheral conversion of T_4 to T_3; the thionamide may be given in a dosage of 200 mg. every 6 hours to ensure continuous action over 24 hours, and 1 hour after the first dose administration of iodide should be started. Since many of these patients also require continuous intravenous fluid therapy, the iodide can be added to the parenteral solution in a concentration to provide 1 mg. per hour. Alternatively, oral iodide may be given as 2 drops of SSKI every 6 hours. Glucocorticoid is commonly also prescribed, but there is no rationale for this unless there is independent evidence of adrenal cortex insufficiency, including, presumably, hypotension.

Ophthalmopathy. This aspect of Graves' disease is seldom of sufficient severity to require direct therapy. A gritty feeling of the eyes may be helped by the periodic (e.g., thrice daily) insertion of "artificial tears" such as 1 per cent methyl cellulose eye drops. Periorbital puffiness can often be helped by raising the head of the bed (not the mattress) 4 inches to reduce nocturnal distribution of dependent body fluids. Chronic, established, external ocular muscle paresis requires surgical section of fibrotic muscles if diplopia is a significant clinical problem. Therapy of the (fortunately) infrequent acutely inflamed condition in which sight is threatened either by retrobulbar pathology or by corneal involvement is much more debatable. Since this is now accepted as a reflection of autoimmune processes, there is no question of trying to inhibit thyrotropic function by the administration of thyroid hormone (although hypothyroidism, if present, must be treated) as was formerly in vogue. Rather, the advantages, disadvantages, and priorities of three distinct but not mutually exclusive modes of therapy must be considered. They are presented in the sequence in which they might rationally be attempted.

1. CORTICOSTEROID THERAPY. In view of the need for high dosage if systemic treatment is initiated and the recognized dangers of such dosage, this approach should be adopted only to save sight in acute inflammatory disease. A typical schedule we have found effective in some patients is prednisone, 100 mg. daily in divided dosage, until improvement occurs or for a maximum of 10 days; if there is a successful response, the dosage may be reduced by sequential reduction to 50 per cent of the preceding dose weekly to, if necessary, a maintenance dose of 10 to 20 mg. per day. If a greater dose of prednisone is required to prevent deterioration of vision or advance of the inflammatory process, alternative therapy is indicated. The need for an acceptable maintenance dose is unlikely to be greater than 3 months.

Instead of hazardous high-dosage systemic corticosteroid therapy the retrobulbar injection of glucocorticoid (40 mg. methylprednisolone in 1 ml. solvent once a month) is advocated by some. Reported experience from North America is limited, but encouraging results have been described elsewhere.

2. EXTERNAL IRRADIATION. Treatment by x-irradiation with conventional sources has not been impressively successful. However, in the acute inflammatory phase, a total of up to 2000 rads delivered to retrobulbar tissues by a linear accelerator that allows adequate "aim" or collima-

tion to avoid damage to cornea, lens, pituitary, and other neighboring tissues has been claimed by some as sightsaving, effective therapy.

3. SURGICAL DECOMPRESSION. Rather than the older supraorbital approach to decompression by craniotomy, the currently advocated—and apparently usually advantageous when required—operation is via the maxillary antrum. It must be emphasized that this treatment reduces pressure on the orbit, particularly the sensitive optic nerve, and thus may save sight; correction of muscle palsy may not be expected and, indeed, diplopia may develop only postoperatively.

Finally, it may be worthwhile emphasizing that there is no general support for the treatment of ophthalmopathy, advocated by some, by total thyroidectomy. The theoretical basis for this approach is inadequate and confirmation of initial apparent success has not been reported.

HYPOTHYROIDISM

method of
LEONARD WARTOFSKY, M.D.,
and KENNETH D. BURMAN, M.D.
Washington, District of Columbia

Etiology

Primary Hypothyroidism. Hypothyroidism is a disorder caused by inadequate circulating levels of the thyroid hormones, thyroxine (T_4) and 3,3',5-triiodothyronine (T_3). The cause may be primary deficiency of the thyroid gland, as may be seen after either radioiodine therapy for hyperthyroidism or total or subtotal thyroidectomy for a variety of indications. Thyroid hypofunction probably occurs most commonly in the general population secondary to an autoimmune destructive process (Hashimoto's thyroiditis), but partial or relative thyroid deficiency may accompany a number of conditions including colloid or nontoxic nodular goiter, and secondary diseases of the thyroid such as amyloid, sarcoid, and metastatic carcinoma, which impair or destroy the functioning mass of the tissue.

Secondary Hypothyroidism. Not infrequently, clinical hypothyroidism with low serum T_4 and T_3 is associated with low or undetectable levels of serum thyroid stimulating hormone (TSH). This indicates either partial to complete pituitary insufficiency or hypothalamic disease. The latter has been termed "tertiary" hypothyroidism and is presumably due to thyrotropin releasing hormone (TRH) deficiency, although this remains to be confirmed. Secondary or "pituitary" hypothyroidism may be due to pituitary insufficiency caused by primary or metastatic tumor, atrophy

(Sheehan's syndrome), or other more unusual disorders. Other signs or symptoms of end-organ failure may be apparent, such as gonadal and adrenal insufficiency, and the diagnostic hallmark is the finding of low levels of both T_4 and thyroid stimulating hormone (TSH). A thyrotropin-releasing hormone (TRH) stimulation test may help differentiate between secondary and tertiary disease, in that the patient with pituitary disease will have an absent to minimal increment in TSH after TRH, whereas the patient with hypothalamic disease and intact thyrotropic function should respond to TRH although the peak increase may be somewhat delayed.

Treatment

Regardless of the cause of the thyroid hypofunction, therapy with thyroid hormone in one of its many dosage forms is essential for reversal of the clinical abnormalities and restoration of euthyroidism. The patient with pituitary or hypothalamic disease will require additional evaluation and consideration for other therapies, the most significant of which is adrenal steroid replacement for partial or complete ACTH deficiency. Rarely, primary thyroidal failure is accompanied by primary adrenal insufficiency (Schmidt's syndrome), which often coexists with diabetes mellitus. Any patient in whom either primary or secondary adrenal insufficiency is suspected may require adrenal steroid replacement therapy prior to initiation of thyroid hormone replacement in order to prevent the potential occurrence of adrenal crisis.

Preparations and Dosage. A large variety of preparations of thyroid hormone are presently available for clinical use, but recent developments in our understanding of the physiology of thyroid hormone secretion and metabolism clearly help to narrow the field to a few specific and more ideally physiologic preparations. Those most commonly employed include:

DESICCATED THYROID. Usually prepared by removing fat and water from hog or beef thyroids with assay standards largely based on iodine rather than T_4 or T_3 content. Depending upon species and batch variation, the content of $T_4:T_3$ ranges from 2 to 3:1 on a molar basis. These preparations tend to be the least expensive and most ubiquitously available. Drawbacks to their use include: (a) variations in potency, (b) relative instability with loss of potency after long shelf storage, (c) inadequate absorption due to incompletely assimilated tablets, and (d) acute relative increases in serum T_3 levels that may produce thyrotoxic symptoms. The usually recommended dosage for full replacement is 2 to 3 grains (120 to 180 mg.) daily, which represents a cost of approximately $1.00 to $1.95 per month.

THYROID EXTRACT (PROLOID). This preparation represents thyroglobulin extracted from hog glands which is standardized as is dessicated thyroid on the basis of its iodine content and also for potency in a goiter prevention bioassay. The $T_4:T_3$ content approximates 2.5:1. In general, it has the same potential disadvantages as the desiccated preparation, and the cost is approximately one third greater.

L-THYROXINE (SYNTHROID, LETTER). Levothyroxine (L-T_4) is supplied as the sodium salt of T_4 and recently has become readily available in a number of convenient dosage forms. Advantages of this preparation include its reliable potency and the absence of wide swings in serum T_4 and T_3 that accompany its use in appropriate dose (see guidelines for therapy below). Although previously more expensive than dessicated thyroid, cost is no longer a consideration since the customary replacement dosage of 0.1 to 0.15 mg. per day represents a cost of only $0.75 to $1.45 per month.

L-TRIIODOTHYRONINE (CYTOMEL). L-Triiodothyronine (L-T_3) is also available as the sodium salt and almost totally absorbed orally. Because of its rapid absorption, large distribution space, rapid metabolic clearance rate, and less avid binding to serum binding proteins, elevated serum T_3 levels obtain within a few hours after ingestion to then rapidly and progressively decrease toward normal by 24 hours. It is of no value to monitor serum T_4 in patients taking L-T_3 and measurements of serum T_3 by radioimmunoassay are less readily available than serum T_4 in most routine hospital laboratories. Hence, use of this agent is attended by problems in interpretation of blood levels at any given time, as well as by a greater potential for induction of signs and symptoms of thyroid excess. It may be prudent to administer T_3 in divided dose to obviate some of these problems but such a recommendation is often associated with less satisfactory patient compliance. For all of these reasons and because the cost is some two- to three-fold greater than any of the preparations above, T_3 is rarely used in our clinics except for specific diagnostic tests.

COMBINATIONS OF L-T_4 AND L-T_3: LIOTRIX (THYROLAR, EUTHROID). These preparations contain the sodium salts of L-T_4 and L-T_3 in a 4:1 ratio and are available in a variety of dosage potencies. The original basis for their formulation and use was to simulate normal thyroid secretion and also permit easier monitoring of routine thyroid function tests. This rationale appears no longer to have any basis in fact (see "Guidelines for therapy" below). Such mixtures approximate desiccated thyroid in content but offer the advantage of greater stability of the synthetic materials. The major disadvantages include: (a) the relatively greater cost and (b) the wide fluctuations in serum T_3 that were described above for L-T_3. In addition, the T_4/T_3 combination represents a minor drawback when adjusting dosage, in that the two constituents obviously must be altered simultaneously and the patient may receive more or less of one than desirable as a consequence.

Which Drug to Use? For several years, advocacy of the use of some of these agents was based on physiologic concepts that have since proved untenable. For example, we believed that patients being treated with L-thyroxine should have serum T_4 or protein-bound iodine (PBI) values that were 2 to 3 micrograms per dl. higher than those in patients receiving desiccated thyroid. The rationale for this was based on the absence of T_3 in the synthetic L-T_4 preparation. With the development of a radioimmunoassay for serum T_3 and the discovery that T_4 is converted to T_3 peripherally, it became apparent that physiologic levels of both T_4 and T_3 can be maintained by replacement with L-T_4 alone. Similarly, there is no indication for combination T_4/T_3 preparations since the patient may derive adequate amounts of T_3 by endogenous conversion from the much less expensive L-T_4 preparations. Indeed, administration of L-T_4 leads to more gradual restoration and maintenance of stable serum T_3 levels, whereas the use of any T_3-containing preparation will be associated with greater lability and fluctuations in serum concentration of T_3, which may in turn produce symptoms. The greatest rationale for avoiding such preparations obtains in the elderly hypothyroid patient or in those with underlying cardiac disease. Thus, L-T_4 is the drug of choice for replacement and most closely simulates thyroidal economy in normal subjects, providing constant concentrations of serum T_4 and T_3 throughout the day with values within the normal range when the patients are clinically euthyroid. In most patients, the ideal replacement dose of L-T_4 correlates directly with weight, with only very large subjects requiring 0.3 mg. or more per day. The physician should beware of dosage recommendations in older articles and textbooks which suggest that 0.1 mg. of L-T_4 is equivalent to 1 grain (60 mg.) of thyroid which would result in an average replacement dose (3 grains) = 0.3 mg. per day of T_4. As indicated, most patients will require only 0.1 to 0.15 mg. per day or approximately 2.2 micrograms per kg. of body weight.

Guidelines to Adequacy of Therapy. The objectives of treatment are reversion of the signs and symptoms to normal and "normalization" of the serum T_4, T_3, and TSH. Within days after initiation of treatment, the elevated TSH levels characteristic of primary hypothyroidism begin falling toward normal but may remain elevated for several weeks. Persistently elevated values of TSH after 8 to 12 weeks of therapy are grounds for either increasing the dosage or questioning the compliance of the patient. Overzealous replacement may produce signs and symptoms of thyrotoxicosis, which may be seen even with T_4 levels at the upper end of the normal ranges. The most sensitive guide to supraphysiologic replacement would be the demonstration that TSH levels fail to increase after administration of TRH. The usual replacement doses listed here are those which will restore serum T_4 and TSH to normal and which will be associated with a normal TSH response to TRH. Whether or not mildly abnormal TRH responses that suggest either under-replacement (a slightly exaggerated response) or over-replacement (an absent response) have any long-term deleterious effects in the absence of clinical signs or symptoms is yet to be proved. Employing any form of replacement with the exception of T_3, one may settle quite satisfactorily for normalization of serum T_4, T_3, and TSH. In secondary or pituitary hypothyroidism, monitoring the serum TSH or the TSH response to TRH is of no value, and replacement is guided solely by serum T_4 and T_3 values and the clinical response. Once the dosage requirement is clearly established, the patient is instructed to return at 6- to 12-monthly intervals for follow-up evaluations, and is strongly advised of the necessity for refilling prescriptions and of the inviolable requirement for thyroid hormone for the rest of his life. At each follow-up evaluation, the patient's clinical status is assessed, and blood is obtained for the measurement of serum T_4 and TSH.

Special Treatment Situations

Children. When hypothyroidism is suspected in the neonate, serum should be drawn for thyroid function blood tests, and therapy initiated immediately and without waiting for the results. The risks of a few days of unnecessary thyroid hormone (should the suspicion not be confirmed) are negligible compared with the potential damage to mental development that may attend an unnecessary delay in treatment. An initial dose of 10 to 12 micrograms per kg. of L-thyroxine (L-T_4) is recommended and can be reduced to 8 to 10 micrograms per kg. after 3 months of life. Between the first and fifth years of life, a dose of 6 micrograms per kg. generally suffices with further adjustments based upon the clinical response (manifested by achievement of normal growth and development), and by serum T_4 and TSH determinations as in the adult. Between the ages of 5 and 15 years, L-T_4 replacement doses are variable but approximate 4 to 6 micrograms per kg. and the usual adult replacement dose of 2.2 micrograms per kg. is generally achieved by age 16. In contrast to the adult patient, children tolerate thyroid hormone well, and full replacement doses can be started from the outset without the need to gradually build up to the final dose. As always, precise adjustments in dosage are based on serial monitoring of serum T_4 and TSH.

Myxedema Coma. This relatively unusual presentation of severe hypothyroidism may have a mortality approaching 50 per cent and hence deserves early and vigorous therapy. Incipient coma may be heralded by the appearance of confusion and stupor in an untreated hypothyroid patient. Such deterioration may be due to CO_2 retention secondary to congestive failure, pneumonia, or the unusual sensitivity to sedatives and narcotics that is characteristic of hypothyroidism. The full-blown syndrome is marked by coma, hypothermia, hypotension, electrolyte abnormalities, and hypoventilation with CO_2 narcosis and respiratory acidosis. Complications include hyponatremia, hypoglycemia, and occasionally gastrointestinal hemorrhage. Hypothermia may be dramatic or suggested by the failure of the patient to manifest fever despite obvious infection. The approach to therapy may be considered a three-pronged attack which includes: (1) thyroid replacement, (2) neutralization of any precipitating cause, and (3) correction of life-threatening hypoxia, hypotension, or hypothermia. Survival demands early and aggressive treatment that cannot await the laboratory determination of T_4, T_3, or TSH. In addition to the usual signs, the clinical diagnosis may be supported by delayed Achilles tendon reflex times and a very low radioactive iodine (RAI) uptake at 3 hours. When suspected on clinical grounds, serum should be drawn and sent for thyroid function studies and then therapy instituted immediately.

Thyroid Hormone Replacement. The only parenteral preparation available for therapy of the comatose patient is L-T_4 (Synthroid). There are differences of opinion among thyroidologists whether the more rapidly acting T_3 should be given (by nasogastric tube if necessary) in preference to T_4, since the latter has to be converted to T_3 in the patient and this introduces some delay in onset of action. Others argue that it is this inherent delay that leads to a more gradual and less dangerous onset of action. If T_3 is given, multiple small doses would be prudent, e.g., 12.5 to 25 micrograms every 6 to 8 hours. When the clinical suspicion of this syndrome is very high, advocates of T_4 therapy recommend one large loading dose to replace the presumably void volume of distribution for T_4 in the patient. This initial dose should be 300 to 500 micrograms (one ampule) intravenously and may be followed by an additional 50 to 100 micrograms intravenously daily. Therapy with either T_3 or T_4 should be discontinued should the initial clinical impression prove incorrect and the thyroid function blood tests return within the normal range. If the suspected diagnosis is confirmed, treatment with parenteral T_4 should be discontinued once the patient is conscious and stable, and an oral preparation begun, e.g., levothyroxine (Letter or Synthroid) 0.1 mg. per day.

Therapy Directed Against Underlying Problems. The underlying precipitating event, such as infection, cerebrovascular accident (CVA), or drug overdose, must be treated.

Correction of Hypoxia, Shock, and Hypothermia. Strict attention to ventilation and pulmonary toilet with frequent monitoring of arterial blood gases is mandatory. Hypotension is corrected with the administration of pressors, while adrenal steroids (hydrocortisone, 100 mg. intravenously every 8 hours, during the initial few days) may also have a beneficial effect and ensures against the supervention of adrenal insufficiency, either on a relative basis or due to coexistent adrenal disease or pituitary ACTH deficiency as discussed above. The principal electrolyte abnormality, hyponatremia, is most often dilutional on the basis of inappropriate ADH secretion and best managed by fluid restriction or cautious use of hypertonic saline solution. Digitalis and diuretics may be indicated if congestive heart failure is present. Finally, the profound hypothermia that often accompanies myxedema coma must be managed conservatively with gradual warming rather than the use of electrical warming blankets. The latter may increase metabolic rate and lead to peripheral vasodilatation, thereby aggravating any tendency toward shock.

Treatment of Patients With Underlying Cardiac Disease

Since thyroid hormone will increase the work of the heart, injudicious rapid replacement in the hypothyroid patient with cardiac disease may precipitate congestive heart failure, arrhythmias, or myocardial infarction. In view of this, in any hypothyroid patient over age 50 (or of any age with a history of cardiac problems), the deficiency should be replaced very slowly under all circumstances except in the presence of life-threatening myxedema coma. In the absence of such urgency, no rate of cautious gradual replacement can be considered too conservative. One could start with 0.025 mg. per day (half of a 0.05 mg. tablet, the smallest available) and increase the dose to 0.05 mg. per day in 2 to 3 weeks. If no symptoms develop during the subsequent 4 weeks, the dose may be increased to 0.075 or 0.1 mg. per day, depending upon the age and general health of the patient. The response to therapy should be monitored (as described above) on clinical grounds and with serial measurement of serum T_4 and TSH. In addition, serial electrocardiograms should be obtained during the period that thyroid hormone doses are being increased. Should symptoms (angina, arrhythmia, etc.) develop at any dosage increment, the dose should be immediately decreased to the previous dosage level which had not been associated with such symptoms. Patients with severe arteriosclerotic cardiovascular disease may not tolerate full replacement to the euthyroid state, and the physician may have to settle for suboptimal replacement accompanied by mild clinical hypothyroidism, and serum T_4 and TSH determinations at the lower and higher ends of their respective normal ranges. (Indeed, until recent years, induction of mild hypothyroidism with radioiodine was an acceptable form of therapy for patients with otherwise intractable angina pectoris.) In contrast to the follow-up evaluations provided for younger, uncomplicated patients described above, the treated hypothyroid patient with heart disease should be seen more frequently, e.g., every 3 months with careful attention paid to cardiac as well as thyroid aspects of the history, physical, and laboratory evaluation.

THYROID GLAND MALIGNANCY

method of
JOEL B. FREEMAN, M.D.,
and FARID SHAMJI, M.D.
Ottawa, Ontario, Canada

Introduction

The most common surgical problem of the thyroid gland is a thyroid nodule. This article does not deal with endocrine or inflammatory disorders of the thyroid. The management of thyroid carcinoma is synonymous with the management of a patient who has a thyroid nodule, which is the most common mode of presentation for thyroid carcinomas. The incidence of thyroid carcinoma is low (2 to 3 per 100,000) as is its incidence as a cause of death (0.4 per cent of total cancer deaths). The reported incidence of carcinoma in thyroid nodules varies from 3 to 25 per cent. Whereas thyroid nodules, particularly those arising in a goiter, are common clinical problems, thyroid carcinoma is a rare malignancy.

Confirming the Diagnosis. When the history and physical examination indicate that a nodule may be malignant, the next step is usually a thyroid scan

with radioactive iodine. This test is predicated upon the fact that most thyroid carcinomas do not take up radioactive iodine and hence appear as cold areas on the scan. The incidence of carcinoma in such nonfunctioning nodules ranges from 10 to 15 per cent. Hypofunctioning nodules with irregular uptake of radioactive iodine usually indicate a goiter. The incidence of carcinoma in functioning or "warm" nodules is less than 1 per cent. Parenthetically, the terms "warm" and "hot" are not synonymous. The decision to operate on a suspicious thyroid nodule is not predicated solely upon whether the nodule is cold or warm. The iodine scan is a two dimensional study, so that a suspicious nodule which is warm may be a carcinoma obscured by functioning thyroid tissue lying anterior to the lesion. Conversely, many benign lesions are cold on iodine scanning. This is particularly common with multinodular goiter, thyroiditis, cysts, or adenomas with degenerative changes. Hence the thyroid scan should complement the history and physical examination but not make the ultimate decision. The uptake of ^{75}Se methionine provides an index of protein synthesis. Hence a nodule which is cold after radioiodine and warm after ^{75}Se methionine scanning should be suspect for carcinoma. However, the incidence of false positives and false negatives is common enough that this test has not supplanted ^{131}I scanning. Neck roentgenographs may reveal stippled calcification, indicating the formation of psammoma bodies by a papillary carcinoma. The calcification in degenerative cysts is more coarse than the stippled calcification seen in papillary carcinoma.

A history of rapid, painful enlargement suggests a cyst. Such lesions are firmer than most thyroid nodules, but not rock hard as in carcinoma. Furthermore, not all cysts are acute in the nature of their presentation. They may arise in any hyperplastic nodule or in a benign adenoma. The key to diagnosis is in appreciating a firm lesion which is easily movable, not fixed to the overlying muscles, and frequently accompanied by other palpable but smaller nodules. Such patients are ideal candidates for needle aspiration.

TABLE 1. **Differential Diagnosis of Thyroid Nodules**

Adenoma:
  Papillary cystic
  Follicular solid: Macrofollicular (colloid)
                  Microfollicular (fetal)
                  Embryonal
                  Hurthle cell
Carcinoma:
  Follicular
  Papillary
  Mixed follicular and papillary
  Undifferentiated
  Medullary
  Epidermoid, sarcoma, lymphoma
  Metastatic
Thyroiditis:
  Hashimoto (Lymphadenoid goiter)
  Subacute (De Quervain)
  Riedel's (Struma)
Colloid goiter

Thyroid Echography.   Most cystic thyroid lesions are benign, whereas most thyroid cancers are solid. The differentiation of solid versus cystic lesions by ultrasound therefore has preoperative diagnostic importance. The incidence of thyroid cysts within solitary thyroid nodules is between 15 and 22 per cent. Purely cystic lesions less than 4 cm. in diameter are almost never malignant and can be satisfactorily treated by needle aspiration. Mixed solid and cystic lesions, especially those larger than 4 cm. in diameter, will not completely resolve with aspiration. In addition, the possibility of a coexisting carcinoma is high enough to justify surgical removal. Also, lesions which appear solid by ultrasound are more likely to be neoplastic.

See Table 1 for differentiation of nodules.

Treatment

Cysts, benign adenomas, hemorrhagic nodules, multinodular goiters, or thyroiditis diagnosed by needle aspiration or biopsy can be treated conservatively. Hypofunctioning nodules under 3 cm. in size which clinically appear to represent a nodular goiter in patients in the proper age and sex bracket may be treated with thyroid hormone. These hyperplastic nodules are under the influence of endogenous thyroid-stimulating hormone (TSH), and secretion of the latter is inhibited by the administration of exogenous thyroid hormone. It is fruitless to use suppressive therapy for large lesions, particularly when they are firm and highly suspect for carcinoma. Suppression is the ideal treatment for the middle-aged female patient who has a small nodule in an enlarged gland. However, nodules which do not regress usually require surgical intervention. Thyroid suppression will seldom be effective for lesions greater than 2 cm. in size.

The first consideration in larger lesions is whether surgical exploration can be avoided by needle biopsy. Needle biopsy of the thyroid gland has been proposed as an accurate diagnostic technique and is widely used by many experienced thyroidologists. However, it is still controversial because the amount of tissue obtained is limited, making it occasionally difficult to distinguish between a benign nodule and a well-differentiated carcinoma. The combination of needle aspiration using rapid fixation and a needle biopsy has increased the yield. Generally, advocates of needle biopsy are those who use the technique frequently and are experienced in interpreting the results. Results are less satisfactory when one is attempting to biopsy small solitary nodules, particularly if the technique is not carried out by an experienced operator. The concern for seeding tumor in the needle track is theoretical, especially if thyroidectomy closely follows a positive needle biopsy. The risk of inserting the needle into benign thyroid tissue adjacent to a tumor is worrisome to many clinicians.

If needle biopsy is not feasible or it has already failed and the lesion does not take up iodine, the chances of carcinoma are approximately 1 in 10. When suspicion for carcinoma is not high and if the patient is reliable enough to return for follow-up examinations, TSH suppression is a reasonable mode of therapy. Of course, nonfunctioning nodules will not regress with exogenous thyroid therapy, and apparent regression simply indicates that the patient had a goiter, previous thyroiditis, or a cyst which resolved coincidentally with thyroid therapy. Additional justification for administering exogenous thyroid to patients with nonfunctioning nodules is as follows: such therapy prevents development of other nodules or cysts if the patient has a TSH-dependent goiter; thyroid suppression is a reasonable treatment for small papillary or follicular carcinomas; and growth of a lesion while on thyroid suppression is an absolute indication for surgical intervention. As mentioned, some thyroidologists feel that thyroid hormone is as effective as extirpation for some types of thyroid carcinoma, although this conservative approach is not shared by all clinicians. The use of observant and/or suppressive therapy for large, firm lesions is mentioned only to be decried. Such patients should be promptly referred to a surgeon. Thyroid scans in these patients are hardly necessary, because the indication for surgical intervention is obvious.

Surgical Management

The majority of thyroid carcinomas are well differentiated and the prognosis is generally excellent, particularly for papillary and follicular carcinomas in the patient under 40 years of age. Patients with medullary carcinoma and lymphoma have a 40 per cent 5 year survival rate. Anaplastic carcinoma, which typically occurs in elderly patients, has a dismal prognosis, and often these patients are not even surgical candidates. However, each patient should have the benefit of a surgical opinion even when the lesion appears to be inoperable. Prior to operation and regardless of age, patients with advanced lesions must be prepared for the possibility of radical surgery. Elderly patients with large fixed lesions tolerate extensive neck surgery surprisingly well. Of even more importance is the confusion which frequently arises between small cell anaplastic carcinoma of the thyroid and lymphoma. Hence if the needle or open biopsy reveals anaplastic carcinoma, the surgeon should not hesitate to remove the bulk of the tumor and to perform an adequate neck dissection if he feels that he can safely do this. Conversely, surgery has no role in patients with advanced anaplastic lesions. Usually a tracheostomy and external irradiation is all that can be offered. Some recent reports indicate that doxorubicin (Adriamycin) may be helpful for advanced thyroid tumors.

The operative approach to thyroid carcinoma commences with the customary curved neck incision, separation of the strap muscles, and a systematic examination of the thyroid gland and surrounding tissues. It is wise to plan the incision so that extension is easily facilitated should a neck dissection be necessary.

When there is a unilateral lesion with a normal contralateral lobe, we perform a lobectomy on the side of the lesion that includes the isthmus and a rim of the contralateral lobe. This may appear to be a somewhat radical approach for a lesion which has a 90 per cent chance of being benign. However, frozen sections of the thyroid gland are notoriously difficult to interpret, and in the event that the pathologist should subsequently change the diagnosis after reviewing the permanent sections, the aforementioned operative procedure will generally eliminate the necessity for reoperation. There is seldom an indication for nodulectomy alone unless the nodule is either very small or located in the isthmus of the gland. The extended lobectomy should suffice for all unilateral benign lesions as well as for most papillary and follicular lesions. If the diagnosis of carcinoma is confirmed at the time of surgery, we leave only a small rim of the posterior portion of the contralateral lobe to assure a euparathyroid state postoperatively. We do not perform total thyroidectomy for low grade lesions. The risks of hypoparathyroidism (11 to 27 per cent) outweigh the benefits derived from doing a total thyroidectomy to remove microscopic foci of cancer in the contralateral lobe. When indicated, it is relatively simple to ablate the thyroid remnants with ^{131}I postoperatively, and the use of ^{131}I is preferred over routine and indiscriminate total thyroidectomy.

When the carcinoma is more extensive, a decision regarding treatment of the lymphatics must be made. Metastases to the internal jugular nodes are treated by a formal neck dissection. This may be modified by preserving the sternomastoid muscle, accessory nerve, and the jugular vein. However, the dissection must not be compromised in the interest of cosmesis. It is difficult to adequately excise the jugular nodes without removing the vein itself. Involved strap muscles must be removed with the thyroid. Extension into the sternomastoid muscle indicates the necessity for a classic radical neck dissection. Node plucking operations are associated with a high incidence of recurrence and should not be performed. Subsequent operations for recurrent disease are difficult and associated with a 10 to 15 per cent incidence of recurrent nerve injury or hypoparathyroidism.

Thyroid carcinoma also metastasizes to the posterior triangle of the neck, the tracheoesophageal groove, and the superior mediastinum. It is particularly important to dissect the entire tracheoesophageal area. This can be difficult if the patient has had previous neck surgery. It is best to identify the recurrent nerve inferiorly and trace it superiorly into the groove before beginning the lymphatic dissection. Despite dense adhesions this area must be adequately explored. Most involved mediastinal nodes can be swept out from under the sternum and included en bloc with the resected thyroid gland. It is seldom necessary to divide the sternum. Total thyroidectomy should always be performed for medullary carcinoma or when there is gross involvement of both lobes by any tumor. When this operation is performed, the presence of viable parathyroid glands must be documented by frozen section and by observing bleeding from the cut surface of the gland. If there is any doubt, the parathyroid gland should be removed, macerated, and reimplanted into the sternomastoid muscle. If the capsule of the thyroid is inadvertently entered, the wound should be irrigated with hypotonic sterile water to lyse any potentially viable tumor cells.

Recurrent neck masses in patients who have had previous partial thyroidectomy for carcinoma seldom respond to ^{131}I therapy, because malignant lymph nodes do not take up radioiodine. Proper therapy consists of reoperation, conversion of the partial to a total thyroidectomy, and an appropriate dissection of the lymph nodes.

The vast majority of patients with thyroid nodules, regardless of histology, require suppression. Those with benign lesions usually have a multinodular goiter with nodules in the contralateral unresected lobe. Without suppression of endogenous TSH, these nodules may undergo compensatory hypertrophy, necessitating a second operative procedure at a later date. As previously noted, this exposes the patient to an unnecessarily high risk. One exception to this general rule would be the young patient with a clearly demarcated adenoma or solitary cyst and a normal contralateral lobe. All patients with thyroid carcinoma require thyroid suppression for life regardless of the histologic type. We withhold exogenous thyroid until the final sections confirm that the uninvolved lobe is not microscopically involved with cancer. This being the case, levothyroxine (Synthroid), 0.3 mg. per day, is prescribed and TSH levels are monitored at 6 month intervals. Most patients with benign disease will be adequately suppressed with 0.125 to 0.200 mg. of Synthroid per day. The higher dose is preferred in patients with cancer, because many thyroid malignancies are TSH dependent. In elderly patients or when there is a history of heart disease, exogenous levothyroxine is given cautiously, beginning with 0.05 mg. per day and gradually increasing over a 4 to 8 week period until the desired dosage is reached. Occasional patients experience symptoms of toxicity and this must be rectified by lowering the dose.

When there is microscopic involvement of the contralateral lobe or if there is residual uptake in the neck after total thyroidectomy performed for a more aggressive lesion, suppressive therapy is withheld for 3 weeks. The patient is then given a therapeutic dose of radioactive iodine and discharged on Synthroid. Six months later, the total body scan is repeated, being certain to instruct the patient to discontinue thyroid hormone 3 weeks prior to the scan. If the neck tissue has been ablated and there are no metastases, the patient resumes suppressive therapy. However, if there is persistent uptake in the neck or if there are metastases, a second ablative dose is administered, Synthroid is reinstituted, and the total body scan is repeated again 6 months later. Radioiodine uptake may be facilitated with exogenous TSH or propylthiouracil. When there is no evidence of persistent tumor in the neck or distant metastases, it is fruitless to perform periodic body scans. They are seldom helpful, and there is a theoretical risk of potentiating growth of the tumor during the 3 week interval when the patient is not taking thyroid hormone.

All patients with thyroid carcinoma should be followed for life—twice yearly for the first 2 years and then yearly. During these clinic visits, the patient is questioned with regard to symptoms of local recurrence, the neck is examined, and a chest roentgenograph is obtained to rule out metastases. The serum calcium and phosphorus are checked for hypoparathyroidism in appropriate patients, and TSH levels are drawn to confirm the adequacy of suppression. Thyroid scans are done as indicated above.

PHEOCHROMOCYTOMA

method of
STEPHEN L. SWARTZ, M.D.,
and ROBERT G. DLUHY, M.D.
Boston, Massachusetts

Although pheochromocytoma occurs in only 0.1 per cent of patients with diastolic hypertension, its potential for complete surgical cure with proper diagnosis and management and possible fatal outcome if unrecognized makes it an important disease to recognize. Approximately 30 per cent of patients with pheochromocytoma have sustained hypertension, 30 per cent have both sustained and paroxysmal hypertension, and 30 per cent have only paroxysmal hypertension, while 10 per cent are normotensive. Therefore, all patients with characteristic symptoms (diaphoresis, palpitations, intermittent headaches) or with severe or paroxysmal hypertension should be evaluated for pheochromocytoma. Twenty-four hour urine collections should be analyzed for free catecholamines and catecholamine metabolites (metanephrines and vanillylmandelic acid); creatinine should also be measured to determine the adequacy of the collection. A diagnosis of pheochromocytoma should be made only after biochemical documentation of catecholamine excess has been established. Localization of the tumor is then attempted by aortography and selective angiography after the patient has first received alpha-adrenergic blockade. In the case of a normotensive patient presenting with a history of characteristic paroxysms, increased urinary catecholamines or its metabolites or both may only be demonstrable during a 6 to 12 hour urine sample obtained at the time of a typical episode. If a patient does not have any episode while under observation in the hospital, it is recommended that fractional urine samples be collected at home during a characteristic paroxysm (Figure 1). Rarely is provocative testing with histamine, glucagon, or tyramine indicated in such patients, since these tests may be hazardous and are associated with both significant false negative and false positive responses. However, if these tests are performed, careful blood pressure monitoring is mandatory, and the alpha-adrenergic blocker phentolamine (Regitine) should be available at the bedside. For a provocative test to be diagnostic of pheochromocytoma, biochemical documentation of elevated levels of urinary catecholamines and its metabolites are required coincident with a hypertensive paroxysm.

Finally, since pheochromocytoma may occur as part of a hereditary familial syndrome in association with medullary carcinoma of the thyroid and hyperparathyroidism (MEA II), serum calcium and calcitonin levels may be indicated.

Medical Management

Adrenergic Blockade. The cornerstone of preoperative and long-term medical management of pheochromocytoma is a thorough understanding of the α-adrenergic blocking agent, phenoxybenzamine. The goal of α-adrenergic blockade is to return the blood pressure to normal levels and to eliminate the clinical symptoms and paroxysms associated with pheochromocytoma by competitively inhibiting tumor catecholamines at peripheral receptors. Since phentolamine (Regitine) is too short-acting to achieve continuous α-adrenergic blockade, its use should be reserved for intravenous administration to control hypertensive emergencies arising during aortography or surgery. Phenoxybenzamine (Dibenzyline) can be administered orally and has a longer duration of

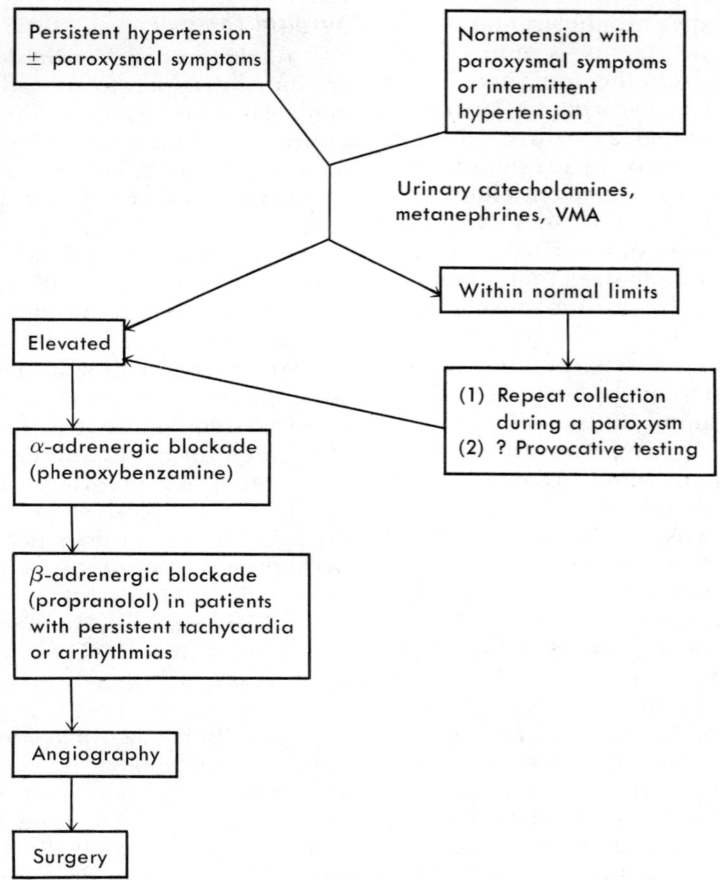

Figure 1.　Preoperative evaluation and medical management of patients with pheochromocytoma.

action since it binds covalently to the α-receptors. With a biologic half-life of 18 to 24 hours, it is best given as the total effective daily dose on a twice daily schedule. Treatment with phenoxybenzamine is usually started with 20 to 30 mg. per day orally and progressively increased by 10 to 20 mg. per day until blood pressure is controlled and symptoms of catecholamine excess disappear. Some patients with pheochromocytoma require as much as 150 mg. of phenoxybenzamine per day, with the average dose ranging from 80 to 120 mg. per day. (This dose may be higher than that listed in the manufacturer's official directive.) The most common side effects of phenoxybenzamine therapy are nasal congestion, sedation, dry mouth, and orthostatic hypotension. The orthostatic hypotension occurs as a result of relaxation of a chronically contracted vascular bed. Subsequently, as the intravascular space is slowly replenished from the interstitial and intracellular fluid compartments, a fall in hematocrit commonly occurs. Concomitant administration of intravenous isotonic saline solution or a high sodium diet with phenoxybenzamine therapy will help correct the intravascular

volume deficit and ameliorate the orthostatic changes in blood pressure. In patients with diminished cardiac reserve, it may not be possible to administer large amounts of sodium; these patients should be confined to bed during phenoxybenzamine therapy.

The duration of preoperative treatment with phenoxybenzamine depends upon the individual patient and the clinical circumstances, but optimally requires 1 to 2 weeks. There has been recent discussion of the advantage of incomplete versus complete preoperative α-adrenergic blockade. Advocates of incomplete blockade argue that the demonstration of a hypertensive episode during exploratory palpation of the abdomen is important in searching for the presence of multiple tumors. We consider this an unnecessary risk and have relied upon careful palpation in a safely blocked patient. Furthermore, the manipulation of a suspicious lesion, even in an adequately treated patient, will usually lead to enough catecholamine release to overcome the adrenergic blockade but without serious blood pressure elevation.

Routine preoperative administration of beta (β)-adrenergic blocking agents is unnecessary. However, β-blockade may be indicated in the presence of persistent tachycardia or cardiac arrhythmia that occurs either as a direct effect of circulating catecholamines or as a result of reflex tachycardia following α-blockade. In either case, bed rest and the addition of 10 to 40 mg. four times daily of propranolol orally usually will control this problem. It is emphasized that β-blocking drugs should *never* be administered until α-adrenergic blockade has first been established. Otherwise, blockade of β-adrenergically mediated vasodilatation will lead to unopposed α-adrenergic vasoconstriction by tumor catecholamines, possibly resulting in a severe hypertensive episode.

In those patients in whom preoperative angiography indicates the necessity of bilateral adrenalectomy, hydrocortisone should be administered intravenously intra- and postoperatively at the rate of 10 mg. per hour, similar to the schedule used in addisonian patients.

Precautions in Patients with Pheochromocytoma. Any patient in whom the diagnosis of pheochromocytoma is strongly suspected or established should adhere to the following precautions: (1) avoid colonic enemas; (2) avoid tyramine-containing foods; (3) avoid catecholamine-depleting antihypertensive medications (such as reserpine, α-methyldopa, clonidine, guanethidine) that may produce a state of denervation hypersensitivity, which is then hyperresponsive to a sudden release of catecholamines; (4) avoid phenothiazines or morphine; and (5) avoid saralasin (P113) infusions and ACTH stimulation tests. The latter agents have the potential to stimulate catecholamine release either directly or indirectly via a decline in blood pressure.

Long-Term Medical Management. Long-term medical management with adrenergic blocking drugs may be necessary in patients who are poor operative risks or who have metastatic malignant pheochromocytoma. Since radiotherapy and cytotoxic agents are generally ineffective in treating patients with malignant pheochromocytomas, chronic therapy with phenoxybenzamine and propranolol has been continued for many years in such patients. Alpha-methyl para-tyrosine, an analogue that blocks the synthesis of catecholamines, was developed in order to reduce catecholamine production on a long-term basis in patients with metastatic pheochromocytoma. Although a significant reduction in blood pressure and urinary catecholamine values occurs with its use, a high incidence of parkinsonian-like symptomatology has also been noted. Alpha-methyl para-tyrosine is presently available only as an investigational drug.

Surgical Therapy

Analgesia and Anesthesia. Prior to administration of preoperative sedatives, intraarterial and central venous catheters should be positioned, and continuous electrocardiographic monitoring should be started. Proper anesthetic management starts preoperatively with sodium pentobarbital to help reduce anxiety. The preferred induction agent is sodium thiopental. Succinylcholine may then be used for intubation. Until recently, halothane had been considered the agent of choice for maintenance of anesthesia because of its ability to suppress sympathoadrenal activity and thereby lower blood pressure. However, its propensity for causing frequent ventricular arrhythmias led to the search for better anesthetic agents. Enflurane (Ethane), a new anesthetic agent from the ether group, is nonexplosive, produces excellent muscular relaxation, and does not result in ventricular arrhythmias. Enflurane is now considered the anesthetic agent of choice.

Intraoperative Management. Intraoperatively, blood pressure elevations should be titrated into the normal range with a continuous infusion of nitroprusside. This is prepared by adding 50 mg. of sodium nitroprusside to 500 ml. of 5 per cent dextrose solution. A microdrip regulator should be used to ensure a precise flow rate. The average adult dose is 3 micrograms per kg. per minute (approximately 200 micrograms per minute); the maximum dose should not exceed 800 micrograms per minute. Nitroprusside has the advantage of a direct effect on the arterial wall, immediate onset of action, and recovery within 1 to 2 minutes. Moreover, blood pressure control is much smoother with this agent than with the short-acting α-blocking agent phentolamine, which cannot be administered as a continuous infusion but rather as intermittent boluses. Another advantage of using nitroprusside is that the infusion can be immediately terminated when the adrenal vein is clamped, thereby preventing exacerbation of falling blood pressure when the tumor is removed.

Replacement of blood lost at operation with whole blood, 5 per cent albumin in saline, or plasma is of major importance in the control of the hypotension seen after removal of a pheochromocytoma. In fact, a fall in blood pressure occasionally seen at the time of removal of the tumor should always be initially treated by expanding intravascular volume, even in the absence of known significant intraoperative blood loss. Only rarely are vasoconstrictor agents required to treat intra- and postoperative hypotension. In general, adequate preoperative α-adrenergic blockade and sodium repletion largely prevent such hypotensive episodes.

To accomplish both systemic transabdominal exploration and removal of the tumor, a thoracoabdominal incision should be used. Careful palpation of the sympathetic ganglia along the vena cava and aorta should be performed prior to any manipulation or exploration in the area of the tumor. Manipulation of the tumor mass should be kept at a minimum while the blood supply of the neoplasm is carefully dissected and ligated. Because of the possibility of malignancy, local fixation of the tumor to surrounding tissues should be dealt with aggressively. This may require excision of part or all of the adherent kidney plus lymphadenectomy.

Postoperative Management. Postoperatively, the intra-arterial and central venous catheters should be maintained for at least 24 hours. Persistent postoperative *hypotension* may be due to (1) inadequate volume replacement, (2) cardiac failure, or (3) intra-abdominal bleeding, which may result from phenoxybenzamine inhibition of vasoconstriction at the time of surgery, leading to persistent oozing of blood from the operative site. Persistent postoperative *hypertension* may be the result of (1) fluid overload, (2) residual tumor, (3) continued release of stored catecholamines from sympathetic nerve endings (due to the previous high circulating levels of catecholamines), (4) underlying essential hypertension or nephrosclerosis, (5) persistent pain, or (6) inadvertent ligation of the renal artery.

It is emphasized that persistent postoperative hypertension does not indicate metastatic disease or an additional unsuspected pheochromocytoma unless it is accompanied by elevated urinary levels of catecholamines. Urinary catecholamines measured within the first few weeks postoperatively after the removal of a pheochromocytoma may be misleading, since they may be elevated secondary to the release of stored catecholamines from the sympathetic nerve endings. Thus, it is recommended that the first postoperative urine catecholamine excretion level be obtained approximately 1 month after removal of the tumor.

Pheochromocytoma and Pregnancy. Although pheochromocytoma occurs very rarely in pregnant patients, the preferred management of this condition remains surgical removal of the tumor as soon as it is discovered, regardless of the duration of pregnancy. If the pregnancy is near or at term when the tumor is discovered, a cesarean section is recommended with tumor extirpation, so as to avoid the stress of vaginal delivery. Labor and vaginal delivery have been followed by maternal or fetal death or both, owing to the sudden discharge of catecholamines into the circulation. Although it is not recommended, some pregnant patients with pheochromocytoma have been successfully controlled with phenoxybenzamine and propranolol therapy. In those patients who were treated with phenoxybenzamine during the first trimester of pregnancy, there have been no reported teratogenic effects.

Long-Term Follow-up

Malignancy, which occurs in approximately 10 per cent of pheochromocytomas, cannot be diagnosed from the histologic appearance of the tumor but rather on the basis of gross or microscopic evidence of local invasiveness or metastatic spread to nonchromaffin tissue. Since recurrent metastatic lesions usually produce catecholamines, urinary catecholamine measurements and clinical assessment at 6 to 12 month intervals afford early diagnosis of recurrent tumor while still potentially removable by operation. Measurement of plasma or urinary dopamine (or its metabolite homovanillic acid) levels may be helpful in patients with documented pheochromocytoma, as elevated levels are most commonly seen in adult patients with malignant disease. On the other hand, following the removal of a benign pheochromocytoma, all patients should have periodic urine collections to rule out the appearance of recurrent pheochromocytoma, since multiple neoplasms occur in some patients.

As many as 25 per cent of patients with pheochromocytomas may have mild sustained hypertension postoperatively without biochemical or intraoperative evidence of residual tumor. This may be the result of irreversible small vessel disease or renal damage or both owing to the previous long-standing hypertension. The hypertension should be managed with the standard medications used to treat patients with essential hypertension.

THYROIDITIS

method of
IAN R. HART, M.D.
Ottawa, Ontario, Canada

Acute Infectious Thyroiditis

Since the advent of antibiotics acute infectious thyroiditis has become a very rare condition. Currently, the usual causative organisms are streptococci, staphylococci, pneumococci, and coliform bacilli. Acute infectious thyroiditis may arise by direct extension of an infective focus in the neck or by hematogenous spread from a distant focus and it may be suppurative or nonsuppurative.

The symptoms are of severe pain and tenderness in the region of the thyroid gland. Often the pain extends up to the ears or angle of the jaw and is accentuated by movement of the neck. It is accompanied by general malaise and fever. Examination of the neck reveals localized swelling and tenderness. The neck uptake of iodine or technetium may be normal but areas of decreased uptake in the scan are usually found.

Although similar in presentation to granulomatous thyroiditis, acute infectious thyroiditis can be distinguished from that condition by the more severe constitutional symptoms, the finding of marked heat or discoloration of the skin over the lesion and the presence of a marked leucocytosis.

Occasionally the early use of a broad-spectrum antibiotic will obviate the need for surgery. More commonly, localized suppuration occurs and requires surgical drainage. The dense fascial planes overlying the thyroid may mask fluctuation and this sign of localized abscess formation should not be waited for before surgical intervention. If the lesion is localized to one lobe, lobectomy is the treatment of choice. Multiple abscesses require incision and drainage. In all cases, appropriate antibiotic treatment is necessary. Complete recovery from this condition is the rule.

Chronic infectious thyroiditis is also exceedingly rare. The usual causes are syphilis, tuberculosis, actinomycosis, and echinococcosis. Treatment is with the appropriate anti-infective agent.

Radiation Thyroiditis (Postirradiation Thyroiditis)

Although all thyroid glands treated with ^{131}I show histologic changes of inflammation, this term is reserved for those cases that become symptomatic. Symptoms include pain, swelling, and tenderness in the gland. A temporary worsening of hyperthyroidism (if this is the reason for treatment) may accompany the local features. Symptoms usually commence about the fifth day after the dose of ^{131}I and subside over the next 7 to 10 days.

The syndrome occurs somewhat more often after the higher doses of ^{131}I given to ablate remaining normal tissue in patients with thyroid carcinoma than it does following ^{131}I therapy for hyperthyroidism.

By definition, symptoms are self-limiting and the only treatment usually required is aspirin, 600 mg. (10 grains) every 8 hours. Occasionally corticosteroids are required and are used as described below for granulomatous thyroiditis, although tapered off somewhat more rapidly.

Granulomatous Thyroiditis (Subacute Thyroiditis, de Quervain's Thyroiditis, Viral Thyroiditis, Acute-Nonsuppurative Thyroiditis)

This condition is generally considered to be of viral cause. Most commonly either Coxsackie or mumps viruses have been implicated, but in various series several other viruses have been the apparent causative agents. Although many cases occur in a sporadic fashion, most cases occur in small epidemics.

The clinical picture can be quite varied, ranging from a mild unilateral aching neck to a severe prostrating acute illness. Most cases lie somewhere between these two extremes and patients present with pain in the neck or throat (often radiating to the ear) accompanied by general malaise and fever. The pain is exacerbated by swallowing and movements of the neck, and the diagnosis is clinically evident by the finding of a tender diffusely swollen thyroid gland.

Occasionally, the disease is localized to one lobe or pole of the gland and may move slowly over to the other side as the original side resolves. This localized form of granulomatous thyroiditis is easily missed if the neck is not carefully palpated, and occasionally it may be difficult to differentiate from hemorrhage into a cyst or nodule.

Most patients who present with diffuse involvement of the gland also develop hyperthyroid symptoms due to the release into the circulation of colloid (and thus thyroxine and triiodothyronine) from damaged follicles.

The disease is self-limiting and, in the usual case, has run its course in 2 to 4 weeks. About 10 per cent of patients run a more prolonged course marked by exacerbations and remissions for as long as 12 to 18 months after the onset.

In addition to general measures, management is aimed at suppressing the inflammatory process and treating symptomatically any symptoms of hyperthyroidism that may occur.

It is important to reassure the patient regarding the benign and self-limiting nature of the condition. Bed rest and mild sedation should be prescribed for those patients with fever and constitutional symptoms.

In the milder cases the only necessary anti-inflammatory (and analgesic) therapy is aspirin in doses of 0.6 to 0.9 gram (10 to 15 grains) every 6 hours. This should be continued as long as pain or local tenderness persists and then tapered off over the next 2 weeks. In all patients who have severe constitutional symptoms and those who fail to respond to or relapse after a course of aspirin, adrenal steroids should be used. Prednisone, in doses of 10 to 15 mg. every 8 hours, is prescribed for the first 10 days. Thereafter, the total daily dose is halved every 5 or so days and finally discontinued after reaching a dose of 2.5 mg. daily. If symptoms recur, the prednisone dose is again raised to the minimum level at which the patient was asymptomatic and the same course of dosage reduction again followed. In the occasional patient who shows a pattern of relapses and remissions over many months it is important to taper the dose of steroids more slowly than described above. Response to steroids is dramatic in this condition and usually complete remission of local symptoms occurs within 24 hours. If marked improvement has not occurred within 48 hours, one should suspect a mistaken diagnosis.

Usually hyperthyroid symptoms are mild and require no treatment. If moderate or severe symptoms of heat intolerance, nervousness, tremulousness or palpitations occur, propranolol, 20 mg. every 8 hours, may be prescribed for 7 to 10 days (see manufacturer's official directive for use of this agent).

During the recovery phase the goiter may persist or clinical hypothyroidism may become apparent. In either case, thyroxine, 0.2 mg. daily, should be prescribed, but this should be discontinued after a 3 month course. Although complete thyroidal recovery following granulomatous thyroiditis is the rule, the occasional patient will develop permanent hypothyroidism.

Chronic Lymphocytic Thyroiditis (Hashimoto's Thyroiditis)

Other terms for this condition, e.g., struma lymphomatosa, chronic thyroiditis, lymphadenoid goiter, autoimmune thyroiditis, lymphoepithelial goiter, and Hashimoto's struma, are now obsolete and to avoid confusion should no longer be used.

Chronic lymphocytic thyroiditis is a common condition that can occur in either sex at any age, but has a predilection for middle-aged women. It is almost certainly autoimmune in origin, although the precise mechanism of gland damage is, as yet, unclear. It occurs with an increased frequency of association with other autoimmune diseases, including pernicious anemia, autoimmune Addison's disease, chronic active hepatitis, and several others. The relationship of this form of thyroiditis to Graves' disease is unclear, there being a close association and possibly even overlap between the two conditions. Hyperthyroidism and even exophthalmos have been reported as occurring in patients who appear to have unequivocal chronic lymphocytic thyroiditis, but this is rare.

Chronic lymphocytic thyroiditis tends to be familial and shows also a close familial association with other forms of thyroid disease. Many cases of what were previously termed familial goiter or simple colloid goiter are now thought, on the basis of biopsy or circulating antibody studies, to represent simply chronic lymphocytic thyroiditis.

This condition usually presents as an asymptomatic, firm, diffuse goiter. Some patients are clinically (or biochemically) hypothyroid at the time of presentation or later become so if left untreated. The frequently made statements that all patients with chronic lymphocytic thyroiditis will eventually become hypothyroid if left untreated and that all cases of primary hypothyroidism represent "burned-out" chronic lymphocytic thyroiditis await definitive proof. Although usually firm (often described as "rubbery") and symmetrically enlarged, the texture and shape of the gland varies widely. In children the gland is often quite soft, and in older people it may be asymmetrically enlarged or even nodular. Occasionally, this form of thyroiditis occurs in one area of the gland and presents as a solitary thyroid nodule. Although usually asymptomatic, chronic lymphocytic thyroiditis can be large and firm enough to cause local pressure symptoms, but these are seldom severe.

All patients with chronic lymphocytic thyroiditis should be treated with L-thyroxine. This will result in a reduction in size of the gland in almost all patients (and disappearance of the goiter in some) and will forestall the development of hypothyroidism. Further, there is some evidence that the earlier the goiter is treated, the greater the reduction of goiter size achieved. In most patients treatment should commence with L-thyroxine, 0.15 mg. daily, which is also the prescribed maintenance dose unless there is no change in gland size or the serum TSH level remains elevated after 3 months of treatment. In such patients the dose may be increased by 0.05 mg. increments every 6 weeks to 3 months till optimum effect or to a maximum of 0.3 mg. daily. In the elderly patient, patients with any evidence of cardiac disease, and in patients with severe hypothyroidism, dosage should start at 0.05 mg. daily, increasing by increments of 0.05 mg. monthly to tolerance or until maximum effect is obtained.

In most patients some decrease in goiter size will be seen in about 6 weeks, although maximum resolution is not achieved for about 6 months and in some patients some improvement may occur up to 12 months. Some smaller goiters may disappear completely, although the usual pattern with larger goiters is a 30 to 50 per cent decrease in size. Often the goiters become more firm and irregular in consistency with treatment. Thyroxine therapy should be continued as long as a palpable goiter persists (and in most patients this means lifelong). In those patients in whom the goiter disappears, thyroxine therapy may be discontinued 1 year after successful resolution. If careful follow-up and testing reveal recurrence of goiter or the development of serum TSH elevation or fall in serum T_4, lifelong thyroxine therapy should be reinstituted.

Surgical removal of thyroid tissue is rarely indicated in chronic lymphocytic thyroiditis. Occasionally subtotal thyroidectomy is required for cosmetic or obstructive reasons when a very large gland is present. Postsurgically it is important in all patients, to institute lifelong thyroxine therapy to prevent recurrence of thyroid swelling and the development of hypothyroidism.

Thyroid extract (desiccated thyroid) and liothyronine offer no advantages (and have some disadvantages) over thyroxine in the management of this condition and their use should be discouraged. Older treatments, such as irradiation to the thyroid gland and the use of adrenal steroids, although effective, are dangerous and should not be used. Iodine or iodides, used in the mistaken belief that the goiter may be due to iodine lack, usually increase the goiter size and may cause the rapid development of hypothyroidism; for these reasons their use is therefore potentially dangerous.

Silent Thyroiditis

A number of reports over the last few years have described a new syndrome of transient hyperthyroidism with or without a palpable goiter. This has been called silent or painless thyroiditis. Some reports suggest that pathologically these represent classic granulomatous thyroiditis, while others report a picture of chronic lymphocytic thyroiditis during a phase of active follicular damage. Probably both are correct and the syndrome represents a heterogeneous group of conditions.

Since most cases of the syndrome present as goiter with hyperthyroidism clinically similar to Graves' disease, it is most important to distinguish it from that condition before prolonged or definitive therapy for the hyperthyroidism is undertaken. The major distinguishing feature is that in the silent thyroiditis syndrome the thyroidal uptake of ^{131}I or technetium is very low during the hyperthyroid phase.

Since the hyperthyroidism is transient, usually all that is required is mild sedation and propranolol, 20 to 40 mg. every 8 hours until symptoms abate (see manufacturer's official directive for this use). The long-term sequelae of this syndrome are as yet unknown.

Riedel's Thyroiditis

This is an extremely rare condition of obscure cause. There is progressive destruction of thyroid gland tissue and its replacement by dense fibrous tissue. The condition is associated with other rare sclerosing conditions, including retroperitoneal fibrosis, sclerosing cholangitis, and mediastinal fibrosis, all of which show a similar pathologic picture.

It presents as a very hard goiter fixed to surrounding structures and is usually accompanied by marked obstructive symptoms. The fibrotic process may spread to include local blood vessels, nerves, and the esophagus and trachea. Hypothyroidism, when it occurs, is late in the disease process.

Diagnosis can be made definitively only at open surgical biopsy, at which time a wedge of isthmus should be removed to alleviate current and prevent further constrictive symptoms. More extensive removal of thyroid or fibrous tissue is usually futile and potentially dangerous. High-dose adrenal steroids may be tried during acute progressive phases of the condition but are of little use and dangerous in the long-term management.

Although it probably does not influence the course of the condition, patients should be put on L-thyroxine, 0.15 to 0.2 mg. per day, in anticipation of the development of hypothyroidism.

MALIGNANT CARCINOID SYNDROME

method of
JOHN S. KAUFMANN, M.D.
Winston-Salem, North Carolina

Introduction

The classic malignant carcinoid syndrome was originally described characterizing clinical manifestations observed in patients with carcinoid tumors arising in the ileum with subsequent hepatic metastases. Typical findings in this syndrome included: episodic attacks of flushing and discoloration over the face and upper body; severe diarrhea, often associated with abdominal cramping and watery, mucus-laden stools; the presence of a distinctive endocardial fibrosis, primarily involving the right cardiac chambers; cutaneous telangiectases; and, less commonly, symptoms suggestive of bronchial constriction.

Subsequently, the syndrome and its variants have been associated with a variety of malignant neoplasms. These tumors characteristically produce and release one or more biologically active compounds capable of causing numerous symptoms, which range in severity from simply annoying to virtually disabling. The clinical course of a patient with carcinoid syndrome may extend for many years; therefore, it is essential that an accurate anatomic and biochemical characterization of the tumor be established so that a rational and effective therapeutic program can be initiated. As a guide to the institution of such a therapeutic regimen, Table 1 depicts the differential clinical manifestations of these tumors according to their sites of origin and predominant endocrine function.

TABLE 1. **Features of Carcinoid Syndrome Based on Site of Tumor**

| FEATURES | CLASSIC (USUAL) PATTERN IN TUMORS OF ILEAL ORIGIN | DIFFERENTIAL CHARACTERISTICS | | |
		Gastric	Bronchial	Gonadal
Flush	Variable; red to violaceous; occurs over head and neck; caused by excitement, exertion, ethanol, eating, and epinephrine	Bright red; widespread or "geographic"	Prolonged, severe; facial edema, tears; anaphylactoid reaction	Usual pattern
Cardiac lesions	Endocardial fibrosis; right side of heart; tricuspid and pulmonary valves involved	Rare	Often left-sided	Usual pattern
Diarrhea	Frequent; may show varying degrees of malabsorption	Less severe	Usual pattern	Usual pattern
Tumor secretion	Primarily serotonin and bradykinin formed by released kallikrein; 5-HIAA makes up >90% of urinary indoles	High levels of 5-HTP* and histamine; <90% urinary indoles as 5-HIAA	High 5-HTP*; ACTH and insulin-like substances occasionally	Usual pattern (not well studied)
Metastases	Hepatic; intra-abdominal	Usual pattern	Widespread; skin and bone involvement	Rarely widespread
Miscellaneous		High incidence of peptic ulcer	Association with other endocrine disorders; pluriglandular adenomas	Association with benign teratomas
Prognosis	Fair; 5–10 year survivals not uncommon	Usual pattern	Poor; tumors often rapidly growing	Very good if surgery done

*5-HTP = 5-hydroxytryptophan

Patient Management and Treatment

Surgery. Complete cure by surgical removal of the tumor can be accomplished only rarely, for the more common ileal carcinoid is usually asymptomatic until hepatic metastases have occurred. Occasionally, the less frequent bronchial or gonadal carcinoid may herald its presence prior to metastasis and complete surgical extirpation is possible if diagnosis is made early. Palliative surgery is justified in patients who develop complications such as intestinal obstruction or infarction of large tumor masses with ensuing hemorrhagic necrosis. Consideration for surgical removal of large tumor masses should also be made in instances in which medical control of incapacitating symptoms is unsuccessful. Prosthetic valve replacement of incompetent or stenotic cardiac valves or both can be accomplished in selected patients with gratifying reversal of progressive right-sided cardiac decompensation.

Radiation and Chemotherapy. In general, carcinoid tumors are resistant to radiation therapy; however, such treatment should be considered for isolated lesions that involve critical areas and for painful osseous lesions.

The response of carcinoid tumors to various antitumor chemotherapeutic agents has been disappointing. Partial remissions, reduction in hepatic tumor mass, and short-term amelioration of symptoms have been observed following: chronic, intermittent intra-arterial infusion of 5-fluorouracil (5-FU); treatment with various alkylating agents such as nitrogen mustard, thioTEPA, phenylalanine mustard (melphalan), cyclophosphamide, and BCNU (1, 3-bis(2-chloroethyl)-1-nitrosourea); and miscellaneous agents including methotrexate, streptozotocin, DTIC (dimethyltriazenoimidazole carboxamide), and doxorubicin (Adriamycin).

In general, the use of any of the currently available anticancer drugs should be reserved for patients with rapidly progressive tumor masses and increasing disability not readily controlled by symptomatic therapy. Treatment with these drugs should be undertaken by physicians familiar with such therapeutic agents. Based upon biochemical evaluation of the tumor and the observed response of the patient to drugs used for symptomatic relief (see following section), appropriate premedication should be undertaken prior to the institution of cancer chemotherapy to preclude severe and prolonged exacerbation of symptoms following massive release of humoral substances consequent to drug-induced tumor cell injury and death.

Hemodialysis should be considered in patients who show progressive manifestations of central nervous system (CNS) depression and hepatic or renal failure or both consequent to such tissue damage following intensive radiotherapy or chemotherapy.

Nutrition. The declining nutritional status that occurs in most patients with large tumor masses may be complicated further in carcinoid syndrome by protein or niacin deficiencies or both. Such deficiencies result primarily from the utilization of dietary tryptophan by the tumor in the synthesis of large amounts of serotonin (5-hydroxytryptamine). The excessive urinary excretion of 5-hydroxyindoleacetic acid (5-HIAA), the oxidative metabolite of serotonin, may be used not only as the diagnostic hallmark of carcinoid syndrome but also as a guide in nutritional therapy. Thus, the daily excretion of more than 150 to 200 mg. of 5-HIAA indicates that excessive amounts of tryptophan are being utilized by the tumor and that a relative niacin deficiency can be anticipated. It is advisable, therefore, that supplementary nicotinamide, 50 mg. daily, be given to such patients. In addition, the associated diarrhea and malabsorption found in many carcinoid patients will require supplementary vitamins of all types (especially lipid-soluble vitamins), and these should be combined with a well-balanced, low-residue diet.

Patients should be encouraged to identify and avoid foods and beverages that are found to provoke flushing or to cause exacerbation of diarrhea.

Symptomatic Therapy. The symptomatic therapy of patients with carcinoid syndrome should be undertaken with positive enthusiasm based on rational evaluation of the biochemical abnormalities observed in the individual patient, for patients with this disease may live in excess of 20 years with known metastases. The physician should strive to individualize therapy so as to decrease the frequency and severity of symptoms and thereby enhance the patient's productivity and mobility.

The persistent diarrhea and abdominal cramps that occur in most patients may respond to any of several antiserotonin drugs. Perhaps the most effective, currently available medication of this type is methysergide (Sansert), which usually decreases the severity of these symptoms (dosage range is 4 to 24 mg. per day in divided doses). (This use of methysergide is not listed in the manufacturer's official directive.) However, the long-term use of this drug in a disease noted for capricious fibrotic tendencies should be undertaken with caution in view of the drug's known association with retroperitoneal fibrosis. Careful follow-up to detect this complication of prolonged methysergide therapy should include comparative intravenous pyelography. Another potentially useful agent is cyproheptadine (Periactin). This agent is a potent antihistamine and antiserotonin compound, and 16 to 32 mg. per day in divided doses may diminish the diarrhea in some patients. (This specific use of cyproheptadine is not listed in the manufacturer's official directive.) These patients should be advised of the usual side effects and necessary precautions associated with the use of potent antihistamine compounds. Opiate derivatives, e.g., paregoric, codeine, deodorized tincture of opium, or diphenoxylate plus atropine (Lomotil), are useful therapeutic adjuncts during episodes of increased intestinal motility and diarrhea. Anticholinergic compounds alone have been disappointingly ineffective.

It should be noted that exercise, emotional stress, ethanol ingestion, or the administration of catecholamines and related substances can evoke the flushing attacks. These episodes, which may or may not be associated with arterial hypotension, usually result from the release of bradykinin as well as other vasoactive compounds. The mechanism of bradykinin release is unclear, but available evidence suggests that stimulation of beta adrenergic type receptors may result in the activation of the tumor's kallikrein system. Thus, flushing attacks mediated by bradykinin may be precipitated by epinephrine, norepinephrine, isoproterenol, and other noncatecholamine adrenergic agonists (apparently much more apt to occur during systemic use). Somewhat paradoxically, however, beta-blocking agents (e.g., propranolol) are not useful in the treatment of these attacks, whereas alpha-blocking agents are often effective in terminating repetitive attacks (phentolamine) and decreasing the frequency and severity of these episodes during long-term therapy (phenoxybenzamine). It is probably through the mechanism of alpha adrenergic blockade that chlorpromazine (Thorazine) exerts its beneficial effect in certain patients with severe flushing attacks. The additional sedative effect of chlorpromazine also would be expected to diminish attacks brought about or augmented by emotional disturbances.

Awareness of the catecholamine-induced release of the kinins and the ensuing flushing and hypotension that result cannot be overemphasized. Thus, in a patient with carcinoid, hypotensive episodes, either spontaneous or those which might occur at the time of surgery, should not be treated with "pressor agents" of the catecholamine type. Use of such agents will only intensify the hypotension. Rapid fluid replacement should be used to combat such hypotensive episodes; however, patients unresponsive to such therapy and those with heart failure may require the cautious use of a pressor agent such as angiotensin (Hypertensin) (if still available) or a directly acting, alpha-agonist such as phenylephrine or methoxamine.

The very debilitating flushing episodes commonly associated with foregut tumors (pulmonary and gastric carcinoids) usually respond more readily to chlorpromazine than other medications. Uniquely, the same type of neoplasms often respond to chronic glucocorticoid therapy, in that the frequency and severity of the attacks are diminished by such treatment.

Complications of endocardial fibrosis usually lead to cardiac decompensation. The usual measures of salt restriction and the judicious use of digitalis and diuretic agents should be employed as indicated. Special attention must be given to evaluation of serum potassium levels in such instances, for diuretic therapy during episodes of severe diarrhea may rapidly precipitate digitalis toxicity secondary to hypokalemia.

The oral administration of the experimental drug, p-chlorophenylalanine (PCPA) in doses of 1.5 to 3.0 grams per day, has been associated with 50 per cent reduction in the frequency of diarrhea and a concomitant decrease in the urinary excretion of 5-HIAA. This drug inhibits the excessive production of serotonin by the tumor, but its long term use has been associated with eosinophilia, pulmonary infiltrates and fibrosis, and behavioral disorders.

The medical management of a patient with incurable malignant carcinoid presents a difficult challenge to the medical practitioner. Treatment based on adequate evaluation and sound pharmacologic principles will prove beneficial to the patient and rewarding to the physician.

The Urogenital Tract

BACTERIAL INFECTIONS OF THE URINARY TRACT (MALE)

method of
WARREN W. KOONTZ, JR., M.D.
Richmond, Virginia

Urinary tract infections in the male may present as a simple, annoying disturbance in voiding, with frequency, dysuria, urgency, and/or incontinence. It also may present as life-threatening sepsis. In the pediatric age group, the only sign of infection may be fever, and in this group congenital abnormalities of the urinary tract are frequently the predisposing factor for urosepsis. When a male child presents with urinary tract infection, he deserves urologic investigation, including intravenous urography and voiding cystourethrography. Prompt therapy with a bactericidal antibiotic agent is indicated for the acutely ill child. The dosage must be based on the weight of the patient, and while waiting for cultures to be obtained, a choice of antibiotic medication would be intravenous ampicillin or a cephalosporin. With a severe infection, a second antibiotic such as gentamicin may be desirable. Sensitivity results on the urine culture will provide a guide as to the final decision of antibiotic therapy.

In the adult male, urinary tract infections may also vary in severity but are more likely to be classified into acute or chronic pyelonephritis, acute or chronic cystitis, acute or chronic prostatitis, acute or chronic urethritis, and acute or chronic epididymitis. Adult male patients with urinary tract infection should have significant structural abnormalities excluded by intravenous urography. If the infection is severe or becomes chronic or recurrent, further urologic investigation to include cystourethrography and cystoendoscopy may be indicated.

Treatment

Acute Infection. Patients who present with an acute infection but no urosepsis can be started on an effective oral antimicrobial agent such as nitrofurantoin macrocrystals, 50 to 100 mg. four times per day, ampicillin, 250 mg. orally four times per day, cephalothin, 250 mg. orally four times per day, or trimethoprim 80 mg.--sulfamethoxazole 400 mg., two tablets orally twice daily. Treatment should be given for 10 to 14 days or continued until the urinary tract infection has been eradicated. This can be determined at the 10- to 14-day interval if a urinalysis does not show bacteriuria or pyuria. After the cessation of treatment, repeat studies of the urine should be obtained to rule out the persistence of low colony counts of the same organism; presence of these organisms would indicate failure of therapy. As reinfection of the urinary tract is common, the knowledge that the previous infections had been completely eradicated is of benefit clinically, as the clinician is better informed if he knows that the reinfection is truly a second urinary infection and not a persistent infection with a reoccurrence of symptoms.

Urosepsis. The patient who presents with urosepsis manifested by chills, fever, and systemic symptoms including hypotension must receive prompt and vigorous antibiotic therapy. Prompt urologic investigation is mandatory to exclude significant underlying causes of sepsis such as urinary obstruction secondary to stone, a congenital anomaly or some other cause of obstructive uropathy. An intravenous urogram is required for diagnosis. After obtaining urine for culture, a colony count, and sensitivity studies, the institution of parenteral bactericidal antibiotics is mandatory. These would include ampicillin, 500 mg. to 1 gram, cephalothin, 500 mg. to 1 gram intravenously every 6 to 8 hours, or gentamicin sulfate, 3 to 5 mg. per kg. per day parenterally in three equally divided doses every 8 hours. The dosage of these drugs should be adjusted to the patient's level of renal function. In addition, restriction of activity, analgesia to relieve discomfort, and an increased fluid intake, usually by parenteral means, are also necessary. The clinician should always remember that either the pediatric or adult patient with urosepsis may have developed an abscess that could be present in the epididymis, the prostate, or the kidney area with subsequent persistent systemic symptoms and signs until surgical drainage of the abscess has been carried out. With acute urinary infections and sepsis from prostatitis and urethritis, the clinician may be forced to do a urinary diversion by means of a suprapubic cystostomy to allow the prostate and urethral area to be free of any foreign bodies such as a catheter while the infection subsides. Upper urinary tract obstruction may also require prompt surgical drainage and temporary diversion.

Chronic and Recurring Infections. The major cause of recurrent urinary infections in men is the persistence of gram-negative bacteria in the prostate. Most antibiotics do not diffuse well into prostatic tissue and, as a result, foci of infection are difficult to eradicate from the gland. Sterilization of the patient's urine however may result in longterm suppression of symptoms. The selected antibiotic can usually be given in reduced dosage but for a prolonged period of time. Nitrofurantoin macrocrystals, trimethoprim-sulfamethoxazole, and tetracycline may be used in half dosage once or twice a day. If low dose chronic therapy is administered with one dose of antibiotic per day, the best time for administration may be just before retiring, e.g., 50 mg. of nitrofurantoin macrocrystals at bedtime so that the antibiotic's maximum urinary concentration would be during the time at which the patient is asleep and therefore has low fluid intake, low urinary output, and infrequent voiding. At night with infrequent voiding by the patient, the bacterial count usually gains its highest level. Similar therapy may be administered for the patient with chronic pyelonephritis, urethritis, or epididymitis.

BACTERIAL INFECTIONS OF THE URINARY TRACT (FEMALE)

method of
EDWIN M. MEARES, JR., M.D.
Boston, Massachusetts

Studies have shown that about 15 to 20 per cent of women will experience at least one bout of urinary tract infection (UTI) during their lifetime; likewise, the prevalence of bacteriuria is about 2 per cent in the 15- to 24-year-old group and increases steadily 1 to 2 per cent per decade until it reaches 10 per cent in the 55- to 64-year-old group. On the other hand, the prevalence of bacteriuria in nuns has been found to be strikingly low (0.4 to 1.6 per cent) in the four decades from 15 to 54 years of age, which clearly suggests that sexual intercourse plays a significant role in the pathogenesis of urinary tract infection in women. Although uncomplicated urinary tract infection seldom progresses to chronic renal disease, renal failure, and death, recurrent urinary tract infection often causes considerable morbidity. The greatest morbidity and mortality occur in patients who experience urinary tract infection in association with pregnancy, "infected" renal or ureteral stones, or congenital or acquired structural abnormalities of the genitourinary tract—especially those causing significant obstructive uropathy, high-grade vesicoureteral reflux, or neurogenic bladder dysfunction.

Current evidence indicates that the fecal flora is the reservoir for urinary tract pathogens and that the usual route of infection in women is ascending infection via the urethra by enteric bacteria that first establish significant colonization along the vaginal mucosa at the introitus. Once established upon the vaginal mucosa, these pathogens gain easy access into the short female urethra and then quickly ascend into the urinary bladder, especially as a result of vigorous physical activity, such as sexual intercourse.

Longitudinal studies of careful bacteriologic cultures of the external vagina, urethra, and bladder urine among healthy, normal, sexually active women with no history of urinary tract infection indicate that they seldom have colonization of the vagina or urethra with pathogenic bacteria. Although vaginal and urethral colonization is seen occasionally in these normal women, this usually rapidly disappears spontaneously without therapy and without causing symptoms. Conversely, similar studies in women who are prone to recurrent bacteriuria indicate that they usually carry large numbers of pathogenic bacteria on the vaginal and urethral surfaces for long periods of time in between bouts of overt urinary tract infection, and that the causative agent of the next bout of bacteriuria is totally predictable from knowledge of the vaginal bacteriology.

These observations clearly suggest that women who are otherwise healthy and have normal genitourinary tract anatomy but who experience recurrent bouts of urinary tract infection must be variably deficient in some form of local defense mechanism that normally protects the female urinary tract from invasion by pathogenic enteric bacteria. Two recent important observations give credence to the notion of a local defense mechanism and offer exciting possibilities for future studies. First, a statistically significant difference has been proved between women with recurrent urinary tract infection and normal women in the adherence of pathogenic bacteria to the surface of vaginal epithelial cells. Specifically, pathogenic strains of *Escherichia coli* have been shown to adhere more readily to vaginal epithelial cells from women with recurrent urinary tract infection than to similar cells from control women who are resistant to urinary tract infection. Second, a significant diminution in local cervicovaginal antibody specific against pathogenic bacteria has been found in women with recurrent urinary tract infection as compared to normal control women who are resistant to urinary tract infection. Although the full significance of these studies awaits further investigation, for the first time significant biologic differences between "anatomically normal" women who are prone to develop recurrent urinary tract infection and normal women who are resistant to urinary tract infection have been observed.

A concept fundamental to the proper management of urinary tract infection is a clear understanding that the cure of uncomplicated urinary infection correlates better with the level of antimicrobial agent achieved in the urine during therapy than with its blood level. Indeed, the main indication for the clinician to design antimicrobial therapy that will assure therapeutic "blood" levels against the urinary pathogen is the suspicion of an associated bacteremia, as in the toxic, febrile patient with an acutely infected and significantly obstructed renal unit. Most uncomplicated urinary tract infections clear rapidly during a short course of therapy with an appropriate drug that achieves bactericidal levels in the urine, regardless of the blood level. When functioning normally, the kidney excretes most antibiotics in urinary concentrations that are at least 50 to 100 times greater than their simultaneous concentrations in blood. Indeed, this is the only rational basis for ever using a drug such as nitrofurantoin, which achieves negligible blood levels, but whose high urinary levels are bactericidal against a wide variety of common urinary tract pathogens.

Although by tradition most uncomplicated urinary tract infections are treated empirically for 7 to 10 days (assuming a favorable clinical response), the optimal duration of therapy has never been clearly defined. Recent studies indicate that a 5-day course of appropriate drug therapy is probably just as efficacious in curing uncomplicated urinary tract infection. Indeed, one recent study showed that 36 of 39 women whose urinary infections were localized to the bladder by means of the Fairley "bladder-washout" test were cured with a single intramuscular injection of 500 mg. of kanamycin sulfate.

Acute Urinary Tract Infections

Acute infections uncomplicated by obstructive uropathy or bacteremia are usually managed on an outpatient basis with oral antimicrobial therapy. Urinalysis aids in diagnosis, but an appropriate specimen of urine should also be obtained for diagnostic confirmation and pathogen identification by means of quantitative bacteriologic culture. If the patient is symptomatic, I usually immediately initiate therapy with an antimicrobial agent; if the patient is essentially asymptomatic, I generally await the culture results and begin therapy only as indicated. Depending upon the clinical response to therapy and the results of initial and follow-up cultures, initial therapy is either continued or altered appropriately. An acute infection acquired outside the hospital in a woman who has infrequent urinary infections most often is caused by a strain of *Escherichia coli* that is sensitive to most of the usual antibacterial agents. Conversely, an infection that is hospital-acquired or occurs in a woman who takes antibiotics frequently for recurrent urinary infections most often is due to a relatively resistant pathogen. For initial therapy, especially in the former type, I generally prefer to use one of the following drugs:

1. *Nitrofurantoin,* 100 mg. orally four times daily. Because of its negligible blood levels but high urinary levels that are highly bactericidal against many common urinary pathogens, nitrofurantoin is indicated only for treatment of uncomplicated urinary tract infections. Another advantage is that this drug is so completely absorbed from the upper gastrointestinal tract that it rarely causes resistant bacteria to emerge in the fecal flora, despite repeated or prolonged usage. I prefer to use nitrofurantoin macrocrystals (Macrodantin) because this form of the drug minimizes gastrointestinal side effects. If other forms of nitrofurantoin are used, the patient must take the medicine with food or milk in order to prevent nausea.

2. *Penicillin G,* 500 mg. (800,000 units) orally four times daily, 1 hour before eating; or *ampicillin,* 250 mg. orally four times daily. Penicillin G is an inexpensive drug, which, when taken as advised, generally achieves high urinary levels that are bactericidal against most strains of *Escherichia coli, Proteus mirabilis,* and enterococcus, and as these bacteria are common urinary pathogens, this drug can be a highly effective agent in the management of uncomplicated urinary infection. The main advantage of the more expensive ampicillin over penicillin G is that its urinary levels become so high that complete absorption from the gastrointestinal tract is a less critical factor. Penicillin G must be taken on an empty stomach to assure complete absorption and resultant full therapeutic urinary levels.

3. A *sulfonamide.* Sulfonamides remain excellent agents for the short-term therapy of uncomplicated urinary tract infection. Although several different types of sulfonamides of about equal effectiveness are currently available, my preference is sulfamethoxazole (Gantanol), 1.0 gram orally twice daily, because patient compliance is generally better when medication must be taken only twice daily instead of four times daily. Sulfisoxazole (Gantrisin), 1.0 gram orally four times daily, and sulfamethizole (Thiosulfil Forte), 500 mg. four times daily, are probably equally

effective. Repeated or prolonged administration of any sulfonamide will likely result in emergence of resistant bacteria in the fecal flora, a distinct disadvantage regarding reinfection.

Other oral antimicrobial agents that are effective in patients with uncomplicated urinary tract infection include nalidixic acid (NegGram), 1.0 gram four times daily; trimethoprim-sulfamethoxazole (Bactrim or Septra), 2 tablets twice daily (or 1 double-strength tablet twice daily), oxytetracycline or tetracycline, 250 to 500 mg. four times daily; amoxicillin (Larotid), 250 mg. every 8 hours; cephalexin (Keflex), 250 to 500 mg. four times daily; and various other cephalosporins. Although these drugs are highly effective, their expense makes them more appealing agents for specific therapy (based on sensitivity testing), rather than for initial therapy prior to sensitivity testing.

Antimicrobial Sensitivity Testing

My preference is always to obtain an appropriate urine specimen for culture to confirm the diagnosis of urinary tract infection and to identify the specific pathogen responsible. I do not, however, advocate the routine ordering of sensitivity testing of the pathogen in all patients. As the isolated bout of non-nosocomial infection that occurs in the woman who infrequently experiences urinary infection most often is due to a pansensitive *Escherichia coli*, routine sensitivity testing in such patients usually is an unnecessary expense. Susceptibility testing becomes more important in the management, however, of patients with nosocomial urinary tract infection or in women who suffer from recurrent bouts of urinary tract infection, since relatively more resistant pathogens are often encountered. More importantly, the proper use of sensitivity testing in management of urinary tract infection demands that the clinician have a thorough understanding of the testing method used by the laboratory and of the possible limitations of this method. The important concept that the cure of uncomplicated urinary tract infection depends upon the urinary (not serum) concentration of the antimicrobial agents has already been emphasized. If the laboratory performs susceptibility testing that actually measures the minimum inhibitory concentrations (MICs) of the various agents against the pathogen and the sensitivity results are, in turn, reported on the basis of urinary concentrations of the agents, then the clinician can use these results with confidence in choosing his therapy. Unfortunately, many laboratories continue to perform sensitivity testing for urinary pathogens by the Kirby-Bauer disc method, in which the disc content of most of the drugs give inhibition zones that correlate with blood levels, not urinary levels. With this method, for example, 100 per cent of strains of *E. coli* will always be reported as being resistant to penicillin G, whereas the urinary levels of standard oral therapy with this drug are bactericidal against 80 to 85 per cent of all strains of *E. coli* that are known urinary pathogens. Hopefully, someday all laboratories will exclusively use methodologies that allow reporting of susceptibility testing in terms of minimum inhibitory concentrations. Until then, the clinician must understand the method used by his laboratory and its relevance to urinary antimicrobial levels.

Post-treatment Follow-up

Assuming that the clinical response is favorable, I prefer to treat uncomplicated urinary tract infection in women with an appropriate antibacterial agent for a total of only 5 to 7 days. The patient then returns for a post-therapy culture 1 to 2 weeks after medication is stopped to assure that the urinary tract is sterile. Failure to respond favorably to therapy both by prompt relief of symptoms and by sterilization of the urine, or a rapid recurrence of either warrants thorough investigation. If the patient had the usual type of urinary pathogen, responded quickly and favorably to therapy, and had normal physical findings and no history suggestive of serious underlying genitourinary tract disease other than a rare, isolated bout of "cystitis," I do not proceed with additional urologic work-up, unless subsequently she develops a tendency to more frequent bouts of recurrent urinary tract infection.

The patient who has infection with an organism that splits urea, especially any species of *Proteus,* warrants careful therapy and follow-up plus at least a plain film x-ray of the abdomen, as these organisms have great propensity to form "infected" struvite or apatite urinary stones.

Recurrent Urinary Tract Infections

Although studies indicate that about 90 per cent of uncomplicated recurrent urinary tract infections in women are "new" infections due to different strains of pathogens and not relapses or persistent infections, I believe that women who experience recurrent infections deserve at least one thorough urologic evaluation to rule out underlying genitourinary tract abnormalities. My evaluation basically consists of determination of the serum creatinine and a chemical screening battery, an excretory urogram, a voiding cystourethrogram, and diagnostic cystourethroscopy with a careful pelvic examination. The patient with recurrent infection due to a urea-splitting organism may also require plain film tomograms of the kidneys to rule out "infected" calculi that cannot be visualized by other means. These studies may or may not indicate the need for additional investigations.

Once an underlying structural or functional cause for the infections has been ruled out, one must assume that the woman is experiencing reinfections via the ascending route from the perineum. In my opinion, the woman who experiences four or more bouts of urinary tract infection per year is a definite candidate for preventive therapy.

Preventive Therapy for Recurrent Urinary Tract Infection

As has been emphasized, about 90 per cent of recurrent urinary tract infections in women are not relapses of persistent infections, but are "new" infections characteristically caused by ascending invasion of the bladder via the urethra by pathogens that have initially established colonization on the vaginal mucosa at the introitus. There is no convincing evidence that periodic urethral dilatation with sounds, the use of showers instead of tub baths, the use of vaginal douching, or other such activities play any significant role in prevention of recurrent urinary infections in women.

Although several studies have shown that "postintercourse" therapy (the woman voids immediately after coitus and takes a single tablet or capsule of an appropriate antibacterial agent) can effectively reduce the incidence of recurrent infections in women, I generally avoid this form of preventive therapy. My main objection is directly linking the antibacterial dosage to the act of sexual intercourse, which surely is not always the cause of the infection. Furthermore, the frequency of sexual activity is highly variable, so that wide fluctuations may occur in dosage schedules (from forgotten pills, to 4 times daily, to 1 per month)—which hardly is a desirable manner in which to administer antibacterial therapy.

In my opinion, the most ideal current preventive therapy against recurrent urinary tract infection in women is for the women to take a single tablet of regular (*not* double-strength) trimethoprim-sulfamethoxazole (Septra or Bactrim) each night at bedtime. During such therapy breakthrough infections are extremely rare; indeed, the high levels of trimethoprim achieved with this dosage in vaginal fluid (several-fold the blood levels) usually sterilize the vagina of bacterial pathogens without affecting the normal vaginal flora, which likely explains why secondary yeast vaginitis rarely occurs as a complication. Furthermore, such therapy seldom has adverse effects upon the fecal flora, and resistant bacterial mutants rarely emerge.

My second choice for preventive therapy is nitrofurantoin macrocrystals (Macrodantin), 100 mg. orally each night at bedtime. Although this drug has no activity on the vaginal flora, its broad spectrum against the common urinary pathogens and its usually insignificant alterations of the fecal flora make it an ideal alternative for preventive therapy.

If the response is favorable, I usually continue preventive therapy for at least a total of 6 months. Cultures should be obtained occasionally during this time to assure that the urine actually is sterile. At the end of 6 months of successful preventive therapy, I prefer to stop all antibacterial therapy and observe what happens. Many patients will remain asymptomatic with sterile urine for several months before experiencing a recurrence of urinary tract infection. Some patients disappointingly rather quickly develop a recurrent infection. Whenever a patient clearly resumes her former pattern of frequent recurrent urinary infection, I recommend resuming another 6 months of preventive therapy, once the urine has been sterilized with full therapy.

Urinary Tract Infection in Pregnancy

The potential consequences of urinary tract infection occurring during pregnancy are significantly more serious than those in nonpregnant women. Studies have shown that the development of acute pyelonephritis from uncomplicated urinary tract infection is uncommon in nonpregnant women; however, about 30 per cent of pregnant women with untreated bacteriuria will develop acute pyelonephritis in association with that pregnancy. This risk can be markedly reduced if the bacteriuria is properly treated and cleared when first diagnosed. For this reason urine cultures should be carefully monitored routinely throughout the course of the pregnancy, especially if the patient has any past history of urinary infection. Any overt infection, whether or not it is symptomatic, should be quickly eradicated with a short course of appropriate medication. If follow-up cultures indicate a tendency for recurrent infection, I prefer to sterilize the urine and then institute continuous preventive therapy with nitrofurantoin macrocrystals (Macrodantin), 100 mg. daily, throughout the remainder of the pregnancy and for 1 month following delivery. Because of their potentially harmful effects upon the fetus, antimicrobial agents must be carefully selected by the clinician for use in a pregnant woman. The safest antibacterial agents for short-term use during pregnancy, especially during the first trimester, are penicillin G, ampicillin, nitrofurantoin, and the short-acting sulfonamides, such as sulfisoxazole (Gantrisin) or sulfamethizole (Thiosulfil). The tetracyclines, nalidixic acid, and trimethoprim-sulfamethoxazole should definitely be avoided.

Urinary Tract Infection in Renal Failure

Alteration in selection of antimicrobial agents and dosage schedules is usually necessary in therapy of patients who are azotemic. In general, the more severe the level of azotemia, the greater the alterations must be in antibacterial therapy. Significantly impaired renal function not only leads to poor urinary concentration of most antimicrobial agents and ineffective antibacterial activity, but also leads to high blood levels that may rapidly reach toxic proportions.

BACTERIAL INFECTIONS OF THE URINARY TRACT (FEMALE CHILDREN)

method of
R. DIXON WALKER, M.D.
Gainesville, Florida

Bacteriuria in the female child is common, whether asymptomatic or symptomatic. In the newborn, bacteriuria is more common in the male, but by age 3 months this changes, and bacteriuria becomes 20 times more common in the female. The prevalence of bacteriuria in preschool age children is 1 per cent and in school age children 2 per cent. By age 12, 4.6 per cent of female children will have exhibited bacteriuria at one time.

Bacteriuria may be classified as follows: symptomatic or asymptomatic, chronic or acute, complicated or uncomplicated. The latter is the most clinically useful classification. Uncomplicated bacteriuria is that associated with no structural or functional abnormalities. These children are at little risk of developing chronic pyelonephritis. Complicated bacteriuria is that associated with structural or functional abnormalities (e.g., hydronephrosis, reflux, neurogenic bladder), and it is these children who are at risk of developing chronic pyelonephritis. Therefore, it is most important to differentiate this latter group, and the purpose of the radiologic evaluation is to do that.

Bacteriuria presents in myriad ways. A significant number of female children have asymptomatic bacteriuria that will be discovered only by routine urinalysis and culture. Many children who present with symptoms in other organ systems or with nonspecific symptoms are found to have bacteriuria on evaluation. Such conditions may include vague abdominal pain, nausea, vomiting, lethargy, failure to thrive, or unexplained fever. Finally, some children will present with specific symptoms related to the upper or lower urinary tract. Children with uncomplicated urinary tract infec-

tion most often complain of urgency, frequency, incontinence, dysuria, or perineal irritation, all symptoms representative of cystitis or lower urinary tract infection. Children with complicated bacteriuria are more likely to have chills, fever, flank pain, nausea, and vomiting, all symptoms associated with pyelonephritis or upper urinary tract infection.

Evaluation of bacteriuria begins with proper collection of the urine specimen. In older children urine can be collected by the midstream, clean-catch method. In newborns and infants urine can be collected with an adhesive bag after careful cleansing of the genitalia. Urine obtained in this way is most significant if it is negative; positive urine cultures may represent contamination. In newborns or infants bacteriuria should be confirmed with a suprapubic needle aspiration of the bladder or by catheterization with a #5 infant feeding tube. In older children three consecutive early morning positive clean-catch urine specimens will correlate well, or positive evidence of bacteriuria can be confirmed with urethral catheterization with a #5 infant feeding tube. Once obtained, the urine should be examined microscopically and always cultured. Additional helpful information may be obtained by Gram staining the spun sediment.

Further evaluation consists of doing studies to tell whether a child has complicated bacteriuria. The intravenous pyelogram (IVP) and voiding cystourethrogram (VCU) should be done after the bacteriuria is eliminated. If the bacteriuria is eliminated easily, I do these studies 6 weeks after a negative urine culture. If the bacteriuria is difficult to eradicate, then the IVP is indicated immediately as the patient may have a severe complicating problem. All children deserve radiologic evaluation after the first documented urinary tract infection. Further evaluations, including cystoscopy and cystometrogram, should be reserved for children with specific indications.

Treatment

Treatment of urinary tract infection should be directed at eradication of the bacteria. It is, therefore, vital that infection be documented by culture and treatment based on appropriate sensitivities. The length of time initial or recurrent infections are treated is controversial with a recommended range of 2 to 14 days. I prefer to treat for at least 10 days. It is important that once treatment is initiated a follow-up urine culture and urinalysis in 1 to 2 weeks be obtained to make sure that the urine is sterile.

In treating initial urinary tract infections I first try to assess whether or not I can wait the 2 days until the culture report is back or need to proceed with treatment. If a child is asymptomatic, then one can wait and treat the patient with the appropriate drug. Most often the bacteriuria will respond to 10 days' treatment with one of the following: nitrofurantoin, 5 to 7 mg. per kg. per 24 hours divided into four doses; sulfisoxazole, 150 mg. per kg. per 24 hours divided into four doses; trimethoprim, 8 mg. per kg. and sulfamethoxazole,

40 mg. per 24 hours divided into two doses. If the patient, when seen in the office, has sufficient lower tract symptoms and I do not want to wait for the initial culture, then I treat with one of the above, changing in 2 days if the culture so indicates. If the patient, when first seen, has a mild fever and minimal symptomatic signs, then I initiate treatment with an antibiotic (usually ampicillin or cephalexin), rather than an antibacterial. Patients with marked fever, chills, systemic symptoms, and costovertebral angle tenderness almost always have pyelonephritis and may well be septic. This latter group will have a high incidence of complicated problems when radiologically investigated. Serious consideration needs to be given to hospital admission and parenteral antibiotic therapy with kanamycin, gentamicin, tobramycin, or carbenicillin, changing therapy after culture results are known. The initial infection then is treated differently, depending on whether the child is symptomatic or asymptomatic and the degree of symptomatology. The goal is to eradicate the bacteriuria with the most inexpensive, best-tolerated drug available. The remainder of the treatment will be based on whether the patient has a complicated or uncomplicated urinary tract infection.

Those patients who have a normal intravenous pyelogram and voiding cystourethrogram will primarily have uncomplicated bacteriuria and recurrent cystitis. After initial treatment of the urinary tract infection, I follow the urine culture at 2 month intervals for the first year and at 4-month intervals for the second year. Any breakthrough infections are treated as the initial infection was. If the patient has 3 breakthrough infections within 6 months, then I continue prophylactic long-term treatment. The most common drug I use for this is nitrofurantoin in a dose of approximately one half the therapeutic dosage: 3 to 5 mg. per kg. per 24 hours in two divided doses per day. Occasionally, the patient's urine can be kept sterile with as little as a single dose of nitrofurantoin daily. I commit these patients to a minimum of 6 months' prophylactic therapy and at the end of 6 months stop all medication. If the urine stays sterile, then the patients are followed as above, but if 3 infections recur within another 6 months, the patients are recommitted to prophylactic medication. Patients can tolerate long-term prophylactic medication for years with very little side effects. Sulfisoxazole and trimethoprim-sulfamethoxazole at one half the therapeutic dosages can also be used for prophylaxis.

Symptomatic treatment of cystitis, particularly the symptoms of dysuria and frequency, may be improved by sitz baths or by alkalinizing the urine with a level teaspoon of sodium bicarbonate taken 3 to 4 times a day.

Patients with complicated bacteriuria first need to have attention turned to the structural abnormality. If the structural problem can be completely corrected, the patients can be changed from a complicated to an uncomplicated urinary tract infection and managed in that fashion. Most often the structural abnormality cannot be completely reversed (e.g., hydronephrotic kidney), is managed medically until it reverses spontaneously (e.g., mild vesicoureteral reflux), or is an ongoing problem that will never be reversed (e.g., neurogenic bladder). In these instances the patients are at risk from developing chronic pyelonephritis. The patients may require prophylaxis with nitrofurantoin, sulfisoxazole, or trimethoprim-sulfamethoxazole to keep the urine sterile. In this group it is vital that the urine be kept sterile or the patients quite likely will develop acute pyelonephritis and may require hospitalization with intravenous fluid therapy and parenteral antibiotics. Drainage of the urinary tract by surgical procedures, catheters, or prosthetic devices may be required. In all patients with complicated urinary tract infection the urine needs to be cultured at 2 month intervals for as long as the problem exists. With close surveillance and vigorous management of infection, chronic pyelonephritis can be prevented.

CHILDHOOD ENURESIS

method of
BETTI JO WARREN, M.D.
Los Angeles, California

Definition

Enuresis is a syndrome of repeated involuntary micturition in otherwise normal children after the age of about 5 years. The frequency of the bedwetting is at least once or more a week. Between ages 2 and 5 years the incidence of bedwetting is approximately 40 per cent, but by age 5 years only 10 per cent are still enuretic. The frequency of this syndrome in older children has been variously reported to range from 13 per cent in 6- to 7-year-olds to 3 per cent in 13- to 14-year-olds. Approximately 60 per cent of children who wet the bed have always done so and are called "primary enuretics." Those who have a dry period between their pretrained wetness and recurrence of wetness are called "secondary" enuretics and comprise the remaining 40 per cent. Within the total population of enuretic children, the proportion of secondary enuretics generally increases with age, with 57 per cent of enuretics reported to be relapsers by age 12. Boys are much more likely to be enuretic than girls.

Contributing Factors

A review of the several hypotheses will serve as an approach to management of this symptom complex. The voluntary initiation or inhibition of bladder contractions requires a certain maturation level of bladder function usually attained in children between 2 and 4 years of age, although the variation among normal children is wide. Some infants under 1 year of age can have consistently dry nights. Prior to attainment of this developmental milestone, a small bladder capacity volume results in higher nocturnal frequency. Cystometrograms of primary enuretics are similar to those of infants in this regard. Those with primary enuresis tend to have smaller functional bladder volumes than those who have the secondary variety. The largest functional volumes are in children who are not enuretic.

Electroencephalographic correlation studies indicate that enuresis does not occur during dreaming, but rather during the predream non–rapid eye movement (nonREM) stage of sleep. During this stage, which occurs just after the deepest sleep, the EEG shows the arousal pattern. This arousal stage, which is associated with mental confusion, autonomic behavior, relative nonreactivity to external stimuli, poor response to efforts evoking wakefulness, and retrograde amnesia, lasts longer in enuretic than nonenuretic children.

Family history is often of diagnostic significance. Monozygotic twins are concordant for enuresis twice as often as dizygotic twins. In 70 per cent of families with an enuretic child, the symptoms occur in more than one member, and in 40 per cent at least one parent is found to have had nocturnal enuresis. Psychologic functioning relates to enuresis at three levels. It may be only one aspect among many of disturbed behavior, or it may be an isolated symptom of emotional disturbance in a child whose behavior is otherwise normal. More commonly, emotional stress is caused by enuresis.

Urologic problems are more likely to be identified in those who wet the bed more than once per week and in those who had never been dry for a sustained period of one month. In one series of adolescents, 75 per cent of those with the high frequency and 83 per cent of those with the more severe symptoms had numerous urologic findings, ranging from chronic infection to urethral strictures or horseshoe kidneys.

Management

Just as this syndrome has an effect on all members of the family constellation, so must the approach to therapy involve all of them. The majority of enuretics have the primary variety, which carries a good prognosis for cure; however, simple reassurance of the anxious parents or of the embarrassed patient does not make it better. The primary care provider is perhaps in the best position for an impartial evaluation and should consider each patient and family individually, in light of the many possible contributing factors. An approach involving both education and active participation by patient and family provides the best opportunity for cure. This parental support ensures a safe and secure environment in which to solve a very threatening problem for the child.

Before deciding on a particular course of therapy, a complete history and physical examination should be done to determine the likelihood of structural abnormality of the urinary tract. The history should be explicit about diurnal enuresis, urine dribbling, involuntary wetness, difficulty initiating a urine stream, secondary vs. primary type onset. and frequency. Knowledge of prior family history of enuresis, adjustment problems of patient and family, other developmental disorders, and sleeping patterns will be important. Physical examination should include assessment of the child's growth and development. If possible, it should also include observation of the urine stream for deviation, caliber, and strength.

Baseline laboratory studies should include routine urinalysis, testing for sugar, specific gravity, protein, and a microscopic examination. Multiple, repeated negative bacterial cultures are more reliable for a diagnosis of a non-infection process than one negative urine culture. Functional bladder capacity should be ascertained by measuring volume following prolonged refraining from voiding. Intravenous pyelogram is indicated in all secondary enuretics and in selective primary enuretics. An electroencephalogram may be helpful when the medical history or physical examination suggests a specific seizure disorder.

It is appropriate to consider children age 4 years and younger as still being in the normal bladder control development stages and parents should simply be properly educated and reassured. Vigorous treatment at this point might have more serious later implications. This allows for separation of enuretics of 5 years and older into basically two categories:

Silent Urologic Disease.   Concern for organic lesions should be entertained in evaluation of the adolescent enuretic and in the child with recurrent enuresis. Enuresis associated with poor urinary stream abnormal physical findings, or diurnal incontinence in adolescents, should be investigated for underlying organic disease. Urologic work-up should include an intravenous urogram with voiding cystourethrogram, and cystoscopy if these studies are abnormal. Other specific tests, including urethral flow and intravesical pressure, are sometimes required in the evaluation of the more chronic secondary enuretic.

Developmental Delay.   A supportive but systematic approach geared to the individual patient should begin with reassurance about the absence of anatomic abnormality, along with explanation of the frequency of the disorder in the general population, and good prognosis for spontaneous improvement. Suggestions for symptom alleviation should be directed toward active participation of both patient and parent, and should be age-appropriate. Suggesting that 5- or 6-year-olds be totally responsible for their symptoms and its inconvenience is inappropriate. The regimen should be practical, reasonable and within the scope of resources of the family.

Bladder training is aimed at gradually increasing bladder functional capacity by forcing fluids both day and night and includes daily recording of voided volumes, fluid intake, and gradual extension of intervals between voiding. Preference for this mode of therapy is based on the documentation of decreased functional bladder capacity. The disadvantages are related to the discomfort of the patient.

Conditioning devices are electrolytically triggered alarms that evoke two responses: awakening of patient and inhibition of micturition. Eventually the child will awaken prior to voiding. The relapse rate may be as high as 79 per cent; however, after relapse, dryness is attained more quickly and permanently with a second course of conditioning. Complications include a perineum or buttock rash thought to be due to electrolysis of sodium chloride in the urine with production of sodium hydroxide at the cathode.

Various *pharmacologic agents* with anticholinergic or sympathomimetic properties have been used; imipramine is currently the most popular. The mechanism of action is either a direct anticholinergic effect on the bladder detrusor muscle or a stimulating effect on the central nervous system, which may relate to a change in the sleep pattern. The imipramine is generally given one half hour before bedtime, and there is no need for multiple daily doses. The initial dose is 25 mg. in children under 12 years, and 50 mg. for children 12 years and older (see manufacturer's official directive before use in children). In some instances dosage may be increased to 75 mg. in children over 12 years. In general, 40 per cent of patients respond with significant improvement. Relapses represent a significant problem with rates of 40 to 60 per cent reported. Gradual discontinuation of the drug is less likely to lead to relapse than abrupt cessation. Tapering to once every other night and then every third night over a period of 4 to 6 weeks is suggested.

Adverse effects of imipramine are nervousness, sleep disorder, and mild gastrointestinal disturbances. A more serious consequence results from overdosage in the patient and the poisoning of a younger sibling. Coma, convulsions, and cardiac disturbance are the sequelae, with death occurring from severe central nervous system depression. There is a very small margin between the therapeutic and toxic doses, and death has been reported with a dose as low as 32 mg. per kg. This mode of therapy should be reserved for those *more chronic* enuretics, comprising only about 3 per cent of the secondary form.

Counseling. All patients and their families will require brief counseling, but only a few will need in-depth psychotherapy. This counseling should be an adjunct to any of the above regimens and is within the capability of the primary care provider.

Goals of counseling are:

1. Parental understanding of multiple contributing factors.

2. Parental acceptance of the child and symptoms to provide maximal emotional support.

3. Instilling optimism in child and family.

4. Acceptance of child and problem as an "individual difference" similar to other illnesses or handicaps.

5. Child's acceptance that he or she is responsible for and can control enuresis.

6. Enhancement of child's social maturity where indicated.

Responsibility plus reinforcement is based on active participation of the child, who keeps a record of successes and who is also able to determine those factors that contribute to bedwetting. He or she receives reinforcement for successes but also learns to be responsible for his or her actions.

EPIDIDYMITIS

method of
MARK S. SOLOWAY, M.D.
Memphis, Tennessee

Acute epididymitis is a common inflammatory process arising usually in the globus minor and progressing to involve the entire epididymis. The overlying fascia is often involved and the scrotal skin may become warm and erythematous. The onset may be sudden or gradual. Concomitant cystitis, urethritis, or prostatitis accounts for the frequently accompanying symptoms of urinary frequency, dysuria, hematuria, urethral discharge, and back pain. An examination early in the disease process may detect an edematous, tender epididymis located posterior and lateral to the testis. With increasing swelling, the delineation between the two structures is lost.

There are numerous causative agents. Gonococcal urethritis was previously the most common organism, but now a number of gram-negative bacteria are more common. Nonspecific urethritis due to Chlamydia or Mycoplasma may antecede the epididymal infection.

Torsion of the spermatic cord must be differentiated from acute epididymitis. This can usually be done by the history of sudden onset, and the lack of fever, pyuria, and bacteriuria. The examination in torsion discloses the altered position of the epididymis in relation to the testis. Elevation of the testicle in epididymitis characteristically reduces the pain; it is unaltered in torsion (Prehn's sign). A Doppler will usually indicate a lack of blood flow to the testis in torsion (normal or elevated in epididymitis). The Tc^{99m} scan has also been utilized to document this discrepancy.

Treatment

1. Bed rest, until symptoms allow ambulation.

2. Scrotal support.

3. Analgesia. Injection of lidocaine hydrochloride into the spermatic cord may be utilized in addition to oral or parenteral medications, e.g., codeine. Ice applied to the scrotum may provide symptomatic relief for the first 12 to 24 hours.

4. Antibiotics. Systemic or oral drugs are indicated if an infectious cause is suspected. Prior to initiation of the drug, blood and urine cultures should be obtained. Broad-spectrum drugs with gram-negative coverage are preferred. A cephalosporin, e.g., cephalexin (Keflex), 500 mg. four times daily; tetracycline, 500 mg. four times daily; or an aminoglycoside, gentamicin (Garamycin), is used depending upon the severity and whether or not nonspecific urethritis (NSU) is suspected.

5. Hydration. Marked fever with dehydration requires parenteral fluids. This is usually important in elderly patients with an indwelling urethral catheter.

6. Anti-inflammatory agents. Oxyphenbutazone or indomethacin have been suggested by some, but their potential side effects (myelosuppression) probably outweigh potential benefits.

7. Surgery. Occasionally the patient will not respond to the above measures and progress to abscess formation or develop a protracted course. Epididymectomy or epididymo-orchiectomy should be considered in these patients. The age of the patient and number of prior episodes are important considerations.

Although the severe pain usually abates within a few days, the edema and induration resolves over several weeks. Careful monitoring of this gradual process is necessary to ensure the absence of a neoplastic process.

BALANITIS AND BALANOPOSTHITIS

method of
ROBERT ROSS, JR., M.D.
Venice, Florida

Definition

Balanitis is an inflammation of the glans penis, posthitis is an inflammation of the foreskin, and balanoposthitis is a combined inflammation of both (this is the usual clinical presentation).

Causes

Phimosis, neoplasms, poor hygiene, increased amount of coagulated secretions (smegma), bacteria, fungus, yeast, and glucosuria secondary to uncontrolled diabetes mellitus are all possible causes.

Management

1. Meticulous hygiene. This consists of two or three times daily foreskin retraction, cleansing with a mild soap and water solution and drying.

2. Topical antibacterials or antimycotic agents, e.g., polymyxin B, neomycin, gramicidin (Neosporin), nystatin (Mycostatin), or other similar preparations.

3. Correction of glucosuria.

4. Specific antibacterials according to culture and sensitivity results in extremely resistant types.

If these methods of treatment are unsuccessful, circumcision is indicated. If possible, it should be carried out after the acute episode has subsided.

GLOMERULAR DISORDERS

method of
GERALD F. DIBONA, M.D.
Iowa City, Iowa

Disorders of glomerular structure and function are one of the major problems encountered in patients with diseases of the kidney. The major clinical manifestations of the glomerular disorders (glomerulopathies) may be grouped according to common patterns of clinical presentations or syndromes. These may occur as primary or idiopathic glomerulopathies in the absence of multisystem organ involvement, specific causative events, or known heredofamilial disorders, or as distinct clinicopathologic entities as a result of known causative processes or part of a multisystem disease. The major clinical syndromes are:

Acute Nephritic Syndrome. Abrupt onset, hematuria, proteinuria, reduced glomerular filtration rate, sodium and water retention, circulatory congestion, hypertension and oliguria; tendency for spontaneous recovery and frequent association with antecedent infection.

Rapidly Progressive Glomerulonephritis. Insidious onset, relentless and progressive loss of renal function with oliguria; spontaneous recovery and antecedent infection unusual.

Chronic Nephritic Syndrome. Insidious onset, protracted course of progressive renal functional impairment with variable amounts of hematuria, proteinuria, and hypertension.

Asymptomatic Hematuria and/or Proteinuria. Mild to moderate amounts of hematuria or proteinuria or both without hypertension, impaired renal function, or edema.

Nephrotic Syndrome. Edema resulting from hypoproteinemia (hypoalbuminemia), which in turn is due to proteinuria, variable tendency for hyperlipidemia, and lipiduria.

The major renal functional and systemic abnormalities which may accompany the glomerular disorders are:

1. Reduction in glomerular filtration rate, which results in a fall in creatinine clearance and a rise in blood urea nitrogen and serum creatinine.

2. Sodium and water retention, which result in circulatory congestion and edema formation.

3. Hypertension, which results in deleterious effects in other organ vascular beds (brain, eye, heart) as well as kidney.

4. Hematuria and proteinuria, which result in hypoproteinemia (hypoalbuminemia) and contributes to sodium and water retention, circulatory congestion and edema formation.

To aid in the assessment of the severity of the patient's illness, in the determination of the need for a specific therapy and in the evaluation of therapeutic effectiveness, a set of uniform criteria for the evaluation of the severity of established renal disease is desirable. Such a set of criteria has been developed by the Council on the Kidney in Cardiovascular Disease of the American Heart Association (Table 1). These criteria provide for classification of severity of signs and symptoms, of renal functional impairment and of performance. They are useful for following the progress of the patient's illness and serve as indicators of potential need for specific therapy as well as effectiveness of therapy.

TABLE 1. **Criteria for the Evaluation of the Severity of Established Renal Disease**

I. Classification of Signs and Symptoms by Severity

Class 1: Requires (a) plus one or more of (b) through (f):
a. No symptoms directly referable to renal disease
b. Fixed proteinuria (>200 mg./24 hours)
c. Repeatedly abnormal urine sediment or bacteriuria
d. Demonstrable radiographic abnormality of the upper urinary tract
e. Hypertension attributable to past or active renal disease
f. Biopsy-proven parenchymal renal disease

Class 2: Any two or more of the following:
a. Symptomatic because of symptoms directly referable to the kidney (e.g., hypoproteinemic edema, dysuria, flank pain, renal colic, nocturia)
b. Radiographic evidence of osteodystrophy
c. Stable anemia attributable to renal disease
d. Metabolic acidosis attributable to renal disease
e. Severe hypertension (diastolic BP>110 mm. Hg)

Class 3: Any two or more of the following:
a. Symptomatic osteodystrophy
b. Symptomatic peripheral neuropathy
c. Nausea and vomiting without primary gastrointestinal cause
d. Limited ability to conserve or excrete usual dietary load of sodium and water; tending to sodium depletion, dehydration, or congestive heart failure
e. Impaired mentation attributable to renal disease

Class 4: Any two or more of the following:
a. Uremic pericarditis
b. Uremic bleeding diathesis
c. Asterixis and severely impaired mentation, with or without convulsion
d. Hypocalcemic tetany

Class 5:
a. Coma

II. Classification of Renal Functional Impairment

Class A: GFR normal	Serum creatinine normal
Class B: GFR 50–80% of predicted normal	Serum creatinine normal to 2.4 mg./dl. (100 ml.)
Class C: GFR 20–50% of predicted normal	Serum creatinine 2.5–4.9 mg./dl.
Class D: GFR 10–20% of predicted normal	Serum creatinine 5.0–7.9 mg./dl.
Class E: GFR 5–10% of predicted normal	Serum creatinine 8–12 mg./dl.
Class F: GFR <5% of predicted normal	Serum creatinine >12 mg./dl.

III. Performance Classification

Class 1: Capable of performing all his usual types of physical activity

Class 2: Unable to perform the most strenuous of usual types of physical activity for that particular patient, e.g., sports activity, fast walking, running, shoveling, lawn mowing

Class 3: Unable to perform all his usual daily physical activities on more than a part-time basis, e.g., household duties, employment, driving an automobile, playing with children

Class 4: Severe limitation of usual physical activity. May need assistance for some facets of self-care, e.g., shaving. Mentation may or may not be impaired. May be confined to bed.

Class 5: Semicoma or coma

General Treatment Measures

Bed Rest. The use of strict bed rest is dependent on the severity of the signs and symptoms and should be instituted when cardiovascular complications exist. Otherwise, physical activity may be permitted as tolerated. There is no evidence that restriction of normally tolerated physical activity influences the subsequent clinical course of these diseases.

Diet. Initially, oral intake should be restricted to 1000 ml. of relatively sodium- and potassium-free liquids containing sufficient carbohydrate calories (400 or more) to prevent ketosis and minimize endogenous protein catabolism. This program permits evaluation of the degree of renal functional impairment and the clinical status while appropriate measurements (electrolytes, acid-base status, blood urea nitrogen or serum creatinine or both) are made. This approach is of particular importance when the disease is acute, symptomatic, and associated with decreased renal function. In patients with the least severe disease, a general diet with free access to liquids and modest dietary sodium restriction (4.0 grams of sodium chloride, 68 mEq. of sodium) is appropriate. In more severe disease, dietary restriction of sodium to 2.0 grams of sodium chloride (34 mEq. of sodium) and of protein to 0.5 gram per kg. body weight per day is appropriate with some restriction of total liquid intake. In the presence of oral intolerance or severe oliguria, intravenous administration of hypertonic dextrose (10 to 20 per cent in water) allows for restriction of the total liquid intake to match the average insensible loss plus an amount equal to the previous 24 hour urine volume.

Treatment of Complications

Edema. Should the combination of bed rest and dietary sodium and water restriction be insufficient, diuretic agents may be used. Hydrochlorothiazide (50 to 100 mg. per 24 hours in two divided doses, orally) is useful for induction of a gradual diuresis. When there is circulatory congestion or anasarca requiring more vigorous diuresis or when the decrease in glomerular filtration rate limits the effectiveness of hydrochlorothiazide (creatinine clearance less than 30 per cent of normal), furosemide in divided doses orally or intravenously may be given in increasing amounts to promote a diuresis. Should congestive heart failure due to underlying primary cardiac disease be present, digitalization can be accomplished by any of the conventional programs with care taken to adjust the dose schedule for the amount of renal functional impairment present and with awareness of the predilection to digitalis toxicity in patients with electrolyte abnormalities, especially hypokalemia.

Hypertension. CONTROL OF ACUTE SEVERE HYPERTENSION (HYPERTENSIVE CRISIS). This is often associated with hypertensive encephalopathy and circulatory congestion. Diazoxide (300 mg. per dose) may be given intravenously over 5 to 10 seconds. Nitroprusside may be given intravenously; although the usual initial infusion rate required is expected to be between 0.5 and 1.5 micrograms per kg. per minute, this dose must be continuously titrated with careful monitoring of blood pressure in each patient. Intravenous furosemide is a useful adjuvant to either of these agents.

CHRONIC LONG-TERM CONTROL OF HYPERTENSION. A stepped-care approach may be used with hydrochlorothiazide or furosemide, depending on the glomerular filtration rate, as the initial baseline agent. As a general principle, agents to control the hypertension should be added one at a time and the dose increased to the maximum acceptable level before another is added. Other agents are: hydralazine (50 to 300 mg. per 24 hours orally in two to four divided doses), methyldopa (500 to 2,000 mg. per 24 hours orally in two to four divided doses), propranolol (40 to 400 mg. per 24 hours orally in two to four divided doses).

Electrolyte and Acid-Base Disturbances. With progressive renal functional impairment, there is a tendency to hyperkalemia and acidosis. The latter, while rarely symptomatic, may be treated with sodium bicarbonate (13 mEq. of Na^+ and HCO_3^- per gram), which may contribute to lowering of hyperkalemia. Intravenous sodium bicarbonate or glucose and insulin will lower hyperkalemia rapidly by shifting potassium into cells, whereas oral or rectal potassium-binding resins with sorbitol and dialysis will lower hyperkalemia less rapidly by removing potassium from the body. Hyperkalemia is a potentially life-threatening emergency and demands immediate and expert treatment.

Anemia. This will not require treatment if the patient is asymptomatic. Only when symptoms are clearly related to the anemia itself should it be treated cautiously with transfusions of packed red blood cells.

Metabolic Bone Disease. Secondary hyperparathyroidism occurs in the hyperphosphatemic patient. Treatment is directed at lowering hyperphosphatemia by restricting dietary phosphorus (protein) and reducing gastrointestinal phosphate absorption with oral phosphate binding agents as well as normalizing serum calcium by cautious use of oral calcium and vitamin D analogues.

The programs outlined address the general treatment measures and the treatment of complications that arise as a result of the predictable functional consequences of progressive glomerular disease. There is relative agreement on the therapeutic approach to the sequelae of glomerular disorders; however, this is not the case for specific therapies of the underlying causes of the glomerular disorders. This is not surprising, as in the majority of instances the underlying cause of the glomerular disorder is not known. Some exceptions are the toxic disorders, in which the offending agent can often be removed, or immunologic glomerular disorders associated with certain neoplasms, in which removal of the neoplasm will generally reverse the glomerular disorder. Other exceptions are the glomerular disorders associated with infections such as bacterial endocarditis or infected ventriculoatrial shunts.

There are three major reasons for advising a specific therapeutic program: (1) it is of proven efficacy, (2) a valid study of efficacy is being conducted, (3) despite intensive treatment a fatal outcome is imminent. For a large number of glomerular diseases, reason 1 is unsatisfied. There is much anecdotal information concerning therapeutic benefits from prednisone, azathioprine, cyclophosphamide, heparin, warfarin, dipyridamole, acetylsalicylic acid, indomethacin, etc., in various glomerular disorders. However, there is no adequately controlled information that any long-term effect whatsoever is achieved by any of these agents, alone or in combination, in any glomerular disorder that does not have a natural tendency to remit or heal. Reason 3 has been supplanted by available dialysis and renal transplantation therapy. The need for prospective controlled studies of efficacy (reason 2) is required both by the intellectual concern for the solution of a serious clinical problem and the physician's desire to justify a still unsubstantiated clinical prejudice.

PYELONEPHRITIS

method of
JOHN N. WETTLAUFER, M.D.
Denver, Colorado

Introduction

Acute pyelonephritis is characterized by a primary interstitial renal parenchymal bacterial inflammation that secondarily involves the tubules and, in later stages, the vessels and glomeruli. Inflammation of the renal pelvis is often part of the same process. In most instances the causative organisms are gram-negative from the bowel flora, with 75 to 85 per cent due to *Escherichia coli,* and less commonly Klebsiella, Enterobacter, *Proteus mirabilis,* Pseudomonas, and *Streptococcus faecalis.*

The most common route of infection is ascending: in the female, introital-urethral-bladder; in the male, prostate-bladder. In children and females ureteral reflux often precedes and accompanies these infections. The following are frequent predisposing factors: congenital anomalies, mechanical or functional obstruction, calculi, diabetes mellitus, pregnancy, neurogenic bladder, and instrumentation.

The clinical manifestations include fever, malaise, back pain, tenderness to palpation in the costovertebral area, leukocytosis, and bacteriuria. The presence of leukocyte casts in the urine strongly supports the diagnosis. Irritable lower urinary tract symptoms are not uncommon. Infants and children may have no localizing signs and symptoms but evidence generalized illness with vomiting, diarrhea, and fever.

Treatment

General Supportive Measures. 1. Bed rest until pain, tenderness, and fever have subsided. Hospitalization may be indicated for patients with diabetes, for pregnant women, for infants, and for patients with obstructive uropathy.

2. Fluids: An intravenous route is indicated for patients with severe or complicated infections, and for those with extensive nausea and vomiting, especially infants and children. In adults a minimum of 3000 ml. orally or intravenously is suggested.

3. Fever: For temperature elevations to 101°F. (38.3°C.) or higher, use acetylsalicylic acid (650 mg. [10 grains]) orally or rectally by suppository (1300 mg. [20 grains]) every 4 hours. Cooling measures may be required for extreme temperature elevations.

4. Pain: Codeine sulfate (30 to 60 mg.) or meperidine hydrochloride (50 to 100 mg.) intramuscularly or orally every 4 hours in severe illness.

Antibiotics. GENERAL CONSIDERATIONS. In the uncomplicated usual case of acute pyelonephritis the causative organism will most often be a highly sensitive *Escherichia coli.* Until culture confirmation, initial therapy should be with a single antimicrobial agent directed against this organism. The urine should culture sterile within 24 hours in the uncomplicated case if the initial antibacterial agent has been appropriate.

More resistant organisms (Proteus, Klebsiella, Enterobacter, and Pseudomonas) should be suspected if the infection is recurrent, and there is a history of calculi, instrumentation, urologic surgery, or recent antimicrobial therapy.

The preferred route of antibiotic administration is dependent upon the severity of the infection and presence of complicating factors. In the less severe uncomplicated infections the oral route may be quite suitable (ampicillin, cephalexin, nitrofurantoin macrocrystals [Macrodantin], sulfisoxazole [Gantrisin], or trimethoprim and sulfamethoxazole [Septra or Bactrim]), whereas initial therapy in patients with more severe or complicated infections should be parenteral. The oral form can then be substituted when the clinical condition permits. Frequent urine cultures with sensitivity studies will allow for any necessary changes in antibiotic therapy (agent and route). The preferred antimicrobial agents for the more severe infections are those available both in parenteral and oral forms.

Pregnancy is an absolute contraindication to the use of tetracycline because of its potential maternal and fetal hepatotoxic effect and discoloration of fetal teeth. Chloramphenicol is to be limited to rare life-threatening infections with sensitivities precluding other medications.

SPECIFIC ANTIMICROBIALS. The following useful drugs are available in a parenteral and oral form:

1. Ampicillin, 1 to 2 grams intravenously over 30 minutes every 6 hours (this dose may be higher than that listed in the manufacturer's official directive), or orally, 250 to 500 mg. every 6 hours. Excellent with aminoglycosides for serious life-threatening infections.

2. Cephalothin, 1 to 2 grams intravenously over 30 minutes every 6 hours or cephalexin orally, 250 to 500 mg. every 6 hours.

3. Carbenicillin, 2 to 5 grams intravenously over 1 hour every 4 hours or orally, 2 tablets (382 mg. per tablet) every 6 hours. To avoid rapid development of resistance, use with an aminoglycoside for serious infections from Pseudomonas, Enterobacter, and indole-positive Proteus.

The following aminoglycosides are useful in complicated or more severe infections and instances of allergies to other agents. They are available only in parenteral form. Patients should be observed closely for ototoxicity and nephrotoxicity and serum concentrations should be monitored when available to ensure adequate levels and avoid toxic levels.

1. Gentamicin sulfate, 3 mg. per kg. of total body weight (total daily dose) in divided doses intramuscularly every 8 hours for 5 to 7 days.

2. Kanamycin, 1 gram intramuscularly immediately followed by 500 mg. intramuscularly every 12 hours for 5 to 7 days.

3. Tobramycin, 1 to 1.5 mg. per kg. of total body weight (total daily dose) in divided doses every 8 hours intramuscularly for 7 to 10 days.

4. Amikacin sulfate, 15 mg. per kg. of body weight per day divided into every 12 or every 8 hour intervals for 7 to 10 days.

The following antimicrobials are available only in oral form and may be useful in uncomplicated infections as initial or long term therapy or both.

1. Nitrofurantoin macrocrystals (Macrodantin), 100 mg. orally three or four times daily. Excellent for long-term suppressive therapy; no effect on fecal flora.

2. Sulfonamides: Sulfisoxazole (Gantrisin), initial dose 2 to 4 grams orally, then 1 to 2 grams every 6 hours, or sulfamethoxazole and trimethoprim (Septra or Bactrim), 1 double strength or 2 regular tablets every 12 hours.

3. Tetracycline, 250 to 500 mg. every 6 hours (uncommonly used in initial treatment).

4. Nalidixic acid (NegGram), 1 gram every 6 hours (uncommonly used in initial treatment).

Duration of Therapy

For initial uncomplicated acute pyelonephritis I prefer 10 to 14 days of therapy. Recurrent or complicated infection may well require several weeks (4 to 6) of aggressive therapy followed by long-term suppressive antimicrobial treatment (Macrodantin, 100 mg. at bedtime or 50 mg. twice daily, is ideal).

Follow-up

Urinalysis may be misleading in following the course of patients with acute pyelonephritis, as pus cells may appear in the urinary sediment for at least 10 days after adequate treatment and sterilization of the urine. Accordingly, periodic urine cultures appear to be the most reliable index as to the response to therapy. In the uncomplicated patient periodic urine cultures should be performed at 6 weeks and then at 3 month intervals for 1 year. Patients with severe or complicated disease should have urine cultures at more frequent intervals. All patients with acute pyelonephritis should undergo urologic evaluation with excretory urography and selectively with cystourethroscopy and cystourethrography. Diabetics and those responding poorly to initial therapy should have prompt excretory urography.

TRAUMA OF THE GENITOURINARY SYSTEM

method of
STANLEY BROSMAN, M.D.
Los Angeles, California

Immediate Evaluation

History taking in the trauma patient is usually perfunctory and obtained more out of curiosity than for any clinical benefit. However, there are some important data that should be elicited if possible. Information should be obtained of past urologic disorders and surgeries. It is helpful to know if the patient has only one kidney. The patient should be asked if the trauma occurred when the bladder was full or empty, since blunt or penetrating trauma is more likely to disrupt a full bladder and produce intraperitoneal leakage of urine. The patient should be asked about the number of urinations since the trauma and if blood was noted in the urine.

The presence of hematuria does not correlate with the severity of the trauma and the absence of hematuria does not rule out the possibility of significant trauma. Patients with disruptions of the ureter or those with renal arterial injuries do not have gross hematuria and may not have any significant microscopic hematuria. Patients with alarming hematuria may have relatively minor contusions within the urinary tract and the bleeding usually stops within a few hours. Patients with seemingly insignificant trauma yet who have evidence of genitourinary tract injury often turn out to have a congenital malformation.

On physical examination abdominal tenderness, bowel sounds, ecchymoses over the flanks, pelvic bone pain, suprapubic pain, a palpable bladder, blood coming from the urethra or dried blood at the meatus, perineal ecchymosis, and the position of the prostate on rectal examination should be noted.

If bleeding has occurred or is occurring from the urethra, the patient should not be catheterized or asked to urinate. This type of bleeding is evidence of a urethral disruption. The management of this problem will be discussed subsequently.

Upper Urinary Tract Injuries

Radiologic assessment of the urinary tract with infusion pyelography, tomography, and renal arteriography will permit an accurate diagnosis of the nature and severity of the injury. The emergency room patient is usually receiving intravenous fluids to which can be added 100 to 150 ml. of contrast solution. There is little point in attempting pyelography in the hypotensive patient, as the kidneys will not be visualized. Angiography should be performed on patients with nonvisualizing kidneys, those in whom the pyelogram is of nondiagnostic quality, and patients allergic to intravenously administered contrast.

With this information the diagnosis can be established and a therapeutic plan initiated.

Renal Contusion. This common injury results from blunt trauma that produces an ecchymosis on the surface of the kidney and a subcapsular hematoma. The kidney is seen well on pyelography, the collecting system is intact, and the renal outlines are clearly seen and not disrupted. The amount of hematuria is variable and

the bleeding usually stops quickly. There is no necessity for surgical therapy. Patients who are undergoing surgery for other injuries do not need to have the kidneys examined. There may be evidence of a retroperitoneal hematoma, but unless this is visibly expanding, Gerota's fascia should not be opened.

Patients with renal contusions may be discharged from the hospital or the emergency room when their condition is stable. They are advised to avoid physical exertion and potentially traumatic situations for at least two weeks.

Renal Laceration. Lacerations can vary from superficial parenchymal disruptions to complete fractures with separation of a renal segment from the main body of the kidney. Lacerations may be stellate in shape and may extend into the collecting system and renal pelvis. Pyelography may disclose a poorly visualizing kidney with a distorted collecting system or poor visualization of a renal segment. The kidney outlines are obscure and may be disrupted. Hemorrhage is often significant and the psoas margins are obliterated by the retroperitoneal bleeding. Extravasation of urine may be present and produces a dramatic picture on x-ray but is not a surgical emergency.

Even though the bleeding can be quite profuse, a tenacious clot forms over the laceration and the bleeding begins to subside within a few hours. Rarely does a patient require emergency surgery for a renal laceration.

Most patients can be managed without surgery. The kidney has an amazing capacity to heal and it is surprising how a seriously lacerated and disrupted kidney can return to normal. Extravasation of urine per se is not an indication for surgery. If the collecting system and ureter are in continuity, the laceration will heal adequately. Patients who are managed without surgery should have their vital signs, hematocrit, and urine monitored at regular intervals. These patients are generally in severe pain and require large amounts of narcotics. The retroperitoneal hematuria produces an intestinal ileus and a febrile response. Patients may be severely ill for 10 days before their condition begins to improve.

Patients who require early surgery are those with extensive parenchymal and collecting system disruption, those with large segments of ischemic kidney, and those with continuing severe bleeding. Kidney hemorrhage can be stopped by injecting autologous clot or absorbable gelatin (Gelfoam) particles into the lacerated arteries at the time of arteriography. This manages the acute hemorrhage and the patient's condition can be stabilized. The need for emergency surgery may be obviated by this technique.

Often, patients are being explored for other abdominal trauma. If the kidney evaluation has been completed, the surgeon may decide to treat the renal injury at the same time. Emergency renal explorations for trauma should be done through a transabdominal, transperitoneal incision because the abdominal contents should be examined.

The first consideration in exploring a severely injured kidney is to obtain control of the vascular pedicle before exposing the kidney. When this is completed, the kidney can be dissected from its bed. Ischemic tissue should be debrided, lacerations sutured with absorbable sutures, and the area drained. An upper or lower pole may be completely transected and can be removed from the wound.

The renal artery can be safely occluded for 20 minutes; for longer periods the kidney should be cooled. Troublesome bleeding areas on the surface of the kidney can be effectively treated by applying microfibrillar collagen hemostat (Avitene).

Kidneys that are extensively lacerated so that there is no longer continuity of the collecting system and vascular system will need to be removed.

Sometimes a surgeon is surprised to find a retroperitoneal hematoma when no renal injury was suspected. Since a kidney evaluation has not been made, a conservative approach is necessary. The kidney should not be exposed unless there is clear evidence of active bleeding from the area of the kidney. Stable hematomas should be left alone. If the kidney must be explored, the vascular pedicle should be secured as the first step. A minor laceration may be the only injury, but these can bleed heavily and frighten the surgeon into performing an unnecessary nephrectomy.

In many patients surgery can be delayed for 3 to 5 days. This allows the patient's condition to stabilize and a therapeutic plan to be developed. A flank approach can be used, but vascular control of the pedicle should be obtained before Gerota's fascia is opened.

The same surgical plan is followed for patients with gunshot wounds involving the kidney. Knife wounds to the kidney may not require surgery, particularly if this is the only organ injured. Even in patients whose abdomens are being explored for knife wounds, the kidney should be left alone unless there is active bleeding. Arteriography is very useful in these patients to assess vascular injuries.

Vascular Injuries.   Trauma to the renal artery is the most serious type of injury because renal preservation depends upon prompt diagnosis and surgical correction. The injury is usually an intimal dissection with thrombosis as a result of arterial compression against a vertebra. These patients have few symptoms related to their injury and hematuria is insignificant. A high degree of suspi-

cion is necessary to detect these injuries. Excretory urography reveals no visualization of the affected kidney, and arteriography demonstrates a blind ending arterial stump.

There is no point in attempting a repair if the renal ischemia time is more than 18 hours. In fact, very few kidneys have had the return of partial renal function if the ischemia time was more than 6 hours. A delayed nephrectomy may be necessary because of the high incidence of hypertension in these patients.

Patients with bilateral renal artery trauma should be explored. The duodenum and pancreas should be carefully examined for injuries because of their close proximity to the renal arteries. The most effective means of repair is a bypass graft. Other forms of therapy include thrombectomy with intimal suturing and autotransplantation.

Ureter

Traumatic injuries to the ureter are rare but can occur with blunt or penetrating trauma. Avulsion of the ureter from the ureteropelvic junction is a result of rapid flexion of the trunk. This type of injury is usually seen in young adults. Penetrating trauma can produce a partial or complete disruption of the ureter.

Excretory urography will demonstrate extravasation of contrast media at the site of injury, establishing the diagnosis. If the diagnosis is equivocal, it can be substantiated by retrograde pyelography. During various operative procedures in the pelvis, the ureter may be injured. Ligation of the ureter, either complete or partial, or transection of the ureter may occur. Although it is preferable to correct these injuries as soon as they occur, the diagnosis may not be made until several days have elapsed. Patients complain of flank pain; a urinary fistula indicates that an injury has occurred.

Treatment.   Ureteral avulsions are managed by prompt reanastomosis of the ureter. A careful closure with fine suture material (5-0 chromic or polyglycolic acid) is preferable. Stents and proximal drainage with a nephrostomy tube or a pelvic vent may be used. Stenting may not be necessary if the area is uncontaminated and the anastomosis is not under tension, but the area should be drained.

Ureters that have been injured by a gunshot wound require debridement. Large caliber bullets produce extensive tissue destruction and a large ureteral gap may be present. If a direct anastomosis without tension cannot be performed, a variety of techniques is available. The proper selection of the procedure depends upon the nature and site of injury, the patient's age, clinical condition, and renal function.

Lower ureteral injuries can be treated with

reimplantation and by moving the bladder out of the pelvis and tacking it to the psoas muscle. A bladder flap can be created that can reach to the midureter. Mid- or lower ureteral injuries lend themselves to transureteroureterostomies. The ureter can be replaced partially or in its entirety by ileum. In desperate situations a nephrostomy or a nephrectomy may be indicated.

Bladder

Pelvic trauma, particularly associated with pelvic fractures, should alert the clinician to the possibility of bladder and urethral injuries. Ten to 15 per cent of patients with pelvic fractures have associated bladder or urethral trauma or both.

The cystogram is the most important diagnostic study. After a catheter has been placed into the bladder, 250 to 300 ml. of contrast media can be introduced with gravity drainage. X-rays should be made in the anteroposterior and oblique positions if possible. The contrast agent should be allowed to drain from the bladder and another film made. Contrast material left behind is diagnostic of a bladder perforation.

Contusion. Contusions result from blunt trauma producing an ecchymosis of the bladder wall without perforation. Usually no treatment is necessary. The hematuria clears in a short period of time, and there is no loss of bladder function.

Extraperitoneal Laceration. This may result from bladder perforation by the bony spicules of a fracture and usually occurs near the bladder neck. There is extravasation of urine into paravesical tissues and retroperitoneally. The classic method of therapy includes surgical repair of the laceration, drainage of urine with urethral or suprapubic catheters or both, and placement of Penrose drains. Selected patients with extravasation confined to the parapelvic tissues have been treated successfully with urethral catheter drainage and no surgery. The catheter is left in place for 7 to 10 days, and the cystogram is repeated before it is removed.

Intraperitoneal Laceration. This laceration occurs in the patient who has a distended bladder at the time of the accident or is the result of a gunshot wound. The laceration involves the dome and superior wall of the bladder, which is the area covered by the peritoneal reflection.

Surgical therapy for these patients includes closure of the laceration on the peritoneal and bladder surfaces. Urine is drained from the bladder with urethral or suprapubic catheters or both.

Combined Intraperitoneal and Extraperitoneal Injuries. These injuries require surgical repair and are treated in a similar fashion to the intraperitoneal lacerations.

Urethra

The diagnosis of urethral trauma can be made on the basis of these clinical findings:

1. Blood coming from the urethra or the presence of dried blood around the meatus.

2. Perineal ecchymosis. This is usually present in patients with straddle injuries.

3. Proximal displacement of the prostate. Disruption of the prostatomembranous urethra is associated with severe pelvic bleeding. This elevates the prostate into the pelvis and is detectable on rectal examination.

4. A desire to urinate, but the inability to do so produces a distended bladder. Patients with prostatomembranous urethral injuries have intense spasm at the bladder neck. Patients with suspected urethral injuries should not be asked to urinate.

5. Fractured pelvis. Because of the high association between pelvic fractures and urethral or bladder trauma, all patients with such fractures should have a cystourethrogram.

Retrograde urethrography establishes the diagnosis by demonstrating extravasation of contrast material. A straight 14 to 16F Robinson catheter can be passed a few centimeters into the urethra and 30 ml. of contrast media instilled by gravity drainage. In some patients a Foley catheter has already been passed into the bladder without evaluating the urethra. An 8F feeding tube can be passed alongside the Foley catheter and contrast injected. This will provide an adequate urethrogram.

Treatment. Injuries distal to the urogenital diaphragm are usually incomplete disruptions. The injuries are caused by straddle or perineal trauma, or a traumatic catheterization. Depending upon the severity of the injury, this type of urethral disruption can be managed by passing a Silastic catheter into the bladder, diverting the urine with a suprapubic catheter, or a primary urethral repair with catheter drainage.

Prostatomembranous urethral injuries are associated with a high degree of morbidity, mortality, and difficulties in management. No attempt should be made to pass a catheter into the bladder of a patient suspected of having urethral trauma until that diagnosis is ruled out with urethrography.

The introduction of a catheter through a traumatized urethra into the bladder is difficult, usually unsuccessful, and unnecessary because immediate surgery is required to divert the urine. A suprapubic catheter is placed, and the urethra is realigned with a stenting catheter if possible. The puboprostatic ligaments, which are often partially separated, should be completely divided to allow greater mobility of the prostatic urethra and reduce tension at the site of the urethral laceration. The perivesical area is drained with Penrose drains. The urethral catheter can be removed after 4 to 6 weeks and the continuity of the urethra determined with urethrography. If the patient's condition is critical, operative time should not be prolonged by attempting to realign the urethra.

Occasionally, a 14 or 16F Foley catheter will successfully traverse the disrupted urethra. When this occurs, the catheter should be left in place and no additional therapy may be necessary.

The most common complication of urethral injuries is stricture formation, which requires some form of urethroplasty for correction.

Genitalia

Penis. Avulsion of the penile skin can be corrected by using a combination of remaining penile skin, scrotal flaps, or skin grafts to cover the defect.

Amputations are most unusual, and a few successful reanastomoses have been reported. Otherwise, the wound is debrided, hemostasis is obtained, and an adequate urethral meatus constructed.

Scrotum. Occasionally clothing and scrotum can be caught in a machine, avulsing segments of each. Fortunately, the scrotum is so redundant that after thorough cleansing and debridement there is usually enough scrotal skin to repair the defect. If not, the testes can be temporarily placed in the thigh or inguinal area and the wound allowed to granulate. Later this area can be covered with skin grafts or abdominal flaps.

Testis. Blunt or penetrating trauma can result in disruption of the tunica albuginea. This may be difficult to diagnose, but if in doubt, the testis should be explored and the lacerations repaired. Open scrotal wounds should be explored and the testis trauma repaired.

Attempts to reconstruct a shattered testis are usually unsuccessful and orchiectomy is indicated.

Minor degrees of blunt trauma produce testicular contusions that are treated with bed rest, ice packs, scrotal support, and analgesics.

BENIGN PROSTATIC HYPERPLASIA

method of
THEODORE H. LEHMAN, M.D.
Portland, Oregon

Benign prostatic hyperplasia, a condition of aging men, is the most common cause of obstruc-
tion of the bladder neck. The incidence, on autopsy studies, is approximately 50 per cent in men over the age of 50, rising to 75 per cent in men past the eighth decade.

When surgical treatment is required, because of related symptoms, is more difficult to ascertain owing to the variability of subjective and objective findings in this patient population. Unfortunately, there is no adequate medical treatment for this condition when it becomes symptomatic, and definitive treatment is primarily surgical.

In hyperplasia, fibrous and muscular tissue have developed from the acini and the stroma of the periurethral gland of the prostatic urethra. With progressive hyperplasia, the true prostate is compressed into a narrow, fibroglandular structure. Between the hyperplastic tissue and the compressed prostatic tissue a well-defined plane of cleavage is found that is known as the surgical capsule of the prostate. This characteristic is a valuable landmark in the surgical treatment of bladder neck obstruction in patients who have benign prostatic hyperplasia.

Evaluation of the Patient

Usually the symptoms of bladder neck obstruction develop slowly and insidiously. Patients commonly minimize the degree of obstructive symptoms, making the assumption that a gradual slowing of their stream, increased urinary frequency, and nocturia are natural components to the process of aging. The symptoms of nocturia, frequency, and slow, hesitant, and interrupted stream are the result of the gradual compression of the bladder neck and prostatic urethra by the hyperplastic tissue, and, in turn, the response of the bladder to the progressive obstruction. As the bladder is a hollow, muscular viscus, the muscle wall of the bladder responds to the progressive obstruction by becoming hypertrophied.

A thick-walled bladder can, for some time, compensate for the increased peripheral resistance, but the urinary stream is ultimately decreased in force and caliber. The bladder becomes thickened and less able to distend, and it becomes more irritable, causing increased urinary frequency and nocturia. If the obstruction is progressive, the detrusor muscle eventually decompensates, and the bladder, which normally should completely empty, does not empty itself, allowing residual urine to remain in the bladder after urination. This may or may not be followed by infection and either acute or chronic urinary retention. Drugs with anticholinergic properties, chilling, prostatitis, and holding urine for prolonged periods of time (e.g., a car trip), may precipitate bladder decompensation and retention.

There are some patients who do not have progressive bladder neck obstruction, whose detrusor muscle seems to compensate and they have fairly stable symptoms of mild urinary frequency and slowing of their stream. These people generally do not require surgical treatment if their renal function remains stable and urinary tract infection does not supervene, but they should be followed closely.

Other secondary effects of bladder neck obstruction may require surgical treatment: bladder calculus, bladder diverticula, hydronephrosis, hydroureter, and azotemia.

The decision to carry out prostatectomy is based on a combination of factors, among which are urinary symptoms, presence of infection, impaired renal function, and other organ system disease.

It is important to mention that prostatic size alone is not an indication for surgery. The size does not correlate well with the degree of obstructive symptoms and objective findings. Many patients with large prostates have minimal symptoms and empty their bladders quite well without deterioration of renal function or the development of a urinary tract infection. They may never require a prostatectomy.

Other patients may have quite small glands on rectal examination and have marked obstructive symptoms with changes in their upper urinary tract. At times, patients are seen with relatively few symptoms in the face of far-advanced bladder decompensation and severe renal damage.

Each patient must be evaluated individually with careful assessment of his general medical condition, especially the cardiopulmonary system, the presence of anemia, and evidence of preexisting renal disease. An attempt must be made to ensure the optimal medical and metabolic condition before surgery is embarked upon.

The alternatives to surgical treatment of prostatic hyperplasia for a patient who is a poor surgical risk would be an indwelling catheter or intermittent self-catheterization.

Preoperative evaluation includes the history and physical examination and generally should include a chest x-ray, electrocardiogram, routine hematologic studies, evaluation of coagulation mechanisms, and 12-channel SMA chemistry screen. An excretory urogram is also of value in assessing the function of the upper urinary tract, and a postvoiding film may give information regarding the amount of residual urine or the presence of bladder calculi or diverticula, in addition to giving some information regarding the size of the prostate. When the presence of symptoms and findings suggestive of abnormal bladder or sphincter function is suspected (e.g., diabetic neuropathy, multiple sclerosis, spinal cord injury), urodynamic studies such as uroflowometry, cystometrogram, and urethral pressure profile studies are indicated. This information is helpful in weighing the indications for prostatic surgery.

Choice of Operation

In general, there are four surgical approaches to the obstructing hyperplastic benign prostatic hyperplasia. The type of operation should be chosen on the basis of the specific needs and requirements of the patient and the training and experience of the surgeon.

Regardless of the type of surgical approach to the prostate, each patient is cystoscoped at the time of the operation to ascertain the degree of obstruction and the amount of obstructing tissue that should be removed.

Transurethral Prostatectomy. In a transurethral prostatectomy the obstructing prostatic tissue is removed through the urethra with a resectoscope. This operation removes the prostatic tissue piecemeal down to the surgical capsule of the prostate, after which any remaining chips of prostatic adenomatous tissue are evacuated from the bladder. This operation probably is the most common type of prostatectomy carried out by American urologists and has the advantages of reduced morbidity and mortality, minimal postoperative pain, early ambulation, and short hospital stay. It is limited primarily by the size of the prostatic hypertrophy. Urologists with different training and experience may limit their transurethral resections to those patients whose resectable tissue can be removed within a 1 hour period of time. It also may not be the operation of choice in a patient who has difficulty assuming the lithotomy position on the operating table or if there are associated conditions such as bladder diverticula or large bladder stones that cannot be removed through the resectoscope.

Suprapubic (Transvesical) Prostatectomy. This is a relatively simple operation, ideally suited for patients who have prostates that are predominantly intravesical and have other complications such as bladder calculi or diverticula that can be removed at the same operative setting. The incision is made through the bladder wall. The adenomatous, obstructing hyperplastic tissue is enucleated.

The disadvantage of the procedure is that the control of bleeding may sometimes be difficult because of inability to gain access to the bleeding vessels in the prostatic fossa. A removable, encircling suture about the bladder neck and around the urethral catheter is sometimes helpful in isolating and tamponading the bleeding from the prostatic fossa. Sometimes a cystotomy tube is used to provide through-and-through irrigation if bleeding is a problem.

Retropubic (Trans-capsular) Prostatectomy. Retropubic prostatectomy is carried out with an incision, either transverse or vertical, in the anterior surface of the prostatic capsule. It is possible to enucleate large prostates by this method that are not amenable to removal though the resectoscope. As bleeding vessels are under direct vision, they can be dealt with more readily. If necessary, the vertical incision can be extended into the bladder for removal of diverticula or stones.

The disadvantage of this type of operation is that it is difficult to carry out in obese patients, and bleeding from the plexus veins that run across the anterior capsule of the prostate may be troublesome. Osteitis pubis is more apt to occur after this operation than with other approaches.

Perineal Prostatectomy. Perineal prostatectomy is suited for patients in whom the amount of tissue is felt to be too large to remove with a resectoscope. It can be done in relatively poor-risk patients who are able to assume exaggerated dorsal lithotomy position. Hemostasis is generally easier than in other methods of open prostatectomy, and usually the postoperative course is smoother in terms of lack of pain. The patient does not splint his abdomen when he coughs, thus avoiding pulmonary complications. The approach is through a curvilinear incision anterior to the rectum.

The disadvantages are that some patients cannot be put into or tolerate the position. There is a danger of injuring the rectum when using this method of exposure, and many urologists who do not do this operation frequently feel uncomfortable in using this exposure because of the variability of perineal anatomy. It is thought by some that the incidence of impotence is higher in perineal prostatectomy when compared to other methods of prostatectomy.

Complications Associated With a Prostatectomy

The patient population that requires prostatectomy is frequently elderly men who are poor surgical risks, especially in terms of their cardiorespiratory status and renal function. Nevertheless, with careful assessment of cardiorenal function and metabolic abnormalities and their correction, the overall death rate of all patients having surgery for benign prostatic hyperplasia is less than 2 per cent.

Some complications are peculiar to the transurethral prostatectomy itself. These include absorption of irrigating fluid that enters the vascular spaces in the prostatic capsule as the prostate is resected. This can result in fluid overload. If a nonisotonic solution is used to irrigate, such as distilled water, intravascular hemolysis may occur. The latter complication can be obviated by giving the patient 250 ml. of a 10 per cent solution of mannitol intravenously during the last half of the operation and 250 ml. in the recovery room, or by the judicious use of furosemide, 20 to 40 mg., intravenously. An alternative is to use an isotonic solution such as sorbitol, which will prevent hemolysis, but some urologists feel that the visibility through the resectoscope is not as good as when distilled water is used.

Extravasation of irrigating fluid may take place through a perforation or a thin area in the prostatic capsule or the area of the bladder neck. Small perforations do not require surgical drainage, but the procedure should be terminated when this condition is recognized. If the opening is larger than 1 cm. and fluid can be seen to run through the area of injury, surgical drainage of the extraperitoneal space should be carried out.

Hemorrhage. All prostatectomies have the associated risk of hemorrhage. This may occur during the surgical procedure or postoperatively. Serious arterial bleeding during transurethral resection of the prostate can usually be controlled by electrocoagulation. The bleeding veins generally are controlled with catheter drainage or with traction against the bladder neck by a 30 ml. balloon Foley catheter, or both.

For an open prostatectomy, the bleeding is usually most readily controlled by suture ligaturing the vessels where they enter the prostate at 5 and 7 o'clock area at the vesical neck and with coagulation or ligature of bleeding vessels in the prostatic fossa or capsule.

Delayed postoperative bleeding most commonly occurs 1 to 4 weeks postoperatively when the eschar begins to slough. This usually is not of a serious nature but can be alarming to the patient. If clots are passed and the patient has difficulty emptying the bladder, he may require catheter drainage and irrigation of his bladder to free it of clots. Occasionally, but not commonly, surgical intervention is necessary.

Infection. Patients who have bacteriuria preoperatively should be treated preoperatively with an antibiotic of choice according to their urine culture bacterial sensitivity. Occasionally, during or following a prostatectomy, bacteremia takes place, resulting in peripheral vascular collapse. A urinary antiseptic such as sulfisoxazole, 1 gram twice daily, is used for the first 2 weeks postoperatively.

Epididymitis is occasionally a complication postoperatively. Although it is the policy of some urologists to ligate each vas deferens at the time of prostatectomy, it is debatable whether or not this procedure is effective in preventing postoperative epididymitis. It is not routinely done by us.

Osteitis pubis, reputed to be a complication of retropubic operation, is actually quite rare.

Urethral Stricture. Urethral strictures can occur in any patient who has an indwelling catheter. It can also be iatrogenic if a resectoscope sheath fits too snugly in the urethra. This can be avoided by either doing a meatotomy or internal urethrotomy during transurethral surgery.

Vesical Neck Contracture. Bladder neck contracture results from circumferential scarring at the bladder neck after prostatectomy. It can occur with any approach, but seems to be most common after a transurethral resection of the prostate. The cause is unknown. It can usually be treated by urethral dilatations but occasionally will require incision of the scar tissue at the bladder neck or resection with the resectoscope.

In severe cases, bladder neck plasty interposing bladder mucosa into the bladder neck is necessary.

Incontinence. Incontinence after prostatic surgery is relatively uncommon, although the urethral sphincter may be damaged during prostatic surgery. Some patients have urgency incontinence because of their hypertrophied detrusor muscle. This usually lasts a few hours to a few days after the catheter is removed and frequently responds to anticholinergic drugs. The bladder usually accommodates to the difference in dynamics, although some patients may continue to have urgency and frequency because of their decreased bladder capacity, the result of a thickened bladder muscle that will not allow the bladder to adequately distend.

Patients who have long-term inflammatory symptoms such as chronic prostatitis, prostatic calculi, and urethral strictures may have difficulty with control because of lack of pliability of the urethral and periurethral structures that do not permit the sphincter mechanism to close adequately. Generally, this can be predicted preoperatively and the patient warned that this might occur.

Patients who have preexisting neurologic disease such as Parkinson's disease, diabetic neuropathy, and spinal cord injury may also have difficulty controlling their urine once the peripheral resistance to urinary flow has been removed.

Impotence. Sexual function is usually not affected by prostatectomy for benign prostatic hyperplasia. Patients are told that they may have retrograde ejaculation after prostatectomy, but their ability to have erections and orgasms should not be made any better or any worse.

Some urologists report that the perineal route is commonly associated with loss of potency in their patients. However, I have found the incidence of this complication in the perineal approach to be no different from that of any other approach but feel obliged to inform the patient that this complication can occur. However, the majority of patients who are selected for the perineal approach usually are elderly, infirm men who are not sexually active.

PROSTATITIS

method of
CRAIG G. HINMAN, M.D.,
and DAVID F. PAULSON, M.D.
Durham, North Carolina

Prostatitis is a physically and psychologically debilitating disease entity with minimal lethal potential, yet it remains a perplexing problem to the practicing physician. Whereas symptomatic prostatitis is a frequently encountered entity, bacterial prostatitis, confirmed by culture, is an infrequently documented event.

Bacterial Prostatitis

Bacterial prostatitis presents as a disease spectrum with symptoms ranging from chronic dysuria, frequency, perineal fullness or pain, urethral discharge, low back or suprapubic ache, hematospermia, and urethral discomfort on ejaculation to the more severe acute presentation with chills, fever, marked vesical irritability, initial and terminal hematuria, severe prostration, and acute toxemia. Edema of the prostate or abscess formation may cause bladder outlet obstruction. Considerable psychologic overlay is not unusual with inordinate anxiety and fears of cancer and loss of potency. Exacerbations are frequently associated with excessive alcohol indulgence, sexual withdrawal, or markedly increased sexual activity.

General measures in treatment include adequate rest without vigorous exercise, good hydration (intravenous if necessary), frequent voiding, avoidance of alcohol and caffeinated beverages, frequent sexual release without overindulgence, and sitz baths of 15 to 30 minutes twice daily.

Antimicrobial treatment of bacterial prostatitis is theoretically quite complex, dependent on a lipid soluble drug with antimicrobial activity at the low pH of prostatic fluid. However, alterations in the membrane permeability and increase of the pH of prostatic tissues with inflammation further enhance antibiotic penetration and efficacy during clinical infections.

Acute prostatitis with prostration and toxemia will require hospitalization, intravenous hydration, and parenteral antibiotics. Two recommended 10 day regimens include:

1. Gentamicin or tobramycin,* 80 mg. every 8 hours (adjust to weight and renal function), with ampicillin, 500 mg. intravenously ever 6 hours, or cephalothin sodium, 500 mg. intravenously every 6 hours.

2. Kanamycin, 1.0 gram per day intramuscularly, and penicillin, 20 to 40 million units per day in divided doses.

Less severe prostatitis is treated with oral medications on an out-patient basis. Treatment needs to be continued for at least 4 to 6 weeks and low dose suppressive antibiotics are often required to prevent recurrence. Multiple antibiotics have been shown to be effective in the therapy of prostatitis.

1. Tetracycline, 250 to 500 mg. four times daily, given 1 hour before meals and on retiring to prevent chelation with dietary calcium. This has long been the mainstay and is still a good initial choice.

2. Minocycline hydrochloride, and doxycycline hyclate, 100 mg. orally twice daily, are both effective with an easier dosage schedule and less drug alteration by dietary intake, but both are expensive.

3. Trimethoprim-sulfamethoxazole, 2 tablets twice daily, has good prostatic tissue penetration. However, clinical trials have shown that prolonged treatment for 4 months might be required, as well as long term suppressive treatment.

4. Ampicillin, 500 mg. four times daily.

5. Erythromycin, 500 mg. four times daily, with sodium bicarbonate, 600 mg. four times daily.

6. Nitrofurantoin, 50 mg. four times daily.

7. Cephadrine, a new semisynthetic cephalosporin, has shown good prostatic tissue levels in preliminary reports and may be a welcome addition to prostatitis treatment.

Parenteral antimicrobials have been used by several in resistant cases with good reported results including:

1. Kanamycin, 1 gram twice daily intramuscularly for 3 days then 500 mg. intramuscularly twice daily for 11 days.

2. Streptomycin, 1 gram intramuscularly every day for 14 days.

Local therapy with direct injection into the peripheral prostate transperineally of cefazolin, 250 mg., and three injections of gentamicin or amikacin, 80 mg., has reportedly given high cure rates, although this has never been used personally. (This use of these agents is not listed in the manufacturer's official directive.)

---

*See manufacturer's official directive which states the dose should not exceed 5 mg. per kg. per day unless serum levels are monitored.

Prostatic massage was once the main modality of treatment, relieving the prostatic acini engorgement. Some patients receive considerable benefit with stripping of the gland two times per week for a 4 to 6 week course. However, increased sexual activity will accomplish much the same results. Stool softeners to prevent the irritation of hard bowel movements over the inflamed prostate are helpful. If considerable bladder irritability is present, small doses of anticholinergics are helpful such as oxybutynin chloride (Ditropan), flavoxate HCl (Urispas), propantheline bromide (Pro-Banthine) or methantheline (Banthine), one tablet daily to four times daily. However, their use is limited if bladder outlet obstructive symptoms are present or develop. For acute urinary retention, a small caliber (#14 F) Foley catheter is inserted or suprapubic drainage accomplished. Cystocath is an easily performed method of bedside suprapubic drainage.

Good success with zinc sulfate, 50 to 150 mg. every day for 2 to 16 weeks, has been reported. Fair and others have recently shown the bactericidal activity of prostatic antibacterial factor to be related to prostatic zinc concentration with normal values of 150 to 1000 micrograms per ml., but all patients with chronic prostatitis have values of less than 150 micrograms per ml. However, Fair could not effectively increase the prostatic level with oral administration of zinc, and could not demonstrate improvement of the clinical course of infections or subsequent cultures.

Anatomic and functional abnormalities that can predispose a patient to prostatic irritation such as benign prostatic hypertrophy, urethral stricture, prostatic carcinoma, neurogenic bladder, and occasionally bladder dyssynergia should be always kept in mind and appropriate evaluation accomplished if suspicion is raised or prostatitis is resistant to treatment efforts. Helpful studies include excretory urogram, voiding cystourethrogram, retrograde urethrogram, cystourethroscopy, and urodynamic studies when indicated.

Surgical intervention is required if a prostatic abscess develops. Transurethral drainage is preferable, although perineal drainage is occasionally necessary. Further surgical manipulation is confined to correcting anatomic abnormalities such as urethral strictures or obstructing prostatic hypertrophy. Bladder neck incisions have been used sparingly in the past. With the definite risk of retrograde ejaculation, it should be reserved only to those patients who show a definite bladder neck obstruction by urodynamic studies.

Abacterial Prostatitis

In some patients with symptoms of chronic prostatitis, significant pus cells may be seen in the expressed prostatic fluid but the bacterial cultures are negative. Many of these will still respond to the antibiotics and other measures discussed for bacterial prostatitis. It has become increasingly apparent that Mycoplasma and Chlamydia organisms, both difficult to culture with even sophisticated media, are frequently involved as causative agents in prostatitis. They are quite sensitive to tetracycline and the synthetic tetracyclines so commonly used for bacterial prostatitis. In addition, the absence of a positive culture does not rule out bacterial prostatitis, since the prostatic antibacterial factor in expressed prostatic fluid often alters culture growth.

Trichomonas vaginalis can infect the prostate and urethra of males and if the organism is seen on wet smear or the patient's consort is infected with trichomoniasis, then treatment with metronidazole (Flagyl), 250 mg. three times daily for 10 days, should be given. The patient's sexual partner can be treated with metronidazole, 2 grams taken once. (The patients should be advised to avoid alcohol while on metronidazole, since it has similar properties to disulfiram [Antabuse]). (The single 2 gram dose is not listed in the manufacturer's official directive.)

Prostatosis is a term applied to a disorder in many patients in which no identifiable organism is present. Passive congestion secondary to lack of ejaculation, or alcohol overindulgence is often present. However, close questioning may reveal a history of infrequent voiding or enuresis as a child with lifelong frequency, urgency, and occasional urge incontinence. Further evaluation may reveal bladder decompensation, large bladder capacity, and neurogenic bladder, all which can force urine into the urethral tissues, causing a chronic inflammatory reaction. Cerny describes a simple regimen that requires the patient to void at least every 2 hours during the day and once at night, plus the use of an anticholinergic agent if a neurogenic bladder is present.

If urodynamic evaluation reveals bladder dyssynergia with high bladder neck and proximal urethral pressures present during voiding, then marked improvement will result with phenoxybenzamine (Dibenzyline), 10 mg. daily to four times daily. Potent side effects of dizziness, tachycardia, hypotension, and loss of ejaculation must be considered. Bladder neck incision or possibly transurethral prostatectomy may be preferable to the potential adverse effects of prolonged treatment with phenoxybenzamine. (This use of phenoxybenzamine is not listed in the manufacturer's official directive.)

In summary, prostatitis is not a single entity. Many factors seem involved and much is yet to be learned. No one regimen will be effective for all patients; therefore, multiple regimens have been discussed. The possibility of underlying anatomic or functional abnormalities must always be kept in mind. The chronic recurrent nature of prostatitis needs to be understood by the patient. Strong psychologic support is often the key to achieving acceptable symptomatic control.

ACUTE RENAL FAILURE
method of
CARL M. KJELLSTRAND, M.D.,
and THOMAS D. DAVIN, M.D.
Minneapolis, Minnesota

Definition

Acute renal failure means a sudden cessation of renal function. Uremia and electrolyte and fluid imbalances, usually acidosis, hyperkalemia, hyperphosphatemia, and hypocalcemia occur. If oliguria (less than 300 ml. urine per day) or anuria (less than 50 ml. urine per day) are present, the syndrome is easily detected. However, good urine output is often maintained and unless blood urea nitrogen and serum creatinine levels are followed, the syndrome can be overlooked and patients may slip into life-threatening homeostatic imbalances, particularly fluid overload, hyperkalemia, and acidosis.

Although acute renal failure is a syndrome with many different causes, the name is frequently considered synonymous with the most common cause of acute renal failure, acute tubular necrosis, also called vasomotor nephropathy. In the rest of this chapter we will not discuss other causes of acute renal failure such as glomerulonephritis, obstructive uropathy, renal artery thrombosis, or embolism, but limit the discussion to acute tubular necrosis (ATN).

ATN is most commonly iatrogenic. It is usually associated with major surgery, prolonged prerenal failure (dehydration) and the use of nephrotoxic antibiotics (especially aminoglycosides such as gentamicin, kanamycin, amikacin, and tobramycin). Most antibiotics have some nephrotoxicity. Most instances of acute renal failure are multifactorial.

As in other acute situations, patients presenting with acute renal failure first need to be resuscitated, then diagnosed, and finally treated with etiologic and symptomatic treatment and watched for special complications.

Cause of Death

Causes of early death are generally cardiac secondary to fluid overload (sometimes iatrogenic), hyperkalemia, and acidosis (often overlooked).

Causes of late death are infections and malnutrition, which are responsible for two thirds of the deaths, gas-

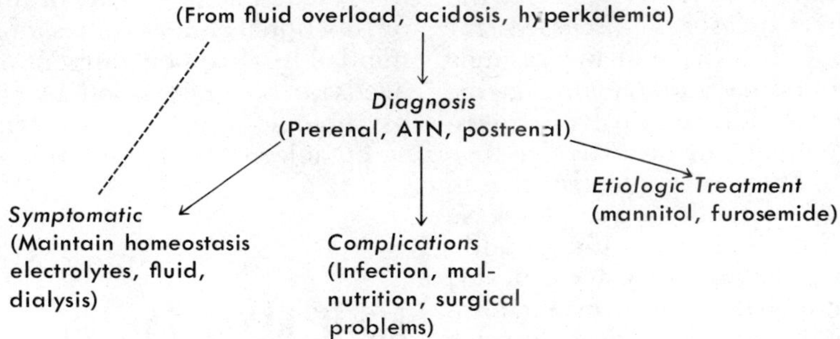

Figure 1. Plan of Attack

trointestinal bleeding from stress ulcers, or incurable underlying disease.

Diagnosis

When acute renal failure occurs, ATN must be differentiated from prerenal and postrenal failure, and acute parenchymal renal disease, e.g., glomerulonephritis and interstitial nephritis.

Post Renal Failure. There are no specific diagnostic tests that can be performed on blood and urine of these patients. Clinical suspicion is the most important factor in making this diagnosis. Renal scan and echo studies of the kidney can be helpful in diagnosing obstructive uropathy and have the advantage of being noninvasive. A plain film of the abdomen can also be of help. Intravenous pyelography is useful if there is sufficient residual renal function. Unilateral retrograde studies become necessary if obstruction is suspected and the above studies are inconclusive. The work-up of obstructive uropathy should be done in cooperation with an experienced urologist.

Differential Diagnosis Between Prerenal Failure and ATN. It is of utmost importance to diagnose immediately prerenal failure due to dehydration or decreased cardiac output, because prolonged prerenal failure is often an important factor predisposing to ATN and because the treatment of prerenal failure is different from the treatment of ATN.

Patients with an acute deterioration of renal function should always be evaluated for clinical signs of dehydration, sepsis or heart failure. Evaluation of skin turgor, orthostatic blood pressure changes, peripheral perfusion, and signs of infection are essential.

Evaluation of urine chemistries can also be helpful in diagnosing prerenal azotemia. During prerenal failure, the body tries to preserve volume by maximal secretion of aldosterone and ADH. The urine therefore is highly concentrated (specific gravity more than 1.018, osmolality in urine more than 600 mOsm. per liter, urine creatinine more than 100 mg. per dl. (100 ml.), urea nitrogen in urine more than 1000 mg. per dl., sodium in urine less than 20 mEq. per liter, potassium in urine more than 30 mEq. per liter, sodium-potassium ratio in urine less than 1.0). In ATN, the tubular cells cannot manipulate filtered urine. Therefore, the urine is usually isosthenuric (specific gravity 1.010, the osmolality is less than 400, creatinine less than 70 mg. per dl., urea nitrogen less than 200 mg. per dl.,

sodium more than 20 mEq. per liter, potassium less than 30 mEq. per liter, sodium-potassium ratio in urine more than 1.0). However, all these tests have a large overlap. Currently, the best way to differentiate from prerenal failure is to measure the fractional excretion of sodium (FeNa). To obtain this, urine sodium is divided by serum sodium and multiplied by the ratio of the serum creatinine over urine creatinine. This is then multiplied by 100 to obtain percentage.

$$FeNa =$$

$$\frac{\text{Urine Sodium (mEq. per liter)} \times \text{Serum Creatinine (mg. per dl.)}}{\text{Serum Sodium (mEq. per liter)} \times \text{Urine Creatinine (mg. per dl.)}}$$

$$\times 100$$

If the FeNa test is less than 1, good tubular function is present and the patient is probably dehydrated. If the FeNa is over 2.0, acute tubular necrosis is probably at hand. The FeNa test should thus be obtained on all patients with acute renal failure in order to help distinguish prerenal azotemia from ATN. In the dehydrated patient, volume must be promptly restored; otherwise, persistent dehydration may lead to ATN. Alternatively, if excessive fluid is given to the patient with ATN, pulmonary edema may result.

Acute Parenchymal Renal Disease. Acute inflammatory disease of the kidney can be responsible for rapid deterioration of renal function. The history and physical examination will often suggest the presence of a systemic disease that might be associated with glomerulonephritis or acute interstitial nephritis. Careful examination of the urinary sediment is, of course, critical if this diagnosis is to be made. (Please see section about glomerular disorders.)

Etiologic Treatment

It is hoped that mannitol and furosemide might alter or reverse the pathologic process within the kidney that causes the renal failure.

When confronted with a patient with acute renal failure, after having eliminated as well as possible on initial laboratory and physical examination those patients with prerenal and postrenal failure, we have generally used one or both of these agents.

Mannitol, 50 ml. of a 25 per cent solution can

be infused, and this can be repeated after 1 to 2 hours. It must not be used in a fluid overloaded patient as the osmotic load will exacerbate the problem. Furosemide (Lasix) can also be given as an infusion of 2 mg. per kg. over 30 minutes. If there is no effect in one to two hours, 5 to 10 mg. per kg. is infused (this dose exceeds the dose recommended by the manufacturer). If diuresis ensues, additional doses of intravenous furosemide can be given as required or an infusion of 100 to 1000 mg. furosemide in 500 ml. of 20 per cent mannitol can be infused at a rate of 10 to 20 ml. per hour. Serum osmolality must be checked so that mannitol intoxication does not ensue and the drugs must not be given if diuresis does not persist. We believe that sometimes these measures will result in return of renal function. At other times, only urine volume increases. This is advantageous, however, because more carrier volume can then be given patients and this eases electrolyte balance, hyperalimentation, and the use of intravenous medications.

The chart should be carefully checked for the use of nephrotoxic drugs and these should be discontinued.

Symptomatic Treatment

Fluid Overload. This is one of the problems contributing to early death. The patient must be weighed daily and careful intake and output recorded. An increase in weight signals fluid overload. The patient will lose approximately 0.3 to 0.5 kg. per day if adequate nutrition is not given. The most dangerous complication of fluid overload is pulmonary edema. Daily auscultation of the heart and lungs, and frequent chest x-rays should be performed. Frequent vital signs, and sometimes central venous pressure and pulmonary wedge pressure should also be monitored in the acute resuscitation period particularly if the physician gives a fluid challenge in the early period before ascertaining how much prerenal failure is at hand.

Fluid overload should be treated with fluid removal, not digitalis. Fluids can be removed by not replacing ongoing losses. If the situation is more urgent and the patient does not respond to furosemide (Lasix), sorbitol can be given to the patient with a functioning gastrointestinal tract as a 70 per cent solution orally, 2 ml. per kg. If vomiting occurs, trimethobenzamide (Tigan), 200 mg., is given intramuscularly and the sorbitol dose repeated after 45 minutes. If there is continued vomiting, sorbitol can be given as a 20 per cent solution 5 to 10 ml. per kg. as a retention enema. The use of a Foley catheter with a large 30 ml. balloon and taping the buttocks helps the patient retain the enema. If the gastrointestinal tract is not functioning, the only way to remove fluids is through dialysis with ultrafiltration.

Hyperkalemia. Hyperkalemia is another cause of early death in patients with acute renal failure. The patient dies because potassium is cardiotoxic. Six mEq. per liter of potassium is dangerous and over 7 mEq. per liter is urgently life-threatening. The ECG goes from mild (tented T wave, high T wave) to moderate (prolongation of the PR interval, depressed ST segment) to severe intoxication (auricular standstill, intraventricular block, ventricular fibrillation with sine wave and ventricular standstill). It is best checked in lead V_3-V_6.

Hyperacute hyperkalemia is treated by infusion of 10 per cent calcium gluconate; 10 ml. is infused every 1 to 2 minutes under ECG observation until signs of only moderate toxicity are present. This may take up to 50 ml. of 10 per cent calcium gluconate infused over 10 to 30 minutes. Sodium bicarbonate infused intravenously also is instantaneously active against potassium intoxication.

In the less acute situation or after the above measures, potassium can be forced back into cells through the use of a glucose, insulin, and bicarbonate drip. A suitable infusion consists of 500 ml. 50 per cent glucose in water with 30 units insulin and 100 mEq. sodium lactate and 20 ml. 10 per cent calcium chloride. The sodium lactate is metabolized to bicarbonate in the body. The infusion rate is 100 ml. the first hour, then 20 to 30 ml. per hour. This shifts potassium to the intracellular space. The effect can be expected approximately one half hour after the start of the infusion and the effect diminishes almost immediately after the infusion is stopped. The solution must be given through a central line. Because the above measures do not actually remove potassium from the body, patients with acute hyperkalemia should be treated concomitantly with a Na-K exchange resin (Kayexalate). Thirty to 60 grams are given either orally together with 100 ml. of 20 per cent sorbitol or in 500 ml. of water as a retention enema. The use of Kayexalate in this setting is not necessary if dialysis is imminent. All these methods of treating hyperkalemia, except dialysis, also aggravate fluid and sodium overload and therefore are unsuitable for a patient who is both hyperkalemic and fluid overloaded.

Acidosis. Another major metabolic complication of acute renal failure is acidosis. Bicarbonate levels should therefore be measured daily and treatment should be initiated if the bicarbonate falls below 15 mEq. per liter. Treatment consists of the infusion of sodium bicarbonate. One can calculate the approximate amount of bicarbonate necessary to correct the acidosis by subtracting the actual measured bicarbonate value from the laboratory's normal value, and then multiply this by half body weight (normal bicarbonate-measured bicarbonate) × body weight × 0.5. This formula increasingly underestimates the bicarbonate need, the more severe and the more long-standing the acidosis is. Correction of acidosis by this method also contributes to fluid overload and in the situation in which fluid overload and severe acidosis coexist, dialysis is the only solution.

Hyperphosphatemia. All patients with renal failure develop hyperphosphatemia. They should be given aluminum hydroxide or calcium carbonate (Amphojel, Alu-Caps, Dialume, Basaljel). The usual starting dose is 30 ml. of Amphojel 4 times daily. Magnesium-containing antacids must never be used because of the possibility of magnesium intoxication.

Calcium. All patients with renal failure have moderate hypocalcemia that usually requires no treatment.

Uremia. Uremia is an invariable consequence of renal failure. It should be combatted through the use of a proper diet with high caloric content and 1 gram of protein per kg. (high biologic value protein) and low sodium (2 grams Na) and potassium (2 grams K). An anabolic steroid, nandrolone phenpropionate (Durabolin, 100 mg. intramuscularly twice weekly), should also be used. The old treatment with butterballs and glucose orally is inappropriate. Patients who can eat should be given a palatable diet and dialyzed rather than put on such severely restricted diets. Multivitamin tablets should also be given.

Frequently, patients cannot eat. When they have been resuscitated, hyperalimentation containing 1 gram per kg. of amino acids, 2 grams of carbohydrates per kg., and 2 grams of fat per kg. daily should be used. Because of inevitable fluid overload, this cannot be given to the oliguric patient without daily dialysis to remove the carrier solution.

Dialysis

Dialysis should be used early in these patients. The blood urea nitrogen (BUN) should not be allowed to rise above 100 to 125 mg. per dl., nor should the creatinine be allowed to rise over 10 to 12 mg. per dl. Hyperkalemia with a potassium over 6 mEq. per liter or acidosis with a bicarbonate value below 15 mEq. per liter should never be allowed. Early and frequent dialysis improves the prognosis in these patients.

Both peritoneal and hemodialysis are effective in correcting the abnormalities of metabolism and fluid balance that occur in acute renal failure. Peritoneal dialysis has the advantage of being more gradual and therefore less stressful to the cardiovascular system. Hemodialysis, however, is more efficient. Patients with acute renal failure should be transferred to a facility that is proficient in the use of either procedure and that also has available surgeons, anesthesiologists, and internists trained in dealing with these desperately ill patients.

Complications of Acute Renal Failure

Infections. Infection is responsible for two thirds of the deaths in patients with acute renal failure. Many sources of infection are iatrogenic. Indwelling urinary catheters are almost never needed after the resuscitation phase and may give rise to urinary tract infection, pyelonephritis and septicemia. Condom catheters for men and special plastic bag catheters are available for children and women to collect urine. It is better to be incontinent in bed than to have an indwelling catheter causing pyelonephritis and septicemia.

Central venous and pulmonary wedge pressure catheters become infected if left in for prolonged periods. Once acute resuscitation is over, all these catheters should be removed.

Patients should be mobilized and receive physical therapy to prevent pulmonary infections. Temperature is an unreliable sign of infection, as urea is a potent antipyretic. Clinical signs of peritonitis are also frequently absent in these desperately ill patients. Repeated cultures of urine, wound drainage, sputum, and feces should therefore be done and appropriate antibiotics used. Surgical complications are very common and must be sought carefully. In patients with acute renal failure after abdominal surgery, reoperation will often reveal an inapparent intra-abdominal infection. Appropriate treatment will sometimes result in recovery of renal function and patient survival. If untreated, such complications are invariably fatal. Nystatin (Mycostatin), 400,000 units every 4 hours, should be given, "swish and swallow," or through a nasogastric tube, as Candida suprainfections are common.

Drug Elimination. Many drugs are eliminated through the kidneys. Before any drug is used, one should therefore consult recent lists of how to modify the dosage of such drugs (Bennett, W. M. et al.: Ann. Intern. Med., *86*:754, 1977; Anderson, R. J. et al.: Clinical Use of Drugs in Renal Failure. Charles C Thomas, 1976).

Many antibiotics and many digitalis preparations are eliminated through the kidneys and need dose modification. No magnesium-containing medications, such as several antacids and milk-of-magnesia, should be used because they may give rise to magnesium intoxication.

Gastrointestinal Complications. Many patients with acute renal failure die because of bleeding stress ulcers. They should therefore receive prophylactic aluminum hydroxide (Amphojel), 30 ml. four times daily, and cimetidine (Tagamet),

300 mg. twice daily. Pancreatitis and perforation of small or large intestines may occur and should be treated appropriately.

Cardiovascular Complications. Cardiac arrhythmias and heart failure, frequently due to electrolyte abnormalities and fluid overload, are dealt with earlier. Pericarditis occurs with extreme uremia and can be cured only by dialysis.

Hematologic Complications. Anemia invariably occurs secondary to renal failure. However, acidosis and hyperphosphatemia increase oxygen delivery. There is usually no need to transfuse these patients unless the hemoglobin level is below 75 to 50 per cent of normal. Watch for fluid overload with transfusions.

Coagulation Complications. With increasing uremia, platelet function decreases. Platelet transfusions are not helpful in this circumstance, as the transfused platelet does not function normally in uremic plasma. Because of the effect of uremia on platelet function, bleeding can be an indication for dialysis in the uremic patient.

Neurologic Complications. Confusion, myoclonus, asterixis, and, in severe cases, seizures are consequences of severe uremia and electrolyte imbalances and thus indicate that the patient has been incorrectly treated. They should be dealt with through dialysis and correction of electrolytes. Particularly dangerous is hyponatremia secondary to fluid overload. Symptomatic seizures are treated through the use of 2 to 5 mg. diazepam (Valium) intravenously while arrangements are being made for dialysis and electrolytes are being normalized.

Recovery Phase

Acute tubular necrosis is usually limited to 3 to 4 weeks. Return of renal function is heralded by an increase in urine output. All patients go through a period in which they are diuresing but cannot by themselves maintain homeostasis. Sodium, potassium, bicarbonate, and weight therefore need to be carefully monitored in this phase and appropriately replaced. Sometimes patients develop significant polyuria. For the first 12 hours, urine should be replaced with fluid, milliliter for milliliter. The patient can then be increasingly deficited (reduction of fluid intake) as the high urine output frequently signifies that the patient is getting rid of extra fluid. Vital signs (blood pressure and pulse rate), and sometimes central venous and pulmonary capillary wedge pressure need to be followed closely during this period.

Almost all patients are left with some slight degree of renal malfunction. However, this is usually not of any clinical consequence and can be detected only through sophisticated renal function studies.

Prognosis

Acute renal failure has an extremely grave prognosis: 20 to 40 per cent of patients with a medical cause, and up to 80 per cent of patients with acute postoperative ATN die. Age is not particularly important prognostically; children with ATN have as high a death rate as the very old. Everyone should therefore be vigorously treated. Again, infection is the most common cause of death.

Prophylaxis

Acute tubular necrosis (ATN) is particularly common in dehydrated patients after major and prolonged operations and in patients who already have defects in homeostatic mechanisms (diabetics, preexisting renal failure, addisonian patients, etc.). It is of utmost importance to see that these patients are not dehydrated when they go to surgery. In high risk patients a drip of 20 per cent mannitol, to which has been added 100 to 500 mg. of furosemide and run at 5 to 20 ml. per hour to maintain a urine output of 100 to 200 ml. per hour, may prevent a decline in renal function. It is very important to replace the urine excreted with 0.45 per cent saline solution to which has been added 20 mEq. of KCl per liter.

Acute Exacerbation of Chronic Renal Failure

Patients with preexisting chronic renal failure are particularly sensitive to dehydration and may develop acute exacerbation. The problems are the same as in patients with acute tubular necrosis, but their management is particularly difficult, as they already have the deranged renal capability to begin with. They therefore need particularly close supervision when being rehydrated (see Chronic Renal Failure).

Conclusion

1. Acute renal failure (due to acute tubular necrosis) (ATN) is usually iatrogenic. Dehydration and nephrotoxic antibiotics are common causes.

2. Through the use of careful clinical investigation and the FeNa test, it is important to differentiate prerenal failure from ATN early. Prerenal failure needs fluids; ATN patients may be harmed by fluids.

3. Early ATN may be reversed through the use of intravenous mannitol and furosemide or at least switched from an oliguric to a polyuric phase, easing management.

4. Early deaths are caused by fluid overload, hyperkalemia, and acidosis.

5. Late deaths are caused by infections, frequently secondary to overlooked surgical complications that should be managed by aggressive

surgery, repeated cultures, and appropriate antibiotics. Nystatin should be given prophylactically.

Gastrointestinal bleeding can be prevented by the use of aluminum hydroxide and cimetidine.

6. Good oral nutrition with a diet of 70 grams of protein, 2 grams of Na^+, 2 grams of K^+ and high in calories or hyperalimentation. Early dialysis and anabolic steroids should be used.

7. Catheters in the bladder and blood vessels must be removed after the patient has been resuscitated.

CHRONIC RENAL FAILURE

method of
MORRIS DAVIDMAN, M.D.,
and FRED L. SHAPIRO, M.D.
Minneapolis, Minnesota

The diseases responsible for chronic renal failure include: primary glomerular disease (glomerulonephritis), chronic interstitial nephritis (including pyelonephritis), polycystic kidney disease, hypertensive nephrosclerosis and renal disease secondary to such systemic diseases as diabetes mellitus, lupus erythematosus, generalized vasculitis, and amyloidosis. Although prevention of chronic renal failure is the ultimate goal, specific prevention or therapy is unknown except for a few renal diseases. However, the rate of progression of renal insufficiency and the tolerance of the disease by the patient may be positively influenced by appropriate medical management.

This chapter will discuss the following principles of management of chronic renal insufficiency: (1) prevention of chronic renal disease, (2) specific treatment of the underlying pathologic process, (3) retarding progressive functional deterioration by treating aggravating complications, (4) maintenance of homeostasis by dietary, fluid, electrolyte and mineral manipulation, and (5) preparation of the patient for dialysis or transplantation.

Prevention of Chronic Renal Disease

Hypertension. Long-standing untreated hypertension is a major cause of cardiovascular morbidity and renal failure. It is now well accepted that the early diagnosis and treatment of hypertension can prevent, or at least delay, the onset of vascular complications, including nephrosclerosis. Malignant hypertension consistently results in rapidly progressive renal failure and its early aggressive management may reverse or arrest most of the underlying renal vascular pathology.

Analgesic Abuse. Analgesics containing phenacetin, when used in large amounts over pro-

longed periods of time, are a common cause of chronic interstitial nephritis and renal failure. In some countries, the addition of phenacetin to analgesic compounds has been prohibited. In the United States, phenacetin-containing analgesic compounds are still widely available. Patients with chronic pain syndromes should be cautioned about the danger of excessive use of phenacetin-containing analgesics. Should the diagnosis of analgesic nephropathy be made when renal function is still adequate, discontinuation of the drug frequently results in improved or stable renal function.

Urinary Tract Obstruction and Infection. Urinary tract obstruction may cause irreversible renal disease. Occasionally, chronic renal parenchymal infection without obstruction may lead to chronic renal failure. The combination of obstruction and infection may be rapidly destructive and should be managed as an urgent problem to prevent irreversible renal damage. Relief of obstruction may improve or at least stabilize renal function.

Other Causes of Chronic Interstitial Nephritis. Long-standing hypercalcemia, hypokalemia, and hyperuricemia have been implicated as causes of progressive interstitial disease of the kidney. These conditions are preventable causes of renal failure. They may also occur as a complicating factor in other types of renal disease and may precipitate acute exacerbations of renal failure.

Specific Treatment of Underlying Disease

It is beyond the scope of this discussion to elaborate in detail about specific treatment of the underlying disease. However, when evaluating a patient with evidence of early renal insufficiency, a specific diagnosis should be established whenever possible, so that definitive treatment may be prescribed. As an example, systemic diseases such as Wegener's granulomatosis and lupus erythematosus may be controlled with steroids or immunosuppressive agents or both. There is recent evidence to suggest that glomerular diseases caused by antiglomerular basement membrane antibody (Goodpasture's syndrome) may be retarded by early immunosuppressive drug therapy and repeated plasmaphoresis if treatment is instituted before oliguria and advanced renal failure have supervened. Obstructive, analgesic, uric acid, and hypercalcemic nephropathy may all respond to specific therapy.

Retarding Progressive Functional Deterioration

The rate of progression of chronic renal disease depends upon the primary disorder. For example, membranous nephropathy usually progresses very slowly, whereas diabetic glomerulosclerosis progresses at a more rapid rate. Therefore, knowing the primary renal disease and its natural rate of progression is very helpful in following patients with renal insufficiency. If unexpected accelerated deterioration ensues, complicating conditions should be sought and treated.

The rate of progression of renal insufficiency may be followed by relatively simple measurements—blood urea nitrogen (BUN), serum creatinine, and creatinine clearance. The BUN concentration is a result of the balance between urea generation and renal urea excretion. Urea generation depends upon dietary protein intake and endogenous production from protein catabolism. Urea excretion depends upon glomerular filtration rate (GFR) and tubular reabsorption. Thus, the final BUN can be modified by many factors in addition to a change in GFR. Normally, the BUN and serum creatinine ratio is about 15:1. If this ratio remains constant, it suggests that the change in BUN results from a change in GFR. A ratio of more than 15:1 indicates increased urea generation or increased tubular reabsorption. Examples of increased urea generation include a very high protein diet, bleeding into the gastrointestinal tract, steroid therapy, and tetracycline therapy. Increased tubular reabsorption of urea occurs in volume depleted states. A ratio of less than 10:1 often indicates a low dietary intake of protein.

The serum creatinine concentration is a better index of renal function than the BUN because creatinine is produced at a constant rate and is excreted mainly by glomerular filtration. In an individual patient, once the serum creatinine is correlated with a creatinine clearance measurement, then further elevations in serum creatinine will be inversely proportional to the filtration rate; i.e., if the creatinine doubles, the clearance halves.

The necessity to compare serum creatinine and creatinine clearance in a given patient results from the fact that serum creatinine is a function of muscle mass. Therefore, females and older patients with somewhat diminished muscle mass will have a lower clearance than more muscular patients with the same serum creatinine concentration.

Clinically, it is useful to divide chronic renal insufficiency into three stages; mild, moderate, and severe. Mild renal insufficiency corresponds to a serum creatinine up to 3 mg. per dl. (100 ml.) and is typically asymptomatic although hypertension may be present. Moderate renal insufficiency corresponds to serum creatinine concentrations between 3 and 8 mg. per dl. Patients with this degree of renal insufficiency notice increasing fatigability, hypertension becomes more severe,

TABLE 1. **Manifestations of Uremia**

GENERAL	CIRCULATORY
Weakness, lethargy*	Heart failure*
Nocturnal sleeplessness	Pericarditis
Pruritus, dry scaly skin, anhidrosis	Hypertension*
Loss of libido	Edema, occasionally dehydration
Bone pain, fractures	
Arthritis	
GASTROINTESTINAL	NEUROMUSCULAR
Anorexia, nausea, vomiting*	Apathy, depression, confusion
Diarrhea	Seizures, coma
Pancreatitis	Tremulousness, cramps
Bleeding	Peripheral neuritis
	Visual and auditory impairment
	Asterixis

HEMATOLOGIC
Anemia*
Hemorrhagic tendencies*

*Most frequent symptoms.

and anemia appears. Severe renal insufficiency is manifested clinically by the uremic syndrome with symptoms referrable to all systems (Table 1) and typically occurs when the serum creatinine exceeds 8 mg. per dl., which corresponds to a GFR of less than 15 ml. per minute. However, when renal function deteriorates rapidly, severe uremic symptoms may appear with serum creatinine level below 8 mg. per dl. On the other hand, patients with very slowly progressive renal failure may be totally unaware of ill health at serum creatinine levels above 10 mg. per dl.

Hypertension. Hypertension is a frequent complication of chronic renal disease and may contribute to the deterioration of renal function in a previously stable patient. Typically, patients with glomerular disease will manifest increasing hypertension as GFR falls. This is mainly due to progressive extracellular volume expansion. Patients with interstitial nephropathy are often salt and water "wasters" and hypertension may be absent even in the late stages of renal insufficiency. Hypervolemia may not be the only mediator of increasing blood pressure in chronic renal disease. In some instances, an increased plasma level of angiotensin II secondary to hyper-reninemia is involved. Recent work suggests that urinary kallikrein excretion is low in renal failure patients, providing a possible role for abnormalities in vasoactive polypeptide metabolism. Patients with polycystic kidney disease may become hypertensive early in the course of their disease without evidence of volume overload or renin hypersecretion.

Irrespective of the pathogenesis, hypertension should be detected and treated to prevent hypertensive renovascular damage. Generally, the therapy of hypertension in renal disease is similar to the management of essential hypertension. Sodium restriction to 2 grams per day plus a diuretic constitutes the first step in treatment. Thiazide diuretics are suitable if the GFR is above 30 ml. per minute. With more severe degrees of renal insufficiency, a loop diuretic, e.g., furosemide, is usually required. The use of diuretics must be modified by the conflicting goals of blood pressure control and maintenance of extracellular volume. Whereas in patients with normal renal function, moderate volume depletion may be tolerated, this is not so in renal insufficiency. Therefore, in hypertensive patients with renal insufficiency, other antihypertensive medications are added to the diuretic rather than attempting to achieve maximum diuresis.

Antihypertensive medications that are highly effective in patients with chronic renal disease include propranolol, methyldopa, and clonidine. In advanced renal insufficiency, methyldopa and clonidine may confuse the assessment of uremic encephalopathy since they both can produce somnolence and lethargy. If the diuretic/antihypertensive drug combination proves inadequate, then the addition of hydralazine or prazosin as vasodilators may be beneficial. With this stepwise approach, blood pressure control with volume preservation can usually be achieved. In a small percentage of patients, accelerated hypertension is resistant to usual antihypertensive regimens. In these patients, minoxidil, a potent vasodilator not yet approved for marketing, has been highly effective when added to a beta blocker, e.g., propranolol, and a diuretic.

Clinically involving the patient in his treatment by having him monitor his weight and blood pressure at home has been highly successful in maintaining optimum control.

Abrupt Change in Renal Function in Previously Stable Patient. DEHYDRATION, INFECTION, OBSTRUCTION. When renal function unexpectedly declines, volume depletion, urinary tract infection, and obstructive uropathy should be considered. Volume depletion is a frequent complicating factor arising from extrarenal salt loss, vigorous diuresis or injudicious salt restriction. The diagnosis is established clinically by the presence of orthostatic hypotension, acute weight loss, poor skin turgor, and possibly mild hematocrit elevation compared to the usual level for the patient. Measurement of the central venous pressure is rarely necessary to confirm the diagnosis. The method of volume replacement is dependent upon the severity of the situation, but intravenous repletion should be closely monitored.

The presence of fever, back pain, and dysuria suggests a urinary tract infection. Pyuria without bacteriuria does not necessarily indicate infection and usually is a consequence of noninfectious interstitial inflammation of the kidney. Urine cultures should be obtained and appropriate antibiotic therapy initiated with consideration of the proper dosage and toxicity of the drug chosen. Tetracyclines (except doxycycline) and nitrofurantoin, are contraindicated in renal insufficiency.

Bladder outlet obstruction should be suspected when the patient complains of hesitancy, thin stream, frequency, and incontinence. The bladder may be palpated clinically, and a residual urine measurement confirms the diagnosis. A voiding cystourethrogram will document the obstruction radiographically as well as demonstrating vesicoureteral reflux. The diagnosis of upper tract obstruction depends upon radiographic demonstration or retrograde studies or both. It should be noted that patients with incomplete bilateral obstruction of the urinary tract, e.g., retroperitoneal fibrosis, may present clinically with polyuria.

RADIOGRAPHIC CONTRAST MEDIA. It has recently been shown that diabetic patients with serum creatinine levels greater than 2 mg. per dl. are at significant risk for abrupt decline in renal function after intravenous pyelography (IVP). If the serum creatinine is greater than 4 mg. per dl., the renal functional deterioration may be irreversible. Patients with multiple myeloma or hyperuricemia are at a greater risk of developing renal failure after an IVP. The use of radiographic contrast material is hazardous in patients with renal disease. If a dye study is indicated, adequate hydration is an important prerequisite. The statement that "a dehydrated kidney is a kidney at risk" is a valid clinical dictum supported by experimental data.

DRUG TOXICITY. All drugs administered to patients with renal disease are potentially dangerous. Phenacetin-containing analgesics, tetracyclines (except for doxycycline), methicillin, aminoglycoside antibiotics, cephaloridine, amphotericin B, and gold are a few drugs that are particularly hazardous in renal insufficiency. (The reader is referred to J.A.M.A., *230*:1544, 1974, for a comprehensive discussion of drug therapy in renal failure.)

CONGESTIVE HEART FAILURE. The development of congestive heart failure in a patient with chronic renal disease will result in a reduction of renal blood flow and GFR. Management of the heart failure with antihypertensive medication, digoxin, and sodium modification can improve renal function. Digoxin is primarily excreted by the kidney and, therefore, dose reduction is necessary. A dose of 0.125 mg. daily is usually adequate. The patient should be followed with plasma digoxin levels.

The Maintenance of Homeostasis

Chronic progressive renal diseases, regardless of cause, pathogenesis, and pathologic expression, have one major common denominator— the relentless destruction of nephrons. The pathophysiologic abnormalities of chronic renal insufficiency begin with the earliest loss of nephrons and the subsequent reduction of GFR. Several pathophysiologic adaptations to maintain homeostasis occur as renal insufficiency progresses. An understanding of these changes is helpful in optimizing treatment. Therefore, a brief description of a few of these adaptations follows.

There is a direct relationship between a decrease in GFR and an increase in parathyroid hormone release. As GFR falls, phosphate retention ensues, resulting in a decrease in ionized calcium. Decreased ionized calcium stimulates an increase in parathyroid hormone release, which in turn suppresses tubular phosphate reabsorption, which restores the serum phosphate to normal. Thus, early in the course of renal insufficiency, the serum calcium and phosphorus remain normal but at the expense of an increasing release of parathyroid hormone. The active metabolite of vitamin D, 1, 25-dihydroxycholecalciferol, is produced by the kidney. As renal disease progresses, the availability of this metabolite decreases, resulting in decreased calcium absorption by the gut and further stimulation of the parathyroid glands to release parathyroid hormone. Finally, when the GFR drops below about 20 ml. per minute, increasing parathyroid hormone levels cannot further increase renal excretion of phosphate and the patient develops hyperphosphatemia and hypocalcemia. Although symptomatic renal osteodystrophy is extremely rare in mild renal insufficiency, the factors that ultimately result in this complication come into play early in the course of the renal disease.

Similar adaptations occur with regard to salt and water homeostasis and acid-base metabolism. As the GFR declines and, if the patient maintains a salt and water intake in excess of his excretory capacity, the consequence is an expanding extracellular fluid volume. This is followed by decreasing tubular reabsorption of salt and water, so that as a renal insufficiency progresses, the fractional excretion of sodium (amount excreted/ amount filtered) continues to rise. The normal person has a fractional excretion of sodium of about 1 per cent; the patient with late renal insufficiency may have a fractional excretion of 10 per cent. Salt and water homeostasis is thus maintained but at the expense of an expanded extracellular fluid volume, hypertension, and possibly heart failure.

As renal mass is lost, the acid excretion per nephron increases and, with moderate renal insufficiency, acid-base parameters are normal. However, when the GFR falls below 20 ml. per minute, total acid excretion no longer balances production and metabolic acidosis ensues. Another consequence of declining nephron mass is the reduction of the capacity of the kidney to produce erythropoietic factor, which contributes to the anemia.

A direct consequence of the fall in GFR is a loss of excretory capacity by the kidney. This leads to increasing accumulation of many compounds in the body fluid. Among these compounds are urea, ammonia, organic acids, phenols, and guanidines. Many of these compounds are the nitrogenous end products of protein metabolism and, when elevated, contribute to the development of uremic symptoms. A specific uremic toxin has not been defined. This increasing plasma solute concentration in the face of declining nephron mass results in solute diuresis and is clinically manifested as polyuria and nocturia. The large urine flow rate provides for adequate potassium excretion in the urine and increasing serum potassium is not usually a problem until the daily urine volume falls below a liter.

In severe renal insufficiency, carbohydrate and lipid metabolism is abnormal. Hyperglycemia in the presence of hyperinsulinemia and hyperglucagonemia occurs. Lipid abnormalities occur in high incidence and, for the most part, are of the Type IV hyperlipoproteinemia type. The carbohydrate abnormalities appear to be improved by dialysis. In contrast, in the diabetic patient with progressive renal insufficiency, the half-life of insulin increases because the kidney is one of the sites of insulin degradation. This probably accounts for the commonly observed clinical fact that as renal failure progresses in a diabetic, insulin requirements fall.

In summary, as renal insufficiency progresses, there ensues a series of adaptive mechanisms that tend to maintain homeostasis until the limits of adaptation are exceeded, at which point biochemical abnormalities and clinical deterioration become identifiable. Because of loss of their further ability to compensate adaptively, patients with advanced renal insufficiency cannot withstand excesses or deficiencies in electrolytes or fluids. Treatment of these patients is directed toward prevention of excesses and deficiencies and intervention with therapy when appropriate.

Dietary Management. SALT AND WATER INTAKE. Patients with advanced chronic renal insufficiency do not conserve or excrete sodium normally. Inadequate sodium intake may result in volume depletion and a decrease in GFR. If sodium intake exceeds renal excretory capacity, then hypertension and possibly congestive heart failure may develop. The objective is, therefore, to determine the sodium intake that regulates the extracellular fluid volume in each patient optimally for maintenance of GFR without cardiac decompensation or severe hypertension. To achieve this may require no sodium restriction, mild to moderate restriction, or possibly even supplemental sodium intake. The clinical guides are a stable body weight and serum creatinine level without evidence of severe hypertension, congestive heart failure, or significant edema. Fluids may usually be allowed ad libitum to satisfy thirst until the patient becomes oliguric. Forcing fluids to patients with advanced renal insufficiency is potentially dangerous because of their inability to excrete the water load.

POTASSIUM INTAKE. Because of the high urine flow of patients with chronic renal insufficiency, potassium balance is usually not a problem until the daily urine output falls below 1 liter. There are, however, some exceptions to this observation. Sudden potassium excesses can result in acute hyperkalemia. If the patient's serum potassium should exceed 5 mEq. per liter, dietary restriction of high potassium foods should be instituted. If hyperkalemia persists after reducing the potassium intake below 70 mEq. per day, the diagnosis of hyporeninemic hypoaldosteronism should be considered. This diagnosis is being made more frequently in patients who are not taking potassium-sparing diuretics who have a GFR of between 20 and 30 ml. per minute and unexplained hyperkalemia. If the plasma renin and urinary aldosterone suggest this diagnosis, then the hyperkalemia can be managed by the institution of 100 to 300 micrograms per day of 9-alphafluorohydrocortisone (fludrocortisone).

NUTRITIONAL MANAGEMENT. The goals of nutritional therapy are to maintain blood urea at a level that does not cause symptoms and at the same time maintain nutritional balance. Dietary manipulation is not required until the GFR falls to about 30 ml. per minute. Usually with this GFR patients are still asymptomatic, and a protein intake of 1 gram per kg. of body weight avoiding high phosphate content foods such as dairy products should be prescribed. This degree of moderate protein restriction is palatable and well accepted by patients, and may prove useful in controlling the serum phosphorus level without the need for phosphate binders.

When the GFR falls below 20 ml. per minute, it is common for uremic symptoms to develop. At that time, further protein restriction, while maintaining a caloric intake, is indicated. Strict protein restriction in a patient with advanced renal insuf-

ficiency is a two-edged sword. The control of symptoms may be accomplished at the expense of negative nitrogen balance and, therefore, patient nutrition. Positive nitrogen balance can be maintained with a protein intake as low as 0.5 gram per kg. of body weight, providing the protein is of high biologic value and dietary calories are adequate. High biologic value proteins are those that contain a high proportion of essential amino acids. These proteins are found in animal food sources such as eggs, milk, cheese, fish, meat, and fowl. The low biologic value proteins include flour, cereals, vegetables, and fruits.

An adequate caloric intake is of major importance in achieving successful diet therapy. In order to prevent endogenous protein catabolism, a minimum of 30 calories per kg. of body weight is required. This must be supplied mostly as carbohydrate and fat when protein is significantly restricted. If the patient is not obese and is reasonably active, his caloric intake should be increased to a maximum of 50 calories per kg. of body weight.

Although a protein-restricted diet is usually low in salt, the salt intake should be assessed periodically and appropriate intake prescribed as described previously. It is also important that protein-restricted renal diets be supplemented with vitamins and minerals, particularly vitamin B complex, calcium, and iron.

In following diet therapy, a BUN to creatinine ratio of less than 10:1 and a serum albumin of over 3.3 grams per dl. are biochemical values that indicate effective compliance and response. If the serum albumin is low, then negative nitrogen balance exists and the protein intake should be increased.

Diets that are predominantly of high biologic value protein are monotonous and patient compliance may be poor. However, the diet is so effective in relieving uremic gastrointestinal symptoms that patients are motivated to follow instructions. Low protein renal diet manuals are available to assist in planning a varied and appetizing diet.

Recent reports have shown that positive nitrogen balance can be achieved with a 20 gram unqualified protein diet if 10 to 20 grams of essential amino acids, including histidine, are added to the diet daily. The 20 grams unqualified protein diet is less monotonous and more palatable than the high biologic value protein-restricted diets. The problem is that there is no readily available essential amino acid preparation that is palatable to all patients. When essential amino acids are available in gelatin capsule form, their use may become more widespread. Recently, ketoacid analogs of essential amino acids have been reported to provide a non-nitrogen source for essential amino acid production and, therefore, may be useful in dietary supplementation.

Dietary therapy has been most successful for long-term management in patients with advanced renal insufficiency whose urine output are in excess of 2 liters daily. In our experience with patients whose urine volumes are less than 1500 ml. daily, dialysis is usually required within 6 months.

Calcium and Phosphorus Homeostasis. Theoretically, dietary phosphorus should be restricted with the earliest decrease of GFR to prevent secondary hyperparathyroidism, which accompanies chronic renal insufficiency. Practically, attempts to control phosphorus metabolism are usually begun when the patient's serum creatinine is approximately 3 mg. per dl. or a GFR of 30 ml. per minute. Initially, decrease in protein intake, particularly of high phosphate foods, such as dairy products, is effective in controlling the serum phosphate at the desired level of 4.0 to 4.5 mg. per dl. If this cannot be accomplished by diet alone, then aluminum hydroxide antacids are added as phosphate binders. It is important to give the aluminum hydroxide either in tablet, capsule, or liquid form with meals to accomplish the phosphate binding. Because of recent concern of aluminum toxicity in patients receiving maintenance dialysis, the smallest amount of aluminum hydroxide possible should be used to control the serum phosphate. Serum phosphate levels lower than 4 mg. per dl. potentially will result in osteomalacia and serum levels much higher than 5 mg. per dl. increase the danger of metastatic calcification when calcium control is achieved.

Once phosphorus control has been obtained, 1 to 2 grams of supplemental calcium is added to the diet daily if the patient is not hypercalcemic. The patient's serum calcium should be maintained at about 10 mg. per dl. to assure maximum suppression of the parathyroid glands and adequate mineralization of bone.

If after phosphorus control and elemental calcium addition to the diet the patient is still hypocalcemic, dihydrotachysterol (Hytakerol), 0.25 mg. daily, is judiciously added to the regimen. This preparation has a shorter half-life than does vitamin D_3 and, therefore, toxicity will be easier to manage. Whenever vitamin D preparations are used, serum calcium should be closely monitored. Soon there will be available on the market for clinical use 1, 25-dihydroxycholecalciferol, the active hormone normally produced by the kidney, and also a synthetic analog, 1-alpha hydroxycholecalciferol. There are still questions to be answered about the appropriate time for inclusion of these active drugs in the management of patients with chronic renal insufficiency. It appears that their proper use will provide a major advance in the prevention of bone disease in this population of patients.

Acid-Base Balance. Patients with advanced renal insufficiency tolerate mild acidosis well and usually maintain a serum bicarbonate level of 15 mEq. per liter or greater. Some patients, however, are bicarbonate wasters and may develop a more severe metabolic acidosis. This problem occurs most frequently in patients with primary interstitial renal disease. In patients whose serum bicarbonate level falls below 15 mEq. per liter, supplementation with either sodium bicarbonate or sodium citrate solution is indicated. Shohl's solution, which consists of 140 grams of citric acid and 90 grams of sodium citrate made up with water to 1 liter, is commonly used to treat acidosis. One ml. of this solution will yield 1 mEq. of base and the usual dose is 15 to 30 ml. by mouth 3 times daily. One gram of sodium bicarbonate yields 12 mEq. of bicarbonate, but patients often complain of abdominal bloating when using bicarbonate preparations. Patients who cannot tolerate the additional sodium contained in the alkalinizing agent will need to restrict further their dietary sodium intake.

Patients with chronic renal insufficiency compensate for their metabolic acidosis by chronic pulmonary hyperventilation. Therefore, acute, severe acidosis can occur if there is interference with pulmonary ventilation. Thus, caution must be taken when prescribing drugs that may depress the central nervous system and thereby cause these patients to hypoventilate. Acute pulmonary hypoventilation may occur during the induction phase of anesthesia just before intubation with a rapid pH fall and secondary abrupt hyperkalemia. Finally, acute disturbances in acid-base balance may also occur if there is a sudden increase in the acid load. This commonly occurs in hypercatabolic states, particularly acute infections. Patients with previous stable hydrogen ion balance should be carefully monitored if any of the above clinical settings occur and prophylactic alkalinization instituted if indicated.

Anemia. A normochromic normocytic anemia is usual in chronic renal insufficiency. A search for correctable causes of anemia such as iron deficiency, folic acid deficiency, and vitamin B_{12} deficiency should be made, but in most instances no cause will be found. Physiologically, because of changes in the oxyhemoglobin dissociation curve, there is almost as much oxygen released into the tissues of the uremic patient as in the normal person, even though the uremic's hemoglobin is low. This may be one reason why the uremics tolerate their anemia well and that even if transfused, their hemoglobin will drop within 7 to 10 days to their pretransfusion level. Repeated blood transfusions in the asymptomatic patient increase the risk of iron overload, suppress the bone marrow, may transmit hepatitis, and may stimulate the development of white cell antibodies. Therefore, repeated blood transfusions should not be administered unless the patient is symptomatic of anemia. The symptoms include angina pectoris, severe lethargy, or cerebral ischemia. If the patient with severe renal insufficiency is to undergo major surgery, it is advisable to elevate his hematocrit to at least 25 per cent preoperatively. Packed red cells, administered slowly, should be used for transfusion unless the patient is actively bleeding.

Preparation of Patient for Dialysis or Transplantation

Renal transplantation, chronic hemodialysis, and chronic peritoneal dialysis are satisfactory modalities of treatment for patients with advanced renal insufficiency who can no longer be well controlled with more conservative medical management. These treatments are now widely available throughout the United States. Although these therapies are expensive, patients who require them are entitled to Medicare insurance benefits which, fortunately, provide for the overwhelming majority of the costs.

Dialysis and transplantation are both physically and emotionally stressful to the patients and their families. Much of this stress can be ameliorated or avoided if the patient and his family are adequately informed as to the treatment options, anticipated results, and financial obligations prior to the time that the treatments are initiated. This can best be achieved if the patients are evaluated when their creatinine clearance is less than 20 ml. per minute at renal centers that employ an experienced, multidisciplinary staff team of physicians, nurses, social workers, financial counselors, and dietitians to assist in this important activity.

Dialysis or transplantation should be initiated prior to the time that the patient suffers severe disabling complications of uremia. The indications to commence dialytic therapy include the onset of pericarditis, psychosis, or bleeding diathesis. Malnutrition, uncontrolled hypertension, persistent hyperkalemia, progression of peripheral neuropathy, and chronic fluid overload, separately or in combination, also necessitate chronic hemodialysis or transplantation. A patient's inability to continue work is the usual indication to begin dialysis. The creatinine clearance at this time usually ranges from 3 to 12 ml. per minute, being generally higher in those patients who have associated medical complications who tolerate renal insufficiency poorly.

GENITOURINARY TUBERCULOSIS

method of
BARRY H. USOW, M.D.
Milwaukee, Wisconsin

Tuberculosis of the urinary tract is generally considered to be secondary to the hematogenesis spread of tubercle bacilli from a primary pulmonary lesion. The diagnosis is based on a stained smear showing acid-fast bacilli confirmed by cultures of *Mycobacterium tuberculosis* from a first voided morning specimen, when the urine is most concentrated. A minimum of three cultures, one per morning, should be obtained. However, occasionally tissue aspiration or biopsy may be necessary to make the diagnosis.

A high suspicion of tuberculosis should be entertained if pyuria or hematuria in an acid urine persists without the finding of bacteria or despite antibiotic therapy. Sulfonamides and tetracycline may interfere with cultures and diagnosis so that antibiotics should be discontinued prior to obtaining cultures.

Before initiating therapy, physical examination of the genitalia and prostate should be done to determine concomitant involvement of these organs and an intravenous pyelogram performed to evaluate the extent of disease in the urinary tract. A significant proportion of patients give no history of pulmonary tuberculosis, but a chest x-ray should be performed and skeletal survey to rule out tuberculosis in these areas.

It is no longer necessary to isolate patients to a hospital, but close contacts should be screened for tuberculosis with skin tests and chest x-rays. Children with positive PPD skin tests should be treated for one year with isoniazid (INH). General supportive measures of adequate rest and nutrition are also important. Chemotherapy is the treatment of choice, with surgery playing a very minor role. Treatment is still recommended for two years with follow-up for life, but several centers are reporting short course therapy of 6 months to 1 year with 2 or 3 drug therapy. Combination chemotherapy is utilized to ensure bactericidal treatment with minimal bacterial resistance. The most important facet of treatment is a discussion with the patient to ensure his understanding of the chronicity of the problem, the ease of transmission to his family and friends, the necessity for taking medication as prescribed, and the maintenance of close contact with the physician.

Specific Chemotherapy

Although specific regimens are followed, therapy is individualized to the patient, depending on extent of disease, presence of other underlying problems (hematogenous, gastrointestinal, or hepatic disease), and the clinical response of the patient. As often as possible, oral drugs are utilized with the initial triple drug therapy used until cultures and x-rays become negative (usually 2 to 6 months), followed by 2 drug therapy. The usual primary regimen consists of:

1. Isoniazid (INH), 8 mg. per kg. per day given up to 300 mg. per day, either as a single dose or two times per day.

2. Ethambutol, 25 mg. per kg. per day by mouth as single dose for two weeks, then 15 mg. per kg. per day.

3. Rifampin, 600 mg. per day as single dose or 300 mg. twice per day by mouth.

4. Pyridoxine (vitamin B_6), 100 mg. daily by mouth.

Give isoniazid (INH) and rifampin for 18 to 24 months after cultures are negative. INH is the least toxic of these agents, with infrequent side effects. These are usually dose-related and consist of peripheral neuropathy, convulsions, psychosis, ataxic dizziness, and optic neuritis. Pyridoxine is given to protect against the neuropathy. Hepatic disease also related to INH can occur but is very rare and is unpredictable in any patient and not dose-related. One should question the patient about the use of other long-term medications such as diphenylhydantoin, meprobamate, or hormones. Excessive stimulants should not be used with INH, as it irritates the central nervous system.

Ethambutol is bacteriostatic, acting on RNA synthesis, and can cause retrobulbar neuritis with reduced visual acuity manifesting initially as the inability to perceive the color green. It may be unilateral. All patients should have visual acuity, color vision, and visual fields checked prior to initiation of therapy and at monthly intervals on therapy by a qualified ophthalmologist. This complication resolves with removal of the drug. If renal impairment is a problem, the dose should be altered accordingly, as 85 to 90 per cent of the drug is excreted by the kidney.

Rifampin is bactericidal and acts by inhibiting RNA polymerase. It is relatively nontoxic but may alter liver function tests and rarely cause thrombocytopenia. It is unaffected by renal impairment, as it is excreted by the liver. It may cause a skin rash or "flulike" syndrome in some patients and colors the urine and other body fluids bright orange.

On this regimen, urinary cultures should return to normal in 6 to 8 weeks. Other parameters to check are urinalysis, to determine absence of pyuria and hematuria, and an intravenous pyelogram, to detect healing. If the medication is taken as prescribed and sediment continues to show *Mycobacterium tuberculosis,* sensitivity studies should be performed to determine which drugs are effective and can replace those that are not. At no time should one drug be added to a regimen; rather, all drugs should be tested as to their sensitivity.

Secondary drugs are:

1. Para-aminosalicylic acid (PAS), 5 grams, three times per day orally. The major side effect is gastrointestinal distress. Sodium PAS may decrease these untoward effects of nausea and diarrhea. Allergic reaction of chills, fever, and skin rash are common. However, it is a valuable drug in pregnant women and small children.

2. Cycloserine (Seromycin), 500 mg. once per day or 250 mg. two times per day if better tolerated. A major side effect is its action as a stimulant to the central nervous system with resulting seizures, somnolence, and muscle twitching. Stimulants (amphetamine sulfate, coffee) should not be consumed when the patient is on this drug. Pyridoxine may prevent these side effects.

3. Ethionamide, 250 mg. three times per day, is highly toxic, affecting the gastrointestinal tract and liver, and causing ganglionic blockade.

4. Pyrazinamide, 20 to 35 mg. per kg. per day to a maximum of 3 grams per day, is excreted by the kidneys and can cause hepatic toxicity and elevation of serum uric acid.

5. Streptomycin is given intramuscularly, 1 gram daily for two to three months, then discontinued. Its major side effect is eighth nerve damage with auditory and vestibular impairment and possible renal failure.

Follow-up care of these patients should include monthly urinalysis, complete blood count, liver and renal function studies, acid-fast stains and culture, and bacterial urine culture. Intravenous pyelograms every 3 months for the initial year, every 6 months for the following 2 years, once a year for the following 3 years, and then at 2 year intervals. The intravenous pyelogram is extremely important as infundibular and ureteral scarring can lead to obstruction and may necessitate surgical intervention.

Surgical Management

The necessity for surgery has significantly diminished with better medical management, so that nephrectomy is not commonly performed. Nephrectomy may be required for intractable pain, persistent fever, and positive cultures despite adequate therapy and ureteral stricture not amenable to dilatation or drug intolerance. Hypertension secondary to tuberculosis of the kidney has not necessarily improved following nephrectomy. Heminephrectomy may be indicated for segmental damage or if a solitary kidney is involved.

Ureteral calibration and dilatation is an important facet of care to prevent complete ureteral obstruction. Ureteral reimplantation may be indicated for this complication. Bladder contracture secondary to disease or healing from treatment may necessitate cystoplasty or diversion. Orchiectomy and epididymectomy are only rarely indicated.

The author thanks Thomas Dee, M.D., and Lori Bennett for their assistance in writing this article.

TUMORS OF THE GENITOURINARY TRACT

method of
CLAUDE E. MERRIN, M.D.
Buffalo, New York

PROSTATE

Benign Tumors

The most frequent benign tumor of the prostate gland is the adenoma, which is most commonly termed benign prostatic hyperplasia. It is treated by surgery. The two best techniques, in my opinion, are the transurethral resection and the retropubic prostatectomy using the technique described by Millin.

Malignant Tumors

Adenocarcinoma

Adenocarcinoma is the most common malignant tumor of the prostate. Its peak incidence is in the seventh and eighth decades, but it has been reported as early as the third decade. A great deal of controversy still exists about the best way to treat this disease. The treatment varies with the stage. Therefore, evaluation of the disease should be complete and precise.

Our evaluation consists of intravenous urography, cystoscopy, perineal needle biopsy, lymphography, metastatic radiographic survey (bone and chest), bone scan, liver scan, brain scan, biochemical and hematologic studies, and biologic markers (acid phosphatase). The results of the evaluation permit the categorization of the patients by stages.

STAGE A. Minimal amounts of tumor present in the gland. It is often an incidental finding after transurethral resection.

STAGE B. Nodular prostate on rectal examination. The tumor is still limited to the gland, but a significant amount of normal tissue is replaced by tumor.

STAGE C. Locally invasive tumor with infiltration of the capsule or the seminal vesicles or both.

STAGE D. Metastatic disease.

STAGE D_1. Metastases limited to the pelvis.

STAGE D_2. Metastases outside the pelvis.

Treatment. Our treatment by stages is as follows:

STAGE A. After initial findings of the tumor, we wait 6 to 12 weeks and repeat transurethral resection (TUR) and perineal needle biopsy to rule out residual tumor. If residual tumor is found, the patient is submitted to radical prostatectomy. If no residual tumor is present, the patient is followed every 3 months (with perineal needle biopsy) for 1 year; then every 6 months for 2 years.

STAGE B. The patient is submitted to radical prostatectomy and orchiectomy. We feel that the orchiectomy at the time of prostatectomy adds to the therapeutic effectiveness of the procedure by its hormonal suppressive action on prostatic tumor cells. This is not detrimental to the patient, because he has already been rendered impotent by the radical prostatectomy.

STAGE C. The patient is treated with multimodal therapy: First, a radical prostatectomy and orchiectomy is performed. The patient is then started on estrogen therapy with diethylstilbestrol (DES), 1 mg. per day, and adjuvant chemotherapy. Our choice, at present, is 5-fluorouracil (5-FU), 8 mg. per kg. per day for 5 days every month; cyclophosphamide (Cytoxan), 4 mg. per kg. per day for 5 days. This combination is well tolerated on a long-term basis.

STAGE D. The treatment varies according to the *sites* of the metastases.

STAGE D_1. Limited to the lymphatics of the pelvis. The treatment is the same as for Stage C patients.

STAGE D_2. The patient undergoes bilateral orchiectomy and is started on estrogen therapy (DES, 1 mg. per day), which is then followed by chemotherapy.

Some areas of metastases require a different approach.

Chemotherapy for Stage D_2 Carcinoma of the Prostate. In our experience, several drugs are effective: cyclophosphamide (Cytoxan), doxorubicin (Adriamycin), 5-fluorouracil (5-FU), and cis-diamminedichloroplatinum (cis platinum).* These drugs are used alone or in combination: 5-FU (8 mg. per kg. per day for 5 days) and Cytoxan (4 mg. per kg. per day for 5

---

*This drug is still experimental. It is available upon request from the National Cancer Institute, Washington, D.C. It will probably be released for community use within 1 year.

days) every month; or cis platinum (1 mg. per kg. per week for 6 weeks) and every 3 weeks thereafter; or cis platinum (1 mg. per kg.) and doxorubicin (Adriamycin) (40 mg. per square meter) every 3 weeks, doxorubicin (Adriamycin) (40 mg. per square meter) and cyclophosphamide (Cytoxan) (250 mg. per m.^{2} daily for 4 days) every 3 weeks.

Spinal Metastases.   When spinal pain is present, a neurologic examination is mandatory, including a myelogram to rule out cord compression. If the myelogram is positive, we perform a decompressive laminectomy followed by local radiotherapy to the area of metastasis, combined with systemic chemotherapy.

Pathologic Fractures and Bone Pain.   Pathologic fractures are treated by surgical pinning and radiotherapy.

Sarcoma of the Prostate

The most common sarcomas of the prostate are the leiomyosarcomas and rhabdomyosarcomas. Their peak frequency is in children and adolescents. They have been observed occasionally in older men. The treatment consists of a combination of surgery with radiotherapy and chemotherapy.

Surgery.   When the tumor is localized to the prostate, radical prostatectomy is performed. If the tumor is invading the bladder or the rectum, anterior or total pelvic exenteration is done. The bed of the tumor and the retroperitoneal lymph nodes are then irradiated. Adjuvant chemotherapy is then administered combining vincristine, 1.5 mg. per square meter weekly for 12 weeks, then every 3 weeks; actinomycin D, 0.5 mg. per day for 5 days every 6 weeks; cyclophosphamide, 500 mg. per square meter every 3 to 4 weeks; doxorubicin (Adriamycin), 30 to 60 mg. per square meter every 3 to 4 weeks. Depending on the degree of spread of the tumor, three drugs (vincristine, actinomycin D, and cyclophosphamide) or the four drugs in combination are used (doxorubicin, vincristine, actinomycin D, and cyclophosphamide).

BLADDER

The most frequent malignant tumor of the bladder is the transitional cell carcinoma. As in the prostate, the treatment is based on a very careful evaluation. The evaluation consists of intravenous pyelography, cystoscopy, transurethral biopsy, bimanual palpation under anesthesia, lymphangiography, hypogastric arteriography, metastatic surveys (bone and chest), liver scan, and bone scan. The clinical classification commonly used has been proposed by Jewett and modified by Marshall.

The treatment is based on this classification.

STAGE 0.   Intraepithelial tumor.
STAGE A.   Tumor invading the submucosa.
STAGE B.   Tumor invading the muscle.
STAGE C.   Tumor in the perivesical fat.
STAGE D.   Distant metastases.
STAGE D$_1$.   Metastases limited to pelvis.
STAGE D$_2$.   Metastases outside the pelvis.

In Situ Carcinoma.   Multifocal neoplastic transformation of the vesical mucosa, initially limited to the transitional epithelium, soon becomes invasive.

Treatment.   STAGE 0.   Forty per cent of these tumors are benign papillomas, which will never become invasive. Sixty per cent represent the early stage of carcinoma. The treatment consists of transurethral resection and fulguration.

STAGE A.   This stage represents an early invasive tumor. The treatment is based on transurethral resection and fulguration of the tumor.

Patients with Stage 0 and A are followed with cystoscopies, biopsies, and cytologic studies every 3 months for 1 year, every 6 months for 2 years, and yearly thereafter. In addition, we perform intravesical chemotherapy by instillations of different drugs.

Triethylenethiophosphoramide (ThioTEPA).   30 to 60 mg. in 60 ml. of water in the bladder every week for 6 weeks.

Bleomycin.   30 units in 60 ml. of water every week for 6 weeks.

Doxorubicin (Adriamycin).   40 mg. in 60 ml. of water weekly for 4 weeks.

Mitomycin C.   30 mg. in 60 ml. of water weekly for 8 weeks. (This use of bleomycin, Adriamycin, and mitomycin C is not listed in the manufacturer's official directive.)

After the cycle of chemotherapy, patients are recystoscoped.

STAGES B AND C.   Patients with these stages are treated by radical cystectomy (cystectomy, prostatovesiculectomy, bilateral pelvic lymphadenectomy) and ileal loop urinary diversion.

Patients are then started on adjuvant chemotherapy for 2 years with the combination of doxorubicin (Adriamycin), 40 mg. per square meter intravenously every 3 weeks up to a total of 500 mg. per square meter; and cyclophosphamide, 250 mg. per square meter a day for 4 days every 3 weeks.

STAGE D$_1$.   Lymphatic metastases limited to the pelvis. These patients are treated by radical cystectomy and adjuvant chemotherapy as Stages B and C patients. Instead of the combination doxorubicin (Adriamycin) and cyclophosphamide, they receive cis platinum (1 mg. per kg. weekly for 6 weeks and every 3 weeks thereafter).

STAGE D$_2$.   Metastases outside the pelvis.

These patients are treated with the combination cis platinum, doxorubicin (Adriamycin), and cyclophosphamide.

Adenocarcinomas and squamous cell carcinomas are more infrequent than transitional cell carcinoma. They are treated following the same approach by stages. In advanced disease, the chemotherapy of adenocarcinomas will include 5-fluorouracil (5-FU) and lomustine (CeeNU). For the chemotherapy of squamous cell carcinoma, bleomycin and methotrexate will be combined with cis platinum.

KIDNEYS

Renal Cell Carcinoma

Renal cell carcinoma constitutes the most frequent renal tumor. Its peak frequency is in the fifth and sixth decades of life, but it has been reported in young adults and children. The treatment is based on the extent of the disease.

Tumor Limited to the Organ or Locally Invasive. Radical nephrectomy is performed. This operation should comprise the removal of the kidney en bloc with its surrounding frames (perinephric fat, Gerota's fascia). The ligation of the renal vessels is recommended before mobilization of the tumor to avoid venous tumoral embolization. As 30 to 40 per cent of the patients present with metastases to the retroperitoneal lymph nodes, a retroperitoneal lymphadenectomy should be performed as part of the operation.

Disseminated Tumor. Renal cell carcinoma is difficult to treat when metastases are present. When resectable, they should be excised. Nephrectomy in the presence of metastases is indicated when these metastases are resectable. In addition, it may be helpful as palliation when bleeding, hypercalcemia, and erythrocytosis are present.

Radiotherapy has been disappointing in our experience. It is of help to control pain secondary to bone metastases. Chemotherapy has also shown to have limited effect. The best drug at present is CeeNU (65 mg. per square meter orally every 3 weeks).

Hormonal Therapy. Medroxyprogesterone (Provera) may be of some help. The dose is 100 mg. given 3 times a day. In rare occasions, testosterone is of therapeutic value.

Wilms' Tumor

Wilms' tumor is the most common renal tumor in childhood. It arises from embryonic cells in the metanephric blastema.

Our treatment is based on the clinical classification and schedules proposed by the National Wilms' Tumor Study Group. It consists of a combination of surgery, chemotherapy, and radiotherapy.

Surgery. The technique is similar to the technique used for radical nephrectomy in other renal neoplasms. The tumor is approached through a midline incision transperitoneally. The vascular pedicle is ligated first, and the kidney is removed en bloc with its surrounding structures (perirenal fat and Gerota's fascia). Retroperitoneal lymphadenectomy is performed, and the other kidney is explored to rule out bilaterality of the tumor.

Chemotherapy. Three drugs are active:

Actinomycin D. 15 micrograms per kg. intravenously daily for 5 days with a total dose of 75 micrograms per kg. per course. No single injection should exceed 500 micrograms. When necessary, smaller doses can be given (10 micrograms per kg. daily for 7 days).

Vincristine. 1.5 mg. per square meter intravenously once weekly. No single injection should exceed 2 mg.

Doxorubicin (Adriamycin). 30 to 60 mg. per square meter intravenously every 3 to 6 weeks.

Radiotherapy. Radiotherapy is given within 10 days of surgery. The tumor bed, the retroperitoneal area, and the metastases are included. The remaining kidney is shielded. Opposing anteroposterior portals are used. The recommended dose varies with age:

Birth to 18 months	1800–2400 rads
19 to 30 months	2400–3000 rads
31 to 40 months	3000–3500 rads
41 or more	3500–4000 rads

The combination therapy is as follows:

Group I (Tumor limited to kidney and completely resected): Radical nephrectomy and chemotherapy with the combination of actinomycin D and vincristine.

Group II (Tumor extends beyond the kidney, but is completely resected): Radical nephrectomy; chemotherapy with the combination actinomycin D and vincristine; radiotherapy to the tumor bed.

Group III (Residual tumor confined to the abdomen): Treated as Group II. Radiotherapy is given to the retroperitoneal area in addition to the tumor bed.

Group IV (Hematogenous metastases [lung, liver, brain, bone]): Surgery is performed as described before. Chemotherapy is administered combining Adriamycin to actinomycin D and vincristine. Radiotherapy is given to the tumor bed and the areas of metastases. This combined modality approach has been successful in controlling patients with advanced disease (in our experience, 50 per cent of Group IV patients are alive free of disease at 2 years).

Renal Pelvic Tumor

These tumors arise from the transitional epithelium lining the pelvis of the kidney. Histologically, they are similar to bladder and ureteral tumors.

Treatment consists of radical nephroureterectomy. The kidney and its surrounding tissues are excised, using the transperitoneal approach as described for renal adenocarcinomas. A retroperitoneal lymphadenectomy is done, and the ureter and a cuff of the bladder surrounding the ureteral orifice are also excised.

If local metastases are present, the patients receive adjuvant chemotherapy with the combination of doxorubicin (Adriamycin) and cyclophosphamide (Cytoxan) (as described for transitional cell carcinoma of the bladder). In addition, radiotherapy to the tumor bed and retroperitoneal areas may be indicated when residual tumor is left behind.

Patients with this tumor should be followed strictly every 3 months during 1 year, every 6 months for 2 years and every year thereafter. Serial cytologies in urine and cystoscopies are mandatory. These tumors are often recurrent in the bladder and may be the expression of generalized malignant transformation of the urothelium.

Renal Sarcomas

Renal sarcomas are rare tumors. They consist mainly of fibrosarcomas, liposarcomas, and leiomyosarcomas. They are treated by a combination of radical nephrectomy (as described previously) and chemotherapy with Adriamycin, cyclophosphamide, actinomycin D, and vincristine. They are relatively radioresistant, but radiotherapy when combined with the other therapeutic modalities may be of help to control local lesions.

Benign Renal Tumors

The only benign epithelial tumor of the kidney is the adenoma. A controversy exists as to its meaning. Many pathologists think that it may represent an early carcinoma. When asymptomatic, no treatment is required. When large in size, it is considered an adenocarcinoma and should be treated as such. The other benign tumors of the kidney are mesenchymal in origin. They are: fibromas, lipomas, lipomyomas, angiomas, rhabdomyomas, neurofibromas, and angiomyolipomas. When asymptomatic, they require no treatment. When symptomatic, surgical excision is recommended. In some instances a differential diagnosis with renal adenocarcinoma may be difficult (angiomyolipoma).

URETER

Benign Tumors

They consist of papillomas, hemangiomas, angiomas, and endometriomas. Their treatment consists of the surgical excision of the area of the lesion with restoration of the ureteral continuity by anastomosis.

Malignant Tumors

They consist of transitional cell carcinomas and squamous cell carcinomas. Their treatment consists of the excision of the ureter with ileal replacement. If the renal pelvis is invaded, the kidney should be removed in the fashion described previously. Removal of a cuff of bladder surrounding the ureteral orifice is also indicated. When the tumor is invasive, adjuvant chemotherapy with doxorubicin (Adriamycin) and cyclophosphamide (Cytoxan) is given for 2 years. If residual tumor is present after surgery, irradiation of the tumor bed is recommended. As in patients with renal pelvis tumor, the follow-up (cytology and cystoscopy) should last a lifetime.

URETHRA

Benign Tumors

The only benign tumor of the urethra is the condyloma acuminatum, which is viral in origin. It is treated by a combination of intraurethral ThioTEPA and fulguration.

Malignant Tumors

The types vary with the affected part of the urethra. The anterior part gives rise to squamous cell carcinomas and the posterior part to transitional carcinoma. They are treated in a different way, according to the degree of invasion and the location in the urethra.

Prostatic Membranous and Bulbous Urethra

Superficial Lesions. Transurethral resections are performed, combined with topical chemotherapy consisting of ThioTEPA, bleomycin, or Adriamycin.

Deep Lesions. These lesions generally invade the prostate and the bladder neck and are treated as bladder carcinoma by radical cystoprostatourethrectomy with ileal loop diversion and adjuvant chemotherapy in the manner described for bladder tumors.

Anterior Urethra

Superficial Lesions.   They are treated by local transurethral resection and topical therapy with bleomycin.

Deep Lesions.   Partial or total penectomy is performed combined with ilioinguinal lymphadenectomy. If the lymph nodes are positive, the patient is then started on adjuvant chemotherapy with a combination of cis platinum, bleomycin, and methotrexate.

PENIS

Benign Tumors

They consist of nevi, hemangiomas, and condylamata acuminatum. They are treated by local excision and in the case of condyloma acuminatum application of a solution of podophyllin or 5-FU cream.

Precancerous Lesions.   They are mainly Queyrat's erythroplasia, balanitis xerotica obliterans, leukoplakia, and penile hypercornification. The treatment consists of local excision and very careful followup.

Malignant Tumors

The most common of these tumors is the squamous cell carcinoma. The treatment consists of a combination of radical surgery and adjuvant chemotherapy.

The first step consists of a partial or total penectomy (depending on the location of the lesion). If the tumor is small, localized, and superficial, no other therapy is considered, and the patient is carefully monitored every 6 weeks, initially; then every 3 months for 1 year, every 6 months for 2 years, and every year thereafter. If the tumor is superficially invasive, bilateral groin dissection is performed in addition to the penectomy. If the tumor is deeply invasive, bilateral ilioinguinal lymphadenectomy is performed at the time of the penectomy. When lymph nodes are invaded by tumor, the patient is placed on adjuvant chemotherapy with a combination of cis platinum, bleomycin, and methotrexate.

TESTIS

Seminoma

Seminoma represents 40 to 50 per cent of all the germ cell tumors of the testis. It is rare in childhood. Its peak incidence is in patients between 35 and 50 years of age.

Our treatment consists initially of radical orchiectomy with clamping of the cord before mobilizing the testicle. After orchiectomy, a thorough evaluation of the patient should be performed to measure the extent of the disease and stage of the patient. This is achieved by lymphangiography; venocavography; aortography; scans of the liver, brain, and bone; chest tomography and alphafetoprotein; and beta subunit of human chorionic gonadotropins in serum. This tumor is extremely radiosensitive and the prime therapy consists of irradiation.

Stage I.   Tumor confined to one testis without evidence of metastases. Irradiation, 2500 to 3000 rads, given to the ipsilateral, inguinal, iliac, and periaortic lymph nodes below the diaphragm. When metastases are suspected on the contralateral side, it is also included in the radiation field.

Stage II.   Clinical or radiologic evidence of metastases to the femoral, inguinal iliac, or paraaortic lymph nodes. No evidence of spread beyond the diaphragm or to visceral organs. The periaortic and inguinal iliac areas are treated with the same doses and techniques of radiotherapy as in Stage I. After a rest period of 3 weeks to 1 month, additional radiation is directed at the mediastinum and left supraclavicular area (2500 rads).

Stage III.   Tumor beyond the diaphragm, but still confined to the lymphatic system. The radiotherapy treatment is the same as for Stage II.

Tumor above the diaphragm with spread outside the lymphatic system with visceral or disseminated metastases. The treatment is the same as for Stage II. In addition, local radiotherapy is administered to the areas of metastases in distant organs.

Patients with Stages II and III tumors receive adjuvant chemotherapy with phenylalanine mustard or cyclophosphamide for a period of 2 years. The doses are as follows: phenylalanine mustard, 2 mg. orally daily; cyclophosphamide, 1 to 1.5 grams per square meter every 3 weeks.

Nonseminomatous Testicular Tumors

In the past 5 years great progress has been achieved in the treatment of nonseminomatous germ cell tumors. This progress is the consequence of multidrug chemotherapy schedules used in combination with aggressive surgery.

Treatment.   Our treatment varies with the different stages of the disease:

STAGE I.   There is no clinical or radiologic evidence of metastases. A retroperitoneal lymphadenectomy is performed using the midline transabdominal approach (from the symphysis pubis to the xiphoid process). The lymphatic tissue and fat bilaterally surrounding the renal vascular pedicles, the aorta and the vena cava are excised to the femoral ligament on the ipsilateral side and to the level of the bifurcation of the iliac vessels on the contralateral side. Care is taken to free the vessels posteriorly and to remove all the lymph nodes. If the lymph nodes are not invaded by tumor, the patient is Stage I (tumor limited to the testes without evidence of metastasis). Adjuvant chemotherapy is given during 2 years with actinomycin D (0.5 mg. per day for 5 days every 6 weeks).

STAGE II. Metastases present in the retroperitoneal lymph nodes below the diaphragm.

1. Microscopic invasion of the retroperitoneal lymph nodes without presurgical clinical evidence.

2. Gross invasion of the retroperitoneal lymph nodes with presurgical clinical evidence.

TREATMENT OF STAGE II. After the retroperitoneal lymphadenectomy, patients receive chemotherapy with cis platinum, bleomycin, vincristine, and actinomycin D during 2 years (see chemotherapy schedule).

STAGE III. Tumor present above the diaphragm or metastases in visceral organs.

TREATMENT OF STAGE III. Patients are started on intensive chemotherapy with cis platinum, bleomycin, vincristine, and actinomycin D (see schedule). After 2 months, they are reevaluated. If a complete clinical remission is obtained, (defined by a total disappearance of the lesions and a return of the biological markers to normal [alphafetoprotein and beta subunit of human chorionic gonadotropins]), the patients are observed and continued on chemotherapy for a period of 2 years. If residual disease is still present, they are taken to surgery and the lesions are excised. After surgery, chemotherapy is continued for 2 years.

Maintenance therapy is continued for 2 years, giving the cis platinum and vincristine every 3 weeks and the actinomycin D every 6 weeks. Toxicity should be monitored, and dosage and schedule modification made according to needs. The overall results of our treatment have shown that 95 per cent of Stage I patients and 60 per cent of Stage III patients are disease free at 2 years.

Nongerminal Testicular Tumors

These tumors consist of Leydig's cell tumors and gonadal stromal tumors. They are usually benign. Surgical excision of the affected testis through the inguinal approach is sufficient to treat them.

Paratesticular Rhabdomyosarcoma

This tumor often originates in the epididymis and initially spreads to the regional and retroperitoneal lymphatics like the germ cell testicular tumors.

Treatment. Treatment consists of a radical orchiectomy through the inguinal approach and retroperitoneal lymphadenectomy as described for the testis tumors.

Chemotherapy. Actinomycin D, vincristine, cyclophosphamide, and Adriamycin are used in the same fashion as in rhabdomyosarcoma of the prostate.

Radiotherapy. Irradiation of the areas with residual disease is performed as a local adjuvant treatment to the chemotherapy.

TABLE 1. **Chemotherapy Schedule**

WEEK 1:	Day 1: Cis platinum,* 1 mg. per kg. mixed with 2000 ml. of dextrose 5 per cent in one-third isotonic saline solution plus 37.5 grams of mannitol and 40 mEq. of KCl. This is infused in 6 to 8 hours Vincristine, 2 mg. intravenously Prednisone, 10 mg. orally twice daily Days 2 to 7: Bleomycin, 30 units in 1000 ml. of dextrose 5 per cent in $^1/_3$ isotonic saline solution infused in 6 hours Prednisone, 10 mg. orally twice daily
WEEK 2:	Day 1: Bleomycin, 30 units (infused intravenously) Prednisone, 10 mg. twice daily Day 2: Cis platinum*, 1 mg. per kg. infusion Vincristine, 2 mg. intravenously Prednisone, 10 mg. twice daily Days 3 to 7: Prednisone, 10 mg. twice daily
WEEK 3:	Same as in Week 1
WEEK 4:	Same as in Week 2
WEEK 5:	Cis platinum,* 1 mg. per kg. infusion Vincristine, 2 mg. intravenously (stop the prednisone)
WEEK 6:	Same as in Week 5
WEEK 7:	Day 1: Cis platinum,* 1 mg. per kg. infusion Vincristine, 2 mg. intravenously Days 2 to 6: Actinomycin D, 0.5 mg. intravenously

Maintenance therapy is continued during 2 years with cis platinum and vincristine every 3 weeks and actinomycin D every 6 weeks.

*Experimental.

SCROTUM

Tumors of the scrotum are usually squamous cell carcinomas. They are rare but represent the first described malignant tumor produced by exposure to chemical carcinogens (tar in chimney sweepers).

Treatment. *When localized and superficial,* partial scrotectomy is performed. *When invasive,* a total scrotectomy is done and the testicles are placed in pouches in the internal aspect of the thighs. If there is evidence of lymph node invasion, bilateral inguinoiliac lymphadenectomy is performed. If the lymph nodes show histologic evidence of tumor, adjuvant chemotherapy is given with the combination of cis platinum, bleomycin, and methotrexate.

URETHRAL STRICTURES

method of
WILLIAM O. MILLER, M.D.
Knoxville, Tennessee

Strictures of the urethra are reductions in the normal luminal size of the urethra and inability of this tubular structure to attain its normal size during the act of micturition. A stricture may occur at any age and in either sex. True anatomic strictures appear to be more common in males than in females. However, relatively large caliber strictures seem to produce more symptoms in females than the corresponding diminution in size in males.

Clinical symptoms of a weak or dribbling urinary stream, persistent or recurrent urinary tract infection with or without pyuria, distended urinary bladder, nocturia, and acute urinary retention should suggest lower urinary tract obstruction with urethral strictures as a prime differential diagnosis.

Before any treatment of a urethral stricture is instituted, a urinalysis with urine culture and bacterial sensitivity should be obtained. In males, particularly before instrumentation is carried out or urethral calibration is attempted, a broad-spectrum antibiotic should be started. The precipitation of a gram-negative bacteremic sepsis, while not common, can occur with minimal instrumentation or trauma and produce a devastating effect on the patient.

Female Urethral Strictures

Management of the urethral stricture in females is difficult because so often the diagnosis of urethral stricture, being an anatomic finding, frequently has symptomatology that is functionally based. Calibration with the bougie à boule sound can define an anatomic stenosis, and often a meatotomy will be of help. In postmenopausal women, local vaginal estrogen creams will be helpful in alleviating the symptoms when used in conjunction with a urinary analgesic. We have not found repeated dilatations of the female urethra or instillations of silver nitrate to be of help to relieve either stenosis or symptoms for any length of time. We have also not found internal urethrotomy to be as helpful as had been hoped. External urethral meatotomy at the time of cystoscopy in young girls seems to be of significant help in alleviating symptoms when the meatus is stenotic to a No. 10 to 12 bougie à boule sound. If no true anatomic stenosis is found in sexually active women, or infection proven, then attempts to control the symptoms by urinary analgesics with vaginal estrogens in postmenopausal women may be helpful.

Male Urethral Strictures

Congenital. 1. Contracture of the bladder neck in association with neurogenic disorders of the urinary bladder may be found and may require incision of the bladder neck either transurethrally or, in some patients, suprapubically in the form of Y-V incision of the bladder neck. We have not found the latter to be necessary.

2. Urethral valves are located in the male prostatic urethra and are diagnosed by voiding cystourethrography or direct urethroscopy or both. These have been reported to be very common but this has not been our experience. These obstructive valves can be corrected by transurethral avulsion or incision, or occasionally by a suprapubic approach.

3. Congenital narrowing of the urethra can be treated by gentle dilatation on occasion. However, if this does not achieve desired luminal size, internal urethrotomy should be attempted.

4. Congenital meatal stenosis, which is a relatively frequent finding in infant males, is easily corrected by a urethral meatotomy.

Acquired Strictures. These are most commonly seen at the membranous or bulbar urethra and usually are secondary to:

1. Pelvic fractures.
2. Straddle injuries to the perineum.
3. Traumatic instrumentation.
4. Infectious processes, either nonspecific infections or gonococcal.
5. Foreign bodies including self-introduced objects and iatrogenic-induced by urethral catheter.
6. Chemical trauma, either self-induced or iatrogenic such as silver nitrate.

Procedures. Initially, if a No. 16 French or Coude catheter cannot be passed with ease into the urinay bladder, the penis is cleansed with povidone-iodine (Betadine) or benzalkonium chloride (Zephiran), grasped behind the glans penis at the coronal sulcus, and then after filling the distal urethra with lidocaine (Xylocaine) jelly, attempts to pass urethral filiforms of varying sizes can be made. Once a filiform is passed into the bladder, a woven Phillips (hollow) catheter can be inserted gently into the urinary bladder to alleviate retention, followed by subsequent sizes up to a No. 18. If retention is not a problem, the same size LaForte solid sound can be inserted. After dilatation, a Foley catheter may be left indwelling for several days to soften a stricture if necessary so that subsequent dilatations may be carried out more easily. If a luminal size to a No. 24 French can be maintained with ease, this should suffice. However, multiple traumatic dilatations are to be avoided for long-term management.

Internal urethrotomy is usually recommended at a first surgical procedure to maintain urethral luminal size. However, if this does not prove successful, it can be followed by appropriate urethroplasty such as a Johannsen type urethroplasty, Turner-Warwick procedure, or a DeVine procedure of a full thickness graft. Vesical neck strictures or contractures that do not respond to periodic dilatations can usually be corrected with quadrant incisions of the contracture with the resectoscope using the cautery knife. This has worked well in our hands, avoiding the necessity of Y-V plasty of the bladder neck.

NONGONOCOCCAL URETHRITIS

method of
R. NICOL THIN, M.D., F.R.C.P.E.
London, England

Definition and Diagnosis

Urethritis is characterized clinically by dysuria and urethral discharge, and in the laboratory by an excess of polymorphonuclear leucocytes (PMN) on a Gram-stained smear of urethral exudate. Urethritis is either gonococcal or nongonococcal in origin, and subclinical infections of both forms occur. Clinical differentiation between the two forms is unreliable, and laboratory investigations are essential. It is bad practice to treat men with urethritis without determining its type.

The following specimens should be collected: a smear of urethral exudate for Gram staining; another specimen for culture for *Neisseria gonorrhoeae*; first 10 ml. of voided urine may be examined microscopically for pyuria. Microscopy for gram-negative intracellular diplococci is quick, simple, and at least 90 per cent accurate in men, but should always be supplemented by culture. Men with nongonococcal urethritis (NGU) show an excess of PMN, at least 20 per high power field using a × 100 objective on the Gram-stained smear and laboratory evidence of pyuria in the absence of intracellular diplococci on microscopy, and negative results to cultures for *N. gonorrhoeae*.

About 50 per cent of cases are caused by *Chlamydia trachomatis*. The cause of the remainder is uncertain, but some may be caused by *Ureaplasma urealyticum* (T-strain mycoplasma). Facilities for culturing these organisms are not generally available at present. It should also be remembered that among the minority of cases due to other identifiable causes a few will be due to upper urinary infections, and it is important that these should be recognized. Postgonococcal urethritis (PGU) occurs when a patient treated for gonorrhoea has persistent urethritis despite the elimination of *N. gonorrhoeae*. The management of NGU and PGU is identical.

Antimicrobial Therapy

The drugs of first choice are the tetracyclines, with erythromycin as second choice. The following regimens are effective:

Oxytetracycline or tetracycline, 250 mg. four times a day for 2 to 3 weeks. Medication should be taken either 1 hour before or 2 hours after meals. Since tetracyclines chelate with calcium, milk, and milk products, ingestion should be prohibited during therapy. For the same reason antacids containing aluminum or magnesium should also be avoided, as should oral iron.

Minocycline, 100 mg. twice daily for 2 to 3 weeks. This drug produces high serum and tissue concentration so dietary restrictions may be less important and patient compliance is better with twice daily dosage. However, a few patients experience vestibular side effects with this drug.

Erythromycin stearate, 250 mg. four times daily for 2 to 3 weeks, is a satisfactory alternative for patients unable to take tetracyclines.

The ideal duration of therapy for NGU is unknown, but a course of less than 2 weeks is probably suboptimal.

Sulfonamides have little effect on NGU; the penicillins, spectinomycin, and metronidazole have no effect and should not be prescribed.

General Measures

Nongonococcal urethritis is sexually transmissible, and patients should refrain from intercourse until they are considered cured. If such restraint is impossible, a condom must be worn.

Alcohol is traditionally prohibited during therapy. The value of this measure is uncertain, but clinical experience suggests that alcohol aggravates urethritis in some patients.

Patients should be encouraged to consume plenty of bland fluids, during the day as well as in the evening.

Assessing Response to Treatment

After completing treatment the patient will need reexamination twice during the following month, the initial diagnostic tests being repeated to confirm that he no longer has urethritis. If, at the end of this time, he is symptom- and sign-free, and there is no laboratory evidence of urethritis, he may be regarded as cured. Men whose progress is favorable may normally resume intercourse a week after finishing therapy, although a condom should be advised for the first 2 weeks after resuming intercourse. It is good practice to see patients once more 3 months after the start of therapy.

Management of Female Contacts

Nongonococcal urethritis is a sexually transmissible disease and many female contacts of men with *Chlamydia*-positive urethritis harbor this organism and other pathogens. Furthermore, *C. trachomatis* causes pelvic infection and it causes ophthalmia neonatorum among babies born to mothers harbouring *C. trachomatis* in the genital tract. Untreated female contacts of men with NGU can reinfect their partners or infect new ones. Therefore, these female contacts should be examined and appropriate cultures taken from the cervical os and vagina. Because of the difficulty of deciding clinically if a woman has nongonococcal genital infection, many authorities recommend epidemiologic treatment with tetracycline or erythromycin (the latter is indicated during pregnancy). Any associated infection should be treated also.

Management of Relapsing Nongonococcal Urethritis

The treatment outlined will cure about 80 per cent of men with NGU, but the remainder either have persistent symptoms and signs of urethritis after therapy or subsequently relapse. NGU persists in a few patients for months and may cause much distress.

Although the causes of relapsing or persisting nongonococcal urethritis are not fully understood, the clinician should consider the following points:

1. Has the patient taken his medication according to instructions?

2. Should a change of antimicrobial be considered or a longer course or both be prescribed?

3. Have regular sexual contacts received treatment? Is there any possibility of infection from a new source?

4. Is the patient perpetuating the urethritis himself by squeezing the urethra?

5. Has he any rare cause of urethritis unresponsive to tetracycline or erythromycin, such as trichomonal, candidal, or herpetic urethritis? Black men more often have trichomonal infection than do white men.

6. Has he developed prostatitis?

7. Has he a urethral stricture or other urologic disease?

Each of these points will require consideration. If after 2 or 3 months the cause of repeated relapse cannot be identified, urologic investigation for prostatitis, stricture, or other urogenital disease is indicated.

Emergency Situations

There may be occasions in which a patient develops acute urethritis under circumstances in which laboratory investigation before treatment is not possible. However, the experienced practitioner prepared to treat urethritis should always equip himself with microscope slides and, if possible, culture media such as Transgrow. Before treatment, a sample of discharge can be smeared on a slide with a matchstick and either kept by the doctor or given to the patient for subsequent examination when this is possible; at the same time, a Transgrow culture may be taken. The drugs of choice in these situations are oxytetracycline or tetracycline, 500 mg. four times a day for 14 days. This will cure most gonococcal infections and is adequate for NGU. The patient should attend a suitable facility as soon as possible when the slide can be stained and examined, and the culture may be processed. A retrospective diagnosis can then be made and treatment adjusted accordingly.

Conclusion

NGU is one of the common sexually transmitted diseases and it is now recognized that in many parts of the world it is more common than gonorrhea. It causes discomfort and anxiety and complications may occur in the men or in their female partners, so thorough and effective treatment with careful follow-up are highly desirable.

RENAL CALCULI

method of
FREDRIC L. COE, M.D.,
and MURRAY J. FAVUS, M.D.
Chicago, Illinois

There are four common types of kidney stones. The most common (75 to 85 per cent) are calcium stones composed of calcium oxalate, calcium phosphate, or both. Stones of struvite, the triple salt of magnesium ammonium and phosphate, compose the next largest group (10 to 15 per cent). Uric acid and cystine stones are least common. Uric acid stones account for 5 to 8 per cent and cystine stones for less than 1 per cent. Calcium and uric acid stones occur more in men than in women; the reverse is true for struvite. Cystine stones occur equally in both sexes.

The major factor that determines whether stones will form is the saturation of the urine with stone-forming salts. Saturation depends upon the daily excretion of stone-forming materials, the volume of urine in which the materials are dissolved, and the extent to which the urine possesses compounds that can bind the materials and hold them in a soluble form. Urine pH may be important when a stone component is a weak acid whose dissociation varies over the physiologic urine pH range of 4.5 to 7.5. Another important factor is the level in urine of substances that can slow or prevent the formation and growth of crystal nuclei.

Diagnostic Evaluation

Stone Type and Activity. Any available stone should be analyzed. Chemical analyses are not a good practice, because crystal types cannot be discerned, and minor but important constituents may go undetected. Excellent crystallographic analysis of stones can be obtained from commercial or university-based laboratories, at a modest price. Certain gross features of stones are helpful clues to their composition. Calcium oxalate stones are usually small and black. Uric acid gravel is orange-red, and the stones may also be red. Struvite stones are like chalk. Cystine stones are lemon-yellow and often have surface crystals that sparkle. Uric acid stones are radiolucent; the others are opaque to the x-ray beam, least so for cystine and most for calcium oxalate.

Clinical activity of stone disease is measured by the growth of existing stones, as estimated by sequential radiographs, or the formation of new stones. Stones that are passed or removed, or are seen on an x-ray can be considered new if they have not been visualized on a previous x-ray. Stone growth and new stone formation connote an active disease that is best treated. When there are no prior radiographs to examine, stone activity cannot be determined. All stones that are seen on a single radiograph or are passed or removed may have formed in some remote, past time when stone-forming conditions were present in the urine.

Metabolic Evaluation

Causes of Stones (Table 1). Uric acid, cystine, and struvite stones each imply a single well-defined pathogenesis and treatment, whereas treatment of calcium stones depends more on the type of metabolic disorder that is present than

TABLE 1. **Major Causes of Nephrolithiasis**

Calcium Stones
    Idiopathic Hypercalciuria
    Hyperuricosuria
    Primary Hyperparathyroidism
    Hyperoxaluria
    Renal Tubular Acidosis
    Idiopathic
Uric Acid Stones
    Gout
    Idiopathic
    Dehydration e.g., climate, ileostomy
    Massive overproduction of uric acid

Cystine Stones Due to Cystinuria
Struvite Stones Due to Urinary Infection With Urea-Splitting
    Bacteria

TABLE 2. **Laboratory Evaluation of Patients with Nephrolithiasis**

Serum:	Calcium ×3
	Phosphorus ×1
	Sodium ×1
	Potassium ×1
	Chloride ×1
	CO₂ content ×1
	Creatinine ×1
	Uric acid ×1
24 hour urine:	Calcium ×3
	Uric acid ×3
	pH ×3
	Creatinine ×3
	Oxalate ×3*
	Phosphorus ×3
	Cystine†
	Sodium ×3

*Usually, this test cannot be obtained except by special arrangement.
†One screening test is sufficient.

upon the specific types of calcium crystals in a stone. Nevertheless, patients with uric acid, cystine, and struvite stones should be evaluated as comprehensively and in the same way as calcium stone formers because they may harbor metabolic disorders that could lead to future calcium stones or require that special precautions be taken during treatment.

Protocol for Evaluation (Table 2). All the disorders in Table 1 can be detected by an out-patient protocol based upon three 24 hour urines and corresponding blood samples, provided the protocol is combined with a thorough clinical evaluation. Urines should be collected in clean containers with tight-fitting caps and a few crystals of thymol as preservative. Creatinine can be determined by autoanalyzer methodology, but calcium and uric acid should be determined by atomic absorption spectrophotometry and the uricase method, respectively, if possible. The latter is especially important for testing urine. The three urine and blood samples give a reasonably reliable picture of the average findings in a patient. Since stone diseases may require treatment for many years, the initial investment in multiple samples is justified.

TREATMENT OF CALCIUM STONES

Idiopathic Hypercalciuria

Definition. Serum calcium is normal. Twenty-four hour urine calcium excretion exceeds 300 mg. (men), 250 mg. (women), or 4 mg. per kg. (either sex). No established cause of normocalcemic hypercalciuria such as sarcoidosis, renal tubular acidosis, Cushing's syndrome, hyperthyroidism, rapidly progressive osteoporosis, malignant neoplasm, immobilization, vitamin D excess, or medicinal calcium supplementation is present.

Diagnosis. Normal people do not exceed these limits, even when dietary dairy products are plentiful, but calcium excretion by patients with idiopathic hypercalciuria is variable. One of three elevated values requires confirmation; two high values are sufficient. Calcium restriction can mask idiopathic hypercalciuria, but a high calcium intake will not cause hypercalciuria in a normal person, so patients should be studied while they are consuming their customary diets. This syndrome is present in 40 to 50 per cent of calcium stone formers.

Special Tests. Intestinal calcium overabsorption and a renal calcium leak both can cause hypercalciuria. They can be told apart by response to fasting and by serum parathyroid hormone (PTH) values. In primary overabsorption, urine calcium per gram of creatinine is below 0.12 after a 14 hour fast; it exceeds this value in renal hypercalciuria. Serum parathyroid hormone (PTH) is low or normal in absorptive and high in renal hypercalciuria. Treatment, however, need not be different for the two forms. Low calcium diet raises urine oxalate so that urine saturation with respect to calcium oxalate does not fall. Cellulose phosphate, a calcium binding resin, also causes reciprocal hyperoxaluria and may, therefore, not be effective in preventing calcium oxalate stones. The compound is not yet available as a drug. Thiazide diuretic agents lower urine calcium in either form of idiopathic hypercalciuria and are the drugs of choice.

Treatment. 1. Trichlormethiazide, 2 mg. twice daily, will reduce urine calcium excretion in most patients. A good alternative is chlorthalidone, 50 mg. each morning. (This use of trichlormethiazide or chlorthalidone is not listed in the manufacturer's official directive.)

2. Sodium intake should be reduced, if necessary, to no more than 100 mEq. per day. A large sodium intake reverses the hypocalciuric action of the diuretic agents, and also promotes excessive urinary loss of potassium.

3. Follow-up measurements of urine calcium and sodium excretion and serum potassium should be made after 8 weeks of treatment and then yearly. Salt intake should be lowered or the drug dose raised if calcium excretion is not within the normal range. Conventional potassium supplementation is used if required.

Hyperuricosuria

Definition and Diagnosis. A daily urine uric acid excretion above 800 mg. (men) or 750 mg. (women) is elevated. This abnormality occurs in 20 to 25 per cent of patients and is associated with idiopathic hypercalciuria in 10 per cent. Serum urate level may be normal or high. How hyperuricosuria causes calcium stones is still uncertain, but it is likely that crystals of uric acid or sodium hydrogen urate act as seed nuclei to promote calcium oxalate crystallization. The main contributor to hyperuricosuria is dietary purine excess, from meat, fish, and poultry. Endogenous uric acid overproduction occurs in a minority of patients.

Treatment. 1. Intake of meat, fish and poultry, as well as other high purine foods, should be reduced. Breads, grains, and starches are a good substitute, as they provide protein and little fat.

2. Allopurinol, 100 mg. twice daily, is useful if dietary alteration is not acceptable to the patient or if reducing dietary purine intake fails to reverse hyperuricosuria because endogenous overproduction is present. Severe stone disease also warrants allopurinol, at least during the first several years of treatment when new dietary patterns are being established. *Note:* Alkalinization of the urine, as for uric acid stones, will not be beneficial in calcium stone formers and may promote precipitation of sodium hydrogen urate. Also, once a day allopurinol administration may not control urine uric acid excretion consistently, because the allopurinol effect wanes in less than 24 hours after a single dose.

3. Uric acid excretion must be evaluated after 8 weeks of treatment, whether dietary or based upon allopurinol, and yearly thereafter. Diet or drug dosage should be adjusted to keep daily uric acid excretion below 700 mg. (men) or 600 mg. (women).

Primary Hyperparathyroidism

Definition. In this disease, a primary enlargement of one or more of the parathyroid glands causes overproduction of parathyroid hormone (PTH). Serum and urine calcium rise, and stones occur. This disease accounts for 5 to 8 per cent of calcium stones.

Diagnosis. Hypercalcemia that is not explained by a malignant tumor, hyperthyroidism, sarcoidosis, vitamin D intoxication, use of a thiazide diuretic agent, or any other cause is sufficient for diagnosis. The serum PTH value will be elevated using some assays, but a normal PTH level need not exclude the diagnosis because many assays cannot reliably distinguish normal from hyperparathyroid subjects. Hypophosphatemia, low tubular phosphate reabsorption and hyperchloremia all may occur in primary hyperparathyroidism but are neither sufficient nor necessary for diagnosis. In the absence of hypercalcemia, the diagnosis of primary hyperparathyroidism is untenable, whatever the serum PTH level.

Treatment. 1. Surgery is the only effective treatment. In 85 per cent of patients a single adenoma is present. The remainder of patients have hyperplasia that usually affects all four glands. In these patients, subtotal parathyroidectomy, leaving one half of one gland, is the usual treatment. A newer approach is total parathyroidectomy and transplantation of portions of one gland to the forearm. Other glands are frozen for later use, if necessary.

Hyperoxaluria

Definition. More than 50 mg. per 24 hours of oxalate excretion is abnormal. There are many causes of this condition. Intestinal hyperoxaluria can occur when more than 22 cm. of ileum has been resected, usually because of inflammatory bowel disease, or when bowel disease has produced severe malabsorption. Inadequate absorption of fat leaves excessive amounts of fatty acids in the bowel lumen, where they can bind dietary calcium to form soaps. Oxalate is absorbed to excess in the colon because it does not combine with calcium and precipitate in the proximal bowel lumen in the normal way. Ileal bypass, in treatment of obesity, can produce the same picture. Dietary oxalate excess can be produced by overconsumption of foods such as black pepper, tea, parsley, nuts, cocoa, rhubarb, and spinach. Carrots, celery, and green peppers have less oxalate but are often used in larger portions. Hereditary hyperoxaluria can arise from deletion of α-ketoglutarate:glyoxylate carboligase (Type I) or D-glyceric dehydrogenase (Type II), enzymes that are related to the metabolism of glycolate and glyoxylate, precursors of oxalate. In type I hyperoxaluria, urine glycolate and glyoxylate excretions are also raised; L-glyceric acid excretion is raised in type II. Ethylene glycol intoxication and the volatile anesthetic methoxyflurane also cause hyperoxaluria.

Diagnosis. Daily urine oxalate excretion above 50 mg. establishes hyperoxaluria. In primary hereditary hyperoxaluria, values range between 100 and 300 mg. per 24 hours. The cause can usually be determined by history and physical examination.

Treatment. 1. General measures. Large fluid intake, at least 2 liters (64 ounces) daily, will help to prevent extreme oversaturation and should be used in all patients. A low oxalate diet also should be recommended. The specific treatment depends upon the cause of hyperoxaluria.

2. Intestinal hyperoxaluria. Low fat diet will reduce soap formation and decrease oxalate absorption. Oral calcium, 10 to 14 grams daily, as the carbonate or lactate salt, will precipitate oxalate. Cholestyramine, a resin that adsorbs oxalate, 8 to 16 grams in two to four divided doses, can be used if low fat diet and calcium supplementation prove ineffective. Vitamin K depletion can result, and supplemental vitamin K may be needed. Intestinal bypass, if present, should be reversed if the risk of stones or nephrocalcinosis seems to outweigh that of obesity, or if azotemia is present.

3. Primary hyperoxaluria. Pyridoxine, 400 mg. daily, may increase conversion of glyoxylate to glycine and reduce oxalate excretion. Very high fluid intake and low oxalate diet are the only other measures available. The disease may produce renal failure so that dialysis becomes necessary.

Distal Renal Tubular Acidosis

Definition. The distal nephron segments, distal convoluted tubules and collecting ducts, are unable to lower the pH of the final urine as far as they normally do because of an hereditary defect. Net acid excretion falls and systemic acidosis appears, but glomerular filtration rate is well preserved. Hyperchloremia is produced because chloride ions must be reabsorbed along with sodium in the distal nephron to compensate for the lack of proton secretion, which normally balances a portion of sodium reabsorption and makes unnecessary the reabsorption of an anion. Hypokalemia and hypophosphatemia occur. Acidosis causes bone mineral loss, osteomalacia, hypercalciuria, hyperphosphatemia, and low urine citrate. Calcium phosphate stones result from elevated urine calcium, low urine citrate and high urine pH.

Diagnosis. Hyperchloremic acidosis and a urine pH that is unduly alkaline, above 5.5 or 6.0, suggest distal renal tubular acidosis (RTA), as do stunted growth, osteomalacia, and papillary nephrocalcinosis.

Special Test. Proof resides in the failure of urine pH to fall with induction of acute acidosis using ammonium chloride (NH_4Cl). The urine must not be infected when the test is done. At 8 A.M., after overnight fast, 1.9 mEq. per kg. of NH_4Cl is given along with 30 ml. of a nonabsorbable antacid, to prevent nausea. Urine is collected at 2 hour intervals for 6 hours, and corresponding arterialized venous blood samples are drawn from a hand has been warmed for 15 minutes. Venous total CO_2 will fall and chloride level will rise. Normally, urine pH will fall below 5.1 during the test. A minimum value above 5.5 establishes the diagnosis; in the fully developed disease, urine pH usually does not fall below 6.

Treatment. 1. Alkali, 0.5 mEq. per kg. body weight is given in 4 divided daily doses. Sodium bicarbonate, 10 grain (0.6 gram) tablets, each provide 7.2 mEq. of base. Shohl's solution provides 1 mEq. per ml.

2. Follow-up measurements of venous CO_2 and urine calcium guide treatment. Venous CO_2 must be increased to 24 mm. per liter, and urine calcium excretion below 4 mg. per kg. body weight per 24 hours.

Idiopathic Calcium Stones

Definition. When all the causes of calcium stones have been sought in vain, one comes to this bleak category. The mechanisms of stone genesis lie beyond our understanding, and treatment is neither selective nor satisfactory.

Diagnosis. This condition is diagnosed by exclusion. A complete clinical and metabolic evaluation (Table 2) must be performed and all of the causes of calcium stone (Table 1) excluded.

Treatment. 1. High fluid intake, 64 oz. (2 liters) of water daily. Precautions should be advised concerning episodes of dehydration.

2. Orthophosphate is given as the neutral salt to provide 1.5 to 2 grams of phosphorus daily. A lower dosage of 1 gram of phosphorus daily has proved completely ineffective in stone prevention in two prospective trials, one placebo controlled. The higher dose of 1.5 to 2 grams phosphorus daily has been found to be effective in a single uncontrolled prospective study.

TREATMENT OF URIC ACID STONES

Definition and Diagnosis. Uric acid lithiasis is established by stone analysis. The stones are radiolucent. In people with gout, average urine pH is low, so that undissociated uric acid (pK 5.47) predominates. Only 200 to 300 mg. of this molecule can be dissolved in a liter of urine, so oversaturation frequently occurs. Some people without gout or hyperuricemia also elaborate excessively acid urine and form uric acid stones. The patients are said to suffer from idiopathic uric acid lithiasis. In either type of patient, hyperuricosuria may be present, from dietary purine excess or endogenous overproduction, and enhance stone formation. Chronic dehydration, from habit, life style, climate or ileostomy causes a concentrated urine of low pH and predisposes to uric acid lithiasis. Massive uric acid overproduction, from myeloproliferative syndromes, Lesch-Nyhan syndrome or chemotherapy of lymphoma or leukemia can cause uric acid sludge or stone at even a normal urine pH.

Treatment. 1. Alkali are needed, whatever the basis for the stones. Two sodium bicarbonate tablets, 10 grains (0.6 gram) each, may be given three to four times daily, one dose at bedtime. The pills should be taken 2 hours after meals. The goal is a urine pH that is above 6 but below 7; excessive alkali can cause phosphate stones. Patients should test their urine using pH paper, at each voiding at first, to monitor therapy and detect over or under treatment.

2. Allopurinol, 200 to 300 mg. daily, is indicated if 24 hour urine uric acid excretion is above 800 mg. or if alkali alone fails to stop new stone formation and dissolve preexistent stones. A higher dose of allopurinol is appropriate when hyperuricosuria is massive.

3. High fluid intake.

4. Thiazide diuretic agents are needed if patients are hypercalciuric or form both calcium and uric acid stones or stones that contain both calcium and uric acid. Calcium stone disease may appear or worsen when alkali are used in a hypercalciuric patient.

TREATMENT OF CYSTINE STONES

Definition. Cystine stones occur only in patients who have cystinuria. Renal and intestinal tract epithelia fail to transport cystine, lysine, ornithine and arginine properly in this autosomal recessive hereditary disease. Cystine is very insoluble and forms stones.

Diagnosis. Stone analysis and the finding of elevated urine cystine excretion are the basis for diagnosis. A positive urine cystine screening test is not uncommon because the heterozygous cystinuric trait has a prevalence of 0.1 to 0.3 per cent in an otherwise normal population; the vast majority of these people do not form cystine stones and should not be treated as if they had homozygous cystinuria. Though elevated, their urine cystine excretion rates will be low (75 to 200 mg. per 24 hours) compared to homozygous cystinuria (above 400 mg. per 24 hours).

Treatment. 1. High fluid intake. Three to 4 liters of urine must be produced daily. At night, patients must arise at least once to void and ingest 16-oz. (480 ml.) of water.

2. Alkali (sodium bicarbonate, 20 grains (1.3 grams) four to five times daily, or oral citrate mixture (Polycitra), 1 mEq. base per ml., 15 ml. four to five times daily) to achieve a pH above 7 throughout the day and night. Alkali must not be used if hypercalciuria of other cause is present, until the hypercalciuria has been controlled.

3. D-penicillamine, 250 to 500 mg. daily, is given when fluids and alkali have failed to control the stone disease; the dose must be sufficient to keep daily urine cystine excretion between 400 and 500 mg. Occasionally, a higher dose may be used to lower cystine excretion below 200 mg. per day when dissolution of a stone is being attempted. Anosmia and loss of taste occur, and can be

treated by supplemental zinc. If nephrotic syndrome occurs, D-penicillamine must be discontinued.

TREATMENT OF STRUVITE (INFECTION) STONES

Definition. Struvite is a triple salt $MgNH_4PO_4$ that is produced in the urinary tract only by the action of bacteria that possess an enzyme, urease, that hydrolyses urea to NH_3 and CO_2. The NH_3 hydrolyses to NH_4^+ and, in the process, raises urine pH greatly. In an alkaline urine, CO_2 is converted to $CO_3^=$, which combines with calcium to form $CaCO_3$. The result is a stone composed of struvite admixed with calcium carbonate. The bacteria usually are proteus species. Abnormal urinary tract anatomy is a common reason for proteus infection. Often, proteus organisms infect preformed stones that have had another metabolic cause.

Diagnosis. Stone analysis is definitive evidence for the syndrome; all struvite stones are of infectious origin. Bacteriologic evidence of a urea-splitting organism in the urine is confirmatory but is not a necessary requirement. Culture of stone fragments may well yield the organism when the urine does not. Urine pH often is high, above 8. The stones are radiopaque and display growth rings or laminations by x-ray. A staghorn appearance is very common. Complete metabolic assessment is critical, as metabolic stone disease often has been the basis in the past for stones in this group of patients.

Treatment. 1. Any metabolic disorder must be treated.

2. Surgical removal should be carried out only when the stones are producing obstruction, serious pain, bleeding, or infection. Recurrence is very frequent, and the risk of nephrectomy rises greatly when a second or third surgery is performed on a kidney. When stone removal is attempted, every fragment must be removed, because even a small bit of stone can regrow.

3. Urine acidification with methenamine mandelate (Mandelamine), which also has modest bacteriostatic properties is of minor, adjunctive value in patients with preformed stones. Chronic antibiotic treatment usually is valueless, because resistant forms emerge.

4. Bactericidal antibiotics may be used for 10 to 14 days to lower the bacterial population, and then chronic suppression can be attempted using trimethoprim and sulfamethoxazole (Bactrim or Septra). An occasional flare-up can be retreated using a second course of bactericidal drugs. This regimen is ideal before and after surgical stone removal; here, suppressive treatment should be continued for at least 3 years after all stone material has been removed.

The Venereal Diseases

CHANCROID

method of
AXEL W. HOKE, M.D.
San Francisco, California

Chancroid, alias soft chancre, is an uncommon, sexually transmitted disease characterized by the appearance of multiple, nonindurated, painful, foul-smelling genital ulcerations several days after contact. Tender inguinal adenopathy, usually unilateral, occurs in approximately half the patients. Smears obtained from an ulcer previously cleansed with saline or from aspirate of a fluctuant lymph node may demonstrate gram-negative streptobacillary organisms in parallel "railroad tracks" or clustered "school of fish" arrangements characteristic of the causative organisms, *Hemophilus ducreyi*. The differential diagnosis must include causes of any painful genital lesion, most commonly herpes or trauma, with secondary bacterial infection. Primary syphilis should be ruled out by darkfield examination prior to initiation of therapy, and follow-up serologic tests for syphilis should be done monthly for 3 months.

Treatment

1. Sulfamethoxazole, 800 mg., with trimethoprim, 160 mg., every 12 hours (this use of this drug combination is not listed in the manufacturer's official directive) or sulfisoxazole 1 gram four times a day, should be given orally for 2 to 3 weeks. If no response is observed after several days of treatment, tetracycline, 500 mg. four times a day for 2 to 3 weeks, should be added. Occasionally, longer courses of therapy are needed. Rarely, resistant cases may require kanamycin, 500 mg. intramuscularly every 12 hours for 1 to 2 weeks. (This specific use of kanamycin is not listed in the manufacturer's official directive.)

2. Local therapy with cool isotonic saline soaks 10 to 15 minutes four times a day is an important adjunct in alleviating discomfort and reducing secondary infection.

3. Fluctuant lymph nodes may be carefully aspirated through a number 19 or 20 needle to prevent rupture and reduce pain.

4. Severe phimosis may require urologic surgical intervention.

5. One must remember that multiple venereal diseases may coexist, so that persistent lesions should be carefully reexamined. At times, a biopsy may be indicated to rule out granuloma inguinale or carcinoma.

GONORRHEA

method of
STEPHEN J. KRAUS, M.D.,
W. DAVID HAGER, M.D.,
and NORMAN F. JACOBS, JR., M.D.
Atlanta, Georgia

General Considerations in Treating Uncomplicated Gonorrhea

Penicillinase-producing *Neisseria gonorrhoeae* (PPNG), first detected in 1976, pose a potential threat to gonococcal therapy. Nevertheless, penicillin remains the drug of choice because PPNG prevalence remains low (less than 1 per cent of *N. gonorrhoeae* isolated in the United States), and a safe, highly effective inexpensive, single-dose alternative antibiotic is not available. Spectinomycin hydrochloride is effective against PPNG and is recommended for this problem but its indiscriminate use in treating all uncomplicated gonorrhea could result in an increase in spectinomycin-resistant gonococci and possibly penicillin/

spectinomycin-resistant strains. Spectinomycin may also be used in patients not cured by recommended first-line regimens or those patients who are at a high risk of having PPNG. The latter are sexual contacts of persons known to have PPNG and patients who contracted gonorrhea in areas of the world endemic for PPNG such as the Philippines. Tetracycline, the nonpenicillin alternative gonorrhea therapy, is relatively ineffective against PPNG. Synthetic penicillins and available cephalosporins active against penicillinase-producing staphylococci are also expected to be relatively ineffective in PPNG infections. The Center for Disease Control is closely monitoring the prevalence of PPNG in the United States and evaluating other antibiotics that could be used in addition to spectinomycin for treating PPNG. If the prevalence of PPNG increases or other antibiotics effective against PPNG become available, the treatments outlined in this chapter may be revised.

Gonococci infecting different mucosal sites are not eradicated with equal facility. Ampicillin-probenecid and spectinomycin regimens effective in treating genital gonorrhea are not adequate for the treatment of gonococcal pharyngitis. The same mucosal surfaces in different populations may also respond differently to the same treatment, as illustrated by the problem of eradicating anorectal gonorrhea in male homosexuals with the ampicillin and tetracycline regimens that are highly effective in treating infections at the same site in heterosexual women.

Single-dose therapy for uncomplicated gonorrhea is preferred because it minimizes problems with patient compliance. This is one reason for favoring penicillin-probenecid over tetracycline. Among the various penicillin regimens, aqueous procaine penicillin G (APPG) is highly effective and remains the standard to which other regimens are compared. It is also the only regimen known to eradicate incubating syphilis. Patients receiving ampicillin, spectinomycin, tetracycline, or erythromycin should have a follow-up serologic test for syphilis 3 months after gonorrhea therapy. Disadvantages of aqueous procaine penicillin G are the neuropsychiatric procaine reactions seen in 0.2 to 1 per cent of patients receiving 4.8 million units intramuscularly and the increased potential of anaphylactic reactions with parenteral penicillin. Provisions for treating anaphylaxis must be available whenever parenteral penicillin is given. Penicillin G benzathine and penicillin V should not be used to treat gonorrhea.

A universally effective gonorrhea therapy is not available and resolution of symptoms is not synonymous with cure. All infected sites should therefore be cultured 3 to 7 days after completion of therapy. Reinfection, in addition to resistant organisms, should be considered in patients with persistent gonorrhea after standard therapy. Failure of therapy to eradicate symptoms or signs attributed to gonorrhea should also raise the possibility that the patient was originally misdiagnosed or has gonorrhea as well as a second disease. In men infected with *Chlamydia trachomatis* as well as the gonococcus, penicillin will eradicate the gonococci but the *Chlamydiae* continue to cause the dysuria and urethral discharge of postgonococcal urethritis. Misdiagnoses of gonorrhea are frequent when the diagnosis is based solely on the clinical picture. Gram stains of urethral and conjunctival exudate and cultures from other mucosal sites are essential for the accurate diagnosis of uncomplicated gonorrhea.

Uncomplicated Genital and Rectal Gonorrhea

The treatment of choice is aqueous procaine penicillin G, 4.8 million units intramuscularly, divided into two doses and injected into each buttock at one visit, together with 1 gram of probenecid by mouth just before the injections. Alternative oral penicillin regimens consist of single doses of ampicillin, 3.5 grams, or amoxicillin, 3.0 grams, together with 1 gram of probenecid. Rectal gonorrhea in male homosexuals responds poorly to ampicillin-probenecid but does respond to the aqueous procaine penicillin G–probenecid regimen.

Patients allergic to penicillin or probenecid may receive tetracycline hydrochloride, 0.5 gram four times per day with a total dose of 9.5 grams. Other tetracyclines are no more effective than tetracycline hydrochloride. Oral tetracycline should be given 1 hour before or 2 hours after meals, because certain foods interfere with absorption; antacids also interfere with tetracycline absorption. A second alternative antibiotic for the allergic patient is spectinomycin, 2 grams intramuscularly in one injection. Rectal gonorrhea in male homosexuals responds poorly to tetracycline and such patients allergic to penicillin should be treated with spectinomycin.

Pregnant patients allergic to penicillin or probenecid may be treated with erythromycin (other than the estolate), 0.5 gram four times a day for 7 days. The high failure rate with this antibiotic demands that cultures be obtained to document cure.

Pharyngeal Gonorrhea

Pharyngeal gonococci may be more difficult to eradicate than genital organisms. The single-dose schedules for spectinomycin, ampicillin-probenecid, and amoxicillin-probenecid described for the treatment of uncomplicated genital gonorrhea are particularly ineffective and are not recommended. The procaine penicillin–probenecid and tetracycline regimens described for genital gonorrhea can be used for pharyngeal infections. Treatment failures with one of these antibiotics can sometimes be managed with the other regimen or a longer course of therapy.

Uncomplicated Gonorrhea in Children

Treatment of uncomplicated genital infection (vaginitis or urethritis) is a single course of aqueous procaine penicillin G, 75,000 to 100,000 units per kg. intramuscularly, and probenecid, 25 mg. per kg. by mouth. Local or systemic estrogens are of no benefit in gonococcal vaginitis. Children allergic to penicillin can be given erythromycin, 40 mg. per kg. per day in 4 doses by mouth for 7 days. Postpubertal children and those weighing more than 100 pounds should be treated with the dosage regimens outlined for adult therapy. Child abuse should be considered when gonococcal infection occurs in young children.

Neonatal Gonococcal Ophthalmia

Prevention of this problem consists of culturing the mother for gonococci during the last trimester and instilling antigonococcal ophthalmic preparations such as 1 per cent silver nitrate into the neonate's eyes; this should not be washed out with saline irrigations. Alternatively, tetracycline or erythromycin ointments may be used. Bacitracin ointment is ineffective, and penicillin preparations should be avoided because of their sensitizing potential.

Treatment of gonococcal ophthalmia neonatorum consists of aqueous crystalline penicillin G, 50,000 units per kg. per day in three doses intravenously for 7 days. Conjunctival exudate is removed with frequent saline irrigations, followed by tetracycline or chloramphenicol ophthalmic drops. Topical antibiotics alone are not recommended for the treatment of gonococcal conjunctivitis. Newborn children with gonococcal ophthalmia are at risk of having gonococcal infection in other body sites and the systemic antibiotics will eradicate these other foci of infection.

Sexual Contacts

All sexual contacts of patients with gonorrhea, regardless of symptoms, must be evaluated and receive appropriate therapy. The signs and symptoms of uncomplicated gonorrhea in women may be minimal or go unnoticed. Urethral gonococci can be recovered from up to 40 per cent of asymptomatic contacts of certain women with gonorrhea. Awareness of gonorrhea in a sexual contact may be the sole clue that the person is infected. Even if the diagnosis cannot be made at the time, all contacts should receive treatment at their first visit because the Gram stain is undersensitive in asymptomatic men, a single cervical culture may not detect 10 to 15 per cent of infected women, and the default rate may be high in patients asked to return for therapy. Epidemiologic treatment regimens are the same as those used for uncomplicated genital gonorrhea.

Test of Cure and Management of Treatment Failures

No therapy for gonorrhea is universally effective and, therefore, all infected sites must be cultured 3 to 7 days after completion of therapy, especially those sites at which gonococci may be more difficult to eradicate such as the pharynx and the male rectum. Gonococci from all treatment failures should be tested by local or state laboratories for penicillinase activity (all state laboratories can perform this test). Patients having PPNG must be reported to the local health department, since therapy failure and subsequent demonstration of penicillinase activity is one mechanism that facilitates monitoring PPNG prevalence. Also, a rapid and thorough epidemiologic investigation of sexual contacts has contributed to PPNG control.

Reinfection should be considered in patients with persistent or recurrent gonorrhea occurring after adequate therapy. Failure of treatment correlates with gonococcal antibiotic resistance whether the resistance is secondary to plasmid-mediated penicillinase production or chromosome-mediated resistance. In the latter mechanism, organisms are frequently resistant to both tetracycline and penicillin but sensitive to spectinomycin. PPNG strains currently identified in the United States originated in the Far East where most gonococci are resistant to tetracycline but sensitive to spectinomycin. Therefore, spectinomycin is the drug of choice for patients with uncomplicated anogenital gonorrhea who are not cured by penicillin or tetracycline.

Salpingitis

It has been estimated that 10 to 15 per cent of women who have gonorrhea will develop gonococcal salpingitis. Gonococci can be cultured from the endocervix of women with their first episode of salpingitis in 50 to 80 per cent. Although it is common practice to define the cause of salpingitis by the pathogen isolated from the endocervix, it may be better to define the causative agents by examining tubal flora. Several studies have shown a poor relation between endocervical culture of the gonococcus and tubal isolation in the same patient. Culturing from the tube or pelvic peritoneal cavity by culdocentesis or through the laparoscope has revealed that salpingitis is often polymicrobial in cause. This information indicates that therapy for salpingitis must be adequate for a number of potential pathogens. Since a large percentage of initial, acute disease is gonococcal in cause, it is helpful to determine whether the patient is having her first acute episode or has a history consistent with recurrent disease.

Many patients may be managed without hospitalization. They should be carefully instructed about the symptoms of progressive disease, told to avoid sexual intercourse, and followed carefully with a return visit at 48 to 72 hours and again at 7 days. Out-patients may be treated with: (1) aqueous procaine penicillin G, 4.8 million units intramuscularly divided into two doses, injected at two sites at the same visit, along with 1 gram of oral probenecid; or (2) ampicillin, 3.5 grams orally in a single dose, plus 1 gram of oral probenecid. Both are to be followed by 2 grams per day of oral ampicillin given in four divided doses for at least 10 days; (3) nonpregnant women with no evidence of renal failure who are allergic to penicillin may be treated with tetracycline hydrochloride, 1.5 grams orally in a single dose to be followed by 2 grams per day orally in four divided doses for at least 10 days. Follow-up test-of-cure cultures and appropriate contact tracing must be done on all women with gonococcal salpingitis.

Salpingitis may be a complication of cervical infection with penicillinase-producing *N. gonorrhoeae* (PPNG). Spectinomycin is the drug of choice in the treatment of this organism, although information about the use of this agent in the therapy of PPNG-related salpingitis is limited. At present, it is best to hospitalize patients with salpingitis caused by PPNG and treat with spectinomycin, 2 grams intramuscularly twice daily, for 5 to 7 days. Many of these organisms are resistant to the tetracyclines as well as the penicillins; therefore, completing a course with oral medication is not indicated. An aminoglycoside may be substituted for spectinomycin in the treatment of these women. All sexual contacts of patients with gonococcal salpingitis must be treated.

Certain patients require hospitalization to treat their disease adequately. There are 7 primary indications for hospitalization: (1) questionable diagnosis (e.g., inability to rule out appendicitis, ectopic pregnancy); (2) nausea and vomiting preventing oral treatment; (3) presence of adnexal mass suggestive of an abscess; (4) evidence of generalized peritonitis; (5) poor response to outpatient therapy; (6) pregnancy (very rare after first trimester); (7) complicating medical disease (e.g., diabetes mellitus, valvular heart disease).

In-patient therapy includes supportive measures such as bed rest, analgesics, and intravenous fluids. In addition, these drug regimens may be used:

1. For patients with initial acute disease and no pelvic abscess: (a) Aqueous crystalline penicillin G, 10 to 20 million units per day intravenously, or ampicillin, 1 gram intravenously every 4 to 6 hours, until there is definite clinical improvement, to be followed by ampicillin, 2 grams per day orally in four divided doses to complete 10 days of therapy. (b) In penicillin-allergic patients without a history of anaphylaxis, a cephalosporin may be used parenterally (such as cefazolin 1 to 2 grams intravenously every 6 hours) (this dose may be higher that that listed in the manufacturer's official directive) until there is definite clinical improvement, to be followed by cephalexin, orally, 2 grams daily in four divided doses, to complete 10 days of therapy.

2. A broad-spectrum type of therapy is advised for patients with recurrent acute disease or an acute exacerbation of chronic disease, or those who have or are suspected of having pelvic abscess or an anaerobic infection, or those who have shown a poor clinical response to out-patient administration of antibiotics. Gonococci, aerobic cocci, and anaerobes are the organisms most frequently isolated from culdocentesis specimens, but aerobic gram-negative rods are also found. No controlled studies have been done to evaluate the need for treatment of each of these organisms. One reasonable approach is to use the same aqueous crystalline penicillin G regimen mentioned above plus clindamycin, 600 mg. intravenously every 6 hours. Some clinicians also recommend adding an aminoglycoside (e.g., tobramycin, 1 mg. per kg. every 8 hours, if renal function is normal). Alternatively, chloramphenicol, 2 to 4 grams per day can be used in conjunction with the penicillin. As soon as definite clinical improvement has occurred, a switch to oral ampicillin should be made to complete 10 to 14 days of therapy, and to oral clindamycin to complete 7 to 10 days of therapy. Since clindamycin has been associated with the development of pseudomembranous enterocolitis, this drug should be discontinued if the patient develops significant diarrhea. The incidence of aplastic anemia among the patients taking chloramphenicol is very low but must be considered when prescribing this antibiotic.

There is a definite role for surgery in the management of patients with severe salpingitis. The decision to intervene surgically in a patient who is responding poorly to medical management is often difficult. The indications for surgery are (1) absence of clinical improvement after adequate antimicrobial therapy; (2) presence of a pelvic abscess that does not respond to medical management; (3) suspected rupture or leakage of a pelvic abscess (a surgical emergency); and (4) a serious question about the diagnosis. The timing of a surgical management in these patients must be individualized.

Disseminated Gonococcal Infection (DGI)

The majority of patients with gonococcal bacteremia suffer from the "arthritis-dermatitis" syndrome. These patients may have tenosynovitis and skin lesions but do not have purulent joint effusions, and they respond readily to a wide variety of antibiotic regimens. However, the occurrence of serious complications of gonococcal bacteremia (e.g., meningitis and endocarditis) points out the need for careful management of DGI. Septicemic gonococci are very sensitive to the antibiotics used to treat gonococcal infections.

Indications for Hospitalization. Although some patients with the arthritis-dermatitis syndrome may be treated as outpatients, any patient with a purulent joint effusion or evidence of meningitis, endocarditis, or osteomyelitis should be hospitalized. If the clinical diagnosis of DGI is in doubt, if the patient cannot be relied upon to adhere to the outpatient regimen, or if marked improvement does not occur within 24 to 48 hours, then hospitalization is necessary.

Therapy for the Arthritis-Dermatitis Syndrome. Treatments of choice: (1) Aqueous crystalline penicillin G, 10 million units intravenously daily for 3 days; this may be followed by ampicillin, 500 mg. orally four times a day for an additional 4 to 7 days. (2) Aqueous procaine penicillin G, 4.8 million units intramuscularly, together with probenecid, 1 gram orally as a single dose, followed by ampicillin (as above) for 7 to 10 days.

Alternative regimen: Ampicillin, 3.5 grams (or amoxicillin, 3.0 grams) orally, together with probenecid, 1 gram orally, followed by 500 mg. ampicillin (or 500 mg. amoxicillin) orally four times a day for 7 to 10 days.

Therapy for penicillin-allergic patients: (1) Tetracycline hydrochloride, 500 mg. orally four times a day for 7 to 10 days taken on an empty stomach. (2) Erythromycin, 500 mg. orally four times a day for 7 to 10 days. Erythromycin stearate must be taken on an empty stomach; the estolate is adequately absorbed in the presence of food, but causes cholestatic jaundice in some patients.

Therapy for Pregnant Patients. One of the penicillin regimens should be used unless the woman is allergic to penicillin, in which case erythromycin should be substituted. Tetracycline should not be used. Spectinomycin has not been proved safe in pregnancy, but doses of 4 grams per day parenterally have been used to treat nonpregnant patients with DGI.

Therapy for Gonococcal Septic Arthritis. Treatment of choice: Aqueous crystalline penicillin G as outlined above. In addition, joint fluid should be aspirated on a daily basis if necessary to prevent exudate accumulation. Painful joints should be immobilized. Open drainage is not necessary, except for hip involvement where repeated aspiration of the joint cannot easily be performed. Intra-articular antibiotics or anti-inflammatory agents are never indicated.

Childhood Disseminated Gonococcal Infection. Postpubertal children and those who weigh more than 100 pounds should receive adult therapy. Younger children can be given aqueous crystalline penicillin G intravenously, 75,000 to 100,000 units per kg. per day in four doses, or aqueous procaine penicillin G, 75,000 to 100,000 units per kg. per day intramuscularly in two doses for 7 to 10 days. In patients with a minor penicillin allergy, intravenous cephalothin may be used in a dose of 60 to 80 mg. per kg. per day in four doses for 7 to 10 days. Children 8 years of age or older and having a major penicillin allergy, such as anaphylaxis, may be treated with intravenous tetracycline in a dose of 15 to 20 mg. per kg. per day in four doses for 7 to 10 days. The use of tetracycline in children less that 8 years of age may cause permanent tooth discoloration.

Therapy for Gonococcal Endocarditis, Osteomyelitis, and Meningitis. Gonococcal endocarditis requires 10 to 20 million units of intravenous aqueous crystalline penicillin G daily for at least 4 weeks. In case of minor penicillin allergy, cefazolin, 6 grams daily in divided doses, may be given parenterally, but close observation is necessary since alternatives to penicillin have not been well evaluated in gonococcal endocarditis. If the patient has had an anaphylactic reaction to penicillin, intravenous erythromycin may be preferable to cefazolin.

For osteomyelitis, the same regimens are used as in endocarditis.

For gonococcal meningitis, one should use the same penicillin regimen as in endocarditis, but for only 10 days. In penicillin-allergic patients, the alternative regimens are chloramphenicol, 1 gram intravenously every 6 hours, or tetracycline, 500 mg. intravenously every 6 hours. Cephalosporins should not be used to treat meningitis.

Therapy for Disseminated Gonococcal Infection Caused by Penicillinase-Producing Neisseria Gonorrhoeae (PPNG). At the time of this writing, PPNG strains are not a major problem in the United States. Clinical studies of antibiotic therapy of PPNG-induced disseminated gonococcal infection (DGI) have not been conducted, but in vitro data suggest that erythromycin and spectinomycin should be effective. Physicians may contact the Venereal Disease Control Division at the Center for Disease Control, (404) 633-3311, for latest information on DGI caused by PPNG.

DONOVANOSIS
(Granuloma Inguinale)

method of
GAVIN HART, M.D., M.P.H.
Perth, Western Australia

Donovanosis is a chronic granulomatous disease caused by *Calymmatobacterium granulomatis.* Although probably sexually transmitted, lesions are rarely detected in casual sexual contacts, but a number of studies have detected infection in 12 to 52 per cent of marital or steady sexual partners.

Therapy

1. Tetracycline, 500 mg. orally four times daily until lesions heal, which may be 3 to 4 weeks. Response to therapy, indicated by shrinking and decreasing redness of lesions, should occur in 7 to 10 days. If lesions are unchanged after this time, an alternative antibiotic should be commenced immediately.

2. Gentamicin, 80 mg. twice daily intramuscularly, or

3. Chloramphenicol, 500 mg. every 8 hours orally. This drug is probably the most effective against Donovanosis but is best reserved for resistant cases.

Lesions often continue to heal if drug therapy is ceased prematurely, but the relapse rate will be increased by this practice.

LYMPHOGRANULOMA VENEREUM (LGV)

method of
GAVIN HART, M.D., M.P.H.
Perth, Western Australia

Lymphogranuloma venereum (LGV) is a systemic, sexually transmitted disease, which may be produced by a number of closely related chlamydia. Primary inoculation may occur at any anatomic site involved in intimate contact. Regional lymphadenitis develops in the nodes draining this site and the disease disseminates further via the lymphatic system. Since the primary lesion is often transient and passes unnoticed, the most common presentation to a physician is lymphadenopathy of the anogenital or neck regions.

The LGV complement fixation test (LGV-CFT) should be used to confirm the diagnosis and monitor therapy. A 4-fold rise in titer is diagnostic, but the titer has often reached a stable level by the time a client presents for treatment. A stable titer of 1:32 or greater in the presence of lymphadenopathy is diagnostic. Tit-

ers may not fall for 3 months (or even 6 months when very high titers have been reached) and should be determined every 3 months for at least 1 year after cure.

Therapy

1. Tetracycline, 500 mg. orally four times daily for at least 3 weeks.

2. Sulfisoxazole, 4.0 grams orally, followed by 1 gram four times a day, for at least 3 weeks.

3. Fluctuant nodes should be aspirated, but surgical intervention should otherwise be minimized. Unnecessary removal of lymph nodes may worsen lymphedema or elephantiasis.

4. Rectal stricture should be managed by dilatation at 2-week intervals. Colostomy should be reserved for the most refractory cases in which conservative management fails.

5. Surgery is contraindicated during active disease and should be covered by antibiotic therapy for 2 weeks before until 2 weeks after operation.

SYPHILIS

CDC RECOMMENDED TREATMENT SCHEDULES, 1976

U.S. Department of Health, Education, and Welfare/Public Health Service

The following recommendations were established by the Venereal Disease Control Advisory Committee* after deliberation with therapy experts.†

Few data have been published on the treatment of syphilis since CDC revised these recommendations in 1968. Penicillin continues to be the drug of choice for all stages of syphilis. Every effort should be made to document penicillin allergy before choosing other antibiotics, because these antibiotics have been studied less extensively

---

*R. H. Henderson, M.D., Chairman, Venereal Disease Control Division, Bureau of State Services, Center for Disease Control, Atlanta, Ga.; J. H. Miller, Executive Secretary, Venereal Disease Control Division, Bureau of State Services, CDC; D. Fouser, WNET-TV, New York, N.Y.; H. Hamilton, Editor, *Urban Health*, Atlanta, Ga.; G. H. Handy, M.D., Department of Health and Social Services, Madison, Wis.; B. Krohn, Barbara Krohn, and Associates, Seattle, Wash.; S. Nixon, M.D., Floresville, Tex.; M. O. Shinn, EOC of Imperial County (Cal.), Inc., El Centro, Cal.

†V. Cave, M.D., Brooklyn, N.Y.; P. E. Dans, M.D., University of Colorado Medical School, Denver, Colo.; N. J. Fiumara, M.D., State Department of Public Health, Boston, Mass.; A. R. Hinman, M.D., State Department of Public Health, Nashville, Tenn.; R. H. Kampmeier, M.D., Central State Hospital, Nash-

than penicillin. Physicians are cautioned to use no less than the recommended dosages of antibiotics.

Early Syphilis (Primary, Secondary, Latent Syphilis of Less Than 1 Year's Duration)

1. Benzathine penicillin G, 2.4 million units total by intramuscular injection at a single session. *Benzathine penicillin G is the drug of choice because it provides effective treatment in a single visit.* OR*

2. Aqueous procaine penicillin G, 4.8 million units total: 600,000 units by intramuscular injection daily for 8 days. OR

3. Procaine penicillin G in oil with 2 per cent aluminum monostearate (PAM), 4.8 million units total by intramuscular injection: 2.4 million units at first visit, and 1.2 million units at each of two subsequent visits 3 days apart. *Although PAM is used in other countries, it is no longer available in the United States.*

Patients Who Are Allergic to Penicillin. 1. Tetracycline hydrochloride,† 500 mg. four times a day by mouth for 15 days. OR

2. Erythromycin (stearate, ethylsuccinate, or base), 500 mg. four times a day by mouth for 15 days.

These antibiotics appear to be effective but have been evaluated less extensively than penicillin.

Syphilis of More Than 1 Year's Duration (Latent Syphilis of Indeterminate or More Than 1 Year's Duration, Cardiovascular, Late Benign, Neurosyphilis)

1. Benzathine penicillin G, 7.2 million units total: 2.4 million units by intramuscular injection weekly for 3 successive weeks. OR

2. Aqueous procaine penicillin G, 9.0 million units total: 600,000 units by intramuscular injection daily for 15 days.

The optimal treatment schedules for syphilis of greater than 1 year's duration have been less well established than schedules for early syphilis. In general, syphilis of longer duration requires higher-dose therapy.

Although therapy is recommended for established cardiovascular syphilis, there is little evidence that antibiotics reverse the pathology associated with this disease.

Cerebrospinal fluid (CSF) examination is mandatory in patients with suspected, symptomatic neurosyphilis. This examination is also desirable in other patients with syphilis of greater than 1 year's duration to exclude asymptomatic neurosyphilis.

Published studies show that a total dose of 6.0 to 9.0 million units of penicillin G results in a satisfactory clinical response in approximately 90 per cent of patients with neurosyphilis. There is more published clinical experience with short-acting penicillin preparations than with benzathine penicillin G. Some clinicians prefer to hospitalize patients with neurosyphilis, particularly if the patient is symptomatic or has not responded to initial therapy. In these instances they treat patients with 12 to 24 million units of aqueous crystalline penicillin G given intravenously each day (2 to 4 million units every 4 hours) for 10 days.

Patients Who Are Allergic to Penicillin. 1. Tetracycline hydrochloride, 500 mg. four times a day by mouth for 30 days. OR

2. Erythromycin (stearate, ethylsuccinate, or base), 500 mg. four times a day by mouth for 30 days.

There are NO published clinical data which adequately document the efficacy of drugs other than penicillin for syphilis of more than 1 year's duration. Cerebrospinal fluid examinations are highly recommended before therapy with these regimens.

Syphilis in Pregnancy

Evaluation of Pregnant Women. *All pregnant women should have a nontreponemal serologic test for syphilis, such as the VDRL or RPR test, at the time of the first prenatal visit. The treponemal tests such as the FTA-ABS test should not be used for routine screening. In women suspected of being at high risk for syphilis, a second nontreponemal test should be performed during the third trimester. Seroreactive patients should be expeditiously evaluated. This evaluation should include a history and physical examination, as well as a quantitative nontreponemal test and a confirmatory treponemal test.*

If the FTA-ABS test is nonreactive and there is no clinical evidence of syphilis, treatment may be withheld. Both the quantitative nontreponemal test and the confirmatory test should be repeated within 4 weeks. If there is clinical or serologic evidence of syphilis or if the diagnosis of syphilis cannot be excluded with reasonable certainty, the patient should be treated as outlined below.

Patients for whom there is documentation of adequate treatment for syphilis in the past need not be re-treated unless there is clinical or serologic evidence of reinfection such as darkfield-positive lesions or a fourfold titer rise of a quantitative nontreponemal test.

1. Patients at All Stages of Pregnancy Who Are Not Allergic to Penicillin. Penicillin is given in dos-

ville, Tenn.; I. Klein, M.D., Grady Memorial Hospital, Atlanta, Ga.; W. Ledger, M.D., University of Southern California Medical Center, Los Angeles, Cal.; W. McCormack, M.D., Boston City Hospital, Boston, Mass.; G. McCracken, M.D., University of Texas Medical Center, Dallas, Tex,; N. B. Nichols, M.D., University of Oklahoma Health Sciences Center, Oklahoma City, Okla.; P. L. Perine, M.D., Virginia Mason Clinic, Seattle, Wash.; M. F. Rein, M.D., University of Virginia, Charlottesville, Va.; J. P. Sanford, M.D., Uniformed Services University of the Health Sciences, Bethesda, Md.; A. L. Schroeter, M.D., Mayo Clinic, Rochester, Minn.; P. F. Sparling, M.D., University of North Carolina, Chapel Hill, N. C.; L. Taber, M.D., Baylor College of Medicine, Houston, Tex.; E. C. Tramont, M.D., Lt. Col., M. C., Walter Reed Army Medical Center Washington, D. C.

*Italics indicate commentary.

†Food and some dairy products interfere with absorption. Oral forms of tetracycline should be given 1 hour before or 2 hours after meals.

age schedules appropriate for the stage of syphilis, as recommended for the treatment of nonpregnant patients.

2. Patients at All Stages of Pregnancy Who Are Allergic to Penicillin. Erythromycin (stearate, ethylsuccinate, or base) is given in dosage schedules appropriate for the stage of syphilis, as recommended for the treatment of nonpregnant patients. Although these erythromycin schedules appear safe for mother and fetus, their efficacy is not well established. Therefore the documentation of penicillin allergy is particularly important before treating a pregnant woman with erythromycin. *Erythromycin estolate and tetracycline are not recommended for syphilitic infections in pregnant women because of potential adverse effects on mother and fetus.*

Follow-up. Pregnant women who have been treated for syphilis should have monthly quantitative nontreponemal serologic tests for the remainder of the current pregnancy. Women who show a four-fold rise in titer should be re-treated. After delivery, follow-up is as outlined for non-pregnant patients.

Congenital Syphilis

Congenital syphilis may occur if the mother has syphilis during pregnancy. If the mother has received adequate penicillin treatment during pregnancy, the risk to the infant is minimal. However, all infants should be examined carefully at birth and at frequent intervals therafter until nontreponemal serologic tests are negative.

Infected infants are frequently asymptomatic at birth and may be seronegative if the maternal infection occurred late in gestation. Infants should be treated at birth if maternal treatment was inadequate, unknown, or with drugs other than penicillin, or if adequate follow-up of the infant cannot be ensured.

Infants with congenital syphilis should have a CSF examination before treatment.

Infants with Abnormal CSF. 1. Aqueous crystalline penicillin G, 50,000 units per kg. intramuscularly or intravenously daily in two divided doses for a minimum of 10 days. OR

2. Aqueous procaine penicillin G, 50,000 units per kg. intramuscularly daily for a minimum of 10 days.

Infants with Normal CSF. *Benzathine penicillin G, 50,000 units per kg. intramuscularly in a single dose. Although benzathine penicillin has been previously recommended and widely used, published clinical data on its efficacy in congenital neurosyphilis are lacking. If neurosyphilis cannot be excluded, the procaine or aqueous penicillin regimens are recommended. Since cerebrospinal fluid concentrations of penicillin achieved after benzathine penicillin are minimal to nonexistent, these revised recommendations seem more conservative and appropriate until clinical data on the efficacy of benzathine penicillin can be accumulated. Other antibiotics are not recommended for neonatal congenital syphilis.* Penicillin therapy for congenital syphilis after the neonatal period should be with the same dosages used for neonatal congenital syphilis. For larger children the total dose of penicillin need not exceed the dosage used in adult syphilis of more than 1 year's duration. After the neonatal period, the dosage of erythromycin and tetracycline for congenital syphilitics who are allergic to penicillin should be individualized but need not exceed dosages used in adult syphilis of more than 1 year's duration. Tetracycline should not be given to children less than 8 years of age.

Follow-up and Retreatment

All patients with early syphilis and congenital syphilis should be encouraged to return for repeat quantitative nontreponemal tests 3, 6, and 12 months after treatment. Patients with syphilis of more than 1 year's duration should also have a repeat serologic test 24 months after treatment. Careful follow-up serologic testing is particularly important in patients treated with antibiotics other than penicillin. Examination of CSF should be planned as part of the last follow-up visit after treatment with alternative antibiotics.

All patients with neurosyphilis must be carefully followed with serologic testing for at least 3 years. In addition, follow-up of these patients should include clinical re-evaluation at 6 month intervals and repeat CSF examinations, particularly in patients treated with alternative antibiotics.

The possibility of reinfection should always be considered when retreating patients with early syphilis. A CSF examination should be performed before retreatment unless reinfection and a diagnosis of early syphilis can be established.

Retreatment should be considered when (1) clinical signs or symptoms of syphilis persist or recur; (2) there is a sustained 4-fold increase in the titer of a nontreponemal test; or (3) an initially high-titer nontreponemal test fails to show a 4-fold decrease within a year.

Patients should be retreated with the schedules recommended for syphilis of more than 1 year's duration. In general, only one retreatment course is indicated because patients may maintain stable, low titers of nontreponemal tests or have irreversible anatomical damage.

Epidemiologic Treatment

Patients who have been exposed to infectious syphilis within the preceding 3 months and other patients who on epidemiologic grounds are at high risk for syphilis should be treated as for early syphilis. Every effort should be made to establish a diagnosis in these cases.

Reported by Venereal Disease Control Division, Bureau of State Services, CDC.

Diseases of Allergy

ANAPHYLAXIS AND SERUM SICKNESS

method of
SAMUEL O. FREEDMAN, M.D.
Montreal, Quebec, Canada

ANAPHYLAXIS

Definition

Human anaphylaxis is an acute, severe, and sometimes fatal reaction occurring within seconds or minutes after exposure to an allergenic agent to which the person is specifically hypersensitive. At present, the bulk of the available evidence suggests that human anaphylaxis is an immunologic reaction primarily mediated by homocytotropic antibodies (reagins) belonging to the IgE class of immunoglobulins, although other mechanisms may be operative under certain circumstances.

The great majority of human anaphylactic reactions result from the injection of therapeutic or diagnostic agents or the ingestion of a drug or food, or they occur accidentally following an insect sting. Historically, the most common antigen provoking anaphylaxis in man has been heterologous serum, such as equine tetanus antitoxin. Horse serum is now a much less frequent causative agent since the introduction of human antitetanus immunoglobulin for passive immunization against tetanus. Perhaps the most common cause of anaphylactic reactions due to biologic material is the injection of allergy extracts during immunotherapy for atopic diseases. Such reactions may take place due to the inadvertent and sometimes unpredictable administration of too high a dose or through accidental intravascular injection.

It has been estimated that anaphylactic reactions to stinging insects of the Hymenoptera family account for 40 to 50 reported fatalities each year in the United States. The actual incidence of insect sting deaths is undoubtedly much higher than reported, because many deaths are erroneously attributed to so-called natural causes such as heart disease, heat stroke, or cerebrovascular accidents occurring outdoors during the summer months.

Prevention of Anaphylaxis

Horse Serum. If the administration of horse serum for passive immunization is contemplated, some attempts must be made to determine whether the patient is hypersensitive to it. Intradermal testing is usually carried out with 0.025 ml. of horse serum in a dilution of 1:100. If this test gives negative results, it should be repeated at a dilution of 1:10 to exclude horse serum sensitivity. Any patient who has a history of rhinitis or asthma due to horse dander or of previous allergy to horse serum should be presumed sensitive to horse serum even if the intradermal result is negative.

Penicillin. At present there is no rapid and reliable method for predicting penicillin sensitivity. Penicillin or one of its homologs is rarely the only available lifesaving drug, except perhaps in certain cases of subacute bacterial endocarditis. Whenever there is any suspicion of a previous adverse reaction to penicillin, it would be prudent to choose a different class of antibiotic. In patients with proved or suspected subacute bacterial endocarditis, skin testing with both penicilloyl-polylysine and crystalline potassium penicillin G may possibly be of assistance. If either of these tests is positive or if there is a convincing history of penicillin hypersensitivity, intravenous penicillin should be administered only after carefully weighing the anticipated risk of an anaphylactic reaction against the anticipated risk of witholding a bactericidal drug.

Insect Stings. Unfortunately, there are no generally available techniques for diagnosing and overcoming this dangerous form of anaphylactic hypersensitivity. For many years water-soluble extracts of whole insect bodies were used for skin testing, with results assumed to be satisfactory on an anecdotal basis. It has recently been demonstrated that skin testing with these materials shows considerable overlap between the various species of Hymenoptera and fails to distinguish adequately between allergic and normal persons. Intradermal tests with commercially available Hymenoptera whole-body extracts are positive, depending on the manufacturer, in 40 to 90 per cent of all persons tested. Recently, it has been suggested that Hymenoptera venom rather that whole-body extract is a more appropriate allergen for skin testing and this material is now commercially available. The effectiveness of immunization with whole-body extracts of stinging insects as a preventive method is at best a questionable procedure, since the evidence is incontestable that it may fail in some patients.

Treatment

The single most effective agent in combating human anaphylaxis is epinephrine. Because it antagonizes edema of the respiratory mucous membranes and constriction of the bronchodial musculature, it reverses many of the pathophysiologic consequences of human anaphylaxis. The action of antihistamines is slower and weaker than that of epinephrine, and this class of drugs has no significant effect on bronchoconstriction. Corticosteroids have little place in the treatment of acute anaphylaxis because of the delayed onset of their therapeutic effect, but they may provide additional symptomatic relief during the recovery period.

1. At the first sign of systemic anaphylaxis, the patient should be placed on his back with his feet elevated to combat shock.

2. If a subcutaneous or intramuscular injection has been given in the arm, a tourniquet should be placed proximal to the injection site to slow further systemic absorption of the drug.

3. Following these measures, the patient should be given 0.5 ml. of 1:1000 aqueous epinephrine subcutaneously. Unless there is profound shock from the outset, the intravenous use of epinephrine should be avoided because of its tendency to cause cardiac arrhythmias in anaphylaxis. If considered necessary because of poor circulation due to hypotension, epinephrine may be administered intravenously by diluting 0.2 ml. of 1:1000 aqueous epinephrine in 5 ml. of isotonic saline solution and injecting it slowly over 2 to 3 minutes.

4. Diphenhydramine hydrochloride, 50 mg., may be given intravenously at the same time as the first dose of epinephrine.

5. Most patients will respond quickly to this relatively simple treatment. Should recovery not occur within 5 minutes after the initial injection of epinephrine, an additional 0.3 ml. of 1:1000 aqueous epinephrine should be given every 5 minutes until the desired effect is obtained or until marked tachycardia and excitability make further administration of the drug unwise.

6. Hypotension that persists despite administration of epinephrine is an absolute indication for the prompt and rapid administration of large volumes of plasma or plasma substitutes. Vasopressor agents are of little value in maintaining blood pressure in acute anaphylaxis.

7. Hypoxia manifested by increasing cyanosis constitutes a life-threatening emergency. If epinephrine fails to relieve bronchial obstruction, aminophylline, 500 mg., should be injected intravenously. Severe laryngeal edema may require intubation or even emergency tracheostomy and assisted respiration.

8. As respiratory failure inevitably leads to cardiac arrest, external cardiac massage may be indicated in extreme situations.

9. Persistent but nonfatal symptoms of bronchospasm, laryngeal edema, and urticaria are best treated with hydrocortisone, 100 mg. intravenously, and diphenhydramine, 50 mg. by mouth every 6 hours, for as long as necessary.

10. The preferred treatment for insect sting anaphylaxis is the self-administration of epinephrine, 1:1000 solution, 0.3 ml. subcutaneously, as soon as possible after the sting. Several commercial laboratories have prepared emergency kits containing plastic syringes, preloaded with epinephrine that are considerably easier for the inexperienced or nervous person to handle at the time of crisis. A somewhat less effective alternative is the use of an epinephrine inhaler by persons incapable of mastering the technique of self-injection. Because only a small amount of epinephrine is absorbed systemically through the lung, the patient should be instructed to inhale 6 times rather than the usual 2 times recommended for the treatment of asthma.

11. If an implanted stinger with its attached venom sac is left behind when a honeybee is brushed off, the stinger should be carefully scraped away with the fingernails without compressing the sac.

SERUM SICKNESS SYNDROME

Definition

Classic serum sickness caused by the injection of foreign serum into human subjects is considerably less common than it was 20 to 30 years ago. Widespread immunization programs, the development of potent antibiotic agents and the increasing use of human antitetanus immunoglobulin have all contributed to the declining incidence of this syndrome. On the other hand, serum sickness-like reactions due to nonprotein drugs, especially penicillin, remain a problem of considerable magnitude. Well-documented serum sickness-like reactions have also been described following orally administered sulfonamides, hydantoin drugs, and piperazine citrate.

Clinical Manifestations

The characteristic clinical picture consists of urticaria, fever, arthralgias, lymphadenopathy and, less commonly, peripheral neuritis. The usual incubation period between the administration of the causative agent and the onset of symptoms varies from 6 days to 3 weeks. In certain persons with low residual titer of antibodies following previous exposure, an accelerated reaction may occur with the onset in 1 to 5 days.

Treatment

1. Milder cases usually respond well to hydroxyzine, 25 mg., four times daily for pruritus, and salicylates for joint pain and fever.

2. More severe attacks may require short courses of prednisone, 20 to 40 mg. daily, in divided doses. As serum sickness is usually a self-limited disease, there should be little hesitancy in prescribing systemic corticosteroids in otherwise healthy persons.

ASTHMA IN ADULTS
method of
SHELDON L. SPECTOR, M.D.
Denver, Colorado

Definition and Background

A useful working definition of asthma is "reversible obstructive airways disease caused by varying degrees of bronchospasm, mucosal edema and excessive mucus." This definition has certain implications:

1. The term wheezing is purposely omitted, since bronchoconstriction can occur without wheezing, and the patient may have chest tightness or cough instead of wheezing.

2. The term reversible is relative, since some asthmatics have an irreversible component to their disease, and only after maximal bronchodilation and long-term administration of corticosteroids can the reversibility be properly assessed.

3. Asthma is not necessarily associated with allergies, particularly those mediated by IgE or reaginic mechanisms.

4. Many patients with so-called chronic bronchitis, i.e., the presence of cough productive of sputum for at least 3 months of the year for 2 consecutive years, also have hyperreactive airways disease, as determined by metacholine and histamine inhalation tests. Since reversibility is almost invariably present, treatment of these patients should also be directed towards maximizing bronchodilation.

5. The cliches "extrinsic" and "intrinsic" asthma have outlived their usefulness. Although the term extrinsic implies a reagin-mediated mechanism, the term intrinsic has come to signify a diagnosis of exclusion. In reality, patients usually have heterogeneous mechanisms responsible for bronchial obstruction. In fact, patients are heterogeneous in the following ways:

The Factors Responsible for Precipitating Attacks. Although truly allergic reactions may trigger an attack, asthmatic patients have hyperreactive airways ("the twitchy lung") and respond to cold air, strong odors, exercise, etc., by other than IgE mechanisms.

The Location of the Major Areas of Obstruction. Some patients have primarily large airway obstruction, others small airway obstruction, and others have both, as delineated by sophisticated pulmonary function measurements.

The Degree of Reversibility of Airway Obstruction. Some patients who are thought to be irreversible by the use of a few breaths of standard aerosolized bronchodilators, will reveal their reversible component only after prolonged around-the-clock bronchodilators, and sometimes daily or alternate day corticosteroid therapy.

The Response to Various Forms of Medications. Although almost all asthmatic patients improve with corticosteroids and respond to theophylline bronchodilators, not all patients respond to other groups of bronchodilators. Some respond dramatically to β adrenergic agents, others to anticholinergic agents such as atropine and their analogues, and a very few respond to α-blocking agents.

The Amount of Medication Necessary to Produce the Desired Effect. Since absorption and metabolism differ in patients, the therapeutic dose often differs as well. A good example is the variable dose of theophylline required to produce a therapeutic effect. Elaboration of some of these concepts will be found under "Long-term Management of the Asthmatic Patient."

Management of Severe Asthma ("Status Asthmaticus")

The following discussion assumes that the diagnosis of asthma has been confirmed and the physician is aware of concomitant problems such as hiatus hernia, diabetes, congestive heart-failure, and pneumonia. Sequelae of severe asthma such as pneumothorax or pneumomediastinum must also be considered. Laboratory tests such as complete blood count, urinalysis, chest x-ray, electrocardiogram, and blood gas analysis should be routine. Sinus x-rays should not be forgotten, since sinusitis is very common and may contribute to persisting asthmatic symptoms. Serum electrolytes are also important, especially in patients on chronic therapy, since many of the medications commonly ingested by asthmatic patients contribute to hypokalemia. Spirometric measurements such as 1-second forced expiratory volume and peak flow can be measured with simple equipment. They are most useful in following the course of an acute asthmatic attack, or in the chronic evaluation of a patient.

The term "status asthmaticus" should really become obsolete, since it implies neglect on the part of the physician, patient, or both, or as Farr says, "The time to treat status asthmaticus is three days before it happens."

The following measures are then taken, depending on the severity of the patient's attack:

1. Repetitive blood gas and pH measurements are necessary to dictate whether the patient needs endotracheal intubation and assisted ventilation. Severe asthma is best handled in a hospital setting, preferably in the respiratory care unit, where continuous monitoring and specialized nursing care are available. The use of oxygen and sodium bicarbonate are dictated by the patient's clinical state.

2. Give intravenous fluids (5 per cent dextrose in water) for hydration and for administration of intravenous medications. More than 2500 ml. per day is preferable if there are no contraindications.

3. Administer 250 to 500 mg. of aminophylline by intravenous route over a 20 minute period, by piggy-back or Soluset. Although this method is personally preferred, a popular alternative is continuous intravenous infusion to obtain a therapeutic blood-level of between 10 and 20 micrograms per ml. Initial doses will depend on whether a loading dose has already been given and if the patient is on maintenance aminophylline at designated intervals.

4. Give intravenous corticosteroids. Although methylprednisolone sodium succinate (Solu-Medrol), 40 to 80 mg. every 4 to 6 hours, might be preferable in older patients due to its minimal salt retaining properties, hydrocortisone sodium succinate (Solu-Cortef) can also be given in doses of 300 to 500 mg. every 4 to 6 hours. Taper the corticosteroids when a definite clinical effect is seen.

5. An aerosolized bronchodilator such as Bronkosol (with isoetharine as its β_2-adrenergic component) or metaproterenol may be administered if there is no previous history of patient abuse.

6. Epinephrine, 1:1000 at 0.2 to 0.3 ml. subcutaneously may be helpful in younger patients but should be given cautiously or avoided in the older age group, due to the production of tachycardia. Terbutaline, 0.25 mg. subcutaneously, works in a similar fashion.

The advantage of intravenous therapy is better control over the administered doses of bronchodilators and more consistent and adequate hydration, thereby mobilizing secretions. After the inspissated secretions are loosened, physical therapy with postural drainage can bring them up more effectively.

A common mistake is to discontinue therapy by the intravenous route too soon! Once the physician feels confident that maximum benefit has been achieved, oral therapy may be instituted as discussed under "Long-term Management".

Long-term Management of the Asthmatic Patient

Avoidance.   Although avoidance is logical, it is often impractical, since precipitants such as airborne pollen, or nonspecific irritants like cigarette smoke, car exhausts, or perfumes are too pervasive. Also such contributing factors as changes in barometric pressure or humidity are often impossible to regulate.

Avoidance of foods, of some value in children, is probably of little importance in the treatment of adult asthmatics, except with potent allergens such as nuts or seafood. Although food allergies are often best detected by elimination diets and double-blind ingestion techniques, elimination diets must be used cautiously, or malnutrition or near starvation can result. Certain environmental precautions can be done with relative ease and may alleviate symptoms in some patients. Feather pillows can be removed or a room can be dustproofed. Patients should stop smoking and avoid smoke-filled rooms.

Aspirin, aspirin-containing compounds, and other analgesics can cause adverse reactions and even death in asthmatic patients. A sub-group of patients develop bronchial obstruction with tartrazine (FD&C #5), a common yellow-coloring found in a gamut of adulterated foods, ranging from frankfurters to oleomargarine, as well as most orange or yellow medications. Aspirin is easy to avoid on an empiric basis. However, oral challenges may be necessary to rule out an adverse reaction to tartrazine.

Theophylline Derivatives

These phosphodiesterase inhibitors are probably the most valuable group of medications for bronchodilatation. Aminophylline (theophylline ethylenediamine) can be conveniently given as a tablet or elixir on an around-the-clock basis. The usual oral dosage for adults is 200 to 400 mg. every 6 hours. Although Fleet's theophylline enemas may occasionally be used, aminophylline suppositories should be avoided due to their erratic absorption.

Longer-acting preparations with known bioavailability characteristics, such as anhydrous theophylline (Slo-phyllin or Theo-Dur) should allow for an every 8 hour or even every 12 hour schedule. Dyphylline is dihydroxypropyltheophylline and does not give measurable theophylline blood levels. It has questionable value in the usual recommended doses. Since the blood half-life of theophylline varies up to eight-fold among different patients, the therapeutic dose of theophylline may vary by at least that much from patient to patient. Blood theophylline determinations can prove helpful not only in determining toxicity, but also in confirming suspicions about a patient who does not take his medications. Although 10 to 20 micrograms per ml. is a typical therapeutic blood level, some patients on long-term theophylline therapy may require higher levels for optimal bronchodilatation, while others, for example, those with a history of convulsion, may require less. The patient should be observed for toxic side effects such as nausea, vomiting, and central nervous system stimulation, including convulsions, hematemesis, cyanosis, albuminuria, and dehydration.

Sympathomimetics Administered by Inhalation

Aerosolized bronchodilators are useful when taken properly and have fewer systemic side effects than comparable orally administered agents. The more selective β_2-adrenergic stimulators, such as isoetharine (usually combined with phenylephrine as in Bronkosol) and metaproterenol are preferred, due to their longer duration of action and minimal cardiac side effects. However, aerosolized bronchodilators such as isoproterenol or epinephrine diluted with sterile water or saline and delivered by either pump (e.g., Maxi-Mist) or bulb nebulizer, are also useful agents in some patients. (There is no proved advantage of administration with positive pressure ventilators, i.e., IPPB.) Commercially available products containing the controversial inert freons are more susceptible to abuse because of their convenient size.

Sympathomimetics Administered by the Subcutaneous Route

Terbutaline and epinephrine given subcutaneously have little value in the chronic management of the asthmatic patients and usually mean that the basic bronchodilator program should be changed. Sus-Phrine is an aqueous suspension of epinephrine tannate 1:200 with slower release that persists for 6 to 8 hours. Although it can be given to supplement and sustain effects of aqueous epinephrine in a dosage of 0.05 to 0.25 ml. given subcutaneously, it should be used infrequently. When employed, it often signifies the lack of an adequate basic bronchodilator program of theophylline and other sympathomimetics. Because of its prolonged action, it inhibits the use of other agents for hours, while the effect dissipates. The side effects of aqueous epinephrine (Sus-Phrine) are similar to those of epinephrine and should be used with caution, especially in adults with cardiac problems or hyperthyroidism.

Sympathomimetics Administered Orally

All sympathomimetics should be used with caution in patients with hypertension, coronary artery disease, congestive heart failure, hyperthyroidism, diabetes, or respiratory failure.

Metaproterenol is marketed as a specific β_2-adrenergic stimulant for bronchial smooth muscle. Like other β_2 stimulators, it is only relatively selective. It has a relatively long duration of action, but patients should be observed for tolerance. Usual adult dosage is 10 to 20 mg. every 6 hours orally.

Terbutaline is another selective β-adrenergic stimulant with side effects and precautions similar to those of metaproterenol. It is presently not recommended for children under 12 years of age. The usual dosage is 2.5 to 5 mg. three times daily.

Ephedrine given concomitantly with xanthine in a round-the-clock manner, can be useful in some patients. However, a combination medication containing a fixed dosage of theophylline and ephedrine should be avoided for initial therapy, since it does not allow individualization of dosage. The usual dosage of ephedrine is 25 mg. every 6 hours.

Cromolyn Sodium (Disodium Cromoglycate)

This agent is used prophylactically and not for quick relief of symptoms. In fact, if it is given during an acute attack, it can make it worse. Since its effectiveness cannot be predicted in an individual patient, a 4 to 6 week trial is often indicated. The usual dosage is 20 mg. by Spinhaler four times daily, and careful instructions are necessary. It is also effective in exercise-induced bronchospasm. Cromolyn sodium may be irritating to the throat or trachea and can produce wheezing or cough. On rare occasions it has been associated with hypersensitivity reactions.

Corticosteroids

When maximally tolerated doses of the previously discussed medications are inadequate to control symptoms, corticosteroids may be used. They are the last to be added to a program and when possible, the first to be removed. The physician should explain the benefit-to-risk ratio prior to the initiation of steroid therapy, along with the other possible side effects. Possible weight gain should be mentioned, so that the patient can watch his diet.

Corticosteroids should be given with caution to patients with a history of peptic ulcer, hypertension, osteoporosis, cardiovascular disease, psychologic disorder, pregnancy, tuberculosis, or bronchial infections. Adverse effects are related to the duration and timing of the steroid therapy, as well as the type of preparation given. Long-acting corticosteroids such as triamcinolone acetonide, dexamethasone, and sustained action intramuscular preparations should never be given for alternate day therapy. If the patient has received corticosteroids during the previous year, or has been on maintenance doses, a substantial amount should be given during periods of stress, such as surgery.

Few side effects occur when large doses are given for short periods, especially when the alternate day program can be quickly resumed. Short-acting preparations such as prednisone, prednisolone and methylprednisolone are preferable to the longer-acting medications. They produce minimal, if any, side effects when given in small doses on an alternate day basis. When an attempt is made to convert a daily dosage schedule to alternate days, three to four times the daily dose may be required initially. Tapering to 15 to 20 mg. every 48 hours in the morning is sometimes a very effective stabilizing dose.

During an upper respiratory infection or other stressful situation, 40 to 80 mg. of prednisone or methylprednisolone can be given every 4 to 6 hours for a few days, and then the previous alternate day program can be resumed. With more severe attacks, procedures listed in "Management of Severe Asthma" should be followed.

Adrenocorticotropic hormone (ACTH) offers no proven advantage over corticosteroid and has certain disadvantages.

Aerosolized Corticosteroids

These agents should also be used prophylactically in patients in whom more than 3 or 4 pills on an alternate day basis of short-acting corticosteroids are necessary. They may produce dramatic benefit in some patients who have required large doses of daily steroids. In fact, the oral dose should not be discontinued too rapidly or adrenal insufficiency may result. Like cromolyn sodium they provide no benefit during an acute attack and occasionally may even be discontinued, since the propellants may exacerbate symptoms.

Beclomethasone dipropionate, 100 to 200 micrograms four times daily, the usual dose, is presently the only commercially available product. These agents are absorbed though rapidly metabolized to by-products that do not suppress the pituitary-adrenal axis. However, overuse can also affect the hypothalamic-pituitary-adrenal axis.

The patients should be cautioned against abuse and observed for oral candidiasis, the most common adverse side-effect. Increased risk factors for oral thrush are concomitant antibiotics, diabetes, large oral doses of corticosteroids and poor dental hygiene. Rinsing the mouth after application is also recommended, but should thrush develop, nystatin mouthwash may be tried. Previously controlled eczema, hay fever, sinusitis, etc., may worsen during oral steroid withdrawal.

Antibiotics

In general, antibiotic therapy should be reserved for asthmatic patients with a particular bacterial infection, such as *Haemophilus influenzae*, which is thought to contribute to bronchial obstruction. The antibiotic is withheld, pending results of studies to identify the causative organisms. Occasionally, chronic sputum producers (asthmatics or bronchitics) may benefit from antibiotic therapy, in the absence of identified pathogenic organisms. In those patients, broad-spectrum antibiotics such as ampicillin or tetracycline can be administered along with good bronchial hygiene.

Expectorants and Mucolytics

Hydration is the best means for thinning secretions and can be accomplished by urging fluids by mouth or intravenously. Hydration by means of a Puritan nebulizer combined with postural drainage and aerosolized bronchodilators can prove very useful for some patients. Occasional patients respond to saturated solutions of potassium iodide for reasons that are not fully understood, but hypothyroidism may develop with chronic use. Guaifenesin (glyceryl guaiacolate) is of questionable value, as is the mucolytic agent acetylcysteine, which may in itself produce bronchospasm.

Less Commonly Used Medications

The antibiotic troleandomycin is useful in a subgroup of asthmatic patients, due to its steroid-sparing properties. Atropine sulfate has been used as an aerosol and is helpful in a subgroup of patients. Although antihistamines may have some drying properties, there are occasional patients who experience relief from asthma with antihistamines. There are even a few patients who respond to α-adrenergic blocking agents such as phentolamine; however, the above agents should not be used routinely and are only tried when the usual measures have failed.

Physical Therapy and Postural Drainage

Postural drainage may be a useful adjunct to therapy, especially when used with adequate hydration and bronchodilatation in patients in whom mucous plugs and secretions are a problem. Certain bronchitics have found this so useful as to prompt recommendation for home therapy, which can be given by a spouse or relative. Some patients actually get worse with this therapy, especially if the bronchospasm is sufficient to impede expulsion of secretions. Thus, it should be reserved for selected patients at selected times. Since some asthmatics have a tendency to tighten their neck muscles and larynx while breathing, physical therapists can help by teaching proper breathing techniques and supervising appropriate conditioning exercises.

Emotional support is essential. The proper explanation of effects and side effects of medication encourages a positive outlook and appropriate cooperation between doctor and patient.

Relaxation training using techniques such as biofeedback may be useful in certain patients as can asthma discussion groups where asthma can be openly discussed.

Immunotherapy (hyposensitization) may be indicated in asthmatics in whom precipitating factors such as pollens or molds play a role, but cannot easily be eliminated from the environment. Hopefully, improved diagnostic techniques, such as bronchial inhalation challenge, when combined with history and skin test information, might distinguish that subgroup in whom immunotherapy may prove most efficacious. More well-controlled studies are needed for asthmatic patients.

Tranquilizers and Sedatives

The asthmatic does not differ from other patients in terms of the caution with which tranquilizers should be prescribed. Occasionally, tranquilizers can counteract the stimulatory effect of sympathomimetic medications. In general, sedatives should be avoided, especially if they are used to allay anxiety. An anxious patient may be manifesting a common sign of hypoxia, at which time oxygen is the treatment of choice.

Future Directions in Therapy

Prostaglandins E_1 and E_2 analogues, oral cromolyn-like agents and atropinelike anticholinergics are a few medications presently undergoing clinical trials. These potential additions to the physician's armamentarium, along with a team approach that considers the heterogeneity of mechanisms, lead to optimism regarding future treatment of asthma.

ASTHMA IN CHILDHOOD

method of
R. MICHAEL SLY, M.D.
Washington, D.C.

Asthma is a chronic pulmonary disease characterized by increased irritability of the tracheobronchial tree and manifested by recurrent episodes of generalized airway obstruction, usually reversible either spontaneously or following appropriate therapy.

Mediator Release

When due to exposure to allergens, allergic symptoms follow interaction between antigen and specific antibody, usually of the IgE class, fixed to the surfaces of mast cells. Bridging of adjacent, specific, IgE molecules initiates a chain of biochemical reactions within the mast cell, causing degranulation of the cell with release of preformed chemical mediators including histamine, eosinophil chemotactic factor of anaphylaxis (ECF-A), a kallikrein (kinin-forming enzyme), and neutrophil chemotactic factor of anaphylaxis (NCF-A). Formation and release of slow reacting substance of anaphylaxis (SRS-A) and platelet activating factor (PAF) are also stimulated.

Histamine can cause increased vascular permeability, vasodilation, bronchoconstriction through direct action upon smooth muscle, and possibly stimulation of secretion by mucous glands. Histamine can also cause cholinergic reflex bronchoconstriction by stimulation of irritant vagal receptors at least in the dog.

Slow reacting substance of anaphylaxis causes bronchoconstriction.

The kallikrein found to be released from basophils, the circulating counterparts of mast cells, can cleave bradykinin from circulating kininogen. Bradykinin may cause bronchoconstriction, vasodilation, and increased vascular permeability.

Platelet activating factor probably causes aggregation of platelets and release of histamine and serotonin, as does the similar factor in rabbits. Serotonin can cause bronchoconstriction in asthmatics.

Eosinophil chemotactic factor of anaphylaxis and NCF-A attract eosinophils and neutrophils to the site of the reaction.

Other bronchoconstrictive agents including certain prostaglandins ($PGF_{2\alpha}$) and thromboxanes may be formed as a result of actions of some of the primary chemical mediators released from mast cells.

Secretion of tracheobronchial mucous glands is enhanced by vagal stimulation or cholinergic agents such as acetylcholine.

Cholinergic stimulation can also cause release of mediators from mast cells without alteration in exposure to antigen. Acetylcholine or methacholine interacts with guanylate cyclase to cause conversion of guanosine triphosphate to cyclic guanosine monophosphate (cyclic GMP), which enhances release of mediators.

Pharmacologic Modification of Mediator Release

Release of mediators from the mast cell can also be modified by the intracellular concentration of cyclic adenosine monophosphate (cyclic AMP), which inhibits release of mediators. The formation of cyclic AMP from adenosine triphosphate can be stimulated by isoproterenol or other β-adrenergic agents, that activate adenylate cyclase. Activation of adenylate cyclase and the consequent increase in concentration of cyclic AMP can also be caused by certain prostaglandins (PGE_1, PGE_2) or by histamine itself, acting upon H-2 receptors.

The intracellular concentration of cyclic AMP can also be increased by inhibition of the phosphodiesterase responsible for its hydrolysis to 5-adenosine monophosphate with a methylxanthine such as theophylline.

Alpha-adrenergic stimulation may cause a decrease in the intracellular concentration of cyclic AMP and enhancement of mediator release possibly through stimulation of adenosine triphosphatase.

Pathophysiology

Chemical mediators released or formed through these pathways cause bronchoconstriction, mucosal edema of the wall of the tracheobronchial tree, and an increase in the rate of production of tracheobronchial secretions. The consequent airway obstruction is followed by hyperinflation, decreased thoracic compliance, and an increase in the work of breathing.

Airway obstruction is not uniform through the lung, and mismatching of ventilation and perfusion occurs. Some regions are well ventilated but poorly perfused, while others are poorly ventilated but well perfused. Segmental or lobar atelectasis may even occur, aggravating further the imbalance between ventilation and perfusion. Whereas the increasing carbon dioxide tension in blood perfusing poorly ventilated lung initially can be compensated for by hyperventilation of well ventilated regions, oxyhemoglobin saturation and the partial pressure of oxygen cannot be substantially improved above normal values while breathing room air. Thus, hypoxemia and metabolic acidosis due to interference with conversion of lactic acid to carbon dioxide and water precede the hypercapnea and respiratory acidosis, which supervene if airway obstruction continues to progress.

MANAGEMENT

Possible approaches to the management of asthma are implicit in the earlier description of mediator release and its consequences. These include prevention of the antigen-antibody interaction, prevention of cholinergic stimulation, use of pharmacologic agents to inhibit mediator release and to reverse bronchoconstriction, and judicious use of physical therapy to facilitate removal of excessive secretions.

Prevention

The most effective form of management is prevention of the asthma before it has even occurred. Asthma is more likely to occur in children with parents or siblings having atopic respiratory diseases than in children in the general population. It has been estimated that allergic rhinitis or asthma can be expected in 60 to 70 per cent of children when both parents have allergic rhinitis or asthma compared with 40 to 50 per cent when one parent has allergy and a frequency of 20 to 25 per cent in the general pediatric population.

Dietary elimination of cow's milk, beef, veal, chicken, egg, wheat, citrus juice, fish, chocolate, and cola drinks for the first nine months is prudent for such infants at risk for atopic diseases. Although the value of such precautions is not confirmed by all pertinent data, sufficiently convincing studies have been published to justify such precautions. Measures to minimize exposure to house dust are also recommended for such infants (Table 1), and neither fur-bearing nor feather-bearing animals should be permitted indoors.

Avoidance of Allergens

The most effective form of management for the child with atopic disease is prevention of exposure to the offending allergen.

House Dust. House dust is probably the most common inhalant allergen. Although complete avoidance is impossible, exposure to house dust and the house dust mites with which most samples abound can be greatly reduced by observing certain precautions in the child's bedroom (Table 1). Because youngsters usually spend so much more time in the room where they sleep than elsewhere in the house, preparation of this room alone is often sufficient to result in substantial clinical improvement when house dust is the major allergen.

Mechanical high-efficiency particulate air (HEPA) filters are highly effective in removing dust, mold, and pollen from air. Both room units and central units are available. Clinical response to installation of such units has been variable, possibly because benefit can be anticipated only when the patient is indoors and because other allergens may also be important.

Danders. Dog and cat danders are also potent allergens. Most patients with allergy to one breed of dog (or cat) are also allergic to other dogs (or cats). Dogs, cats, and other implicated fur-bearing animals and birds must not be permitted indoors at all, because the offending allergen is then distributed throughout the house by the heating and cooling system, resulting in continual exposure, even when the patient has no direct contact with the animal.

Other inhalants of allergenic significance include cattle hair, horse hair, sheep wool, goat hair, rabbit fur, feathers, kapok, cottonseed, flaxseed, and pyrethrum, which is found in many insec-

TABLE 1. **Preparation of a Dust-Free Bedroom**

1. Remove everything, including rugs, curtains, and venetian blinds, from the room.
2. Clean both the room and closet thoroughly. Wax the floor.
3. Use tire tape or adhesive tape to seal shut hot air vents if the room temperature will not fluctuate too widely without their use. If a central heating or cooling system must be used, change the furnace filter at least once each month and even more often if frequent inspection shows it to be dirty. Disposable filters are preferable to permanent filters unless a central electronic filter or HEPA filter (Air Techniques, Inc., 1717 Whitehead Road, Baltimore, Maryland 21207) is installed. Clean wall or floor heating units thoroughly with a vacuum cleaner weekly.
4. Encase all mattresses and box springs in the room in air-tight, dustproof covers (Allergen-Proof Encasings, Inc., P.O. Box 5236, 1450 East 363rd Street, Eastlake, Ohio 44094). If plastic covers are used the seams must not be stitched. Seal with adhesive tape at the point where the zipper ends. Seal air vents in the sides of plastic-covered crib mattresses. Vacuum the covered mattress at least once each week.
5. Use quilted mattress pads, comforters, quilts, or pillows only if filled with a synthetic stuffing such as Dacron or polyester.
6. Avoid chenille bedspreads.
7. Use as little furniture as possible and none that is padded or upholstered. Clean all furniture before returning it to the room.
8. The floor should be wooden or tile. Use no carpet.
9. Bare windows are best, but curtains may be used if they can be washed at least weekly.
10. Opaque windows shades can be used. Do not use venetian blinds.
11. Dust the room daily and clean it completely at least weekly, including door tops, window frames, and sills. Use a vacuum cleaner or a cloth or mop sprayed with Endust.
12. Air the room thoroughly during and after cleaning; otherwise keep doors and windows closed.
13. Only toys stuffed with polyester or other synthetic materials are permitted.
14. Store only clothing in current use in the closet.

---

ticides. Pyrethrum is obtained from a plant related to ragweed and is a frequent source of allergic symptoms in patients with hypersensitivity to ragweed.

Food. Food allergy is much more common in infants than in older children, and it may cause allergic respiratory symptoms with or without gastrointestinal symptoms. Foods most frequently implicated include cow's milk, egg, wheat, corn, chocolate, citrus fruit, legumes, nuts, berries, and shellfish. When allergy to a food has been established by definite production of symptoms following challenge three times, the only treatment of established value is dietary elimination.

Soybean formulas are satisfactory for most infants with allergy to cow's milk, but less satisfactory than human milk because allergy to soybean can also occur. Pregestimil or Nutramigen is almost always tolerated by infants with allergy to cow's milk, but they should be offered initially at half strength and then only gradually increased over several days to full strength to minimize the possibility of diarrhea due to a sudden increase in osmolar load.

Highly restricted diets must not be continued for more than a few days without assessment for nutritional adequacy. Supplemental vitamins, calcium, or iron may be necessary.

Fungi. When allergy to fungi has been found exposure in the home can be reduced by removal of potted plants, old books, and old furniture. Mold growing in shower stalls, on shower curtains, in sinks and laundry rooms, in garbage pails, and in refrigerator drip trays can be cleaned off with a solution of sodium hypochlorite. Captan can be used to spray rooms, closets, and basements or crawl spaces beneath houses. Use of a dehumidifier may be helpful. The patient with allergy to molds should avoid contact with fallen leaves, hay, ensilage, and mulch piles.

Avoidance of Irritants

Precautions should also be observed to minimize exposure to irritants when possible. Asthmatic residents of areas subject to industrial or vehicular air pollution should especially avoid sprays, fumes, fresh paint, and smoke during periods of intense air pollution. Remaining indoors in an environment protected by an HEPA filter or at least by air conditioning may occasionally be necessary. When an asthmatic youngster lives especially close to a source of intense air pollution it may be necessary to consider a move to another neighborhood.

Cigarette smoke is the most common cause of localized air pollution. Smoking should not be permitted in the asthmatic's home. Restaurants and other indoor facilities where smoking is not permitted should be sought for dining or entertainment when away from home.

Pharmacologic Therapy

Pharmacologic agents most useful in the treatment of asthma include methylxanthines, sympathomimetics, cromolyn sodium, and adrenal corticosteroids.

Methylxanthines. Methylxanthines such as theophylline (1-3 dimethylxanthine) and aminophylline (theophylline ethylenediamine) inhibit the phosphodiesterase responsible for conversion of cyclic AMP to 5-AMP. The resultant increase in cyclic AMP in the mast cell inhibits release of chemical mediators, and the increase in cyclic AMP in the smooth muscle cell causes bronchodilation.

Both effectiveness as a bronchodilator and toxicity are closely correlated with serum theophylline concentrations. Concentrations of 5 micrograms per ml. cause demonstrable bronchodilation in some patients, but most require serum concentrations of at least 10 micrograms per ml. for optimal response. A few patients complain of side effects at concentrations of 15 micrograms per ml. and most experience side effects when serum concentrations exceed 20 micrograms per ml. Accordingly, a goal of 10 to 20 micrograms per ml. is usually reasonable.

The serum theophylline concentration is determined by the anhydrous theophylline content or equivalent of the dose administered (Table 2), the size of the patient, the nature of the preparation, and the rate of metabolism and elimination of the drug. Peak serum concentrations are usually found 1½ to 2½ hours after administration of the usual theophylline tablet or capsule, and administration of the next dose is usually necessary 6 hours later. After administration of a liquid preparation or a tablet or capsule containing micronized theophylline (Bronkodyl, Theolair) peak concentrations may occur as early as ½ to 1½ hours later. Peak concentrations are usually found 4 to 8 hours after administration of a sustained release preparation (Aerolate capsules, Slo-Phyllin Gyrocaps, Theo-Dur), permitting adequate control with administration of doses at 8 to 12 hour intervals.

Oral administration of theophylline at doses of 20 to 24 mg. per kg. per 24 hours is safe and effective for most children less than 12 years old,

TABLE 2. **Selected Oral Theophylline Preparations**

PREPARATION	GENERIC NAME	CONTENT (mg.)	ANHYDROUS THEOPHYLLINE EQUIVALENT (mg.)
Aminophylline Tablets	Aminophylline	100	85
Brondecon Elixir	Oxtriphylline	100/5 ml.	64
	Glyceryl Guaiacolate	50/5 ml.	
Brondecon Tablet	Oxtriphylline	200	128
	Glyceryl Guaiacolate	100	
Elixophyllin	Theophylline (anhydrous)	80/15 ml.	80
Elixophyllin Capsules	Theophylline (anhydrous)	100,200	100,200
Marax Syrup*	Theophylline (anhydrous)	32.5 mg./5 ml.	32.5
	Ephedrine	6.25	
	Hydroxyzine	2.5	
Marax Tablet	Theophylline (anhydrous)	130	130
	Ephedrine	25	
	Hydroxyzine	10	
Quibron Capsule or Elixir	Theophylline (anhydrous)	150/cap or 15 ml.	150
Slo-Phyllin Syrup*	Theophylline (anhydrous)	80/15 ml.	80
Slo-Phyllin Tablets	Theophylline (anhydrous)	100,200	100,200
Somophyllin Oral Liquid*	Aminophylline	105/5 ml.	90
Tedral Elixir	Theophylline (anhydrous)	32.5/5 ml.	32.5
	Ephedrine	6	
	Phenobarbital	2	
Tedral Suspension*	Theophylline (monohydrate)	65/5 ml.	58.5
	Ephedrine	12	
	Phenobarbital	4	
Tedral Tablet	Theophylline (anhydrous)	130	130
	Ephedrine	24	
	Phenobarbital	8	
Theophyl Chewable Tablet	Theophylline (anhydrous)	100	100
Micronized Theophylline			
Bronkodyl Capsules	Theophylline (anhydrous)	100,200	100,200
Theolair Tablets	Theophylline (anhydrous)	125,250	125,250
Sustained Release Preparations			
Elixophyllin SR Capsules	Theophylline (anhydrous)	125,250	125,250
Slo-Phyllin Gyrocaps	Theophylline (anhydrous)	60,125,250	60,125,250
Theo-Dur Tablets	Theophylline (anhydrous)	100,200,300	100,200,300
Theophyl-SR Capsules	Theophylline (anhydrous)	125,250	125,250

*Nonalcoholic liquid preparations.

while children older than 12 tolerate somewhat smaller doses (16 to 20 mg. per kg. per 24 hours). It is prudent to start therapy with the smallest dose indicated and gradually increase the dose only if necessary. For infrequent, intermittent episodes of asthma a rapid-acting preparation is preferred at least for the initial dose (liquid preparation or micronized theophylline), but a sustained-release preparation (Slo-Phyllin Gyrocaps, Theo-Dur) is preferred for continual treatment. Treatment is started at the first symptom and continued for at least 3 to 5 days after overt symptoms have subsided because airway obstruction can persist several days after symptoms or even auscultatory abnormalities have subsided.

There are wide variations in rates of metabolism and elimination of theophylline in different patients. Serum half life in children is known to vary at least from 70 minutes to 10 hours. Thus, an ineffective dose for one child may be a toxic dose for another. Consequently, safe, effective therapy is assured only by determination of serum concentrations following a given dose. Effective monitoring is possible, even in outpatients, by obtaining a specimen at the anticipated trough (6 hours after the usual preparation, 8 to 12 hours after a sustained-release preparation) and peak (2 hours after most preparations, 6 hours after sustained-release preparations). Monitoring of serum theophylline concentrations is indicated whenever clinical response to the usual dose has been inadequate or when signs or symptoms of theophylline toxicity occur. These include restlessness, nausea, vomiting, irritability, headache, epigastric pain, hematemesis, twitching, convulsions, pallor, fever, coma, dehydration, and albuminuria. Deaths have occurred.

Among factors known to affect the rate of metabolism of theophylline, tending to shorten the serum half-life, are smoking and high protein diets. Congestive heart failure, liver disease, fever, high carbohydrate diets, and administration of troleandomycin or erythromycin cause prolongation of the serum half-life, necessitating reductions in dosage of theophylline.

An earlier impression that alcohol was necessary for adequate absorption of theophylline from the gastrointestinal tract has not been substantiated by more recent study. Accordingly, there seems to be no reason to prescribe the drug in elixirs that often reduce compliance. Slo-Phyllin Syrup and Somophyllin Oral Liquid are among the very few nonalcoholic liquid preparations containing only theophylline that are available.

Although numerous oral preparations containing both theophylline and a sympathomimetic are available, use of such a preparation limits the adjustment in theophylline dosage that may become necessary. There is evidence of a partially additive effect of ephedrine and theophylline, however, and for many patients with average rates of theophylline metabolism use of a preparation with an appropriate theophylline/ephedrine ratio (4 to 6:1) offers the convenience of both drugs in a single preparation.

Intravenous aminophylline is the treatment of choice for status asthmaticus. Most children can safely receive 4 to 5 mg. per kg., diluted and infused over 10 to 20 minutes if previous theophylline dosage has not been excessive and if the usual dosage interval has elapsed. This same dose can then be repeated at 8 hour intervals or the serum concentration can be maintained with a constant infusion of 0.5 to 1.0 mg. per kg. per hour. The specific infusion rate is that found to maintain the serum concentration at 10 to 20 micrograms per ml. Larger doses should be reserved for the few patients in whom adequate serum concentrations are not achieved.

Rapid, accurate determination of theophylline concentrations in serum specimens of 0.1 ml. or less is now possible utilizing high pressure liquid chromatography or enzymatic immunoassay. Availability of these methods permits the rapid adjustment of the dosage of intravenous aminophylline essential for optimal therapy.

Theophylline can also be administered rectally, but because of the considerable uncertainty regarding absorption and optimal dosage by this route and the numerous reports of toxicity, it should probably be reserved for the very rare patient unable to tolerate any oral preparation, and serum theophylline concentrations should be monitored closely.

Sympathomimetics. Aqueous epinephrine (1:1000) usually elicits bronchodilation within a few minutes after administration of an appropriate dose (Table 3) by subcutaneous injection during an acute asthmatic attack. If necessary, this same dose can be repeated twice at 20 minute intervals. Failure to respond to three doses administered at 20 minute intervals would establish the diagnosis of status asthmaticus. When satisfactory improvement has followed injection of 1:1,000 aqueous epinephrine, 1:200 epinephrine suspension (Sus-Phrine) can be administered 30 minutes later for more sustained relief.

Although the maximal adult dose of 1:1000 aqueous epinephrine is 0.5 ml., 0.25 ml. usually affords relief even in adolescents, and larger doses more frequently cause side effects such a tachycardia, hypertension, precordial discomfort, headache, nausea, vomiting, vertigo, muscle tremor, nervousness, excitement, pallor, or drowsiness. Subarachnoid hemorrhage and hemiplegia have followed subcutaneous injection of 0.5 ml. of 1:1,000 aqueous epinephrine in young adults.

Ethylnorepinephrine is an effective bron-

TABLE 3. **Sympathomimetic Bronchodilator Dosage**

DRUG	DOSE	ROUTE
Epinephrine, 1:1,000, aqueous	0.01 ml./kg. (max 0.25 ml.) every 20 min. × 3 if necessary May repeat in 4 hours	Subcutaneous
Epinephrine, 1:200, aqueous suspension (Sus-Phrine)	0.005 ml./kg. (max. 0.15 ml.) May repeat in 8 hours	Subcutaneous
Ethylnorepinephrine (Bronkephrine)	0.01–0.02 ml./kg. (max. 0.5 ml.) May repeat in 20 min	Subcutaneous
Ephedrine	0.5–1 mg./kg. every 4–6 hours	Oral
Isoproterenol 1:200	0.25–0.5 ml. in 1.5–8.5 ml. Saline every 8 hours	Inhalation
Metaproterenol	0.5 mg./kg. every 6–8 hours (max. 20 mg. 4 times daily)	Oral
	> 12 y.o.: 1.3–1.95 mg. every 4–8 hours	Inhalation
Terbutaline*	12–15 years: 0.075 mg./kg. or 2.5 mg. every 6 hours 3 times daily Adult dose: 5 mg. every 6 hours 3 times daily	Oral
	0.01 mg./kg. (max. 0.25 mg.)	Subcutaneous

*Not approved by Food and Drug Administration for use in children below the age of 12 years.

chodilator with less alpha adrenergic activity than epinephrine. It may be safer for use in infants or patients with hypertension than is aqueous epinephrine.

Ephedrine is effective as a bronchodilator following oral administration, and its effects are partially additive with those of methylxanthines when both drugs are used. Side effects of ephedrine are the same as those of epinephrine, but insomnia, irritability, and increased activity due to central nervous system stimulation are especially common.

Isoproterenol is a very effective bronchodilator but one with several drawbacks, including a short duration of action of only 1 to 2 hours following inhalation. It is rapidly metabolized by catechol-o-methyltransferase to a weak beta adrenergic blocking agent, 3-methoxyisoproterenol, which tends to block further bronchodilating action of isoproterenol itself. Following oral administration it is also inactivated by intestinal and hepatic sulfatase, so it must usually be given by inhalation, although it may also be effective following sublingual absorption.

In some asthmatics a temporary improvement in ventilation after inhalation of isoproterenol has been followed within one hour by more severe airway obstruction than was present before treatment. The reason for this paradoxical response in occasional patients is unknown.

Inhalation of isoproterenol has often elicited decreases in arterial Po_2 despite lessening of airway obstruction, probably because of reversal of compensatory pulmonary vasoconstriction with the result that the ventilation-perfusion imbalance typical of acute asthmatic attacks has been further aggravated. Similar decreases in arterial Po_2 have also followed subcutaneous injection of epinephrine and intravenous administration of aminophylline. The changes have not usually been more than 5 to 10 mm. Hg, but rarely they have been as great as 25 mm. The larger decreases have usually occurred in patients with a relatively high initial Po_2, and the response can be prevented by simultaneous administration of supplemental oxygen or inhalation of an aerosol containing phenylephrine as well as isoproterenol.

Overuse of isoproterenol has been implicated as a possible factor contributing to deaths from asthma, especially in adolescents and young adults, whether due to some of its inherent limitations or to the poor judgment of patients who overused the only bronchodilator convenient to them in a futile attempt to reverse airway obstruction that was no longer responsive. A rapidly effective, short-acting drug seems particularly subject to abuse.

Despite these limitations of isoproterenol, its inhalation often elicits bronchodilation in asthmatics who have become refractory to aqueous epinephrine. Because of its shortcomings, however, its use is best restricted to the hospitalized patient or out-patients in whom its use can be closely monitored by a reliable parent. Side effects include tachycardia, palpitations, excitation, flushing, weakness, headache, tremor, and insomnia.

Excessive doses of isoproterenol can cause

tachycardia and extrasystoles, ventricular fibrillation, or bradycardia followed by asystole. Fatalities following its use in conjunction with epinephrine have occasionally been reported, so it is prudent to avoid administration of the two drugs within two hours of each other.

The limitations of isoproterenol have stimulated a search for safer, more effective bronchodilators with less cardiac activity relative to their activity upon the smooth muscle of the tracheobronchial tree. Isoetharine was one of the first, but it, too, has a very short duration of action and probably offers no substantial advantage over isoproterenol.

Metaproterenol is an effective bronchodilator with a longer duration of action of at least 4 hours after inhalation. It is less susceptible to inactivation by intestinal sulfatases, so it is active following oral administration. Side effects include those that can be elicited by isoproterenol and drowsiness. They have been much more common following oral administration than after inhalation. Side effects after inhalation of metaproterenol have been less frequent than after inhalation of isoproterenol. Oral metaproterenol is probably a more effective bronchodilator than ephedrine.

Terbutaline is an effective bronchodilator with an even longer duration of action than metaproterenol following inhalation (5 hours), oral administration (7 hours), or subcutaneous injection (4 hours). Inhalation of therapeutic doses causes no tachycardia or other side effects and appears to be the route of administration of choice, but it has not yet been approved by the Food and Drug Administration for use by this route. Tachycardia follows oral administration or subcutaneous injection, but this may possibly be due to a baroreceptor response to the decreased diastolic blood pressure which it causes rather than to a direct cardiac effect. Other side effects that may follow oral or subcutaneous administration include nervousness, headache, nausea, and muscle tremor. Tremor is the most common side effect, and it may be intense enough to necessitate discontinuation of the drug in some patients.

Cromolyn Sodium. Cromolyn sodium (disodium cromoglycate) prevents release of chemical mediators from sensitized mast cells following the antigen-antibody reaction. Although it has seemed more effective for the treatment of extrinsic asthma than intrinsic asthma, it has also been found to inhibit airway obstruction induced by exercise or inhalation of cold air.

It must be administered by inhalation because of poor absorption from the gastrointestinal tract and is supplied as a crystalline powder in capsules containing 20 mg. A special inhaler permits administration after perforation of the capsule.

Children less than 5 years old can rarely be taught how to inhale the drug properly.

Since cromolyn is not a bronchodilator it is not helpful during an acute asthmatic attack. In fact, temporary discontinuation during acute attacks, status asthmaticus, and during bronchial infections is recommended because of a possible adverse effect upon the consistency of tracheobronchial secretions. Inhalation of the contents of one capsule 4 times each day often is followed within 2 to 4 weeks of treatment by a lessening in the frequency of asthmatic attacks. If there has been no improvement within 4 weeks, the drug is discontinued as a failure. If improvement is observed it is often possible to reduce the frequency of use of cromolyn to 3 times each day without loss of effect.

Throat irritation due to deposition of powder can be obviated by following each treatment with a few swallows of water. Coughing or wheezing provoked by inhalation of the powder is usually prevented or minimized by pretreatment with a bronchodilator. Other side effects have been very rare, but these have included maculopapular and urticarial eruptions, nausea, vomiting, nasal congestion, and pulmonary infiltrates. Rare hypersensitivity reactions have included polymyositis, eosinophilic pneumonia, and systemic anaphylaxis.

Adrenal Corticosteroids. Adrenal corticosteroids are of well-established efficacy in the treatment of asthma, but their use is limited by numerous side effects. The most common side effect is one of the most serious — suppression of the hypothalamic-pituitary-adrenal axis. Its extent is closely related to dosage and duration of treatment. Evidence of adrenal suppression has been found after single doses of corticosteroids, and as little as 2.5 mg. prednisone daily can maintain adrenal suppression in children. Recovery usually occurs within 9 months , at least after discontinuation of steroid therapy but adrenal insufficiency has been known to persist for as long as 24 months after daily treatment with steroids had been stopped. Consequently, it is prudent to prescribe steroids at times of stress for children who have received continual steroid therapy within the previous 9 to 12 months. A severe asthmatic attack is among the types of stress for which such therapy would be indicated.

Sudden discontinuation of steroid therapy in a patient who has been receiving it for more than a few days can also precipitate potentially fatal adrenal insufficiency with symptoms that include vomiting, abdominal pain, shock, and coma.

Oral administration of a corticosteroid with intermediate duration of action as a single morning dose on alternate days has often been found to provide adequate symptomatic control without adrenal suppression in the rare asthmatic whose response to other therapy is not satisfactory. Prednisone, prednisolone, and methylprednisolone are suitable steroids for such regimens, while dexamethasone or betamethasone is not suitable owing to the longer duration of action of these last two steroids.

When severe asthmatic symptoms are present despite optimal use of other forms of therapy, administration of prednisone or prednisolone at a dose of 2 mg. per kg. per day (minimum dose 20 mg., maximal dose 80 mg.) in 3 or 4 divided doses for 3 days may afford adequate symptomatic control that may continue even if steroids are then discontinued. For the rare patient in whom more prolonged steroid therapy is necessary, prednisone or prednisolone is continued at the lowest single morning dose on alternate days consistent with adequate control. This dose is determined by adjustment of dosage at intervals of 1 to 2 weeks, reducing the dose by 2.5 to 5 mg. when possible, and discontinuing therapy as soon as possible. A severe exacerbation of asthma within 9 to 12 months after discontinuation of therapy would be an indication for prompt treatment with steroids again because of possible adrenal suppression.

Inhalation of beclomethasone dipropionate (Vanceril) at doses that often afford adequate control of asthmatic symptoms (50 to 100 micrograms three or four times daily, maximum total daily dose in children 500 micrograms) causes no demonstrable adrenal suppression. Larger doses can cause adrenal suppression. As the drug is supplied in a convenient, self-propelled, Freon nebulizer, its use must be closely supervised by a responsible adult to forestall abuse, which could cause adrenal suppression.

It must be recognized that patients treated with beclomethasone aerosol who have previously received oral corticosteroids may already have some adrenal suppression. Severe exacerbations of asthma in such patients constitute indications for temporary treatment with oral corticosteroids.

Occasionally, oral or pharyngeal candidiasis has occurred as a complication of inhalation of beclomethasone dipropionate, but this has responded to treatment with nystatin or has subsided even without treatment.

Beclomethasone dipropionate is approved for use in children who are at least 6 years old. Younger children are usually unable to learn how to inhale the drug properly.

Expectorants. Only one controlled study has indicated that potassium iodide is efficacious as an expectorant in asthmatics. Because of the numerous associated side effects, including hypothyroidism and thyroid enlargement, its use cannot be encouraged.

There is no conclusive evidence that guaifenesin (glyceryl guaiacolate) is an effective expectorant, and N-acetylcysteine cannot be recommended for inhalation in asthmatics because of the frequency with which it provokes bronchospasm.

Oral fluids have been found to reduce the viscosity of sputum and are certainly of importance in preventing the adverse effect of dehydration upon tracheobronchial secretions, but overly enthusiastic efforts to increase oral fluids can cause vomiting. Inhalation of nebulized saline solution can provoke bronchospasm in asthmatics and only very small volumes of water delivered by nebulization reach the lower airways, so treatment of the asthmatic child with mist is less likely to be beneficial than harmful. Intravenous fluids are indicated in status asthmaticus, but evidence of an increased rate of secretion of antidiuretic hormone in such patients indicates the importance of constant reassessment to prevent water intoxication.

Antihistamines. Antihistamines are contraindicated in status asthmaticus because of their potential inspissating effect upon tracheobronchial secretions, although this has never been substantiated by experimental evidence. Ambulatory asthmatics can safely receive diphenhydramine, tripelennamine, or chlorpheniramine for the treatment of allergic rhinitis, however. Maintenance of nasal breathing in asthmatics is probably important when possible, to minimize delivery of allergens and irritants to the lower airways.

Atropine. Inhalation of atropine or ipratropium bromide (Sch 1000), a synthetic atropine analogue, has been found to elicit bronchodilation in many asthmatics at doses that do not cause frequent side effects. Their use is still experimental, but it is likely that such an anticholinergic agent will be available commercially in the near future, permitting another approach to treatment of the asthmatic child.

Physical Therapy

Gravity-assisted postural drainage with cupping or percussion over the chest is effective in increasing sputum production and in improving pulmonary function. It may be especially helpful in the treatment of lobar or segmental atelectasis due to retained secretions but is recommended for the patient recovering from an acute asthmatic attack even when atelectasis is not present. It should not be attempted when severe, generalized, airway obstruction is present, but is usually well tolerated when only mild or moderate obstruction is present.

For most effective drainage, successive use of several different positions is necessary to permit gravity to assist drainage of the various bronchopulmonary segments with cupping for 1 to 2 minutes over each segment 2 to 3 times each day. Diagrams of specific positions recommended are published elsewhere.* Nurses and parents are easily taught the necessary technique when therapists are not available.

Immunotherapy (Hyposensitization)

When frequent or severe asthmatic attacks continue despite measures to minimize exposure to offending allergens and adequate bronchodilator therapy and when hypersensitivity to inhalant allergens that cannot be avoided has been demonstrated — allergens such as pollens, molds, or house dust — a trial of immunotherapy is indicated. Treatment should include only those inhalant allergens to which allergy has been demonstrated by a careful history and positive immediate skin tests with antigens of appropriate concentrations applied with appropriate controls.

Most controlled studies of immunotherapy with bacterial vaccine have shown no beneficial effect upon children with asthma, and immunotherapy is of no proven value in the treatment of food allergy.

Controlled studies of immunotherapy with inhalant allergens for the treatment of asthma have usually disclosed improvement in approximately 80 per cent of patients compared with improvement in about 30 per cent of patients receiving injections with placebo. Improvement has been dose related. The results of therapy with low doses have been indistinguishable from those of placebo controls.

Immunotherapy has often been associated initially with an increase in total serum IgE concentration, but as therapy continues, serum IgE concentrations decrease and the seasonal increase in IgE in patients with seasonal allergy is suppressed. Immunotherapy also causes an increase in specific IgG blocking antibody and a decrease in release of histamine following antigenic challenge of basophils. An associated decrease in the proliferative response of T lymphocytes to challenge with specific allergen has also been found. Thus, multiple factors appear responsible for the clinical improvement that has been observed.

Therapy is started with small doses of aqueous extracts of the offending allergen and gradually increased by 50 per cent increments at intervals of 3 to 7 days. Maintenance doses of 0.5 ml. of 1:60 to 1:100 are usually reached within 4 to 6 months. Intervals between injections are then gradually increased to 3 to 4 weeks if tolerated.

Immunotherapy is continued until the patient has been free of allergic symptoms for 1 to 2 years or until only minimal symptoms have been present for 3 years. Some patients who show no benefit during the first year improve during the second year. Initial improvement followed by increased symptoms during another season suggests acquisition of allergy to additional antigens.

Doses are not usually increased when the interval since the last injection has exceeded 1 week, and the dose is not increased if the last injection has been followed by a local reaction larger than 2 cm. in diameter. The next dose is decreased when the local reaction has been more than 2.5 cm. in diameter. If a systemic reaction occurs, the next dose is decreased to 10 per cent of the previous dose by administering the same volume of the next weaker serial 10-fold dilution. This is then followed again by gradual increases in dosage.

It is prudent for allergy injections to be administered only at a physician's office because of the possibility of a systemic reaction. The child should remain in the office for at least 20 minutes after the injection because of the possibility of such a reaction and to permit inspection of the arm at 20 minutes to determine whether the size of the local reaction indicates a need for modification of the next dose.

Allergy injections are not given when significant airway obstruction is already present because of the severe airway obstruction that might then result from a systemic reaction. Strenuous exercise should be avoided for at least 1 hour after the patient has received the allergy injection and the injection site should not be massaged.

Systemic reactions may consist of sneezing, coughing, wheezing, pruritus, generalized urticaria or even anaphylactic shock. Vomiting or abdominal pain may occur. Treatment must be initiated immediately.

1. Mild systemic reactions usually respond promptly to subcutaneous injection of 1:1,000 aqueous epinephrine into the arm that did not receive the allergen (see Table 3 for dose).

2. Application of a tourniquet above the site of the allergen injection and injection of half the previous dose of 1:1000 aqueous epinephrine at the site of the injection are effective in delaying further systemic distribution of the allergen.

3. Establishment of an airway, administration of oxygen, or ventilation may be necessary.

4. Rapid administration of intravenous fluids (5 per cent glucose in isotonic saline solution) may be necessary if shock supervenes.

5. Intravenous aminophylline may be necessary if airway obstruction persists. This can be administered over 10 to 20 minutes at an initial dose of 7 mg. per kg. after dilution.

---

*Sly, R.M.: *Pediatric Allergy,* Flushing, New York, Medical Examination Publishing Company, 1977.

6. If urticaria or angioedema is present, diphenhydramine (Benadryl) can be administered (2 mg. per kg. by intravenous injection or 5 mg. per kg. per 24 hours in four divided doses by mouth).

7. If necessary, hydrocortisone can be administered by intravenous infusion (7 mg. per kg. followed by 4 mg. per kg. every 4 hours). No immediate effect of hydrocortisone is expected, but it is helpful because of the anti-inflammatory effect anticipated a few hours later.

8. Addition of metaraminol bitartrate (Aramine), 0.4 mg. per kg. (0.5 to 5.0 mg.), to the intravenous fluids may become necessary to maintain blood pressure.

Treatment of Asthmatic Attacks

Treatment of asthmatic attacks is most effective if started at the onset of symptoms. Therapy is started with the onset of coughing or even with rhinorrhea in the child in whom this is known to be followed usually by wheezing, and therapy with oral bronchodilators is continued for at least 3 to 5 days after overt symptoms have subsided. Such a regimen necessitates continual treatment for the child symptomatic as often as once or twice each week.

1. Theophylline is initially prescribed at the anticipated appropriate dose of 5 to 6 mg. per kg. every 6 hours for the child less than 12 years old (4 to 5 mg. per kg. every 6 hours for an older child), starting with the lower dose and gradually increasing the dose if necessary. If response is inadequate, serum theophylline concentrations are obtained to determine whether even larger doses are necessary. A liquid preparation or micronized theophylline is preferred for the initial dose because of more rapid onset of action, but a sustained-release preparation is preferred for continued therapy, especially in the child who will need continual drug therapy. Measuring spoons, calibrated droppers, or syringes must be used for accurate measurement of liquid preparations. Although most toddlers are unable to swallow the sustained-release tablets or capsules, Slo-Phyllin or Aerolate capsules can be opened and their contents administered in a spoonful of applesauce or ice cream without loss of potency. The granules must not be chewed or dissolved, however. The contents of a capsule cannot be divided accurately for adjustment of dosage, because some of the granules do not contain theophylline.

2. In patients who do not respond adequately to an appropriate theophylline preparation found to produce an adequate serum concentration, a sympathomimetic should be added. Terbutaline, the most effective oral sympathomimetic available in the United States, is approved for use in children at least 12 years old. Metaproterenol can be used in younger children.

3. If use of both theophylline and terbutaline fails to afford adequate control, a trial of cromolyn is indicated in the child who is at least 5 years old. Some recommend a trial of cromolyn even before addition of the sympathomimetic to the regimen. Within 4 weeks it will be known whether cromolyn has been beneficial. If not, it is discontinued.

4. In the few patients who have failed to respond to appropriate avoidance, immunotherapy, and all of these pharmacologic agents, treatment with adrenal corticosteroids is indicated. If the youngster is at least 6 years old, inhalation of beclomethasone dipropionate is indicated, 50 to 100 micrograms 3 or 4 times daily (not more than a total of 500 micrograms per day). In the child in whom adequate control is still impossible, prednisone given as a single morning dose on alternate days can be added after careful discussion with the parents of possible side effects. The goal of steroid therapy is not complete freedom from symptoms but reduction of symptoms to a tolerable level, which will permit regular school attendance and some semblance of a normal life. Oral steroid dosage should be adjusted at 1 to 2 week intervals to the smallest dose consistent with this goal and should be discontinued as soon as possible.

If moderate or severe wheezing does not improve within 30 to 60 minutes after administration of an appropriate oral bronchodilator, prompt, further treatment is needed. Subcutaneous injection of terbutaline or 1:1000 aqueous epinephrine usually affords relief. Failure to respond to these measures would be diagnostic of status asthmaticus.

Inhalation of isoproterenol or metaproterenol can be an effective alternative to subcutaneous injection of terbutaline or epinephrine. Parental supervision is necessary to minimize the possibility of overuse, and this possibility can also be reduced by administration by a nebulizer driven by an air compressor or a hand nebulizer rather than a Freon self-propelled nebulizer. There is no evidence that delivery by intermittent positive pressure offers any advantage over these methods.

Exercise-induced Asthma. Exercise-induced asthma can be diagnosed in many asthmatics by measurement of pulmonary function before and after exercise, even when it has been unsuspected by the parents or child. Physical activity should not be restricted unnecessarily in those who are not highly susceptible to exercise-induced asthma, and in the others it can be prevented or minimized by administration of an oral bronchodilator 30 to 60 minutes before exercise or inhalation of cromolyn sodium 15 to 60 minutes before exercise. In many children exercise may occur at any time throughout the day. Exercise-induced asthma is most conveniently inhibited in them by administration of a sustained-release theophylline preparation in the morning.

With appropriate management it is probably possible for almost all asthmatic children to participate safely in physical exercise despite the potentially adverse effect of exercise.

Treatment of Status Asthmaticus

Status asthmaticus is a medical emergency necessitating hospitalization and treatment as soon as possible after its diagnosis has been established by persistence of severe wheezing, despite 2 or 3 adequate doses of 1:1000 aqueous epinephrine or 2 doses of terbutaline given by subcutaneous injection. Some authors include failure to respond to intravenous aminophylline in their definition of status asthmaticus.

Factors implicated as possible causes of status asthmaticus include mucosal edema, inspissated tracheobronchial secretions, infection, acidosis, and overuse of nebulized isoproterenol or epinephrine.

Details concerning recent oral intake of fluids, vomiting, frequency and volume of urination, recent changes in weight, and the usual clinical signs of dehydration are useful in assessing the state of hydration.

The presence of fever or purulent nasopharyngeal or tracheobronchial secretions suggests infection, but fever, possibly due to dehydration, may be present without other evidence of infection, and secretions may appear purulent because of an abundance of eosinophils.

Information concerning previously administered drugs is essential to safe effective therapy and must be sought, although measurement of serum theophylline concentration often discloses values that have been unsuspected from the history.

Assessment of the adequacy of ventilation is facilitated by use of a clinical scoring system (Table 4).

Initial laboratory procedures necessary include a complete blood count, serum electrolytes, arterial pH, Pco_2, and Po_2, and serum theophylline concentration. Lateral and posteroanterior chest roentgenograms should be obtained as soon as possible without delaying therapy and examined for evidence of atelectasis, pneumonia, pneumomediastinum, and pneumothorax. Frequent additional determinations of arterial blood gases, pH, and serum theophylline concentration are often necessary to assess response to therapy, depending upon the clinical response.

Hypoxemia and metabolic acidosis are often present initially with a decrease in arterial Pco_2 due to hyperventilation. As airway obstruction continues, the Pco_2 gradually returns to normal and may than quickly become elevated, resulting in respiratory acidosis.

1. Fully humidified oxygen must be administered at a rate sufficient to maintain the arterial Po_2 at 65 to 100 mm. Hg.

2. With moderate or severe dehydration intravenous fluids (5 or 10 per cent glucose in 1 to 4 or 1 to 3 isotonic saline solution or 5 per cent glucose in isotonic saline solution) are administered at a rate of 360 to 400 ml. per square meter of body surface during the first 45 to 60 minutes. After renal flow is established, a polyionic, hypotonic solution containing potassium is given at a rate of 2400 to 3000 ml. per sq. meter per 24 hours. Subsequent fluid and electrolyte needs are determined by frequent clinical evaluation and measurement of serum electrolytes. If no dehydration is present initially, maintenance with 1500 ml. per sq. meter per 24 hours may be adequate.

3. Intravenous aminophylline is the treatment of choice for status asthmaticus. If previous dosage has not been excessive and the usual dosage interval has elapsed, 4 to 5 mg. per kg. is diluted and infused over 10 to 20 minutes. The initial dose can be followed by a constant infusion of 0.5 to 1.0 mg. per kg. per hour *or* the initial dose can be repeated at 8 hour intervals. The specific infusion rate or subsequent doses are adjusted as indicated by serum theophylline determinations

TABLE 4. **Clinical Asthma Score**

	0	1	2
Po_2 or	70–110 in air	≤70 in air	≤70 in 40% O_2
cyanosis	None	In Air	In 40% O_2
Inspiratory breath sounds	Normal	Unequal	Decreased or absent
Use of accessory muscles of respiration	None	Moderate	Maximal
Expiratory wheezing	None	Moderate	Extreme or none because of poor air exchange
Cerebral function	Normal	Depressed or agitated	Coma

Total score of 5 suggests respiratory failure. Score of 7 with arterial Pco_2 ≥65 mm. Hg indicates respiratory failure.

to maintain a concentration of 10 to 20 micrograms per ml. This may necessitate use of more rapid infusion rates or larger doses.

4. Isoproterenol, 1:200, 0.25 to 0.5 ml., diluted to 2 to 10 ml. with sterile saline solution, is nebulized, and administered by inhalation. Intermittent positive pressure, which can cause increased airway resistance in asthmatics, is avoided. The isoproterenol can be repeated at 4 hour intervals if necessary. It is not used within 2 hours of administration of epinephrine. Inhalation of a longer-acting beta adrenergic agent with less cardiac activity—an agent such as terbutaline—would be expected to be safer and more effective, but terbutaline is not approved by the Food and Drug Administration for use by nebulization and inhalation.

5. Hydrocortisone, 4 mg. per kg., is administered by intravenous injection if substantial improvement has not occurred within 1 hour after intravenous administration of aminophylline or immediately if the patient has received continual therapy with adrenal corticosteroids within the previous 9 months. This same dose is then repeated at 4 hour intervals to maintain a plasma cortisol concentration of at least 100 micrograms per ml. Hydrocortisone is discontinued after substantial improvement has occurred. Clinical response to hydrocortisone is not anticipated for several hours.

6. Sodium bicarbonate, 1.5 to 2 mEq. per kg., infused intravenously over 20 minutes may be helpful in correcting metabolic acidosis. Subsequent similar doses can be repeated at hourly intervals as long as metabolic acidosis persists with arterial pH < 7.35, plasma bicarbonate < 20 mEq. per liter, and serum sodium < 145 mEq. per liter *or* the extracellular base deficit (negative base excess) can be corrected with 0.3 mEq. of sodium bicarbonate per kg. of body weight times base deficit infused over 20 to 60 minutes. The treatment for respiratory acidosis is improvement of ventilation rather than administration of sodium bicarbonate, and administration of too much sodium bicarbonate to a patient with poor ventilation can cause hypercapnea. Furthermore, too rapid infusion of sodium bicarbonate can cause a sudden osmolar shift from the brain to extracellular fluid with the risk of brain injury. Nevertheless, cautious correction of acidosis may restore responsiveness to epinephrine.

7. Responsiveness to aqueous epinephrine may have been restored after hydration and improvement in acid-base balance. If improvement follows administration of 1:1000 aqueous epinephrine, Sus-Phrine can be administered 30 minutes later for a more sustained effect. If unresponsiveness to aqueous epinephrine persists,

however, continued administration can only cause adverse side effects, and its use should be abandoned until improvement has occurred.

8. Antibiotics are administered when there is evidence of superimposed bacterial infection but are not necessary in most episodes of status asthmaticus.

9. Sedatives, tranquilizers, and other opiates are contraindicated because of their potentially fatal depressant effect upon the respiratory center except during mechanical ventilation. The restlessness and agitation often interpreted as indications of a need for sedation are usually signs of hypoxemia that should be treated with supplemental oxygen and measures to improve ventilation. In the rare child for whom sedation becomes necessary, chloral hydrate, 15 mg. per kg., can be administered by mouth or rectum if ventilation can be monitored by frequent determinations of arterial blood gases and if facilities for mechanical control of ventilation are immediately available.

10. Antihistamines are contraindicated because of their potential inspissating effect upon tracheobronchial secretions as well as a possible depressant effect upon the respiratory center.

11. Controlled mechanical ventilation is indicated in the rare child who fails to respond to the foregoing measures, progressing to respiratory failure (Table 4), coma, or apnea. If gasping or apnea is evident, humidified, 100 per cent oxygen is administered manually by bag and mask while preparations are made for nasotracheal intubation under direct vision laryngoscopy. If the child is conscious, sodium pentobarbital, 1 mg. per kg., is given intravenously to facilitate intubation. The anesthesiologist responsible for intubating the child should have been consulted initially when impending respiratory failure was recognized (Table 4). Oxygen is again administered after placement of the nasotracheal tube, tracheal secretions are aspirated quickly with a sterile catheter, and the endotracheal tube is connected to a volume-cycled ventilator set for moderate hyperventilation. A slight expiratory resistance is applied.

Continuous muscle paralysis is maintained with tubocurarine chloride, 0.2 to 0.4 mg. per kg. every 3 to 6 hours, or with gallamine triethiodide intravenously if renal function is normal, or pancuronium bromide. Light sleep or sedation is maintained with pentobarbital, 1 to 2 mg. per kg. every 3 to 6 hours.

After mechanical ventilation has been started, a chest roentgenogram is obtained to verify proper placement of the tube. If the tube passes the carina, ventilating only one lung, it must be withdrawn to the proper position.

Continuous electrocardiographic monitoring and frequent blood gas determinations are indicated, and frequent notations of vital signs, skin color, and ventilator pressures and volumes are made. Tracheal secretions are aspirated at 30 to 60 minute intervals, using aseptic technique.

The ventilator is readjusted periodically as dictated by blood gas determinations and clinical findings to maintain arterial Pco_2 at 30 to 35 mm. Hg and arterial Po_2 between 65 and 100 mm. Hg.

Manual hyperventilation for 5 to 10 breaths at 30 minute intervals helps to minimize possible atelectasis, but some ventilators automatically supply deep breaths periodically.

After restoration of normal acid-base balance and sufficient clinical improvement the muscle relaxant can be discontinued (usually within 24 to 48 hours). When spontaneous ventilation has recurred the ventilator is set to assist, and if blood gases remain normal it can be disconnected, and the patient can be extubated. Other therapy for status asthmaticus is continued during mechanical ventilation.

Possible complications of endotracheal intubation and mechanical ventilation include unrecognized hypoventilation or hyperventilation, impairment of venous return to the heart causing hypotension, tension pneumothorax or pneumomediastinum, iatrogenic pulmonary infection, accidental extubation, and subglottic stenosis following extubation.

Intravenous Isoproterenol. Intravenous administration of isoproterenol as a constant infusion has been reported effective in the treatment of children with respiratory failure or impending respiratory failure and has sometimes obviated the need for mechanical ventilation (see manufacturer's official directive before using). Cardiac arrhythmias and cardiac arrests have resulted from this form of therapy, and deaths have occurred in adolescents and adults.

Continuous electrocardiographic monitoring is necessary, and the isoproterenol is administered with a slow infusion pump at an initial dose of 0.1 microgram per kg. per minute. This dose is increased by 0.1 microgram per kg. per minute every 15 minutes until arterial Pco_2 has begun to decrease or until pulse rate has reached 200 or some other persistent cardiac arrhythmia has occurred. Constant observation by the physician is recommended while the dose is being increased. Other precautions include constant monitoring of arterial pulse and pressure with a strain gauge through a radial artery cannula flushed constantly with a heparin solution (1 unit per ml.), also delivered by a constant infusion pump. This cannula also serves as a source for frequent specimens for blood gas determinations (initially every 15 to 30 minutes; after response to therapy, every 2 to 4 hours).

After restoration of acid-base balance and clinical improvement the dose of isoproterenol is reduced by 0.1 microgram per kg. per minute at 1 to 2 hour intervals if blood gases remain normal and if the clinical condition otherwise remains stable.

The required maximum dose has varied at least from 0.10 to 1.70 micrograms per kg. per minute. Treatment with intravenous isoproterenol has usually been necessary for at least 36 hours and has sometimes been necessary for as long as 6 days.

It seems likely that intravenous administration of a beta adrenergic agent with less intense cardiac activity would be safer for the treatment of status asthmaticus, and intravenous administration of such an agent, albuterol, has been reported effective and safe from England.

ALLERGIC RHINITIS DUE TO INHALANT FACTORS

method of
JERRY DOLOVICH, M.D.,
F. E. HARGREAVE, M.D.,
and JOSEPH GREENBAUM, M.D.
Hamilton, Ontario, Canada

About one person in six will have allergic rhinitis at one time or another. The diagnosis is usually simple and the treatment can be highly satisfactory in most cases if the patient learns how to utilize an adequate and flexible system of treatment.

General Principles

The most important single message to convey to the patient is that appropriate treatment can bring excellent relief of symptoms. The patient equipped with this information and with easy access to the therapist can be expected to look for help when it is needed.

The various medications presently available permit considerable flexibility in finding the best treatment regimen for each patient. No single treatment regimen is best for everyone. The physician and patient should understand that a trial-and-error process is required to identify the minimum level of treatment required to keep the patient comfortable. Generally, no side effects from medications should be accepted except for mild transient irritation from topical nasal medication and a small local reaction at the site of injection in allergen injection treatment, if this therapy is used.

The approach to treatment presented here includes (1) avoidance of the offending allergens to the extent that this can be accomplished by reasonable measures, (2) medical treatment, with emphasis upon careful monitoring and a trial-and-error approach, and (3) allergen injection treatment (immunotherapy, hyposensitization) when the other measures do not conveniently produce a good result.

Avoidance of Offending Allergens

Seasonal air-borne allergens include the pollens of trees, grasses, and weeds and the spores of numerous molds. These originate mainly outdoors. Keeping windows and doors closed in the appropriate season keeps out virtually all particles that originate outdoors. An air conditioner permits this, by keeping the home cool. It is to be remembered that an air conditioner recirculates the air indoors and releases the heat to the outdoors; it does not generally bring in air from the outdoors. Air cleaners probably are much less effective; they cannot keep up with a constant new supply of allergen that is introduced if the windows are kept open. However, in the presence of an important household allergen such as a pet, there is a dilemma; measures that reduce ventilation from the outdoors tend to increase the level of exposure to the household allergen. The obvious solution is to eliminate indoor allergens to the extent possible.

Tree pollens are in the air mainly in the spring. Exposure to grass pollen is mainly in the summer and pollens of weeds, including ragweed, mainly in the fall. Ragweed pollen is a particularly important air-borne allergen in eastern and central North America. It is released at midday. The sensitive person venturing outdoors in the early morning or late evening hours has less exposure. After a rainfall, the air is cleaned of all particles for a short period of time. There are manuals that indicate geographic locations where exposure to particular air-borne allergens may be reduced. Pollen counts are reduced over bodies of water and at high altitudes.

Important perennial allergens include house dust and animals. For house dust allergy, a more intensive than usual cleaning of the bedroom including vacuuming of the mattress when sheets are changed and avoidance of feather pillows and old comforters can be useful. The room with the television is another place where considerable time may be spent. Sometimes the television set is in a room away from the main part of the house and the room may be less well maintained and excessively dusty; this should be corrected. In general, recommendations that would require a major revision of the household are probably not justified.

In instances where an animal contributes to symptoms, it is most important to make provision for removal of the animal from the home, followed by careful cleaning. It is axiomatic that when there are (1) respiratory symptoms, (2) a positive allergy skin test to a particular animal, and (3) the presence of the animal in the home, the conclusion can be drawn that this animal is contributing to the symptoms. Other sources of animal products include felt rug under-pads, which contain horse hair, and feather pillows. Synthetic pillows do not generally harbor allergens.

Medical Treatment

Patients need to be reminded that there are no known incompatibilities among the various classes of medications discussed in this section or between the various types of medications and the simultaneous use of allergen injection treatment. When needed, the most useful approach is to combine a number of modalities of treatment in doses of each that are known to be free of side effects.

Antihistamines (H_1 Receptor Antagonists). For most people, chlorpheniramine (Chlor-Trimeton) or bromopheniramine maleate (Dimetane) provide as good a result as can be obtained. Sometimes, switching from one antihistamine to another can improve results, but this strategy is usually useless. A key consideration in the use of antihistamine is the person-to-person variation in the dose required and the dose tolerated. If there are any side effects, such as drowsiness or unsteadiness, the dose should be reduced until these effects disappear; it is generally not necessary to stop the medication. The use of a larger dose before sleep than during the day is often a good strategy. The intent is to determine the minimum dose that controls symptoms and to vary the dose, within limits of complete tolerance, according to need. The antihistamine, in a dose free of side effects, should be taken *at least once a day* during the period of allergic nose or eye symptoms.

If avoidance measures (environmental control) and antihistamine do not sufficiently control symptoms, there should be an addition to the treatment regimen without delay.

Cromolyn Sodium. Cromolyn sodium (Rynacrom) is administered with a special insufflator as a powder from a 10 mg. capsule into each nasal cavity. This medication has also been shown to be effective when applied topically in the form of an aqueous solution. The spray is synchronized with a sniffing maneuvre. Cromolyn sodium is mainly preventative. It can be started in a dose of one capsule on each side four times daily and then reduced to the minimum required dose. It is often ineffective in allergic rhinitis and should be discontinued if it does not prove helpful. Sometimes treatment with adrenocortical steroid (topical ± systemic) opens the nasal cavity and renders cromolyn sodium more effective. In the United States cromolyn sodium is available for inhalation use in asthma but is not yet available in a form designed for nasal use.

Topical Adrenocortical Steroid. Beclomethasone (Beconase), a topical steroid aerosol, has an excellent local effect without apparent systemic effects when used at the recommended dose. In the United States beclomethasone has been approved only for use in asthma. This inhaler can also be adapted to nasal use; one or two sprays is used on each side up to four times daily. However, this treatment has not received approval in the United States. It is nevertheless probably preferable to ingested steroid in patients in whom it suffices. A sniffing maneuvre is used at the same time as the topical steroid is sprayed into the nasal cavity. It can be used on a trial basis as an alternative or addition to cromolyn sodium and is more consistently effective than cromolyn sodium in the control of rhinitis. In the event of nasal dryness, crusting, burning, or nose bleeds, the daily dose should be reduced. There appears to be no evidence of serious side effects. Antihistamines should be used at the same time.

Flunisolide (Rhinalar) is a topical corticosteroid prepared in aqueous solution and has been found to be locally effective for nasal use without systemic effects in clinical trials in the United States. It is presently available only in Canada. It appears to have a usefulness that corresponds to topical beclomethasone.

Topical dexamethasone (Decadron Turbinaire) has been available for many years; a disadvantage is the demonstrated systemic effects that are produced by its regular topical use.

Ingested Adrenocortical Steroid. Prednisone tablets are recommended. Steroid injections do not provide sufficient flexibility in individual variations of dose and duration of treatment; as a result, there would seem to be no indication for steroid injections in the treatment of allergic rhinitis. Other modalities of treatment should be continued to minimize the dose and duration of required prednisone; prednisone should be the last drug started and the first discontinued. It is indicated if the patient cannot function or sleep normally. These effects are most likely to result from seasonal allergic rhinitis. The dose used is the minimum, in addition to other medications, needed to restore normal function or permit normal sleep. Often, in the adult, 4 to 6 prednisone (5 mg.) tablets, taken as a single dosage after breakfast for a few days, are sufficient to control the symptoms. This can then immediately be changed to a single dose after breakfast every second day and then gradually reduced on an alternate-day basis at a rate permitted by the symptoms, until discontinued. The usual contraindications to steroids apply.

Allergen Injection Treatment (Hyposensitization, Immunotherapy). Allergen injection treatment has proved effective in allergic rhinitis, particularly due to pollen sensitivity. However, not all patients benefit, and those who do benefit do not necessarily become asymptomatic. If there are symptoms, symptomatic treatment with medications should be included in the treatment program.

Injections are given subcutaneously on the lateral side of the upper arm below the shoulder. Treatment begins with a low dose of an extract of the offending allergen. The dose is gradually increased according to a standard schedule, but the rate of increase varies commensurate with the development of reduced reactivity to the injected allergens.

The authors take a conservative approach to the use of allergen injection treatment of allergic rhinitis. This is largely because alternative modalities that have become available provide a reasonable alternative treatment.

Advantages of allergen injection treatment include (1) it is preventative, (2) it may reduce the requirement for medications, and (3) it may help other symptoms including asthma and conjunctivitis.

Disadvantages include (1) distraction of the therapist from effective symptomatic treatment, (2) distraction of the patients from making provision for adequate symptomatic treatment since "my allergies are being treated with shots", (3) inconvenience to the patient, (4) inconsistent results, (5) dependence upon accurate identification of the major offending allergens, and (6) the risk of adverse reactions including anaphylaxis to the injected antigen.

The guidelines followed by the authors in the use of allergen injection treatment are as follows:

1. A trial of avoidance of allergens (environmental control) and medications is used first; allergen injection treatment is then added if necessary.

2. Injection treatment is currently withheld in the presence of coexisting disease such as rheumatic disease, which may have an immunologic origin. Since there is no proof that in-

jection treatment aggravates these diseases, this avoidance is on a speculative basis.

3. Clear identification of responsible allergens by history and allergy skin tests by the prick or puncture method is required before injections are considered.

4. If the conditions are appropriate for a consideration of injection treatment, the advantages, disadvantages, probabilities, and alternatives are explained to the patient and it is the patient (family) who decides whether to embark upon a trial of injection treatment.

5. The dose of antigen is increased if the interval from the last injection is two weeks or less and there was no generalized reaction or excessive local reaction (see below). The dose of antigen remains the same if the interval is 2 to 6 weeks. The dose of antigen is reduced proportionately to the time interval after 6 weeks. If the time interval elapsed from the previous injection is more than 3 months, a "starting schedule" is utilized.

6. If there is a swelling at the site of injection, greater than 2 inches (5 cm.) in diameter or lasting more than 24 hours, the dose is decreased.

7. The dose is decreased or injection treatment is discontinued if there are any distant side-effects such as respiratory symptoms or urticaria.

8. If the situation is stable for 2 years and, particularly if there is no benefit after 2 years, the injection treatment is stopped.

Associated Conjunctivitis

Ingested antihistamine is helpful and should be used regularly in a dose that produces no side-effects at the time of symptoms. A topical vasoconstrictor-antihistamine preparation such as naphazoline-antazoline preparation (Vasocon-A or Zincfrin A) as an additional treatment is used, if needed. Cromolyn sodium in an ophthalmic preparation has been shown to be effective in allergic conjunctivitis but is not as yet approved for use in the United States. We sometimes use it by dissolving the contents of two capsules for inhalation (each containing 20 mg. of cromolyn sodium) per 1 ml. of a commercial methyl cellulose eye drop preparation and then having the patient apply 1 or 2 drops in each eye up to 4 times daily. It is to be remembered that there is no approval for use of ophthalmic cromolyn sodium in the United States. With this regimen, the topical use of steroid eye drops has proven entirely unnecessary. If steroid is needed, a nonabsorbable preparation such as medrysone (HMS Liquifilm) is recommended.

Associated Chest Symptoms

In persons with allergic rhinitis, recurrent or persisting chest symptoms such as cough, breathlessness or wheeze at any time of year, are likely to be related to the allergic process. The authors believe that it is well demonstrated that cough and other chest symptoms in persons with allergic rhinitis are due to coexisting endobronchial disease and not due to postnasal drip. Many of these patients have readily demonstrable increase in nonspecific bronchial reactivity. The type of treatment that almost invariably is effective is the type of treatment used in asthma; that is, bronchodilators, inhaled cromolyn sodium and, if necessary, inhaled and ingested steroid. Antibiotics are generally useless and cough medicines do not deal with the primary problem.

Complications

These include infective sinusitis, otitis media, nasal polyps, and rhinitis medicamentosa (from the chronic use of nose drops). In all of these, the most important component of treatment is the effective treatment of rhinitis by methods outlined. Antibiotics are required as an additional component of treatment for sinusitis or otitis media due to bacterial infection. Nasal polyps initially receive medical treatment by the methods cited above, including ingested prednisone if needed. It is often possible to restore comfort and maintain a remission with a medical regimen that avoids the use of long-term ingested prednisone. If continuing prednisone appears necessary, surgical excision is utilized as an alternative.

ADVERSE REACTIONS TO DRUGS: HYPERSENSITIVITY*

method of
HAROLD S. NELSON, M.D.
Denver, Colorado

A minority of untoward reactions occurring during drug therapy is due to an allergic reaction to the drug (see Table 1). However, other reactions are frequently confused with drug allergy, especially in the mind of the patient, and account for a surprisingly high proportion of the histories of drug allergy recorded in patients' records.

---

*The opinions or assertions contained herein are the private views of the author and are not to be construed as reflecting the views of the Department of the Army or the Department of Defense.

TABLE 1. **Classification of Adverse Drug Reactions**

TYPE OF REACTION	EXAMPLE
1. Nondrug related:	
a. psychogenic	Vasovagal reaction with injections
b. coincidental	Viral exanthema in patients receiving antibiotics
2. Drug-related, dose related:	
a. toxic	Respiratory depression with sedatives
b. side effect	Vomiting with opiates
c. secondary effects	Superinfection with antibiotics
3. Drug-related, nondose related:	
a. idiosyncratic	Primaquine-induced hemolytic anemia in patients deficient in glucose-6-PD
b. allergic	Anaphylactic reaction to penicillin

Critical evaluation of the history is vital in cases of possible drug reaction since the diagnosis of drug allergy is essentially clinical. With the exception of skin testing for immediate hypersensitivity to high molecular weight compounds such as vaccines or to penicillin, no tests are available that can confirm or exclude a clinically significant immunologic reaction to a drug.

The diagnosis of drug allergy is suggested by the occurrence of symptoms consistent with an immunologic reaction (Table 2). Additional support is provided if the clinical picture has been previously reported with that particular drug. Clearing of the symptoms on discontinuing the drug provides partial confirmation. Prompt re-

TABLE 2. **Clinical Manifestations of Drug Allergy**

1. CUTANEOUS ERUPTIONS
   Urticaria
   Maculopapular-morbilliform rashes
   Contact sensitivity
   Fixed drug eruptions
   Erythema multiforme
   Purpura
   Exfoliative dermatitis
   Photosensitivity eruptions
2. ANAPHYLACTIC REACTIONS
3. HEPATITIS AND OBSTRUCTIVE JAUNDICE
4. PULMONARY
   Nitrofurantoin reaction
   Pulmonary infiltrate with eosinophilia
5. LUPUS-LIKE SYNDROME
6. INTERSTITIAL NEPHRITIS
7. HEMATOLOGIC
   Hemolytic anemia
   Thrombocytopenia
   Granulocytopenia
8. DRUG FEVER
9. VASCULITIS
10. SERUM SICKNESS

currence with readministration of the drug provides additional evidence but is rarely indicated. This should be considered only where there is a clear indication for use of the drug and no alternative therapy is available.

Management of Suspected Drug Reactions

In most instances, it is sufficient to discontinue the drug. Depending on the severity of the symptoms, supportive therapy including antihistamines or corticosteroids may be indicated.

In instances in which symptoms of an immediate hypersensitivity reaction occurs, more vigorous treatment is usually required (see Table 3).

Management of Patients with a History of Penicillin Allergy

It has been repeatedly demonstrated that the majority of patients who give a history of a previous allergic reaction to penicillin can be treated with penicillin without an adverse reaction.

Selection of patients with a history of penicillin allergy who can presently tolerate penicillin without danger of an immediate or accelerated allergic reaction depends on the availability of three skin test reagents:

Penicillin G   10,000 units per ml. (10^{-2}M)
Penicilloyl polylysine   (10^{-6}M)
   (Pre-Pen, Kremers-Urban Co.)
Minor Determinant Mix
   Benzylpenicilloate (10^{-2}M)
   Benzypenilloate   (10^{-2}M)

If the patient has negative immediate prick and intradermal skin tests to these three agents, it is possible to proceed with therapeutic doses of penicillin despite a history of a previous allergic reaction. Under these circumstances, only isolated delayed urticarial reactions occurred in two large series.

If only penicillin G and penicilloyl polylysine are available for skin testing, these skin tests will detect 90 per cent of those at risk for an immediate allergic reaction. That leaves 10 per cent of those actually allergic or approximately 1 per cent of those with a positive history of penicillin allergy who are at risk for immediate or accelerated reactions despite negative skin tests to the two commercially available skin test reagents.

Recommended Management. 1. If a rash occurs during the course of penicillin treatment, it is prudent to stop the penicillin and substitute another antibiotic.

If the indications for continuing penicillin are very strong, and the patient is hospitalized, it is possible to continue the drug. In many cases the rash will subside during the continued treatment.

TABLE 3. Emergency Measures for Management of Anaphylaxis

1. If the patient with an anaphylactic reaction is pulseless or appears moribund, immediately ventilate mouth to mouth or bag to mouth, intubate as soon as possible, start external cardiac massage, start an intravenous infusion, and institute cardiac resuscitation.
2. The drug of first choice in treating anaphylactic reactions is aqueous epinephrine. Any other drug is secondary. While epinephrine is being obtained, if the medication was given subcutaneously or intramuscularly in an extremity, apply a tourniquet proximal to the drug injection site.
3. 0.2 to 0.3 ml. 1:1000 aqueous epinephrine should be administered subcutaneously. This may be repeated every five minutes, three times if necessary.
4. If the drug causing the reaction was injected subcutaneously, give 0.1 ml. aqueous epinephrine 1:1000 directly into the drug injection site. Do not inject epinephrine into the drug site if it was given intramuscularly.
5. Slow intravenous administration of diluted epinephrine (e.g., 0.3 ml. 1:1000 diluted in 10 ml. saline solution) is indicated *only* in extreme cases of profound shock and cardiac arrest.
6. Start intravenous fluids.
7. 50 mg. diphenhydramine (Benadryl) may be given slowly intravenously (at least over a 1 minute period of time). More rapid administration may cause vomiting or fall in blood pressure.
8. If the blood pressure falls below 90 mm. Hg systolic or below 100 mm. Hg in a hypertensive patient and does not respond promptly to epinephrine and recumbency, pressor agents may be indicated; however, the hypotension of an anaphylactic reaction is better treated with brisk administration of intravenous volume expanders and epinephrine.
9. If persistent wheezing is a problem, aminophylline, 6 mg. per kg., may be administered intravenously over a period of 15 to 20 minutes.
10. If laryngeal edema is suspected and it persists or progresses despite epinephrine, the treatment of choice is endotracheal intubation. Cricothyroidostomy with a 14 or 16 gauge needle may be employed as a temporary measure.
11. Corticosteroids do not act for several hours and there is no evidence that they are necessary in the treatment of most acute anaphylactic reactions.
12. Patients should be hospitalized and observed following resuscitation from a significant anaphylactic reaction, as symptoms may recur when the effect of the medication wanes.

2. If a patient with a history of penicillin allergy has a clear indication for penicillin therapy, and an alternative equally effective therapy is not available, penicillin skin testing should be performed. If the three skin test antigens (penicilloyl polylysine, penicillin G and the minor determinant mix) are available and negative, penicillin therapy may be administered beginning with normal therapeutic doses. If only penicillin G and penicilloyl polylysine are available, and both are negative, a small risk of an immediate or accelerated allergic reaction still exists, and penicillin should be administered beginning with graded doses (Table 4). If any of the skin tests is positive, a high risk of an immediate or accelerated allergic reaction exists, and penicillin should be employed only if the likelihood of an allergic reaction, which could conceivably be fatal, is acceptable. In this instance, a slow, desensitization regimen should be followed (Table 4).

3. A high incidence of cross allergenicity exists between penicillin G and the semisynthetic penicillins, all of which share the 6-aminopenicillanic acid nucleus, and also with cephalosporins, all of which share with penicillin the beta lactam ring. Therefore, a history of penicillin allergy should be considered equally a contraindication to treatment with these drugs as with penicillin itself, until skin testing has been performed.

4. The maculopapular rash that occurs in 9 per cent of patients given ampicillin need not be considered an indication for stopping the drug, provided the rash is not urticarial, is nonpruritic, and is not accompanied by systemic symptoms. Continuation of the ampicillin is not usually associated with progression of the rash, and evidence of an allergic basis for the rash is lacking.

Radiocontrast Materials

Radiocontrast studies are followed in 1.7 per cent of patients either immediately or within minutes, by symptoms suggesting an allergic reaction. In about 1 in 50,000 studies, this reaction is fatal.

Patients who have had an immediate systemic reaction to radiocontrast materials are significantly more prone than others to have a recurrence with readministration of the same or a similar agent. Usually the second reaction is no more severe than the initial reaction.

Evidence suggests that these are not true allergic reactions. Indeed, recent studies appear to explain these reactions by the nonimmunologic release of mediators from basophils and also through activation of the alternative complement pathway.

When patients who have previously experienced an immediate systemic reaction to radiocontrast dyes require a repeat contrast study, it has generally been possible to accomplish this by following the protocol outlined in Table 5. Although the incidence, and hopefully the severity, of recurrent reactions are reduced by this procedure, repeat studies are still associated with a higher than the normal incidence of symptoms attributable to mediator release.

TABLE 4. **Penicillin Desensitization Regimen**

A. GRADED ADMINISTRATION OF PENICILLIN (Positive history, negative skin tests to penicillin G and penicilloyl polylysine)

Concentration	Amount	Dose
1. 10,000 units/ml.	0.02 intradermally	200 units
2.	0.2 subcutaneously	2000 units
3. 100,000 units/ml.	0.2 subcutaneously	20,000 units
4.	1.0 subcutaneously	100,000 units

Administer at 20 minute intervals
If no reaction to dose number 4, proceed with routine therapy with penicillin C
If a reaction occurs, either abandon use of penicillin or proceed using desensitization schedule B beginning with last dose tolerated.

B. DESENSITIZATION SCHEDULE
1. Positive prick test

Concentration	Amount (unit, subcutaneously)	Dose (units)
1 unit/ml.	0.1	0.1
	0.3	0.3
10 units/ml.	0.1	1
	0.3	3
100 units/ml.	0.1	10
	0.3	30

2. Positive intradermal, negative prick test

Concentration	Amount (unit, subcutaneously)	Dose (units)
1000 units/ml.	0.1	100
	0.3	300
10,000 units/ml.	0.1	1000
	0.3	3000
100,000 units/ml.	0.1	10,000
	0.3	30,000
	0.6	60,000
1,000,000 units/ml.	0.1	100,000
	0.2	200,000
	0.3	300,000
	0.5	500,000

Administer at 20 minute intervals
Twenty minutes following last dose, begin continuous intravenous therapy with penicillin G.
If a local reaction larger than 3 cm. occurs, repeat dose until local reaction decreases.
If systemic symptoms occur, treat as outlined in Table III, repeat last tolerated dose three times and resume progression.
Schedule A or B should be administered only in a setting with resuscitation equipment readily available.
Schedule B should be administered only in an intensive care unit with intravenous fluids being administered.

TABLE 5. **Procedure for Readministration of Radiocontrast Medium to Patients with a History of Previous Reactions, but Compelling Indications for Repeat Studies**

---

1. Administer prednisone, 50 mg. orally every 6 hours beginning 18 hours prior to study.
2. Diphenhydrazine, 50 mg. intramuscularly one hour prior to study.
3. In those with a history of a particularly severe reaction, graded administration may provide a margin of safety. Administer intravenously at 10 minute intervals:

0.1 ml.	1:100 dilution
0.1 ml.	1:10 dilution
0.1 ml.	full strength
1 ml.	full strength
5 ml.	full strength
20 ml.	full strength
full dose	

Local Anesthetic Reactions

The incidence of true allergy is particularly low among those patients who have been labeled sensitive to local anesthetic agents.

1. An approach to the management of this problem is based first on the existence of two groups of agents that are chemically dissimilar and that have been shown in limited studies not to cross react (Table 6). If the putative reaction is to a member of one group, and a representative of the other group is available, then use of this alternative agent is indicated.

2. If identity of the implicated agent is in doubt, or representatives of both groups are implicated, use of diphenhydramine 1 per cent, or similar local anesthetics has been suggested. In

TABLE 6. **Management of Adverse Reactions to Local Anesthetic Agents**

I. USE OF CHEMICALLY UNRELATED AGENTS

Esters of Benzoic Acid		*Amides*	
Generic	*Proprietary*	*Generic*	*Proprietary*
Procaine	Novocain	Lidocaine	Xylocaine
Tetracaine	Pontocaine	Mepivacaine	Carbocaine
Ethyl aminobenzoate	Benzocaine	Prilocaine	Citanest
		Dibucaine	Nupercaine

II. USE OF Diphenhydramine (Benadryl) 1 per cent (10 mg. per ml.)
III. SKIN TESTING AND PROGRESSIVE CHALLENGE
    a. Prick test with 1 per cent solution diluted 1:100
    b. Prick test with 1 per cent solution full strength
    c. Intradermal skin test with 0.02 ml. of 1 per cent diluted 1:100
    d. Intradermal skin test with 0.02 ml. of 1 per cent full strength
      (Ignore reactions less than 10 mm. and without pseudopods)
    e. Subcutaneous injection of 0.1 ml. of 1 per cent
    f. Subcutaneous injection of 0.5 ml. of 1 per cent
      (Injections to be at 20 minute intervals unless the history suggests a delayed reaction; in the latter case, there should be a delay of 24 hours between steps d and e, and a similar delay after step f before further administration of a local anesthetic)

general, these are more satisfactory for local infiltration in the skin than in dental work.

3. When the agent responsible for the reaction is unknown, or representatives of the other chemical group are not available, an alternative approach is to perform skin testing and progressive challenges with lidocaine. In doing this, the history should be reviewed with particular attention to the time relationship between the previous injection and the onset of symptoms. If symptoms were delayed in onset, both the intradermal test to undiluted drug and the subcutaneous injection of 0.5 ml. of undiluted drug should be observed 24 hours for late reactions (local or systemic) before any further drug is given. An occasional patient will have an irritative reaction to the injection of undiluted 1 per cent local anesthetic. If this skin reaction is less than 10 mm. and there are no pseudopods, it probably represents an irritative reaction and may be ignored.

Aspirin Sensitivity

The ingestion of aspirin will precipitate severe bronchoconstriction in some patients with bronchial asthma. This reaction is more common in patients with severe, nonallergic asthma, in whom its incidence may reach 20 per cent, but it also occurs in patients with mild allergic asthma. Evidence suggests that this reaction is not immunologically mediated, but rather related to inhibition of prostaglandin biosynthesis, with the resultant shunting of arachnidonic acid into pathways leading to increased production of bronchoconstrictors.

The precipitation of bronchoconstriction in these patients is not limited to aspirin. Indeed, all of the nonsteroidal anti-inflammatory drugs that inhibit cyclo-oxygenase similarly provoke asthma attacks in these patients (Table 7).

In addition to drugs, certain azo dyes and food preservatives that probably have some action on prostaglandin biosynthesis also have been reported to induce asthma in some aspirin-sensitive patients.

A number of patients with chronic urticaria appear to have whealing precipitated by the same analgesics, dyes, and preservatives that cause bronchoconstriction in the aspirin-sensitive patient. This suggests that derivatives of arachnidonic acid are important in producing the urticaria in these patients.

Two additional groups have been identified among patients with chronic urticaria who are ad-

TABLE 7. **Drugs Causing Asthma or Urticaria in Aspirin-Sensitive Patients**

GENERIC	PROPRIETARY
Predictable	
Aspirin	
Indomethacin	Indocin
Mefenamic acid	Ponstel
Flufenamic acid	
Phenylbutazone	Butazolidin, Azolid
Fenoprofen	Nalfon
Ibuprofen	Motrin
Diclofenac	
Naproxen	Naprosyn
Noramidopyrine	
Occasionally	
Acetaminophen, Paracetamol	Tylenol and others
Tartrazine & other azo dyes	
Benzoic acid preservatives	
BHA AND BHT?	
Usually Tolerated	
Sodium salicylate	
Propoxyphene hydrochloride, dextroproxyphen	Darvon
Chloroquine	

versely affected by aspirin. In one large group, comprising perhaps 30 per cent of patients with chronic urticaria, aspirin appears to aggravate urticaria by a pharmacologic route, and does so only when the underlying disease process is active. In the second and much less common group with chronic urticaria, there appears to be a true immunologic reactivity to impurities in the commercial aspirin. This reaction appears to be IgE mediated, and urticaria is precipitated by small amounts of the drug. In this latter, immunologically mediated type of chronic urticaria, unrelated drugs that inhibit prostaglandin biosynthesis do not cause cross reactions.

ALLERGIC REACTION TO INSECT STINGS

method of
J. ANDREW GRANT, M.D.,
and DAVID O. THUESON, Ph.D.
Galveston, Texas

TABLE 1. Management of Systemic Allergic Reactions in Insect Stings

I. Diagnosis
  A. Symptoms beginning within minutes of sting
    1. Respiratory—dyspnea, cough, wheezing
    2. Cardiovascular—dizziness, shock, unconsciousness, arrhythmias
    3. Cutaneous—itching, redness, urticaria, angioedema
    4. Gastrointestinal—nausea, vomiting, diarrhea, cramps
  B. Confirmation of sensitivity
    1. Skin testing with insect extracts; venoms preferred to whole body extract
    2. Leukocyte histamine release test
    3. RAST
II. Therapy
  A. Immediate management
    1. Epinephrine—drug of choice
    2. Antihistamines—of some value
    3. Aminophylline—for bronchospasm
    4. Corticosteroids—to reduce later reactions
    5. Maintenance of vascular volume in shock
    6. Maintenance of adequate ventilation in respiratory failure
  B. Long-term management
    1. Avoidance of future stings
    2. Identification bracelet
    3. Emergency drug kit for self-administration
    4. Immunotherapy ("desensitization")

Stinging insects cause more deaths each year than venomous snakes. However, unlike snakes, the adverse effects generally are not due to the venom of the insect but to an allergic response to the toxin. It is estimated that about 1 million Americans are susceptible to systemic life-threatening allergic reaction to insect stings. This sensitivity to venoms is due to reaginic IgE antibodies, produced in response to a previous sting. The symptoms of anaphylaxis are probably caused by histamine, slow reacting substance, and other mediators that are released by basophils and mast cells during the allergic reaction. The symptoms of systemic reactions usually appear within minutes and may involve one or more of the following systems: respiratory, cardiovascular, cutaneous, or gastrointestinal (see Table 1).

Insects of the order Hymenoptera, which most frequently cause allergic reactions, include honeybees, yellow jackets, wasps, and hornets. In the southeastern United States, the imported fire ant is also a major contributor to these reactions. The type of insect to which a patient is allergic can be objectively determined by means of skin testing. Extracts made from the whole body of insects contain large quantities of irrelevant proteins and indeterminate amounts of venom. A number of investigators have shown that skin testing with venom-rich extracts more accurately identifies allergic persons. Commercial suppliers are in the process of securing approval of venom preparations for use in skin testing and immunotherapy in the United States. A number of medical centers also offer the leukocyte histamine release test and radioallergosorbent test (RAST) to confirm immediate hypersensitivity to stinging insect venoms.

The immediate therapy for systemic reactions to insect stings is similar to that described in the article on Anaphylaxis and Serum Sickness. Subcutaneous epinephrine (0.3 to 0.5 ml. of 1:1,000 for adults; 0.1 to 0.3 ml. for children) is the drug of choice. In patients with vascular collapse, epinephrine can be given cautiously by the intravenous route using 1:10,000 dilution. Epinephrine can be repeated in 5 to 30 minutes, as needed. Antihistamines (e.g., diphenhydramine, 25 to 75 mg. orally or intramuscularly) are of secondary importance. Aminophylline (250 to 500 mg. given intravenously over 15 to 30 minutes) may be beneficial in reversing bronchospasm. Corticosteroids will not be effective for the immediate allergic symptoms but may reduce the degree of delayed reactions. Expansion of intravascular volume with saline or dextrose solutions may be used in cases of shock reactions. Intubation and use of a mechanical ventilator is indicated for patients with respiratory failure.

After recovery from an allergic reaction, the patient should be counseled to avoid situations in which a repeat sting is likely. Light clothing is preferable and shoes should always be worn outdoors. An identification bracelet can be obtained from the Medic Alert Foundation, Turlock, California.

The patient should have an emergency stinging insect kit with a prefilled syringe containing epinephrine and oral antihistamines available at all times for therapy. The Ana-Kit (Hollister-Stier Laboratories) is widely available. The thigh is the preferred site for self-administration of epinephrine. Inhaled epinephrine should be prescribed where injectable drugs are not practical, such as for children.

Immunotherapy using gradually increasing doses of insect extracts followed by periodic maintenance injections has been recommended for several decades to stimulate production of blocking IgG antibodies. It has recently been demonstrated that enriched venoms are more effective than the currently available whole body extracts. Desensitization therapy should probably be continued indefinitely.

Delayed reactions to insect stings often resemble serum sickness reactions. Appropriate management of this condition is outlined in the article on Anaphylaxis and Serum Sickness. Immunotherapy is not indicated for serum sickness reactions or any condition other than an immediate systemic reaction.

Diseases of the Skin

ACNE VULGARIS

method of
ALAN R. SHALITA, M.D.
Brooklyn, New York

Acne vulgaris is the single most common skin disease. It affects approximately 80 per cent of the teenage population and, contrary to popular belief, may persist well into the third and fourth decades of life. Acne is a disease of the pilosebaceous follicle with a multifactorial cause. The pathogenesis includes an androgen-dependent increase in sebum production, proliferation of the follicular microflora (principally *Propionibacterium acnes*), and alterations in follicular keratinization. This results in the clinical lesions of acne—namely, open comedones (blackheads), closed comedones (whiteheads), papules, pustules, and nodulocystic lesions. Current therapy is directed toward suppression of these lesions and is usually remarkably effective.

Topical Therapy

Many acne patients may be successfully treated with topical therapy alone. For comedonal and mild inflammatory acne, therapy is initiated with tretinoin cream 0.05 per cent daily. The patient should be advised that an initial erythema and exfoliation may occur, that an exacerbation of inflammatory lesions is possible during the first month of therapy, and that an increased sensitivity to sunburn is likely. For the sunburn, judicious exposure combined with a para-aminobenzoic acid (PABA)–containing sunscreen is advisable. Patients with a pronounced seborrhea or those refractory to the 0.05 per cent tretinoin cream may tolerate a 0.1 per cent cream or the 0.05 per cent tretinoin swabs or liquid—all of which have a tendency to produce more pronounced erythema and desquamation. An alternative dosage form is the 0.025 per cent gel, which is particularly useful in treating inflammatory acne. Significant therapeutic improvement does not usually occur before 4 to 6 weeks, and 12 weeks are normally required for optimal therapeutic benefit. Topical tretinoin appears to exert its effect on the keratinizing epithelium of the follicle. Salicylic acid 5 per cent in a hydroalcoholic gel may be a useful alternative to tretinoin in those patients who do not tolerate the erythema produced by the latter.

Benzoyl peroxide gels are very good topical antibacterial agents. Therapy is usually initiated with a 5 per cent gel applied daily. Refractory cases may require the 10 per cent concentration or more frequent application. Although little erythema occurs, there may be considerable desquamation.

Many patients benefit from the combined use of topical tretinoin and a benzoyl peroxide gel, one applied in the morning and the other at night. The effects of the two drugs appear to be additive. Some patients, however, will not tolerate the "dryness" produced by this regimen. One may then try therapy with each drug on alternate days.

Topical antibiotic solutions such as those containing erythromycin and clindamycin offer promise as additions to the therapeutic armamentarium. At the time of this writing, however, they are still experimental, and there are few data available on the stability of extemporaneous preparations.

Preparations containing various combinations of sulfur, resorcin, and salicylic acid, particularly in tinted lotions and creams, may be useful when used judiciously. They accelerate the resolution of inflammatory lesions while providing cover.

Systemic Therapy

Broad-spectrum antibiotics remain valuable tools in the treatment of inflammatory acne. Therapy is usually initiated with 500 to 1000 mg. of tetracycline hydrochloride or erythromycin. The dose is decreased at appropriate intervals according to the therapeutic response. Minocycline, 50 mg. daily to three times daily, is occasionally useful in patients who appear to be refractory to the aforementioned agents. An alternative is larger doses of tetracycline. One thousand five hundred to 3000 mg. of tetracycline is effective in patients with severe nodulocystic acne who have not responded to lower doses. The safety of the long-term use of these antibiotics for acne treatment is now well established.

In resistant acne in women, systemic estrogen therapy is beneficial. This can be administered in the form of oral contraceptives. Most useful are those containing 80 to 100 micrograms of ethinyl estradiol or mestranol. Those containing norgestrel as the progestational agent appear to be contraindicated because of their apparent mildly androgenic effect.

Systemic steroids are frequently useful for short periods in recalcitrant nodulocystic acne. Doses of 30 to 40 mg. of prednisone per day may be used if rapidly tapered.

Local Therapy

Intralesional injections of triamcinolone acetonide or triamcinolone hexacetonide (2.5 to 5 mg. per ml.) are most useful in achieving the prompt resolution of inflammatory lesions, particularly those of the nodulocystic variety. No more than 0.5 mg. should be injected into any single lesion of the face in order to minimize local atrophy. The hexacetonide salt should be limited to lesions of the chest and back, because it may produce more pronounced and prolonged atrophy.

Cryotherapy with liquid nitrogen probes, liquid nitrous oxide, or solid CO_2 is also useful in treating large inflammatory lesions. An initial edematous reaction is followed by relatively prolonged resolution of nodulocystic lesions.

The physical removal of comedones with a comedo extractor is frequently of benefit. Incision and drainage of inflammatory lesions rarely accomplishes more than intralesional steroids or cryotherapy.

PSEUDOFOLLICULITIS BARBAE

method of
A. PAUL KELLY, M.D.
Los Angeles, California

Pseudofolliculitis barbae (PFB) is a common, chronic disorder that occurs most often in black males. It has been described by many authors under different names, such as folliculitis barbae traumatica, scarring pseudofolliculitis of the beard, chronic sycosis barbae, "ingrown hairs," and "shaving bumps."

Shaving is the precipitating factor and stiff, strongly recurved hairs provide the diathesis for PFB. Since most blacks have a genetic predisposition for curved hairs, they are more susceptible to this condition than whites. Not only the beard but also the scalp, axilla, pubis, and legs of those with short, thick, curly hair may have similar lesions if shaved. The chin and neck, where hair grows in various directions and often exits the follicles parallel to the skin, are the areas most often affected.

Pseudofolliculitis barbae lesions are produced when strongly recurved hairs are shaved and the distal end of the hair is cut at an oblique angle, creating a sharp tip. As the hair continues to grow in its curved manner, it may penetrate the skin 1 to 2 mm. from where it exits the follicle, producing a foreign body reaction manifested by papules and pustules. The symptoms may vary from mild (fewer than a dozen papules or pustules) to severe (hundreds of papules and pustules and some abscesses caused by secondary bacterial infection). If shaving is discontinued, these sharp embedded tips will reach a maximum depth of 2 to 3 mm. and, thereafter, the external segment of the hair will form a loop which in 2 to 3 weeks will function like a spring to pull the tip out. Once the embedded hairs are out, clinical manifestations of PFB usually resolve spontaneously. Thus, termination of shaving and growing a beard would prevent PFB. However, in many instances patients find this impractical or impossible. Fortunately, alternatives are available and must be selected on an individual basis because there is no one best method for all patients.

Before any therapy is initiated, the patient should be given a candid explanation about the cause of PFB and the methods to keep it under control. It should be stressed that the only way to cure the disease is to stop shaving.

Acute Management

Except for very mild cases, PFB requires medical intervention during its acute phase when it is often painful or pruritic or both. The following therapeutic approach is recommended:

1. Shaving should be discontinued for a minimum of 1 month for mild cases, 2 to 3 months for moderate cases and from 6 to 12 months for severe cases. During this time, the beard may be trimmed with scissors or electric clippers to a minimum length of 0.5 cm.

2. Warm tap water, saline, or Burow's solution compresses are used 10 minutes three times daily to soothe the lesions, remove any crust, stop drainage secondary to inflammation or excoriation or both, and to soften the epidermis to allow easier release of "ingrown hairs."

3. With daily use of a magnifying mirror, the patient should search for "ingrown hairs" and release them with a sterile needle. These hairs should not be plucked because regrowth may be fraught with irritation and penetration of the follicular wall.

4. After compressing and freeing embedded hairs, a topical corticosteroid lotion should be applied.

5. When secondary bacterial infection is present, the appropriate systemic antibiotic should be given.

6. In resistant cases, 1 to 2 weeks of systemic corticosteroids, 30 to 50 mg. of prednisone or its equivalent a day, may be necessary.

7. Shaving should not be resumed until all the inflammatory lesions have cleared and all "ingrown hairs" have been released.

Shaving Methods

For those who shave, the following is recommended:

1. Remove any preexisting beard with electric clippers, leaving approximately 1 to 2 mm. of stubble.

2. Wash the beard area with a nonabrasive acne soap and rough washcloth. In areas with "ingrown hairs," gentle massaging with a soft toothbrush may be helpful.

3. Rinse the beard area with water and then compress the face with warm tap water for several minutes.

4. Use the shaving cream of your choice and massage a moderate amount of lather in the area to be shaved (do not allow the lather to dry; if it does so, reapply).

5. Using a sharp blade of a type that seems to cut the best but not too closely (most prefer an adjustable razor at one of the midsetting levels), shave with the grain of the hair, using short, even strokes with minimal tension. Twice over one area is usually sufficient, although in hard-to-shave areas one may occasionally shave against the grain.

6. After shaving, the face should be rinsed with tap water and then compressed with cool to cold water for 5 minutes.

7. Then, using a magnifying mirror, the patient should search for and dislodge any embedded hairs with a sterile needle or toothpick.

8. The least irritating, but most soothing, aftershave lotion of the patient's choice should then be applied. However, if excess burning or pruritus ensues, then a topical corticosteroid lotion should be used as the aftershave preparation.

Chemical Depilatories

The chemical depilatories (Ali, Magic Shave, Royal Crown, Jaybra, etc.) have had greater patient acceptance during the past few years with the advent of "odorless" preparations. Before using a depilatory on the face, the patient should be instructed to apply a small amount to a 2 to 3 cm. hair-bearing area on the forearm. If moderate or marked irritation appears in the area within 48 hours, the depilatory should not be used on the face. However, if either mild or no irritation is appreciated, then the depilatory should be used as follows:

1. Follow the instructions on the product information sheet because the prescribed use of each product may vary.

2. Patients with a beard should be instructed to trim it as short as possible without irritating or traumatizing their skin, prior to using the depilatory.

3. The depilatory may be removed with a table knife, spatula, spoon, or tongue blade, after which steps 5, 6 and 7 of the above shaving techniques should be followed.

4. In order to prevent excessive irritation, depilatories should not be used more often than every third day.

Topically Applied Tretinoin

Tretinoin (Retin-A) solution, gel, or cream may be used as an adjunct to shaving in patients with early mild to moderate PFB. However, those with severe and chronic PFB usually have only slight improvement. It is thought to work by alleviating hyperkeratosis and "toughening" the skin. Initially, tretinoin is applied every night. The patient should be told to expect some stinging, burning, and peeling. Depending on the response, the dose may be changed to twice a day or once every second or third day. The shaving methods outlined above should still be followed.

Other Therapeutic Modalities

Temporary x-ray epilation, although out of vogue with most younger practitioners, has been used to relieve the severe symptomatology of PFB, giving the skin a chance to recover before instituting other therapy. Weekly use of Cryospray to cause a light peel is sometimes a helpful adjunct to shaving. Antibiotics, topical or systemic, are of no benefit unless secondary infection is present.

ALOPECIA

method of
HENRY MAGUIRE, JR., M.D.
Philadelphia, Pennsylvania

"Alopecia" denotes an abnormal lack of hair. It is a descriptive term, not a diagnosis. When alopecia is observed, proper management requires that a diagnosis be made of the condition causing the absence of hair. Often, therapy consists of discontinuing a specific drug or of avoiding a damaging cosmetic procedure. The emotional impact of hair loss, particularly in women, should not be underestimated. Successful treatment requires wise counsel; occasionally, psychiatric referral is necessary.

Common Male Baldness

Male-pattern or androgenetic alopecia appears as a progressive, symmetrical, diffuse loss of hair. It begins in the temporal and frontal areas and is entirely asymptomatic. To some degree, nearly all adult males are affected. Pathologically, there is a characteristic noninflammatory degeneration of the affected hair follicles.

The development of common male baldness requires three factors: sufficient male hormone, genetic predisposition, and age. Normal postpubertal levels of androgens in the male are fully permissive; the appearance of early extensive baldness (alopecia prematura) does not connote an excess of male hormone. We lack a genetic analysis of common male baldness; however, men who develop patterned alopecia early and rapidly are usually related through one or both parents to similarly affected males. Age increases the susceptibility of scalp hair follicles to the toxicity of androgen; on the average, older men have fewer hairs.

There is no medical treatment for male-pattern alopecia. Topical testosterone, topical or intralesion estrogens, topical anti-inflammatory steroids, and local rubrifacients are without demonstrated value. Massage and other physical therapies fail to regrow hair or to prevent its loss. Clearing a coincident seborrhea or dandruff does not alter the progress of the alopecia.

In a few patients with ample side hair a cosmetically agreeable redistribution of scalp hair follicles can be accomplished by free autografting. Full thickness grafts are transplanted, with a 3.5 or 4 mm. Orentreich biopsy punch, from haired lateral donor sites to appropriate bald recipient sites in the frontocentral area of the scalp. The cylinder-shaped grafts contain viable hair follicles, which, when revascularized, synthesize hair in the recipient site just as they did in their site of origin.

Although usually an outpatient procedure, the surgical technique is tedious and requires experience, planning, and a meticulous attention to detail if a high percentage (90 per cent plus) of transplanted follicles are to retain function.

Common Female Baldness

Female-pattern alopecia is a forme fruste of common male baldness; exposed to less androgen, the genetically equally susceptible hair follicles of women degenerate more slowly. Clinically, the hair loss is diffuse and concentrates in the frontocentral area; usually, there is no temporal recession. The pathologic findings are the same as those of common male baldness. There is no acceptable medical treatment for this physiologic alopecia. Because the hair loss is milder and tends to be less patterned than that of common male baldness, grafting is rarely useful. Exogenous androgens or androgen-secreting tumor or hyperplasia can precipitate a male-type common baldness in the genetically predisposed woman. In such instances, menstrual abnormalities and signs of masculinization are usually seen. With correction of the hyperandrogenism, the progress of the alopecia stops; however, restoration of the bald areas is, at best, only partial.

Postpartum Alopecia

Beginning in the weeks after delivery, there is an increased shedding of scalp hair, from an average of about 80 to several hundred hairs each day. This may last for many months. The lost hairs are normal club (telogen) hairs. The resultant, generally mild alopecia is diffusely distributed. No bald patches are seen, the scalp is normal, and there are no symptoms. This postpartum telogen effluvium represents a physiologic change. Curiously, in a given patient it may be severe after one pregnancy and almost imperceptible following another. There is no specific therapy; the excessive hair loss gradually and spontaneously ceases.

Alopecia of the Newborn

In the first few months of life there is a normal shedding of large numbers of scalp hairs; these are telogen hairs. A diffuse alopecia of variable degree results. The process may be precipitated by the abrupt withdrawal of the same maternal hormones whose loss is responsible for postpartum alopecia in the mother. The shed hairs are soon replaced, usually by somewhat thicker hairs. There is no specific treatment.

Drug-induced Alopecia

Heparin, heparinoids, and coumarin frequently cause a mild reversible alopecia. Antimitotic cancer chemotherapeutic drugs such as colchicine, cyclophosphamide, methotrexate, doxorubicin (Adriamycin), 5-fluorouracil, and actinomycin D regularly cause loss of scalp hair. The alopecia is often severe; however, regrowth occurs when the drug is stopped. Alopecia is occasionally seen with quinacrine, quinine, thiouracil compounds, allopurinol, and trimethadione (Tridione). Prolonged treatment with high doses (250,000 units daily) of vitamin A may cause hair loss. Generally, the hair regrows when the particular drug is stopped. Systemic androgen given to women induces common baldness; this alopecia, for the most part, persists even after the androgen is discontinued.

Radiation-induced Hair Loss

X-ray or other ionizing radiation causes alopecia. In low (epilating) doses, the hair loss is transient. With x-ray in amount sufficient to cause a radiation dermatitis, the hair loss is generally permanent. In a few selected patients autografting is feasible; however, x-irradiated skin generally does not accept grafts well.

Alopecia Areata

Alopecia areata presents as a patchy loss of hair, usually confined to the scalp but occasionally involving other hairy areas. The bizarre distribution of the alopecia frequently makes it a major cosmetic and emotional problem. The general health is unaffected. Histopathologically there is a diagnostic aseptic inflammation, which probably has an autoimmune origin.

Anti-inflammatory corticosteroids temporarily suppress the inflammation and allow for normal hair growth. Systemic corticosteroids, in equivalents of 20 to 30 mg. of prednisone daily, may suffice to allow satisfactory regrowth of hair, although some of the new hairs will be poorly pigmented, lusterless, and thin. An every other day schedule of twice (or slightly less) the amount of steroid is equally effective and may reduce steroid side effects. Unfortunately, the maintenance dose of steroid for the acceptable control of the disease is almost always in excess of the equivalent of 15 mg. per day of prednisone. Rarely should alopecia areata be treated on a long-term basis with systemic steroids.

Patients with alopecia areata, in which there are a few patches of alopecia on the scalp, eyebrows, or face can be treated with intralesional depot corticosteroid, thereby a therapeutic local concentration of steroid is obtained without appreciable toxic side effects of systemic steroid administration. (Small amounts of steroid are absorbed systemically.) In a typical patient a patch is treated with multiple injections of 0.1 ml. of 0.5 to 1.0 per cent triamcinolone acetonide suspension (or equivalent depot corticosteroid). The injection sites are 1.5 to 2.0 cm. apart; a disposable 1 ml.

syringe with 25 gauge needle is convenient. Sites should not be reinjected any more often than every 6 weeks. Excessive doses of intralesion corticosteroid will lead to local cutaneous atrophy, which is usually reversible.

Topical anti-inflammatory steroids are ineffective by usual application. Sometimes a therapeutic concentration can be obtained with an occlusive dressing; however, this method is very clumsy and rarely practicable. A variety of other topical and systemic medications have been advocated, but none have shown any definite value.

In moderate or severe cases of alopecia areata, particularly in women, wigs should be used. The wearing of a wig does not compromise hair growth or make recovery less likely.

Secondary Syphilis

A patchy alopecia of moth-eaten appearance may occur in the early stages of secondary syphilis. Appropriate antiluetic therapy is curative (see Syphilis, treatment of secondary stage).

Tinea Capitis

The infecting fungi proliferate in the hair shaft. The fungus utilizes the dead hard keratin as substrate, thereby producing a biologic dissolution of hair. The baldness is patchy. Diagnosis is confirmed by identifying the fungus (1) on microscopic examination of an infected hair, or (2) in the culture of a specimen on Sabouraud's media. In children in the United States most cases of tinea capitis are caused by fungi that produce a characteristic bright green fluorescence when the scalp is examined under Wood's (long ultraviolet) light. A pet dog or cat with ringworm may be the source of some of these infections. Treatment is with griseofulvin, 20 mg. per kg. body weight with meals, once daily, for about 6 weeks, or until at least 2 weeks after the scalp has become negative for fungi. The average adult dose of griseofulvin is 1 gram daily. If microsize rather than regular griseofulvin is used, the dosage is halved. Frequent shampoos and the application of topical antifungal preparations to the infected areas will reduce contagion. However, tinea capitis does *not* respond to any topical antifungals.

Cicatrizing Alopecia

Formation of new hair follicles does not occur in the human; thus, any lesion that destroys follicles will cause irreversible alopecia. Common examples of destructive processes that produce cicatrizing alopecia are malignant neoplasms of the skin (especially basal cell epithelioma, squamous cell epithelioma and melanoma), keloids, third degree burns, syphilitic gummas, deep bacterial infections (especially furuncles and carbuncles), severe foreign body reactions, x-ray dermatitis, pseudopelade (of Brocq), and scleroderma. Therapy is directed toward cure of the cicatrizing disease. In some patients in whom there is no active disease, autografts containing hair follicles can be transplanted from unaffected sites into the cicatricial bald spots.

The inflammatory stage of discoid lupus erythematosus (erythema, scaling) usually responds to intralesional triamcinolone acetonide (or comparable depot-corticosteroid) used in the same way as in the treatment of alopecia areata. Topical corticosteroids are helpful if the activity is mild. Systemic corticosteroids or antimalarials may be useful, particularly during the summer. However, the several hazards (especially eye and bone marrow) of the long-term administration of these drugs must be borne in mind. (This use of antimalarials is not listed in the manufacturer's official directives.) Of course, avoidance of natural or artificial ultraviolet light is essential.

Injurious Cosmetic Procedures

Setting lotions, permanent wave solutions, bleaches, epilating creams or waves, etc., when applied too long, in too high a concentration, or too frequently, can damage hair. A nylon brush with bristles having ragged tips or a comb with sharp edges also may injure the hair, as can teasing and, occasionally, hair weaving. The weakened hair fiber breaks more easily, and cuticular damage causes the hair to lose its sheen. If the damage is limited to the hair shaft, discontinuing the injury is curative; new normal hair replaces the damaged hair.

More serious is the follicular damage caused by the frequent use of tight braids, tight rollers, hot irons with oil (for straightening the hair), hot curlers, hot hair dryers, etc. Permanent follicular injury and irreversible alopecia often result. Treatment consists in stopping the particular traumatizing procedure.

Toxic Alopecia

Certain endocrine disorders sometimes are associated with alopecia, i.e., hyperthyroidism, hypothyroidism, hypopituitarism, and hypoparathyroidism. Correction of the endocrine abnormality restores normal hair growth. Hyperandrogenism may cause severe patterned alopecia in genetically predisposed women; this hair loss is *not* reversible.

Alopecia is *not* a typical feature of human vitamin deficiencies. Hair loss frequently occurs with kwashiorkor and is reversed by an appropriate treatment. Iron deficiency, with or without anemia, is occasionally responsible for mild diffuse alopecia in women; treatment is that of the iron deficiency.

Fever (particularly typhoid fever) or any serious stressful disease may produce a diffuse hair loss. Toxic alopecia is particularly frequent during the acute stage of systemic lupus erythematosus; generally, normal hair growth follows resolution of the acute disease.

Trichotillomania

Trichotillomania, the compulsive pulling out by the patient of his own hair, is often the explanation of an otherwise mysterious case of patchy alopecia. Trichotillomania is more common and has a better prognosis in children; in adults it is often a sign of serious psychiatric disease. Repeated plucking over many years leads to permanent follicular damage and irreversible alopecia.

CANCER OF THE SKIN
method of
WILLIS I. COTTEL, M.D.
Dallas, Texas

There are approximately 500,000 skin cancers diagnosed each year in the United States. These cancers are more prevalent in persons who live in areas of the country that receive the largest amount of ultraviolet irradiation. Since the most important single cause of skin cancer is sun exposure, it is important that skin cancer patients protect themselves from the sun.

Ultraviolet Protection

A sun screen should be applied every day, 365 days a year. In most patients one application will last the entire day. However, with excessive exposure to the sun, as occurs while playing tennis, golf, or fishing, the sun screen should be reapplied. At these times it is important for patients to wear a large hat and to protect their arms, chest, and back with clothing. The patient is allowed to swim; however, it must be remembered that sun screen agents will wash off with water and will need to be reapplied. With heavy exercise perspiration will have the same effect. Sunbathing is prohibited.

The most common and most cosmetically acceptable sun screening agents are those that contain para-aminobenzoic acid (PABA) or its esters. Some of the newer agents tend to resist the effects of water and perspiration. These include Sundown and Sunguard. Other sun screening agents include Pabafilm, Maxifil, Eclipse, and Pre-Sun. It should be remembered that all of the pure PABA preparations will tend to stain clothing. The esters do not have this problem.

Treatment

The treatment of skin carcinoma is varied according to the type of tumor and its location on the patient. Small nodular basal cell carcinomas, superficial basal cell carcinomas, superficial squamous cell carcinomas, and Bowen's disease (squamous cell carcinoma in situ) may be cured by a variety of methods. These include excision and primary closure, electrodesiccation and curettage, radiotherapy, and cryotherapy. The cure rate of all primary previously untreated tumors is approximately 95 per cent, regardless of which method is used. The cure rate in certain difficult areas is much less, as shown in Figure 1. Recurrent tumors are cured less than 50 per cent of the time by conventional methods. Mohs' surgery (chemosurgery) is the treatment of choice for skin carcinomas in difficult locations. It is also the treatment of choice in recurrent skin carcinomas.

Electrodesiccation and Curettage. Following local anesthesia with lidocaine and epinephrine, the mass of tumor is removed with a curette. The tumor is soft in comparison with the underlying normal tissue. This allows the operator to determine the extent of the tumor. Following this, a smaller curette will ferret out small extensions. With a Bantom Bovie or Hyfrecator, he destroys a small margin of normal tissue and the base of the lesion. This desiccated material is then removed by curettage. The procedure is repeated three times. The last desiccation is used for hemostasis.

Excision and Primary Closure. Care should be exercised to place the line of excision in the appropriate skin folds. An adequate margin of tissue should be removed. The specimen should be sent to the pathologist and an attempt should be made to tell whether the tumor has been totally excised. Tumors have statistically been proved to extend a full radius past their clinical margins. This is true of primary lesions and those in "nondifficult" locations (see Figure 2).

Radiotherapy. This should be reserved for patients over 60 years of age.

Cryotherapy. Cryotherapy has become practical since the development of efficient closed spray liquid nitrogen systems. There are many such units on the market. The least expensive is the Foster Froster. Other units such as the Brymill, Cryac, and Zacarian are more expensive but are more sturdy. A cotton tipped applicator dipped in liquid nitrogen has no place in the treatment of carcinomas. Cryosurgery should not be used in the management of scalp lesions because of the high recurrence rate.

THERMOCOUPLE METHOD. 1. Implant the thermocouple under the deepest margin of the tumor.

2. Direct spray at the center of the tumor until thermocouple registers $-25°C.$ and the ice ball extends an appropriate distance past the tumor margin.

3. Repeat the freeze thaw cycle.

HALO THAW TIME METHOD. Infiltrate the lesion with lidocaine. Freeze the lesion until the surface ice ball expands an appropriate distance beyond the margin of the tumor. Allow the lesion to thaw, noting the time required for the halo of frozen normal tissue to disappear. This is called the halo thaw time. Repeat the freeze thaw cycle. If the halo thaw time is less than one minute use a third freeze thaw cycle.

5-Fluorouracil. This drug is often the treatment of choice for actinic keratoses, as it destroys them adequately and gives the patient an excellent cosmetic result. At this time, it has little place in the treatment of skin cancer. The treatment is too time-consuming and messy, and yields an inadequate cure rate.

Mohs' Chemosurgery. This is a highly specialized method of excision of skin carcinoma with microscopic control. The technique has been used

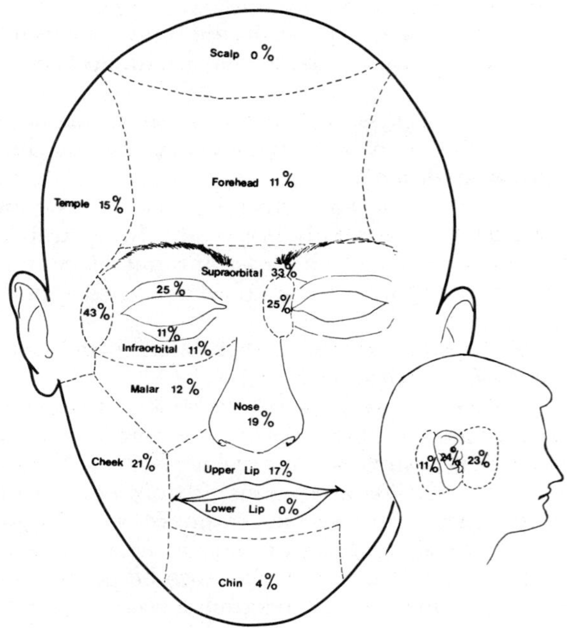

Figure 1. Percentage of recurrent lesions (out of 1168 treated basal cell carcinomas) on various areas of face. (From Shanoff et al.: Basal cell carcinoma. A statistical approach to rational management. Plast. Reconstr. Surg., *39*:619, 1967.)

Primary and recurrent basal–cell epitheliomas (BCE)	TOTAL (72)		PRIMARY (27)		RECURRENT BCE (45)	
	7.6 ± 4.5		5.5 ± 3.0		8.9 ± 4.8	
CASE HISTORY	1 year	2 years		3–5 Years	more than 5 Years	
	4.6 ± 2.3	6.3 ± 3.4		8.3 ± 3.4	8.9 ± 5.0	
LOCATION (Face)	LIPS	NOSE	CHEEK	EYE–NOSE–CHEEK–ANGLE	TEMPLE and SCALP	FOREHEAD
	4.8 ± 3.0	5.4 ± 2.5	8.1 ± 5.6	8.2 ± 2.2	9.5 ± 5.0	9.7 ± 5.0
DIAMETER (Clinically)	Less than 20 mm			More than 20 mm		
	6.2 ± 3.9			10.2 ± 4.2		
NUMBER OF PREVIOUS TREATMENTS	One previous treatment			More than one previous treatment		
	7.2 ± 3.5			9.4 ± 5.1		
KIND OF PREVIOUS TREATMENTS	Surgery			X–ray		
	8.2 ± 5.1			8.2 ± 4.9		
HISTOLOGY	Solid BCE			Morphea–like BCE		
	6.5 ± 3.8			9.3 ± 5.5		

Figure 2.   Subclinical extensions given in millimeters in primary and recurrent basal cell carcinomas. (From Gunter Burg et al.: Histographic surgery: accuracy of visual assessment of margins of basal cell epithelioma. Journal of Dermatologic Surgery and Oncology, *1*:3, 1975. Copyright 1975, The Journal of Dermatologic Surgery and Oncology, Inc.)

for 35 years by Frederic Mohs and has become widely accepted as the most accurate method for removal of skin carcinomas. The name chemosurgery is confusing. Thirty-five years ago when it was coined by Mohs this was not the case. He applied the chemical zinc chloride paste to fix the tissue in the patient much as formaldehyde would do after excision. The chemical fixative is now rarely used, but the name chemosurgery remains.

TECHNIQUE.   Following local anesthesia, the mass of the tumor is removed. Following this, a thin saucer-shaped piece of tissue encompassing the area involved by tumor is excised. A map is drawn corresponding exactly in size and shape to the patient's defect. The tissue is cut into 1 cm. pieces. The edges are color coded. Frozen sections are done on the undersurface of these 1 cm. pieces of tissue. These sections are then stained with toluidine blue or hematoxin and eosin. The sections are then examined beneath the microscope. Wherever the tumor is found, it is marked on the map and another layer of tissue is removed. This procedure is repeated until the patient is free of disease. Mohs' surgery cures 99 per cent of all basal cell carcinomas and 94 per cent of all squamous cell carcinomas. It cures 95 per cent of all recurrent basal cell carcinomas and 85 to 90 per cent of recurrent squamous cell carcinomas.

THE INDICATIONS FOR MOHS' SURGERY.   1. All recurrent basal and squamous cell carcinomas.

2. All primary lesions in the inner and outer canthus, nasolabial fold, the ear canal, and about scar tissue.

3. All aggressive skin carcinomas that have already shown their destructiveness by size and depth of invasion.

4. Primary lesions in areas in which cosmetic appearance is extremely important, for example, the tip of the nose. The least amount of normal tissue is removed by this method as the exact margins of tumor are known.

5. Sclerosing basal cell carcinomas and other tumors with indistinct margins.

A special note is necessary for squamous cell carcinomas, as these tumors occasionally metastasize. This is unusual for primary lesions of small size in the sun-exposed areas. It does occur with more aggressive tumors and tumors of the mucous membrane. Because of this, it is necessary that an adequate lymph node examination be performed on every patient with a squamous cell carcinoma. This should be repeated on each follow-up visit as clinically unapparent nodes may become positive. A lymph node dissection is done when palpable nodes are present.

CREEPING ERUPTION

method of
JOHN VAN DE ERVE, M.D.
Charleston, South Carolina

Larva migrans, caused by skin contact with animal droppings in warm moist soil at the time of larval hatching, is becoming a rare condition. This may be due to the widespread use of thiabendazole by veterinarians and pesticide spraying of land (fire ants, etc.). The condition is found mainly in the southern states, and is usually due to *Ancylostoma braziliense* and *caninum* from cats and dogs. The larva chews and tunnels through the skin, causing a remarkable amount of pruritus. The larva is usually about 1 cm. beyond the end of the visible burrow.

Prevention

Prevention is by covering sandboxes and by spreading a plastic dropcloth under cars or houses before working under them. Massive infestations of the past are rare now.

Topical Therapy

Wash and clean infested areas, opening pustules. Apply thiabendazole (Mintezol oral suspension) thickly on the areas and seal in with plastic film (Stretch and Seal Food Wrap) morning and night (this use of thiabendazole is not listed in the manufacturer's official directive). Even large areas can be covered in this way. Single burrows may be coated and sealed also, or the suspension may be coated over all areas 4 times daily without occlusion for a week or more if needed. Relief of the intense pruritus often occurs in 24 hours, and 3 to 4 days treatment is usually sufficient.

Systemic Therapy

Except in massive infestation this is rarely needed. Thiabendazole (Mintezol) in tablets or the marshmallowy oral suspension is given at 10 mg. per pound (22 mg. per kg.) of body weight twice daily for 3 days. Common side effects are nausea, dizziness, and stomach distress. Children tolerate it better than adults.

Other Measures

Parents or patients should be told that the worms do not multiply in the human skin and rarely penetrate the anal opening.

Diphenhydramine (Benadryl) or hydroxyzine (Atarax) will help control the itching. Severe itching may be relieved by ice cold wet compresses used as needed over topical thiabendazole. Antibiotics for secondary infection and topical erythromycin (Ilotycin) ointment help.

Older methods of "blistering" the larvae with liquid nitrogen or ethyl chloride are painful and effective in only a third of patients, and are not now recommended.

DECUBITUS ULCER

method of
WILLARD D. STECK, M.D.
Cleveland, Ohio

Decubitus ulcers occur in patients who remain too long in the same position. Pressure necrosis develops in areas where blood supply is easily compromised by prolonged weight bearing. These are the bony prominences of the sacrococcygeal and scapular areas, the heels, elbows, and scalps of patients who are chronically ill, comatose, paraplegic, or restricted from normal weight shifting by injuries or therapeutic requirements such as orthopedic traction. The lateral malleolar, trochlear, and trochanteric areas are subject to abnormal pressures that may lead to ulceration in certain physically and mentally ill patients who remain too long in a fetal position.

Decubitus ulcers will heal only if the pressure that caused them can be relieved. The ulcer that can be cured is one that probably could have been prevented, given adequate nursing care and medical supervision. The same pressure-relieving techniques necessary for successful treatment are effective as preventive measures.

Decubitus Ulcer Program

The program has two phases. Phase one is general skin care, carried to meticulous extremes. It should be invoked immediately upon identifying a patient at risk, and it will usually prevent the development of an ulcer. Phase two incorporates specific therapy for an ulcer that already exists. It operates in conjunction with phase one and cannot succeed independent of it.

Phase One: Minimizing the Effects of Pressure

1. The entire body must be searched daily for evidence of pressure damage. Either pallor or redness in any weight-bearing area should signal the need for special care.

2. Weight must be shifted frequently. The more difficult it is to move a patient from one position to another, the more necessary it is. A Turning Record should be established, with the shifting of weight recorded every 2 hours at a minimum.

3. No rubber or stiff plastic undersheets should be used. Mattresses may be protected by thin, soft plastic film under the regular, cotton sheet.

4. Weight dispersion devices may be useful but do not relieve the need for frequent shifting of weight. Sheepskins are helpful under the back and hips. Foam rubber heel boots and elbow pads are very helpful. Special foam mattresses, air mattresses, and water mattresses may be employed but may increase the effort required to turn the patient—still the most important step. A Stryker Frame or a Stryker Circ-o-Lectric bed may help solve the problem of weight shifting.

5. The skin should be kept clean and dry with as little irritation as possible. It is not necessary to use strong soap or germicidal detergents. When the skin tends to be too dry, as is generally the case, a bath oil is helpful. One teaspoonful of Alpha Keri bath oil in one or two quarts of lukewarm water for a bedbath will have ample cleansing effect without drying the skin. If some areas of skin are too wet, from excretory soilage or wound seepage, 1 teaspoon of povidone-iodine (Betadine) solution in 1 quart of water provides good cleansing and is drying. For skin areas that are moist from sweating, simple rubbing alcohol is good for cleansing and drying.

6. Skin that is subject to excretory soilage may be protected, to some degree, with films. Tincture of benzoin may be painted on clean, dry skin and dusted with talcum powder to relieve its tackiness. Its color, however, does tend to obscure an area that should be examined frequently. Skin Prep is a resinous substance that can be sprayed on the skin to leave a dry, transparent, protective film. It can be reapplied every day or so as necessary. Colored substances such as gentian violet and Castellani's paint should be avoided, because they interfere with close observation.

7. Impending or incipient ulceration, betrayed by erythema or exudation in weight-bearing areas, may be treated with paste dressings, as described in Phase Two.

Phase Two: Treating an Ulcer

1. Continue general skin care, inspection of all ulcer-prone areas, and all efforts to minimize the effects of pressure, as in Phase One.

2. Treat any apparent infection with appropriate systemic measures.

3. Cleanse the ulcer. Soap and water, povidone-iodine (Betadine) solution and water, Burow's solution, and many other agents may be used for soaks or wet dressings, but gravity limits their effectiveness, since most decubitus ulcers are in dependent positions. Hydrogen peroxide 3 per cent is probably easiest to use and as effective as any cleansing agent.

4. Surgically debride the ulcer of any grossly necrotic tissue. Exuding or suppurating wounds may be treated for a few days with dextranomer (Debrisan), a granular powder composed of dextran beads. When packed in a wound, these beads draw out fluids and tissue degradation products by intense capillary action. They can be removed and replaced in a wound several times a day until it appears to be clean. Debrisan is nontoxic and apparently nonallergenic (unlike some enzymatic debriding agents). It is quite effective but also quite expensive. Somewhat similar effects can be obtained with a paste of magnesium hydroxide-aluminum hydroxide (Maalox) that has been boiled to reduce its volume by about one half.

5. Treat the ulcer to prevent infection and to stimulate the formation of new granulation tissue. Benzoyl peroxide is best for this. This organic peroxide releases oxygen when in contact with tissue fluids. It is antibacterial, especially effective against anaerobic organisms, and is a powerful stimulant to fibroblasts, histiocytes, and endothelial cells, the elements of granulation tissue. It is commercially available in suitable lotion form as Benoxyl 10 per cent lotion. Benoxyl 20 per cent lotion is available in Canada and may work even better.

Cover the skin surrounding the ulcer with Norwegian cod liver oil, zinc oxide in a petrolatum base (Desitin) ointment, zinc oxide ointment, or petrolatum. Cut a piece of terry cloth (ordinary towelling) to fit exactly into the ulcer, including any undermined edges but not to overlap onto normal skin. Moisten the terry cloth with isotonic saline solution and then cover one side with the benzoyl peroxide lotion. Place the terry cloth in the ulcer with the Benoxyl in close contact with all ulcerated areas. Cover the area with a plastic sheet (Saran Wrap), which will adhere to the protective ointment on the skin edges. Then pad the dressing well with a soft overdressing such as an ABD pad. Change the benzoyl peroxide dressing every 8 hours, cleansing between dressings with hydrogen peroxide. If granulation tissue becomes exuberant to the degree that it rises above the surrounding skin, reduce it to that level with applications of silver nitrate. Continue treating the ulcerated area with benzoyl peroxide dressings just large enough to cover the granulating areas until the entire wound has reepithelialized. Continue all Phase One practices to prevent recurrence.

For the 3 to 5 per cent of patients who do not tolerate benzoyl peroxide for reasons of allergy or irritation, the ulcer may be treated with 10 per cent ichthammol in Lassar's paste. Lassar's paste contains 50 per cent particulate matter (equal parts of zinc oxide and starch) in petrolatum. It is absorptive and nonmacerating. With the ichthammol it has the color of putty and the consistency of peanut butter.

Spread the paste very liberally on several thicknesses of gauze sponge large enough to cover the ulcer and surrounding skin. Press the paste dressing into firm contact with the ulcerated areas. Use an ABD pad as an overdressing. Change the paste dressing daily. The paste is sticky and cannot be washed away with water. It can be removed easily by gently wiping with a gauze sponge soaked with mineral oil. After the ulcer has healed continue Phase One practices to prevent recurrence.

For the rare patient who does not tolerate ichthammol, which is a shale tar, Lassar's paste may be used by itself, following the steps outlined above.

CONTACT DERMATITIS

method of
DAVID E. PAYNE, M.D.
Columbia, Missouri

There are two kinds of contact dermatitis: primary irritant contact dermatitis and allergic contact dermatitis. It is necessary to differentiate between these, as the diagnosis affects both the prognosis of the patient and the type of treatment used.

Primary irritant contact dermatitis, for all practical purposes, is usually hand eczema. In this case there is considerable scaling, thickening, and cracking. Often, circular or nummular areas are on the backs of the hands and the anterior parts of the lower arms. The palms are often spared, but if the patient is a sweaty-palmed person, small, palmar vesicles will accompany this picture. The classic example of this diagnosis is dishpan hands.

Treatment, in this case, must be more conservative, because the assumption is the patient cannot totally avoid the conditions that cause the dermatitis. With this in mind, heavier superficial steroid preparations such as betamethasone (Valisone) or fluocinonide (Lidex) ointment are used for their maximum local effect without systemic steroid effect and for the extra protection given by the ointment base. Systemic steroids, such as 60 mg. of triamcinolone intramuscularly, should only be used to control severe discomfort because this is not a permissible long-term treatment. In very acute stages that involve some weeping eczematous changes, soaks in Burow's solution are helpful. One Domeboro tablet per pint of cool water for soaking, 20 minutes, twice daily, is very helpful.

Acute allergic dermatitis classically presents with a more acute eczematous change, including vesicles and considerable erythema and edema. Very often, bizarre configurations are present such as streaks of blisters with poison ivy or involvement of particular parts of skin such as upper eyelid dermatitis from eyeshadow.

Of prime importance is the identification of the allergenic substance, as treatment will be unsuccessful until it is removed. In identifying the allergen, the pattern of the dermatitis is the best clue, but three rules must be kept in mind.

First, a patient may become allergic to items to which they have been exposed for a long period of time. Therefore, the suspected substances include anything that fits the clinical pattern.

Second, allergic dermatitis represents a disproportionate response to the allergen. Therefore, agents must be considered that were given limited exposure to the patient. An example is make-up worn only on social occasions.

Third, there is classically a delay from 18 to 72 hours between exposure and full appearance of the rash. This explains the clinical observation of a case of poison ivy getting worse for 2 to 4 days following the exposure and must be kept in mind to identify the original cause.

With the agent identified, the treatment can be more vigorous than in the case of primary irritant dermatitis, with the assumption that this will be a self-limited episode and that the more severe symptoms can be treated adequately to control the patient's discomfort. Systemic steroids such as triamcinolone (Aristocort), 60 mg., intramuscularly, or prednisone (Deltasone Dosepak) are useful. Soaks, such as Domeboro's solution, are more useful than in chronic dermatitis for controlling the vesicular stage. The steroid preparations are better used with the creams rather than ointments to avoid occluding acutely weeping lesions.

A final category of contact dermatitis is photocontact dermatitis, which involves a combination of a contactant to the skin associated with sun exposure. There are two important clinical presentations of this. The first is a very widespread photocontact dermatitis that is associated with antibacterial soaps containing salicylanilides. The second is photocontact dermatitis in areas of applications of perfumes containing oil of bergamot. In addition to the treatment of these two conditions as described for allergic contact dermatitis, it is also necessary to protect the patient for a period of time with sunscreens to avoid further activation of the rash even after the contactant is removed. In addition, photocontact dermatitis from perfumes very often leaves a disproportionate amount of postinflammatory pigmentation that is distressing to the patient but always clears in time.

DERMATITIS HERPETIFORMIS
(Duhring's Disease)

method of
WILLIAM J. SAHL, JR., M.D.
Oklahoma City, Oklahoma

Introduction

Dermatitis herpetiformis is a disease of the skin, often the gastrointestinal tract and, rarely, the mucous membranes. Skin lesions tend to be symmetrical and polymorphic, i.e., urticarial, vesicular, bullous, erythematous, papular, and pustular. They typically elicit an intense burning, itching, and stinging sensation that drives the patient to fierce excoriation.

Areas of predilection are the scalp, scapulae, sacrum, elbows, knees, and flanks. Here one finds deep excoriations, scars, and postinflammatory hyperpigmentation, but rarely the typical grouped primary lesions.

Approximately two thirds of these patients also have a gluten-sensitive enteropathy. Those with both skin and gut pathology share the HL-A8 histocompatibility locus. Typical lesions may occur in the mouth, but are rare.

Routine diagnostic procedures should include biopsy of a primary lesion if possible. Also helpful, if available, is direct immunofluorescence to demonstrate IgA and complement at the dermal-epidermal junction. Intestinal biopsy is rarely needed for diagnosis. A favorable and rapid response to a therapeutic trial of sulfapyridine or dapsone (Avlosulfon) favors a diagnosis of dermatitis herpetiformis. (This use of dapsone is not listed in the manufacturer's official directive.)

Treatment

Dermatitis herpetiformis lasts for years and follows a natural course of remissions and exacerbations. The goal of therapy is to suppress the skin lesions and to relieve the symptoms of pruritus and diarrhea.

I begin treatment using dapsone (Avlosulfon) and dietary restrictions.

Dapsone (Avlosulfon). Dapsone is commonly used to treat dermatitis herpetiformis in spite of the fact that, officially, dermatitis herpetiformis is still not listed as an indication for treatment with dapsone by the manufacturer. Reports also show that dapsone can cause cancer in a certain species of male (not female) laboratory animals. Despite these problems, dapsone is frequently favored in the treatment of dermatitis herpetiformis. Before therapy with dapsone, the physician should obtain a white blood count and hematocrit and red cell morphology (searching for Heinz bodies), as well as liver function tests. Glucose-6-PD-deficient cells produce large numbers of Heinz bodies. If either sulfapyridine or dapsone (Avlosulfon) are given to a G-6-PD-deficient patient, a hemolytic crisis may be precipitated. Other possible side effects include aplastic anemia, agranulocytosis, methemoglobinemia, peripheral neuropathy, and hepatic and renal damage, as well as headache, gastrointestinal upset, and skin rash. Caution should be exercised when giving dapsone with other drugs, especially probenecid (because of competition for excretion).

Usually treatment is begun with 200 mg. (two 100 mg. tabs) of dapsone per day. Symptomatic relief of itching and reduction of lesions are noted within 2 days. Reduction to the maintenance dose is accomplished in 1 to 2 weeks. Usually 25 to 75 mg. (25 mg. tablets) daily is required. Follow-ups every 2 to 4 weeks with a complete blood count and methemoglobin level should continue throughout therapy.

Sulfapyridine. This drug may be used as an alternative to dapsone (Avlosulfon). It is more expensive and treatment is accompanied by crystalluria. Therapy is begun with 2 to 6 grams daily (0.5 gram tabs). After 2 to 3 weeks, a maintenance dosage of 0.5 to 2 grams is achieved. Patients should be advised to increase oral fluids to prevent crystalluria when taking sulfapyridine.

Halogens. Both iodides and bromides should be avoided, since exacerbations of dermatitis herpetiformis have been associated with ingestion of these halogens.

Diet. If a gluten-sensitive enteropathy is present with dermatitis herpetiformis, gluten-containing foods should be eliminated from the diet. The dietary restriction should be continued for at least 14 months. Occasionally, both gastrointestinal and cutaneous involvement may be controlled with dietary restriction alone. A list of gluten-free foods may be obtained from: CPC International Corp., Best Foods Research Center, Union, N.J. 07083.

Lymphoma. Dermatitis herpetiformis and lymphoma may occur concurrently, and therapy for lymphoma may improve the dermatitis. A careful search for lymphoma should be pursued in the older patient with dermatitis herpetiformis.

ATOPIC DERMATITIS

method of
PAUL S. PORTER, M.D.
Pittsburgh, Pennsylvania

Atopic dermatitis is a genetically determined disorder of the skin associated with an increased ability to form IgE (reagin), decreased cell-mediated immune response, and decreased chemotactic abilities of the neutrophil during periods of generalized infection.

Therapy for the disease is largely determined by two factors: the age of the patient and the stage of the disease. Acute, subacute, and chronic forms of atopic dermatitis occur and may occur intermittently in the same patient. In general, fluorinated, topical, and systemic steroids should be avoided in the prepubertal patient.

There is no scientific evidence that dietary factors are causative in this disease. There is also good scientific evidence that the immediate humoral and T cell type allergic responses that may be elicited by intradermal or scratch testing play no role in the pathogenesis of the disease. Numerous positive skin tests of the wheal and flare type are, however, a characteristic of the patient with atopic dermatitis. Individual cases in specific situations (e.g., season flares) do respond to desensitization.

Therapy for the acute stage of the disorder, which is characterized by weeping lesions that are often secondarily infected with staphylococcus or streptococcus or both, should consist of rest, antipruritic systemic therapy such as hydroxyzine hydrochloride (Vistaril) or cyproheptadine hydrochloride (Periactin) or both, bland wet dressings that are antiseptic such as Domeboro solution, frequent application of hydrocortisone lotion (e.g., Nutracort lotion) to which can be added topical antibiotics such as erythromycin, chloramphenicol (Chloromycetin) or clindamycin (Cleocin); short courses of systemic antibiotics such as erythromycin can also be used, infrequent bathing with a mild soap, e.g., Lubriderm soap with a bath oil added, e.g., Nutraspa, particularly in the winter months. Humidifiers are also ameliorating in winter.

The subacute phase of the disease requires the elimination of wet dressings; continuation of frequent applications of topical steroids having cream bases is indicated, with or without added antibiotics, depending on the presence of secondary infection. At this stage of the disease, various forms of coal tar may be introduced such as Cutar Bath Oil, bland soaps should be continued, and patients may begin to resume near normal activities.

The chronic stage of atopic eczema is by far the most difficult therapeutically. Long-term use of topical steroids results in tachyphylaxis, which is characterized by a diminishing therapeutic efficacy of the topical steroid. Alternating topical steroids with topical tar therapy, e.g., Estar gel, is a practical solution to the problem of tachyphylaxis. Occlusive-dressing techniques utilizing fluorinated steroid ointment such as triamcinolone acetonide (Aristocort) ointment covered with plastic of a suitable type can be used intermittently on localized areas of the disorder in the chronic

phase, particularly when lichenification occurs. Tars should not be used with occlusive-dressing techniques. Bland soaps and bath oil are to be continued in this phase. Salicylic acid can also be added to topical creams, e.g., 3 per cent salicylic acid in triamcinolone acetonide (Aristocort) cream, for frequent use during the daylight working hours when occlusive-dressing techniques are impractical. Short courses of low-dose oral prednisone can be used in the healthy adult without side effects. Systemic steroids should not be given daily for longer than 10 days; the dose of prednisone can vary from 20 to 40 mg. per day.

In general, all cutaneous irritants should be avoided during all phases of the disease. These include deodorant soaps, wool clothing, excessive bathing, lower humidity, and excessive overheating in addition to exposure to irritating chemicals such as detergents, turpentine, grease, and industrial oils. The patient should avoid exposure to other persons with herpes simplex infection and those that have been vaccinated; because of diminished immune response, Kaposi's varicelliform eruption can occur and become a serious complication in a patient with atopic dermatitis.

Patient and parent education is essential in this disorder, as guilt feelings are often part of the parental side of the relationship, and passive-aggressive behavior often develops in the child. Booklets are often helpful; however, there is no substitute for good medical counseling in the family constellation.

Several manifestations of atopic dermatitis require careful differential diagnosis; atopic dermatitis of the hands and feet can be confused with contact dermatitis or fungal infection. The distribution of the lesions often rules out contact dermatitis; fungal culture and examination of the scales from the diseased area in potassium hydroxide solution under the microscope should rule out fungal infection. Chronic atopic dermatitis of the scalp can be confused with either seborrhea or psoriasis; however, thorough examination of the entire integument, and a detailed medical history should differentiate these disorders. In the hairy areas of the adult, a steroid lotion such as fluocinolone acetonide (Synalar) solution or a keratolytic lotion such as phenol, paraffin oil and water (Baker's "P & S") should be used with a daily shampoo with a keratolytic shampoo, e.g., zinc pyrithione (Zincon).

Atopic dermatitis is often attributed to nerves and is referred to as neurodermatitis; in its present usage this is a misnomer. Emotional stress and anxiety can make disease control more difficult and can result in a very specific form of atopic dermatitis, which is more specifically designated lichen simplex chronicus. This form of the disorder is often aggravated by the vicious itch-scratch cycle, which can be broken using the methods described for therapy of the chronic phase.

Another complication is prurigo nodularis. These pruritic, sometimes tender, and often infected nodules frequently require intralesional therapy with long-acting depository forms of intralesional steroids. A concentration of 4 mg. per ml. of intralesional steroids, e.g., triamcinolone hexacetonide (Aristospan) mixed with lidocaine, should not be exceeded, as the danger of steroid atrophy of the skin at higher concentrations is great.

Hay fever, asthma, drug sensitivity, migraine headaches, acute urticaria, vitiligo, and alopecia areata are also said to be more common in the patient with atopic dermatitis, and the index of suspicion of these complications should be high. Rarely, keratoconjunctivitis can occur in the atopic and if untreated leads to blindness. Atopic cataracts are seen in 10 per cent of those with atopic dermatitis and are not due to steroid therapy. Ocular disease is best managed by an ophthalmologist.

In summary, patient education and the avoidance of irritants and other factors, as well as good hydration of the skin, are the best therapies as the morbidity from the disease can thus be considerably reduced.

NEURODERMATITIS

method of
RICHARD D. BAUGHMAN, M.D.
Hanover, New Hampshire

Neurodermatitis is a term that should always be modified by an adjective — localized or generalized. The localized form is now better classified as lichen simplex chronicus, discussed here, while the generalized neurodermatitis is better referred to as atopic dermatitis (see p. 584). The initial derivation of the term neurodermatitis was appropriate, because it emphasized the peripheral neurovascular abnormalities that characterize the person with atopic dermatitis. However, today the term "neuro" carries a psychosomatic implication which may not be scientifically supportable or therapeutically in the patient's best interest.

Lichen simplex chronicus is the localized expression of the itch-scratch cycle, consisting of individual or confluent lichenoid, papules grouped into thickened plaques with exaggeration of the normal skin markings. The surface is rough, with variable amounts of redness and scale. The process often occurs in persons with the atopic diathesis. It may occur on any part of the body. Common areas include periorbital, anogenital, nuchal, and ankles. Histopathologically, the findings are those of chronic eczematous inflammation with spongiosis and thickening of all layers of the epidermis. Peripheral nerve trunks may show hypertrophy.

Lichen simplex may be superimposed on a variety of processes such as allergic or irritant contact dermatitis, psoriasis, or atopic dermatitis. The diagnostic signs of the initiating dermatosis may be obscured by the lichen simplex or may have long since disappeared. Prurigo nodularis is an extreme expression of lichen simplex with an intense focal proliferative process.

Treatment

The recognition of the itch-scratch cycle by physician and patient is essential, i.e., the itchy eruption produced by chronic frictional trauma is perpetuated by the scratching. "Internal causes of pruritus" should be sought as appropriate in each patient. It is useless to say simply "don't scratch," when the effort must be coupled with breaking the itch by recognition of any specific underlying dermatosis and topical, systemic or physical antipruritic measures at the same time.

Diagnostic measures may include scrapings for tinea, biopsy to rule out other dermatoses, and patch tests to rule out a concomitant allergic contact dermatitis.

Antihistamines probably work more because of sedation than specific interference with histamine as a chemical mediator. Within the limitations of drowsiness and other side effects of antihistamines, hydroxyzine (Atarax), 10 to 25 mg., cyproheptadine (Periactin) or chlorpheniramine, 4 mg. every 4 to 6 hours, are indicated. It is important to remember that itch, like pain, is better *prevented* by regular administration than treated episodically once the cycle is reestablished. Barbiturates and "tranquilizers" are less effective than antihistamines.

Topical corticosteroids, such as fluocinolone (Synalar) or betamethasone valerate (Valisone), in a cream base should be applied at least 3 times daily. Occlusion with a plastic film such as Saran Wrap, usually at bedtime, enhances penetration and provides protection. The cream base is preferred to the newer gels, which often sting. It must be emphasized that prolonged corticosteroids should be avoided in acne areas, especially in young women.

If topical corticosteroid fails, intralesional injection of triamcinolone acetonide (Kenalog), 2.5 mg. per ml. through a #30 needle or pressure injector (Dermajet), is useful. Atrophy, infection, and syncope can be problems with intralesional therapy. Systemic corticosteroids are rarely indicated unless all other measures fail and the process is debilitating.

Physical modalities such as ultraviolet light and Grenz rays may be employed in the most resistant cases. Lichen simplex chronicus is probably the disorder best suited for Grenz rays if ionizing radiation is to be used in "benign disease," because often as few as 3 treatments of 200 R each will break the itch-scratch cycle in resistant cases.

Topical anesthetics (benzocaine) and topical antihistamines (diephenhydramine, triplennamine) are to be condemned as ineffective and likely to perpetuate the process by inducing allergic contact dermatitis.

POISON IVY DERMATITIS

method of
ALEXANDER A. FISHER, M.D.
Woodside, New York

General Prophylaxis of Rhus Dermatitis

Patients should be taught to recognize and avoid the poison ivy group of plants. When a poison rhus plant is present in the garden or cannot be avoided, its chemical destruction or physical removal is indicated. Farmer's Bulletin No. 2158 Chemical Control of Brush and Trees, issued by the United States Department of Agriculture, should be consulted for information on specific chemicals for destroying poison ivy or poison oak.

Unfortunately, no topical measure is effective in the prevention of poison ivy dermatitis. Barrier creams and chelating, detoxicating, and oxidizing agents are of no value. All persons exposed to these plants should thoroughly wash the entire body with ordinary soap and water. Complete change of clothing is also advisable, and, whenever possible, contaminated clothing should be washed with soap and water.

The poison ivy antigen enters the skin so rapidly that the oil must be totally removed within 10 minutes of exposure. When such early washing is not feasible, however, it is worthwhile to wash at the first opportunity to remove any oleoresin remaining on the skin and thereby prevent it being transferred to other parts of the body.

Management of Mild Poison Ivy Dermatitis

Mild poison ivy dermatitis usually consists of papules and vesicles, often in linear streaks. Treatment with an antipruritic "shake" lotion, such as one consisting of 1 per cent menthol in equal parts of alcohol and calamine lotion is often sufficient. Corticosteroid sprays may be effective.

Topical preparations containing benzocaine, zirconium, or antihistaminics should be avoided, because these substances are notorious sensitizers. Preparations containing iron salts should also be avoided because they can produce a permanent tattoo. Most steroid creams and ointments are not very effective in poison ivy dermatitis. However, a combination of a topical corticosteroid and lidocaine may be quite soothing. Some patients find that either very cold or moderately hot water gives temporary relief from the pruritus. Antihistamines may be given orally, but never topically.

Baths or showers, with a bland soap, are permitted in mild poison ivy dermatitis.

Management of Moderately Severe Poison Ivy Dermatitis

In this stage, in addition to papules, vesicles, and bullae, edematous swellings of various parts of the body may be present. Large vesicles or bullae should be opened under sterile conditions and with preservation of the roof of the lesion if possible. Cool compresses of Burow's solution (1:10) may be applied to edematous areas. Edema of the eyelids can be treated with wet dressings of cold boric acid.

On the face, lotions should usually be avoided in acute allergic dermatitis, because they tend to cake, making the skin uncomfortably stiff. Application of wet dressings followed by zinc oxide ointment or petrolatum are better tolerated. Men with facial involvement should be allowed to shave, because the trauma of shaving causes less discomfort and irritation than does the accumulation of crusts and debris in the beard.

Baths with potassium permanganate are valuable, after vesicles or bullae are opened, for their quick-drying effect and when there is the possibility of secondary infection. One teaspoonful of potassium permanganate crystals is dissolved in a tube of lukewarm water. The patient may sit in the tub from 15 to 20 minutes. In the absence of infection, a bath with a cupful of plain colloidal oatmeal (Aveeno) to a tub of water is also cleansing and soothing.

For antipruritic and sedative effects, antihistamines may be given before retiring to help ensure a good night's sleep.

Management of Severe Poison Ivy Dermatitis

This stage is characterized by widespread involvement and marked edema of the extremities and the face. Often the eyelids are so swollen that they cannot be opened. Any male with edema of the prepuce, even if there is no severe involvement elsewhere, should be given systemic corticosteroids. Systemic corticosteroid therapy is dramatically beneficial, provided there are no contraindications. Topical therapy is similar to that given for moderately severe cases.

Schedule of Corticosteroid Therapy for Severe Poison Ivy Dermatitis. 1. First and second days: Two 5 mg. prednisone tablets or the equivalent every 4 hours for five doses.

2. Third and fourth days: Two tablets (5 mg.) every 4 hours for four doses.

3. Fifth and sixth days: Two tablets (5 mg.) every 5 hours for three doses.

4. Seventh, eighth, ninth, and tenth days: One tablet (5 mg.) four times daily.

5. Eleventh, twelfth, thirteenth, and fourteenth days: One tablet (5 mg.) three times daily.

6. Fifteenth to twenty-first days: One tablet (5 mg.) twice daily. (In children, the doses are proportionately reduced.)

The corticosteroid therapy is spread over a 3 week period. In many patients who receive this therapy for a few days, the poison ivy dermatitis seems to be under control. If the therapy is stopped at this time, the patient often has a rebound reaction with return of the dermatitis to its original intensity. Such a reaction is prevented by gradually tapering off the steroid dosage over a 3 week period.

Occasionally, the patient is suffering so much when first seen that the physician may give an initial intramuscular injection of 40 mg. of triamcinolone (Aristocort or Kenalog) suspension or the equivalent of a more quickly acting corticosteroid such as betamethasone (Celestone solution).

SEBORRHEIC DERMATITIS

method of
C. H. WINGERT, JR., M.D.
State College, Pennsylvania

Seborrheic dermatitis is characterized by erythematous scaling patches. The borders of the patches are indistinct and the scale is oily and slightly yellow. The cause is not known, but apparently is associated with activation of the sebaceous glands at puberty and in infants still under the hormone influence of the mother.

The disease occurs most frequently on the scalp and face but can involve the axilla, groin, perianal region, and can, on rare occasions, become generalized. It is estimated that seborrheic dermatitis occurs in up to one third of the population of the United States.

Seborrheic dermatitis may be associated with Parkinson's disease, mental deficiency, diabetes, and obesity.

It is frequently complicated by secondary bacterial and *Candida* infections. It is associated at times with other skin diseases such as severe acne, acne rosacea, and psoriasis.

Treatment

The treatment of seborrheic dermatitis depends on the location and severity. It can range from a very mild scaling eruption to an extensive generalized exudative acute dermatitis. It must be carefully explained to the patient that the disease can be readily controlled but not cured.

Scalp

For mild involvement of the scalp, frequent shampooing with commercial shampoos such as Head and Shoulders, Sebulex, or Zincon is usually effective. These shampoos can be used daily if necessary for control. For more severe involvement, the use of shampoos containing selenium sulfide such as Selsun shampoo is effective. These shampoos work best when applied to the scalp for several minutes, then washed out completely. The patient must be instructed to rub in the shampoo and loosen the scale, then wait five minutes before rinsing well. Failures occur when the patient washes the hair but does not treat the scalp. Shampoos such as Selsun should be used initially no more than twice weekly, then, after control is obtained, the frequency decreased to weekly or even every other week to maintain control. If this type of shampoo is used too frequently, the hair will become excessively oily.

If there is considerable scaling, a preparation such as cetyl trimethyl ammonium bromide and stearyl dimethyl benzyl ammonium chloride (Scadan) is helpful if applied to the wet scalp after the shampoo. Fluocinolone acetonide (Synalar) solution or halcinonide (Halog) solution are very helpful for control of the erythema and pruritus if 2 to 3 drops are applied and rubbed in well daily.

Face

The involvement is usually in the eyebrows and nasolabial folds but may occur in the cheeks and chin. The eyelid margins are commonly involved. Acne rosacea and lupus erythematosus are the two most common entities that must be differentiated from seborrheic dermatitis. This differentiation is usually by clinical appearance, distribution, and areas of involvement with typical seborrheic dermatitis.

A preparation containing 15 grams of cetyl alcohol–coal tar distillate, sulfar, and salicylic acid in oil-water emulsion (Pragmatar) cream mixed with 15 grams of betamethasone valerate 0.1 per cent cream (Valisone), applied twice daily is very effective. This mixture should be used only for short periods because of the possibility of producing a rosacea-like syndrome, telangiectasia, and atrophy with chronic use. If the seborrhea is mild, hydrocortisone 1 per cent cream or desonide cream (Tridesilon) is reasonably effective.

Occasionally, especially in the nasolabial folds and perioral region, secondary bacterial infection occurs that is manifested by small pustules, erythema, and scaling. When this occurs, tetracycline, 250 mg. orally two times daily for one month, is helpful.

Intertriginous Areas (Including Posterior Auricular, External Ear Canals, Axilla, Inframammary Region, and Groin)

The area surrounding the ears and the external ear canals are the most commonly involved areas in this group. A good treatment is a mixture of 10 grams of Pragmatar cream and 5 grams of triamcinolone acetonide (Aristocort-A) 0.5 per cent cream. This should be rubbed in well twice daily until control is obtained and then discontinued until the next flare occurs. Between flares desonide cream (Tridesilon) can be applied 2 times daily to help maintain remission. Occasionally, secondary bacterial infection occurs that should be treated with systemic antibiotics.

In intertriginous areas the seborrheic dermatitis can occur as mild erythema and scaling up to a very acute weeping dermatitis. If weeping occurs Burow's solution (Domeboro soaks—1 powder packet to 1 pint of water) is used 20 minutes two to three times daily. A mixture of 15 grams of iodochlorhydroxyquin (Vioform) cream and 15 grams of betamethasone valerate (Valisone) 0.1 per cent cream applied two to three times daily until control occurs is helpful. This preparation should not be used continually in these areas because of the possibility of producing striae.

Occasionally intertriginous seborrheic dermatitis is complicated by secondary bacterial and *Candida* infections. This is manifested by weeping, pustules, tenderness, and regional lymphadenopathy. Cultures should be taken for both bacteria and *Candida* and then appropriate treatment initiated. If a bacterial infection is present, systemic antibiotics are indicated. If a *Candida* infection is present, a topical nystatin-containing preparation such as nystatin, neomycin sulfate, gramicidin with triamcinolone acetonide (Mycolog) cream is useful. Be aware of the possibility of a contact dermatitis from either the neomycin or ethylenediamine contained in Mycolog cream. A preparation that is also effective is a mixture of 15 grams of miconazole nitrate (Mica-Tin) 2 per cent cream and 15 grams of desonide (Tridesilon) cream. This should be applied spar-

ingly two times daily for at least 2 weeks after complete clearing occurs.

Occasionally, seborrheic dermatitis becomes generalized and acute and a short burst of steroid administration is indicated. Prednisone is started at 60 mg. daily until reasonable clearing occurs then decreased by 5 mg. every other day.

STASIS DERMATITIS AND STASIS ULCERS

method of
HENRY H. ROENIGK, JR., M.D.
Chicago, Illinois

General Principles of Management

Stasis dermatitis develops in an extremity because of interference with the return of venous blood flow with resultant edema and extravasation of serum and cells into the surrounding tissue. Minor trauma to an edematous leg usually leads to stasis ulceration that often becomes secondarily infected. Moreover, the patient's neglect of the lesions or indifference to them may delay effective treatment and the many proprietary preparations that may be applied to the leg before he seeks professional help may complicate it.

Bed rest with the affected leg elevated will usually produce rapid disappearance of edema. Diuretics such as hydrochlorothiazide (HydroDiuril), 50 mg. twice daily, may help, especially when it is necessary for the patient to be ambulatory. A 3 to 4 inch Ace elastic bandage should be applied when the patient is not at bed rest, to prevent recurrences of edema.

Acute Stasis Dermatitis

The weeping acute dermatitis superimposed on stasis dermatitis is best treated with bed rest and wet compresses. The compresses should be changed every 2 to 3 hours. Never enclose the wet dressing in a plastic sheet because this leads to maceration of tissue and prevents evaporation of the compress solution. Evaporation of the solution helps the healing process. The following solutions are suggested for compresses: (1) aluminum acetate (Burow's solution) 0.5 per cent, (2) isotonic saline solution 0.9 per cent, (3) potassium permanganate solution 1:10,000 in saline, or (4) acetic acid solution 1 per cent.

Between compresses a drying anti-inflammatory lotion or cream containing a topical corticosteroid such as fluocinolone (Synalar cream) 0.025 per cent, betamethasone (Valisone) cream 0.1 per cent, or triamcinolone (Kenalog cream) 0.025 per cent will have a further drying effect on the acute dermatitis.

Subacute Stasis Dermatitis

When the acute phase of the dermatitis has subsided and the patient becomes more ambulatory, recurrence of edema after prolonged standing must be prevented. If this is not done, the acute dermatitis will promptly recur. The use of a modified Unna paste dressing is ideal in this situation. A commercially prepared Unna boot is Dome-Paste bandage. These flesh-colored roll bandages are impregnated with a uniformly spread paste of zinc oxide, calamine, glycerin, and gelatin. Unna boots also contain a mixture of bacteriostatic hexachlorophene and dichlorophene. They are available in 3 or 4 inch wide rolls.

The leg is elevated and cleansed of any debris or previous medication with tepid water or mineral oil. Any of the following topical medications may be applied to the leg: (1) Terramycin, oxytetracycline and hydrocortisone (Terra-Cortril) ointment, (2) fluocinolone acetonide (Synalar) cream or ointment 0.025 per cent (or any other topical corticosteroid preparation), (3) topical antibiotics alone, such as ointments containing polymyxin B, bacitracin, and neomycin (Polysporin, Neosporin).

The modified Unna boot is applied from behind the first metatarsal to just below the popliteal space. The foot should be kept at a right angle to minimize chafing. Make a circular turn with the bandage around the foot, and direct the bandage obliquely over the heel. Repeat until the leg has been adequately covered as with the Unna boot. The bandage is then cut to ensure a flat surface. The first layers of the Unna boot should be snug. The bandage roll should be cut at each turn, gauze being brought in an upward manner to lock in place and to ensure a contoured fit with proper support. The boot should be applied in a "pressure gradient manner"; that is, the greatest pressure should be applied at the ankle and lower third of the leg with progressively diminishing pressure over the upper two thirds of the leg. At no time is the bandage given any reverse turns because the ridges thus turned could cause discomfort as the bandage hardens. Care should be taken not to apply the dressing too loosely or too tightly on the patient's leg. Each turn should overlap the preceding turn, covering the leg about two or three times. A double layer of Tubegauze is placed over the Unna boot and secured at the upper and lower limits with tape. Do not place the tape directly on the skin. The dressing is usually changed at weekly intervals unless there is drainage from the ulcer, which may necessitate a new Unna boot every 3 to 5 days.

Chronic Stasis Dermatitis

After the acute and subacute stages have subsided, the treatment of stasis dermatitis must be continued. The physician must impress the patient with the fact that because he has a problem of venous stasis, continuous supportive measures will be necessary to prevent recurrences of acute dermatitis. Elastic bandages and proprietary elastic stockings are usually not satisfactory for most patients. Individually measured "pressure-gradient" supportive stockings such as the Jobst stocking (Jobst Institute, Box 653, Toledo, Ohio 43601) are preferred. Jobst stocking measurements should be made only after all edema has subsided. The patient should put the supportive stockings on the legs before arising and remove the stockings when he is ready to retire. In general, patients are encouraged to walk without restriction. The following lubricant may be applied to the legs at bedtime; phenol 1 per cent, menthol 0.25 per cent, cocoa butter 5 per cent in ungua aqua rose to make 120 grams.

It is often necessary for the patient to purchase new Jobst stockings every 4 or 5 months because they become stretched and lose their effectiveness in preventing edema.

Because of lichenification and "habit scratching," an associated neurodermatitis of the legs may develop. If this occurs, the application of fluocinolone acetonide (Synalar) or flurandrenolone (Cordran) cream 0.025 per cent under Saran Wrap at bedtime will be helpful. Intralesional injections of triamcinolone acetonide (Kenalog-10 Injection) suspension (10 mg. per ml.) into localized neurodermites may bring more prompt relief of the pruritus.

Complications of Stasis Dermatitis

Bacterial Infections. 1. Tepid compresses, as mentioned previously, facilitate removal of pyogenic crusts.

2. Culture of the organisms and tests of antibiotic sensitivity of any open drainage should be done before administering antibiotic therapy.

3. Topical antibiotic ointments or sprays may be used between compresses.

4. If cellulitis, lymphangitis, regional adenopathy, or septicemia develops, systemic antibiotic therapy is indicated. The choice of antibiotic should be dictated by results of cultures and sensitivity tests.

5. Systemic antibiotics are often not necessary for ulcers that do not have associated cellulitis or lymphangitis. Cultures of ulcers often show organisms in which systemic antibiotic therapy in-

volves significant risk of systemic toxicity. Local therapy will often remove the bacteria and exudate.

Stasis Ulcers

Stasis ulcers often follow minor trauma to a region of chronic stasis dermatitis. Neglect on the part of the patient often results in infection and extension of the ulcer. The general principles of management of stasis ulcers are the same as for stasis dermatitis.

General measures will include clearing the surrounding skin (stasis eczema) with compresses, topical corticosteroids, and occasionally topical antibiotics. Bed rest and reduction of edema will speed up healing in all types of ulcers.

1. Local treatment of the ulcer is important in clearing the infection and stimulating granulation tissue that can accept either a skin graft or epithelial regrowth from the borders of the ulcer. Debridement of the ulcer may be done with enzymes and other chemicals. Another excellent method of local debridement is the use of a small sharp curette after topical application of viscous lidocaine (Xylocaine). Curettement will remove the moist eschar that frequently inhibits reepithelialization.

2. If there is considerable secondary infection, the ulcer should not be occluded. Bed rest and continuous compresses, as mentioned previously, should be applied until the infection subsides.

3. Benzoyl peroxide, a potent oxidizing agent widely used in the treatment of acne vulgaris, can promote granulation tissue in ulcers.

The method of application of the 20 per cent benzoyl peroxide lotion involves cutting terrycloth in the exact shape of the ulcer, moistened with isotonic saline solution, impregnated with benzoyl peroxide lotion (20 per cent) and then applied to the ulcer. The normal skin margins of the ulcer are protected with petroleum jelly, and the padded ulcer is then occluded with plastic film. The dressings are changed every 8 to 12 hours. Excessive granulation tissue at epithelial borders may be cauterized with 10 per cent silver nitrate solution.

The mechanisms of action of benzoyl peroxide are probably multifold, consisting of: (1) bactericidal, (2) granulation tissue stimulation, (3) hyperbaric oxygen production, and (4) debridement.

4. Dextran polymer beads (Debrisan) are a new medication for cleansing infected ulcers. The treatment consists of applying a thick layer of small, porous beads, 0.1 to 0.3 mm. in diameter, composed of a three dimensional network of dextran polymer (DPBs), to the ulcer. The DPBs are highly hydrophilic and in the presence of a water-containing fluid they absorb the fluid until saturated, swelling in the process. When placed on a discharging ulcer surface DPBs promptly absorb the exudate, bacteria, and tissue degradation residues from the ulcer surface. The DPBs are pharmacologically inert and their action is entirely physical.

5. The following preparations may be applied to a clean ulcer to encourage reepithelialization: (1) gentian violet solution 3 per cent, (2) Castellani's paint, (3) brilliant green solution, (4) gold foil (six to eight layers of autoclaved 23 K XX deep gold leaf, obtained at a paint or art supply store; the ulcer is first cleansed with ethyl alcohol).

6. Topical antibiotic ointment or corticosteroid ointment is applied to the surrounding stasis dermatitis.

7. An Unna boot is then applied from the base of the toes to just below the popliteal space and covered with a double layer of Tubegauze.

8. The patient is encouraged to be ambulatory, but is told to report any persistent pain, swelling, or discoloration of the toes.

9. The dressing is changed every 3 to 7 days until the ulcer has healed. If serous drainage seeps through the Unna boot, the dressing should be changed.

10. A pressure-gradient Jobst stocking should be worn after the ulcer has healed.

11. Large ulcers, or smaller ulcers that fail to respond to conservative therapy because of poor surrounding tissue should be referred to a plastic surgeon for split-thickness skin grafting.

DERMATOMYOSITIS-POLYMYOSITIS

method of
KENNETH E. GREER, M.D.
Charlottesville, Virginia

Polymyositis is an inflammatory disease of striated muscle that is characterized by symmetrical, proximal muscle weakness, fairly characteristic muscle biopsy and electromyographic changes, and an elevation of muscle enzymes in the serum (especially creatine phosphokinase but also serum glutamic oxalacetic transaminase and aldolase). The disorder is called dermatomyositis when the muscle changes are associated with the typical skin lesions, which include a dusky erythematous eruption on the face (including the heliotrope around the eyes), erythematous, scaly or scarred lesions over the extensor surfaces of the joints, and dilatation of the capillaries of the proximal nailfolds.

The disorder can begin in childhood, but occurs most frequently in adults.

After defining the disorder in a fairly simple fashion, as has been done here, the confusion begins. There is controversy with respect to pathogenesis (although it seems most likely that the myopathy is mediated through hypersensitivity mechanisms), classification (especially of polymyositis), criteria for diagnosis, and treatment. Although there is no statistical evidence to support it, there does seem to be an association of this disease with internal malignancy (predominantly the stomach and ovary), almost exclusively in patients over 40 years of age.

Treatment

The type of and the response to therapy vary with (a) the age of patient at onset, (b) how soon therapy is begun in the course of the disease, (c) the acuteness or severity of the onset, and (d) whether or not the disease is associated with an internal malignancy. The symptoms appear to resolve more quickly when therapy is begun early in the course of the disease. Children may have a lower mortality than adults, but the morbidity, especially with severe muscle wasting, contractures, and calcinosis cutis, may be severe.

Glucocorticoids (prednisone preferably), either alone or in conjunction with immunosuppressive or cytotoxic drugs (such as methotrexate, cyclophosphamide and azathioprine) provide effective control but not cure in a significant percentage of patients. However, the natural history of polymyositis-dermatomyositis is not well defined, and there have been no real prospective controlled studies with or without therapy. Spontaneous remissions can occur. The majority of patients are begun on prednisone, 1 to 2 mg. per kg. per day in divided dosage, and are kept on moderate high doses until the therapeutic response is evident by (1) clinical improvement and (2) a drop in the level of the muscle enzymes in the serum. If the patient responds, the dose of steroids should be tapered very gradually (a decrease of 5 mg. at 1- to 2-week intervals), yet kept at a maintenance level (usually 7.5 to 15 mg. daily) for months or years, depending upon the clinical course. When exacerbations occur, the steroid dosage must be raised accordingly. Antacids should be given concomitantly. Acutely ill patients must be kept at bedrest and receive only passive physical therapy, but as symptoms subside, more active programs should be instituted, primarily for the prevention of permanent musculoskeletal deformities.

Experience with the immunosuppressive or cytotoxic drugs has been limited and the drugs are reserved frequently for patients with a more severe form of the disease and who have not responded to glucocorticoids. The drugs may be useful in providing a "steroid-sparing" effect. Methotrexate is usually given intravenously on a daily or weekly basis (doses up to 0.5 to 0.8 mg. per kg. of body weight), whereas azathioprine (50 to 150 mg. daily, or a sufficient dose to produce mild leukopenia) and cyclophosphamide are given orally. The results with these drugs are difficult to evaluate, but there are responders, and, in some situations, the side effects may be less severe than with long-term high dose prednisone. (This use of methotrexate, azathioprine, and cyclophosphamide is not listed in the manufacturer's official directives.)

The cutaneous lesions may be extensive and severe (especially in childhood dermatomyositis) and may not respond as the muscle weakness is being controlled. Bland lubricating creams are helpful in mild cases, but topical steroid creams (1 per cent hydrocortisone or 0.1 per cent triamcinolone) are usually beneficial for patients with more inflammatory skin disease. The lesions may show a better response to therapy if the skin is moistened with tub soaks or wet compresses before the creams are applied. The more potent steroids must be used for short intervals only, due to their tendency to produce cutaneous atrophy.

One of the dreaded complications of this disease, calcinosis cutis, is seen in the majority of patients with onset during childhood and in a much smaller percentage of adults. Therapy is disappointing, despite occasional reported success with chelating agents, such as $CaNa_2EDTA$, biphosphonates, aluminum hydroxide, and a low calcium diet. Surgical excision of calcium deposits is often necessary for relief of pain and for local infection. Contractures, another complication not infrequently seen in children, may require surgery in addition to intense physical therapy.

THE ERYTHEMAS

method of
MAURAY J. TYE, M.D.
Haverhill, Massachusetts

Classified under the erythemas is a group of delayed hypersensitivity reaction disorders. The antigen may be of viral, bacterial, rickettsial, or fungal origin, or a chemical or protein substance. It is manifested pathologically by vasodilation and a lymphocytic perivascular infiltrate.

Toxic Erythemas

The eruption is usually generalized and may vary from pinpoint erythematous macules (scarlatiniform) to diffuse erythema. Although the morphologic appearance may be similar, diverse disorders, such as lymphoma, collagen abnormalities, autoimmune mechanisms, infections, and drugs, may be the cause. The reaction must be differentiated by concomitant clinical symptoms or laboratory findings from such diseases as scarlet fever, measles, infectious mononucleosis, etc. (See management of erythema multiforme for therapeutic approaches.)

Erythema Multiforme

This acute inflammatory disease shows erythematous lesions with marginate, arciform or iris configuration, or both. In addition, there may be papules, macules, wheals, vesicles, or bullae. There may be localized involvement (especially on the hands), or it may be widespread. A severe form known as Stevens-Johnson syndrome also involves the mucous membranes. Erythema multiforme may be idiopathic or may be a sign accompanying a bacterial, fungal or viral infection (especially herpes simplex), internal malignancy, or allergies due to a food or drug.

Management. 1. Cultural, agglutination, blood, urine, and x-ray studies for establishing or eliminating specific causes. Biopsy and immunofluorescence study of lesions to eliminate pemphigus, pemphigoid, or dermatitis herpetiformis.

2. Many outbreaks are asymptomatic and spontaneously resolve (e.g., an erythema frequently noted in newborns soon after birth at pressure sites.)

3. Appropriate antibiotics if of bacterial genesis or secondarily infected.

4. Withdrawal of a nonessential drug (or drugs) suspected of being a possible factor and replacing it with a chemically unrelated drug.

5. Lidocaine (Xylocaine Viscous), as a mouth rinse, can be helpful before meals if there is mucous membrane involvement. Most mild or moderately severe cases require no treatment.

6. Pruritus, if present, may be relieved by 0.5 per cent menthol in calamine lotion, or a full strength corticosteroid cream may be helpful. One to two antihistamine tablets, diphenhydramine hydrochloride (Benadryl), 50 mg. or dexchlorpheniramine (Polaramine), 6 mg. four times a day, or hydroxyzine hydrochloride (Atarax), 10 mg. four times a day, probably because of their sedative effects, may be useful in relieving the discomfort.

7. Only in the severe bullous forms are corticoids used. Prednisone, 40 to 80 mg. daily, orally with gradual tapering over a 10 to 14 day period, is generally used. If the outbreak is severe and life-threatening, 160 to 240 mg. daily is indicated and the dosage should be decreased over a longer period, depending on the clinical response. Also taken into account is the clinical state of the patient, e.g., diabetes, high blood pressure, peptic ulcer, mental disease, and tuberculosis, which may contraindicate its use or require appropriate concomitant therapy.

Erythema Nodosum

Erythema nodosum is manifested by more or less symmetrical tender, red nodules, up to 5 cm. in diameter located usually on the anterior aspect of the legs. They last classically 7 to 10 days, although frequently longer. This disturbance represents a panniculitis that may be associated with vasculitis. It often is idiopathic, but may be related to such associated diseases as sarcoidosis, post-streptococcal syndromes, autoimmune diseases, deep mycoses, drugs, and others. If erythema nodosum occurs in association with sarcoidosis, there may be marked hilar adenopathy on the chest films. (It is to be differentiated from erythema induratum, subacute nodular migratory panniculitis, Weber-Christian disease, and a nodular panniculitis associated with pancreatic disease.)

Management. 1. Chest x-ray, antistreptolysin or streptozyme titers, SMA profile, electrocardiogram (ECG), sedimentation rate, and tuberculin sensitivity tests are among the most valuable laboratory data in evaluating concomitant provocative diseases.

2. Among the drugs that may produce this reaction are birth control pills, halogens, and sulfonamides.

3. The pain may be relieved and the resolution of the lesions accelerated with the use of more potent fluorinated corticosteroid creams, e.g., fluocinonide (Lidex), halcinonide (Halog), or desoximetasone (Topicort) cream 3 times a day covered by plastic wrap (Saran) and held in place by Ace bandages over a period of 7 to 10 days.

4. Oral prednisone in doses of 10 to 20 mg. per 24 hours, for 7 to 10 days may produce a prompt response if not contraindicated by an associated disease. Recurrences are common and this therapy is only rarely indicated.

Figurate Erythemas

Erythema chronicum migrans, or erythema annulare centrifugum, shows one or several lesions characterized by arcuate borders that are migratory or fixed. Typically, one sees an advancing border that is slightly raised, with scaling on the inner margin with clear centers. Sensitivity to benign or malignant tumors and inflammatory diseases due to infections, drugs, or bites are among the major causal factors. A syndrome of erythema chronicum migrans associated with cryoprecipitates, neurologic signs and arthritis has recently been described as Lyme arthritis. Its cause remains uncertain, though a tick bite has been associated with some cases.

If due to a tick bite, penicillin, erythromycin, or tetracycline in full doses given over 10 days is helpful.

Erythema gyratum repens consists of parallel red bands with annular and serpiginous borders presenting a woodlike grain pattern over most of the body, the pattern changing from day to day as the bands advance. It is always associated with an underlying visceral carcinoma. (A familial, persistent form occurring fairly early in life, is recognized.)

Erythema marginatum occurs with rheumatic fever and is characterized by ring lesions with raised margins spreading peripherally, leaving pale and sometimes a slightly pigmented inactive center.

Erythema dyschromicum perstans appears in Latin Americans and is probably the result of liquefaction degeneration of the basal cell layer and the accumulation of mononuclear cells and melanophages in a perivascular pattern. These lesions start as erythematous areas but assume a blue-gray color. The macules coalesce to form polycyclic patches. The cause is unknown.

Management. The lesions, per se, require no treatment, the delineation, if possible, of the underlying causal factor being the prime approach.

SUPERFICIAL FUNGUS INFECTIONS OF THE SKIN

method of
EDGAR B. SMITH, M.D.,
and EDUARDO H. TSCHEN, M.D.
Albuquerque, New Mexico

Superficial fungus infections of the skin include dermatophytosis, tinea versicolor, tinea nigra, and candidiasis. These conditions can be mimicked by a variety of other dermatoses and misdiagnosed, and the resulting treatment of nonfungal conditions with antifungal medications is a common cause of treatment failure. We believe the mycologic confirmation of clinically suspected superficial fungus infections should always be obtained before antifungal therapy is initiated. The identification of fungal hyphae on microscopic examination of scales from the suspected lesion in a potassium hydroxide preparation is the quickest and most useful means of obtaining this confirmation. Culturing of lesion material on mycologic media such as Sabouraud's, Mycosel or DTM is essential when it is desirable to identify accurately the causative organism. However, some organisms, such as *Pityrosporum orbiculare,* do not grow in the usual media for fungi and others grow quite slowly. The potassium hydroxide preparation can be done when the patient is initially seen and is a most valuable guide to choosing appropriate therapy. Wood's light examination is a useful confirmatory test in some dermatophyte infections of the scalp and can help to differentiate erythrasma from tinea cruris but is not useful in identifying fungus infections of the nonhairy skin.

Many quite effective antifungal preparations are available over-the-counter. Most of these contain undecylenic acid or its derivatives or tolnaftate. Since a large proportion of patients have used these relatively available preparations prior to seeking medical advice and have thus eliminated the less refractory infections, we shall limit our discussion to the use of antifungal agents available by prescription.

Dermatophyte Infections

Dermatophytosis of the Scalp and Beard Area. Fungus infections of the scalp and beard area are caused by organisms in the *Microsporum* and *Trichophyton* groups which invade hairs. This leads to broken hairs and alopecia as well as varying degrees of inflammation in the adjacent epidermis and dermis. Hairs from suspected lesions should be selected for potassium hydroxide preparations and cultures. These infections rarely respond to topical therapy and orally administered griseofulvin is the treatment of choice. We use the microcrystalline form of griseofulvin in the following dosages: for very small children, 125 mg. of griseofulvin suspension daily; for children from 30 to 50 pounds, 250 mg. daily; for children over 50 pounds, 500 mg. daily; for adults, 1 gram daily. The total daily dosage is divided into two equal doses and is best given after meals. Griseofulvin should be continued for approximately 2 weeks after the infection is clinically clear and laboratory examinations are negative. In most cases, the usual course of therapy is 6 to 8 weeks. Concomitant use of a topical antifungal agent such as clotrimazole (Lotrimin), 1 per cent solution or miconazole (MicaTin), 2 per cent lotion may reduce dissemination of the organisms. Siblings and pets should be examined and treated if infected to prevent reinfection of the patient. With modern therapy, it is not necessary to require children to remain home from school.

Occasionally, a severely inflammatory fungus infection of the scalp, or kerion, is seen. This represents an immunologic response to the fungi in hair follicles. Mild cases will respond to the use of topical steroids. In very severe cases, short (1 to 2 weeks) courses of systemic steroids are useful in suppressing the inflammatory reaction and reducing the risk of scarring and permanent hair loss.

Dermatophytosis of the Nonhairy Skin. These infections can be caused by many *Microsporum* and *Trichophyton* species and *Epidermophyton floccosum* and result in the classic ringworm. Most such infections can be managed successfully by topical treatment with clotrimazole (Lotrimin), 1 per cent solution, miconazole (MicaTin), 2 per cent lotion, or haloprogin (Halotex), 1 per cent cream. The medication should be applied sparingly twice daily to all involved areas and a 5 to 6 cm. area of normal skin surrounding the clinically evident infection. The medication should be continued for about 1 week after the lesions have cleared. The usual duration of treatment is 4 to 6 weeks. Oral griseofulvin, microcrystalline forms, 500 mg. twice daily for 1 month, is indicated in patients with extensive cutaneous involvement, lesions at hard-to-reach sites, and those with chronic or recurrent infections.

Dermatophytosis of the inguinal folds, or tinea cruris, is a common variant that occurs frequently in young athletically active patients and is frequently associated with dermatophyte infections of the feet. Patients should be advised to reduce sweating and chafing in the groin area by avoiding tight or highly occlusive synthetic material underclothing. The treatment is otherwise the same as that of other dermatophyte infections of the glabrous skin.

Dermatophytosis of the Feet. There are two main variants of foot infection with the dermatophytes. The most common involves the toe webs and the instep of the sole, is most frequently due to *Trichophyton mentagrophytes* and responds more readily to therapy. Most infections of this type can be successfully treated with clotrimazole (Lotrimin), 1 per cent solution or miconazole (MicaTin), 2 per cent lotion applied twice daily. Treatment should be continued for about 4 weeks. This type of infection is often complicated by secondary bacterial infection, usually with the streptococcus or staphylococcus. If pustules or purulent exudate are present, cultures should be taken and the patient started on a program of bed rest, elevation of feet with compresses or soaks with warm tap water for 15 to 20 minutes three times daily, and systemic antibiotics. After the bacterial infection resolves, appropriate antifungal treatment should be initiated.

The dry, scaly diffuse type of infection of the soles is usually due to *Trichophyton rubrum* and tends to be chronic. However, most infections will respond at least temporarily to topical treatment with clotrimazole or miconazole. The treatment should be continued for 5 to 6 weeks, and sometimes even more prolonged therapy is necessary. More refractory infections of this type are treated with a combination of a topically applied imidazole such as clotrimazole and orally administered griseofulvin. Relapses are quite common even with such combined therapy.

The warm, moist environment within shoes and the presence of thicker skin on the soles to provide abundant amounts of keratin as nutrient for the dermatophytes explains the refractoriness of superficial fungus infections of the feet. Patients should be advised to keep the feet cool and dry, and to wear cotton socks rather than the rather more occlusive nylon or other synthetic fabrics. Wearing of sandals or perforated shoes is also useful. Prophylactic use of tolnaftate powder (Tinactin) will also reduce the frequency of recurrences.

Dermatophytosis of the Hands. Dermatophytosis of the hands is usually unilateral and clinically resembles the dry, scaly, diffuse type of infection of the feet with which it is frequently associated. These chronic infections of the palmar skin usually require combination therapy with topical agents such as clotrimazole and oral griseofulvin.

Dermatophytosis of the Nails. Infections of the hands and feet are frequently accompanied by infection of the nails. Nail infections rarely respond to topical therapy. Infections of the fingernails usually can be treated successfully with griseofulvin, microcrystalline type, 500 mg. twice daily. Therapy should be continued until the nail appears completely normal and usually requires 4 to 6 months. Toe nail infections can also be treated with griseofulvin, but cure rates are quite low even with very prolonged therapy. Because of the poor response rate and concern about possible oncogenicity of long-term griseofulvin therapy, we do not recommend treatment of toe nail infections unless the resulting thickening of the nail plate produces pain and mechanical problems in the wearing of foot wear. In these relatively rare cases, we avulse the affected nails and treat with oral griseofulvin for 6 to 8 months as the new nail is growing out.

Tinea Nigra

Tinea nigra is a superficial fungus infection caused by *Cladosporium wernecki* and presents as asymptomatic brown or black macules on the palms or soles. This infection responds well to older keratolytic antifungal agents such as Whitfield's ointment as well as the newer agents such as clotrimazole.

Tinea Versicolor

Tinea versicolor, caused by *Pityrosporum orbiculare,* is quite common in areas of warm temperatures and high humidity. It is characterized by asymptomatic, scaling patches on the upper trunk and neck that vary from slightly red to brown and white. Since a few organisms can be found on the normal skin of most persons, this condition can be considered the result of overgrowth of this yeast in more susceptible persons. Tinea versicolor responds well to a variety of topical antifungal agents, but relapses are common with all. Since infections are often extensive, we consider selenium sulfide (Selsun), 2.5 per cent suspension, to be the treatment of choice. Following the bath or shower, the suspension is applied as a lather to all of the skin of the neck and upper trunk, allowed to dry for 10 to 15 minutes, and then washed off well with a washcloth. This treatment is repeated each day for one week. This treatment will usually eradicate active infection characterized by the presence of scaling, but hypopigmented spots may remain for several months. For very susceptible patients who have frequent relapses, we recommend repeating the above regimen once or twice monthly as a form of maintenance therapy. The newer antifungal agents such as haloprogin (Halotex), 1 per cent cream, miconazole (Mica-Tin), 2 per cent lotion or cream, or clotrimazole (Lotrimin), 1 per cent solution or cream are quite effective in treatment of tinea versicolor, but the expense of these agents limits their usefulness to those patients with relatively small areas of involvement.

Candidiasis

Cutaneous candidiasis, caused by the yeast *Candida albicans*, occurs frequently in young, active persons who work or play in hot, humid environments and most frequently involves intertriginous areas such as the groin, perineum, axillae, and inframammary areas. Older patients who are obese or who have diabetes mellitus are also predisposed to infections with this organism. Acute infections are quite inflammatory and should be treated with moist compresses of cool tap water for 10 to 15 minutes three times daily. After the compresses are removed, the skin should be allowed to dry and either a broad-spectrum antifungal agent such as miconazole (MicaTin), 2 per cent lotion or clotrimazole (Lotrimin), 1 per cent solution or the more specific nystatin lotion (Mycostatin) should be applied. Concomitant application of a topical steroid with the anticandidal agent will suppress the inflammation and hasten resolution. We do not recommend use of commercially available nystatin-steroid combinations containing ethylenediamine or parabens because of their potential sensitizing properties. The compresses can be discontinued when weeping and erosions have resolved, but the medications should be continued until the eruption is completely clear. This usually occurs within 1 to 2 weeks. The patient should be instructed to keep the involved area cool and dry. Loose cotton underclothing is useful in achieving this goal.

Candida albicans can also cause chronic infections of the nail folds (paronychia) and separation of the nail plate from the nail bed. These infections most frequently occur in persons whose work involved continuous wetting of the hands. The patient must be instructed to keep his hands out of water as much as possible. Paronychial infections are treated with applications of an anticandidal agent four times daily, nystatin cream (Mycostatin) or one of the newer agents such as clotrimazole (Lotrimin), 1 per cent solution, miconazole (Mica-Tin), 2 per cent lotion, or haloprogin (Halotex), 1 per cent cream are all quite effective. Response is slow and treatment must be continued for 2 or 3 months. When onycholysis and infection of the nail bed are present, the overlying nail plate should be trimmed back as far as possible, then thymol, 4 per cent, in ethanol, is applied thoroughly under the nail three times daily until the nail grows out in a normal fashion.

DRUG ERUPTIONS

method of
JEFFREY P. CALLEN, M.D.
Louisville, Kentucky

Rashes caused by drugs are common in the practice of medicine. In general, removal of the offending agent will lead to eventual resolution of the eruption. Occasionally, the eruption is severe and requires emergency treatment, or at other times symptoms may persist and require therapy.

Almost all drugs have the propensity to produce a rash and many times the diagnosis of a drug eruption is not easily made. After the recognition of a possible drug-induced rash, all nonessential drugs should be discontinued. In patients on multiple medications that may be essential to their care the drugs should be replaced by agents of a different class with a similar action. An example of this would be replacement of a penicillin antibiotic with a cephalothin.

Although treatment of the particular eruption is important, prevention of a recurrence is equally important. Proof of involvement of a particular agent is desirable, but in many patients the proof would require a rechallenge, which is impractical. In severe eruptions the reaction may be life-threatening and is unwarranted. In the case of possible drug involvement, the best approach is avoidance, except when the drug would be required for life maintenance.

Further management of drug rashes depends on the type and severity of the eruption.

Erythema Multiforme and Stevens-Johnson Syndrome. Erythema multiforme is a skin eruption characterized by "target" or iris lesions. The mucosal surface may be involved on occasion. In approximately 25 per cent of cases of erythema multiforme the cause is a drug and another 25 per cent is related to infectious agents. In general, the eruption is mild and produces pruritus or burning. This may be controlled with antipruritics such as cyproheptadine hydrochloride (Periactin), 4 mg. orally four times daily, or hydroxyzine hydrochloride (Atarax), 10 to 50 mg. orally four times daily. Weak topical corticosteroids such as 1 per cent hydrocortisone cream may also help control pruritus. Mucosal involvement should be treated symptomatically as well. Saline mouth washes, diphenhydramine hydrochloride elixir (Elixir of Benadryl), or viscous lidocaine (Xylocaine) have been used effectively. Patients with more severe cases of cutaneous or mucosal disease respond well to systemic corticosteroids (prednisone in a tapering course over 2 to 3 weeks or intramuscular triamcinolone). Hospitalization is usually not required.

Stevens-Johnson syndrome is a severe form of erythema multiforme characterized by bullous cutaneous lesions, multiple mucous membrane involvement and systemic symptoms (fever, malaise, hypotension, etc.). Stevens-Johnson syndrome requires intensive medical management in a hospital setting. Supportive care is often necessary. Symptomatic therapy for pain, fever, and myalgias is warranted. Careful monitoring of fluid and electrolytes is indicated. Usually systemic corticosteroids are used until clearing of the lesions is seen and then a slow tapering course is followed. Local skin care consists of drying solutions for vesiculobullous lesions (Burow's solution soaks for 15 minutes three times daily), and protective care for denuded skin with a water-oil emulsion (Eucerin cream). Secondary bacterial infections and septicemia are not uncommon and should be treated promptly. Oral hygiene is important; mouth washes should be used to cleanse the oral cavity. Often *Candida albicans* will overgrow in the mouth; this may be treated with nystatin (Mycostatin) mouthwash. Ocular involvement may be severe and can lead to blindness. Early ophthalmologic consultation is strongly recommended. Irrigation, lysis of adhesions, topical antibiotics, and corticosteroids are the usual forms of therapy.

The majority of cases of erythema multiforme and Stevens-Johnson syndrome resolve without sequelae in 2 to 4 weeks. Stevens-Johnson syndrome has had a mortality of up to 20 per cent. Recurrences are seen in about 20 per cent of patients with erythema multiforme or Stevens-Johnson syndrome; some may be prevented if a drug cause can be isolated and avoided.

Toxic Epidermal Necrolysis. Toxic epidermal necrolysis is a rare but severe rash. In adults it is almost always drug related. In children a similar eruption may be due to staphylococcal infections. Lately, the most commonly involved drug has been allopurinol. Mortality may be as high as 80 per cent. The rash is characterized by loss of sheets of skin. Often the epidermis may be moved over the dermis with pressure (Nikolsky's sign). Hospitalization is required, with careful monitoring of fluids and electrolytes. Denuded skin must be protected as detailed for the Stevens-Johnson syndrome. Secondary bacterial infections are common and must be treated promptly. Systemic corticosteroids are used in high doses (60 to 120 mg. of prednisone or equivalent per day).

Urticaria and Angioedema. Severe urticaria with pharyngeal or laryngeal edema may be life-threatening and requires emergency treatment. Epinephrine (1:1000) may be given subcutaneously. Prednisone, 40 mg., is then used in a tapering course over a 7- to 10-day period. In less severe cases, antihistamines and antiserotonins may be used. Cyproheptadine (Periactin), 4 mg. orally four times daily, hydroxyzine (Atarax), 10 to 50 mg. orally four times daily, or methdilazine (Tacaryl), 8 mg. orally four times daily, may be beneficial in both suppression and prevention of the hives. Often the urticaria will persist for 7 to 10 days following the withdrawal of the drug, and requires continued therapy.

Morbilliform Reactions. These reactions are generally not life-threatening and may be treated symptomatically. Oatmeal baths often help relieve pruritus, and the application of 0.25 per cent menthol in an oxycholesterin compound (Lubriderm Lotion) is also effective. Patients with more severe reactions may require antihistamines as given for urticaria. Only rarely are systemic corticosteroids indicated.

Drug Induced Photosensitivity. Eruptions in

light-exposed areas are generally due to increased sensitivity to sunlight induced by a drug, rather than a true allergy. Commonly involved drugs include tetracyclines (particularly demeclocycline), sulfonylureas, sulfonamides, phenothiazines, thiazides, and quinidine. These drugs should be discontinued if possible and the patient should be removed from the light or protected by clothing and sunscreens (PreSun, Uval). Topical therapy with triamcinolone in a cream base (Aristocort-A) is generally effective. Persistent reactions may require systemic corticosteroids for suppression (prednisone, 20 to 30 mg. per day tapered over 5 to 7 days).

HERPES SIMPLEX

method of
ALVIN E. FRIEDMAN-KIEN, M.D.,
and RICHARD J. KLEIN, M.D.
New York, New York

Infections with herpes simplex virus type 1 and type 2 are among the most prevalent infections in man. Apparently 80 to 90 per cent of the general population has demonstrable antibodies to either or both of these viruses, which are closely related.

Herpetic infections produce a broad spectrum of clinical manifestations. The primary herpetic infection usually occurs within the first few years of life as an oral-pharyngeal gingivostomatitis. Mucous membrane vesicles and shallow ulcerations are accompanied by fever, malaise, and lymphadenitis, which lasts about 8 to 14 days. Most often, the infection is merely diagnosed as a "viral illness" and is treated symptomatically. In some patients infection may occur as a primary vulvovaginitis or as a severe, localized vesicular eruption at the site of direct virus skin inoculation.

Unlike other viral infections, despite the presence and persistence of humor and cell-mediated immunity to the herpes virus that develops after the primary infection, a large number of persons may be subject to localized herpes simplex virus-induced recurrent lesions throughout life or only for a limited period of time. The antibody titers do not seem to change in these patients before, during, or after the recurrent attacks. It is generally accepted that the virus ascends sensory nerves and establishes latent infections in spinal root ganglia or the ganglion of the trigeminal nerve. Periodically or at irregular intervals latent virus is "reactivated" or "derepressed" and descends the involved sensory nerves to the mucocutaneous surface where it causes a self-limited, localized, painful vesicular-ulcerating eruption lasting from 5 to 10 days. The most common form of these recurrent infections is the "cold sore" or "fever blister" involving the lips, oral mucosa, or perioral skin area; however, the nasal mucosa or facial skin, and, less commonly, any other regions of the skin such as the trunk, genitalia, buttocks, or limbs may be involved. Although not absolute, most cases of herpes infections occurring above the waist are caused by herpes simplex virus type 1, whereas the infections below the waist, especially on the genitalia, are mostly caused by the type 2 virus. These two viruses are very closely related antigenically. Recurrent herpes progenitalis has increasingly become one of the most frequent infectious venereal diseases observed in the past few years, second only to syphilis and gonorrhea. Transmission between sexual partners is common. Aside from the widespread publicity of a possible relationship between herpes progenitalis and cancer, the discomfort and psychologic factors associated with this form of the disease have brought it to the attention of physicians because of the increased incidence of patients seeking medical advice. Penile lesions occur as one or more well-circumscribed clusters of vesicles and superficial ulcers on the shaft or glans often associated with inguinal adenopathy. Involvement of the vulvovaginal region may be localized to one or more lesions on the external labia and intravaginal mucosa. A mucopurulent vaginal discharge is frequently associated with intravaginal involvement. Lesions on the cervix appear as inflamed, shallow ulcerations observed by intravaginal speculum examination. A Papanicolaou ("Pap") smear will demonstrate multinucleate giant cells and with intranuclear inclusions similar to those seen in the Tzanck smear described below. Lesions on the perineal skin, pubic region, and perirectal area are now seen with increased frequency in both males and females. Although herpes progenitalis is suspected as a possible cause of carcinoma of the uterine cervix, there is at present no definite epidemiologic or other evidence that herpes simplex virus type 1 or type 2, alone, or in conjunction with some unknown factors, are involved in human cancer.

Herpetic keratoconjunctivitis is a peculiar unilateral recurrent viral infection of the eye; rarely, both eyes may be involved. The characteristic, clinical manifestations involve minute ulcerated vesicles on the conjunctiva and cornea that rapidly coalesce to form a distinct superficial dendritic ulcer. In certain patients, the superficial recurrent keratoconjunctivitis may involve deeper stromal tissue, causing permanent damage to the cornea and uveal tract. This condition is a major cause of blindness in the United States today.

Recurrent cutaneous lesions are usually characterized by prodromal symptoms of itching, tingling, or burning of the imminent recurrence followed by the development of discrete localized clusters of clear vesicles a few millimeters in diameter superimposed on an erythematous base. The untreated herpetic vesicles usually reach maximum size by 3 days after onset and then begin to dry up and form crusts with total clearing within 7 to 12 days. Lymphangitis or lymphadenitis or both may accompany recurrent lesions. The pain subsides with healing, but a mild erythema and tenderness may persist for several weeks after resolution. Permanent scarring is not commonly seen, although post-inflammatory pigmentation may occur following many repeated bouts at the same site. Secondary purulent bacterial infections may develop, superimposed on the viral-induced lesions. Staphylococci or streptococci are most frequently isolated in these patients. Monilia (yeast) vaginitis is often associated with intravaginal herpetic disease.

TREATMENT

Primary Mucocutaneous Infection

Gingivostomatitis. The primary infection with herpes simplex virus usually occurs in children or less frequently in young adults. The widespread vesicles that form erosions of the lips, buccal mucosa, gums, tongue, and pharynx are usually associated with a fever, malaise, lymphadenopathy, and pronounced discomfort. The pain may be so severe as to limit the ingestion of oral fluids and nutrition. The erosions heal spontaneously in about 10 to 14 days. No specific antiviral therapy is currently available. Treatment consists of supportive measures.

TOPICAL ANESTHESIA. 1. Diphenhydramine hydrochloride (Benadryl Elixir) used as a mouthwash and gargle for 2 to 3 minutes prior to meals and whenever the discomfort is in need of palliation will effectively anesthetize the mucosa and alleviate the pain. This preparation has a pleasant cherry flavor.

2. Other topical oral anesthetics such as viscous lidocaine (Xylocaine) or dyclonine hydrochloride (Dyclone) are also effective but unfortunately are not especially palatable.

3. Acetylsalicylic acid (aspirin), 600 mg., dissolved in cool or lukewarm water used as a mouthwash and gargle for a few minutes has proved very soothing.

Cleansing with over-the-counter mouthwashes will help reduce the fetid mouth odor that usually accompanies this kind of infection.

1. Sodium bicarbonate diluted in cool or lukewarm water can be used as a mouthwash as often as necessary.

2. Mouth rinses with 3 per cent hydrogen peroxide diluted equal parts with water can be used as a mouthwash and gargle to help debride the ulcerations.

ANALGESICS. (1) Propoxyphene napsylate (Darvon), (2) codeine phosphate, (3) oxycodone and aspirin (Percodan), or (4) meperidine (Demerol) may be used cautiously in patients who require stronger pain relief.

FLUID-ELECTROLYTE BALANCE. Intravenous fluids and electrolytes may be required to maintain those patients, especially infants and young children, who are unable to take oral feedings or who cannot use topical oral anesthetics as a mouthwash or gargle.

ISOLATION OF CAUSATIVE ORGANISMS. Proper virus cultures should be performed if a diagnostic virus laboratory is available. Isolation takes about 2 to 3 days. Other viruses such as coxsackie or echo viruses can also cause pharyngitis and gingivostomatitis.

Secondary bacterial infection may become a problem. Isolation of the bacteria and the testing for antibiotic sensitivity would be helpful should this complication arise.

CONFIRMING THE DIAGNOSIS. If possible, samples of acute and convalescent sera should be taken in order to confirm the diagnosis, as measured by a rise in specific antibody titers. The paired serum samples should be sent to local public health laboratories. Such information would help epidemiologic studies on the incidence and natural course of this disease in man.

Primary Herpetic Vulvovaginitis. Primary herpetic vulvovaginitis is usually considered a venereally transmitted disease seen mostly in adolescents and young adults. The entire perineal region including the labia majora, labia minora, pubic region, and perianal skin, as well as the intravaginal mucosa and cervix may be involved. Vesicles and erosive ulcerations develop accompanied by sensations of severe burning pain, inflammation with erythema, edema, and inguinal lymphadenitis. A foul-smelling, mucopurulent vaginal discharge may be present. Monilia infection is often found to be present as well.

1. No specific antiviral therapy is currently available, although *topical antiviral agents* in ophthalmic preparations such as IUdR (5-iodo-2-deoxyuridine) 1 per cent solution, or 0.5 per cent ointment (Stoxil, Herplex, Dendrid), a 3 per cent adenine arabinoside (Ara-A, Vira-A) ointments are being used by some clinicians. Controlled experimental clinical studies using these preparations have not demonstrated that such treatment alters the natural course of the infection in a favorable way.

2. Topical compresses with an aqueous aluminum acetate solution (Burow's, Domeboro, Bluboro) applied intravaginally by inserting a saturated ball of cotton every few hours can be soothing and helpful in resolving the vaginitis.

3. Cool or lukewarm water sitz baths for 15 minutes are very soothing and taken as frequently as possible are very effective in alleviating the symptoms.

4. Topical anesthetics such as lidocaine (Xylocaine) or benzocaine (Americaine) in an aqueous gel or in aerosol spray may be used to relieve the great discomfort that accompanies this condition. Topical anesthetics do tend to cause contact allergic reactions, especially on inflamed mucosal surfaces; therefore, if the condition is aggravated or worsens, use of topical anesthetic therapy should be discontinued.

5. Oral analgesics. Oxycodone (Percodan), codeine, or meperidine (see above) may be used at the discretion of the attending physician to alleviate the considerable pain and discomfort that accompanies this acute infection.

SECONDARY SUPERIMPOSED INFECTIONS. 1. Secondary monilia (yeast), vaginal infection is associated with purulent, milky discharge and can be combatted with the use of nystatin (Mycostatin) intravaginal suppositories, inserted every 12 hours for 7 to 12 days.

2. Secondary bacterial infections of herpetic vulvovaginitis may also occur. This condition is best treated with intravaginal antibiotic ointments such as combined neomycin, bacitracin, polymyxin, gramicidin (Polysporin).

STEROIDS. Neither topical nor systemic steroids should be used during the acute phase of the vaginitis. Once the infection has subsided and the ulcerations have begun to heal, the residual erythema associated with local tenderness, burning, or itching sensations responds to frequent cool tap water compresses as well as topically applied steroid creams or ointments such as triamcinolone acetonide (Kenalog 0.025 per cent, Aristocort 0.1 per cent) or fluocinolone acetonide (Lidex, 0.05 per cent, Synalar 0.25 per cent, Cordran 0.05 per cent) can be used.

Recurrent Cutaneous Infection

Herpes labialis ("sun blisters," "fever blisters," "cold sores"): mucocutaneous involvement of the mouth.

Herpes progenitalis or *genitalis* (venereal) herpes): skin of penis, scrotum, glans, or prepuce in males; external skin of vagina in females.

Herpes involving any portion of the glabrous skin such as on the buttocks, trunk and face.

Herpetic whitlow starts as a direct viral inoculation infection of the skin of a finger, often involving the deeper tissues such as the tendon sheath and producing marked swelling and considerable pain. This condition is often seen as an occupational hazard in dentists and nurses. This localized infection may recur periodically.

Herpes labialis involving the lips is, anatomically, the most common form of the recurrent herpetic disease seen in man. The frequency of recurrences and time required for healing varies with each patient. Lesions may occur as often as every 2 or 3 weeks or as infrequently as every few years lasting from 4 days up to 2 weeks. Recurrent lesions are usually single but may be multiple and can occur at different sites simultaneously or at relatively different times. Most often the same sites are repeatedly involved in any one patient.

Treatment. There is no specific, effective, antiviral therapy available at this time which can abort a recurrent infection, alter the healing time, or prevent future recurrences. A wide variety of treatment modalities is, however, recommended by physicians for the treatment of these recurrent infections. Some forms of therapy border on "witchcraft." The more conservative treatments are concerned with helping to dry up the blisters and ulcerations more quickly and to provide some palliative effect on the discomfort associated with the "sores."

1. Aqueous compresses with aluminum acetate (Burow's, Domeboro, Bluboro), applied at regular intervals can be used with some soothing effect that promotes healing.

2. *Potassium permanganate* compresses (1:30,000 in water) are drying and also provide prophylaxis against secondary bacterial infection. Cool compresses are always more soothing than warm or hot compresses.

3. *Spirits of camphor* applied topically at regular intervals is an "old fashioned," but still popular, treatment that seems to provide comfort for some patients.

4. *Topical ether* (diethyl ether), a lipid solvent known to disintegrate the envelope of the herpes virus, has recently been promoted as an anesthetic and as a healing agent. Presumably, early treatment four times a day with ether, at the onset of a recurrent episode, provides symptomatic relief and shortens the expected duration of the lesions. Ether is a highly volatile and explosive substance that must be handled with extreme caution.

5. *Chloroform*, another lipid solvent, has been used to treat early herpetic lesions and the same caution should be taken in handling this highly inflammable agent. Chloroform applications dry up the lesions and eliminate the virus present in the skin vesicles by disintegrating the virus envelope. Neither ether nor chloroform penetrate the deeper layers of the skin.

6. *Topical glutaraldehyde*, a 2 per cent aqueous solution buffered with sodium bicarbonate to pH 7.5, is currently under investigation. The solution is applied twice a day. It is unstable and must be made up fresh every 2 days.

7. *Liquid nitrogen* lightly applied with an applicator tip to "freeze" early recurrent lesions is reported to suppress the progression of a lesion.

8. *Corticosteroids.* There are many testimonials concerning the efficacy of topical and even intralesional steroid injections for the treatment of recurrent herpes of the skin. Such therapy is absolutely contraindicated in herpetic keratoconjunctivitis. Our impression is that steroids have little or no positive effect on the natural course of recurrent, mucocutaneous herpes. Once the lesion has healed, the persistent erythema, which remains at the lesion site, may resolve more quickly with the use of a topical steroid cream

with mild vasoconstrictor properties. We do not recommend intralesional steroids for recurrent herpetic disease.

9. *Nucleotide analogs.* The first successful topical antiviral agent used in the treatment of herpetic keratoconjunctivitis was IUdR (Stoxil, Herplex, Dendrid). This compound is available as an ophthalmic, 1 per cent aqueous solution or 0.5 per cent ointment and acts by competitive inhibition of thymidine incorporation into the viral nucleic acid. Topically applied to mucocutaneous lesions it has not proved any more effective than simple compresses with Burow's solution. However, if one pricks the herpetic vesicles and applies this agent four to six times a day, following compresses with potassium permanganate or Burow's solution, lesions seem to resolve somewhat more rapidly. No measurable effect on the rate of recurrences has been observed. IUdR-resistant strains of herpes simplex virus type 1 and type 2 have recently been isolated from treated lesions.

The basic biochemical approach to attacking viral replication makes sense; however, the superficial chemotherapeutic application to the cutaneous or ocular viral-induced lesion does not attack the reservoir of virus that is sequestered in the dorsal or trigeminal root ganglia.

Other antiviral agents under investigation such as *adenine arabinoside* 3 per cent ophthalmic ointment (Ara-A, Vira-A) and, more recently, *adenine arabinoside monophosphate* (Ara-AMP) have been shown to be as effective as IUdR in the topical treatment of recurrent herpes in the eye. The use in cutaneous lesions has not proved any more effective than IUdR. No Ara-A resistant strains of herpes simplex virus has been reported to date. Various experimental studies using solvents such as *dimethyl sulfoxide* (DMSO) and dimethyl acetamide (DMAC) facilitating the penetration of IUdR or Ara-A into the skin and deeper tissues are under way. The results are highly varied but are overall not very promising. Both DMSO and DMAC are not approved for general clinical use.

More recently it was shown that *phosphonoacetic acid* (PAA) and some of its analogs exert excellent antiherpes activity in vitro and in experimental animal model infections by interfering with the activity of virus specific enzymes. This agent penetrates the skin but unfortunately has been shown to be deposited in the bone as well as to have teratogenic effects in rabbits. The clinical use in man seems unlikely unless an analogous compound without potential harmful side effects can be found.

Another new compound under investigation is acyclo-guanine [9-(2-hydroxyethoxymethyl) guanine]. The compound can prevent the development of skin lesions and the establishment of

latent infections in sensory ganglia after primary infection in experimental animals. Human studies have not yet been conducted.

10. The use of immune stimulators such as *levamisole,* a drug that increases cell mediated immune (CMI) responses in animals, has been evaluated in a recent double-blind controlled study concerning the prevention of recurrent herpes simplex lesions in man and has shown that the rate of recurrences was not different from the placebo-treated patients. The drug is not approved for human use in the United States.

11. *Smallpox vaccination.* For many years many dermatologists have used multiple repeated vaccinations with smallpox (vaccinia) to prevent recurrences of herpes simplex infections. There is absolutely no rationale for this form of treatment since the vaccinia and herpes viruses are unrelated. A double-blind controlled study in man demonstrated no differences in recurrences in either the vaccinated or placebo-treated groups. It should be stressed that vaccination is not a totally benign procedure. In some patients encephalitis or localized pyoderma gangrenosum has occurred following smallpox vaccinations.

12. *Bacille Calmette-Guérin* (BCG) has been reported to "potentiate the immune response" and prevent recurrences in patients with recurrent herpes simplex lesions. A double-blind study revealed no significant effect on the recurrence rate or severity of the attacks. Furthermore, BCG inoculation caused an abscess formation at the infection site in some patients. This treatment is not recommended.

13. *Photodynamic inactivation* ("dye and light treatment"). It has long been known that heterocyclic dyes such as neutral red or proflavine in the presence of visible light (incandescent or fluorescent) inactivate the herpes simplex virus in vitro.

The clinical application of this observation in treating human recurrent herpes simplex lesions enjoyed a brief vogue a few years ago. It was claimed that use of topical photoactive dye and exposure to light sped up the healing of recurrent lesions and decreased the recurrence rate. A recent, double-blind, controlled study showed no clinical differences between placebo and the dye-treated groups. It should be emphasized that photoinactivated herpes virus particles are biologically inactivated; however, they retain an oncogenic capacity which in tissue culture causes cell transformation, and transformed cells have been shown to produce malignant tumors when transplanted in animals. The possible risks of this kind of treatment are obvious and its use has been abandoned.

VACCINATION WITH HERPES SIMPLEX VI-

RUS. Since patients with recurrent herpes infections do not show any measurable variation in their humoral antibodies to the herpes simplex virus before, during, or following an attack, the use of a specific vaccine for preventing recurrences is not clear. Antibodies do not penetrate living cells such as neurons, the most likely site of the latent herpes virus infection. The virus can spread from cell to cell without coming in contact with the circulating high titered antibodies. The presence of antibodies likely controls the localization of recurrent herpes infection and probably prevents its systemic spread. A herpes vaccine for humans (Lupidon-G and Lupidon-H) has been used only *outside* of the United States. Neither the therapeutic efficacy nor the long-term safety of this vaccination procedure, which is given in multiple doses, has been established by carefully controlled studies.

Eczema Herpeticum (Kaposi's Varicelliform Eruption)

Patients, especially children, with atopic dermatitis, ichthyosis, Darier's disease, or other generalized excoriated diseased skin are susceptible to widespread infection with herpes simplex virus. In severe cases with high fever, fluid and electrolyte imbalance, systemic spread to internal organs, and even encephalitis may occur. Secondary bacterial infection can also occur and cause septicemia.

1. Topical compresses with aluminum acetate or potassium permanganate.

2. Supportive measures such as *intravenous fluid* and electrolytes.

3. Proper antibiotics, if needed, are instituted.

4. The intravenous administration of *adenine arabinoside* (Ara-A, Vidarabine), 10 to 20 mg. per kg. per day, seems to be the only definitive antiviral therapy that is currently available in emergencies under careful investigational study. The therapeutic success so far and the low level of toxicity makes the systemic use of this agent the most promising new development in clinical antiviral therapy in current use.

Disseminated Infection of the Newborn

If a mother has active herpes simplex of the cervix or vagina at the time of delivery it is highly likely that the newborn infant delivered through the infected birth canal will contract a fulminant form of generalized herpes involving the skin, internal organs, and central nervous system. The newborn infant does not yet have the necessary defense mechanisms to combat a severe infection other than the mother's passively transferred humoral antibodies. The morbidity and mortality are extremely high. In this situation, heroic life-saving measures are, therefore, justified. It is recommended that if the mother has herpes progenitalis at or about term, the child should be delivered by caesarean section. Prior to rupture of the amniotic membranes it is not usual for the fetus to become infected.

With the appearance of the first signs of infection, the child should be treated with systemic intravenous adenine arabinoside 10 to 15 mg. per kg. per day. This antiviral agent, although still experimental, has shown promise as a fairly safe therapeutic agent with relatively low toxicity. It is available under careful surveillance from Parke-Davis Co., Ann Arbor, Michigan, for emergency life-threatening situations.

Single volume exchange blood transfusions may be helpful to supplement the newborn's deficient immune responses, the donor being a person who has a recurrent history of herpes type 1 or type 2 or who has recently recovered from a primary herpetic infection. Administration of type specific hyperimmune globulin might also be considered.

Topical applications of compresses with aqueous aluminum acetate solution (Burow's solution, Domeboro, Bluboro) can help dry up the diffuse cutaneous lesions of vesicles and ulcerations that may be present. Cleansing with povidone-iodine (Betadine) will help minimize secondary bacterial infection, which often occurs. In such patients proper systemic antibiotic therapy should be given.

Herpes Simplex Encephalitis

Herpetic infection of the central nervous system especially involves the temporal lobes of the brain and is a severe disease with very high mortality. To date, the only truly successful and fairly safe systemic treatment available is intravenous adenine arabinoside (Vidarabine), 15 to 20 mg. per kg. per day. This antiviral agent, which is still under strict investigational control, can be obtained from Parke-Davis Co., Ann Arbor, Michigan, in emergency situations. At this time the protocol for the use of this agent requires a brain tissue biopsy for viral culture to confirm the viral diagnosis. Samples of cerebrospinal fluid may not contain virus while the brain tissue will. Other therapeutic measures consist of supportive therapy, especially intravenous fluids and electrolytes and anticonvulsive drugs such as phenytoin, (Dilantin), 50 mg., and carbamazepine (Tegretol), 200 mg., or phenobarbital.

Neuralgia Related to Recurrent Herpes Simplex Infections

Some patients with recurrent herpes infections develop an intermittent and somewhat persistent neuralgia involving the nerves serving the anatomic site of recurrences. There may be an aching, throbbing sensation or severe recurrent stinging pains not unlike that seen with the neuralgia that frequently accompanies herpes zoster (shingles). The neuralgic pain usually subsides with cutaneous healing but may persist for several weeks after resolution.

Analgesics such as propoxyphene (Darvon), aspirin, oxycodone (Percodan), meperidine (Demerol), and codeine may be useful. More recently the use of anticonvulsants such as phenytoin (Dilantin),* 50 mg., two or three times a day or carbamazepine (Tegretol),* 200 mg., two or three times per day, will help to alleviate the neuralgia. These agents work by elevating the pain threshold in most patients. Should allergic reactions to these drugs develop, their use should be discontinued.

Recurrent Herpetic Keratoconjunctivitis

Recurrent herpetic keratoconjunctivitis is a serious condition that is one of the major causes of blindness in the United States. Type 1 herpes simplex virus is most frequently seen affecting the eye. The most common form of this ophthalmologic infection causes a characteristic dendrite shaped ulceration of the superficial corneal epithelium. The infection may last up to 2 to 3 weeks. Involvement of the deeper stromal tissue of the cornea can develop an ameboid-shaped ulceration which may progress to permanent damage with scarring and, in some cases, blindness. Chronic deep stromal disease may cause a discoform keratitis that is believed to be host immunologic or an allergic reaction to the viral protein. Involvement of the uveal tract often causes glaucoma to develop.

Several treatment modalities are available and should be only administered by an experienced ophthalmologist.

Mechanical Debridement. Prior to the availability of successful, topical antiviral chemotherapy, the only effective treatment for herpetic keratoconjunctivitis consisted of careful surgical debridement of the diseased superficial layers of the conjunctiva and corneal epithelium. This method is not used when deeper stromal tissue is involved. Debridement can also be accomplished by using a "freezing" technique, employing liquid nitrogen with an instrument called a "cryoprobe." The eye is then covered with a patch to allow for reepithelialization. This type of treatment has gained popularity and is now used in conjunction with topical antiviral agents, especially in difficult cases.

---

*This use of this agent is not listed in the manufacturer's official directive.

Antiviral Chemotherapy. Topical treatment with nucleoside analogs, such as IUdR (0.1 per cent aqueous solution or 0.5 per cent ointment) is extremely effective in the treatment of recurrent herpetic keratoconjunctivitis. The solution is applied to the conjunctival sac every hour; the ointment is applied at least six times a day to the infected eye until the inflammation and dendritic ulceration is totally cleared. The diseased eye should be followed carefully by periodic ophthalmologic examination until healed. Although this treatment is highly effective in resolving each herpetic episode, the therapy has no influence on the incidence of further recurrences. Allergic reactions to IUdR have been reported on occasion. IUdR-resistant strains of herpes simplex virus have been isolated in recent years.

Adenine arabinoside (Ara-A, Vira-A) 3 per cent ointment is a newer nucleoside antiviral agent that is not approved and readily available for use in human ophthalmic infections. The ointment is topically applied to the diseased conjunctiva four to six times a day until healing. Careful follow-up by an ophthalmologist with a slit lamp observation is essential to ascertain total healing of the dendritic corneal ulcer. Ara-A is as effective as IUdR in the treatment of each recurrent herpetic episode of the eye. Like IUdR, Ara-A does not affect the rate of recurrences. No allergic reactions to Ara-A have been reported to date. Unlike IUdR, Ara-A resistant strains of herpes virus have not evolved at the present time.

5-Tri-fluoromethyl-2-deoxythymide (T-F-3) in human studies appears to be as good as either IUdR or Ara-A in the treatment of herpetic keratoconjunctivitis. Again, no influence upon recurrences has been observed. This compound is not available in the United States at this time.

Interferon. Human interferon, a naturally occurring antiviral substance which plays a role in the normal body defenses against viral infections has been prepared, purified, and concentrated in the laboratory and is currently being evaluated as another topical antiviral agent in herpetic keratoconjunctivitis in man. It shows promise as a therapeutic agent by itself and may prove to be helpful as an adjuvant with other antiviral chemotherapeutic agents.

Other antiviral substances such as phosphonoacetic acid (PAA) and its related derivative compounds and acyclo-guanine are under laboratory investigation in tissue culture and in animal models. They seem promising and will perhaps be available for human evaluation.

Corticosteroids. Herpetic infection of the uveal tract with inflammation of the iris and the choroid may occur with or without the superficial ulceration. In such patients, the secondary glaucoma that may develop is best treated with atropine drops. In the rare patient with uveal tract involvement without superficial ulceration, steroids are sometimes used but under very careful observation. In the presence of dendritic or ameboid ulceration corticosteroids are contraindicated. Steroids are known to worsen superficial epithelial lesions, causing perforation of the cornea with resulting herniation of the vitreous body of the eye.

The allergic discoform keratitis is also treated with steroids; however, only an experienced ophthalmologist should provide such treatment.

HIDRADENITIS SUPPURATIVA

method of
FRED F. CASTROW II, M.D.
Houston, Texas

The lesions of hidradenitis suppurativa are caused by a blockage of the apocrine sweat glands with subsequent secondary infection. The term apocrinitis applies to the acute stage and is characterized by nonsuppurative, tender, nodular lesions. Apocrinitis and hidradenitis occur where there is an abundance of apocrine glands, such as the axillary region, genitocrural region, buttocks, umbilicus, breast, and occasionally aberrant sites. The early nodular lesions are tender, but not of the exquisite nature of a furuncle. The lesions are often misdiagnosed and treated as furunculosis or perirectal abscesses. In the early stage of the disease the lesions are confined principally to the dermis but later dissect toward subcutaneous tissue and form multiple sinus tracts which erupt to the surface. Hypertrophic scars occur frequently. The lesions have the tendency to become very resistant to all types of conservative treatment. In cases of advanced hidradenitis suppurativa, the lesions dissect laterally to form pockets filled with pus and a characteristic gelatinous material. It should be noted that as these lesions advance and spread laterally, they rarely or never break into the deep subcutaneous tissue.

If there are a few isolated lesions only, they can be treated under local anesthesia, but treatment of the more extensive eruption must be performed under a general anesthetic. The steps of the method are as follows:

1. A probe is inserted into each sinus tract, and the superficial tissue is incised so as to effect complete exteriorization. The multiple interconnecting sinus tracts often give the lesion a honeycomb appearance. Any redundant tissue is removed during this stage of the procedure.

2. The multiple cavities containing pus and the sticky gelatinous material are adequately drained, and the lining is thoroughly curetted with a dermal or uterine curette.

3. The entire exteriorized area is extensively coagulated with a bipolar current. The bipolar electrocoagulation serves to stop the bleeding, helps destroy the lining of the cavity, and minimizes postoperative pain by temporarily sealing the nerve endings.

4. Starting on the first postoperative day, hot compresses or sitz baths are utilized three times daily, and antibiotics, such as the combination of neomycin-polymyxin-bacitracin, are applied locally. Immediate postoperative discomfort is negligible and is tolerated better than the preoperative pain inherent in the hidradenitis.

Many patients are cured by the operation; in others, a few new lesions develop. These new abscesses are treated early in the same manner as the original ones. Complete healing in severe cases occurs within 3 weeks to 2 months after the operation. The average time required for complete healing varies from 4 to 6 weeks.

The precursor lesions of hidradenitis, comedones, may be treated with the use of vitamin A acid locally. The vitamin A acid should be applied sparingly and only frequently enough to produce minimal erythema. Systemic antibiotics, especially tetracycline, are of adjunctive benefit to control the secondary bacterial infection but should not be relied upon to bring about complete resolution of the hidradenitis. Superficial x-ray therapy and various other surgical approaches have been used effectively in the treatment of hidradenitis suppurativa, but these methods require either special equipment or specialized surgical skills.

KELOIDS

method of
ERVIN EPSTEIN, M.D.
Oakland, California

When treating keloids, one must be very conservative in discussion of the prognosis. It is true that none of the methods described are universally successful, and even after the most efficacious therapy, the results are limited. In other words, the patient must realize that he will still have a scar. Although it may be thinner and narrower than previously, his skin will not revert to its prekeloidal state. The more deforming the keloid, the more apparent the improvement will be. The converse is true also; however, the more minimal the deformity, the less obvious will be the benefit.

Although hypertrophic scars may regress spontaneously in contradistinction to true keloids, the therapy of the two entities is identical. Therefore, in this discussion the two terms are employed interchangeably.

The cause of keloids is not well understood. They occur more commonly in blacks but are certainly not confined to that group. Certain areas of the body develop these hypertrophic lesions more frequently than others. For instance, surgical procedures on the chest and feet are notorious for resulting in this complication. Keloids tend to be multiple, but the presence of these tumors does not indicate that keloidal formation will occur after another surgical procedure in the same person. These lesions are common following intraperitoneal surgery but tend to be minor. Dermabrasion may result in these changes, especially if the skin around the chin should slip while the operator is applying the whirling brush. This can be avoided by holding the skin firmly in place during the procedure. Electrosurgical removals are more apt to produce hypertrophic scars than those performed with cold steel excision.

In treating keloids or hypertrophic scars, combinations of modalities may be necessary to obtain a satisfactory result.

Surgery

Surgery is probably the most successful approach, especially if combined with postoperative radiotherapy or the intralesional injection of corticosteroids, or both. Certain principles must be adhered to in the attempt to eradicate the keloid. The entire scarred area must be excised peripherally and deeply. Tension must be relieved by undercutting the surrounding tissues and the employment of subcutaneous sutures. The excision should be followed by the local applications or, even better, the intralesional injection of corticosteroids. If a hypertrophic scar shows evidence of development, radiation therapy should be instituted promptly. The wound should be approximated expertly. If the defect is too large to close per primum, skin grafting should be enlisted. There are many applicable methods of closure, but a commonly employed one is the use of a subcutaneous stitch employing 5-0 catgut or 6-0 silk. The edges of the wound are approximated with 6-0 silk or nylon or another nonabsorbable suture. Clips and adhesive tape (Steri-Strips) do not produce adequate approximation. Retention sutures are unnecessary if the wound is mobilized sufficiently.

Another procedure that may be adequate is shaving off the neoplasm under local anesthesia. The bleeding may be controlled by the application of a hemostatic preparation such as absorbable gelatin (Gelfoam) or by the use of trichloroacetic acid. This will convert an old keloid into a new one and make it more responsive to x-ray therapy or corticosteroid injections or both.

Corticosteroids

There is no evidence that the local application of corticosteroid creams or liquids to the unbroken skin exerts a favorable effect on keloids. If the surface is removed, as in the shaving technique described, steroid application may furnish a beneficial effect in preventing the recurrence of the scarring process. Systemic administration of these therapeutic agents is ineffective in controlling keloid formation therapeutically or prophylactically. On the other hand, the intralesional injection of these preparations may be helpful in flattening such a cicatrix or in making it more radiosensitive. The dosage ranges from 2 mg. per ml. to 10 mg. per ml. The preferred diluent is isotonic saline solution, as it minimizes complications due to local anesthetics and, surprisingly, the injection of such a mixture causes *less* discomfort than if a procaine or lidocaine solution is employed as the diluent. Depending on the size of the lesion, one may inject 10 to 30 ml. in a single session without encountering undue complications. This should be administered under considerable pressure, through a pressure syringe with three finger holes. The injection, however, should be administered comparatively superficially. The purpose of the therapy is to produce atrophy of the fibrous tissue. The injection may be repeated as often as desired, and as many treatments as are necessary to produce the desired result may be given. An intralesional steroid may be employed as the only therapeutic agent or may be combined with surgical therapy, radiation or cryosurgery.

Radiation Therapy

Although clinical evidence supports the contention that x-ray therapy can be applied safely, especially in adults, current thought has made the use of this modality in benign conditions unpopular in many quarters. However, it is a valuable procedure for the control of these scars. The usual dosage ranges from 75 R once a week for 12 weeks to 200 R every 3 weeks for 4 treatments. The latter seems to be the more effective regimen. The beam selected depends on the thickness of the neoplasm. As a general rule, we employ one with a kilovoltage of 120, milliamperage of 5, a distance of 8 inches and a half-value layer of approximately 4.5 mm. of aluminum. The area around the keloid should be carefully shielded with lead and a cone used to prevent stray rays from reaching the patient or the operator. These lesions tend to lose their radiosensitivity with time, so this ionizing radiation is effective only during the first 6 months after the appearance of the keloid. The sensitivity can be restored by surgical removal of the growth or by the intralesional injection of corticosteroids.

Other Measures

Cryotherapy with liquid nitrogen or carbon dioxide slush may flatten keloids. Unfortunately, at times, it may increase the scarring. One can apply the liquid nitrogen by spray or with a cotton applicator stick. Carbon dioxide slush may be made by pounding dry ice with a hammer, adding enough acetone to give it the consistency of a sherbet and applying it to the skin with a cotton-tipped applicator. The treatment time required varies with the thickness of the scar. One can avoid freezing the surrounding normal tissue by cutting out an aperture the size and shape of the cicatrix in a piece of cardboard and placing this over the scar so that the uninvolved tissue will be protected. In my experience, cryotherapy is less effective than the other methods described.

Proteolytic enzymes injected intralesionally have not been beneficial in my experience.

WARNING. To avoid having disappointed patients and medicolegal entanglements, be conservative in predicting and promising the benefits to be gained from the treatment of keloids and hypertrophic scars.

LICHEN PLANUS

method of
HARRY L. WECHSLER, M.D.
McKeesport, Pennsylvania

Lichen planus is an occasionally occurring papular scaling eruption, usually pruritic, at times acute and generalized, but more often chronic and localized to selective areas. Such sites of predilection are volar aspect of the wrists, small of the back, medial aspect of the thighs, anterior tibial areas, dorsa of feet, and ankles. The scalp is rarely involved and the palmar-plantar areas and nails infrequently. Mucous membrane lesions are not uncommon, particularly on the sides of the buccal mucosa, but lesions of the glans penis and vulva occur less frequently.

The primary lesion is a shiny, flat-topped, violaceous polygonal-shaped papule that, on close inspection, shows fine whitish lines known as Wickham's striae. The lesions are usually discrete but may coalesce to form plaques. Linear arrangement is indicative of a Koebner or isomorphic phenomenon. The papular lesions at times may be atrophic or hypertrophic. The latter may be verrucoid, particularly on the legs. Although the characteristic lesion is a papule, it can be vesicular, bullous, and consequently erosive. This is usually true of palmar-plantar involvement, in which eroded erythematous patches are difficult to distinguish clinically and histologically from lupus erythematosus. Characteristic buccal mucosal lesions are whitish lacelike plaques. However, any of the oral membranes may be involved by a bullous-erosive eruption that can be quite tender and disabling. These have been reported on occasion to undergo malignant degeneration. Scalp involvement may lead to a scarring alopecia. Nail involvement may vary from focal change to complete destruction with scarring of the nail bed. Typical skin lesions resolve with residual pigmentation.

The cause is usually unknown, but a small percentage of cases is caused by such drugs as antimalarials, quinidine, gold, arsenic, para-aminosalicylic acid, bismuth, phenothiazine, thiazide, streptomycin, and methyldopa. A clue that may indicate a drug cause, e.g., quinacrine hydrochloride (Atabrine) and quinidine, is the appearance of lesions over photolocalizing areas such as the sides of the neck and dorsa of the hands. This suggests that some drug eruptions are due to photosensitization. A lichen planus-like contact dermatitis results from exposure to color film developers. Lichen planus may be associated with dermatophytosis and also may be a manifestation of chronic graft-versus-host-disease.

Treatment

1. If caused by a drug, discontinue the drug.

2. When dermatophytosis is present, treat with griseofulvin ultramicrosized and microsized (Fulvicin-U/F, Grifulvin V, Grisactin, and Gris-PEG). These usually beneficially affect the lichen planus.

3. The most effective form of therapy, particularly for the acute and generalized types, is systemic corticosteroids given orally as prednisone, 20 to 30 mg. daily for about two weeks, then taper the dose over the next 4 to 5 weeks.

4. Topical corticosteroids are of little benefit, except under occlusion (Aristocort, Kenalog, Cordran, Synalar—all regular strength). Apply at bedtime and wrap with a plastic sheet (Saran Wrap). Remove the wrappings in the morning. Plastic gloves for the hands and plastic bags for the feet can be used.

5. For oral involvement, a topical preparation consisting of prednisone, 20 mg., crushed to a powder and added to 60 ml. of an antihistamine elixir may be useful. Before meals and at bedtime a teaspoonful should be swished about in the mouth for 2 minutes and then swallowed.

6. If only a few lesions of the skin are present, intralesional injection of 2 to 3 ml. of triamcinolone acetonide (Kenalog-10 diluted two to

three times with isotonic saline or diluting solution) is effective.

7. Antihistaminic drugs and mild tranquilizers may offer some symptomatic relief.

PHOTOSENSITIVITY AND SUNBURN

method of
JOHN A. PARRISH, M.D.
Boston, Massachusetts

Introduction

The sun is the energy source of all life on earth and emits a wide range of electromagnetic energy extending from radiowaves through infrared, visible, and ultraviolet to x-rays. It is the ultraviolet (UV) component (290 to 400 nm.) of sunlight which causes most skin reactions. Because shorter wavelengths are absorbed by atmospheric ozone and longer wavelengths are much less effective, it is the middle ultraviolet (UV-B, 290 to 320 nm.) which primarily causes sunburn, suntan, and skin cancer. However, long wavelength ultraviolet (UV-A, 320 to 400 nm.) may augment these cutaneous reactions, and it is this waveband that is primarily responsible for most drug- or chemical-induced photosensitivity reactions. Sensitivity in certain diseases may extend into the visible portion of sunlight or artificial light.

Photoprotection

Tanning. Melanin, the pigment naturally occurring in skin, is unquestionably a good sunscreen. Genetic factors, however, determine the constitutive (base-line) skin color of a person, as well as the ability to tan in response to UV exposure. Cautious graduated exposures permit progressive tanning without sunburn in all but the poorest responders. Both the ability to tan and its final extent may be increased by PUVA (oral psoralen, e.g., methoxsalen [0.6 mg. per kg.], followed by exposure to artificial or solar UV-A). Great care with exposure times is essential, as severe phototoxicity can result from the steep dose-response curve. Ideally a radiometer should be used to monitor the UV-A dose.

Sun Avoidance. Any measures that reduce exposure of the skin to strong sunlight should be exploited. Outdoor activities should be timed to avoid the peak UV-B times (10:00 A.M. to 2:00 P.M.). Long hair growth helps shade the ears and neck. Broad-brimmed hats and long-sleeved clothing significantly reduce the impact of harmful ultraviolet rays, but it should be remembered that light-textured materials, especially when wet, only partially block the passage of UV-B. Beach umbrellas, although protecting against direct sunlight, may not prevent sunburn from UV-B scattered from the sky or reflected from sand. Windowglass blocks UV-B but not UV-A. This may be relevant in the management of certain photosensitivity states (see below).

Sunscreens. Sunscreens occupy a position in the borderline between medications and cosmetics, and the subject is clouded by misconceptions and folklore. The most common incorrect belief is that certain preparations can promote a tan. Since tanning and sunburn both result from the same ultraviolet waveband, one cannot be promoted independently of the other. Many of the innumerable commercially available preparations that claim to promote tanning provide no protection whatsoever. The most effective and cosmetically acceptable sunscreens are those which contain para-aminobenzoic acid (PABA), PABA esters, benzophenones, and cinnamates (Table 1) in suitable vehicles that promote adherence to the skin. Drug-induced and endogenous photosensitivity reactions (e.g., polymorphic photodermatitis) require screens effective against the longer ultraviolet wavelengths (Solbar, Uval, Piz Buin Exclusive Extrem). In the treatment of certain light-induced pigment disorders (e.g., melasma), opaque sunscreens must be used (Reflecta, Covermark). Ideally, sunscreens should be applied 30 to 60 minutes before the onset of sun exposure and must be reapplied after swimming or excessive sweating.

Treatment of Sunburn

1. Cold compresses of isotonic saline or Burow's solution 1:40 or plain tap water.

2. Tepid tub baths with or without nonirritating additives (e.g., bath oils).

3. Topical fluorinated steroids such as triamcinolone cream 0.025 per cent three or four times daily and under compresses. Steroid-induced vasoconstriction may reduce erythema, itching,

TABLE 1. **Topical Sunscreens**

ABSORBING AGENT	EXAMPLES
PABA	PreSun, Pabanol
Esters of PABA	Sea & Ski, Pabafilm, Block Out
Benzophenones	Solbar, Uval
Combinations (cinnamates and benzophenones)	Piz Buin

and general discomfort. However, there is no evidence that corticosteroids diminish cell damage.

4. Severe sunburn or dangerous accidental overexposure may be treated with systemic corticosteroids. In normal, healthy persons a brief course (e.g., oral prednisone, beginning with 40 to 60 mg. and tapering over 4 to 8 days) will abort severe sunburn.

Photosensitivity Disorders

Solar Urticaria. Solar urticaria is a rare disorder, probably of several different pathogenic mechanisms, in which hives appear within minutes of exposure to sunlight. If the threshold is high enough, some patients can be controlled simply by avoiding prolonged unprotected sun exposure. Other very sensitive patients must avoid any daytime exposure. Most patients are not helped by antihistamines. It is possible to slowly build up sun tolerance by using carefully metered, graduated exposure to artificial light which stimulates pigmentation and possibly depletes the UV-induced mediators of urticaria.

Polymorphous Light Eruption. Severe reactions may be managed as outlined for sunburn, but chronic use of systemic corticosteroids is not recommended. If patients anticipate an unavoidable intense or prolonged sun exposure, they may take a short course of hydroxychloroquine sulfate (Plaquenil), 200 mg. once or twice a day beginning 2 or 3 days prior to exposure. (This use of Plaquenil is not listed in the manufacturer's official directive.) A potential adverse effect of long-term use is deposition in the retina and occasionally irreversible retinal damage. Ocular examinations are advisable once or twice a year, depending upon frequency of use.

Long-term management of mild cases can be achieved by simply avoiding midday sun and using sunscreens. Those more photosensitive patients can also be treated by a careful course of PUVA which tans, depletes mediators, or diminishes lymphocyte capabilities. Beta-carotene (120 to 180 mg. orally per day) is occasionally beneficial. Usually no treatment is required in winter.

Porphyria Cutanea Tarda. The precipitating agents, commonly ethanol or estrogens, should be sought and withdrawn. Phlebotomy has proved to be the most useful treatment to date. Remove 300 to 500 ml. of blood every 3 to 4 weeks until urine porphyrins are normal, or until the hematocrit falls to 85 per cent of its original value. Alkalinization of urine and small doses of antimalarials are still experimental, require close supervision, and may be dangerous, but are sometimes effective.

TABLE 2. **Contact Photosensitizers**

Cosmetics
  Perfumes, colognes, after-shave lotions (essential oils and psoralens)
  Lipsticks (fluorescein derivatives)
  Creams and hair preparations (coal tar derivatives)
Plants (phytophotodermatitis)
  Persian limes
  Pink rot-infected celery
  Many plants of the Umbelliferae and Rutaceae families (These problems are primarily due to psoralen compounds)
Therapeutic Agents
  Phenothiazines and sulfonamides (usually used therapeutically)
  Halogenated salicylanilides
  Sunscreens
  Blankophores (usually photoallergic)
  Diuretics

Erythropoietic Protoporphyria. The most impressive symptom is burning pain within minutes of light exposure, followed by edema and itching if the patient remains in the sun. Oral beta-carotene (Solatene), 60 to 240 mg. daily, decreases subjective symptoms dramatically in some patients. It often requires 6 to 8 weeks of therapy before significant symptomatic relief is noticeable.

Lupus Erythematosus. Sunburn or chronic sun exposure may precipitate or aggravate lesions of chronic discoid lupus erythematosus. Moderate sun exposure often is not harmful to uninvolved skin. Sunscreens are suggested, and hydroxychloroquine (Plaquenil) and topical steroids may be used during times of disease activity. Patients with systemic lupus erythematosus should avoid being sunburned.

Drug-Induced Photosensitivity. Many drugs and chemicals can cause phototoxic or photoallergic reactions upon sun exposure. Examples include thiazide diuretics, antibacterial sulfonamides, sulfonylurea antidiabetic drugs, phenothiazines (especially chlorpromazine), griseofulvin, demethylchlortetracycline, and psoralens (methoxsalen). As soon as is practical, the drug should be discontinued. Otherwise, sun avoidance and clothing are necessary. Sunscreens should block the UV-A as well as UV-B.

Contact Photosensitivity Dermatitis. Table 2 lists contact photosensitizers. Patients photosensitized to halogenated salicylanilides may remain photosensitive for several years, even after the offending chemical is removed. Exposure to psoralens occurs in agriculture workers handling pink-rot celery or carrots. Treatment is to avoid exposure to both sun and the offending agent and treat as for any contact dermatitis.

LUPUS ERYTHEMATOSUS

method of
JAMES C. STEIGERWALD, M.D.,
JOHN ASSINI, M.D.,
and MICHAEL SILVERMAN, M.D.
Denver, Colorado

Lupus erythematosus (LE) is a disease with varied clinical manifestations, ranging from involvement limited to the skin (discoid lupus erythematosus) to multisystem involvement (systemic lupus erythematosus). Since the cause or causes is unknown, the goal of any treatment program is to suppress the symptoms and signs of the disease. The majority of patients with LE do experience spontaneous or drug-induced remissions with some patients (10 to 20 per cent) sustaining long periods of inactive disease on no medication. Once a diagnosis of LE is made, however, the patient is at some risk for disease exacerbation for the remainder of his or her life.

Discoid Lupus Erythematosus

Since 5 to 10 per cent of patients with discoid lupus erythematosus (DLE) will eventually develop systemic lupus erythematosus (SLE), and since approximately 80 per cent of patients with SLE do have skin manifestations (25 per cent with discoid-like lesions), all patients with LE require the following evaluations:

1. A complete history and physical examination.

2. Complete blood count, platelet count, Westergren sedimentation rate, urinalysis, and chest x-ray are part of our routine evaluation. In addition a Venereal Disease Research Laboratories test (VDRL) and a test for the presence of antinuclear antibodies in the serum should be performed at the initial evaluation.

Once the diagnosis of discoid lupus erythematosus (DLE) is confirmed, the following treatment plan is used.

General Measures. 1. The diagnosis and prognosis of DLE should be discussed with the patient. The fact that 90 to 95 per cent of patients with DLE do not develop other organ system involvement should be stressed. The chronicity of the disease and the need for long-term follow-up are also emphasized.

2. If the rash is photosensitive, the patient should be counseled on the use of wide brim hats and clothes that provide a maximum of skin coverage outdoors. Regular window glass filters out the sun's rays that are harmful to the photosensitive LE patient.

3. Cosmetic agents (for example, Lydia O'Leary Covermark) are available to hide prominent skin lesions. If alopecia is significant, a wig is also useful.

Local Therapy. Since the majority of DLE lesions are exacerbated by sun exposure, a sun screen should be used when the patient plans to spend more than brief periods outdoors. Preparations containing para-aminobenzoic acid (PABA) in an alcohol base (Presun, Pabanol, Eclipse) should be applied one hour before and every 4 to 6 hours during sun exposure.

2. Small inflammatory lesions generally respond quite well to one of the fluorinated corticosteroid creams or ointments. Fluocinonide (Lidex) cream or ointment 0.05 per cent applied four times a day has been very effective in our experience, although other preparations including halcinonide (Halog), triamcinolone (Kenalog), fluocinolone (Synalar), triamcinolone (Aristocort), flurandrenolide (Cordran), and betamethasone (Valisone) may be equally as useful.

3. More resistant inflammatory lesions not responsive to simple application of the fluorinated corticosteroid creams or ointments may require the use of a flurandrenolide impregnated tape (Cordran Tape) for small areas or a plastic wrap (Saran Wrap) after applications of the creams or ointment for larger areas. These tapes or wraps may be kept on for 12 to 24 hours and allow for increased penetration of the fluorinated compounds.

4. Occasionally, a lesion will be so refractory to the other local treatment that an intralesional injection of triamcinolone acetonide (Kenalog-10) may be warranted. Using a No. 25 needle, 0.1 ml. is injected into a 1 to 2 cm. lesion. Although this technique is effective, temporary or permanent atrophy of skin and subcutaneous tissue at the site of injection is fairly common. Because of this side effect, we rarely resort to intralesional injections.

5. For areas of involvement that do not respond well to ointments or creams, such as hair or mucous membrane areas, other preparations are available. Corticosteroid solutions (Synalar, Cordran) work well in hairy areas, while a corticosteroid preparation with a special base triamcinolone acetonide (Kenalog in Orabase) works best for mucous membrane areas.

Systemic Therapy. If the local measures discussed above have not adequately controlled the discoid lesions, systemic therapy should be begun.

ANTIMALARIALS. These drugs are currently the systemic drugs of choice for the skin lesions of DLE. Although both hydroxychloroquine (Plaquenil) and chloroquine (Aralen) are effective (this use of chloroquine is not listed in the manufacturer's official directive), we use only hydroxychloroquine since the ocular side effects from chloroquine are more common. After an ophthalmologic examination, which should include slit lamp, funduscopic and visual field examinations, hydroxychloroquine is begun at a dosage of 200 mg. twice daily. This dosage schedule is maintained for up to 3 to 4 months, at which time it is reduced to 200 mg. per day. If the lesions have responded to this treatment program, an attempt should be made to discontinue the hydroxychloroquine after the patient has been stable for 2 to 3 months. While on the hydroxychloroquine, the patient should have complete ophthalmologic examinations every 4 months. If any signs of retinal toxicity are noted, the medication should be stopped immediately. Further eye examinations are still mandatory, for the retinal lesions may progress even after the medication has been discontinued.

If the skin lesions have not responded to hydroxychloroquine, quinacrine (Atabrine), 100 mg. per day, may be added to the treatment program (this use of quinacrine is not listed in the manufacturer's official directive). While we have found this to be quite helpful in improving the discoid skin lesions, the yellow discoloration of the skin caused by quinacrine has been a side effect generally unacceptable to the patient.

CORTICOSTEROIDS. In severe, scarring DLE unresponsive to other forms of therapy, a trial of 5 to 10 mg. of prednisone once daily is warranted.

Systemic Lupus Erythematosus

Systemic lupus erythematosus (SLE) in its full blown stage can involve any organ system in the body.

Our general approach to therapy is to assess each organ system for disease activity. The appropriate overall therapy is then determined, using the least toxic therapy that should benefit all involved systems. The general well-being of the patient is considered an "organ system" for the purposes of this discussion.

General Measures. Certain general measures are worthwhile incorporating in the treatment of any lupus patient. Foremost among these is sun avoidance, since sun exposure in certain patients will cause not only a skin rash but also a flare of systemic disease. Sun avoidance measures are outlined earlier.

Rest is another important feature in the treatment of SLE patients, particularly when fatigue is a prominent complaint. This poorly understood feature of the disease may at times be incapacitating. When such is the case, prednisone at a dose of 10 to 20 mg. every other day usually brings gratifying results.

Another constitutional symptom that can be quite distressing is fever, which often occurs at night. If fever does not respond to the usual antipyretics, indomethacin, 50 to 200 mg. daily, can be quite effective. (This use of indomethacin is not specifically listed in the manufacturer's official directive.)

Since SLE is, by-and-large, a disease of young females, the physician is often faced with a patient who is, or who would like to become, pregnant. As a general rule, we discourage pregnancy while the lupus is active. If the disease should flare during pregnancy, the corticosteroid dose may be adjusted accordingly with minimal danger to the fetus. Therapeutic abortion is not indicated and may in fact exacerbate a flare. Finally, we increase corticosteroids to cover the stress of delivery and maintain them at this elevated level for two months before tapering is undertaken.

Skin. The treatment of skin lesions is discussed in the section on discoid lupus erythematosus. Local therapy is generally still indicated, even when systemic treatment is used for other organ system involvement.

Musculoskeletal. Arthralgias and arthritis are the most common clinical manifestation of SLE. Salicylates are the initial drug of choice beginning at 900 to 1200 mg. four times a day and adjusting the dosage depending on the patient's response. If further anti-inflammatory therapy is needed, one of the nonsteroidal anti-inflammatory drugs (NSAID) is added to salicylates. Our preference is indomethacin, 25 mg. three or four times daily, although any of the NSAID may be effective. If musculoskeletal problems persist after an adequate (4 week) trial of the combination of salicylates and a NSAID, we would then stop the NSAID and add hydroxychloroquine, 200 mg. twice daily. This drug is most effective in suppressing skin and musculoskeletal disease activity.

Hematologic. A normochromic, normocytic anemia of chronic disease is seen in 50 to 80 per cent of patients, its severity usually correlated with disease activity.

Although a positive Coombs' test is not uncommon in SLE, less than 5 per cent of patients will demonstrate significant hemolysis. If evidence of a Coombs' positive hemolytic anemia is present, we recommend daily oral corticosteroid therapy (equivalent to 40 to 80 mg. of prednisone), the higher doses being used for the more severe hemolytic reactions (less than 10 grams of hemoglobin).

Thrombocytopenia occurs in 5 to 25 per cent of patients and thrombocytopenia purpura may be the presenting manifestation of SLE. Qualitative defects such as decreased platelet aggregation are not uncommon but generally do not require therapy. Thrombocytopenia often responds to oral daily corticosteroid therapy (equivalent to 40 to 80 mg. of prednisone). We recommend therapy with 80 mg. of prednisone for platelet counts below 30,000 per cu. mm.; treatment for platelet counts above 30,000 per cu. mm. is dependent upon the rate of decrease and the presence of bleeding. In more refractory cases, splenectomy may be curative. A small percentage of patients may also require oral immunosuppressive therapy (cyclophosphamide or azathioprine, 1.5 to 2.5 mg. per kg. per day). (This use of these agents is not listed in the manufacturers' official directives.)

Although leukopenia may occur in up to 80 per cent of patients, neutropenia is uncommon and therapy is not required.

In addition to quantitative and qualitative platelet defects, hemostatic abnormalities include circulating anticoagulants, hypoprothrombinemia, and acquired von Willebrand's syndrome. Although approximately 10 per cent of patients will demonstrate a circulating anticoagulant, these gamma globulins rarely, if ever, cause serious bleeding; thus therapy is usually not required unless coexistent thrombocytopenia is present.

Pleuropulmonary.   Pleuritis, with or without pleural effusion, occurs in as many as 30 per cent of patients with SLE. While it may be self-limiting, pleuritic pain is often severe enough to warrant symptomatic therapy. Nonsteroidal anti-inflammatory agents, particularly indomethacin, 75 to 150 mg. per day in divided doses, are efficacious in milder cases. When pleurisy accompanies skin rash and arthritis, hydroxychloroquine may ameliorate all symptoms. In more severe, refractory cases, or in patients with large recurrent effusions, we give prednisone, 20 to 40 mg. once a day, although this treatment is not uniformly successful.

Acute lupus pneumonitis must be differentiated from other causes of pulmonary infiltrates and hypoxemia. Patients invariably require such supportive measures as oxygen and fluid therapy. Once the diagnosis of acute lupus pneumonitis is made, prednisone, 60 to 100 mg. daily or its parenteral equivalent, should be given. Patients who are slow to respond to this regimen are begun on azathioprine, 1.5 to 2.5 mg. per kg. per day. (This use of azathioprine is not listed in the manufacturer's official directive.)

Cardiac.   Pericarditis is the most frequent cardiac abnormality in SLE, occurring in approximately 30 per cent of cases. If the pain is mild, we first recommend salicylates (3600 to 4800 mg. daily in divided doses). With more severe pain, indomethacin (100 to 150 mg. daily in divided doses) is often effective. In refractory cases, we recommend oral daily corticosteroid therapy (equivalent to 20 mg. of prednisone). Intravenous steroid preparations may be necessary when the danger of tamponade is imminent. Rarely, pericardiocentesis or pericardiectomy may be required.

SLE myocarditis is often associated with pericarditis and endocarditis. If congestive heart failure is present, we recommend, in addition to the standard therapy, a course of oral daily corticosteroids (20 mg. of prednisone).

In any patient with SLE who develops valvular lesions, verrucous endocarditis (Libman-Sacks) must be suspected. Once infective endocarditis has been ruled out, we recommend a trial of oral daily corticosteroids (60 mg. of prednisone). In our experience, response to steroid therapy is unpredictable, with some patients eventually requiring valve surgery.

Central Nervous System.   Central nervous system involvement may be manifested by seizure disorders, which generally respond well to anticonvulsant medication and moderate doses of corticosteroids (10 to 20 mg. per day of prednisone). Cerebral vasculitis, psychosis, or transverse myelitis respond less well to treatment and may require very high doses of prednisone (80 to 200 mg. per day). If there is confusion as to whether a psychosis is related to disease activity or is steroid-induced, we increase steroids if other aspects of the disease are flaring and taper them if the patient is otherwise doing well.

Renal.   Our initial therapy of lupus nephritis, when possible, is guided by the findings on renal biopsy. During follow-up, however, changes in treatment are most often based on laboratory findings. The most useful of these are creatinine clearance, activity of urinary sediment, amount of proteinuria, anti-DNA antibody titer, and total hemolytic complement level.

Mesangial lupus nephritis does not require treatment. Likewise, patients with focal proliferative nephritis generally pursue a mild course and are given corticosteroids only in doses needed to control non-renal manifestations.

The diagnosis of *diffuse proliferative glomerulonephritis* carries with it a poor prognosis and necessitates aggressive therapy. Patients are begun on prednisone, 40 to 60 mg. daily in a single dose. This is maintained for 4 to 6 months. If no improvement is seen or if glucocorticoid side effects are unacceptable at this dose, we then add azathioprine or cyclophosphamide at a dose of 1.5 to 2.5 mg. per kg. per day. (This use of these agents is not listed in the manufacturers' official directives.) Once clinical improvement occurs, the drugs may be tapered slowly. It is important that, except in the case of drug toxicity, azathioprine be tapered very gradually.

Only a minority of patients with *membranous nephropathy* and nephrotic syndrome will respond to corticosteroid therapy. Nevertheless, selected patients with large amounts of urinary protein may be tried on prednisone in doses similar to those used in diffuse proliferative disease. If, after 4 months, no decrease in proteinuria occurs, we judge the patient to be steroid-unresponsive and the drug is withdrawn.

Patients with significant lupus nephritis require the same types of general therapy as do other patients with chronic renal disease. End-stage renal failure may be treated with dialysis and renal transplantation.

Drugs. When treating patients with SLE, it is imperative that one be familiar with the side effects and complications of the drugs used, since these may occasionally mimic the manifestations of the underlying disease.

SALICYLATES. In addition to the well-recognized gastrointestinal and auditory side effects, there is an increased incidence of hepatotoxicity and nephrotoxicity. Liver damage may present as a toxic hepatitis or as elevated transaminases on routine screening. An elevated serum creatinine that falls to normal upon salicylate cessation may be the only evidence of nephrotoxicity. We recommend that both liver and renal function tests be monitored when SLE patients are receiving salicylates.

NONSTEROIDAL ANTI-INFLAMMATORY DRUGS. The most commonly used, indomethacin (Indocin), is an indole derivative whose well known side effects involve the gastrointestinal and central nervous systems. Generally, we do not recommend it in children under the age of 14 because of its hepatotoxicity. The other NSAID have similar actions and side effects, but their efficacy in SLE has not been clearly established. Phenylbutazone (Butazolidin) is recommended only for short-term therapy because of its potential bone marrow toxicity (see manufacturers' official directives before using these agents).

ANTIMALARIALS. The antimalarial we use in the treatment of SLE is a 4-amino-quinolone derivative, hydroxychloroquine (Plaquenil). The major toxicity is ocular. Fine deposits of the drug may occur in the corneal epithelium, but this keratopathy is often asymptomatic. If visual complaints do occur, the most common are halos around lights and photophobia, but visual acuity is rarely affected. Unless the symptoms are severe, the drug may be continued. The primary toxic effect is pigmentary retinal degeneration. We recommend careful routine ophthalmologic examination every 4 months, since the retinopathy is usually irreversible and may progress after the drug has been stopped.

In addition to the ocular toxicity, hydroxychloroquine has been known to cause respiratory depression in young children, and thus we avoid its use in the pediatric population. Other side effects include skin rashes, muscle weakness, and gastrointestinal distress.

The other antimalarial we use is quinacrine (Atabrine). (This use of quinacrine is not listed in the manufacturer's official directive.) Its retinal toxicity is less than that of hydroxychloroquine, but pigmentation changes of the skin, nails, and mucous membranes may be significant. We recommend yearly ophthalmologic evaluation as well as a complete blood count (CBC) every 1 to 2 months.

CORTICOSTEROIDS. Corticosteroid therapy is usually reserved for patients with involvement of vital organs or severe multisystem disease. Since daily therapy is often necessary to control symptoms, toxicity from long-term steroid use can be significant. When steroid therapy is employed, we recommend that it be given as a single morning dose and be changed to alternate day dosage as soon as the clinical setting permits.

The complications of steroids are multiple, increasing in frequency as the dose and duration of therapy increase. Complications that are particularly pertinent when treating SLE patients include myopathy, osteoporosis, and aseptic necrosis of bone. Chronic corticosteroid therapy may also promote and accelerate the atherosclerotic process.

Once the therapeutically desired effect has been obtained, tapering of the steroids should be attempted, tapering no more than 10 per cent of the dose at any one time. Rapidity of tapering is dependent upon the original dose and the length of therapy—the lower the dose and longer the therapy, the slower the tapering. We recommend tapering to an alternate day regimen first, if clinically feasible.

CYTOTOXIC AGENTS. Cyclophosphamide (Cytoxan) and azathioprine (Imuran) are the two most commonly used cytotoxic drugs. (This use of these agents is not listed in the manufacturers' official directives.) Daily doses of 1.5 to 2.5 mg. per kg. per day are often effective when major organ involvement is present. Because of their bone marrow toxicity, we recommend the complete blood count (CBC) be monitored regularly (every 1 to 2 weeks) to detect early changes.

Adequate hydration should be stressed to the patient on cyclophosphamide to decrease the chances of hemorrhagic cystitis. In addition, regular urinalysis is recommended to detect hematuria. With azathioprine, we regularly monitor liver function tests to detect any transaminase elevation.

DISORDERS OF THE MOUTH (BENIGN)

method of
MANUEL G. BLOOM, M.D.
Houston, Texas

Benign disorders of the oral mucosa include not only the oral manifestations of systemic and cutaneous diseases but also a host of processes related to the physiologic, histologic, anatomic, and mechanical conditions peculiar to the mouth. Consequently, correct diagnosis of oral problems, which must precede definitive therapy, also requires careful examination of the skin and, occasionally, a general medical evaluation.

In diagnosing oral disease it must be remembered that mucosal lesions are rapidly altered by chewing, nibbling, rubbing with the tongue, and irritation from malfitting dentures or carious teeth, as well as by the persistent use of tobacco, snuff, betel nut, and hard candies. Vesicles, bullae, and pustules rupture rapidly to leave erosions and ulcers. Poor dental hygiene permits rapid overgrowth of organisms and results in secondary infections.

Maximal therapy of oral disease frequently requires close cooperation between physician and dentist. The presence of plaque, calculus, periodontitis, caries, ill-fitting dental appliances, and malocclusion must be treated by a qualified dentist. Maintenance of good oral hygiene is the first step in treatment of oral disease. The patient should be instructed in the proper use of the tooth brush, unwaxed dental floss, interdental stimulation (rubber tip on a tooth brush or Stimudents), and perhaps use of an irrigation instrument such as the Water-Pic.

General Therapeutic Considerations

1. Correct dental disorders and maintain good dental hygiene by cooperation with the dentist, as previously mentioned.

2. Frequent mouth rinses with dilute hydrogen peroxide (teaspoonful to glass of water) or a mild alkaline mouthwash such as a solution of one half teaspoonful (2.5 grams) of sodium bicarbonate to a 6 ounce (180 ml.) glass of warm water.

3. Relieve discomfort and pain, especially before eating, by swishing one fourth teaspoonful, or less, of viscous lidocaine (Xylocaine Viscous) in 2 teaspoonfuls of water around the mouth for 2 to 3 minutes. In patients with allergy to lidocaine, one teaspoonful of diphenhydramine solution (Elixir Benadryl) with a tablespoonful of crushed ice, held in the mouth for 4 to 5 minutes, produces satisfactory anesthesia. Swallowing the solution gives added sedative effect.

4. When the mouth is extensively involved with oral ulcerations, the diet should be limited to cool, bland soups, milk shakes, ice cream, and pureed or baby foods. Frequent small snacks are better tolerated than full meals. Attention should be directed to adequate hydration. If the patient is unable to swallow fluids, intravenous fluids and perhaps parenteral nutrition are indicated.

5. Alleviate the anxiety that accompanies oral disease. Changes in oral functions such as eating, tasting, or speaking or in facial appearance produce exaggerated concern. The patient worries about permanent disability or the presence of a malignancy. If specific therapy and alleviation of pain are not adequate, it may be necessary to administer antidepressants or even to request psychiatric consultation.

6. Oral lesions may be malignant or premalignant. Approximately 24,000 new cases of oral carcinoma were diagnosed in the United States during 1978 and more than one third died from the disease. Early recognition while the lesion is small and before metastasis occurs is the most important therapeutic consideration. Adequate, excisional biopsies from one or more areas should always be made when the diagnosis is questionable or if the process does not respond rapidly to therapy. This principle is especially important when dealing with chronic, keratinizing, white lesions, chronic red lesions, and infiltrative masses.

7. When the oral symptoms are part of a systemic or cutaneous disease, treatment must be directed to the basic disorder, as discussed elsewhere. In this section therapy will be limited, primarily, to the local manifestations.

Halitosis

Halitosis, or foul-smelling breath, is a minor but common complaint that has been magnified by advertising campaigns for mouthwashes, troches, and chewing gums. Usually, the problem is more noticeable to associates than to the patient. Most oral odors arise from the bacterial decomposition of food particles, desquamated mucosal cells, and salivary protein. Poor dental hygiene, carious or malpositioned teeth that collect food debris, xerostomia, mouth breathing, chronic periodontitis, and ulcerative oral processes contribute to such bacterial digestion. Bacterial decomposition of diseased oral tissues (severe bullous disease, necrotic tumors, noma, etc.) produces an extremely foul odor.

About 10 per cent of the causes are of extraoral origin, deriving from aromatic compounds circulating in the blood. Allyl disulphides (from garlic), aromas of alcoholic drinks, ketones (fruity odor of diabetic ketoacidosis), paraldehyde, and aromatic products from incompletely digested fats pass from the blood across the alveolar membrane and are exhaled. Rare cases of halitosis are due to inflammatory diseases of the nose, throat, lungs, and stomach.

Treatment. 1. Refer to a dentist for examination and correction of any dental problem.

2. Maintain good dental hygiene with frequent tooth brushing and use of dental floss.

3. Antiseptic mouthwashes are of some value. However, the effect lasts only a few hours and prolonged use may damage oral mucosa.

4. Reduce or eliminate ingestion of aromatic, odor-releasing compounds.

5. Evaluate cause of any associated xerostomia. Treat as indicated.

6. Correct any associated inflammatory or metabolic disease.

Xerostomia

Dryness of the mouth is not a disease but a sign of impaired salivary gland function, which may be temporary or permanent. Various drugs and infectious diseases of the salivary glands produce a transient xerostomia. When the drug is stopped or the primary disease resolves, the salivary flow returns to normal. Atrophic changes in salivary glands, such as found in Sjögren's syndrome, senile atrophy, and post-radiation atrophy, produce irreversible changes.

The principal conditions producing xerostomia are:

1. Mouth breathing: excessive speaking, exercise, adenoids, deviated septum, nasal polyps, hypertrophic rhinitis, respiratory infections.

2. Agenesis of salivary glands.

3. Senile atrophy of the mucous glands.

4. Psychologic: tension (speaking or performing before an audience), menopause, depression, anxiety states.

5. Major salivary gland dysfunction: uncontrolled diabetes, diabetes insipidus, severe uremia, severe dehydration, radiation therapy atrophy, bilateral mumps, infection or fibrosis, chronic hypochromic anemia, systemic lupus erythematosus.

6. Drugs: sedatives, hypnotics, narcotics, tranquilizers, nicotine, atropine and related drugs, propantheline and related drugs, antiparkinsonian drugs, antihistamines, phenothiazines, tricyclic antidepressants, epinephrine or ephedrine and related drugs, amphetamines.

7. Syndromes with xerostomia as an important symptom: Sjögren's syndrome, Mikulicz's syndrome, Waldenström's syndrome.

Ptyalism

Excessive salivary flow is not a disease but a sympton of many conditions, varying from simple local processes or drug reactions to serious organic lesions of the stomach, jaw, or brain. If the cause is not obvious, extensive diagnostic work-up is necessary before specific therapy can be given. The principal conditions producing ptyalism are:

1. Any form of general stomatitis, including thermal and chemical burns.

2. Parkinsonism.

3. Drugs: mercury, iodides, bromides, pilocarpine, expectorants, phosphorus, arsenic, antimony, cantharides, digitalis intoxication, anticholinergic intoxication (roach poison), nicotine (excessive smoking).

4. Reflex stimulation of fifth nerve: sucking on small hard objects; impacted foreign body (fishbone, etc.) in gingiva; periodontal disease including parulis and epulis; new partial dentures, especially when ill-fitting; jagged caries and rough fillings; fungating oral lesions; expanding lesions of the jaws.

5. Esophageal-gastric and hepatic reflex: carcinoma of the distal esophagus, peptic esophagitis, acute gastritis, dilatation of the stomach, gastric ulcer or carcinoma, duodenal ulcer or carcinoma, hepatitis, pancreatitis.

6. Organic lesions of the uncinate gyrus (one symptom of uncinate attacks).

7. Ptyalorrhea (functional?): tension, etc.; facet of a psychogenic aberration (manic-depressive neurosis, etc.); functional affection of the fifth nerve, analogous to tic douloureux; associated with pregnancy; associated with cerebral arteriosclerotic changes.

8. Pseudoptyalism (normal saliva production): mechanical difficulties in swallowing—mumps, acute infections of oral cavity or pharynx; tumors of jaws, tongue, palate, or pharynx; actinomycosis of jaws or tongue; fracture or dislocation o jaw; osteoarthritis or other dysfunction of the temporomandibular joint; painful conditions of pharynx, larynx, or esophagus; inability to swallow—botulism, myasthenia gravis, facial paralysis, bulbar and pseudobulbar paralysis, hypoglossal nerve paralysis; lack of cerebral control (slobbering)—cerebral injury or inadequacy, epileptic convulsions, rabies.

Abnormalities of Taste

The sensation of taste is based on so many interacting factors that abnormalities are difficult to classify. Taste is related to (1) visual response to food, (2) psychogenic response to thoughts of food or drink, (3) taste bud stimulation, (4) olfactory component, (5) physical consistency of food, (6) passage of food over oral structures, (7) thermal stimuli, (8) integrity of nerves and central receptor sites for taste, (9) ability to masticate properly, (10) sufficient saliva, and (11) general health. In addition, numerous local conditions, systemic diseases, metabolic dysfunctions, drugs and trophic processes may affect taste. Therapy must be directed to the underlying factors:

1. Local conditions (loss of taste, foul taste): stomatitis, glossitis, coated tongue, gingivitis, severe caries, oral tumors, gummatous infiltration of tongue, xerostomia.

2. Gastrointestinal disease (foul taste): gastritis, pyloric stenosis, gastric ulcer or carcinoma, regurgital esophagitis.

3. Septic lung disease (foul taste): bronchiectasis, tuberculosis with cavitation, abscess.

4. Perverted taste: pregnancy (various complaints), menopause (altered salt or metallic taste), senility (decreased stimulation by sweets), hysteria.

5. Vitamin deficiencies (decreased taste associated with burning of the tongue): pernicious anemia, nutritional macrocytic anemia, pellagra, chronic vitamin B complex deficiency.

6. Drugs: gymnemic acid, present in leaves of gymnema sylvestre (abolishes sweet and bitter but has no effect on salt or sour); stovaine (abolishes sweet and bitter); local anesthetics (abolish all taste); penicillamine effect (decrease to loss of all taste), possibly related to copper or zinc deficiency produced by chelation with penicillamine.

7. Trophic processes (decrease to loss of taste): peripheral lesions of lingual nerve (distal two thirds of tongue); chorda tympani lesions (distal two thirds of tongue); peripheral lesions of glossopharyngeal nerve (proximal one third of tongue); syringomyelia; migraine (temporary component); organic lesions involving the tractus solitarius or adjacent area of the medulla (tumors, local anemia, hemorrhage, syphilis, multiple sclerosis, etc.); organic lesions of the uncinate gyrus.

Macroglossia

Enlargement of the tongue results from hyperplasia of normal structures, neoplastic involvement, inflammatory and infectious processes, or infiltration of the tissues by fluids or abnormal cells. An unusually enlarged tongue associated with thick speech and a lowered pitch suggests cretinism or myxedema. Edentulous patients who do not wear dentures have a broad flat tongue that may be mistaken for macroglossia. The tongue returns to normal shape after dentures are constructed.

As with any symptom complex, therapy depends upon the underlying cause.

1. Trauma: bites, penetrating wounds, insect stings, corrosive agents and burns, jaw fractures.

2. Allergic reactions: stomatitis venenata, allergic stomatitis, urticaria, angioneurotic edema, dermatitis medicamentosa.

3. Vitamin deficiencies: ariboflavinosis, pellagra, scurvy, beriberi.

4. Congenital syndromes: congenital macroglossia, mongolism (Down's syndrome), gargoylism.

5. Endocrine abnormalities: cretinism, myxedema, diabetes, amyloidosis, acromegaly, glycogen storage disease.

6. Tumors: epithelioma, fibroma, neurofibromatosis, lipoma, hemangioma, lymphangioma, myeloma, sarcoma, rhabdomyoma.

7. Cysts: mucocele, thyroglossal duct cyst, ranula, suprahyoid cyst.

8. Hemorrhage into tongue: scurvy, leukemia, rupture of lingual varicosity, rupture of blood vessel by trauma, purpura (many factors).

9. Infections: syphilis (gummata), actinomycosis, histoplasmosis, zoster, thrush, tuberculosis, smallpox, Ludwig's angina, leprosy.

10. Inflammations: erythema multiforme, pemphigus, bullous pemphigoid, severe glossitis.

11. Miscellaneous disorders: plumbism, mercurialism, cardiac decompensation, progressive muscular dystrophy, superior vena cava syndrome, sarcoidosis.

Hypomobility of the Tongue

Hypomobility of the tongue is so often a symptom of serious systemic disease that diagnostic procedures should be initiated at once if the cause is not immediately apparent. Consider the following differential diagnoses:

1. Physical disorders: ankyloglossia or traumatic glossitis.

2. Neoplastic diseases: infiltrative lingual malignancies or sublingual neoplasms.

3. Cysts: thyroglossal duct cyst, sublingual mucous gland cyst, ranula.

4. Oral infections: glossitis or sublingual infection.

5. Scleroderma.

6. Miscellaneous disorders (concomitant finding): pernicious anemia (loss of muscle tone), myasthenia gravis, amyotrophic lateral sclerosis, myotonia congenita, cerebrovascular accident, bulbar paralysis, syringomyelia, cardiac glycogen disease, severed hypoglossal nerve, bulbar poliomyelitis, hysteria, infiltrative processes listed under Macroglossia.

7. Senility (loss of muscle tone).

Dysphasia

Difficulty in swallowing is also a serious complaint. As with other oral dysfunctions due to multiple causes, the underlying pathology must be determined before definitive therapy can be started. Differential diagnosis is extensive.

1. Pharyngitis, tonsillitis, and lingual tonsillitis.

2. Iron deficiency anemia: Plummer-Vinson syndrome and chronic gastrointestinal bleeding.

3. Pharyngeal muscle dysfunction.

4. Cricopharyngeal muscle hypertrophy.

5. Esophageal spasm (esophagitis, senility, etc.).

6. Conditions listed under pseudoptyalism.

7. Macroglossia.

Infectious Diseases

Those diseases not primary to the oral cavity are only noted with a few pertinent clinical findings. The reader is referred to appropriate sections for definitive therapy and general management. Local treatment has been discussed under general therapeutic considerations.

Bacterial Diseases. *Impetigo* may involve the vermilion surfaces and oral commissures.

Furuncles are common on the lip margins. Large furuncles of the upper lip may eventuate in cavernous sinus thrombosis.

Erysipelas can extend from the face into the oral cavity. Primary intraoral erysipelas is very rare.

Malignant pustule or malignant edema of *anthrax* occurs on the lips and occasionally on the tongue, palate, and pharynx. Involvement of the lips by the pustulous form has been reported a few times.

Cutaneous *diphtheria* of the upper lip is secondary to involvement of the nasal mucosa. Pharyngeal diphtheria may spread to the palate and rarely to the buccal mucosa.

Gingival abscess (parulis) results from the fistulous extension of a periapical or periodontal infection through the cortical plate to the gingival surface. Diagnosis is confirmed by x-ray examination. After several days of systemic therapy with penicillin or broad-spectrum antibiotics, adequate drainage is instituted by the dentist (e.g., apical curettage, apicoectomy, endodontic drainage, extraction of retained root). Today's dentist reserves tooth extraction as a last resort. The antibiotics are continued until the process has cleared. If the infection persists, culture and sensitivity tests are run to determine the more effective antibiotic. Frequent, hot mouth rinses give relief of discomfort. The extraoral dental fistula (sinus) results from extension of the periapical or periodontal infection through the intervening tissue to the cutaneous surface of the maxillary-facial region. The resulting abscess and subsequent draining granulomatous lesion are frequently confused with a local infection. Local therapy and antibiotics are ineffective. After diagnosis is confirmed by x-ray examination of the teeth and culture to eliminate deep fungus or acid-fast bacillus infection, dental therapy is indicated as for the gingival abscess. Hot compressing of the cutaneous lesion promotes drainage and hastens healing. Occasionally, surgical debridement of the sinus tract is necessary.

In *glanders* the acute, primary ulcer often spreads from the nose to the oral cavity. Chronic glanders may present a granulomatous, ulcerative, and destructive process involving especially the lips, palate, and alveolar process. Definitive treatment has not been established. In view of the serious nature of the disease, it is suggested that treatment with large doses of a sulfonamide or tetracycline in combination with intramuscular injections of streptomycin be started as soon as diagnosis is made. Careful sterile technique should be followed in the handling of dressings, bed clothes, and other personal effects.

Gonorrhea of the oral cavity has been reported very rarely. Increased incidence of oral sex and awareness of the problem should result in diagnosis of more cases. Clinically, the oral mucosa presents a fiery red appearance with scattered areas of epitheliitis partially covered by a yellow-white pseudomembrane. The patient complains of a burning sensation.

Granuloma inguinale occasionally develops on the lips and in the oral cavity. As with oral gonorrhea, the increasing incidence of oral sex should lead to more common occurrence.

Almost one half of all patients with *leprosy* present facial and oral lesions. Nodular infiltrations of the lips, tongue, and gingiva are fairly common. Perforation of the palate and severe faucial adhesions occur. Involvement of the trigeminal and facial nerves is common.

Lingual tonsillitis results from inflammation of the lymphoid, foliate papillae located on the sides of the base of the tongue. The process usually responds to hot saline gargles. Antibiotics are indicated for severe cases. A biopsy should be taken if there is a question of diagnosis.

Ludwig's angina is usually due to a hemolytic streptococcal infection of the floor of the mouth and submental areas. Most patients respond to adequate doses of appropriate antibiotics. If the airway is compromised, emergency treatment (tracheotomy, etc.) is necessary.

Melkersson-Rosenthal syndrome (cheilitis granulomatous) is characterized by recurrent swelling of the lips, recurrent facial paralysis, and fissured tongue. This process is listed here because it may be an allergic reaction to various organisms. The course of the disease is recurrent and progressive. Intralesional corticosteroids (triamcinolone, 5 to 10 mg. per ml., not over 0.2 ml. per cubic cm. of tissue) injected into the enlarged lip or tongue may be of value. Surgical revision of chronically enlarged lips has been successful in a few patients. Decompression of the facial nerve has been recommended for persistent paralysis of over 2 months.

Noma (cancer oris) is a very rare disease, occurring most commonly in severely malnourished and debilitated persons. The exact role of constantly present Vincent's organisms is obscure. The disease is characterized by a rapidly spreading, extremely destructive, gangrenous process on the cheek or alveolar process or both. Differential diagnosis must include rapidly growing malignancies and ulceronecrotic lesions associated with leukemia, uncontrolled diabetes, or severe chronic neutropenia. Without treatment, the disease is frequently progressive and fatal. Massive doses of penicillin or broad-spectrum antibiotics or both until all activity has cleared is lifesaving. Local therapy is limited to soothing wet compressing (saline, boric acid solution, prophyllin solution) and careful debridement. A full diet, high in protein, and multivitamin preparations, is important but may not be available in situations wherein the disease occurs. When the infection is brought under complete control, dental restoration and extensive surgical reconstruction may be undertaken.

The severe coughing of *pertussis* frequently causes a fairly pathognomonic ulceration of the lingual frenum.

Rhinoscleroma may slowly spread from the nostrils to the upper lip, and even lower lip, producing keloidlike hardness and adhesions to the alveolar process. Extension to the alveolar process, palate, and tongue is reported. After biopsy confirmation and identification of *Klebsiella rhinoscleromatis* by appropriate culture, sensitivity tests should be run to determine sensitivity of the particular species. Most strains are sensitive to chloramphenicol, tetracycline, and streptomycin. Antibiotic therapy is continued until bacteriologic cure is obtained. In severe cases, tracheotomy is necessary to maintain an adequate airway. Supportive therapy with adequate diet, multivitamin preparations, and attention to secondary systemic, pyogenic infections is utilized as indicated. When the active process is cleared it may be necessary to reconstruct the respiratory tract or repair the cosmetic deformities.

An infectious cause for *sarcoidosis* has not been proved. Nonulcerating nodular infiltrates may extend from the lips to the oral mucosa. Repeated intralesional injections of dilute triamcinolone solution (5 to 10 mg. per ml.) at 3 to 4 week intervals, frequently clears lip and mucosal infiltrates.

The chancre of *syphilis* occurs on the lips, tongue (especially the tip), gingiva and less often on the oral mucosa and palate. Mucous patches appear on the lip, tongue, and cheeks. Split papules suggesting angular cheilitis may occur at angles of the mouth. Gummata develop on and around the lips and in the oral cavity. Gummatous infiltration of the tongue produces macroglossia. Diffuse interstitial glossitis first enlarges the tongue and then produces shrinkage. Painless perforation of the palate is almost pathognomonic. Congenital syphilis is stigmatized by Parrot's radial scars (rhagades) around the lips, an ill-defined vermilion-cutaneous line, Hutchinson's teeth, mulberry molars, and other dental abnormalities.

In *tuberculosis*, the primary tuberculous chancre (Ghon lesion) occasionally develops on the lip and in the oral cavity. Lupus vulgaris may extend to the lips and oral mucosa. The tuberculous ulcer of the lips and oral cavity must be differentiated from squamous cell carcinoma. Scrofula has occurred on the tongue with drainage to the submandibular area.

In *tularemia* oral involvement by the primary complex is fairly common in Europe. In Turkey and southern Russia, the mouth is the most common site for inoculation.

Vincent's disease (trench mouth, acute necrotizing ulcerative gingivostomatitis) is probably due to change in host resistance, permitting *Fusobacterium plauti-vincentii* and *Borrelia vincentii* to become pathogenic. Poor dental hygiene, stress, fatigue, and heavy smoking are predisposing factors. The disease presents as a necrotizing, ulcerative gingivitis that may become chronic and produce extensive alveolysis and bone necrosis. In severe cases the process extends to the buccal mucosa and pharynx but in most instances the adjacent mucosa shows surprisingly little change. The acute, painful, bacterial stage is controlled by frequent mouth rinses with warm 1.5 per cent solution (50 per cent dilution with warm water) of hydrogen peroxide. The solution is forced between the teeth by action of the cheeks and tongue. Necrotic tissue on the interdental papillae is removed by very gentle rubbing with a hydrogen peroxide–moistened cotton swab. Local antibiotics such as polymyxin-bacitracin-neomycin mixtures (Neosporin) may be of some value. Do not use for more than 1 week because of potential hazard of nephrotoxicity and ototoxicity due to the neomycin. Caustic preparations should not be used. Pain and discomfort are controlled by analgesics. In severe infections, especially when associated with ulcers on the fauces and tonsils, systemic antibiotic therapy with penicillin, tetracycline, or erythromycin is indicated. After the acute, painful stage has subsided, the dentist must instruct the patient in proper dental hygiene. The teeth are gently scaled and periodontal pockets are opened. All dental defects, especially gingival caries and malocclusion points, must be corrected. If local predisposing causes are not corrected by the dentist, recurrences and unnecessary loss of gingival tissue are to be expected.

The primary lesion of *yaws* is rare on the lips. The secondary stage frequently involves the perioral areas and lips. Tertiary stage lesions of the lips and oral cavity are similar to those found in tertiary syphilis but present much more destruction of the skin and adjacent bone.

Candida albicans, and to a lesser extent other species of Candida, are almost universal in distribution and can be found in most healthy mouths.

The organism is an opportunistic pathogen and may produce overt infection when stimulated by various factors such as debilitation, chronic infections, pregnancy, and hypovitaminosis B. Hypoparathyroidism, hypothyroidism, diabetes mellitus, thymoma, and low serum iron levels may be associated with chronic Candida infections. Long-term administration of antibiotics, corticosteroids, and estrogens increases the susceptibility to oral (and vaginal) infections. Immunosuppressed patients and children with immunodeficiencies may develop chronic, recalcitrant infections. Local factors such as severe caries, sharp tooth edges, ill-fitting dentures, and cheek nibbling promote and maintain the infection. *Candida cheilitis* of the vermilion border is almost never an isolated finding. *Angular cheilitis due to candida infection* has been previously discussed. *Thrush* (moniliasis) is characterized by the presence of a somewhat adherent, coagulated milklike pseudomembrane on the tongue, cheeks, or pharynx. Removal of the membrane by rubbing with a gauze pad leaves a raw, oozing surface. Oral candidiasis must be considered in every case of glossodynia, even when the tongue appears normal. Treatment consists of the following:

1. Identify and eliminate, if possible, all systemic factors. Correct nutritional deficiencies.

2. Discontinue antibiotics and contraceptive pills.

3. Nystatin solution (Mycostatin Oral Suspension), 1 teaspoonful as a prolonged mouthwash, four times a day, before swallowing; or nystatin oral tablet or nystatin vaginal suppository as an oral troche, 3 times daily. Nystatin cream may be applied under the denture for resistant palatal infections in edentulous patients. Nystatin in Orabase may be released shortly and should prove to be an excellent therapeutic modality.

4. Dilute hydrogen peroxide mouth rinses for oral discomfort.

5. Gentian violet, 1 per cent solution, is messy but effective.

6. Dental prophylaxis. Dental restorative work including attention to ill-fitting dentures and dental appliances.

7. A new product, clotrimazole tablet (Gyne-Lotrimin), may prove very effective as an oral troche but has not been approved by the Food and Drug Administration for this purpose.

Occasionally, the Candida invade beneath the mucosa to produce a chronic, recalcitrant, submucosal infection. This appears as a pale, thickened, macerated, boiled-looking, firmly adherent, pseudomembrane that is crinkled, rugose, and frayed. Characteristically, the areas remain soft and do not develop the firmness found in thickened leukoplakia. Recent investigative work indicates that some patients with recalcitrant and re-

current mucocutaneous candidiasis have a deficiency of an $alpha_2$ globulin, anticandidal factor in their serum and that others lack the enzyme, myeloperoxidase in their leukocytes. Other recent works suggest a deficiency in the enzyme that cleaves β carotene. At present, we have no specific therapy for such deficiencies. Many patients with submucous thrush respond satisfactorily but slowly to the routine for simple thrush. Failure to respond to therapy or rapid recurrence emphasizes the need to reevaluate the case for underlying systemic disease and immunodeficiencies. Chronic, recalcitrant thrush and mucocutaneous candidiasis present a serious problem in therapy. Therapeutic procedures include:

1. Amphotericin B and 5-fluorocytosine, intravenously, as individual drugs or at the same time for their synergistic action. (The intravenous use of 5-fluorocytosine is not listed in the manufacturer's official directive.)

2. Bone marrow transplants

3. Leukocytes from HL-A–compatible sibling

4. Transfer factor in large doses

Mycotic Diseases. Oral lesions of the deep fungus infections (e.g., *actinomycosis, aspergillosis, blastomycosis, coccidioidomycosis, cryptococcosis, histoplasmosis, mucormycosis, nocardiosis, rhinosporidiosis,* and *sporotrichosis* are usually, though not always, part of the general infection. Cervicofacial localization is the most common manifestation of *actinomycosis.* South American *blastomycosis* almost always begins in the oral cavity.

Viral Diseases. Oral lesions may be present in *chickenpox, cat-scratch disease, hand, foot, and mouth disease, Kaposi's varicelliform eruption, infectious mononucleosis, lymphogranuloma venereum, measles, paravaccinia, variola, vaccinia,* and *zoster.* Symptomatic local measures are instituted as indicated by the severity of the oral disease. Systemic therapy is directed to the primary disease.

Herpes simplex is so common as to warrant additional comment. *Primary herpes gingivostomatitis* may be so severe in debilitated infants and children that it is sometimes fatal. This rare variant, *Pospischill-Feyrter disease,* develops principally after whooping cough, measles, and scarlet fever. Extensive vesiculonecrotic lesions involve the oral cavity, pharynx, upper esophagus, perioral areas, finger tips, and genitalia. Treatment is supportive with careful attention to hydration, electrolyte balance, nutrition, and secondary infection. *Recurrent, intraoral, herpes simplex infections* are not uncommon. Grouped, small, vesicular lesions appear on one quadrant of the oral mucosa, persist for 7 to 10 days, and heal spontaneously. Symptomatic treatment as noted under therapeutic considerations is advised.

Coxsackie Group A viruses are the causative

agents for several viral infections that present oral mucous membrane lesions. The typical, discrete, gray-white, papulovesicular lesions of *herpangina*, on the pharyngeal and posterior oral areas, are clinically different from the raised nodules of acute *lymphonodular pharyngitis*. There is no specific therapy for Coxsackie virus infections. Treatment is symptomatic and the prognosis is excellent.

Warts are one of the most common skin diseases. Small, papular and filiform warts of the lips and mouth are not uncommon. Frequently, they are the result of autoinoculation from the fingers. Confluent patches of cauliflowerlike papules, similar to genital condyloma acuminata, occasionally develop on the oral mucosa. Autosuggestion and hypnosis have not been effective in treatment of oral warts. Small warts are best treated by careful and superficial destructive measures with electrodesiccation or liquid nitrogen. It is better to repeat the procedure a second or even third time than to leave an unnecessary scar on the lips. Occasionally, the use of trichloracetic acid or cantheridin (Ver-Acid) is effective. The condylomatous variety frequently responds to local application of 5 per cent solution of podophyllin in tincture of benzoin. This drug should be used very carefully in the mouth because of possible toxicity from absorption. One drop of 5 per cent solution contains 333 mg. of podophyllin. Taken orally, 660 mg. acts as a purge. Coexisting finger or hand warts should be treated at the same time by appropriate measures.

Lip and oral lesions of *molluscum contagiosum* have been described. The easiest form of treatment is flicking off the lesions with a sharp curette. For patients who are not allergic to the drug, local application of lidocaine (Xylocaine Viscous) or 25 per cent solution of benzocaine (Gingocaine) usually gives adequate anesthesia.

Parasitic Infections. Mucocutaneous lesions of *leishmaniasis* occur in both the cutaneous and visceral forms but are most common in American leishmaniasis. Organic antimonials are the drugs of choice. Exact dosage and method of administration (intramuscularly or intravenously) vary with the preparation. As a general rule, the medication is given daily until the lesions have cleared or for a maximum of 30 days. Sodium antimony gluconate may be obtained from the Center for Disease Control, Atlanta, Georgia 30333. Mucous membrane lesions frequently show a chronic progressive course and have a tendency to relapse after apparent cure with antimonials. Resistant or relapsing oral lesions are treated with amphotericin B (Fungizone). Amphotericin B is administered intravenously, as alternate day doses of 0.3 to 0.75 mg. per kg. (maximum of 50 mg.), dissolved in 500 ml. of 5 per cent dextrose solution, very slowly over a minimum of three hours. Usually, 1 mg. is given on day 1, 10 mg. on day 2, and 25 mg. on day 3 before the alternate day course with full dose is begun. A total of 1800 to 2000 mg. may be given, depending upon size of patient and therapeutic response. Carefully monitor patients on amphotericin B for electrolyte balance, especially for hypokalemia.

Trichinosis has been identified in oral structures, especially the tongue.

Nematode infections. Infestation with *Gongylonema hominis* has been reported as occurring in the submucosal tissue of the lower lip, palate, and buccal mucosa. The 1 mm. wide by 30 mm. long worm can be seen beneath the mucosa. Removal is fairly easy through a small incision.

Oral myiasis is very rare. Invasion of dental sockets and necrotic oral tissue by the larvae of dipterous flies has been reported from India and Pakistan. The mature larvae are carefully teased out through small incisions, after local anesthesia. Suture of the wound and administration of broad-spectrum antibiotics may be indicated.

Lips

Fordyce's Disease. These very common (80 per cent of population), asymptomatic, tiny, symmetrically grouped, yellowish tumors, lying flush with the surface are due to hypertrophy of anomalous sebaceous glands of the mucous membrane. The lips as well as buccal mucosa and retromolar areas may be involved. No treatment is indicated except to assure the patient that the process is neither malignant nor premalignant.

Lip Pits. Congenital lip pits are bilateral, symmetrically located depressions occurring on the vermilion surface of the lower lip, one on each side of the midline. On occasion, the pits may be unilateral or present a nipplelike elevation. These blind sinuses represent persistence of developmental sulci. Occurrence is about 1 in 200,000 individuals.

The commisural lip pit, occurring at the angle of the mouth, is a relatively common developmental defect and is found in 12 per cent of whites and 20 per cent of blacks. Twenty-five per cent of the cases are bilateral. Lip pits are usually asymptomatic and require no treatment. Large or constantly draining lesions may be carefully excised for cosmetic reasons.

Cleft Lip and Cleft Palate. These occur in about 1 per 1000 white and 1 per 2500 black births. The clefts may be median, lateral, oblique, or bilateral and may vary from small depressions to extensive, deforming and mutilating processes that involve the nostrils and the hard and soft palate. On rare occasions, the lower lip, tongue, and mandible may be involved. Associated anomalies of other organ systems are not uncommon. Surgical correction of cleft lip is started at 4 to 8 weeks of age. Palatal repair is usually deferred to avoid damage to growth centers and tooth buds. Specially designed nipples and palatal obturators are important for adequate nutrition, prevention of nasal or pulmonary infection and overcoming speech problems. Extensive anomalies, especially with palatal or mandibular involvement, require long-term management by specialized teams of pediatricians, plastic surgeons, dentists, and speech therapists. If possible, infants with extensive clefts should be referred very early to a center specializing in long-term management of this defect.

Vascular Tumors.   *Capillary hemangiomas* of infancy may involve the lips as well as other oral structures. Characteristically, most of the lesions involute spontaneously in several years and do not require treatment. However, the resolution may be slow and not completed until puberty. *Cavernous hemangiomas* are usually not apparent at birth but develop during childhood and may either reach a static size or show progressive enlargement. Mixed lesions occasionally occur. Management requires careful evaluation and frequent reexamination. Rapid growth, especially when vital functions are compromised, requires surgical intervention. Radiation therapy, if utilized, must be of such quality and quantity that the teeth buds and bone growth centers are not harmed. Large lesions may involve such extensive areas of tissue that removal results in severe disfigurement and impairment of function. Malignant transformation is extremely rare. *Venous ectasia (lakes)* and sublingual varices are common among the elderly. No treatment is required. Large venous ectasia can be destroyed by electrolysis for cosmetic reasons.

Mucoceles.   Mucoceles arise from mucous extravasation into the adjacent tissue, usually with a pseudoenclosure of granulation tissue. Less commonly, they represent a true mucous retention cyst with surrounding epithelial sac, due to obstruction of the excretory duct. They occur most often on the lower lip and occlusal line of the cheek. Some lesions drain spontaneously and involute. Persistent lesions are carefully deroofed under local anesthesia. The underlying granulation tissue or enlarged glandular tissue or both is carefully teased and squeezed out through the opening. The base is not desiccated. Postdesiccation granulation tissue may promote recurrence. Absorbable gelatin (Gelfoam) is used to control bleeding. Patients should be reassured that the lesions are not malignant or premalignant.

Trauma.   *Traumatic lesions* of the lip are very common in contact sports and accidents. Lip lesions require careful debridement of devitalized tissue and accurate apposition of the vermilion border to preserve the lip line and prevent unnecessary scar formation. Nodules on the mucosal surface and even nodules deep in the lip tissues are a constant source of irritation. Radiographic examination is indicated when the wound is contaminated or associated with fractured teeth. Face bars on helmets and mouth guards reduce the incidence of injury to the lips and teeth in contact sports.

Mild *thermal, electrical, and chemical burns* of the lips respond to cool boric acid solution, compressing and simple emollients such as 1 per cent hydrocortisone ointment (1 per cent Hytone; 1 per cent Cort-Dome, and others). Thermal burns of the lips, tongue, and especially the palate from hot foods are usually minor and heal uneventfully in about a week. One of the local anesthetic preparations lidocaine (Xylocaine Viscous, and others) will relieve the pain and promote healing. Dry ice burns (seen in children who place dry ice in their mouths) can produce a severe slough. Deep and extensive burns require symptomatic and supportive therapy until definitive reconstructive surgery can be carried out. Severe cold urticaria is a very rare reaction that usually responds to antihistamines (Periactin) and perhaps a short course of corticosteroids. The dry and desquamating lips of severely ill patients should be kept greased with petrolatum or lanolin.

Acute sunburn of the lips is treated by frequent compressing with ice cold Burow's solution, containing one fourth teaspoonful of bath oil (Alpha Keri Bath Oil, Lubath) per pint, followed by application of 1 per cent hydrocortisone ointment. Further occurrences may be prevented by use of sunscreening lip pomades (Sun Stick Lip Protectant; PreSun Sunscreen Lip Protection; RVPaba Lipstick). Windburn and cold chapping of the lips responds to the same routine.

Sucking-Licking Cheilitis.   Some children and an occasional adult have the habit of constantly licking or sucking the lips and adjoining skin. Chapping (dryness and scaling) of the areas is soon followed by fissuring and secondary infection. Thumbsucking, with associated drooling, may produce a similar picture. After secondary infection is brought under control by an antibiotic ointment, the use of a silicone preparation (Silicote Ointment) protects the skin from further masceration. Nighttime lipsucking may be partially alleviated by the wearing of mouth guards when sleeping. However, liplicking or sucking is a "tension" habit and is very difficult to cure. Psychotherapy for the parents is probably more important than treatment of the child.

Fissures.   Lip fissures are chronic tears of the mucous membrane due to dryness following sunburn, windburn, freezing, contact dermatitis, and so on. Secondary infection may modify the picture. The fissures are treated with warm saline compress and an antibiotic ointment. If the lesion does not heal, press the margins of the fissure together and fix them in place with a wisp of cotton coated with flexible collodion. This is a tricky procedure and may require several attempts to carry out successfully. The fissure usually heals in several days. On rare occasions it is necessary to approximate the edges with 8-0 silk suture.

Biting and Chewing. Severe destruction of the lips and cheeks may result from involuntary biting and chewing in brain-damaged patients. If the brain damage is permanent, extraction of the teeth may be necessary to control the problem.

Loss of Vertical Dimension Dermatitis. Marked loss of vertical dimension and shortening of the face is found in all edentulous persons. Severe attrition of the teeth produces a similar but less severe condition. The lips overlap at the commissures to form intertriginous areas. Constant moisture leads to maceration, splitting, and secondary infection, producing the picture of perlèche. In edentulous patients, the wearing of properly constructed dentures will correct the loss of vertical dimension. Severe attrition is corrected by capping the teeth, or extraction and full dentures. Local treatment is the same as for angular cheilitis.

Actinic Cheilitis and Keratoses. These are potentially malignant. Sudden growth of a keratosis, prickly sensation when scratching the lesion or induration of the base or both suggests malignant transformation. Large lesions should be surgically removed for biopsy evaluation. Local application of 5-fluorouracil solution (Efudex, Fluoroplex) for 2 to 4 weeks is effective in many early lesions and does not leave scars but is exceedingly painful. The concomitant use of a corticosteroid ointment may decrease the discomfort without interfering with the action of fluorouracil. Note that after inadequate fluorouracil therapy, extensive squamous cell carcinoma may develop unnoticed beneath normal appearing skin. Cryosurgery and electrosurgical destruction are effective but likely to leave undesirable scars. Severe, chronic lesions are best treated by a lip shave. All persons with active cheilitis should avoid unnecessary sun exposure and should carefully protect the lips with a sunscreen pomade.

Allergic Reactions. *Allergic contact cheilitis and stomatitis* are due to an exogenous allergen reaching the lips or mucosa by direct contact. Virtually any substance can produce the reaction in a susceptible person. Definitive treatment requires the identification and elimination of the allergen. This is not always possible. Whenever a contact allergy is suspected, eliminate lipstick, sunscreening pomades, local applications and medications, mouthwashes, toothpastes, chewing gums, hard candies, cough drops, spicy foods, acid foods, and sucking on citrus fruit, pencils, or vegetation. Contact dermatitis from reed mouthpieces of musical instruments has been described. Consider also substances used by the dentist before onset of the problem, such as antiseptics, antibiotics, phenolic derivatives, volatile oils, and cold sterilizing solutions used on instruments and denture materials. Allergic reactions develop occasionally to prosthetic materials and denture adhesives as well as to nickel, cobalt, and chrome used in dental appliances. Local therapy is symptomatic. Inflammation is relieved by frequent, cool Burow's solution compress for the lips and cool saline mouth rinses for the oral cavity followed by a corticosteroid ointment (0.5 per cent) (Lidex, Kenalog, Aristocort) for the lips and Kenalog in a protective oral paste (Orabase) for mucosal surfaces. Note that Orabase is applied by gently pressing against the mucosa with a fingertip; it should not be rubbed in. Shreds of mucosal tissue are best removed by occasional rinsing with a glass of warm water containing one teaspoonful of sodium bicarbonate. Systemic antihistamines and even systemic corticosteroids are indicated for severe cases. Compromise of the airway is very rare.

Allergic cheilitis and stomatitis are due to blood-borne allergens. The response may be cicatricial, eczematous, or combined. *Urticaria* of the lips and oral cavity is usually associated with a generalized reaction. Elimination of the causative factors and systemic treatment are discussed on p. 661. Cold compressing and cold mouth rinses help in reducing the edema and inflammation. The general term urticaria includes idiopathic, hereditary, and allergic forms of angioedema. All of these varieties may involve the oral tissues, esophagus, and trachea. If the airway is compromised or the patient presents other life-threatening symptoms, immediate injection of epinephrine (0.3 to 0.5 ml. of 1:1000 solution) and, occasionally, a quick-acting corticosteroid, dexamethasone sodium phosphate (Decadron phosphate, 4 to 16 mg.) are indicated. Severe laryngeal edema may require tracheotomy. *Eczematous allergic cheilitis and stomatitis* are rather rare allergic reactions due to blood-borne allergens that present clinical manifestations almost identical with the contact variety. Every substance listed as a possible cause of acute urticaria may also produce an eczematous allergic reaction. Differentiation is made on the basis of history, negative patch test findings, or exposure to the suspected allergen or all three. Treatment requires search for and elimination of the causative factors, if possible. Local treatment is identical with that used for the contact variety.

Macrocheilia. Many of the factors producing

macroglossia may also cause enlargement of the lips. The most common causes of acute enlargement of the lips include trauma, angioedema, and infectious processes. Recurring lip swelling may be part of the Melkersson-Rosenthal syndrome or due to recurrent angioedema. Chronic macrocheilia is usually due to developmental defects, tumors, sarcoidosis, infectious processes, or interference with lymph drainage. In all these conditions, treatment is directed to the underlying cause.

Cheilitis Glandularis Apostematosa.   This is a chronic, idiopathic hypertrophy of groups of the vermilion border mucous glands and their ducts. Occasionally, mucous glands of the oral cavity, pharynx, and nose may be involved. Mild cases are relatively common. Everting and stretching the lower lip reveals erythematous duct openings, up to several millimeters in diameter, scattered irregularly over the vermilion and adjacent mucosal surfaces. In severe cases, the hypertrophied glands evert the enlarged lip. The patient must be assured that the condition is not malignant. Intralesional injections (0.2 to 0.3 ml.) of a dilute triamcinolone solution (5 mg. per ml.) may be of some benefit. Surgical excision is reserved for very severe cases.

Angular Cheilitis (Perlèche).   This is primarily an intertrigo and fissuring due to maceration of the corners of the mouth, frequently complicated by chronic infection with *Candida albicans* or other organisms or both. Underlying factors include loss of vertical dimension, flaccid sagging cheeks, chronic riboflavin deficiency. Sjögren's syndrome, hypochromic anemia, and oral candidiasis. Primary treatment is directed to the underlying factors. Frequent applications of a nystatin, neomycin, gramicidin, triamcinolone (Mycolog) ointment are usually helpful.

Tongue

Glossodynia (painful tongue) or *glossophyrosis* (burning tongue) is usually a complaint of older adults, especially postmenopausal women. As with other subjective complaints, a variety of local and systemic factors must be evaluated. Obvious painful abnormalities such as allergic glossitis, vesiculobullous processes and pyodermas are relatively easy to diagnose. Glossodynia may accompany macroglossia, xerostomia, and perversions of taste. Before making a diagnosis of idiopathic glossodynia, a thorough search must be made for underlying pathology. Dental problems to be considered include poor oral hygiene, periodontal disease, and referred pain from an occult dental abscess. Occasionally, an undiagnosed disease such as mild Candida glossitis (postantibiotic therapy), pernicious anemia, subclinical pellagra, dia-

betes mellitus, hypovitaminosis B, iron deficiency, or gastric reflex can be identified. Rare factors to be considered are trigeminal neuralgia, zinc deficiency, vascular disturbances in the central nervous system, and temporomandibular joint disease. It is reported that glossodynia has followed trigeminal nerve injury resulting from mandibular block injections. When there is definite evidence of nerve entrapment or neuroma formation, surgical intervention may be of value.

Unfortunately, no cause is discovered in most patients. The tongue appears normal except, perhaps, for the presence of mild asymptomatic conditions such as furring, migrating glossitis, or congenital fissures. Management is very difficult. Estrogens, vitamins (including vitamin B_{12}), and various other therapeutic agents are of little or no value. The patient's complaint must not be taken lightly. Assurance and reassurance that the problem is neither serious nor malignant, perhaps combined with judicious use of mild tranquilizers, is important. Good dental hygiene and adequate nutrition should be maintained. If the patient remains unduly disturbed or incapacitated or both, psychiatric consultation is indicated.

Coated tongue is due to more or less retention of normal desquamation of the filiform papillae. Mild coating is normal. The amount varies from day to day and from morning to night in the same person. Increased coating is associated with respiratory disease, fever, and smoking. It may be part of the "morning-after" syndrome. Gentle brushing with a soft-bristled toothbrush followed by thorough rinsing is usually effective therapy.

Smooth tongue is due to atrophy or absence of the filiform papillae. The finding is frequently associated with nutritional deficiencies such as iron deficiency anemia, Plummer-Vinson syndrome, malabsorption states (celiac disease, tropical sprue), pellagra, pernicious anemia, and nutritional macrocytic anemia. Treatment of the underlying process is indicated.

Fissured tongue (scrotal tongue) is a congenital anomaly that appears in 4 to 5 per cent of the population. Usually, the process occurs as an isolated defect. Fissured tongue is also part of the symptom complex of mongolism, Sjögren's syndrome, and Melkersson-Rosenthal syndrome. No treatment is necessary. However, the fissures should be pulled open and the bases carefully palpated. Small, asymptomatic carcinoma have been discovered in deep folds on rare occasions.

Geographic tongue is a benign, superficial, asymptomatic, migrating glossitis of unknown cause, occurring in about 2 per cent of the population. The tongue lesions of Reiter's syndrome are clinically and histologically identical. The patient is assured that the process is benign and self-limited. Gently cleansing the tongue with a soft toothbrush may be of value. Long-term corticosteroid therapy occasionally clears the process but such potentially dangerous treatment is inadvisable for this minor condition.

Moeller's glossitis (glazed or slick tongue) is a very rare, chronic, symptom complex, characterized by appearance of one or more discrete, glazed, beefy red, painful lesions on the tongue. Causative factors include all the conditions listed under glossalgia plus nonulcerative galvanism if such a condition really exists. In most cases no cause can be identified and no definitive treatment is available. Estrogens, androgens, corticosteroids, vitamins, trace elements, hydrochloric acid, and thyroid, individually and in combinations have been tried with varying degrees of unsatisfactory response. Pain is controlled by the use of mild mouth rinses and anesthetic preparations.

Hairy tongue is usually black in color but cases of yellow, dirty-gray, brown, blue, and even green have been reported. The cause for elongation of the filiform papillae is unknown. There is some evidence that activity of chromogenic bacteria or fungi produce the elongation and coloration. Suppression of competing organisms by long-term antibiotic therapy may be a predisposing factor. After local anesthesia with viscous lidocaine (Xylocaine Viscous), the elongated papillae can be carefully snipped away with sharp scissors. The area is then painted with 5 per cent trichloracetic acid. Several such treatments usually clear the process. The patient is advised to brush the tongue gently when he brushes his teeth. The application of 40 per cent urea followed by vigorous brushing is also effective. A thin application of 25 per cent podophyllin in tincture of benzoin clears the process but is rather painful.

Median rhomboid glossitis is usually accepted as a developmental defect due to persistence of the tuberculum impar on the surface of the tongue. The process rarely appears before the age of 30. Median rhomboid glossitis is benign. Although squamous cell carcinoma has been reported to occur on the dorsal surface of the midtongue, this site is rarely affected by cancer. Recent work suggests that chronic infection such as chronic hyperplastic candidiasis may be a causative factor. On this basis, anticandidal preparations could be tried for a month or so. If the lesion shows change in size, shape, or consistency, a biopsy is indicated to exclude carcinoma.

In *bifid tongue* incomplete fusion of the lateral prominences of the embryonic tongue may leave a cleft at the tip of the tongue. A central tag consisting of muscle may be found in the cleft. The fissure requires no treatment. Occasionally, it is advisable to snip off the central tag under local anesthesia.

Oral Mucosa

The oral mucosa heals rapidly after acute trauma, usually without a scar. Chronic trauma frequently produces hyperplasia.

Denture stomatitis is a fairly common inflammatory process occurring beneath the dentures. Removal of the denture for a few days and then leaving the denture out only at night usually relieves the condition. If Candida are found on mucosal scrapings, nystatin ointment applied to the oral mucosa and the denture itself is of value.

Papillary hyperplasia is the hyperplastic response of palatal and gingival mucosa to chronic irritation from ill-fitting dentures. Mild cases regress spontaneously when the dentures are left out for 3 to 4 weeks. Severe cases require surgical removal of the lesions. When the mouth is healed, new, properly fitting dentures are made. Reworking old dentures usually fails. Well-documented instances of carcinoma arising in papillary hyperplasia are exceptionally rare.

Nicotine stomatitis (smoker's palate) is a very common, reactive squamous metaplasia of the palatine ducts and a sialadenitis of the palatine glands due to smoking. Previously considered a premalignant condition, the process is now classified as benign. The tissues revert to normal when the patient stops smoking.

Leukoplakia and Leukokeratosis. There has been much confusion in use of the word leukoplakia. Originally, it meant any white plaque. We feel that the term leukokeratosis should be reserved for white lesions that show no dyskeratosis on histologic examination. Leukoplakia is a histopathologic diagnosis implying premalignant potential. Unless the diagnosis is obvious (thrush, typical lichen planus, etc.) all keratotic lesions should be biopsied and treated on the basis of the histopathologic report.

Leukokeratoses are benign white plaques usually caused by chronic trauma such as cheek-biting or nibbling, sucking mucosa between the teeth, sharp margins of carious teeth, malpositioned teeth, and ill-fitting dental appliances. Diagnosis should be confirmed by biopsy. Correction of dental abnormalities, good oral hygiene, and avoidance of tobacco are frequently followed by definite improvement. The inveterate cheek chewer is helped by a mouth-guard–like dental appliance that he wears at night to prevent cheek chewing while asleep. Most dentists are familiar with this appliance. As a rule of thumb, a biopsy must be taken if the process does not show marked clearing within 6 weeks after irritating factors are removed. The best site for the biopsy is a thin flaky margin or an erythematous area within the white lesion. Furthermore, any change in shape, consistency or configuration, or the development of ulcers or erythroplasia-like areas is indication for additional biopsies.

Leukoplakia is a histopathologic diagnosis of premalignancy. It may be difficult for the pathologist to exclude carcinoma in situ, and multiple biopsies may be necessary to reach a definite diagnosis. Inasmuch as only a small percentage of these lesions develop into overt squamous cell carcinoma, they are treated as outlined for leukokeratoses. Resistant plaques are destroyed by cryosurgery. Frequent reevaluation and additional biopsies are important. Histologic evidence of carcinoma in situ indicates the need of immediate complete surgical excision. Persistent lesions of the tongue and floor of the mouth have the greatest potential for malignant transformation. They should be excised early for histopathologic evaluation of the entire lesion.

Snuff dipper's keratosis (snuff-induced leukoplakia) develops in constant users of this tobacco combination. Development of snuff dipper's carcinoma must be kept in mind and biopsies should be taken in all cases. The prognosis of this problem has not been definitely established. If the process does not resolve after termination of the habit, the lesion should be completely excised or destroyed by cryosurgery.

Pigmented Lesions of the Oral Cavity. *Physiological pigmentation* is found routinely in blacks and other dark-skinned persons. No therapy is indicated.

Amalgam tattoos result from the submucosal inclusion of amalgam particles that spilled into periodontal tissues during filling of a gingival cavity or were thrown into the tissues by a slipped disc or bur. Soft tissue x-ray examination will reveal the metal within the dermis. No treatment is indicated. Occasionally, it may be necessary to take a biopsy to eliminate the possibility of melanoma. Similar areas of pigmentation follow accidentally introduced materials from lead pencils, ink, charcoal, dirt, asphalt, and so on. Pigmentary disfigurement of the vermilion borders of the lips may be improved by a lip shave and careful picking out of the foreign particles.

Cellular nevi are the most common human tumors. However, less than 0.1 per cent are intraoral. All varieties are found. Most lesions occur in dark-skinned persons and many are not pigmented. Clinical differentiation between nevi and melanoma is frequently difficult. It is probably advisable to remove any suspected oral nevus for histopathologic examination. Excisional biopsy must be carried out on any lesion that becomes ulcerated or changes in color, size, shape, or consistency.

The presence of the mucocutaneous melanin pigmentation of *Peutz-Jeghers syndrome* necessitates search for concomitant intestinal polyps. Gastrointestinal roentgenograms should be taken every two years in order to detect developing polyps. Radical surgical procedures should be avoided in absence of overt malignant change.

Oral lesions may be present in *acanthosis nigricans, pityriasis rosea, psoriasis, amyloidosis, Rendu-Osler-Weber syndrome, Sturge-Weber syndrome,* and *Gardner's syndrome.* Therapy, when available, is directed toward the primary disease.

Recurrent Aphthous Stomatitis (RAS). This is one of the most common diseases in the world, affecting up to 60 per cent of the affluent population. On the average, aphthae affect at least 20 per cent of young adults. RAS is classified in three types. The common (80 per cent) minor aphthous ulcers recur as crops of one to five lesions, less than 1 cm. in diameter, on the movable oral mucosa. Attacks remit within 5 years in about half the patients. Major aphthous ulcers recur as single (occasionally several) deep, slowly healing lesions, over 1 cm. in diameter, also on the movable oral mucosa. Attacks remit within 15 years in about one third of patients. Herpetiform aphthous ulcers recur as a large patch of a hundred or more, 1 to 2 mm. lesions, on one quadrant of the mouth, frequently involving the palate. Thirty per cent of the cases persist for 10 to 15 or more years.

The exact cause is unknown. Some cases are associated with a deficiency in the supply, absorption or utilization of Vitamin B_{12}, folic acid, iron, or zinc. This may account for the occurrence of aphthae in chronic ulcerative colitis, Crohn's disease, and celiac sprue. The oral lesions of Behçet's syndrome are typical aphthous ulcers. Other cases may represent an autoimmune phenomenon. Unexplained factors that may aid in management include: (1) recurrent attacks related to tension, the menstrual cycle, administration of progestins, and mild trauma from sharp-surfaced foods or dental manipulation; (2) remission of attacks with pregnancy, contraceptive pills, and heavy smoking; (3) rare occurrence in edentulous mouths until the patient begins to wear dentures; and (4) occurrence in several members of the same family.

Treatment. 1. Correct any deficiency status.

2. Treat any associated systemic disease.

3. Reduce all sources of trauma to the oral cavity: (a) Polish rough tooth edges; (b) correct malocclusion; (c) check prosthetic appliances for proper fit; (d) advise avoidance of sharp-surfaced foods such as peanuts, potato chips, or tacos; (e) advise patient not to talk and chew at the same time to avoid biting tongue or cheek; (f) teach patient proper, gentle, tooth-brushing technique with a soft brush.

4. Cauterization of very early lesions with silver nitrate or negatol (Negatan) decreases pain but frequently delays healing. Topical fluorinated

corticosteroids are of value during the first several days of the disease, but should be avoided once the lesion has become fully established. Topical antibiotics are indicated in the latter stages.

5. Local application of lidocaine (Xylocaine Viscous) or similar local anesthetic relieves the pain for short periods. This is of special value to relieve pain before meals.

6. Carbamide peroxide (Gly-oxide or Proxigel), applied locally, may relieve discomfort in some patients.

7. One teaspoonful of tetracycline (Achromycin) oral suspension used as a prolonged mouth rinse, four or more times daily and then swallowed, is of definite value. Each rinse is followed by the application of triamcinolone acetonide dental paste (Kenalog in Orabase). Herpetic aphthous ulcers often respond very well to this routine.

8. Very large or painful aphthae respond well to sublesional injections of 0.2 to 0.5 ml. of triamcinolone solution (5 mg. per ml.).

9. Occasionally, major aphthae are so painful and persist for so long that surgical excision may be considered.

10. Estrogens or estrogen-dominated oral contraceptives may control attacks associated with the menstrual period.

11. *Lactobacillus acidophilus* or *L. bulgaricus* preparations are of questionable value.

12. Autogenous vaccines from nose and pharynx cultures have been tried with equivocal results.

Gingivae and Periodontal Membrane

Normally, the eruption of deciduous and permanent teeth is associated with only local irritation and increased salivation. *Primary dentition* requires no treatment except reassurance of the parents, cold liquid foods and, occasionally, application of a topical anesthetic lidocaine (Xylocaine Viscous). Other symptoms associated with teething should be investigated for underlying respiratory or gastrointestinal causes.

Eruption cysts usually rupture spontaneously. When they do not, a wedge of gum tissue is removed to expose the crown of the tooth. A single incision may lead to scar formation and recurrence of the cyst.

Pericoronitis is the inflammatory reaction surrounding a partially erupted tooth, particularly a mandibular third molar. Warm saline mouth rinses suffice as treatment. Severe pericoronitis with facial or submaxillary swelling, cervical lymphadenopathy, elevated temperature or trismus should be treated with systemic antibiotics. Extraction of the third molar and opposing third molar is indicated if x-ray examination reveals either tooth to be impacted.

Chronic marginal gingivitis and *periodontal disease* indicate the need for dental prophylaxis, correction of dental or occlusal abnormalities, and construction of proper fitting prosthetic appliances. Severe cases require gingivectomy for complete removal of calculus, debris, granulation tissue, and periodontal "pockets." When the process has resulted in loosening of the teeth, temporary or permanent (expensive) splinting by appropriate dental appliances may save the teeth. Full dentures are never as satisfactory as permanent prosthetics. Patients with rapidly progressing periodontal disease should be examined carefully for the presence of diabetes mellitus, hyperparathyroidism, hyperthyroidism, and collagen disease.

Chronic desquamative gingivitis is a diffuse inflammatory reaction limited to the attached gingiva. There is some question as to whether this condition is a specific disease or a variant of benign mucosal pemphigoid, bullous pemphigoid, or pemphigus. The histopathologic findings are not diagnostic and serve only to exclude other diseases. Management, as discussed under general therapeutic considerations, will give symptomatic relief. Application of a topical fluorinated corticosteroid may be of value. A gel preparation, fluocinonide (Topsyn Gel), is preferable to an adhesive oral paste (Orabase), which may strip the thin friable epithelium. Systemic corticosteroids and estrogens have been used with limited success.

Simple hyperplastic gingivitis has many causes. Some cases develop without apparent cause; others follow chronic irritation or inflammation (poor dental hygiene, ill-fitting dentures, extraction sites). Occasionally, the constant sucking of hard candies or sweet cough drops precedes severe hyperplastic gingivitis. The gingival hyperplasia associated with vitamin C deficiency is one variant of this condition. *Pubertal hyperplastic gingivitis* is related to a disturbed hormonal balance, probably associated with subclinical scurvy superimposed on poor dental hygiene. *Pregnancy gingivitis* occurs in about 10 per cent of pregnancies. The relative ascorbic acid deficiency associated with pregnancy is possibly an underlying cause.

Treatment consists of:

1. Careful dental prophylaxis and maintenance of good oral hygiene.

2. Multivitamin preparations. Vitamin C, 500 to 1000 mg. daily for 7 to 10 days, then slowly decreased to a maintenance dose of 100 mg. daily. Smaller doses for children.

3. Eliminate use of hard candy and cough drops.

4. Gingivectomy for severe recalcitrant cases.

5. Remove pregnancy tumors by electrocautery if severe ulceration or annoying hemorrhage

occurs, but be conservative. Most of the pregnancy hyperplasia regresses spontaneously several months after parturition.

Phenytoin hyperplasia occurs in 6 per cent of patients who take phenytoin (Dilantin) to control their epilepsy. Poor dental hygiene underlies most cases. Treatment consists of:

1. Careful dental prophylaxis should be carried out and good dental hygiene maintained as soon as phenytoin is started because occurrence of hyperplasia does not justify stopping the drug.

2. Epileptic patients must be taught proper dental care and a member of the family must oversee home treatment.

3. Early, local dental treatment may clear the process; later, gingivoplasty is indicated, especially if the hyperplastic tissue interferes with mastication or becomes an esthetic problem.

Leukemic gingivitis does not occur in edentulous patients. Local irritation, secondary to calculus, is probably necessary for development of clinical manifestations. Treatment includes:

1. Systemic therapy.

2. Local therapy: (a) Maintain best possible dental hygiene; (b) relieve pain with anesthetic preparations and soothing, warm, saline mouth rinses; (c) treat any associated bacterial or Vincent's infection; (d) be very careful when doing extractions, deep scaling, and biopsies, as serious hemorrhage may follow minor trauma; (e) treat pulpitis by adequate drainage.

Hereditary fibromatosis is a rare, congenital, gingival hyperplasia. Gingivoplasty is usually necessary. Severe cases may require extraction of several teeth to ensure complete removal of all hyperplastic tissue.

Teeth

Dental agenesis is diagnosed by x-ray evidence of absent tooth buds. The open space should be maintained by an orthodontic appliance until the jaw has reached adult size, at which time a permanent bridge can be constructed. Partial or complete *anodontia* of one or both dentitions is rare but may occur as an isolated defect or may represent a facet of *anhydrotic ectodermal dysplasia*. Untreated anodontia leads to marked facial deformity. Removable and fixed dental appliances should be constructed as soon as the child will cooperate. Continuous modification of the appliance is necessary as the child grows. Every erupting tooth is saved to serve as a fixed abutment.

Early removal of *supernumerary teeth*, either erupted or impacted, is indicated. *Impacted teeth* should be removed because of the danger of pathologic fracture, infection, or development of a follicular cyst. Impacted third molars should be removed in order to prevent forward displace-

ment of the teeth. The opposing third molar should be removed at the same time. Multiple, unerupted, and impacted permanent teeth, and multiple supernumerary teeth are present in *cleidocranial dysostosis*.

Pigmentation of the teeth may result from neonatal jaundice, post injury hemorrhage into the tooth pulp, or ingestion of excessive amounts of fluoride or tetracycline during the development of enamel. The pregnant mother should not be given tetracycline after the first trimester. Prolonged treatment with tetracycline should not be given to children before the age of eight years. Children taking tetracycline for one year (such as for cystic fibrosis) present a 5 per cent incidence of staining. Attempts to bleach heavily pigmented teeth with oxidizing agents and ultraviolet light are only partially successful. Small areas can sometimes be corrected by carefully grinding out the stain and restoring the defect with a composite resin onlay. Only prosthetic replacement of the enamel with a ceramic or resin full crown gives good cosmetic results.

Developmental anomalies of the teeth in form, position, texture and color are not uncommon. Orthodontics and prosthodontia afford excellent improvement for these patients. *Malposition* and *malocclusion* of the teeth can also be corrected by orthodontic treatment. However, severe overbite, underbite, or open bite requires orthognathic surgery. Orthodontic therapy is prolonged, time consuming, and expensive. Except in those patients in whom the deformity compromises the patient's appearance or oral function, advice on such treatment should be tempered by consideration of cultural, esthetic, and financial factors.

Posteruptive Dental Defects. *Dental caries* is the most common posteruptive dental defect. Treatment of caries belongs in a textbook on restorative dentistry, a field which is beyond the scope of this section. Maintenance of good dental hygiene and dietary restriction of refined carbohydrates are proven methods of reducing the incidence of caries. Gum chewers and hard candy devotees should be switched to sugarless products. Fluoridated drinking water (2 ppm.) decreases caries approximately 50 per cent. Fluorinated toothpaste is also beneficial in reducing decay. *Rampant caries* develops in cases of extensive dental hypoplasia, systemic lupus erythematosus, juvenile diabetes, chronic xerostomia, very poor oral hygiene, and in children with high susceptibility to caries. Treatment requires maintenance of excellent dental hygiene, daily use of a fluoride gel (King's Gel-Tin), dietary control, and correction of underlying xerostomia if possible, in addition to restorative dentistry.

TRAUMA. Loosened teeth are checked for vitality and stabilized by orthodontic bands. Occasionally, the root of a fractured tooth can be preserved by endodontic therapy and used as the base for an orthodontic appliance. Reimplantation of dislodged teeth may be attempted with a fair chance of success.

TOOTH SUBSTANCE LOSS. *Attrition* is the wearing away of tooth substance by mastication. *Tooth brush abrasion* is the loss of tooth substances in V-shaped notches at cervical margins of teeth due to horizontal brushing. *Acid decalcification* may follow long-term drinking of lemon juice in hot water, administration of hydrochloric acid in liquid form, and chronic vomiting. *Loss of tooth substance due to habits or occupation* is seen in persons who open bobby pins with their teeth, the tailor who bites threads, and the carpenter who holds tacks or nails in his mouth. The patient with toothbrush abrasion is taught proper, vertical-stroke, brushing techniques. Other self-induced injuries are explained to the patient and an attempt is made to break the habits. Restorative dentistry can correct the defects, if expense is not a consideration.

Complications of Dental Extractions. Extraction of teeth is usually followed by uneventful healing. However, excessive bleeding, osteitis, perforation of the maxillary sinus, injury to the inferior alveolar nerve with resulting paresthesia, and even fracture of the mandible and osteomyelitis may occur. *Bleeding* and *osteitis* respond to accepted dental treatment and are seldom, if ever, seen by the physician. Patients with severe bleeding should be examined for clotting defects. *Paresthesia* usually resolves spontaneously. A *ruptured maxillary sinus* will probably heal spontaneously if the opening is small (1 to 2 mm.). Large openings are closed by surgical intervention. Tooth roots pushed into the sinus must be surgically extracted to prevent sinusitis. Broad-spectrum antibiotics are given during the healing stage.

Jaws

Jaw fractures are immobilized by orthodontic bands or wiring of the mandible, depending upon the type and severity of the fracture.

Osteomyelitis may occasionally follow simple extractions but usually develops from chronically infected teeth or from organisms that enter the oral cavity from an external source, such as from pulmonary tuberculosis or Actinomyces infection. Treatment requires identification of the causative organism and administration of appropriate antibiotics determined by sensitivity tests. *Chronic actinomycotic osteomyelitis* requires large doses of penicillin or tetracycline continued for 2 to 3 months. Drainage is maintained; radiographically identified sequestra are removed. The patient should also be examined for abnormal glucose metabolism.

Jaw cysts may be of odontogenic or nonodontogenic (fissured and epidermoid cysts) origin. All jaw cysts should be completely removed and examined histologically for confirmation of the diagnosis and identification of possible malignant metaplasia. Multiple jaw cysts may represent one component of the basal cell nevus syndrome.

Some jaw tumors present a typical radiographic picture; others require histopathologic identification. Most *odontogenic tumors* are not aggressive and the initial curettage for biopsy tissue may be adequate to prevent recurrence. Should the biopsy reveal marked immaturity of the cells or should the lesion recur, more extensive surgery is indicated. *Ameloblastomas* are aggressive and require block resection or even hemisection of the mandible. Surgical removal of *periapical cementoma* is not necessary unless enlargement of the tumor causes deformity of the face or jaw. *Fibrous dysplasia* is treated conservatively by shaving off the dysplastic bone as necessary to prevent cosmetic deformity. The *giant-cell reparative granuloma* is usually cured by thorough curettage. After histopathologic confirmation, the blood calcium level should be determined to rule out hyperparathyroidism.

Temporomandibular Joint

The temporomandibular joint may show *arthritic changes* as a result of trauma or as one facet of any rheumatoid disease. Treatment is similar to that available for other similarly affected joints. Intracapsular injection of corticosteroids may be of value. Limitation of jaw movement produces special problems in eating and oral hygiene. *Trismus* of the jaw muscles usually responds to physical therapy and muscle relaxants. Any underlying dental infection is treated with appropriate antibiotics.

Temporomandibular joint syndrome is a symptom complex consisting of recurrent, usually unilateral, clicking, limited movement, pain on movement or pressure over the joint, and tender areas in the masticatory muscles. Other symptoms include headache, tinnitus, and neuralgia in the jaw and neck areas. Suggested causative factors include a low-grade fasciitis and tendinitis, muscle spasm due to "tension," bruxism, occlusal abnormalities, and degenerative changes in the joint. Diagnosis is confirmed by elimination of trigeminal neuralgia, tic douloureux, other temporomandibular joint diseases, and diseases of the adjoining structures. Until the cause is determined, treatment is limited to local application of heat, analgesics, and muscle relaxants (diazepam [Valium], chlorzoxazone [Paraflex], methocarbamol [Robaxin]). Improperly fitting dentures and gross occlusal abnormalities are corrected. In rare cases, extensive occlusal equilibration may be helpful. Corticosteroids, locally or systemically, are of no definite value. Meniscectomy is contraindicated.

Salivary Glands

Sialolithiasis. Salivary calculi are not uncommon. Prompt removal of the blockage is necessary to prevent sialadenitis and eventual obliteration of the gland. Small, superficial stones of the submandibular gland may be milked, probed, or surgically removed from the duct. Large or inaccessible stones may necessitate excision of the gland. Obstruction of the parotid gland is more frequently due to inspissated mucous secretion. A diagnostic retrograde sialogram occasionally dislodges the obstruction.

Acute sialadenitis usually is due to obstruction of a major duct by a mucous or bacterial plug. Most cases clear within several weeks on a routine of systemic antibiotics and oral rinses with dilute, hot lemon juice. If the symptoms persist, incision and drainage of a localized abscess or removal of the gland may be indicated.

DISORDERS OF THE MOUTH (MALIGNANT)

method of
VERNE C. LANIER, JR., M.D.
Durham, North Carolina

Oral cavity malignancy accounts for 5 per cent of all cancer and 90 per cent of this is of the squamous cell variety. Although the incidence of intraoral malignancy is decreasing, 20,000 new cases will be diagnosed this year, and of these, less than half will survive 5 years. The point of origin, size of primary lesion, and presence or absence of metastatic disease are major considerations in determining methods of treatment and evaluating the prognosis. Extensive use of alcohol and tobacco are frequently associated with multicentric carcinoma and should be considered in certain patients.

The method of evaluation should include a thorough history and physical examination with endoscopy. Multiple biopsies may be of value in establishing the extent of disease. Facial roentgenograms are useful in determining bone and sinus involvement. Tomography is useful in delineating involvement of such areas as the base of the skull, temporomandibular joints, and cervical spine.

After these studies are completed, classification can then be established based on the tumor,

TABLE 1. **TMN Classification System for Squamous Carcinoma of Head and Neck Proposed by the American Joint Committee for Cancer Staging and End Results Reporting (1967)**

T:	Tumor
T_{1s}:	Carcinoma in situ
T_1:	Tumor 2 cm.
T_2:	Tumor 4 cm.
M:	Metastases (distant)
M_0:	None
M_1:	Distant metastases
N:	Regional lymph nodes
N_0:	No palpable nodes
N_1:	Ipsilateral lymph nodes (not fixed)
N_2:	Contralateral lymph nodes (not fixed)
N_3:	Fixed
Stage I:	$T_1N_0M_0$
Stage II:	$T_2N_0M_0$
Stage III:	$T_3N_0M_0$
	$T_1N_1M_0$
	$T_2N_1M_0$
	$T_3N_1M_0$
Stage IV:	Remainder

nodes, and metastases (TNM) system for squamous carcinoma of the head and neck (Table 1). This system of classification is beneficial in determining the modality of treatment and predicting prognosis.

A multidiscipline approach is then applied to each patient, whereby a "team" composed of a plastic surgeon, otolaryngologist, oral surgeon, oncologist, and radiotherapist evaluate and establish a course of therapy based on the above information. Stages I and II have a good prognosis regardless of method of treatment (surgery, radiotherapy, and adjunctive chemotherapy), but it is in the Stage III and IV lesions that all disciplines must be involved to ensure the patient the optimal chance for survival.

Tumor growth and routes of metastases differ considerably, depending on the anatomic location within the oral cavity. Therefore, division of the oral cavity into the following sections is necessary to adequately discuss treatment methods and prognosis: (1) lips, (2) tongue, (3) floor of mouth, (4) buccal mucosa, (5) gingiva and alveolar ridge, and (6) hard palate.

Lips

Carcinoma of the lower lip accounts for 1.1 per cent of all malignant tumors in males. The upper lip is infrequently involved. Prolonged exposure to sunshine and wind result in hyperkeratosis, which becomes indurated and later ulcerates, eventually leading to a carcinoma. The onset is most frequently in the fifth to seventh decade. Three distinct types of carcinoma are recognized: (1) exophytic, (2) ulcerating, and (3) verrucous. The exophytic is the most common variety, while the ulcerating form is the more aggressive. Verrucous carcinoma is very rare. Metastasis is uncommon, with regional node involvement occurring in 6 to 8 per cent. Patients with submental lymph nodes greater than 2 cm. in diameter should be suspected of having metastases. Treatment can be either external radiotherapy or surgery. The prognosis is excellent with an 80 to 95 per cent 5 year survival rate.

Tongue

Carcinoma of the tongue accounts for 1.1 per cent of all cancer in males. The onset most frequently occurs in the sixth and seventh decades. Alcohol, tobacco, and poor oral hygiene have been incriminated as causative factors. Carcinoma of the anterior two thirds (mobile position) most frequently occurs on the lateral borders. The base of the tongue (posterior third) is involved in 24 per cent. Metastatic disease manifested by cervical adenopathy is noted in 40 per cent of all patients on admission. Bilateral metastases are present in 20 per cent on admission and are more common in midline lesions. Treatment can be either radiotherapy or surgery or combinations of the two. Small lesions (less than 2 cm. in diameter) can be treated by either excision or radiotherapy. Lesions greater than 2 cm. should be treated with surgical excision and a composite radical neck dissection combined with radiotherapy. Such lesions may require resection of tongue, floor of mouth, and mandible. More extensive lesions, which may be unresectable or in which there is an inadequate surgical margin, should be treated with radiotherapy and adjunctive chemotherapy.

Prognosis is dependent upon the presence or absence of metastases. The overall 5 year survival is 46 per cent. In patients without cervical node involvement the 5 year survival rate is 64 per cent, while with metastatic disease the rate is 33 per cent. Carcinoma involving the posterior third is associated with a poor prognosis.

Floor of Mouth

Carcinoma of the floor of the mouth constitutes 15 per cent of oral cavity carcinoma. Males account for 80 per cent of the total incidence. Tobacco, alcohol, and poor hygiene are considered causative factors. The carcinoma usually presents as a fissure or ulcer in the floor of the mouth and may directly involve the tongue, mandible, and submaxillary gland. Lymph node metastases are most often noted in the submandibular region. Diagnosis is established by biopsy and treatment consists of en bloc removal of the primary lesion in continuity with a radical neck dissection combined with radiotherapy. The resection may need to include tongue and mandible. Adjunctive chemotherapy may be useful in advanced cases. Prognosis is somewhat better than in carcinoma of the tongue, with an overall 5 year survival of 55 per cent.

Buccal Mucosa

Carcinoma of the buccal mucosa is less common than that of the tongue and floor of the mouth. The incidence is highest in males in the sixth decade and is frequently associated with the chewing of tobacco. The onset may be insidious, with pain, bleeding, trismus, and adenopathy as the presenting symptoms. The carcinoma may extend throughout the cheek and metastasize to the upper cervical lymph nodes. Treatment consists of surgical excision combined with radiotherapy. In many instances an en bloc resection of the entire cheek, a portion of the mandible, and combined radical neck dissection may be required. Prognosis is determined by the size of the primary lesion, involvement of bone, and presence of lymph node metastases. The overall 5 year survival is 43 per cent.

Gingiva and Alveolar Ridge

The upper gingiva is formed by tissue covering the alveolar ridge of the maxilla while the lower gingiva is formed by tissue covering the mandibular alveolar ridge. The lower gingiva is more frequently involved with carcinoma. Most gingival carcinoma occurs in older persons beyond the fifth decade. The lesion consists of three types: exophytic, ulcerative, and verrucous. The ulcerative is the more aggressive type and bone invasion is a frequent occurrence (53 per cent). Bleeding, trismus, and difficulty fitting dentures may be the presenting complaints. Diagnosis is established by biopsy and roentgenograms can be of aid in determining bone involvement. Treatment is surgical excision, usually including a portion of the mandible in continuity with a radical neck dissection combined with radiotherapy and adjunctive chemotherapy in advanced cases. As in other forms of intraoral malignancy, prognosis is determined by the size of the primary lesion, the local extent, and presence of metastases. The overall 5 year survival is 34 to 47 per cent.

Hard Palate

Squamous cell carcinoma of the hard palate is relatively rare and usually occurs in older men. Due to the slow growth of these lesions, they may be of considerable size when initially seen. Diagnosis is established by biopsy. Treatment is surgical excision, which may involve a radical resection of the maxilla. Radical neck dissection combined with radiotherapy is included for patients with cervical metastases. In view of the age of presentation and extent of local involvement, the prognosis is usually not good, with a 5 year survival rate of 24 per cent.

Summary of Therapy

In spite of improved surgical techniques, better understanding of tumor biology, and advances in radiation and chemotherapy, the overall result of treating carcinoma of the oral cavity has not been good. The multidiscipline approach affords the patient the benefit of each specialty to not only provide the best opportunity for survival but to also enhance the quality of life.

It is in the advanced cases (Stages III and IV) that the "team" is most applicable to decide on the role of surgical intervention, radiation, and chemotherapy.

1. Surgical intervention is designed to remove en bloc the primary lesion and lymph node bearing area. This may require resection of units containing tongue, floor of mouth, mandible, and radical neck dissection. Primary reconstruction is initiated immediately following the extirpation and may require bone grafting, skin grafting, and the use of distant pedicle flaps. In certain instances reconstruction may be delayed to permit pathologic evaluation to ensure that adequate margins have been obtained.

2. Postoperative radiation is given, using a Cobalt-60 unit, whereby 5000 rads is administered to those patients without cervical node involvement and 6000 rads is given to those with positive nodes. The dosage is given in fractions of 200 rads in five treatments each week.

3. Chemotherapy is used as adjunctive therapy and is initiated 3 weeks following surgery or radiation in six 28 day cycles. Agents employed for oral carcinoma include bleomycin, methotrexate, vinblastine, and lomustine (CCNU). Each of these has been demonstrated to be effective against squamous cell carcinoma. Bleomycin is administered subcutaneously in 10 unit aliquots on the first and fourth days of the course, then repeated at a dosage of 2 units on the same days in successive cycles. Methotrexate is given orally at a dosage of 10 mg. per square meter of body surface on days 1 and 4 of each course. Vinblastine is given intravenously at 8 mg. per square meter on the first day of each course. CCNU is effective when administered in conjunction with other agents and is given orally at a dosage of 75 mg. per square meter only on the first day of the course. Bone marrow suppression must be carefully monitored and with vinblastine neurotoxicity must be watched for and, if it occurs, the dosage reduced by 50 per cent.

4. Nursing care involving dietitian, speech therapist, and social service agency should be an integral part of any therapeutic program to assist both the patient and his family to accept, treat, and obtain a satisfactory quality of life.

DISEASES OF THE NAILS

method of
LARRY E. MILLIKAN, M.D.
Columbia, Missouri

Nail Changes

While often considered minor and of no serious import, the nail is of considerable cosmetic importance to the patient and deformities or changes in the nail plate may often bring them in for care. In addition to this, nail changes may often be a valuable indication of systemic disease and the treatment of that disease may spontaneously resolve the offending nail problem. The slow rate of nail growth (0.1 mm. or less per day) should always be kept in mind when following therapy. Appropriate treatment of a disorder in the nail matrix may take in excess of 3 months to allow the regrowth of a completely normal nail. In the elderly patient it takes even longer. A careful examination of the nail plate, cuticle, nail bed, and the paronychial tissue, should be a part of every complete examination. While certain conditions present involving primarily the nail plate, matrix, bed, or cuticle, they seldom involve one structure alone and therefore we will deal with disorders of the nail and surrounding tissues as a whole rather than subdividing them by the primary structure involved.

Infections

Tinea.   Leading the list of infections are those caused by fungi. The dermatophytes are the most common in this group, especially those of the genera *Trichophyton* and *Epidermophyton*. It is not unusual to see tinea unguium accompanying tinea cruris or tinea pedis/manum. One should carefully differentiate tinea unguium from psoriasis and some of the other skin diseases that cause significant nail changes (vide infra). Confirmation using fungal culture is usually easiest because the thickened dystrophic nail plate requires prolonged clearing to get a satisfactory KOH (potassium hydroxide) examination. Heavily infected nails with extensive crumbling subungual debris can be examined by potassium hydroxide, much as is done in tinea infections elsewhere on the body. Griseofulvin is the primary treatment for tinea, but a prolonged course is usually necessary. Some practitioners recommend avulsion of the heavily affected and severely deformed nails prior to the initiation of griseofulvin. This is not routine in my practice, but is done on rare occasions where the distorted nail causes significant discomfort or cosmetic problems. Griseofulvin is indicated in dermatophyte infections and has no therapeutic effectiveness against candidiasis. The newer forms of griseofulvin of smaller particulate size (Gris-PEG, Fulvicin P/G) are preferred because of better absorption. While the recommended dosage is 500 mg. per day for nail infections, we have generally used one (125 mg.) tablet three times daily with meals with satisfactory results. It must be stressed to the patient that treatment is prolonged, usually in excess of 3 months.

Candida. Candidiasis of the nails is often associated with Candida elsewhere on the body, and perhaps the most common presentation is that of the chronic paronychia, in which the lateral nail plate and paronychial tissues are the site of a prolonged low-grade infection. This may be secondary to previous trauma or chronic exposure to moisture from thumb sucking in children and from occupational sources in adults. The paronychial tissue is usually moderately inflamed and quite tender. Culture is helpful in these patients in separating out bacterial infections. Treatment of a chronic paronychia may again require removal of the infected nail plate. In most patients, treatment using liquid anticandida preparations is sufficient. Four per cent thymol in chloroform is a very effective substance that penetrates, is drying, and has antifungal properties. The newer broad spectrum antifungal preparations including clotrimazole (Lotrimin), miconazole (MicaTin), and haloprogin (Halotex) can be applied two to three times daily, and often penetration is adequate enough to eradicate the infection. Chronic paronychias can often be secondarily infected, resulting in rapid coloration of the nail plate. With sudden change, giving a green appearance to the nail plate, one should suspect Pseudomonas and treat it accordingly. The otic solutions containing neomycin and polymyxin (Polysporin and others) are very effective in treating secondary Pseudomonas infections. It has been reported that Proteus can do the same thing, but often the characteristic pigment is then brown. Treatment is again the same as for Pseudomonas.

Bacterial Infections. Staphylococcal infections of the nail usually present acutely as the classical acute paronychia. Here, large amounts of purulent fluid accumulate under the nail, often requiring incision and drainage. With limited involvement in the paronychial area often topical therapy is quite successful in controlling the infection. We use polymyxin B, bacitracin and neomycin (Neosporin Otic) drops on the nail or again use 4 per cent thymol in chloroform, for the drying characteristics of the chloroform often will rapidly clear the infection. With recurrent infections a prolonged course of antibacterial therapy may be necessary and attention must be made to primary factors that allow secondary bacterial invasion. Various eczematous changes and traumatic changes to the paronychial area may often be causative. In these cases iodochlorhydroxyquin (Vioform), which has broad-spectrum antibacterial, antifungal, and anticandidal activity, is very useful. The primary skin disorder associated with the infection will respond to hydrocortisone solution and the ideal preparation for chronic treatment in our hands is hydrocortisone and iodochlorhydroxyquin (HEB-Cort V) lotion. This lotion can be applied two to four times daily and carefully rubbed into the infected area. This will spontaneously clear the underlying structural problem and prevent secondary bacterial colonization.

Viral Infection. Herpes simplex can involve the nail and its surrounding tissues as the classical herpetic whitlow. This can be extremely painful and sometimes strong analgesics such as codeine are required to make the patient comfortable. We routinely use either ether soaks on the acute vesicular stage or the urea lotions (Carmol, Aquacare HP). We have had success also treating recurrent lesions early by freezing them with liquid nitrogen. This seems to hasten clearing and in our estimation may decrease the recurrence rate. Many other techniques have been reported as successful, but we feel these approaches are the most consistently successful ones.

Ingrown Toenails. Ingrown toenails are a chronic problem, sometimes considered infectious in origin, but in reality they are nearly always a foreign body reaction with secondary infection. Trauma to the lateral nail plate and nail groove sets the stage for the problem. Often, tight-fitting shoes are the initiating factor. Control of secondary infection should be done and the drug of choice is one of the tetracycline group because of their capability to concentrate in the inflammatory site. Surgical removal of the edge of nail plate protruding into the granulation tissue then should be done. Often, cotton can be placed in the nail groove under the edge of the nail plate to allow the nail to grow out without causing a recurrence of the problem. In severe and recurrent cases the lateral one third of the nail plate must be surgically excised. If the problem recurs after this, then the lateral one third of the nail plate and the lateral nail matrix will have to be removed totally to eliminate the possibility of regrowth of the lateral portion of the nail.

Nail Changes Associated With Other Disease

Psoriasis. Chronic nail changes are often associated with underlying cutaneous or metabolic diseases, the most common of which is psoriasis. The classical changes seen in psoriasis are the thickening of the nail plate and the extensive build up of subungual debris, or onycholysis. In addition, the nail plate has multiple irregular pits on the surface that result from defective keratinization associated with the accelerated epithelial turnover and parakeratosis of psoriasis. One should always differentiate carefully between psoriasis and dermatophyte infection, for there often can be diagnostic confusion because of the similar appearance between the two. The treatment for dermatophyte infection (vide supra) is very specific, as is that for psoriasis. The nail defects result largely from abnormalities in the nail matrix, and this is the area that should be treated to correct the nail deformity of psoriasis. Injection of steroids into the nail matrix will often remarkably improve the appearance of the nail over the ensuing few months as it grows out. However, this is quite painful and an alternative includes the use of the Dermajet. The newer, more potent steroid gel formulations fluocinonide (Topsyn), betamethasone benzoate (Benisone, Fluorobate), and triamcinolone (Aristogel) may penetrate sufficiently in many cases to give the patient some relief. Treatment of the psoriasis with near complete clearing of the skin by various modalities including the Goeckerman-U.V. therapy and the psoralen and long wave length ultraviolet light (PUVA) treatment also may result in clearing of the nail. Therefore, one should direct therapy not only at the nail matrix but also at the patient's generalized disease. The cytotoxic drugs occasionally used in severe generalized psoriasis are never indicated for nail disease alone.

Alopecia Areata. Nail pits are also seen in alopecia areata. Here, one sees numerous pits in the nail plate generally in a gridlike pattern. This finding should alert one to the possibility of alopecia areata and investigation of the history is in order. There is no specific treatment for this, although the severity of the nail involvement tends to parallel the hair loss. Treatments aimed at correcting the hair loss, often secondarily, result in improvement in the nail. Eczematous disorders involving the nail matrix can result in a wide variety of changes in the nail plate, including pitting, ridging, grooving, and splitting. Careful examination of the cuticle for the changes of eczema establishes the diagnosis. Treatment with

hydrocortisone and iodochlorhydroxyquin (HEB-Cort V) lotion three to four times a day is usually the most satisfactory approach. Other disorders of cutaneous turnover and differentiation may be associated with nail changes, and these include the grooving seen in Darier's disease. Other epithelial disorders are associated with abnormalities of the nails such as pachonychia congenita, and untreated patients with acrodermatitis enteropathica may have profound nail changes with extensive loss of nails. Zinc levels should be evaluated carefully in patients with acrodermatitis enteropathica, for zinc therapy has been shown to be specific treatment with cure in many patients and nearly complete clearing of the disease in most.

The nail may mirror mere systemic disease at a very early stage and appropriate early treatment will correct the nail and underlying disease before it becomes fully manifest.

Anemia. *Koilonychia or spoon nails* has historically been associated with iron deficiency anemia and is the primary underlying condition to be evaluated in such patients. Therapy with iron will often reverse the nail changes. For those patients who have koilonychia of an unknown cause there is no good specific treatment at the present time.

Onycholysis. The regression of the nail bed from the nail plate proximally can be due to a number of causes. It has been associated with thyroid disease and any other signs of hyper- or hypothyroidism should dictate the appropriate laboratory studies and then therapy for the underlying thyroid condition is curative. Onycholysis can result from low-grade chronic infection similar to that seen in chronic paronychia, and here we find hydrocortisone and iodochlorhydroxyquin (HEB-Cort V) a very useful form of therapy to minimize the inflammation of the nail bed as well as treating the underlying infection with iodochlorhydroxyquin (Vioform). Recently, patients on the tetracycline antibiotics have been found to have a photo-onycholysis resulting from tetracycline deposition and secondary photosensitivity. Discontinuing the drug corrects the deformity. Trauma is another significant cause of onycholysis, especially in young typists with long tapered nails. The chronic trauma of the nails hitting the typewriter keys separates the nail plate from the nail bed and results in a progressive onycholysis. We strongly encourage patients with symptomatic onycholysis of occupational origin to trim the nails short and often use an anti-inflammatory agent if significant erythema is present in the nail bed.

Changes in the Nail Plate

Certain classical changes in the nail plate have had diagnostic importance. These include the transverse grooving known as Beau's lines, Mee's lines, Hellers canaliform dystrophy, other miscellaneous linear grooves, and patchy or diffuse leukonychia. Beau's lines have been associated with severe systemic illness that causes a decrease in production of nail matrix. This is reflected in a transverse groove present in almost all the nails. The same decrease in production of keratin is reflected in the hair with a constriction of the hair shaft causing fragility and breakage of the hairs. This finding temporarily documents severe disease and was seen commonly in the past with typhoid fever and other febrile illnesses. Noninfectious severe systemic diseases can also cause the same findings. No treatment is necessary or indicated. Hellers medialcanaliform dystrophy nail is usually associated with an abnormality in the nail matrix and, in some instances, this is an area of mucous degeneration. This localized nail dystrophy usually responds to steroids. They can be given intralesionally using triamcinolone acetonide (Kenalog-10) (10 mg. per ml. diluted with equal parts of sterile saline to make final concentration 5 mg. per ml.) and a small amount injected into the matrix, proximal to the area of the linear deformity. Mee's lines are white transverse lines representing arsenic deposition in the nail.

Leukonychia or white areas of the nail can be seen in both a patchy and diffuse distribution. Those patients with small punctate areas of leukonychia usually have them on the basis of trauma or localized areas of nail abnormalities. There is no specific therapy for this, nor is there generally any concern of systemic causes of serious nature. In contrast, patients who develop a diffuse leukonychia involving all fingers and affecting sometimes more than half of the nail plate of each nail may have this abnormality on the basis of systemic disease, usually related to liver or kidney disease in the cases described in the literature. These nail changes are a clue to investigate further and may be reversible when the primary defect is corrected. Lastly, an asymmetrical or isolated nail deformity may be associated with trauma to the nail on the basis of habit, tics, or overly aggressive manicure. Some of these localized abnormalities have been closely associated with certain activities and occupations and serve as occupational marks. In all of these patients the diagnosis is the result of careful detective work and, once the inciting event is discovered, education of the patient to try to avoid a future trauma of the nail will be corrective.

Tumors

Warts are the primary benign tumor affecting the nail. Periungual warts are perhaps the most difficult type of wart to treat. This is because the infected tissue often extends under the nail plate and easy removal of the wart in total is almost impossible without removing the nail plate. Perhaps the most effective single modality for the treatment of periungual warts is the use of liquid nitrogen, for here, freezing will extend under the nail plate without any significant decrement in activity. In contrast, most destructive agents used for warts elsewhere on the body, including salicylic acid preparations and cantharidin (Cantharone), often have no effect under the nail plate. With failure of usual therapy, more aggressive means may be indicated. However, before going to these, one should always remember that a high percentage of warts clear spontaneously with the passage of time. This perhaps explains the beneficial results sometimes obtained with the various types of treatment that can only be considered suggestive therapy at best. Often, careful hygiene and compulsive cleansing may hasten clearing of the warts. In some instances, I will have the patient wash the periungual infected tissue two to three times a day with povidone-iodine (Betadine) skin cleanser in very hot water using a surgical scrub brush. Often this tends to clear them. The patient should also be advised to be careful about manicuring and biting the nails, for this may have a tendency to spread the wart virus from finger to finger. When all this fails, it is sometimes necessary to remove part of the nail plate to get at the remaining wart tissue and destroy it. It is usually best, when most routine treatments have failed, to refer the patient for further care, and some centers are doing forms of immunotherapy for warts that is promising.

The significant malignant tumors involving the nails are Bowen's disease, basal cell carcinoma, and malignant melanoma. Bowen's disease is becoming more common in my practice and any unusual ulcerated or eczematous patches that are resistant to therapy should be considered as possible Bowen's disease. Diagnosis here is established by biopsy of any lesion of the nail or periungual tissue that does not heal with routine therapy. Bowen's disease can be very successfully treated with the use of topical 5-fluorouracil (Efudex or Fluoroplex). Basal cell carcinoma also presents as a problem of a persistent nodule or nonhealing ulcer and, here again, diagnosis is established on the basis of biopsy and treatment is surgical removal.

Finally, malignant melanoma may present with the initial findings of linear pigmented streaks within the nail. In black patients melanin is present in the nail bed and under these circumstances, linear pigmented streaks do not have as serious a prognosis. However, with the caucasian patient, the appearance of pigment in the nail should immediately lead to a careful examination and biopsy of the affected nail matrix to determine if the pigment is from merely a nevus of the nail matrix, or malignant melanoma. Amputation is the treatment of choice for malignant melanoma.

NEVI
(Common Moles)

method of
CHESTER M. SIDELL, M.D.
Sherman Oaks, California

The two methods most often used in removing pigmented nevi are: (1) excision and closure, and (2) shave (partial excision) and coagulation. Considerable controversy surrounds the treatment of these lesions, just as it does other aspects of the subject of nevi and melanomas. The physician who will be diagnosing and treating them should be familiar with the various classifications and their therapeutic and prognostic implications. A common classification is as follows:

1. Simple lentigo
2. Junction nevus
3. Compound nevus
4. Intradermal nevus
5. Blue nevus (Jadassohn)
6. Juvenile melanoma
7. Lentigo maligna
8. Malignant melanoma
9. Giant congenital nevus

Removal of pigmented nevi is usually done for one of three reasons:

1. To remove a possibly hazardous lesion. This would include: (a) suspected melanoma—lesions with sudden change in pigmentation, size and shape; with irritation or inflammation; very black lesions, particularly in light skinned, blue eyed persons; (b) juvenile melanomas; (c) clinically active junction nevi; and (d) nevi in high-risk areas such as lip, nail, mucosa, and genitalia. Lesions in this category should be excised with a border of normal tissue and submitted in toto for histologic evaluation.

2. To remove a lesion subject to chronic irritation. This would include those benign appearing compound and intradermal nevi which, because of location, would be subjected by clothing, shaving, or other factors to repeated trauma. Lesions in this category may be totally or partially excised and submitted for histologic examination.

3. To remove lesions that are cosmetically objectionable. This group constitutes the majority of lesions removed. They are usually intradermal,

occasionally compound nevi, elevated, dome-shaped or sessile, flesh-colored to lightly pigmented lesions, most often presented for treatment because of location on face or neck and are frequently multiple. Lesions in this category may be partially excised (shaved and coagulated), which gives the best cosmetic result, or totally excised. In either case, the specimen is sent for histologic evaluation.

Excision and "Partial" Excision with Coagulation

Excision. Although there is some opinion in the literature that total excision is the only proper method for removal of pigmented nevi, many physicians disagree with this with respect to Group 2 and especially Group 3, where cosmesis is the primary consideration for removal. Excision of nevi notoriously produces a scar that tends to stretch, leave punctate suture marks, and dehisce. These complications can be minimized by using absorbable buried sutures, intradermal running sutures, and supplementary tape reinforcement of the suture line, both at the time of surgery and after removal of cutaneous sutures. Patients will accept a cosmetic defect if the removal method was dictated by considerations of safety, but they are unhappy with a defect that is less attractive than a "mole" that was removed for cosmetic improvement.

Shave (Partial Excision) and Coagulation. In categories 2 and 3 above, shave with coagulation is easier, faster, and usually gives a considerably better cosmetic end result. Using this technique, elevated portions of the "mole" are shaved off cleanly with a new No. 10 or No. 15 scalpel blade or a flexible safety razor blade, slightly bent between the thumb and first or second finger tip. Shave removal is made as nearly as possible flush with the skin surface. This provides a specimen for microscopic examination that includes the dermal-epidermal junction. Bleeding is controlled chemically with 30 or 50 per cent trichloroacetic acid, a styptic pencil, epinephrine (Adrenalin) and absorbable gelatin (Gelfoam) powder or electrocoagulation. If the high frequency cautery is used, monopolar current is best at a very low setting to minimize deep coagulation, which would impair the scar. The best method for control of bleeding and one that also permits modeling the surface to precisely the level and contour of the skin, is the hot wire cautery, using a small unit, such as the National, with a wire tip heated to a bright cherry red. If the tip is wiped rapidly and lightly over the surface, bleeding will be instantly controlled. Using a gauze sponge saturated with water and a few drops of 10 per cent Duponol (or other wetting agent, not alcohol), wet the area and cauterize the surface using a light rotary motion. A thin layer will carbonize, and the entire area will shrink due to dehydration. When it is sponged lightly with a gauze saturated with water and wetting agent, the carbonized layer will be removed and the tissue rehydrated. Cauterization and sponging are repeated until, after thorough moistening, the surface of the lesion is flush with the surrounding skin. With this procedure it is necessary to anesthetize a narrow zone around the nevus, as the cautery tip radiates considerable heat. When the surface has been brought to the desired level and contour, a bandage may be applied for 2 to 3 hours, then removed, and the area left open. Bathing and ordinary activities are permitted. After getting wet, the area is dried, and rubbing alcohol is applied. Healing is usually complete in 10 to 12 days, leaving a pink macule that eventually turns flesh-colored or a little paler. If the area is elevated after healing, it can be anesthetized and cauterized slightly or more deeply if desired. Occasionally, repigmentation may occur. If this becomes stationary, it may be observed or treated with a single application of 50 per cent trichloroacetic acid. If it is progressive, it should be excised and reexamined.

Blue nevi (Jadassohn) and small hairy pigmented nevi are rarely dangerous but, if treated, should be excised.

The management of congenital giant pigmented nevi is a special problem and will not be discussed here, except to say that it now is considered safe to do wedge or punch biopsies for evaluation of significant areas in these massive lesions.

Removal of lentigo simplex is rarely done. These pigmented macules are benign and of little cosmetic significance. Removal by any method that permits adequate material for biopsy usually leaves a cosmetic defect worse than the lesion.

Management of ientigo maligna (see p. 643) and melanoma (see p. 578) is discussed elsewhere in this volume.

OCCUPATIONAL DERMATOSES

method of
JAMES S. TAYLOR, M.D.
Cleveland, Ohio

Occupational skin disorders still account for almost half of all reported work illnesses, despite the fact that they are almost fully preventable. No industry, whatever its size, scope, or location, is immune to their occurrence. Occupational skin diseases are produced from old chemicals in processes both old and new, new chemicals in new processes, and a wide variety of biologic and physiologic agents. The major categories of work-related skin disorders are contact dermatitis (allergic, irritant, and photosensitivity), acne and follicular eruptions, and pigmentary abnormalities.

Contact Dermatitis

In this category are most occupational dermatoses. They may be caused by some of the hundreds of thousands of chemicals used in industry. About 80 per cent of contact dermatitis is produced by irritants, 20 per cent from allergic sensitization, and a small percentage, often overlooked, from photosensitivity. Most affected are the hands, but any part of the body may be involved.

Acute Contact Dermatitis. 1. Avoid contact with the offending agent. This may require several days away from work or temporary transfer to another job.

2. Avoid contact with potential aggravating factors such as excessive soap and water, alcohol, thimerosal, and sensitizers such as topically applied antihistamines, antibiotics (neomycin or nitrofurazone), and anesthetics ("caine" preparations). Other contributing factors to be avoided are heat, friction, and radiant energy.

3. Apply cool wet compresses to weeping and blistered areas 15 minutes two to three times daily. Isotonic saline solution may be used. With commercial preparations of Burow's solution (Bluboro powder or Domeboro powder or tablets), 1 packet or tablet per 500 ml. (pint) of water makes approximately a 1:40 dilution. Make certain the mixture is completely dissolved before application. A soft cloth such as Kerlix gauze, an old, clean thin white handkerchief, or a towel is immersed in the solution. The cloth is wrung slightly and applied to the affected area of the skin. When the cloth begins to dry, remove it completely and resoak in the solution before reapplying. Do not pour the solution directly on the dressing; a fresh solution should be prepared before each treatment.

As an alternative the patient may soak the affected part, such as a hand or a foot, directly in the solution for the same period of time.

For generalized involvement hospitalization may be necessary. Compresses may be applied to all affected areas of the body, and in some cases baths such as with Aveeno colloidal oatmeal may be preferable.

Treatment should be continued for no more than a few days (usually 3 to 4) to avoid excessive drying of the skin.

4. Immediately following the compresses, soaks, or baths, apply a topical corticosteroid spray

(triamcinolone [Kenalog] spray or betamethasone [Valisone] aerosol). A 2 or 3 second spray to each affected area is sufficient. One of the many topical corticosteroid creams such as betamethasone valerate (Valisone), triamcinolone (Kenalog), or fluocinolone acetonide (Synalar) may be used when the acute dermatitis is not extensively vesicular. Avoid ointments in the acute stages.

5. Oral antihistamines such as cyproheptadine (Periactin), hydroxyzine (Atarax), or diphenhydramine (Benadryl) help relieve itching. It is imperative that workers be warned not to drive or operate dangerous machinery while taking antihistamines.

6. Systemic use of corticosteroids is indicated in patients with severe, localized dermatitis, such as a vesiculobullous eruption of the hands or feet, or with severe, generalized dermatitis. An injection of triamcinolone acetonide suspension (Kenalog-40 injection) may be given, or oral corticosteroids such as prednisone (Deltasone), 30 mg. to 60 mg. daily in two or three divided doses, is begun initially and tapered over 10 to 30 days.

Subacute and Chronic Contact Dermatitis. 1. Avoidances as outlined in (1) above.

2. Do not compress or soak.

3. Use a topical corticosteroid cream or ointment two to three times daily and continue treatment for 2 to 3 weeks after the skin appears normal.

4. Oral antihistamines as in (5) above.

5. I wish to emphasize that frequently recurring cases of acute contact dermatitis should be considered "chronic," and frequent use (more than once every 3 months) of short courses of systemic corticosteroids should be avoided. In these patients a tireless search for precipitating and aggravating factors is necessary.

Secondarily Infected Contact Dermatitis. In my experience this is infrequent. A low grade bacterial infection such as from a coagulase-positive Staphylococcus may occur. In these patients compresses or soaks with povidone-iodine (Betadine Solution) are helpful, followed by application of oxytetracycline-hydrocortisone spray or ointment (Terra-Cortril). Bacterial cultures should be taken, and antibiotic therapy such as erythromycin stearate (Erythrocin), 250 mg. three to four times daily for 10 days, is initiated. Acute cellulitis with accompanying chills, fever, and lymphangitis may require more aggressive and closely supervised antibiotic therapy.

Ancillary Measures in Treatment of Occupational Contact Dermatitis

Resources to Identify Causative Agent(s). It is imperative that the causative agent(s) be identified in every patient. Unless this is done, treatment may be doomed to failure and the patient will experience recurrences of the dermatosis. A careful work history should be obtained to determine in detail all the patient's industrial contacts. Inquiry into exposures from second jobs, hobbies, and household contactants is essential. In this regard I have found it most helpful to consult the following sources:

1. Occupational Diseases of the Skin, by L. Schwartz, L. Tulipan, and D. J. Birmingham. 3rd ed. Philadelphia, Lea & Febiger, 1957.

2. Occupational Contact Dermatitis, by R. M. Adams, Philadelphia, J. B. Lippincott Co., 1969.

3. Contact Dermatitis, by A. A. Fisher. 2nd ed. Philadelphia, Lea & Febiger, 1973.

4. Occupational Dermatoses, by G. A. Gellin. Chicago, American Medical Association, Department of Environmental, Public and Occupational Health, 1972.

5. Chapters 14 and 15 on contact dermatitis by N. Hjorth and S. Fregert, *in* Rook, Wilson, and Ebling: Textbook of Dermatology. 2nd ed. Oxford, Blackwell, 1972.

6. Industrial Hygiene Toxicology, F. A. Patty (ed.). 2nd ed. New York, Interscience, 1958–63.

7. Division of Technical Services, National Institute for Occupational Safety and Health, United States Public Health Service, 4676 Columbia Parkway, Cincinnati, Ohio 45226.

8. The patient's employer (with the consent of the patient), such as the plant manager or industrial research department.

Together these resources may provide lists of chemicals contacted in various occupations, information on cutaneous and systemic toxicity of chemicals, suggested patch testing concentrations, and information on sources of products and processes which contain a particular chemical. The latter is extremely important, because a worker may be exposed to the same chemical at home and at work (e.g., rubber, metal, chromates, dyes, plastic resins) or in several sources at work.

Diagnostic Patch Testing. Patch testing, when properly performed and correctly interpreted, is unquestionably of great value in identifying the causative agent(s) of allergic contact dermatitis. Initial testing is usually done with the most frequent contact allergens (nickel, chromates, rubber, medicaments, preservatives, dyes, and resins). Other materials, found at home or work, may also have to be tested in appropriate concentrations in order to distinguish occupational and nonoccupational factors. Patch testing should be employed only by physicians highly experienced with this technique. Pre-employment patch testing should generally be avoided. The same recommendations and precautions apply to photopatch testing which is used to diagnose photoallergic contact dermatitis.

Preventive Measures. It is impossible to separate treatment from prevention. Personal measures such as wearing protective clothing may be required when they can be used safely. Barrier or protective creams should only be used as a last resort and should never be applied to inflamed skin. Environmental control such as good housekeeping, engineering controls, and removal of physical and chemical hazards is also important.

Fiberglass Dermatitis

This special form of papular, eczematous, and occasionally purpuric dermatitis is produced by mechanical irritation from glass fibers. Body folds and areas of tight-fitting clothing are common sites of involvement. Hardening usually occurs after several weeks of exposure.

Treatment. 1. Limitation of further exposure to fiberglass.

2. Wearing of loose-fitting clothing which is changed daily.

3. Frequent skin cleansing.

4. Topical corticosteroid creams (see Contact Dermatitis, above).

5. Workers with dermographism or urticaria should not work with fiberglass.

Oil Acne

Most cutting fluids used today are synthetic or semisynthetic and most frequently produce contact eczema. Treatment of these patients should follow measures described previously for contact dermatitis. However, exposure to insoluble, straight cutting fluids may produce folliculitis ("oil boils") in areas uncommon for acne vulgaris, usually the extremities.

Treatment. 1. Avoidance of contact with oils and grease.

2. Daily changes of work clothing.

3. Frequent cleansing of the skin with soap and water.

4. The worker should avoid cleansing his skin with his fabric waste, which is intended only for cleaning machines and tools.

5. Local acne medications (benzoyl peroxide 5 per cent lotion or gel or retinoic acid cream 0.05 to 0.1 per cent).

Chloracne

This extremely refractory form of industrial acne is produced by exposure to various chlorinated aromatic compounds, such as chloronaphthalenes, polychlorobiphenyls, polychlorodibenzofurans, and chlorophenol and aniline herbicide intermediates.

Treatment. 1. Absolute avoidance of chemical exposure through a totally enclosed manufacturing process.

2. Appraisal of possible systemic toxicity, including liver, kidney, and porphyrin analyses.

3. Work clothing should be laundered at work.

4. Double locker rooms (clean and dirty) with adequate shower facilities.

5. Protective creams should not be used.

Pigmentation Disorders

Staining. A number of chemicals stain the skin by direct external contact. The stain usually responds to attempts at cleansing, avoidance of chemical exposure, and the passage of time.

Hyperpigmentation. Exposure to tar, pitch, and chemicals such as psoralens in combination with ultraviolet light may produce increased pigmentation of the skin. Protective clothing and/or sunscreens may be helpful. Hydroquinone (Eldoquin), applied twice daily, may help reduce the pigmentation.

Hypopigmentation. Exposure to monobenzyl ether of hydroquinone (rubber industry), paratertiary butyl phenol or catechol, or paratertiary amyl phenol (germicidal disinfectants, oils, plastics, paints, or resins) may produce occupational leukoderma. Treatment involves avoiding chemical exposure and using stains for the skin (Vitadye, Dy-O-Derm). Photochemotherapy with oral psoralens (methoxsalen [Oxsoralen]) and black ultraviolet light is usually not effective in this form of leukoderma.

Other Dermatoses

Microbial infections, granulomatous reactions, ulcerations, and neoplasms may occasionally occur. The spectrum of these and other occupational dermatoses is wide, and therapy varies depending upon cause. The hallmarks for the successful treatment of occupational dermatoses are identifying the causative agent(s), early therapy, and prevention of further chemical exposure.

PEDICULOSIS

method of
THOMAS N. PAIGE, M.D.
Walnut Creek, California

One per cent lindane (gamma benzene hexachloride) has been used in the United States for nearly 3 decades to control lice. Until recent years this chemical was applied to the integument without regard to possible ill effects from percutaneous absorption. It is now known that 10 per cent of lindane can be absorbed from the skin into the blood after extensive or prolonged topical application and can have possible neurotoxic effects. Lindane is still an effective treatment for lice, but the amount and duration of its use on the skin should be carefully monitored.

Pediculosis Capitis

Pediculosis capitis (head louse) is seen frequently in children but can also infest the scalp of adults. Factors that seem to promulgate the disease are overcrowding, sharing of combs, brushes, or headwear and a lack of appropriate scalp cleanliness. The diagnosis is established by finding a scalp hair with a nit firmly attached to it. Hair spray concretions and seborrheic scales can masquerade as nits, but unlike the egg, they are easily removed from the hair shaft.

Treatment. 1. Lather two tablespoons (30 ml.) of lindane shampoo into the scalp for four minutes. Rinse the hair thoroughly and rub with a dry towel.

2. Don a clean set of clothing.

3. Contaminated washable clothing and bed linens should be machine laundered or dried, using a 20-minute hot cycle. Woolen garments may be dry cleaned or stored in a plastic bag for 30 days.

4. Treat any coexistent bacterial infection from scratching and poor scalp hygiene with appropriate systemic antibiotics.

5. Examine all family members for head lice and those infested should be promptly treated.

Pediculosis Pubis

Pediculosis pubis (crab louse) has a proclivity for infesting the hairy regions of the pubic and anal skin. Although this is their main habitat, these lice can also be found on other hairy areas of the body. Special attention should be given to the eyelash and hairline zones of the scalp in children. The diagnosis is easily established by plucking an infested hair and observing the attached louse nit with a hand magnifying lens.

Treatment. 1. Before initiating therapy instruct the patient to take a warm soapy bath or shower. After towelling dry the skin, apply a thin layer of 1 per cent lindane lotion to the infested areas and surrounding integument. No more than 1 ounce of the medication need be prescribed.

2. The lotion should remain on the skin for 12 hours and then the bath or shower repeated.

3. Wear freshly laundered clothing. A change of bed linen and clean pajamas will lessen the possibility of treatment failure.

4. Lindane treatment may be repeated in 8 days if viable lice or nits are observed.

5. All sexual contacts should undergo a similar treatment. (By ordering a VDRL and taking cultures for gonorrhea on the index case, any associated venereal diseases will not be missed.)

6. If the eyelashes are infested, apply petrolatum thickly twice a day for 8 days followed by mechanical removal of the nits and lice.

Pediculosis Corporis

Pediculosis corporis (body louse) occurs when personal hygiene is neglected and clothing is worn for prolonged periods without being laundered. Although called a body louse, it is really a clothing louse, which only visits the skin to feed. The eggs are laid on clothing fibers, especially in the seam portions, but may be found on body hairs where infestation is quite severe. The body louse is the only human louse capable of transmitting the systemic diseases of typhus, relapsing fever, and trench fever.

Treatment. 1. Instituting a regimen of proper hygiene with a warm soapy bath and a change of clothing and bedding will bring about a cure.

2. If nits are found on the body, apply 1 per cent lindane lotion for 12 hours, then wash it from the skin.

3. Particular attention must be given to eradicating the lice and eggs from the clothing. Simply washing the infested garments with detergent and water will only produce cleaner lice. It is necessary to machine wash or dry at high heat for 20 minutes to kill the parasites. Woolen garments should be dry cleaned or stored in a plastic bag for 30 days.

PIGMENTARY DISTURBANCES
method of
MARGUERITE R. LERNER, M.D.
New Haven, Connecticut

Disorders of melanin pigmentation are numerous. In practice, patients seek treatment and physicians provide help for only a few common disorders.

HYPERPIGMENTATION

Melasma, Freckles, and Postinflammatory Pigmentation

Melasma, diffuse darkening of the forehead and cheeks, occurs primarily in women who are pregnant and in those who use oral contraceptives. Melasma also occurs, although less frequently, in nonpregnant healthy women and in men not taking drugs. The same type of hyperpigmentation of the face is seen in patients with endocrine abnormalities such as Addison's disease and a pituitary tumor producing excess melanocyte stimulating hormone (MSH).

Postinflammatory pigmentation can result from burns or from rubbing and scratching following contact dermatitis and atopic eczema.

Treatment. 1. Prevention of further darkening.

2. Avoid sunlight.

3. Immediately after washing the face or shaving in the morning apply a sunscreen such as para-aminobenzoic acid (PABA) 5 per cent in 70 per cent ethanol (see later). Reapply the sunscreen every 2 to 4 hours.

ACTIVE TREATMENT OF MELASMA AND POSTINFLAMMATORY PIGMENTATION. Apply directly to darkened skin small amounts of the following three medications in sequence, rubbing each one into the hyperpigmented areas: 0.1 per cent triamcinolone acetonide, 0.1 per cent tretinoin (Retin-A) cream, and 20 per cent monobenzyl ether of hydroquinone (Benoquin). The order of application is unimportant, as long as the patient rubs in a small amount of each of the three creams or ointments once a day. If there is no adverse reaction after using the three medications once daily for 2 weeks, then the patient could increase the use of the three medications to twice daily.

If the hyperpigmentation is of recent onset one might be able to decrease the hyperpigmentation simply by applying 0.1 per cent triamcinolone acetonide cream or ointment twice daily.

If a corticosteroid of lower potency is desired, try 1 per cent hydrocortisone cream. *Caution:* Long-term application of topical corticosteroids will result in telangiectasia and increased hair growth on the face.

A 2 per cent hydroquinone cream (Artra) is available over the counter. It should be rubbed into the dark spots twice daily. Treatment must continue for several months.

The strongest topical cream for counteracting hyperpigmentation is 20 per cent monobenzyl ether of hydroquinone (Benoquin). *Caution:* Monobenzone 20 per cent is a potent depigmenting agent and it is difficult to control the degree of depigmentation, particularly in people with naturally dark skin. Monobenzone can cause a contact dermatitis. Fifteen to 20 per cent of patients get a sensitization reaction. While using depigmenting preparations one should use concomitantly a sun protective agent. Dark skinned patients, especially blacks, must use hydroquinone and not monobenzone. In blacks the treatment is often unsuccessful. The duration of therapy is measured in months or years.

Freckles. Use monobenzyl ether of hydroquinone (Benoquin).

Nevi. One should not attempt to lighten dark nevi. Excision of the nevus is recommended. Arsenical hyperpigmentation is uncommon. (See Nevi, p. 634.)

Adrenocortical Insufficiency and Pituitary Tumors. Hyperpigmentation may develop in Addison's disease, following bilateral adrenalectomy or in the presence of a pituitary tumor producing melanocyte-stimulating hormone (MSH). If the patient receives enough cortisone, usually 37.5 mg. daily, to suppress the excessive output of MSH by the pituitary, the skin will become lighter. In some patients a higher dose of cortisone is required.

Tattoos. The best treatment of marks resulting from injection of carbon, metals, or ink into the skin is excision and grafting if necessary.

Sun Screens. Many sun screens are available over the counter. Several contain para-aminobenzoic acid (PABA), which protects against burning and tanning rays in the spectrum of 290 to 320 nanometers. They are packaged as lotions, creams, ointments, and gels; for example: PreSun, Eclipse, Pabafilm Gel, Sundown.

If one needs protection against long-wave ultraviolet rays coming through a window, UVAL is helpful, as it contains sulisobenzone.

HYPOPIGMENTATION

Vitiligo

The depigmentation of vitiligo occurs after birth, without preceding skin lesions, and is most common in the exposed areas (face and hands), around the body orifices (eyes, nose, mouth, nipples, umbilicus, and genitalia), in the body folds, and over bony prominences. Treatment of vitiligo requires determination and persistence.

Treatment. REPIGMENTATION. There is no easy or excellent method of inducing repigmentation. The currently acceptable procedure consists of oral administration of psoralen drugs followed by exposure of the skin to sunlight. Treatment is long-term, being carried out during the summer months from May through September and extending for a period of 2 to 6 years. Two psoralen drugs are available: 8-methoxypsoralen (8-MOP) in 10 mg. capsules and tablets (derived from plants); and trimethylpsoralen in 5 mg. tablets (synthetic). Trimethylpsoralen is more potent than 8-MOP for pigment darkening.

1. Trimethylpsoralen (Trisoralen) 5 to 15 mg. or 8-MOP (Meloxine, Oxsoralen) 10 to 30 mg. Take psoralen 1 to 2 hours before exposure to sunlight.

2. On the first day the patient should be exposed to sunlight for only 15 minutes. For the next

10 days exposure time can be increased each day by no more than 5 minutes. After reaching a total exposure time of 1 hour daily, the patient can be in the sun as long as he wishes but should avoid sunburn. Repigmentation may begin about the hair follicles in 2 to 4 months. If the patient complains of nervousness on 1 capsule of 8-MOP, therapy should be changed to trimethylpsoralen.

3. Discontinue treatment during the fall and winter and resume in the spring.

4. Ingestion of the drug without exposure to sunlight is of no value.

5. Side effects of 8-MOP are nervousness and gastrointestinal upsets. No side effects have been reported with trimethylpsoralen.

Depigmentation. When more than 50 per cent of an exposed surface such as the face or arms is affected by vitiligo, the patient may prefer to attempt depigmentation of the remaining normally pigmented areas. If total depigmentation is desired, monobenzyl ether of hydroquinone can be applied topically while avoiding exposure to sunlight.

Gray Hair. There is no medical treatment for reversing gray hair. Indeed, gray hair may represent vitiligo or vitiligo of hair bulbs.

Cosmetic Covering. Make-up can be used to hide the depigmentation.

1. Covermark (Lydia O'Leary) applied once daily.

2. Walnut juice stain (Depelle Laboratories).

3. Dihydroxyacetone (Man Tan, Q-T, Chromelin) combines with amino acids in the epidermis to give a tan shade.

PEMPHIGUS AND BULLOUS PEMPHIGOID

method of
SAMUEL BEAN, M.D.
Houston, Texas

Systemically administered corticosteroids have long been the mainstay of the treatment of pemphigus and bullous pemphigoid. In the majority of patients, the use of corticosteroids results in adequate control. Because of the life-threatening nature of these diseases, particularly pemphigus, the dosage of corticosteroid is usually large, and untoward effects are frequent. Because of the undesirable side effects associated with corticosteroids, alternative methods of treatment have been explored. The immunologic characteristics of both pemphigus and bullous pemphigoid have prompted the use of immunosuppressives such as azathioprine, methotrexate, and cyclophosphamide. In selected cases, the use of these drugs in combination with corticosteroids achieves control with a resultant decrease in the amount of corticosteroid required. While a number of studies have indicated that the combination of corticosteroids and immunosuppressives is an effective method of treatment for pemphigus and bullous pemphigoid, it should be stressed that they should be used judiciously and that these immunosuppressive agents have not been approved for treatment of these diseases in the United States.

Corticosteroids

Pemphigus vulgaris and its variant, pemphigus vegetans, are initially treated with 100 to 120 mg. of prednisone daily, either in a single morning dose or divided doses, until disease activity is suppressed, i.e., no new blisters appear and older lesions resolve. In the usual patient, this is about 2 to 3 weeks. In severe cases, 180 to 240 mg. of prednisone may be required for adequate control. In my opinion, alternate day or injectable corticosteroids should not be used in the initial treatment of pemphigus vulgaris.

After adequate control is achieved, the dosage of prednisone may be tapered slowly until a satisfactory maintenance level is reached. The reduction schedule depends on the response of the disease, but in general, 5 to 10 mg. of prednisone per week is permissible. If activity recurs during reduction, the dose should be doubled or increased half again until activity ceases. An occasional abortive vesicle or bulla does not necessitate a radical increase in dosage as a rule, however. This is particularly true with regard to oral lesions, which are difficult to suppress completely. When a dose of 15 to 20 mg. of prednisone per day is achieved, an attempt may be made to convert the daily dose to an alternate day schedule. In most patients with pemphigus vulgaris, alternate day therapy can be achieved satisfactorily.

In patients who are particularly difficult to control, even with a high dosage of oral corticosteroids, the concurrent use of an intravenous infusion of 40 to 60 units of ACTH daily may prove successful.

Pemphigus erythematosus and pemphigus foliaceous, variants of the same basic disease process, can usually be controlled with lower doses of prednisone; 80 to 100 mg. of prednisone daily are adequate for most patients. The general philosophy of dosage reduction described in pemphigus vulgaris is applicable to pemphigus erythematosus and foliaceous. In my experience, it is easier to convert patients with pemphigus foliaceous and pemphigus erythematosus to an alternate day schedule. Some patients may respond to treatment with topically applied corticosteroids alone. In patients with low-grade activity or localized involvement, the disease process may be controlled with periodic injections of intramuscular corticosteroid.

A few patients with pemphigus vulgaris or foliaceous may be treated successfully with dapsone or sulfapyridine orally. These patients may present with an eruption that appears to be dermatitis herpetiformis but is pemphigus, histologically and immunologically. Fifty to 100 mg. of dapsone daily, or 1.5 to 2 grams of sulfapyridine per day may be used as initial treatment. (This use of dapsone and sulfapyridine is not listed in the manufacturers' official directives.) If the eruption responds, the dose may be increased or decreased as indicated.

Bullous pemphigoid can usually be controlled with an initial dose of 80 mg. prednisone daily, although occasionally 200 mg. or more of prednisone may be required. It should be administered either in a single morning dose or in divided doses. As with pemphigus, I feel that alternate day corticosteroids should not be used in the initial treatment of bullous pemphigoid. When activity ceases, the prednisone dosage should be reduced as described in the section on pemphigus vulgaris, although as a rule it may be decreased more rapidly. Generally, bullous pemphigoid is more easily controlled and the maintenance level of prednisone is more rapidly achieved. A severe flare should be followed by a dosage increase of at least 50 per cent. Many times it is possible to control the disease with a dose of 10 to 15 mg. prednisone daily and often the prednisone may be tapered or discontinued completely. Some patients will require maintenance therapy indefinitely, however.

Immunosuppressants

For the treatment of pemphigus and bullous pemphigoid, I prefer to use azathioprine in conjunction with prednisone. Using the combination of the two agents, I have been successfully able to control the disease in those patients who fail to respond to large doses of corticosteroids alone, those patients in whom I was unable to achieve a reasonable and fairly safe maintenance dose, and those patients who were having severe or multiple or both untoward effects from corticosteroids. Initially, I use a dosage of 100 to 150 mg. of azathioprine.* As control is achieved and a maintenance dose of prednisone is established, the dosage of azathioprine is slowly decreased. I attempt to elim-

inate prednisone and maintain the patient on 25 to 50 mg. of azathioprine daily.

Before therapy is started, the patient should have a comprehensive physical examination with appropriate laboratory studies. Periodically, a complete blood count, urinalysis, and Sequential Multiple Analysis (SMA 12) should be performed.

Methotrexate* and cyclophosphamide* have also been reported useful in the treatment of pemphigus and bullous pemphigoid. Recently, gold compounds* have also been suggested as effective alternative therapy for pemphigus. I have had no experience with the use of these medications, but reports in the literature seem to indicate they are efficacious.

Adjunctive Therapy

In widespread pemphigus and bullous pemphigoid, local therapy is for symptomatic relief only. However, in some patients with localized pemphigus and bullous pemphigoid, topically applied corticosteroids may be used as primary treatment. If the eruption is severe, with much blistering and weeping, wet dressings applied without occlusion are most effective. Plain tap water, isotonic saline solution, or Burow's solution 1:32, may be applied to affected areas four times daily for 30 to 45 minutes or longer. More important than the particular solution used is that the dressings be kept wet and not allowed to dry. Between applications of the wet dressings and before bedtime, a shake lotion such as calamine lotion or zinc oxide lotion may be used. Cool baths, two to four times daily for 20 minutes with colloidal oatmeal (Aveeno), may be substituted for wet dressings in patients with extensive involvement of the skin. As the blistering and erosions heal, lubricating creams are useful.

When oral involvement occurs, it may be treated by using 2 per cent viscous lidocaine (Xylocaine), tetracycline syrup, or dyclonine hydrochloride (Dyclone) solution as a mouthwash. For isolated lesions of the oral mucosa, I have found topically applied fluorinated corticosteroid gels useful.

For relief of itching, diphenhydramine hydrochloride (Benadryl), 50 mg. four times daily, methdilazine hydrochloride (Tacaryl), 8 mg. every 8 hours, cyproheptadine hydrochloride (Periactin), 4 mg. four times daily, or trimeprazine (Temaril), 2.5 to 5 mg. four to five times daily may be effective. If a sedative effect is also desired, hydroxyzine hydrochloride (Atarax), 10 mg. four times daily, or promethazine hydrochloride (Phenergan), 12.5 mg. every six hours, may be used.

---

*This use of this agent is not listed in the manufacturer's official directive.

*This use of this agent is not listed in the manufacturer's official directive.

PITYRIASIS ROSEA

method of
DAVID A. BYRNE, M.D.
Bloomington, Indiana

Pityriasis rosea is a common cutaneous eruption that affects all races, both sexes, and all ages (with a predominant group in the late second and third decades). It is clinically distinctive, nonscarring, and self-limited. Its cause is unknown. No other organ systems are known to be involved. Except for pruritus or minimal fever, the disorder is asymptomatic and usually resolves in 6 to 8 weeks.

The onset is frequently announced by the "herald patch," a 2 to 7 cm. oval-shaped lesion that is normally flat, erythematous, or fawn-colored with fine scales peeling peripherally (forming a "collarette" of scales). In a few days or weeks, the "herald patch" is followed by a shower of similar smaller lesions located on the trunk and proximal extremities. The long axis of the oval-shaped lesions may parallel the skin wrinkle lines, such that the back lesions may collectively resemble a "Christmas tree" figure when they occur in large numbers.

While differential diagnosis includes tinea versicolor, tinea corporis, secondary syphilis, psoriasis, lichen planus, and drug eruption, the progression and appearance of pityriasis rosea and other distinct differences usually allow a confident diagnosis. Potassium hydroxide (KOH) examination of the scale for the hyphae of tinea corporis or tinea versicolor is advisable if the patient is seen during the early single-lesion stage. If fever and malaise occur with the findings of lymphadenopathy and a pityriasis rosea-like eruption, secondary syphilis should be considered and serology obtained.

Treatment

Treatment is symptomatic, utilizing (1) topical corticosteroid preparations and (2) oral antihistamines for significant pruritus. Daily exposure to erythemal doses of artificial or natural ultraviolet light (which results in a slight erythema 24 hours after exposure) can clear the eruption in 2 to 3 weeks. The patient should be reassured that pityriasis rosea is not contagious, resolves without scarring, and lacks systemic sequelae.

If the eruption persists past 8 weeks, dermatologic consultation is desirable.

POLYARTERITIS

method of
W. LEROY GRIFFING, M.D.,
and GENE G. HUNDER, M.D.
Rochester, Minnesota

Polyarteritis nodosa is a necrotizing vasculitis in which focal inflammatory lesions are found predominantly along medium-sized muscular arteries, especially at points of branching or bifurcation. Although knowledge of the mechanisms underlying the inflammatory processes has increased, the cause of polyarteritis is not known. Clinical symptoms result from ischemia, infarction, and hemorrhage, depending upon the location and extent of the vascular lesions. Making the diagnosis early in the disease is often difficult, as the only symptoms may be vague constitutional complaints of weakness, anorexia, weight loss, myalgias, arthralgias, and fever. There are no specific serologic tests, but the use of angiography to visualize the multiple small aneurysms in an involved organ may aid in establishing the diagnosis. Biopsy of a clinically involved area such as skin or muscle is the best method of confirming the diagnosis, and should be performed as soon as the diagnosis is suspected. Due to the segmental nature of the inflammatory lesions, examination of multiple serial sections is frequently necessary.

Treatment

Prior to beginning therapy, it is important to document carefully the extent of clinical organ involvement and to obtain baseline laboratory data, including hemoglobin, leukocyte count, erythrocyte sedimentation rate, serum glucose, electrolytes, globulins, urinalysis, and creatinine clearance. In order for therapy to be maximally beneficial, it must be started early. In addition, it should be aggressive prior to the development of overt evidence of widespread vessel involvement and significant complications of vital organ infarction or failure. Renal involvement and hypertension indicate a worse prognosis.

General measures include bed rest, close monitoring of vital signs, especially blood pressure, and daily weights to help follow fluid balance. Hypertension should be treated by lowering sodium intake in the diet and using additional drug therapy if necessary.

Corticosteroids. Corticosteroids are considered the most effective available therapy. Prednisone (or an equivalent dose of a related steroid) is initiated at a dose of 1 to 2 mg. per kg., given in two or three divided doses spaced evenly throughout the day. This dose is continued until there is evidence of suppression of disease activity as judged by lack of newly developing clinical features, and concomitant stabilization or improvement in laboratory studies. The total daily dose may then be reduced by 10 to 15 per cent at 1 to 2 week intervals as long as disease activity remains suppressed. Generally, as the total dose reaches lower levels, reduction is carried out at smaller decrements at longer intervals.

Throughout the gradual tapering process, relapse of the disease must be watched closely. The development of new clinical symptoms or evidence of continued disease activity in organs previously affected (such as continuing reduction in creatinine clearance) requires reinstitution of higher doses of prednisone. In addition, one must be aware of complications such as bowel infarction, which can be masked by steroid therapy. The total dose should be slowly tapered until therapy can be discontinued, if possible.

When the total dose reaches 15 to 20 mg. per day, conversion to a single morning dosage schedule may be tried if the clinical course has been favorable. In some instances, alternate day corticosteroid therapy appears to be effective in polyarteritis nodosa, but we know of no reliable way to predict who will respond. In non-life–threatening disease, alternate day therapy may be tried in an effort to minimize steroid side effects.

Since high doses and prolonged treatment are often required, patients should be advised at the start of steroid therapy about possible side effects of insomnia, nervousness, alteration of mood, change in body habitus, and the development of osteoporosis, cataracts, and peptic ulcers. Blood sugar and potassium should be monitored periodically. Hypokalemia should be treated cautiously in the presence of renal failure. The development of hypertension should be noted and treated appropriately.

Immunosuppressive Drugs. Treatment using immunosuppressive agents alone or in conjunction with steroids has not been studied on a well-controlled basis and their use is considered investigational in the United States. However, the employment of this class of drugs has been advocated when there is continued disease activity despite high-dose corticosteroids, or when the dose required to maintain suppression is high and one is faced with significant steroid toxicity.

The two immunosuppressive drugs most often used are cyclophosphamide (Cytoxan) and azathioprine (Imuran). (This use of these agents is not listed in the manufacturers' official directives.) There is no evidence that one is superior to the other in the treatment of polyarteritis nodosa. In Wegener's syndrome, cyclophosphamide should be tried first. Cyclophosphamide is usually given in a dose of 2 to 5 mg. per kg., although up to 30 mg. per kg. can be given. Giving cyclophosphamide in a dose sufficient to cause a mild leukopenia of 2500 to 4000 per cu. mm. has been advocated as a means of monitoring the dosage in oncologic uses; however, clinical studies determining the optimum dose for polyarteritis nodosa are not yet available. Azathioprine is given in a dose of 1.5 to 3 mg. per kg. Prednisone is continued with either immunosuppressive agent and disease activity is monitored as before. The duration of use and dose depends on the effectiveness and tolerance. If no therapeutic effect is observed in one month, the drug can be stopped. Even if the drug is helpful, the dose should be tapered slowly at 1 to 2 week intervals to find the minimum effective amount.

Patients should be cautioned about side effects, especially with cyclophosphamide, which include gastrointestinal intolerance (such as nausea and vomiting), alopecia, gonadal atrophy, and a sterile hemorrhagic cystitis (which can be minimized by high fluid intake and frequent voidings). Careful attention to the development of leukopenia (and thrombocytopenia with azathioprine) is necessary with both drugs. It is often necessary to follow blood counts weekly. Both drugs are associated with an increased incidence of unusual infections and the development of malignancies. However, in the patient with life-threatening polyarteritis whose disease is unsatisfactorily controlled with steroids, cyclophosphamide or azathioprine are justifiable additions to the therapeutic regimen.

PRECANCEROUS LESIONS OF THE SKIN AND MUCOUS MEMBRANES

method of
JANICE W. YUSK, M.D.
Louisville, Kentucky

Certain skin lesions have the potential for becoming malignant, although not all of them will do so. Such lesions are (1) actinic keratoses, (2) arsenical keratoses, (3) leukoplakia, (4) Bowen's disease, (5) erythroplasia of Queyrat, (6) chronic radiation dermatitis, and (7) lentigo maligna. All of these lesions show microscopic cellular atypia; entities such as Bowen's disease, erythroplasia of Queyrat, and lentigo maligna are actually cancer in situ.

Other lesions, although lacking cellular atypia, may develop squamous cell carcinomas. Included in this group are lichen sclerosis et atrophicus of the female vulva, oral florid papillomatosis, and chronic draining sinus tracts. Basal cell carcinoma may arise in the congenital nevus sebaceous of Jadassohn. Such lesions should be followed closely for malignant degeneration. The nevus sebaceous of Jadassohn warrants prophylactic excision.

Actinic (Senile, Solar) Keratoses

These lesions, which develop following chronic sun exposure, show a small tendency to develop squamous cell carcinomas. If such malignant degeneration occurs, metastasis is unlikely.

Treatment. 1. Small numbers of lesions readily respond to liquid nitrogen topically. A cotton-tipped applicator dipped in the nitrogen and applied to the lesion for 20 to 30 seconds, or a 10- to 15-second spray with a Cryospray unit, is adequate.

2. Equally satisfactory for such lesions is light curettage (the specimen then may be submitted for microscopic examination) followed by electrodesiccation.

3. Thick lesions and those surmounted by a cutaneous horn are best removed by curettage and electrodesiccation, followed by microscopic examination of the entire lesion (including the base).

4. Multiple lesions are best treated by topical 5-fluorouracil. This treatment selectively destroys the actinic keratoses.

FACE. One or 2 per cent 5-fluorouracil (I prefer the solution instead of the cream form) is applied twice daily to the involved skin (avoid the eyes, nasolabial folds, and vermilion border) for 3 to 4 weeks. The hands should be washed after each application. Sunlight should be avoided during this time. An extremely vigorous and uncomfortable inflammatory response follows, some of which may be alleviated by application of a topical steroid. I use 0.1 per cent betamethasone valerate (Valisone) cream twice daily. The topical steroid should be continued after 5-fluorouracil therapy is complete, until all inflammation is gone.

FOREARMS, DORSA OF HANDS. Tretinoin (Retin-A) cream, 0.1 per cent, may be applied twice daily to the areas for 1 to 2 weeks, then 2 to 5 per cent 5-fluorouracil may be used twice daily for 3 to 4 weeks. Topical steroids may also be used as described.

Any lesions remaining after completion of 5-fluorouracil therapy should be surgically removed for histopathologic examination.

Prophylaxis for future actinic keratoses requires protection from sunlight and the use of a PABA-containing sunscreen (e.g., PreSun, Eclipse, Sundown, Block-Out).

Arsenical Keratoses

These lesions may follow ingestion of inorganic arsenicals (e.g., Fowler's solution, Asiatic pills) as medicines. The presence of these may herald later development of cutaneous or visceral carcinomas. Such patients should be closely followed.

Treatment. 1. Keratolytics such as tretinoin (Retin-A) cream or salicylic acid (Keralyt) gel may be applied twice daily to horny palmar or plantar lesions. Occlusion with plastic gloves or another plastic film may be necessary. Twice weekly 5 per cent 5-fluorouracil applied under occlusion for 3 to 4 weeks may be helpful after the horn has been removed.

2. Following biopsy of any lesions suspected of malignant change, destruction by cryosurgery, local excision, or curettage and electrodesiccation should be performed.

Erythroplasia of Queyrat

This presents as a red velvety patch on the glans penis, oral mucosa, or vulvar mucosa. Histologically identical to Bowen's disease, this lesion requires microscopic examination to confirm the diagnosis. Such lesions may develop invasive squamous cell carcinoma, which shows a ready tendency to metastasize.

Treatment. These lesions may be treated in a manner similar to Bowen's disease. Topical 5-fluorouracil on penile lesions may preserve valuable tissue and prevent or decrease scarring from treatment. Follow-up is mandatory.

Chronic Radiodermatitis

Irreversible changes may occur. If squamous or basal cell carcinoma develops, these lesions may be very aggressive. The squamous cell carcinomas metastasize more readily than do those arising from actinic keratoses.

Treatment. 1. Small lesions may be excised, frozen with liquid nitrogen, or curetted and electrodesiccated, unless scarring in the area from the previous radiation prevents adequate determination of the tumor's borders. If radiation damage is severe, healing may be so slow that these procedures should not be used.

2. Excision and skin grafting in the area will often provide satisfactory results.

3. Moh's chemosurgery offers the best chance of ensuring removal of the cancer. Healing in areas badly damaged by radiation will be slow.

Lentigo Maligna (Melanotic Freckle of Hutchinson)

This lesion begins as an unevenly pigmented freckle on sun-exposed areas. Its irregular borders show progressive peripheral enlargement. About one third of these progress to an invasive malignant melanoma after several years.

Treatment. 1. *Surgical excision.* This is the best method, if it is possible to remove the lesion in this manner.

2. *Cryosurgery.* This therapy has been used successfully in some instances.

3. *Electrodesiccation and curettage.* Care must be taken to remove the entire lesion. Follow-up is mandatory.

Leukoplakia

This term is best reserved for early anaplastic changes in the oral or vulvar mucosa; such a designation requires a biopsy to separate the disorder from other benign leukokeratoses. Squamous cell carcinoma arising in an area of leukoplakia has a poor prognosis.

Treatment.   1. Such irritants as tobacco and ill-fitting dental appliances should be avoided. Jagged or broken teeth must be repaired. Lesions on the lower lip may represent sunlight damage; protection by the use of a sunscreen is necessary. Cigarette smoking should be discontinued.

2. Topical cortisone creams, e.g., desonide (Tridesilon) ointment or triamcinolone acetonide in emollient dental paste (Kenalog in Orabase) may alleviate some inflammation.

3. Early lesions failing to respond to these conservative measures should be treated with liquid nitrogen or curettage and electrodesiccation.

4. Advanced or persistent lesions should be biopsied and removed surgically.

Bowen's Disease

This presents as a slowly enlarging red eczematous patch, which fails to resolve. Biopsy is necessary to make the diagnosis. Bowen's disease is squamous cell carcinoma in situ. If the lesion progresses to an invasive squamous cell, distant metastasis is very likely. Therefore such lesions should be removed completely.

Treatment.   1. Curettage and electrodesiccation.

2. Cryosurgery with liquid nitrogen.

3. Two to 5 per cent 5-fluorouracil, often combined with occlusion with a plastic film, twice daily for 6 to 8 weeks.

4. Local excision.

Follow-up is necessary to ensure complete destruction of the lesion. Suspicious areas that remain should be biopsied.

MILIARIA
(Prickly Heat)

method of
HENRY K. BUTLER, JR., M.D.
Murfreesboro, Tennessee

Miliaria is the clinical manifestation of the anatomic obstruction and rupture of the eccrine sweat duct. The level of eccrine duct occlusion determines the clinical presentation. **Miliaria crystallina** is the most superficial form of miliaria, in which sweat duct occlusion and rupture occurs at the level of the inert stratum corneum. The lesions are asymptomatic clear vesicles. **Miliaria rubra** occurs when the level of obstruction is the innervated epidermis. It presents with very pruritic (prickly) small erythematous macules associated with papular and vesicular lesions. **Miliaria profunda** (the deepest form) usually follows repeated attacks of Miliaria rubra and is caused by obstruction of the duct at a level below the epidermis with extravasation of fluid into the dermis. This is a rare nonfollicular papular disorder found primarily in the tropics.

Miliaria tends to occur in an environment of high temperature and humidity. It is often accentuated in intertriginous areas or at sites of friction from occlusive clothing. Antecedent injury from a preexisting dermatitis, sunburn, or bathing in salt water may be contributory to the occlusion of the sweat ducts with resultant miliaria.

Complications of miliaria include: secondary infection by bacteria (usually staphylococcal) or fungi (usually *Candida albicans*), exacerbation of other dermatoses (e.g., atopic eczema or neurodermatitis), and postmiliarial anhidrosis, which may lead to severe thermoregulatory deficits (heat distress syndrome).

Treatment

1. The sine qua non of therapy is cool the patient. Air conditioning, an electric fan, rest, a shaded environment, and cool baths or showers in plain water are means to this end.

2. Clothing should be nonocclusive and light.

3. Avoid salt water, harsh soaps, detergents, occlusive ointments, and cholinergic drugs.

4. A thin application of a dusting powder (Johnson's Baby Powder or ZeaSORB Powder) may be adequate topical therapy in mild cases.

5. Calamine lotion, U.S.P. with menthol 0.25 per cent, may be used in more extensive cases.

6. Erythromycin, 250 mg. orally four times daily, or cloxacillin, 250 mg. orally four times daily, for secondary staphylococcal infection (usually pustular), which may be proved by appropriate cultures.

7. Nystatin lotion (Candex) or powder (Mycostatin) are indicated for *Candida albicans* infection, which may be proved by skin scrapings for microscopic and cultural studies.

8. Other topical antifungal agents include clotrimazole (Lotrimin), miconazole (MicaTin), and haloprogin (Halotex) preparations.

9. In secondarily infected fissured intertriginous areas, it may be difficult to assess the importance of the bacterial or fungal components. Treatment of both possibilities with appropriate systemic antibiotic and topical antifungal therapy is reasonable in these situations.

10. Patients with postmiliarial anhidrosis and heat distress syndrome may require permanent change to a cooler environment.

PRURITUS

method of
JOHN R. BERTRAM, M.D.
Madison, Wisconsin

Pruritus, or itching, is a frequent symptom encountered in dermatology, as well as in all medical fields. It may be an insignificant complaint or it may be an important clue to the uncovering of an unsuspected internal malignancy. The purpose of this article is to briefly discuss the common causes of generalized pruritus, and the appropriate diagnostic measures and treatments that can be used.

The natural response to itching is scratching, and most patients will be seen with secondary skin lesions—excoriations, lichenification, and scarring—sometimes to a mutilating degree. It appears that pain is preferable to the itch sensation, or perhaps, that scratching is more pleasurable. "Scratching is one of nature's sweetest pleasures, and nearest at hand." (Michel de Montaignes' Essays, Book III, Chapter 13.) Unfortunately, to scratch the itch compounds the problem, and will often introduce a vicious cycle of heightened epidermal inflammation and sensitivity, with continued pruritus and further scratching. The teleologic value of a beneficial "scratching reflex" can be debated, i.e., that scratching fatigues the nerve endings and dilutes the mediators or removes the offending epidermis and its nerve endings (or perhaps scabies mites); but this theory is purely speculative.

Pathophysiology of Pruritus

The pathophysiology of pruritus is complex (the reader is referred to Herndon, J. H., Jr.: Int. J. Dermatol., *14*:465, 1975). Basically, there is a sensory stimulus to the epidermis that is received by chemical mediators and neuronal receptors. It is then transmitted by a peripheral nerve pathway to the central nervous system where sensory perception and associative processes occur. Higher centers have a marked effect upon the perception of itching—particularly important are emotional states of anxiety, or excitement, as well as levels of distracting or competing alternate sensory stimuli. A prime example is the anxious person who itches in bed at night when other competing stimuli and daily activities are at a low ebb; on the other hand, the scabies mite will diligently do its best burrowing in this warm comfortable environment.

General Aspects of Diagnosis and Therapy

The approach to the therapy of pruritus should be threefold: First, to identify the specific cause or causes, and correct or remove the cause if possible; second, to alleviate the itch sensation with topical or systemic therapy or both; and third, to stop the scratching response, often the most difficult aspect of therapy, especially if the patient has a long-term problem with a well-established scratching habit.

A careful history and physical examination will help to differentiate localized from generalized pruritus, and usually, to establish whether there is a primary cutaneous disease, or possibly an underlying systemic disease. The symptom of pruritus must be treated with respect. Many patients with generalized pruritus will simply have dry skin or an anxiety state. However, if there is no obvious cutaneous condition to account for the pruritus, then a work-up for systemic disease is indicated. This should include a complete blood count (CBC), sedimentation rate, chemistry panel, urinary analysis, chest x-ray, and a thyroid function test as a screen. Other measures, such as stool guaiacs, or gastrointestinal x-rays, can be done if signs and symptoms warrant. Many anxious patients have generalized pruritus but the diagnosis of psychogenic or psychophysiologic pruritus must be a diagnosis of exclusion. Some general principles of therapy include the following:

1. Rest and relaxation are important factors to control pruritus. Stress, anxiety, and fatigue will aggravate the itch. A vacation from an aggravating job will often work wonders. In addition, a discussion with the patient of a change in lifestyle can often be helpful. For example, the harassed businessman who has two jobs, a large family, and is performing additional community activities, may change to a more relaxed pace if he were to realize that his pruritus is a signal of emotional stress and fatigue.

2. On the other hand, physical activity, exercise, and recreation can be beneficial. Scratching is a physical response often used as a means to release emotional stress and energy. The patient should be counseled to release this energy in a more constructive manner.

3. Climate control can be helpful. Overheating contributes to vasodilation and can aggravate pruritus.

4. Mechanical irritants, such as rough or tight clothing, should be avoided.

5. Avoid excessive amounts of caffeine (coffee, tea, and cola drinks), nicotine, and alcohol. These are not only central nervous system (CNS) stimulants but are also vasodilating. Also note that certain systemic chemicals and drugs can cause the nonimmunologic liberation of histamine in the skin which can result in pruritus. In this category are large molecules such as dextran, polypeptides, various biogenic polymers (e.g., chemical structures in seafoods, food-fruits, bacterial toxins), radiographic dyes, and histamine-liberating drugs such as polymyxin, neomycin, morphine, codeine, d-tubocurarine, thiamine, atropine, and quinine. Many patients who give a history of "allergies" to different foods and drugs (notably codeine compounds) are probably not allergic but rather have experienced the transient urticaria and pruritus due to the nonimmunologic liberation of histamine by these substances.

6. A very important aspect of controlling pruritus is combating overdrying and providing lubrication for the skin. Simple xerosis is a common cause of pruritus, particularly in cold, dry

climates. Water is a solvent that strips away natural skin oils and produces further drying through evaporation. Contrary to Ann Landers, a bath a day for all should not be part of the great American dream. Bathing frequency in the winter-time should be limited to every other day. Numerous bath oils are available, and these should be added to the bath or applied directly to the moistened skin after a shower. This will provide emolliency for the skin, as well as produce an occlusive barrier to reduce water loss from the epidermis. Apparently, simply adding a cup of ordinary table salt to the bath will help retain the skin water content. Examples are: Alpha Keri, Nutraspa, Lubath, Johnson's Baby Oil, and Aveeno (colloidal oatmeal). Oilated soaps are of some help, e.g., Aveeno Bar, Dove, Camay, Alpha Keri, Oilatum, Lubriderm, and Emulave. Finally, dry skin creams and lotions should be used on a regular daily basis, paying particular attention to the areas where overdrying occurs the easiest, i.e., the hands, arms, legs, cheeks, and flanks. Safe, nonsensitizing dry skin products include: Lubriderm, Nutraderm, Nivea, Alpha Keri, Johnson's Baby Lotion, Aquaphor, Eucerin, *plain* petrolatum, Aquacare, Carmol, Nutraplus, and LactiCare (these last four products contain additional chemicals, such as urea and lactic acid, which help to further retain water in the epidermis).

7. Again, caution and counsel the patient against scratching, rubbing, or further irritating his skin.

Localized Pruritus

The problem of localized pruritus is often due to various forms of dermatitis or eczema, such as seborrheic dermatitis, dyshidrotic dermatitis, or intertrigo. A discussion of these conditions is beyond the scope of this article, but many of the treatment measures outlined would be appropriate.

Generalized Pruritus—Categories

In differentiating generalized pruritus, it is helpful to categorize the clinical syndrome:

1. No cutaneous disease. Often this is a psychophysiologic problem, but a work-up to rule out systemic disease should be done. Studies indicate that about 20 to 30 per cent of these adult patients will have an underlying systemic disease. Children with generalized pruritus, on the other hand, usually show no underlying disease. In most of these patients with idiopathic pruritus (or psychogenic), the condition is self-limiting and disappears spontaneously. General skin therapy should be instituted.

2. Cutaneous disease that is secondary, but no primary cutaneous disease. The rules of Cat-

egory 1 apply. The patient has scratched and produced excoriations, lichenification, scarring, and often urticarial lesions (pressure-dermagraphism). Obviously, it may be difficult to detect a primary skin lesion (e.g., a scabies burrow) if the patient has extensively damaged his skin. General and specific skin therapy should be instituted.

3. Primary cutaneous disease. There are a few common dermatoses that cause generalized pruritus, and these will be briefly discussed. If the correct diagnosis is made, then a systemic work-up is not necessary.

DRY SKIN, XEROSIS, ASTEATOSIS, NUMMULAR DERMATITIS, "WINTER ITCH." This condition primarily affects the limbs and produces a diffuse, dry scaling, fissuring, and mild erythema. Often, small circular scaling patches are noted (nummular, "coin-shaped"). A KOH examination may be necessary to rule out tinea corporis. Often xerosis is a problem with older patients, since there is a loss of normal sebaceous lubrication with aging. General and specific treatment measures, as outlined, should be instituted. Scabies and atopic dermatitis are two other common skin diseases that can cause generalized pruritus and should be considered in the diagnosis. The reader should refer to discussions of these conditions elsewhere in this book.

Specific Therapy Measures

More specific measures of therapy can be used, depending upon how much inflammation and scratching are present.

1. Topical steroid ointments or creams can be used on a three times daily as necessary basis. Steroid sprays or lotions can be used if a drying effect is desired. If the patient has a secondary neurodermatitis, he can be told to apply the steroid more often; i.e., any time he wants to scratch the itch, he should apply the medication instead. This may not increase the percutaneous absorption of the steroid at all (for various reasons concerning epidermal barrier function and transport), but it will help to break a habit. Examples of steroid creams and ointments (usual strengths 0.025 to 0.1 per cent) are: Triamcinolone (Kenalog, Aristocort), fluocinonide (Lidex), flurandrenolide (Cordran), betamethasone (Valisone, Benisone, Diprosone), desonide (Tridesilon), and halcinonide (Halog). Use the lowest strength steroid that is appropriate. These are potent (and more expensive) fluorinated steroids used for inflamed dermatitis. Plain hydrocortisone products (such as Dermacort, Hytone, Nutracort) can be used for mild inflammation or on an *as necessary only* basis for facial dermatitis. The physician should familiarize himself with the usage, cost, etc. of a few of these

steroids, rather than "run the gamut" with the multitude of brands that are available. If the diagnosis is uncertain, it may be best not to use topical steroids at all, since they may be of no benefit or they may worsen the condition (e.g., promoting tinea growth), or they may produce side effects such as atrophy.

2. Antihistamines may also be helpful in controlling pruritus. Additionally, their sedative and tranquilizing effects may be the primary benefit in some patients. These side effects, however, should be discussed with the patient. Hydroxyzine hydrochloride (Atarax), 10, 25, and 50 mg. tablets, or a syrup (10 mg. per 5 ml.), at a four times daily dosage, has both antihistamine and mild tranquilizing effects, and is effective in controlling pruritus. Other antihistamines include diphenhydramine (Benadryl), 25 to 50 mg. four times daily, and cyproheptadine (Periactin), 2 to 4 mg. four times daily. Periactin reportedly has both antihistamine and antiserotonin effects. Sometimes, a combination of two different medications (e.g., hydroxyzine [Atarax] and cyproheptadine [Periactin]) given simultaneously, is very effective.

3. Tranquilizers are of considerable benefit in patients with psychogenic pruritus, agitation, or a significant emotional overlay to their primary cutaneous disease. Examples are: chlordiazepoxide hydrochloride (Librium), 5 to 10 mg. four times daily, or diazepam (Valium), 2 to 5 or 10 mg. four times daily.

4. Sedatives, such as barbiturate, or flurazepam (Dalmane), 15 to 30 mg. at bedtime as necessary, may be helpful in providing rest, but are usually an unnecessary (and potentially addicting) measure in addition to the other therapies mentioned.

5. Aspirin and other salicylates are sometimes advocated as an anti-inflammatory and antipruritic medication, but they have complex metabolic effects, some of which may worsen pruritus (e.g., enhance histamine liberation). Also, aspirin compounds are often implicated in producing hypersensitivity reactions.

6. Systemic steroids should be reserved for use in patients with severe and extensive inflammation or for those who do not respond adequately to the other therapeutic measures. Check the patient for any contraindications (e.g., peptic ulcer disease), and stress to the patient the need to take this potent medication correctly. A helpful short course steroid regimen would be prednisone or its equivalent, beginning at 50 mg. daily and then tapering gradually to discontinue over a 2 week period. Avoid using systemic steroids routinely, as patients can easily become steroid addicts, where they simply take their pills and not bother with any of the other effective, safe therapeutic measures.

7. Compressing or soaks for inflamed skin is helpful if there is an exudative or crusting component. The aim of compressing is to soften the crust as an aid to debridement and also to "draw-out" the weeping exudate and thereby produce a cleansing and drying effect with the aid of evaporation. The cooling effect of evaporation is also helpful in relieving pruritus. Obviously, on normal skin or already xerotic skin compressing will only produce further drying. A recommended regimen would be a 30 minute compress three times daily with gentle cleansing debridement, until the exudate or crusting has ceased. The compress should be soaking wet (not just damp) and cool or room temperature. A soft rag, wash cloth, or towel can be used. Ordinary tap water is usually sufficient, although small amounts of boric acid or hydrogen peroxide can be added for their bactericidal effect. If necessary (e.g., on markedly eczematous skin), a greater astringent effect can be achieved by adding Burow's solution (Domeboro, Bluboro), 1 packet or tablet to a pint of water. Finally, a compress can be applied directly over a layer of a topical steroid—this moist occlusion will produce a greater (approximately four-fold) percutaneous absorption of the steroid.

8. Nonsteroid antipruritic lotions can be helpful and safe to use as necessary (PRN basis). Examples include calamine lotion (caution—a drying effect), Noxzema, and Schamberg's Lotion (menthol, phenol, zinc oxide, calcium hydroxide solution in peanut oil). Phenol, menthol, and camphor all have some cooling, anesthetic, and antipruritic effects and can be incorporated in concentrations from 0.25 to 1 per cent in various vehicles.

Pruritus and Systemic Disease

Generalized pruritus in the absence of primary cutaneous disease may be a symptom of various systemic diseases, including neoplasms, endocrine and metabolic disorders, and intestinal and tissue parasites, or an altered physiologic state, such as pregnancy. Appropriate screening tests, as previously mentioned, may detect the underlying disorder. However, only about 20 per cent of these patients will have a systemic illness definitely associated with their pruritus.

1. Some metabolic disorders, such as diabetes, gout, and anemia, have been reported to be associated with pruritus, but there is no convincing evidence.

2. Rarely, generalized pruritus may be an important signal of hyperthyroidism, and it has also been associated with the carcinoid syndrome. The pathogenesis of the symptom may be related to vasodilatation or to excess levels of histamine or serotonin, but this is unclear.

3. Pruritus due to hepatic disease usually implies some biliary obstruction, e.g., primary biliary

cirrhosis, or ductal blockage by tumor or stone. However, pruritus may also occur in the prodrome phase of viral hepatitis. In the young patient, infectious mononucleosis (with or without hepatic inflammation) may also present with a mild generalized pruritus and urticarial exanthem. Intrahepatic cholestasis, whether due to drugs (e.g., phenothiazines, testosterone derivatives, birth control medication) or to pregnancy, can commonly result in pruritus. Cholestatic itching appears to be due to levels of bile salts in the skin—these may activate lysosomal proteases. Therapy with cholestyramine, which acts to bind and promote excretion of bile salts, has been reported to have some success.

4. Chronic renal disease with azotemia may have a feature of intractible pruritus. Dialysis and low-protein diets will often alleviate this pruritus. On the other hand, patients with chronic renal disease have also been reported with hypercalcemia and secondary hyperparathyroidism, whose pruritus has been relieved by subtotal parathyroidectomy. The mechanism of action may involve the calcium ion's regulatory effect on numerous enzymatic processes, including aspects of histamine release.

5. Malignant disease may be associated with generalized pruritus. The classic example is polycythemia vera where heat associated pruritus is often present (10 to 30 per cent of patients), although this symptom complex may also occur in Hodgkin's disease, myeloid metaplasia, and other disorders. Hodgkin's disease has about a 30 per cent incidence of pruritus, with or without skin lesions (lymphonia cell infiltrates or "id" reactions). Other lymphomas and leukemias are much less commonly associated with pruritus, the exception being, of course, mycosis fungoides. Rarely, a solid malignancy is associated with generalized itching.

PRURITUS ANI AND VULVAE

method of
HENRY W. JOLLY, M.D.
New Orleans, Louisiana

Pruritus ani and vulvae, rather than a true disease, is an anatomic reaction pattern for many stimuli. As the name implies, pruritus is the main, and frequently only, symptom. Its occurrence may be intermittent or continuous, the reaction may be mild to severe, and it is frequently intractable and resistant to therapy. The condition may be painful if edema is excessive or if infection, either primary or secondary, is present.

The pruritus may be caused by single or multiple factors, and in long-standing cases the latter is frequent.

Causes of Pruritus Ani and Vulvae

1. Infection
    a. Fungal (particularly *Candida albicans*)
    b. Bacterial
    c. Parasitic
2. Intertrigo
3. Manifestation of systemic disease
    a. Diabetes
    b. Lymphoma, systemic malignancy
4. Other local diseases process
    a. Lichen sclerosus et atrophicus (LS&A)
    b. Extramammary Paget's disease
    c. Hemorrhoids
    d. Leukoplakia
    e. Atrophic changes-vulvae
5. Contact dermatitis
6. Neurogenic reactions

Clinical findings vary from none to erythema, edema, vesiculation, fissuring, excoriation, exudation, and lichenification. The lesions have varying types of borders, depending on the cause, secondary factors, severity, and duration of the problem. In general, the clinical signs may be any reaction process of which the skin is capable.

Diagnosis is usually obvious, with pruritus in and frequently limited to the anogenital region, with any of the clinical findings listed above. If a specific underlying cause is found, the treatment is directed to correct it.

Treatment

Infection. KOH (potassium hydroxide) and culture for yeast and fungi are frequently initial procedures in diagnosing the cause of pruritus ani and vulvae. The vagina and lower intestinal tract should be thoroughly examined for infection and parasitic infestation.

If yeast is found, topical nystatin/amphotericin B, usually in a drying lotion, is effective. If reinoculation seems to be occurring, eradication of the focus, by means of nystatin vaginally or orally, or both, is essential.

If fungi are present, oral griseofulvin alone or with topical miconazole nitrate or clotrimazole should be effective.

Bacterial infection may be treated with antibiotics, topically or orally or both.

Intestinal parasites should be treated with the proper vermifuge.

Intertrigo. Simple, uncomplicated intertrigo may be treated by nonsoapy cleansing using Burow's solution or boric acid solution two to three times daily followed by application of a drying agent, such as cornstarch or a drying lotion (zinc oxide 24.0 grams, talc 24.0 grams, glycerin 12.0 ml., distilled water added to make 120.0 ml.). Warning: Long-term use of zinc oxide may cause low-grade folliculitis.

Manifestation of Systemic Disease. Systemic disease, particularly diabetes and malignancy, should be considered in the differential diagnosis. If none of the other causes is found, these conditions should be searched for and treated accordingly.

Other Local Disease Processes. Lichen sclerosus et atrophicus is best treated with topical steroids on a short-term basis and at as low an effective potency as possible to prevent atrophy, striae, and telangiectasia in these self-occluding areas. Pruritus associated with lichen sclerosus et atrophicus is frequently alleviated by oral antimalarials, hydroxychloroquine, 200 to 400 mg. per day. Long-term use of that drug is usually not necessary, and eye complications are minimal. (This use of hydroxychloroquine is not listed in the manufacturer's official directive.)

Paget's disease requires expert surgical removal and long-term follow-up.

Hemorrhoidectomy may or may not help the condition.

Leukoplakia should be managed surgically, with regular follow-up examination.

Atrophic (senile) changes of the vulvae respond little, if at all, to any therapy. Care should be exerted to prevent overuse of topical steroids.

Contact Dermatitis. A primary contact dermatitis may be due to factors such as clothing, cosmetics, or hygienic preparations, but it is most frequently due to topical medications. The physician should always keep that fact in mind if the patient's condition worsens with good treatment. The base of the topical medication itself, one of the contents of the base, or the active ingredient may be the sensitizer. Treatment is the same as for any contact sensitization dermatitis.

Neurogenic Reactions. A neurogenic background alone or in combination with other causes may be a difficult problem to handle. Oral antihistamines and oral tranquilizers, either separately or in combination, may be tried. Therapeutic trials are frequently needed to determine the best drug or combination of drugs. Antihistamines or ataractic drugs are possibly the most effective treatment for many patients, unless the neurogenic factor is deep-seated.

General Comments

Because pruritus ani and vulvae is usually characterized by eczema, lichenification is the end result if the condition becomes chronic. In such situations, physical occlusion is needed to break the itch-scratch-lichenification cycle. A thick, folded towel applied like a diaper with firm, moderate pressure at night and held in place by underpants or safety pin attachment to a pajama top or t-shirt is helpful. In spite of what the patients say, they do scratch, and most scratching is done during the semiconsciousness of falling asleep or awakening, or during full sleep. Most patients balk at the suggestion of such physical occlusion, but it often spells the difference between therapeutic success and failure when the problem is chronic.

PSORIASIS

method of
ELIZABETH A. ABEL, M.D.,
and EUGENE M. FARBER, M.D.
Stanford, California

Psoriasis is a relatively common papulosquamous disorder characterized by erythematous papules and plaques topped by silvery, micaceous scales.

Clinical forms of this chronic disorder may vary from a few localized plaques on elbows and knees to widespread geographic plaques or total body involvement with erythroderma. An acute guttate form occurs in which numerous "droplike" papules and small plaques are scattered over the entire cutaneous surface. Pustular lesions may develop within localized plaques or become generalized as in the von Zumbusch type. Palmar plantar psoriasis represents another variety in which chronic scaling or vesicopustular lesions occur on the palms and soles, sometimes in association with psoriasis elsewhere on the body.

Psoriasis is known to represent a hyperproliferation of the epidermis; however, the basic cause is unknown. Although many treatments are directed at interference with DNA synthesis and interruption of cell division, quite different mechanisms may be operative as well.

General Measures

Patient Education. The establishment of good rapport between physician and patient is of utmost importance in the treatment of this lifelong disorder with visible lesions that may be emotionally, socially, or physically disabling. Adequate communication with the patient regarding the nature and course of psoriasis as well as the goals of therapy, as follows, is essential in promoting a favorable outlook and adjustment to the disorder.

1. Psoriasis is a noncontagious, benign disorder limited to the skin except for an association with arthritis in certain patients.

2. Exacerbations alternating with periods of relative quiescence are characteristic. Spontaneous remissions are common. Climate has an influence, as most patients improve in the summer with increased sun exposure and increased humidity.

3. The concept of "latent psoriasis" is consistent with the knowledge that certain triggering factors may precipitate the onset or a flare of the disorder in persons with the genetic predisposition to develop psoriasis. In the Koebner phenomenon cutaneous injury, either physical, mechanical, or thermal in nature, results in a delayed scaling erythematous plaque appearing at the exact site of injury. Viral infections or bacterial infections such as acute streptococcal pharyngitis are frequently associated with a flare of the disease, especially the acute guttate form. Severe exacerbation of psoriasis may follow the institution and withdrawal of systemic steroid therapy. Contact dermatitis and drug eruptions may be responsible for a flare of psoriasis. Antimalarials in particular are to be avoided in patients with known or suspected psoriasis. Although sunlight is usually beneficial, some patients have photo-aggravated psoriasis, which may be on the basis of a Koebner phenomenon. Such factors as stress and anxiety may be involved in an exacerbation of psoriasis, although they are not causally related.

4. There is no cure for psoriasis. Present treatment is palliative and aimed at controlling the epidermal growth rate. Control of known aggravating agents constitutes good preventive medicine.

Therapy

General Principles. Topical therapy, including tars and ultraviolet light (see also Goeckerman regimen), anthralin (see also Ingram regimen), and topical glucocorticosteroids, is generally preferred over systemic treatment because of fewer side effects.

Hospitalization is frequently required for the more severe forms of psoriasis or for treatment of ordinary psoriasis with extensive topical therapy under the Goeckerman or Ingram regimens. An alternative approach allowing for intensive topical therapy on an out-patient basis is the Psoriasis Day Care Center.

For the severe disabling psoriasis that has not responded to conventional forms of therapy, systemic treatment with antimetabolites may be indicated. The relatively new approach of psoralen-photochemotherapy (PUVA), a systemic treatment with local effect, is presently under investigation.

Adjunctive Therapy. In any treatment regimen nonspecific or adjunctive therapy is extremely important. Daily tub baths with a lubricating oil (Alpha Keri, Lubath, Domol, Nutraspa) are useful for relief of dryness and for mechanical debridement of scales. Following bathing and repeated as necessary, the application of bland emollients aids in hydration of the skin and relief of pruritus. Generally, the greasier preparations in an ointment base (e.g., Aquafor or white petrolatum) are most effective; however, different vehicles such as creams (Nivea cream, Albolene, Eucerin) or lotions (Keri lotion, Lubriderm) may be preferred for cosmetic reasons or in certain body areas. Ointments are poorly tolerated in intertriginous areas where they may cause maceration of skin. For treatment of acute flares of psoriasis including the acute guttate form and psoriatic erythroderma, treatment is usually commenced with bland emolliating agents along with bed rest, as more "active" medications may further exacerbate the psoriasis. Specific topical medications are cautiously introduced to small areas initially with gradual application to other areas if no adverse effects occur.

Nonspecific systemic measures include the use of tranquilizers for control of anxiety, which might exacerbate the disease, and systemic antipruritics such as hydroxyzine (Atarax), 10 to 25 mg., or diphenhydramine (Benadryl), 25 to 50 mg. three to four times daily.

Topical Therapy

Keratolytics. Salicylic acid ointment in a concentration of 1 to 20 per cent, depending on the degree of clinical hyperkeratosis is useful in the removal of scales. Six per cent salicylic acid in a gel base (Keratyl gel) may be used under occlusion for several hours on very thick plaques, on palms and soles, or on the scalp covered with a plastic cap overnight. Phenolated saline preparations such as Baker's "P & S" promote the removal of thick scales especially on the scalp. Urea creams, 10 to 20 per cent, are alternative topical preparations for the control of hyperkeratosis.

Topical Glucocorticosteroids. Several dozen topical glucocortiscosteroid preparations are available in a variety of vehicles including creams, ointments, gels, lotions, and solutions. Occlusion of any of these agents under plastic wrap such as Saran Wrap, with resultant increased temperature and humidity, leads to enhanced percutaneous absorption and greater anti-inflammatory and antimitotic effect. Although topical steroids are highly efficacious, prompt rebound ordinarily occurs once treatment is stopped. Significant systemic absorption with consequent pituitary adrenal suppression may occur when large areas of the body are treated. Adverse local effects may occur following the continued use of topical steroids, especially the newer fluorinated preparations when applied to intertriginous areas or under occlusion. Atrophy, telangiectasia, ecchymoses, and striae have all been reported complications.

The choice of steroid preparation and the vehicle depend on the clinical state of psoriasis as well as its location. Hydrocortisone cream or ointment 0.5 to 1 per cent is a commonly used preparation for intertriginous areas or on the face as it has not been associated with adverse chronic cutaneous changes. Examples of the newer fluorinated steroids, which have a more rapid effect, perhaps because of increased penetration, include: triamcinolone acetonide 0.1 per cent (Aristocort, Kenalog), fluocinolone acetonide 0.025 per cent (Synalar, Fluonid), betamethasone valerate 0.1 per cent (Valisone), and flurandrenolide 0.05 per cent (Cordran). Also available are lower strength preparations of triamcinolone acetonide 0.025 per cent and of fluocinolone acetonide 0.01 per cent. High-strength preparations include halcinonide 0.1 per cent (Halog), fluocinonide 0.05 per cent (Lidex), and betamethasone dipropionate 0.05 per cent (Diprosone). Flurandrenolide is also available as Cordran tape for occlusive effect.

Our policy has been to restrict the use of topical steroids. Nonfluorinated steroids may be prescribed for treatment of facial lesions or intertriginous areas. Fluorinated steroids are useful on a short-term basis for treatment of resistant, highly inflamed, or irritated plaques but are not advisable for treatment of widespread psoriasis.

Tar and Ultraviolet Light. Both coal tar preparations and ultraviolet light have been used for centuries in the treatment of psoriasis. Each is effective alone but both have greater benefit when used in combination, as in a Goeckerman type of regimen. Crude coal tar, a complex mixture of hydrocarbons obtained by the destructive distillation of coal, may be prepared in creams, ointments, solutions and gel-base vehicles in concentrations of 1 to 10 per cent. These preparations are often messy to use and have an odor. They should not be used in intertriginous areas, where they may cause irritation and maceration. Folliculitis and allergic contact dermatitis are other occasional complications. Recently introduced refined tar products (Estar gel, psoriGel) are more cosmetically acceptable but may be drying and are best used in conjunction with emollients.

Phototherapy may range from exposure to natural sunlight or artificial light with a single sunlamp bulb to multiple ultraviolet sunlamp tubes (Westinghouse FS40) installed in a walk-in light unit.

Although the action spectrum of coal tar lies in the UVA range, most conventional light sources are of insufficient UVA intensity to produce a photosensitizing action of tar. The effective wavelength in the Goeckerman regimen is thought to be within the UVB spectrum, the mechanism of which is unknown.

A typical modified Goeckerman regimen consists of tar baths (Zetar, Polytar, Balnetar) and exposure to ultraviolet light once or twice daily. In addition, crude coal tar ointment 1 to 5 per cent is applied for several hours daily and is removed in a bath or with mineral oil prior to light exposure. Liquor carbonis detergens (L.C.D.), an alcoholic solution of coal tar, 5 to 10 per cent in a cream base, may be prescribed for overnight use. Tar shampoos (Zetar, Polytar) are frequently prescribed for scalp psoriasis. Five per cent liquor carbonis detergens in Nivea oil may be applied to the scalp overnight. Remissions lasting weeks to many months may be induced by the Goeckerman method of treatment over a 3 week period.

Anthralin. A synthetic compound related to chrysarobin incorporated into a stiff paste will cause more rapid flattening of psoriatic plaques as compared to tar. Disadvantages include difficulty of application, irritation, and staining of the skin. The latter is minimized by incorporation of salicylic acid with the paste, which retards oxidation. A modified Ingram regimen combining the use of anthralin and ultraviolet light was initially popularized in Europe and is being increasingly used in this country in hospitalized patients and selected ambulatory patients. Remissions can be induced in 2 weeks, lasting from several weeks to one year or more. Unlike tar, anthralin is applied to individual lesions, which are then covered with stockinette to prevent spread to uninvolved skin areas. Anthralin preparations used at Stanford for treatment of plaques on the body and for scalp psoriasis are given below:

ANTHRALIN HARD PASTE		ANTHRALIN SCALP POMADE	
Anthralin	0.1 to 0.4%	Anthralin	0.4%
Salicylic acid	0.4%	Salicylic acid	0.4%
Hard paraffin	10 to 15%	Mineral oil	76.0%
Lassar's paste	qs 100%	Cetyl alcohol	21.9%
		Na lauryl sulfate	2.1%

It is important to initiate treatment with 0.1 per cent anthralin with a gradual increase in concentration to prevent undue irritation. Commercially available anthralin preparations include Anthra-Derm ointment (0.1 per cent, 0.25 per cent, 0.5 per cent, 1 per cent), Lasan Unguent (0.4 per cent anthralin), and Anthera.

Systemic Therapy

Systemic Corticosteroids. Although initially effective, these preparations are generally contraindicated, as cessation of systemic steroids is usually accompanied by rebound worsening of the disease.

Intralesional Steroids. Although effective in the treatment of resistant plaques of psoriasis or for severe nail involvement, the intralesional route of administration is equivalent to a parenteral dose. Systemic effects may result, depending on the total dose and frequency of administration. The usual method consists of triamcinolone acetonide suspension 10 mg. per ml. diluted with isotonic saline solution or lidocaine 1 per cent to a concentration of 2.5 to 5 mg. per ml. injected into the mid-dermis with a 25 gauge needle. An amount necessary to raise a small wheal (0.1 ml. or less) is injected in multiple areas within a plaque or at the base of a nail. The lower the concentration of steroid, the less chance there will be of atrophy developing at the site of injection.

Methotrexate. This folic acid antagonist, which interferes with DNA synthesis, is an extremely effective agent in controlling the hyperproliferative psoriatic apidermis. The use of cancer chemotherapeutic agents in psoriasis with their associated risks must be weighed against the benefits in carefully selected patients. Strict guidelines as advanced by the National Program for Dermatology have been published for the use of methotrexate (Arch. Dermatol., *105*:363, 1972, and *108*:35, 1973). Indications for treatment are limited to severe disabling psoriasis that has not responded to conventional treatment, psoriatic erythroderma, and generalized acute pustular psoriasis of von Zumbusch. Assessment of liver and renal function and hematologic studies must be made initially and at intervals during the course of treatment because of the risk of systemic toxicity to the liver, kidneys, and bone marrow. In addition, gastrointestinal toxicity may produce aphthae, nausea, vomiting, and diarrhea. Methotrexate is also teratogenic.

Insufficient data exist to determine the ideal dosage schedule designed to produce the maximum therapeutic effect with least toxicity. Dosage schedules generally preferred in psoriasis include the single weekly oral dose of 7.5 to 20 mg. or three 2.5 to 7.5 mg. doses at 12-hour intervals over a 24-hour period.

Azarbine. This antimetabolite was removed from the market in 1976 by the Food and Drug Administration because of the risk of thromboembolic phenomena associated with treatment of psoriasis.

PUVA-Systemic. PUVA is the acronym for psoralen (P) and long wave length ultraviolet light A (UVA), a systemic treatment with local effect. This relatively new chemotherapeutic approach consists of the ingestion of 8-methoxypsoralen, a photosensitizing furocoumarin, at a dose of 0.65 mg. per kg. followed in 2 to 3 hours by exposure to UVA. Two multicenter clinical trials have established the efficacy of this new approach to the treatment of psoriasis in which clearing occurs in an average of 25 treatments given two to three times weekly. Serious acute side effects requiring discontinuation of therapy are rare. These include phototoxicity with erythema and blistering, pruritus, and nausea. Erythema is related to the dosage of both drug and light and can be prevented by careful dosimetry. Eyes must be protected with opaque goggles during light treatment and with UVA blocking sunglasses during psoralen treatment programs. Potential chronic side effects such as actinic damage and aging of the skin, carcinogenesis, and cataract formation, suggested by in vitro and animal toxicity studies, remain a great concern. PUVA therapy is still investigational; 8-methoxypsoralen, which is available for the treatment of vitiligo, has not yet been approved for use in psoriasis by the Food and Drug Administration. This treatment is best carried out in selected patients with disabling psoriasis under the careful supervision of physicians and specially trained technicians with standardized light sources and adequate precautions taken to prevent side effects. Further studies are necessary to determine the place of PUVA therapy in the psoriasis treatment regimen.

INFLAMMATORY ERUPTIONS OF THE HANDS AND FEET

method of
JAMES E. RASMUSSEN, M.D.
Buffalo, New York

Many diseases have manifestations on the hands and feet as well as on the rest of the body—secondary syphilis, atopic dermatitis, erythema multiforme, scleroderma, photoreactions, and psoriasis. This section, however, deals only with those diseases in which the primary or most important manifestation is on the palms and soles.

Specific Diseases

Tinea Pedis. Occurs in three distinct patterns, which often overlap—a dry scaling hyperkeratotic dermatitis in the "moccasin" distribution of the feet, an acute vesicular dermatitis of the arch of the foot (which may produce an id reaction on the hands), and a white macerated intertriginous dermatitis. Any of these three patterns can be associated with fungal infection of the nails. Tinea pedis is exceptionally rare in prepubertal children.

Dishydrotic Eczema. Crops of clear discrete vesicles on the palms, soles, and sides of the digits accompanied by severe burning and pruritus are the hallmarks of this paroxysmal disease.

Pustulosis Palmaris et Plantaris (Pustular and Vesicular Eruptions of the Palms and Soles, Pustular Bacterid). Clear vesicles rapidly evolve to pustules and then dry, forming characteristic red-brown crusts on the arch and soles of the feet and the palms of the hands. Severe and intractable burning and pruritus make this a most difficult disease to manage.

Allergic Eczematous Contact Dermatitis. Usually due to a chemical contained in the rubber component of insoles, arch supports, and other padded areas of the shoes. The erythema, scale, and vesicles usually occur on the arch, pressure areas of the sole, heel cap, and dorsum of the foot.

Primary Irritant Dermatitis. More common on the hands, features extreme dryness, erythema, hyperkeratosis, and deep fissures. The web spaces are characteristically involved when the irritant is a soap or other liquid.

Atopic Winter Foot. A very characteristic disease of children and young adults with xerosis, erythema, scale, and fissures on the great toes of both feet and to a lesser degree the other toes and the fingers of the hands. It characteristically is much worse in the winter time and better in the summer.

Symmetric Lividities. A red-purple pruritic dermatitis more commonly occurring on the feet. It basically represents an immersion foot and is seen in cold weather in people whose sweaty hands or feet are confined in shoes or gloves.

General Rules of Treatment

Wet or Vesicular Dermatoses. Soaks or wet compresses 3 to 4 times a day for 5 minutes apiece should be the initial therapy. Macerated intertriginous areas should be constantly exposed to the air and small cotton balls can be used to prop the toes apart. Use topical steroids in lotion vehicles only.

Dry (Xerotic). If the disease is primarily xerotic or becomes so following soaks or compresses, then the ultimate goal is lubrication—the feet tolerate ointments and creams quite well, but on the hands it is necessary to use plastic or cotton gloves for obvious functional reasons.

Specific Treatment

Tinea Pedis. The diagnosis should always be established by either potassium hydroxide preparations or appropriate cultures or both, as tinea pedis can appear quite similar to many of the other diseases discussed here. Begin with topical antifungals such as haloprogin, tolnaftate, or miconazole. Topical therapy is frequently ineffective, and it may be necessary to use griseofulvin (the newer suspensions, ultramicrosized griseofulvin, [Gris-PEG and Fulvicin-P/G] are better absorbed). It is frequently impossible to clear these fungal infections.

Dishydrotic Eczema. Potent topical steroids under occlusion are sometimes effective. If the disease is severe, systemic corticosteroids should be the first choice.

Pustular/Vesicular Eruptions of the Palms and Soles. Potent topical steroids applied under occlusion are sometimes successful. Some of these patients probably have a pustular bacterid, and a diligent search should be made for "occult foci of infection" (cystitis, dental abscess). The empirical use of long-term systemic antibiotics (tetracycline, erythromycin) is sometimes successful when nothing else seems to work. Systemic corticosteroids can be used for short periods, but only to gain initial control, *not* for chronic use.

Allergic Eczematous Contact Dermatitis. This usually presents as a vesicular eruption on the soles (and may also produce an id on the hands). If this reaction is severe use systemic corticosteroids (prednisone, 30 to 60 mg. per day). Milder cases respond well to topical corticosteroids. Use patch tests to define the allergen but not while the disease is flaring. Wooden shoes (clogs) are helpful. Ten per cent glutaraldehyde (investigational) soak twice daily or dusting with fluffy tannic acid will prevent the hyperhidrosis that contributes to this problem (see Fisher, A.: Contact Dermatitis. 2nd ed. Lea and Febiger, 1973).

Primary Irritant. Avoidance of the irritant if it is known and lubrication of the xerotic areas are most important. Patients who do physical work with their hands should be required to wear heavy gloves at all times.

Atopic Winter Foot. Simple lubrication is dramatically effective. Occasionally, topical corticosteroids may be necessary.

Symmetric Lividities. The feet must be kept exposed to the air as much as is possible. Antiperspirants used at night will reduce the sweating. Fluffy tannic acid or 10 per cent glutaraldehyde (investigational) twice daily solution will also achieve the desired dryness.

BACTERIAL INFECTIONS OF THE SKIN
method of
ALFRED D. HERNANDEZ, M.D.,
and JOSEPH W. BURNETT, M.D.
Baltimore, Maryland

Superficial Infection

Impetigo (Nonbullous). Nonbullous impetigo is caused by Group A beta-hemolytic streptococci. As lesions become older, *Staphylococcus aureus* may be isolated in combination with streptococci. In long-standing lesions removal of the crust results in an ulcerative lesion known as ecthyma. Although penicillinase producing *S. aureus* may be isolated from lesions, they appear to be a secondary bacterial colonization and antibiotic therapy directed against the streptococci is curative. Impetigo may be complicated by acute glomerulonephritis, although the cutaneous infection has been adequately treated. Scarlet fever has also been reported as a complication of impetigo.

THERAPY. 1. Systemic antibiotics directed against streptococci are the treatment of choice. Oral penicillins (Pen · Vee K) or erythromycin at doses of 250 mg. every six hours for 7 to 10 days is effective in 90 to 100 per cent of the patients. Benzathine penicillin, 600,000 to 1,200,000 units given intramuscularly, is recommended when the patient is unable to take oral antibiotics.

2. Nonspecific topical therapy, such as frequent washing with soap, is a useful adjunct to systemic therapy, helping to remove adherent crust and scales. Topical antibiotics are of little value when systemic antibiotics are used. Prolonged treatment with topical antibiotics may result in allergies and resistant bacterial overgrowth and are not recommended.

Bullous Impetigo. Bullous impetigo is most frequently caused by a Group II type 71 staphylococci that liberates an epidermolysin. Infection results in bullae with fluid that is initially clear but may quickly become purulent. Cultures taken from bullous impetigo usually show the growth of only *S. aureus* over 80 per cent of all staphylococci recovered from the lesions of bullous or nonbullous impetigo are penicillin resistant.

THERAPY. 1. Systemic antibiotics are the treatment of choice. Since most isolates of *S. aureus* recovered are penicillin-resistant, treatment should be initiated with a penicillinase-resistant penicillin, erythromycin, or cephalosporin.

2. Topical therapy with antibiotics such as neomycin and bacitracin have been shown to be ineffective against staphylococci. Other topical antibiotics should also be avoided for the reasons given above.

Bacterial Folliculitis. Bacterial folliculitis is most frequently caused by *S. aureus*. Occasionally, other gram-positive and gram-negative bacteria have been isolated from such lesions. Demonstration of the causative bacteria by Gram stain and culture is important for appropriate therapy, since a similar folliculitis may also be induced by fungi (tinea barbae), drugs (halides and steroids), or lubricating oils.

THERAPY. Systemic antibiotics are frequently required to treat bacterial folliculitis. The antibiotics and doses used are similar to those used

for treating bullous impetigo if *S. aureus* is the causative organism. Culture and sensitivity is helpful in determining therapy especially in lesions caused by nonstaphylococcal bacteria. Topical therapy is identical to that mentioned for impetigo.

Erythrasma. Erythrasma, caused by *Corynebacterium minutissimum*, is a chronic localized infection of the intertrigenous areas and toe webs. Depending on the site of involvement, it may clinically be confused with tinea versicolor or a dermatophyte. Irradiation of affected areas with a Wood's lamp shows a coral-red fluorescence and, along with culture, helps in the diagnosis.

THERAPY. Erythromycin, 250 mg. four times daily for 7 to 10 days, is the treatment of choice. Lesions respond in 1 to 2 weeks. Topical keratolytics and antibiotics have not been curative. Antibacterial soaps may help prevent recurrences.

Toxic Epidermal Necrolysis Due to Staphylococci (Staphylococcal Scaled Skin Syndrome). Staphylococcal scaled skin syndrome (SSSS) is caused by a toxin elaborated by a group II type S1 or 71 staphylococci. Thus, this disease is not due to a direct cutaneous infection. The organisms are most frequently isolated from the nasopharynx and rarely from the cutaneous lesions. The disease primarily affects children under the age of 10 years, although a few cases have been reported in adults.

THERAPY. Systemic antibiotics directed against *S. aureus* should be given (see bullous impetigo), although there is controversy as to whether or not antibiotics influence the course of the disease. Several untreated patients have resolved despite the continued presence of toxin-producing bacteria in the nasopharynx or other foci. There are at least two reasons to give systemic antibiotics: a small percentage of patients have been shown to have bacterial septicemia, and to decrease possible spread of these strains of staphylococci.

2. Systemic steroids, although recommended in the past, are not indicated and there is controversy whether they may actually enhance the disease.

3. Supportive topical skin care consisting of wet dressings and lubricants is advised.

Atypical Mycobacterial Infections

In the United States, the most common cause of cutaneous atypical mycobacterial disease is *Mycobacterium marinum*. This organism has been isolated from various aquatic sources, including brackish water, lakes, swimming pools, and fish tanks. The infection begins by inoculation of the organism, usually by an abrasion or puncture of the skin. Single or multiple nodules are produced that may ulcerate or become verrucous. Not infrequently, the lesions may resemble sporotrichosis.

THERAPY. 1. Untreated lesions may heal spontaneously in months to years.

2. If lesions are small, surgical excision may be curative. Recurrence may occur adjacent to the surgical scar.

3. Various antituberculosis therapeutic agents have been used with varying degrees of success. These include isonazid, ethambutol and rifampin, which have been used separately or in combination (see manufacturers' official directives).

4. The tetracyclines have been shown to suppress growth in vitro, and clinical trials have been encouraging. Of the tetracyclines, minocycline, 100 mg. twice daily, has enjoyed the greatest success.

Other Infections. Other less frequent cutaneous atypical mycobacterial infections have been caused by *M. kansasii, M. fortuitum* and *M. chalonei (abscesses). Mycobacterium kansasii* has produced lesions similar to those seen with *M. marinum* while *M. fortuitum* and *M. chalonei* produce subcutaneous abscesses.

THERAPY. 1. *Mycobacterium kansasii* is treated in the same manner as *M. marinum.*

2. *Mycobacterium fortuitum* and *chalonei* are treated by surgical excision or drainage or both. Both of these organisms are resistant to most antimicrobial agents.

Gram-negative Infection of the Toe Webs

Gram-negative infection of the toe webs and adjacent skin in its mildest form presents as a macerated boggy lesion similar to toe web infection caused by *Candida albicans.* In more severe forms, the lesion (or lesions) progresses to denudation, at times, of the entire plantar surface. Lesions often have a seropurulent discharge and may be quite painful. *Pseudomonas aeruginosa* or *Proteus mirabilis*

Springfield, Illinois

are the most frequent isolates, but other gram-negative bacteria are seen in combination with these.

THERAPY. Because of the localized nature of this disease and the potential hazardous side effects of the antibiotics used for the treatment of Pseudomonas and Proteus, this disease is treated topically.

Bed rest and frequent soaks are recommended to decrease colony counts of bacteria. Some success has been achieved using silver nitrate. Gentamicin cream should be reserved for severe cases.

ROSACEA

method of
STEPHEN P. STONE, M.D.
Springfield, Illinois

Rosacea, sometimes incorrectly referred to as acne rosacea, is a chronic disorder occurring on the face of middle-aged or older persons. Although it most commonly occurs in women, it is usually of greatest severity when occurring in men. The cause of rosacea is entirely unknown, but it is generally believed that afflicted persons are constitutionally predisposed to blushing and flushing of the facial skin. Stimuli which elicit such flushing are those which normally evoke vasodilatation: emotional stress, alcohol, and food or drink that is hot either in temperature or in taste. Patients predisposed to rosacea seem to flush more easily, more intensely, and for a longer period of time than do normal persons.

The primary lesion of rosacea is erythema with telangiectasia located on the central portion of the face (nose, malar eminences, and the point of the chin). Often there is an associated component of papules and pustules, giving a somewhat acneform appearance, and leading to the inappropriate characterization of this disease as "acne rosacea."

Involvement of the nose with extensive soft tissue hyperplasia is known as rhinophyma, a form of the disease that occurs more commonly among men. Rhinophyma is often thought by the lay public to represent intemperance in ingestion of alcohol, and although this is not always true, there may be some validity to this perceived association.

Clinical Manifestations

Rosacea usually begins insidiously with transient dilation of the blood vessels of the blush area of the cheeks and nose. Eventually, the erythema in this area becomes persistent and is accompanied by telangiectasia. Subsequently, papules and pustules may appear, giving the central face an acneform appearance. In contrast to true acne, the appearance of comedones is quite rare.

Rhinophyma usually begins with irregular thickening of the skin of the lower portion of the nose, with widening of the follicular orifices. The skin may appear red to violaceous, and this change in color may spread to the adjacent cheeks. Extensive telangiectasia is often present. Rhinophyma may accompany severe rosacea, or may occur in the absence of other signs of the disease.

Chronic gastritis, demonstrated histologically, and often of no clinical significance, has been reported to occur in many rosacea patients. Abnormal histologic patterns in the proximal intestine have also been noted. It is unclear what role is played by these gastrointestinal changes in the pathophysiology of the disease.

Eye changes, including blepharitis, conjunctivitis, iritis, and keratitis, occur in association with rosacea and may occasionally occur without the associated skin disease. Although these lesions may respond to the systemic treatment of rosacea, ophthalmologic consultation is recommended in the presence of keratitis, which may result in loss of vision.

Treatment

General Measures. Although not well documented, it is advisable to recommend avoidance of things that will result in vasodilatation of the facial blood vessels. Hot food or drink, whether to the taste (highly spiced foods) or in temperature, should be avoided. Alcoholic beverages should be proscribed, and excessive exposure to sunlight and environmental heat and cold, should also be avoided. Prevention of blushing due to emotional factors is, unfortunately, beyond our ability.

Systemic Medications. Tetracycline is remarkably successful in the treatment of rosacea. Treatment should be instituted with 500 mg. twice daily, and the patient should be carefully instructed to take the antibiotic on an empty stomach. As improvement occurs, the dose may be gradually reduced to 250 mg. daily and then 250 mg. every other day before it is discontinued. Reduction in dosage should not be accomplished in a cookbook fashion, but should be carefully titrated against the patient's improvement. Remissions following discontinuance of antibiotic therapy may be quite prolonged, although some patients will require several courses of antibiotic treatment. In view of the relative safety of tetracycline, I do not hesitate to continue low dose tetracycline therapy for a year or more, in order to provide a sustained remission.

In patients sensitive to tetracycline, erythromycin may be utilized in the same dosage. Recent experience suggests that erythromycin (2 per cent) or clindamycin (1 per cent) in a topical lotion (as follows) may be useful in treating rosacea:

To a solvent such as E-solve lotion (Syosset Laboratories, Syosset, New York) or 40 ml. of 70 per cent alcohol and 15 ml. of propylene glycol is added erythromycin base to make a 2 per cent solution, or clindamycin to make 1 per cent. The clindamycin capsules may be opened and emptied into the solvent, but the erythromycin base tablets must be crushed, the film removed, and the powder then mixed well with the solvent.

Local Treatment. The skin of the rosacea patient is more sensitive than it would appear, and the use of harsh topicals is contraindicated. For the patient with oily skin, precipitated sulfur 1 to 10 per cent in hydrocortisone cream is usually satisfactory. Commercially available preparations such as sulfur and polyoxyethylene lauryl ether in a greaseless base with zinc oxide and bentonite (Fostril) and with hydrocortisone added (Fostril HC) are also useful.

For the patient with drier, more sensitive skin, hydrocortisone cream alone may be used.

Fluorinated corticosteroids are capable of producing a rosacealike eruption when used on the face and will give transient improvement followed by a more severe rebound when used for the treatment of rosacea. Their use is, therefore, contraindicated.

Telangiectatic blood vessels and hypertrophic sebaceous glands may best be treated electrosurgically, using an extremely fine electrode (such as a 30 gauge needle) to coagulate the dilated vessels.

For severe rhinophyma, the nose may be sculpted to a normal shape by the use of the cutting current with excellent cosmetic results. Although some dermatologists and plastic surgeons recommend scalpel surgery for removal of redundant tissue in rhinophyma, the extreme vascularity of the nasal tissues makes this a technically difficult procedure and one that cannot be recommended for the inexperienced surgeon.

SCABIES

method of
WILLIAM H. SMOOT, M.D.
Billings, Montana

Scabies, a worldwide, highly contagious disease, continues at its cyclic apogee. The reason for these cycles is not completely understood. Epidemics of scabies usually last 15 years and are followed by a 15 year interval of reduced activity. Our current epidemic began in the mid 1960s and should begin to decrease by 1980.

Treatment

There are multiple chemical and treatment schedules to eradicate scabies. Lindane (gamma benzene hexachloride, U.S.P.) 1 per cent cream or lotion is the treatment of choice. Recently, the safety of this agent in infants has been questioned. It also appears that resistance to gamma benzene hexachloride is being noted. Ten per cent crotamiton (N-ethyl-o-croton-otolmide) cream is a very acceptable substitute, with no toxicity in infants or resistance from the scabies organism being noted. This chemical also appears to decrease pruritus as well. Either gamma benzene hexachloride or crotamiton is applied after a bath, left on for 24 hours and removed by bathing, then reapplied (see manufacturers' official directive before using). It should be reapplied in 3 to 7 days. Often, one reapplication is all that is needed, although two reapplications may be given. It is recommended that all family members and close contacts be treated. It is also recommended that the clothing worn that day and the bedsheets be washed in conjunction with the initial application of the scabicide. It must be stressed that the entire body be covered with the cream or lotion from the chin down. In infants, the entire body should be treated with crotamiton, face and scalp included.

Prognosis

The patient should be told he may continue to itch for days, even though the organism has been eradicated. These eczematous allergic reactions can usually be controlled with oral antihistamines or topical cortisone. Rarely, systemic cortisones are needed to control the patient's itching. Should the pruritus continue after 2 or 3 weeks, the patient should be reevaluated. Most persistent pruritus is either of an eczematous allergic nature or the patient has not applied the creams properly and the disease persists.

SCLERODERMA
(Progressive Systemic Sclerosis)

method of
JAMES F. FRIES, M.D.
Stanford, California

Scleroderma (progressive systemic sclerosis) is a generalized microvascular disease characterized by tightening of the skin with atrophic scarring binding the skin to underlying tissues. Morphea and other "localized" forms of scleroderma with similar histopathology are separate entities; neither require nor respond to specific therapy, and are not discussed here. Systemic sclerosis classically involves skin proximal to the metacarpal phalangeal joints as well as the digits, allowing its ready separation from a variety of conditions which lead to atrophic, bound-down skin over the fingers alone.

While usually grouped with the "autoimmune," "collagen-vascular," or "connective tissue" diseases, systemic sclerosis usually does not have a pronounced immunologic or inflammatory component. The basic pathologic lesion appears to be microvascular, with arteriolar and microvascular intimal fibrosis leading to ischemic atrophy and replacement fibrosis of various organs.

Prognosis is better than frequently described, with published studies representing patients selected for greater than average severity. Stable courses over many years in most patients underscore the inappropriateness of the adjective "progressive." Some disease subgroups, notably those with calcinosis and telangiectasia as prominent features (CREST), almost invariably have benign and long-term courses. Appreciation of the likelihood of stabilization and even partial remission, even in patients with apparent rapid progression in early months of the disease, is the key to successful management, since ill-chosen aggressive pharmacologic approaches to the uncomplicated basic disease offer far more chance of harm than benefit. No therapeutic agent has been shown to alter the underlying disease process. Penicillamine, relaxin, colchicine, cyclophosphamide, chlorambucil, EDTA, potassium p-aminobenzoate, sympathectomy, DMSO, and many other agents have enjoyed brief fads and nearly every year a new agent is added to the long list of treatments whose initial enthusiastic reports cannot be validated in subsequent studies.

On the other hand, certain disease complications respond to specific therapy, and the non-pharmacologic basic program offers benefits in prevention of disability, realistic adaptation to the disease, and prevention of complications. These considerations dictate the therapeutic strategy, which is founded on the basic program and employs specific reactions to specific complications.

Basic Program

Positive Expectation. The ominous diagnostic term "progressive systemic sclerosis" implies for many patients a relentless progression to a fixed, fibrotic, mummylike state. The patient may understand that the disease is mysterious, untreatable, progressive, and fatal; these adjectives are well-calculated to increase a state of despair. In fact, such progression is unusual, and the pessimistic prognosis is inaccurate. Moreover, the continuing popularity of new therapeutic agents and the marked efficacy of placebo treatments in some trials suggest a major therapeutic role for the delivery of hope and positive expectations to the patient. At this time, the "art" of medicine may be more important than the "science" in the management of the patient with scleroderma.

Full Activity and Employment. Following the positive expectation of patient and physician, major lifestyle changes should not be made in anticipation of future disability. Rather, the patient should be encouraged to seek social outlets, to continue to work, to continue schooling plans, and to continue full activities. While modifications must occasionally be made for particular circumstances, such activities provide incidental physical therapy equivalents, promote a feeling of health rather than illness, and act to increase circulatory reserve.

Habit Moderation. Nicotine and caffeine have theoretical adverse effects upon the underlying microvascular and ischemic condition and we counsel avoidance. Gastrointestinal motility problems may develop, and a diet adequate in fresh fruits and vegetables, low in refined carbohydrates, and high in fiber is a useful prophylactic. Alcohol in excess promotes depression and should be avoided, although moderate use of alcohol promotes vasodilatation and relaxation and may even be encouraged.

Warm Clothing and Hand Protection. Vasoconstriction in response to cold accentuates the disease process, and dermal ulcers develop most frequently during the winter months. Minor injuries to the fingers and fingertips heal slowly and potentially may develop into recalcitrant ulcers. Thus, avoidance of cool environments, including air conditioning, and the wearing of adequate clothing are important. Reflex vasoconstriction occurs when the trunk or neck is cooled, hence warm clothing centrally is at least as important as warmth promoted by gloves over the more obviously affected portions of the body.

Active Range-of-Motion Exercises. Contractures are a potential hazard in scleroderma, particularly of the fingers. Stiffness secondary to the disease makes extreme motion uncomfortable, and gradually fibrous and finally bony contractures develop. Clinical experience strongly suggests that these contractures may be minimized by stretching affected body areas through their entire range of normal motion several times daily. The stretching of skin and fibrous tissue not only limits contracture development and helps regain lost mobility, but it also provides circulatory reserve both by the lymphatic and venous pumping afforded by activity and by decreasing the tightness in the very limited anatomic compartments of the digits. We are not enamored of formal physical therapy except as an educational device. Range-of-motion exercises in systemic sclerosis must be performed many times daily as a developed habit and once-or-twice-weekly formal sessions are simply inadequate. Additionally, the patient gains confidence from assuming personal responsibility for the therapeutic program.

Early Symptomatic Response to Heartburn. Loss of peristalsis in the lower two thirds of the esophagus is the rule in scleroderma. Since gravity performs this portion of the swallowing activity quite well, aperistalsis per se is asymptomatic or only modestly symptomatic. However, loss of tone at the lower esophageal sphincter and absence of the swallowing wave, frequently combined with slow gastric emptying, promote the development of reflux esophagitis. Esophageal stricture, when it occurs, is the result of chronic scarring secondary to reflux esophagitis, not directly from the underlying aperistalsis. These strictures can be prevented. Any symptoms suggestive of reflux esophagitis are aggressively treated with standard measures, including antacids, avoidance of foods for two or three hours prior to reclining, and the placement of blocks underneath the head of the bed. Cimetidine is a promising addition but has not yet been adequately studied.

Complications

Dysphagia. When frank dysphagia, usually at the level of the lower sternum, has developed, the first approach is again an aggressive approach to presumed reflux esophagitis. Usually, this will be successful, and further measures are not required. In extreme cases, procedures that dilate the esophagus may be needed. In our experience, this requirement arises in less than 1 of 100 patients.

Malabsorption. Loss of circular smooth muscle and replacement fibrosis results in an atonic bowel throughout its length, with the more proximal portions generally affected more severely than the distal. The resulting intermittent stasis favors bacterial colonization of the small bowel, with a resulting "blind loop" syndrome. This can result in a frank and severe malabsorption syndrome that is dramatically responsive to antibiotic treatment. Tetracycline, ampicillin, and chloramphenicol have been successfully used to treat this syndrome. Nonabsorbable sulfonamide drugs or neomycin, which do not attain tissue levels, have been much less satisfactory. Some patients have been successfully managed for many years with continual antibiotic treatment, switching from tetracycline, 250 mg. four times daily, to ampicillin (in the same dosage) and back again at 6 week intervals to minimize development of resistant organisms. Complicating Candida colonization with malabsorption has been reported.

An occasional patient will show more marked lower intestinal obstruction, usually intermittent. These syndromes, when severe, may require nasogastric suction, intravenous fluids, and even hyperalimentation maneuvers. The avoidance of codeine and other narcotic pain relievers that aggravate the situation, maintenance of physical activity in the patient, and a diet with adequate fiber intake appear to be useful preventive measures. A psyllium hydrophilic mucilloid (Metamucil), 1 teaspoonful in a glass of water followed by a second glass of water twice daily has been helpful in some patients.

Myositis.   Between 5 and 15 per cent of patients with definite scleroderma have a complicating polymyositislike problem. These patients will have elevated creatine phosphokinase or aldolase levels, definite myositis on muscle biopsy, or both. The myositis responds to corticosteroids, begun at 1 mg. per kg. and tapered to a maintenance level of 0.33 mg. per kg. or less as the condition permits. This is the only definite indication for corticosteroids in progressive systemic sclerosis. Although the myositis usually shows a predictable response, the dermal condition may continue or progress at the same time. Corticosteroids are presumed to work either through anti-inflammatory or anti-immunologic mechanisms and should not be expected to improve patients who show evidence of neither of these disease features. Clinical speculation has linked corticosteroid use in scleroderma with subsequent development of a hypertensive/renal crisis, discussed later.

Digital Ulcers and Gangrene.   The ischemic microvascular lesion of scleroderma, even when progressive, is usually slow and stable in its development. Conservative therapeutic approaches in patients with severe involvement are usually rewarded with a slow autoamputation of the distal tuft and even the terminal phalanx, entirely consistent with good hand function and minimal discomfort. In a few patients, digital ulcers or distal gangrene will develop. The natural history of such a lesion is to heal, although the process may extend over many months. Therapeutic trials, such as intra-arterial reserpine versus intra-arterial saline, strongly suggest that either the natural history or a placebo effect are responsible for healing. We soak such lesions in a mild solution of sodium bicarbonate (1 teaspoonful in a cup of warm waer) for 5 minutes twice daily and avoid creams, antibiotic ointments, or other materials that either serve to occlude the area or to sensitize potentially for local reactions. We are similarly unhappy with the use of vasodilatory agents, which, if they give any discernible effect at all, do so only for a period of 1 to 3 weeks. The ineffectiveness of these agents may be related to loss of placebo effect with time or may represent the tachyphylaxis known to develop to each of these agents over approximately this time period. Skin grafts will sometimes successfully "take" over malleolar ulcers but should not be attempted over the distal digits because the blood supply is insufficient to permit success. Skin ulcers begin most commonly in the winter months, and healing frequently begins with the onset of spring.

Pruritus.   Some patients show a most vexing and persistent itching in regions of involved skin. Usually this condition extends for only a portion of the period of illness but may last for 2 or 3 years. No treatment is consistently effective. Alpha Keri bath lotion, sodium bicarbonate (2 to 4 tablespoons per bath), and lanolin creams have helped some. Diphenhydramine hydrochloride (Benadryl) and other antihistamines may be worth trying but are seldom effective.

Dyspnea.   Fortunately, the bilateral lower lobe pulmonary fibrosis and decreased pulmonary diffusing capacity so common in scleroderma patients is seldom progressive or disabling. No specific treatment is available. Home oxygen therapy should be used as a last resort for very few patients.

Hypertensive/Renal Crisis.   The most ominous syndrome in clinical rheumatology is the development of malignant hypertension and acute renal failure in the scleroderma patient. The syndrome involves very high renin levels and cortical infarction and has been widely held to be universally and rapidly progressive. Patients may present with hypertensive seizures, decreased vision with papilledema, or sudden onset of proteinuria and azotemia. We are now following three patients who have survived such crises with medical management for periods of 3, 4, and 10 years. The common element in their survival was aggressive, early antihypertensive management with a goal of reducing the blood pressure to *low normal* levels. Massive amounts of as many as five antihypertensive agents have been required in the initial treatment stage, and guanethidine and propranolol have appeared to be the most important antihypertensive agents. It appears likely that such treatment will be successful in some patients encountering this syndrome and should be attempted in all.

Irreversible Renal Failure.   Patients whose hypertensive/renal crisis does not respond medically may be considered for nephrectomy, dialysis, and transplantation. Dialysis has sometimes been rendered difficult by the severe hypertension with consequent damage to other organs and by congestive heart failure; these problems have been obviated by bilateral nephrectomy, rendering the management on dialysis much less complex. Renal transplantation has been performed in a few patients, with results nearly as good as that in the overall renal transplant registry. Elusive reports suggest that at least some patients on long-term renal management improve their skin disease while on dialysis or after transplantation. We feel that these "heroic" treatment measures should be considered despite the presence of the underlying disease.

Mixed Connective Tissue Disease.   Mixed connective tissue disease (MCTD) is not a complication, but is a diagnostically confusing clinical entity with different management implications. Hence, its exclusion should be a part of the initial evaluation of a patient with presumed scleroderma. MCTD is characterized by marked immunologic abnormalities, notably the presence of antibody to the extractable nuclear antigens, specifically ribonucleoprotein. Corticosteroid treatment may be considered in such patients.

Eosinophilic Fasciitis (Shulman's Syndrome). This rare, recently described syndrome also deserves exclusion, since the therapeutic implications are different. These patients have onset of edema and sclerodermatous changes, frequently most marked over the forearms, and frequently following a period of extraordinarily heavy lifting or physical exertion. Raynaud's phenomenon is generally absent. Peripheral eosinophilia usually ranges from 5 to 30 per cent and on skin biopsy the epidermis and dermis are relatively normal but collections of inflammatory cells are found in fascial layers, sometimes with eosinophils present in such inflammatory cell accumulations. Good response to corticosteroid treatment has been observed in most patients and the condition does not progress to the internal organ complications of progressive systemic sclerosis.

Speculation

We think of systemic sclerosis as a disease of failed peripheral vasoregulatory mechanisms, resulting early in increased arteriolar and capillary pressures, tissue edema, subsequent fibrosis, structural damage (as evidenced by telangiectasis formation, nail-fold changes, and Raynaud's phenomenon), and progressing to anatomic lesions analogous to those of systemic hypertension or primary pulmonary hypertension, with decreased flow, loss of small vessels, ischemic change, and atrophy. This scenario is consistent with the disappointing effects of "vasodilating" agents, sympathectomy, and anti-inflammatory or immunosuppressant medications. It suggests a possible role for agents such as propranolol, which modulate peripheral perfusion by central effects and act to minimize the renin cycle complications sometimes seen. It further suggests the direction in which an underlying defect might lie and that a dramatic therapeutic agent effective against the underlying process may not be soon available. Theories of scleroderma pathogenesis have cycled from the hormonal to the collagen to the immunologic to the microvascular without overwhelming evidence in any direction. The speculations offered here are, however, consistent with a therapeutic approach that has proved clinically rewarding.

URTICARIA AND ANGIOEDEMA
method of
J. C. REED, M.D.
Elkhart, Indiana

Definition

Urticaria occurs as localized areas of swelling and redness in the skin. The size may vary from that of a mosquito bite to a large wheal several inches across. It is identified by the transient and migratory nature of individual lesions. Synonyms include hives and nettle rash.

Urticaria may be acute (lasting days to weeks) or chronic (months to years). In acute cases the causes are frequently apparent and more likely to be allergic. In chronic urticaria the cause is obscure and in the majority of instances never detected.

Angioedema is a variant of urticaria and occurs as subcutaneous swelling often in the head and neck regions. A familial type exists that, although rare, may be life-threatening if laryngeal involvement occurs.

Causes

The possible causes of urticaria include a wide spectrum of immunologic and nonimmunologic factors (see Table 1).

When questioning the patient each area should be explored in detail in a stepwise fashion. As this inquiry is carried out, the patient will be alerted to the types of things that may be responsible. It should be emphasized that the cause need not be anything new but that it is more likely to be something to which they have had repeated exposure.

Treatment

Antihistamines. Most episodes are of short duration and do not require medicines other than antihistamines. They may be used singly or in

TABLE 1.　**Causes of Urticaria**

Drugs: Antibiotics, salicylates, thiazides, phenothiazines, barbiturates, antihistamines, heavy metals, azo dyes, endocrine preparations, x-ray contrast media, narcotics, enzymes, vaccines, heparin, horse serum.
Foods: Eggs, dairy products, fruits, vegetables, meats, fish, cereals, spices, alcoholic beverages, food coloring, shellfish, nuts.
Inhalants: Pollens, dust, molds.
Contactants: Plants, medicines, cosmetics, animal dander.
Infections: Dermatophyte fungus, *Candida,* viral hepatitis, intestinal parasites, teeth, sinus, urinary tract infections.
Physical Agents: Cold, heat, physical exertion, specific wavelengths of light.
Internal Diseases: Collagen vascular disease, lymphoma, gallbladder disease, endocrine disorders.
Miscellaneous: Stings or bites from bees, spiders, jellyfish, snakes, and other organisms belonging to the same genera.

TABLE 2. **Antihistamine Dosages**

TRADE	GENERIC	GROUP
Benadryl 25–50 mg. 3–4 times daily	Diphenhydramine	(Ethanolamines)
Chlor-Trimeton 4 mg. 3–4 times daily 8,12 mg. Repetabs twice daily	Chlorpheniramine maleate	(Alkylamines)
Pyribenzamine 25–50 mg. 4 times daily or every 4 hours	Tripelennamine	(Ethylenediamines)
Phenergan 12.5, 25 mg. 2–4 times daily	Promethazine	(Phenothiazines)
Periactin 4 mg. 3–4 times daily	Cyproheptadine	(5 hydroxy-tryptamine and histamine antagonist)
Atarax 10–25 mg. 3–4 times daily	Hydroxyzine HCl	(Unclassified)

combination. It may be necessary to change from one drug to another during the course of treatment. When combining two drugs the doses of each should be reduced. When changing drugs or using them in combination each should be from a different pharmacologic group.

Table 2 lists an example of one antihistamine from each group.

Vasopressors. If the response to antihistamines alone is unsatisfactory, ephedrine sulfate, 25 mg. three times daily, may be added.

Corticosteroids. In difficult cases it may be necessary to resort to steroid therapy for short periods of time. Prednisone, 30 to 40 mg., should be taken in a single oral dose before breakfast daily and tapered over 1 to 2 weeks. The use of long-term steroid therapy for chronic urticaria should be avoided.

Hospitalization. Hospitalization allows the physician more complete control over medicines, diet, contactants, and environmental factors and is particularly useful in the management of chronic urticaria. It is also indicated for patients whose hives are severe, disabling, or refractory to treatment.

Diet. When foods are suspected as causes of recurrent episodes of hives, the patient is instructed to keep a detailed record of the meal eaten prior to each flare-up. This is kept for a 2-week period and then checked for some ingested substance common to each episode.

The use of elimination diets, except during hospital confinement, does not achieve sufficient compliance by the patient to be useful.

Drug Substitution. When a drug is suspected as the cause and the patient is taking several medicines I prefer to substitute or eliminate as many of them as is possible at the outset rather than attempting to eliminate them selectively. In patients with diabetes in whom urticaria from an insulin preparation is suspected, the insulin can be changed to a single peak or single component type from a different animal source.

Topical Therapy. Modified calamine liniment is prescribed to be applied four times daily for itching.

Rx	Menthol	½%
	Phenol	½%
	Calamine lotion	
		a a q s oz. viii (240 ml.)
	Nivea oil	

Colloidal oatmeal baths may also be used.

All patients with hives should be discouraged from taking salicylates or using alcohol during the course of their illness. Physical activity should be limited, and if anxiety appears to be a significant factor, some attempt should be made to modify it.

WARTS

method of
RICHARD C. GIBBS, M.D.
New York, New York

All skin warts in man are caused by the papovavirus and no virocidal agent has proved practical for use against this virus. Therefore, therapy for warts revolves around crude destructive methods, often with sacrifice of surrounding normal tissue and sometimes with scar formation.

Specific destructive therapy for warts varies according to the type of wart treated.

Verrucae Vulgares.   These common, whitish, hard viral tumors usually occur on digits, especially in children, but are often seen in other skin areas.

Single or few warts are best treated with electrosurgical methods, employing either electrocautery or electrodesiccation. The base of the lesion is infiltrated with 1 per cent lidocaine with or without epinephrine (depending on location) and the lesion is destroyed. Care should be taken to avoid going deeply into dermis or fat because the virus is superficially located histopathologically in epidermis. I prefer to insert an electrocautery tip into the warty mass and char it until it "bubbles" or until the base seems to balloon out into a blanched edematous mass. I then simply snip off the warty mass circumferentially from surrounding normal skin. If there is any bleeding at this point, I apply pressure with dry gauze and dab Monsel's solution (ferric subsulfate solution) into the bleeding area. A dry dressing or Band-Aid is applied after the site of surgery is anointed with erythromycin (Ilotycin) ointment.

When the wart is periungual or subungual, I remove overlying or adjacent nail plate, depending on the configuration of the wart. I use a decent-size nail clipper and remove enough nail so that I can actually visualize the extent of the wart in the nail bed. Postoperative bleeding may be more profuse than in ordinary warts but is rarely a problem.

Cotton-tipped applicator sticks saturated with liquid nitrogen, or other applicators delivering the liquid, as well as sticks of solid carbon dioxide snow can be used to treat warts.

In children, when surgery seems inadvisable, I recommend home-use of keratolytics such as 10 per cent salicylic acid and 10 per cent lactic acid in flexible collodion, cautiously applied nightly and secured with a small piece of Scotch Tape or clear adhesive tape to encourage maceration. This method of therapy is especially valuable in children when warts are palmar in location and myriad in number. Pretreating hyperkeratotic warts by carefully paring with any sharp instrument, pumice stone, or commercially available callus remover "facilitates" eradication of the growths. Occasionally, severe inflammatory reaction results from use of a keratolytic, and the reaction should be treated with warm soaks of saline and application of antimicrobial-containing ointment and even incision and drainage of any bullae.

Verrucae Filiformis.   These slender-stalked warts are commonly found on the head and neck. They are best and easily treated by obtaining local anesthesia with lidocaine (when necessary), snipping off the tumor near its base, and lightly destroying the remaining base with electrosurgical means.

Verrucae Planae.   Flat warts commonly appear on the dorsa of the hands and on the face (particularly around the chin), and on the neck in adults and on the knees and shins of children. These seemingly minor growths should be treated cautiously, lest scarring occurs. Without first obtaining local anesthesia, I prefer to curette them lightly and rapidly with a small chalazion or dermatologic curette. Generally, bleeding is minimal. Very light electrocautery used simply to "sear" the surface of the warts can be used as can liquid nitrogen on a cotton-tipped applicator stick. Sometimes topically applied keratolytics will work; I prefer retinoic acid gel (0.025 per cent) or liquid (0.05 per cent), but other preparations can be used.

Verrucae planae may theoretically be transferred to other areas of the face if, when shaving, the infected area is not shaved last.

Verrucae of the Oral Mucosa and Lips.   Tiny warts of oral mucous membrane should be destroyed electrosurgically after obtaining local anesthesia with 1 per cent lidocaine with epinephrine. One need not curette off the residual charred mass because the site usually heals well. In children, one may have to administer a general anesthetic if the warts are numerous.

Condylomata Acuminata.   Warts of the anal area or penis are frequently the most difficult types of warts to eradicate permanently. Persistence in therapy is essential, but it seems more than that is often needed to obtain cure.

For anal warts, I use 25 per cent resin of podophyllin in compound tincture of benzoin or, less commonly, in 70 per cent alcohol, either preparation made fresh every 3 to 4 months. I treat with chemicals only deep warts in the anus or warts that will become macerated by compression from the buttocks. Condylomata acuminata on the skin of the buttocks or on skin near the anus but not ordinarily occluded by the buttocks are treated exactly as ordinary verrucae elsewhere by electrosurgical means.

When podophyllin is applied, it is dabbed over the entire wart, as the patient, physician, or an assistant holds the buttocks widely separated. Be careful to avoid using cotton-tipped applicator sticks that are drenched in the podophyllin preparation because such therapy may result in flooding of the anus with the corrosive medication. If applied carefully, I have found that there is usually no need to protect the surrounding unaffected tissue as some dermatologists suggest. Have the patient wash the medication off with ordinary soap and water 4 to 6 hours after application, depending on circumstances. Prescribe anodynes, especially for the first treatment or when medication is applied thereafter, because reaction to the chemical may be painful and severe. I also recommend application of ice packs or cool saline solution if pain occurs. Most important, warn the patient about the possibility of pain occurring. Successful therapy requires months of weekly visits and diligence and persistence in therapy. A sexual mate should be examined in chronic recalcitrant cases. Even proctoscopic examination should be done with recurrent anal disease. A strongly positive serologic test for syphilis will easily separate the similarly exuberant (but flat) condyloma latum of the anus occurring in syphilis; repository penicillin is curative in the syphilitic variety.

It may be necessary to resort to hospitalization and administration of general anesthesia before a large mass of condylomata of the anal area or extensive condylomata involving rectal mucosa can be removed successfully.

Penile condylomata are treated in the same manner as anal warts, namely, using electrosurgery for cutaneous lesions of the shaft and resin of podophyllin in an appropriate vehicle for mucosal lesions. Be careful in applying podophyllin to the uncircumcised patient, because the macerating influence of the foreskin may be greater than one would like or anticipate.

Condyloma can also be treated by the application of liquid nitrogen, but the application of 25 per cent resin of podophyllin in compound tincture of benzoin still remains the time-honored treatment of choice.

Verrucae Plantares. There are different types of plantar warts.

Multiple and Small. This type is generally encountered in children. It is best treated with daily swabbing with diluted formalin (1:2 or 1:4) or 3 per cent unbuffered glutaraldehyde solution (investigational). The feet will be kept dry with these preparations and such reduction in moisture is coveted. Powders can also be used to reduce moisture. If patients are wearing nylon or other synthetic socks or stockings, have them switch to predominantly cotton or woolen ones. Bear in mind that multiple and small plantar warts in children frequently and inexplicably disappear.

Single Nonpainful Plantar Wart. In most cases, single nonpainful plantar warts can be left alone. If the patient desires treatment, or if the wart rapidly enlarges, begins to be painful, or multiplies in number, one can recommend daily swabbing with 10 per cent formaldehyde solution. Frequently, this simple 5 to 10 minute swabbing in the evening will be sufficient after weeks of treatment to cause drying of the area and "popping" out of the warts. Often as effective is the application of 10 per cent lactic and salicylic acids in flexible collodion to the wart after it has been pared down with almost any sharp clean tool, pumice stone, or commercially available corn and callus remover.

The patient should visit the office periodically to have the wart pared down as much as possible, after which 50 per cent trichloracetic acid or 75 per cent silver nitrate (by stick) is swabbed onto the base. A 40 per cent salicylic acid plaster can then be applied and then taped securely and left in place for a few days after which the patient replaces it again after paring the area and applying the keratolytic or drying agent.

Single Painful Plantar Verruca. Painful plantar warts are frequently found over weight-bearing areas of the sole and as such require expert care. If one is unable to properly examine an exquisitely painful plantar wart, local anesthesia should be considered before the examination or the patient should be told to use soaks with Johnson's Foot Soap or other commercially available foot powder before the next office visit. One then hopes that enough maceration of overlying hyperkeratosis will occur with soaks that pain will lessen at least on walking and that treatment will be facilitated when the patient returns to the office. Also, one can apply to the proximal circumference of the wart a horse-shoe shaped $\frac{1}{8}$-in.-thick felt padding with an adhesive back so that weight is not born on the painful site. Rubber cement can be brushed on the sole before the pad is stuck on to provide several days adherence to the sole (even when showering).

When the patient returns in a week or so, if pain persists, local anesthesia with 1 per cent lidocaine can be administered sublesionally or a posterior tibial block can be used. I prefer local anesthesia, but recognize that the patient does feel a brief sensation of a burning stick even if the 30 or 27 gauge needle is very rapidly flicked into the skin. Also and most importantly, I try whenever practical to stick the patient initially on the relatively painless dorsal skin of the feet and creep plantarward with anesthetic to the site of the lesion. Such method of obtaining anesthesia requires more time but is worthwhile when operating on an anxious patient or one with a "low" pain tolerance. Once anesthesia is obtained, I pare the warty site with a #10 or #15 blade on a scalpel and delineate the perimeter of the mass. Any pin-point bleeding that interferes with visualization of the wart can be stopped with pressure with gauze plus use of Monsel's solution. I then bluntly dissect a few millimeters beyond the visible border of the wart with a small Gradle stitch or iris scissors until I have encircled the mass. Finally, I remove the wart in toto with the help of a dermatologic curette and *lightly* curette or electrocauterize the crater edges and base.

I do not destroy or remove any further tissue. Bleeding is stopped with digital pressure applied to an ordinary gauze pad or with application of Monsel's solution. Erythromycin (Ilotycin) ointment is applied before the bandaging and the patient is encouraged to elevate the legs as much as practical and return in 3 to 4 days. At that time, the wound is inspected and a felt padding is applied to divert pressure from the surgical site. The patient is instructed to continue nightly application of erythromycin (Ilotycin) ointment until full healing has occurred.

The surgical method described is not foolproof, but morbidity is usually minimal. Recurrences do occur, but in less than 15 per cent of patients. One can destroy plantar warts by using electrocautery and curettage or electrodesiccation and curettage. I prefer electrocautery. The method is really identical to that described for destruction of ordinary verrucae but one is admonished to avoid going into deep dermis or fat because a painful scar may result. The method seems to work well for most dermatologists, but the alternative method using blunt dissection and light electrocautery and curettage is also used.

A nonsurgical method of dealing with painful plantar warts is to apply acids such as 50 per cent trichloroacetic acid or bichloroacetic acid crystals or 75 to 100 per cent silver nitrate solution or sticks to previously pared warts. Then 40 per cent salicylic acid plaster is taped over the treated site and the patient told to return weekly for treatments. The method usually works well, but is often quite costly to the patient in terms of time and money because the method is tedious. A more rapid response entails similar preparatory paring and acid application but use of a 60 per cent salicylic acid paste thereafter. The pared site is covered by an ordinary adhesive tape whose center has been cut out to conform to the shape of the wart. The nonwarty underlying skin is prepared with tincture of benzoin or rubber cement or other glue. Overlying the adhesive tape one applies an identical felt pad of ⅛ or ¼ in. thickness. Sixty per cent salicylic acid paste is then stuffed into the central opening, covering the well to its brim and then a cover of Saran Wrap or felt padding is applied and the entire bandage taped in place. The patient returns in a week and the paring and chemotherapeutic process is repeated, going as deeply as possible. This sequence is repeated until the wart pops out. Frequently, with use of macerating acids, an edematous, even hemorrhagic inflammatory response occurs and the patient experiences discomfort. If the patient is seen at this stage, the painful mass can be nicked and serosanguineous fluid may gush forth. Clipping off the overlying warty tissue usually results in cure, although the remaining "hole" is frightening to the patient and takes weeks to fill in.

Given to selected patients, x-ray therapy of recalcitrant plantar warts is said to be quite successful.

Only as a last desperate resort in exceptional cases should one surgically excise a recurrent wart.

Immunotherapy with a vaccine prepared from the patient's own warty tissue seems promising, but in order to obtain a suitable vaccine the amount of warty tissue removed should be *enormous*.

MOSAIC WARTS. These are the most recalcitrant warts of all. Surgery is really not advisable because of the extremely high rate of recurrence. Therapy should be avoided if the patient is comfortable and unaffected by the growth. If treatment is undertaken, I would recommend use of paring and cautious application of acids as described for single painful plantar warts.

If surgery is decided upon because of failure of other therapies, the method is no different from that for removal of single painful plantar warts, although the recurrence rate will probably be higher.

XANTHOMA

method of
DONALD B. HUNNINGHAKE, M.D.
Minneapolis, Minnesota

Xanthomas are lesions that may occur in skin, subcutaneous connective tissue, or deeper structures such as tendon sheaths or bone. They result from the deposition of lipids, especially cholesterol and its esters, and may or may not be associated with elevated plasma lipid and lipoprotein levels. They have been described in all types of genetically determined hyperlipoproteinemia (HLP) and may occur in HLP secondary to biliary cirrhosis, diabetes mellitus, dysproteinemias, hypothyroidism, nephrosis, and pancreatitis. Superficial lesions are yellowish in color, while xanthomas arising from deeper structures do not discolor the skin. A true xanthoma is generally hard while the majority of skin lesions that may be confused with xanthomas are generally soft or spongy. The following are the major types of xanthomas: tendon xanthomas, tuberous xanthomas, planar xanthomas, eruptive xanthomas, and tuberoeruptive xanthomas.

Initial Evaluation of Patient with Xanthomas

The following are the major considerations in the initial evaluation:

1. Are the xanthomas associated with an elevation of plasma lipid and lipoprotein levels? A plasma cholesterol and triglycerides test should be performed initially after a 12 hour fast. If either or

both are elevated, one can proceed to a more comprehensive work-up.

2. What is the type of the lipoprotein disorder? Characterization of the lipoprotein disorder is essential for instituting appropriate diet and drug therapy. Quantitative lipoprotein analyses that are now available in larger diagnostic laboratories should be performed for identification of the lipoprotein disorder and for future assessment of the efficacy of the treatment regimens.

3. Is the lipoprotein abnormality primary or secondary? Laboratory evaluations to determine the presence of diabetes mellitus, dysproteinemias, hypothyroidism, renal or liver disease, and pancreatitis should be performed, depending upon the type of lipoprotein abnormality present. Hyperuricemia is common in lipoprotein abnormalities. Obesity, excess ethanol intake, estrogens, and thiazide diuretics may be contributing factors.

4. Is there associated arterial vascular disease? Patients presenting with xanthomas are generally at a higher risk for arterial vascular disease and should be carefully evaluated for the presence of coronary, cerebral, or peripheral arteriosclerosis.

5. Adequate baselines. The decision to treat a patient with xanthomas indicates that treatment will be for a prolonged period of time, possibly a lifetime. A sufficient number of plasma lipids (three after appropriate diet) to evaluate the efficacy of future drug treatment should be performed. Adequate baseline laboratory work is also essential to evaluate potential future toxicity from therapy.

Treatment of Specific Lipoprotein Disorders

Type I HLP. This is an extremely rare disorder characterized by a deficiency of lipoprotein lipase and elevated plasma triglycerides in the form of chylomicrons. Diet is the only form of therapy. Dietary fat should be restricted to less than 25 grams per day. Medium chain triglycerides may be added to the diet to make it more palatable. They are taken up directly into the portal circulation and do not aggravate the hyperchylomicronemia. Type I HLP is frequently first manifested in childhood and is associated with abdominal pain, pancreatitis, and eruptive xanthomas. The xanthomas will completely disappear if the triglycerides are returned to normal or only moderately elevated levels.

Type II HLP. This lipoprotein disorder has now been divided into Type IIa characterized by an elevation of plasma cholesterol and LDL cholesterol only, and Type II b, which additionally has an elevation of plasma triglycerides and very low-density lipoprotein (VLDL). Tendon, tuberous, and planar xanthomas are associated with this disorder. Treatment is occasionally either for

cosmetic reasons or the disabling effect of these xanthomas but is frequently instituted because of the increased risk of arteriosclerosis. It is especially important to rule out hypothyroidism, dysproteinemias, and liver disease.

DIET. Treatment should begin with restriction of cholesterol intake to less than 300 mg. per day, decreasing the saturated fats and increasing the polyunsaturated fats. Practically, this means deletion of egg yolks, butterfat, lard, and organ meats. Soft margarine is substituted for butter, vegetable oils and shortening for lard, skim milk for whole milk, and egg whites for whole eggs. Meat intake is reduced to 6 to 8 oz. (180 to 240 grams) per day and total fat and cheese consumption are limited. A more detailed account of these diets is readily available from many sources. An attempt should be made to achieve ideal body weight and this is especially important in the Type IIb, where ethanol intake may also have to be restricted or eliminated.

DRUGS. The bile-acid sequestering agents, cholestyramine and colestipol, which are described later, are the most effective agents for reducing plasma cholesterol and low density lipoprotein (LDL) concentrations. Cholestyramine is generally administered in a total daily dose of 16 to 24 grams, and colestipol at 20 to 30 grams per day. A twice daily schedule is generally preferred. These drugs are the most likely to reduce the size of xanthomas, but their cost is prohibitive for many patients and their administration poses some problems. Nicotinic acid in a daily dose of 3.0 to 6.0 grams per day is the second choice in terms of efficacy in reducing plasma cholesterol and low density lipoprotein (LDL) cholesterol, but this drug has many side effects. If the xanthomas are cosmetically disfiguring or disabling, one should concentrate on the previous two drugs, if possible. One will rarely see a complete regression of the xanthomas but may see a significant decrease in size. Combinations of the preceding drugs as well as ileal bypass surgery have been employed. The following drugs have not yet been reported very effective in terms of xanthoma regression, but are used principally on the assumption that they will decrease the risk of arterial vascular disease. They include clofibrate, in a daily dosage of 2.0 grams, probucol, in a daily dose of 1.0 gram, or dextrothyroxin, 4.0 to 6.0 mg. per day.

Type III HLP. This is a rare type of lipoprotein disorder that may be associated with a variety of xanthomas, including planar (palms), tuberous, tuboeruptive and rarely tendon xanthomas. It is a primary genetic disorder, but the plasma lipid levels may be significantly increased by the presence of other conditions such as hypothyroidism, obesity, and excess ethanol intake, which should be corrected, if present. Type IIb was frequently misdiagnosed as Type III in the past. It is one of the easiest lipoprotein disorders to treat. Adequate treatment is generally associated with complete disappearance of xanthomas. Premature arterial vascular disease is another reason for treatment. Dietary therapy should concentrate primarily on getting the patient to ideal body weight and eliminating or restricting ethanol intake. If the plasma lipid levels are still elevated, clofibrate, 1.0 gram twice a day, will generally normalize the plasma lipids. If clofibrate is not effective, the patient is probably not adhering to diet. Nicotinic acid in a total daily dose of 3.0 grams per day is the second choice drug which is rarely necessary and is associated with many side effects.

Type IV HLP. This disease is characterized by the presence of elevated levels of plasma triglycerides and very low-density lipoprotein (VLDL). Eruptive xanthomas generally do not appear unless the plasma triglyceride concentration is considerably above normal. Pancreatitis may be associated with the more severe elevations of plasma lipids and it is frequently difficult to assess whether the hyperlipoproteinemia preceded the pancreatitis or vice versa. A large number of patients seen with Type IV hyperlipoproteinemia and eruptive xanthomas will have uncontrolled diabetes mellitus, gross obesity, pancreatitis, or excess ethanol intake as a major contributing factor. Estrogen or thiazide administration as well as dysproteinemias and renal disease may also be contributing factors. The major dietary emphasis should be on returning the patient to ideal body weight and the elimination of ethanol. Clofibrate, in a dosage of 1.0 gram twice a day, may be a useful adjunct in patients who do not respond or adhere to diet. Nicotinic acid, in a total daily dose of 3.0 grams per day, may occasionally be necessary in patients who do not respond to clofibrate. Its many adverse effects including deterioration in carbohydrate tolerance and hyperuricemia make it a second choice drug.

Type V HLP. This disorder is associated with elevated plasma levels of triglycerides, chylomicrons, and VLDL and eruptive xanthomas may occur. They usually do not appear unless the plasma triglyceride levels are greatly elevated and effective treatment will cause them to completely disappear. Pancreatitis, obesity, excess ethanol ingestion, and uncontrolled diabetes mellitus are frequently seen in patients with this disorder who have eruptive xanthomas. These conditions must be corrected first. Diet is primarily concentrated on decreasing total fat, total calories, and ethanol. Clofibrate has been reported helpful in terms of reducing plasma lipid levels and episodes of pancreatitis. Diet is the most important therapy. Other forms of therapy including progestins have been reported as efficacious but are beyond the scope of this presentation.

Specific Drugs

Bile-acid Sequestering Agents. Cholestyramine and colestipol are the two drugs in this class. They interfere with the reabsorption of bile acids from the intestine and increase the conversion of cholesterol to bile acids. They also increase the catabolism of LDL. They reduce plasma cholesterol and LDL but may increase triglyceride and VLDL levels. Their use is limited to Type II HLP. They are nonabsorbable resins and are not associated with systemic side effects. They must be suspended in a vehicle such as juice or water. The inconvenience of administration and cost limit their use. Gastrointestinal complaints may include gas, belching, bloating, heartburn, or constipation. The latter is usually transient and is frequently a complaint of increased size and consistency of the stools. Increased fluid, fruit, or fiber in the diet as well as stool softeners may alleviate this problem. Laxatives should not be used. The majority of patients will tolerate 24 grams of cholestyramine or the equivalent dose of colestipol if the dose is gradually increased. The absorption of fat-soluble vitamins should be monitored but is rarely a problem in the adult patient. Digitoxin, thiazide diuretics, thyroxine, and warfarin are examples of drugs whose absorption may be decreased if administered at the same time as cholestyramine. Until more information is available it is prudent to separate the time of administration of other drugs from the resin. Colestipol does not appear to interfere with the absorption of drugs as much as cholestyramine.

Clofibrate. This drug is primarily effective in reducing plasma triglycerides and VLDL. In the Type IIa patient without xanthomas it produces an average reduction in plasma cholesterol and LDL of approximately 10 per cent and a somewhat lesser effect in the Type IIb patient or the patient with xanthomas. Its use is primarily in the Type III and IV patient. Minor gastrointestinal complaints and rarely myalgia are reported. Prolonged use has been associated with an increased incidence of cholelithiasis, thromboembolism, and a variety of cardiac arrhythmias. The usual dose is 1.0 gram twice a day. The dose may have to be reduced in the presence of low serum albumin or uremia. Clofibrate may potentiate the effect of the coumarin anticoagulants because of alterations in the protein binding of these drugs.

Nicotinic Acid. This drug has had rather limited use because of the number of side effects reported. It has the advantages of being cheap and lowering plasma cholesterol, triglycerides, and both the LDL and VLDL fractions. The upper limits of recommended dosage are 3.0 grams per day, but we have occasionally used as much as 6.0 grams per day in patients with very high lipoprotein concentrations. We use the 500 mg. tablet. The first week we give half a tablet or 250 mg. per day. If the flushing has significantly abated, we increase the dosage to 250 mg. twice daily for one week and then progressively increase the dose by 500 mg. per week until a total daily dose of 3 grams per day is achieved. Flushing occurs in all patients treated with this drug, but patients usually become tolerant of the flushing produced by these increments in dosage within approximately one week. Other major side effects of nicotinic acid are gastrointestinal complaints, hyperuricemia, decreased carbohydrate tolerance, and abnormal liver function studies including elevated SGOTs and alkaline phosphatases. The abnormal liver function studies will sometimes disappear if the dose of drug is reduced. If the liver function abnormalities persist in spite of progressive decreases in dose, the drug should be discontinued.

Dextrothyroxine. This drug should not be used in patients with known arteriosclerotic heart disease or patients with multiple premature ventricular contractions. It will lower plasma cholesterol and LDL, but will not affect the major triglyceride-containing lipoproteins unless there is an associated weight loss. It is recommended that the dose not exceed 6 mg. per day. The side effects are similar to those observed in hyperthyroidism, and a mild hyperthyroid state must be induced in some patients to effectively lower cholesterol. We currently rarely use this drug because of the adverse cardiac effects described in previous secondary intervention trials. This drug has the advantage of ease of administration.

Probucol. This drug is primarily effective in lowering plasma cholesterol and LDL, with reductions of around 15 per cent being reported. The usual dosage is 500 mg. twice a day. It is easy to administer and there are few reported side effects. It was recently marketed, and the total clinical experience is still limited.

HERPES ZOSTER

method of
EDWARD SCHOTLAND, M.D.
Kansas City, Kansas

Herpes zoster (zoster, shingles, zona) is an acute painful unilateral vesicular eruption of adults caused by infection of the sensory nerve ganglia with the varicella-zoster virus. Presumably zoster represents a reactivation of the virus lying dormant in the dorsal root or cranial nerve ganglion cells by aging, trauma, malignancies, radiation, and immunosuppressive agents. Furthermore, reinfection with resultant viremia seems likely in patients with altered immune states such as in leukemia-lymphoma. The presence of grouped vesicles on an erythematous base in a dermatomal or zonal distribution accompanied by burning pain is distinctive for the disease.

Uncomplicated Zoster

The course in healthy patients is usually benign, with healing and freedom from symptoms for most within 3 to 5 weeks; the duration is age-related. One treats with a view towards rapid drying of vesicles and erosions, relieving pain, and combating secondary bacterial infection.

1. Burow's solution compresses diluted to 1:20 or 1:40, aluminum chloride hexahydrate 2 per cent (AluWets), or sodium propionate-chlorophyllin (Prophyllin) four times daily during the waking hours for 10 to 15 minutes.

2. Acetaminophen with codeine (Tylenol #3) or ASA with 15 to 30 mg. (0.25 to 0.5 grain) codeine once or twice daily as needed for pain.

3. Culture and sensitivity studies of pustules with appropriate systemic antibiotic therapy.

4. Systemic corticosteroids administered in the earliest stages of the disease to reduce morbidity and possibly prevent postherpetic neuralgia have their advocates. In the absence of contraindications such as peptic ulcer disease, tuberculosis, chemical or overt diabetes, hypertension, or psychosis, an initial morning dose of 60 to 80 mg. of prednisone orally with gradual tapering over 3 to 4 weeks may be tried.

5. Polyamine SP-54 (sodium pentosan polysulfate) is under investigation in West Germany.

Trigeminal and Facial Zoster Syndromes

The appearance of vesicles on the nasal tip indicates involvement of *N. nasociliaris,* one of the three branches of *N. ophthalmicus* V 1, and demands:

1. Immediate ophthalmologic consultation to rule out keratitis and uveitis.

2. Systemic corticosteroids to prevent corneal ulceration and scarring.

3. Topical mydriatics such as 5 per cent homatropine ophthalmic solution twice daily to prevent synechiae, with daily monitoring in the acute stages for secondary glaucoma.

4. Analgesics.

Zoster of the external ear with tinnitus, lingering facial paralysis and severe postherpetic neuralgia (Ramsay Hunt syndrome) may be made more tolerable with early institution of systemic corticosteroids.

Dissemination is to be expected in patients with advanced underlying disease, especially Hodgkin's disease. Predisposing factors in this group seem to be age, recent radiation therapy, and anergic states. This severe variant with high fever, malaise, poor appetite, and pain merits a trial at the onset of vidarabine (ara-A, adenine arabinoside), 10 mg. per kg. of body weight intravenously per day for 5 days (investigational) according to the original National Institute of Allergy and Infectious Diseases (NIAID) paper. Liver and bone marrow studies monitored every 5 days showed no dysfunction, according to the authors.

Postherpetic neuralgia, because of its lingering and, at times, debilitating features, especially in the elderly, has generated interest in an array of remedies, listed below. In many cases zoster is not an approved indication for their use, although these modalities are already widely employed.

1. Systemic corticosteroids are useful as a prophylactic measure. Once severe neuralgia becomes established, the following measures may be undertaken:

2. Triamcinolone, 200 mg. in 100 ml. of isotonic saline solution injected intralesionally or at cutaneous sites of pain daily for 1 to 2 weeks. Complications include tenderness at the treated site, sterile abscesses, subcutaneous atrophy, and thrombophlebitis.

3. Epidural injection of 8 to 12 ml. of bupivacaine 0.25 per cent (Marcaine) is considered by anesthesiologists to be the treatment of choice. Pain relief for the majority is almost immediate. Effective remedies in isolated cases include:

4. Chlorprothixene (Taractan), 50 mg. intramuscularly initially, followed by 50 mg. orally every 6 hours for 7 to 10 days. (This use of chlorprothixene is not listed in the manufacturer's official directive.) This phenothiazine must be used cautiously in combination with barbiturates, narcotics, and atropinelike drugs.

5. Carbamazepine (Tegretol), 600 to 800 mg. per day, together with nortriptyline (Aventyl), 50 to 100 mg. per day orally in divided doses. Side effects involving the central nervous system, including dizziness and tremors, are common. (This use of these agents is not listed in the manufacturers' official directives.)

HERPES GESTATIONIS

method of
MICHAEL FISHER, M.D.
Bronx, New York

Herpes gestationis is a pruritic, polymorphous, vesicobullous eruption having its usual onset during the second and third trimesters of pregnancy. The eruption may begin, exacerbate, or resolve in the postpartum period and recur with subsequent pregnancies. It occurs in approximately 1 of 10,000 deliveries and is associated with an increased risk of maternal morbidity and fetal morbidity and mortality. Immunofluorescent and histopathologic findings suggest a relationship to bullous pemphigoid. The severity of the disease may be correlated with the titer of circulating antibodies to basement membrane zone and peripheral blood eosinophilia.

Treatment

1. Prednisone, 20 to 40 mg. per day orally, in single or divided doses, usually leads to cessation of new blister formation within 48 hours and clearing of lesions within 1 to 2 weeks. Gradual tapering of prednisone by 5 mg. every 2 to 3 days to a maintenance level should be continued until after delivery.

2. Hydrocortisone sodium succinate, 100 mg. should be administered intravenously during delivery.

3. Topical application of corticosteroids three times daily may be tried in mild cases.

4. Open wet dressings of cool tap water, saline, or 5 per cent Burow's solution may be applied to blisters for 10 to 15 minutes three times daily to promote drying of lesions.

5. The efficacy of pyridoxine, progesterone, and sulfapyridine therapy in this disease is questionable.

PAPULAR DERMATITIS OF PREGNANCY

method of
MICHAEL FISHER, M.D.
Bronx, New York

Papular dermatitis of pregnancy is a rare condition characterized by extremely pruritic, generalized, erythematous papules occurring any time during pregnancy and clearing rapidly after delivery. The lesions are discrete, soft, become crusted, and heal within 7 to 10 days with hyperpigmentation and no scarring. The eruption usually recurs with subsequent pregnancies and is associated with increased fetal mortality. A significant number of patients is Rh negative. Other associated maternal findings include elevated urinary chorionic gonadotropin during the last trimester, lower plasma hydrocortisone, and shortened hydrocortisone half-life.

Treatment

1. Prednisone is the treatment of choice, and doses of up to 100 mg. per day orally may be necessary to control the disease and reduce the fetal mortality.

2. The efficacy of progesterone, pyridoxine and sulfapyridine therapy in this disease is questionable.

The Nervous System

BRAIN ABSCESS

method of
WILLIAM A. SHUCART, M.D.
Brooklyn, New York

Brain abscess remains a disease with a high mortality rate and significant morbidity. Prompt and aggressive therapy is essential for good results. Computed tomography affords the most accurate delineation of brain abscesses and allows good observation of the results of the various forms of treatment. There is no single form of therapy considered best for all abscesses and, as further information is gained, there will no doubt be continuing evolution in the current treatment regimen.

When the diagnosis of brain abscess is made, attention is directed to:

1. Identification and treatment of the source of infection.

2. Treament of the abscess.

3. Treatment of the secondary effects of the abscess.

Identification and Treatment of the Source of Infection

The majority of brain abscesses are metastatic, coming most commonly from the lungs, heart, and generalized sepsis; on occasion, no primary source is found. The most susceptible patients are those with cyanotic congenital heart disease, chronic lung disease, and those having increased susceptibility to infection because of underlying debilitating disease or metabolic disorder. Direct extension from an infected focus in the skull such as the paranasal sinuses or the sinuses around the ear may be another source. There may also be direct contamination secondary to penetrating wounds or intracranial surgery.

Regardless of the primary site, intravenous antibiotic therapy should be started as soon as the diagnosis of brain abscess is made. The most common causative organisms are *Staphylococcus aureus,* microaerophilic and anaerobic streptococci, and *Bacteroides.* Since therapy is started before the specific pathogen has been identified, antibiotics giving a broad spectrum of coverage are used. Our usual schedule is:

1. *Penicillin G.* Adults, 24 million units per day in four to six divided doses; children, 250,000 units per kg. per day in four to six divided doses, administered for at least 4 and up to 6 weeks.

2. *Chloramphenicol.* Adults, 1.0 gram every 4 hours for 1 week, 1.0 gram every 6 hours for 3 weeks, 0.5 gram every 6 hours orally for 2 weeks (optional depending on patient's condition); children, 100 mg. per kg. per day in divided doses given for 4 weeks, may be decreased to 50 mg. per kg. per day for last 2 weeks.

3. *Gentamicin.* May be added to above drugs when focus of infection is a cranial sinus because of high incidence of *Proteus* and *Pseudomonas* infections. Adults, 3 to 5 mg. per kg. per day in three divided doses for 7 to 14 days; children, 4 to 6 mg. per kg. per day in three divided doses for 7 to 10 days.

In patients who have an identifiable primary site, cultures should be taken from that source and when the organisms are identified antibiotics can be appropriately changed.

If the abscess is secondary to an infected cranial sinus, not only antibiotic therapy but surgical drainage will be required. The sinus should be drained as soon as possible, but the timing depends on the patient's condition. If the major clinical problem is swelling and mass effect in the brain, attention should be initially directed toward relief of those problems, with the required sinus surgery performed as soon thereafter as practical. If the patient's clinical status is good, treatment of the abscess and drainage of the sinus can be performed at the same operation. In penetrating wounds or postoperative infections that have led to abscess formation the debridement of the focus of infection is carried out as part of the treatment of the abscess itself.

Treatment of the Abscess

Treatment of the abscess with administration of antibiotics only has been associated with an unacceptably high mortality rate. In the patient whose clinical status is good, it is feasible to administer intravenous antibiotics for several hours or a day or two prior to surgical treatment. There is good evidence that systemically administered antibiotics enter the abscess cavity. There are two major techniques available for surgery of the abscess:

Aspiration. Aspiration of the abscess to diminish bulk is used by most surgeons as preliminary treatment and by some as the sole treatment of brain abscess. A burr hole is placed in the skull over the center of the abscess and a small cannula passed into the abscess to remove the purulent contents. The aspirated material is studied with Gram stain and cultures, both aerobic and anaerobic. Following evacuation of the abscess, 0.5 to 1.0 ml. of a micropaque barium sulfate solution is instilled; the particles are phagocytized in the wall of the abscess and permit easy follow-up of abscess size using plain skull radiographs. In the acute phase aspiration is generally adequate for treatment and if the mass shows a continuing decrease in size, the patient's general clinical condition improves, and only one or two further aspirations are required to keep the size of the abscess small, there may be no further treatment required. If there is no significant decrease in the size of the abscess, multiple aspirations are required to keep the size down, or if the patient manifests a persistently septic course, complete excision of the abscess should be performed within 2 or 3 weeks.

Excision of the Abscess. Primary excision is advocated by some surgeons regardless of the stage at which the patient is seen. We feel that primary excision should be avoided in the acute stage. Surgery performed in the acute stage requires dealing with a swollen brain and to provide adequate decompression, normal brain may have to be sacrificed. If the abscess is in an area where excision of brain tissue would lead to a significant neurologic deficit, primary excision should not be done unless aspiration and systemic antibiotics are ineffective. If the patient with an acute abscess shows signs of herniation or no improvement in his clinical state following aspiration and the use of ancillary agents (to diminish brain swelling), primary excision may have to be performed.

Whether aspiration, late excision, or primary excision is used, antibiotic therapy must be continued for at least 4 to 6 weeks.

Treatment of the Secondary Effects of the Abscess

The cerebral edema and increased intracranial pressure associated with a cerebral abscess may pose the most acute threat to life. The edema is treated with two major types of drugs.

Diuretics. We most commonly use the osmotic diuretic mannitol in the patient with increased intracranial pressure and particularly in those patients whose clinical course is rapidly deteriorating. Mannitol rapidly lowers intracranial pressure, but the effect lasts only 4 to 6 hours. Repeated doses can be given, but it generally becomes less effective with repetition. The dosage used is 0.5 to 1.0 gram per kg. given intravenously over 10 to 20 minutes.

Corticosteroids. Corticosteroids have an antiedema effect, but this is not rapid in onset and they do not have the same degree of dehydrating ability as do the osmotic diuretics. They tend not to lose their effectiveness and can be given over several days. We give all patients with brain abscess large doses of corticosteroids and have found no deleterious effects or increased difficulty in treating the infection. We most commonly use dexamethasone. In adults and children the dosage is 0.3 to 1.0 mg. per kg., depending on the patient's clinical status, with larger doses being used for the most seriously ill patients.

All patients with a brain abscess, regardless of location, are treated with anticonvulsants, at least through the period of time they are receiving antibiotic therapy. If the abscess is located in a nonepileptogenic area, the anticonvulsants are discontinued after 6 weeks. If the abscess is located in an epileptogenic area, anticonvulsants are continued indefinitely. There are two major drugs used: Phenobarbital, 3 to 5 mg. per kg. per day in two divided doses, or phenytoin (Dilantin), 5 to 8 mg. per kg. per day in two divided doses.

Other Considerations

Fungal infections, including tuberculosis, once diagnosed should be treated with appropriate antifungal agents. If the patient is known to have tuberculosis, there has been fair success in treatment with only chemotherapy without removal of the abscess. If there are signs of increased intracranial pressure or a progressive neurologic deficit, surgery should be performed.

Follow-up with computerized tomography will give excellent information as to the course of the abscess and may demonstrate hydrocephalus, which on occasion complicates intracranial infections.

INTRACEREBRAL HEMORRHAGE

method of
EUGENE S. FLAMM, M.D.
New York, New York

A 52-year-old man is brought to the hospital following the sudden onset of intense headache, left hemiparesis, and decrease in his level of consciousness. The sudden headache bespeaks intracranial hemorrhage; the focal deficit implies parenchymal involvement and not just subarachnoid hemorrhage. The decrease in level of consciousness makes this an urgent situation.

Although intracerebral hemorrhage may occur in many situations, ranging from blood dyscrasias to brain tumors, three common causes account for the vast majority of intracerebral clots: trauma, hypertension, and vascular lesions such as aneurysms and arteriovenous malformations. The patient described here might have a primary intracerebral hemorrhage due to hypertension or to the rupture of a vascular lesion. In this case, the history will rule out trauma as the cause.

Emergency Treatment

Certain emergency measures must be instituted to protect the patient and gain some time to establish the diagnosis. Immediate treatment must be aimed at correcting life-threatening situations before a definitive diagnosis can be established. If the level of consciousness is depressed or frank evidence of transtentorial herniation is present, such as a dilated pupil or decerebrate posturing, the increase in intracranial pressure must be rapidly reduced. Mannitol, given at 1 to 1.5 grams per kg., should be administered intravenously over a 15 to 30 minute period after a catheter has been placed in the bladder.

Although evidence for the efficacy of steroids in such situations is less clear, corticosteroids should be begun. Methylprednisolone (2 to 5 mg. per kg. per 24 hours), dexamethasone (1.5 mg. per kg. per 24 hours), or their equivalent can be used. This may control the edema that develops over the first few hours around the lesion. The other major emergency measures that must be taken before proceeding with diagnostic tests are the establishment of an adequate airway and measurement of blood gases. Obstruction of the airway, or hypercapnia, can significantly offset any gains made in lowering intracranial pressure. An endotracheal tube should be inserted and blood gases monitored and corrected by assisted ventilation when necessary. A goal should be a Pco_2 of 35 mm. Hg and a Po_2 above 80 mm. Hg.

Diagnosis

Clearly, the easiest and most accurate way to establish the presence of an intracerebral hematoma is with computed tomography (CT) scanning. If there is a history of trauma, the cause of the clot is obvious. If the initial ictus occurred spontaneously in a known hypertensive patient, and the clot is in one of the usual sites associated with hypertensive bleeds, namely the basal ganglia, pons, or cerebellum adjacent to the fourth ventricle, the diagnosis can be safely established. Should the clot be found more superficially in the cerebral hemispheres or within the sylvian fissure, a rupture of an arteriovenous malformation or aneurysm must be considered. If CT scanning is not available, one must rely on other studies to establish the diagnosis. A lumbar puncture will verify the presence of blood in the cerebrospinal fluid, and angiography will define the location of the mass. The patients in whom an aneurysm or arteriovenous malformation may be the source of the intracerebral clot seen on CT scan, angiography must be carried out to plan appropriate management.

Medical Management

Surgery can be avoided, or at least postponed to a nonemergency basis, if increased intracranial pressure can be controlled. This is carried out by the use of corticosteroids and mannitol, or other diuretics, such as furosemide (Lasix), 20 to 40 mg. every 12 hours. Attention must be given to the maintenance of serum electrolytes and osmolality in a normal range. Maintenance of the Pco_2 below 35 mm. Hg also aids in reducing intracranial pressure. The effectiveness of these measures, aimed at lowering intracranial pressure, can be quantitated by the use of an intracranial pressure monitoring device.

Other important medical measures must include control of blood pressure and prevention of seizures. If the elevation of blood pressure is due to the increased intracranial pressure (Cushing reflex), the reduction in blood pressure should not be achieved by specific antihypertensive drugs, but rather through a reduction in the intracranial pressure. To ignore this would reduce cerebral perfusion pressure (the difference between mean arterial blood pressure and intracranial pressure) and risk further neurologic damage. In a known hypertensive patient, or in a patient who has bled from an aneurysm, blood pressure should be controlled with appropriate drugs, such as alpha methyl-dopa (Aldomet, 250 to 500 mg. every 6 hours) or hydrochlorothiazide (HydroDIURIL, 50 mg. every 6 hours). The reduction should be in the order of 30 per cent below the patient's stable pressure, that is, the blood pressure not elevated secondary to increased intracranial pressure. This applies both to the hypertensive as well as the normotensive patient.

Prevention of seizures, which would increase intracranial pressure should they occur, can be achieved with phenytoin (Dilantin), 400 mg. per day after a loading dose of 1000 mg. given intravenously or by nasogastric tube. The intramuscular administration of phenytoin does not produce reliable blood levels. Phenobarbital, 30 mg. three times a day, may also be used, but this may add to the depression of the patient's level of consciousness.

Antifibrinolytic Therapy

The introduction of blood into the cerebrospinal fluid or brain parenchyma produces significant levels of fibrinolytic activity not normally present. This may increase the dissolution of clots occluding the ruptured vessel and lead to secondary hemorrhage. The administration of epsilon aminocaproic acid (Amicar) can reduce the incidence of rebleeding as a result of its potent antifibrinolytic activity. This has been most clearly demonstrated with aneurysms but may also be used for intracerebral hemorrhage. Epsilon aminocaproic acid is given intravenously at 36 grams per day in hourly doses for the first 48 hours (this dose may be higher than that listed in the manufacturer's official directive) and then reduced to 24 grams per day. This is important during the preoperative period and particularly after the evacuation of an intracerebral clot from a hypertensive bleed, since the most common cause of deterioration of such a patient following surgery is the reaccumulation of the hematoma. If an aneurysm is the source of the bleeding, epsilon aminocaproic acid can be discontinued once the aneurysm is clipped.

Surgical Treatment

The indications for evacuation of an intracerebral clot are based on the cause, the location of the clot, the neurologic and general medical condition of the patient, and the progression of neurologic signs after appropriate medical therapy has been instituted.

If the patient's neurologic status is stable, that is, there is no progression of focal neurologic deficit or serious decrease in the level of consciousness, surgery can be delayed and perhaps avoided by the use of medical therapy. If the diagnostic studies show that a clot is large enough to produce a midline shift or significant displacement of normal structures, surgical evacuation is best performed before more serious neurologic compromise develops. The exception to this latter point would be a patient with a clot from an aneurysm. If the patient's clinical picture permits, surgery should be delayed two weeks for elective repair of the aneurysm and removal of the clot at the same time.

This program applies to clots within the cerebral hemispheres. Hypertensive, intracerebellar hemorrhages account for 10 per cent of primary intracerebral hemorrhage. The clinical picture of sudden headache and mild cerebellar and lower cranial nerve deficits, associated with a lateral gaze palsy, requires more urgent attention because of the proximity of such a clot to the brain stem and outflow of the ventricular system. Sudden, irreversible neurologic deterioration may develop in a seemingly stable patient. If this syndrome is suspected, the diagnosis should be rapidly confirmed and the clot evacuated.

As with any intracranial mass lesion, the strongest indication for surgical intervention is deterioration of the neurologic picture in spite of appropriate medical therapy. In patients with massive intracerebral hemorrhages and profound neurologic deficits from the moment of the hemorrhage, the prognosis is obviously poor. The surgeon must decide, on an individual basis, whether this type of salvage surgery should be undertaken.

ACUTE ISCHEMIC CEREBROVASCULAR DISEASE

method of
WILLIAM K. HASS, M.D.
New York, New York

The hallmark of acute ischemic cerebrovascular disease is the sudden onset of focal cerebral or brainstem dysfunction in a defined cerebrovascular territory usually reaching full development in minutes to hours. Computed tomographic (CT) brain scanning and/or cerebrospinal fluid examination performed acutely will assure the investigator that the problem is not a result of cerebral hemorrhage. In the elderly the incidence of ischemic events is 10 to 100 times greater than in patients under the age of 40. Further, in the elderly the range of diagnostic possibilities is more limited; most often ischemia is secondary to cholesterol, fibrinoplatelet, or mixed clot emboli arising from extracranial arteries, particularly from the origins of the carotid arteries in the neck.

The Transient Ischemic Attack

This most common form of acute ischemia may present as one or many transient episodes of dysfunction referable to the carotid or vertebrobasilar arterial territories, usually lasting several minutes or, rarely, several hours. These episodes are now called transient ischemic attacks (TIAs). TIA diagnosis is aided by the identification of an appropriate bruit in a carotid arterial territory in the neck, ophthalmoscopic evidence of cholesterol or fibrinoplatelet embolization, and lack of evidence of cardiac arrhythmia or valvular disease. *The basic aim of treatment in TIA patients is the prevention of a catastrophic stroke causing profound and persistent focal neurologic dysfunction.*

The usual therapeutic modalities employed have been anticoagulants, platelet inhibitory drugs, and carotid endarterectomy. Only aspirin has demonstrated a clear superiority in the prevention of stroke after TIAs; nevertheless, reasonable benefit-to-risk ratios can be achieved by the judicious application of one or more of these treatments in specific patient categories.

1. In the elderly patient with evidence of widespread arterial occlusive disease, a history of arteriosclerotic heart disease, and other risk factors, including diabetes and moderate hypertension, initial treatment with aspirin, 325 mg. four times daily, is preferred if TIAs are in the carotid arterial territory. If there is a history of peptic ulcer or aspirin intolerance, concurrent use of cimetidine, 300 mg. four times daily, has proved effective in our studies.

2. When transient symptoms in the vertebrobasilar territory appear, aspirin should be used as described above as primary treatment. Other investigators favor immediate use of warfarin at dose levels sufficient to increase the prothrombin time to 1½ to 2½ times control prothrombin time for a period of at least 6 months if the patient is free of episodes.

3. When transient ischemic attacks occur in patients in the age group of 45 to 65 who are otherwise healthy or who suffer from at most mild diabetes and/or systolic hypertension, primary treatment with aspirin is suggested, parallel with cerebral angiographic studies designed to demonstrate a surgically treatable arterial lesion if such is present. Stenosis of up to 99 per cent of the lumen of the carotid artery at its origin in the neck can now be successfully treated at recognized medical centers with a less than 3 per cent incidence of mortality and morbidity by the technique of thromboendarterectomy with or without vein patch. This procedure is suggested if an irregular or ulcerated arterial lesion is demonstrated in the *symptomatic vascular territory*. If no lesion is present in the symptomatic vascular territory, continuing therapy with aspirin only is indicated. If there is complete occlusion of the carotid artery in the symptomatic arterial territory and symptoms continue on platelet antiaggregant therapy, or if the occlusive disease is intracranial, consisting of either high grade stenosis or occlusion of the intracranial carotid or the primary stem of the middle cerebral artery, bypass microsurgery linking the superficial temporal artery to a branch of the middle cerebral artery can give excellent results with little risk. This procedure, however, is still considered innovative and should be performed only at major centers where appropriate microneurosurgical techniques are available.

4. In uncommon situations in patients in the age group of 50 to 70, TIAs may evolve into stepwise or progressive, increases in focal deficit related to a specific vascular territory over a period of several days. When such an event occurs in the vertebrobasilar territory, the consensus is that angiography should *not* be performed. If a small cerebral hemorrhage has been ruled out (CT scan, CSF examination) therapy should be begun in a hospital with anticoagulants—e.g., intravenous heparin, 5000 units four times a day for several days, followed by oral warfarin at dose levels sufficient to increase the prothrombin time to twice the control value.

5. When a stepwise or progressive focal neurologic deficit appears in the carotid territory in younger patients who are considered to be good surgical risks, cerebral angiography is indicated. More often than not, high grade stenosis or frank occlusion of the appropriate carotid artery is disclosed. If progression has occurred during platelet inhibitory treatment with aspirin, treatment with intravenous heparin, 5000 units four times daily for a period of 2 weeks, is indicated, followed, if the patient has largely recovered, by an appropriate endarterectomy or bypass procedure.

6. As seizures are an extremely rare presenting symptom in this group of patients, it is usually necessary to employ only anticonvulsants, i.e., phenytoin, 100 mg. three or four times a day (sufficient to provide a phenytoin [Dilantin] blood level of 10 to 20 micrograms per ml.) for a period of at least 6 months after a superficial temporal artery–middle cerebral artery bypass procedure.

7. Concurrent hypertension should be initially treated with methyldopa (Aldomet), 250 mg. three times a day, and/or hydrochlorothiazide (HydroDIURIL), 50 mg. daily.

8. TIAs are rare in patients who present with a cardiac arrhythmia. More commonly a cardiac arrhythmia is associated with episodes of global cerebral ischemia, characterized as Stokes-Adams attacks. Attention in these instances is most properly directed toward the treatment of the arrhythmia with appropriate drugs or with a pacemaker.

The Catastrophic Stroke

When a catastrophic stroke occurs with permanent and persistent deficit in the carotid–middle cerebral arterial territory in the absence of demonstrable cardiac disease, angiography and surgery are contraindicated in the acute period, especially if there is depression of the state of consciousness. Further, there is no compelling evidence that anticoagulant or platelet inhibitor therapy is of value in these patients. The use of corticosteroids—e.g., methylprednisolone, 160 to 320 mg. intravenously daily for 10 days—has been suggested, but no clinical or experimental studies clearly support the use of steroids. The use of glycerol as a 10 per cent solution intravenously for this type of edema is currently under investigation.

During the period of acute catastrophic focal cerebral ischemia, feeding and administration of drugs by parenteral routes only is indicated. Frequent turning from side to side at 1 to 2 hour intervals and careful attention to skin care are mandatory. Tracheal suctioning with sterile tracheal tubes as necessary is indicated. Passive range of motion exercises of the paralyzed extremities should be begun as soon as possible. A sterile indwelling catheter connected to a sterile receptacle bag may be necessary for several days to weeks. Uncommonly after a period of several days unexpected significant recovery of function may appear. After 2 to 3 weeks in the hospital it may be determined that the patient is now able to care for himself and make his needs known adequately. At this time prevention of subsequent episodes should again be a major concern of the physician. Platelet antiaggregant therapy with aspirin should be begun, and cerebral angiography should be considered as described previously under item 3.

Cerebral Embolization from the Heart

Although TIAs often precede catastrophic strokes in patients with carotid or vertebrobasilar atherosclerotic disease, they are uncommon precursors of acute focal cerebral infarction secondary to embolism from the heart. When classic rheumatic heart disease with mitral stenosis and atrial fibrillation are present and acute massive cerebral hemispheric ischemia occurs, concern about recurrent embolization is matched by concern about the effect of breakup of a proximal large occluding embolus in the presence of anticoagulation within the first 48 hours, leading to lethal hemorrhagic changes in the established infarct. In these patients, therefore, initial attention should be restricted to the conservative measures described for catastrophic focal ischemia and appropriate antibiotic treatment if there is evidence of concurrent subacute bacterial endocarditis. Should significant recovery occur after the first 2 weeks, warfarin in doses sufficient to maintain the prothrombin time at twice the control value should be considered even if there is concurrent evidence of subacute bacterial endocarditis for which the patient is receiving antibiotic therapy. When there is evidence of only partial nonhemorrhagic hemispheric involvement giving rise to a limited, noncatastrophic stroke and there is no evidence of endocarditis, warfarin therapy is indicated on the first day of hospitalization. In such a situation the therapeutic aim is prevention of further embolization.

Unlike persistent partial or severe focal ischemic episodes related to carotid arterial disease, those caused by emboli from the heart may evolve with apoplectic rapidity. There is often associated loss of consciousness. Not infrequently focal and/or generalized convulsive seizures occur. Seizures at onset require immediate treatment, because they further compromise brain tissue viability by increasing metabolic demand from a limited blood supply. Seizure treatment is always parenteral. If the seizures have persisted for 15 minutes or more at the time the patient is seen, phenobarbital, 200 mg., should be given intravenously, followed by the same dose at 20 minute intervals if seizures persist. When seizures cease, treatment may be maintained with phenobarbital, 45 mg. subcutaneously four times a day. When the patient is more alert, phenytoin may be added at a dose of 300 to 400 mg. a day by mouth to achieve a blood level of 10 to 20 micrograms per ml. Continuing lethargy may require the reduction of the phenobarbital dose or cessation of phenobarbital therapy when adequate phenytoin blood levels are established. Alternative initial treatment with intravenous phenytoin, 100 mg. per minute for 5 to 6 minutes, is of value.

When attacks of transient or persistent territorial ischemia are seen in patients with neoplasms, tumor embolus may be suspected. More commonly the cerebral embolus will consist of fibrinoplatelet material from cardiac valves demonstrating nonbacterial thrombotic endocarditis which often accompanies disseminated neoplastic disease. A concurrent chronic or acute disseminated intravascular coagulopathy may be present. It should be appropriately treated after a blood coagulation profile is obtained.

Perhaps the most common source for cerebral emboli from the heart now seen in large centers is the artificial prosthetic heart valve, particularly prosthetic mitral valves. Present evidence favors prophylactic therapy after surgical valve implantation, with warfarin, sufficient to maintain a prothrombin time at twice control values. There is evidence that addition of dipyridamole, 50 mg. four times daily, may provide an additional factor of safety. (This use of dipyridamole is not listed in the manufacturer's official directive.) When cerebral embolization occurs in patients with prosthetic heart valves, there is strong evidence that a bland infarction may quickly turn into a hemorrhagic infarction. If this occurs, anticoagulants should be stopped. If the area of hemorrhagic infarction is accessible, i.e., in the cerebellum, appropriate emergency neurosurgical decompression measures should be taken. Satisfactory recovery of a patient with either a bland or hemorrhagic infarction should raise the question of replacement of the artificial prosthetic heart valve with a glutaraldehyde-treated porcine heart valve. There is evidence that the incidence of cerebral embolization is reduced when these valves are used. Their limited supply prevents their universal employment as primary valve replacements. Up to one third of patients with emboli from artificial heart valves may exhibit a complicating endocarditis. As in the case of cerebral embolus in patients with subacute bacterial endocarditis with rheumatic heart disease and atrial fibrillation, there is still controversy about the concurrent administration of antibiotics and anticoagulants. At present, initial treatment with antibiotics only is suggested. After evidence of eradication of the infection in patients who show significant recovery, the physician should weigh a return to anticoagulant therapy against consideration of replacement of the artificial prosthetic valve with a porcine valve.

There is, in conclusion, little evidence to support the use of vasodilator drugs or carbon dioxide inhalation in the treatment of either transient ischemic attacks or completed strokes. In the rare patient in whom thrombocytosis is discovered alone or in association with polycythemia, the use of aspirin, 325 mg. four times daily, is recommended. Anemia when present should be treated but should not be considered causal in the vast majority of patients. When hypoglycemia is present at the onset of transient or persistent focal cerebral ischemia, it should be appropriately treated.

REHABILITATION OF THE PATIENT WITH HEMIPLEGIA

method of
J. DONALD EASTON, M.D.
Columbia, Missouri

Hemiparesis or hemiplegia is a common neurologic disability and it requires early and intensive treatment, regardless of its cause, if the patient is to achieve optimal self-sufficiency or even total independence. The following guidelines for the acute and convalescent phase of rehabilitation are recommended.

Acute Phase Management

Most acute treatment is aimed at the specific pathologic process causing the hemiplegia and at avoiding medical complications that threaten further brain injury or even the patient's life.

Respiratory Complications. Impaired swallowing and coughing plus immobility frequently result in atelectasis, pooling of bronchial secretions, and aspiration with resultant pneumonia and hypoxemia. These complications are more likely to occur in obtunded patients or those with impaired bulbar function. The patient should be encouraged to cough regularly. He should be turned frequently into a high lateral position, and intermittently into a deep Trendelenburg position, so that effective bronchial drainage will occur. In obtunded patients with no cough reflex, deep tracheal suction is necessary. It is important that this be done *gently*, with a soft, sterile, fenestrated catheter, turning the head to one side and then the other so that the catheter enters both mainstem bronchi. Deep, gentle, sterile suctioning, along with proper positioning for intermittent pulmonary drainage, is usually the single most important aspect of medical care in the obtunded patient who does not cough. Most such patients who ultimately succumb do so as a result of pulmonary complications. Oral fluids should be avoided until the patient can take small sips of clear water easily. Nasogastric feeding should be carefully monitored for gastric overloading so that esophageal regurgitation and the threat of aspiration are avoided.

Tracheobronchial humidification is important, but oxygen should be given only to patients who have clinical or laboratory evidence of hypoxemia. Endotracheal intubation or tracheostomy are reserved for those patients requiring actual ventilatory assistance for a brief or prolonged period of time, respectively. Antibiotics should be used only if clinical infection results and the choice of antibiotic will be dictated by the clinical circumstance, the Gram stain of tracheobronchial secretions, and culture and sensitivity results.

Circulatory Complications. Blood pressure problems are usually associated with specific intracranial or systemic processes and attention must be directed at an accurate assessment of the cause (e.g., expanding intracranial mass or malignant hypertension on the one hand and occult systemic hemorrhaging, myocardial infarction, sepsis, or hypoxia on the other). Mild hypertension or hypotension should not, of itself, be altered. Strict bed rest in the first few days is desirable.

Skin Complications. The skin must be protected from pressure-induced necrosis in any patient with immobility of any body part. The skin must be kept clean and dry and abrasions and injections into the paretic part must be avoided. Redness over bony protuberances warns of impending skin necrosis. This can be minimized by moving the patient frequently and padding these areas with foam rubber. Sheepskin padding of the sacrum is desirable along with a pressure mattress.

Urinary Bladder Complications. Bladder function is usually normal but incontinence is common. Since incontinence is frequently transient, absorbent padding in women and condom catheters in males are often all that is necessary to prevent the skin maceration that may result. Urinary retention with resultant bladder atony and infection should be anticipated. Since it too is usually transient, bethanechol chloride (Urecholine), 5 mg. subcutaneously, may be used as necessary, or sterile catheterization can be carried out every 6 to 8 hours until normal voiding returns. If retention persists for more than 2 or 3 days, an indwelling catheter should be inserted and drained in a closed system. Hydration should be adequate to maintain 1500 to 2000 ml. urine output daily. Methenamine mandelate (Mandelamine), 1 gram orally four times daily, plus acidification of the urine with ascorbic acid, 500 mg. orally twice daily, should be given to minimize the likelihood of infection. Antibiotics should be given only if there is clinical infection of the urinary tract.

Thromboembolic Complications. Acutely hemiplegic patients confined to bed are at risk for developing venous thrombi and pulmonary embolism. Well-fitting elastic stockings and active foot flexion exercises against a bedboard or passive exercising and massage of the lower extremities, along with low dose heparin will minimize this likelihood. Three thousand units of heparin should be given subcutaneously or intravenously every 8 hours if no contraindication exists.

Bowel Complications. Constipation is a common but usually transient problem in the acute hemiplegic. Regular bowel movements may not occur until the patient is eating regularly, but an ileus or fecal impaction must be considered. Prune juice and a stool softener such as dioctyl sodium sulfosuccinate (Colace) should be given and adequate hydration maintained. Milk of magnesia or a gentle enema may be necessary if constipation is persistent. Mineral oil or castor oil should be avoided in any patient likely to aspirate.

Muscle Contractures. Physical therapy should begin as soon as possible. Passive and active range of motion exercises can be initiated by the nursing staff or physical therapist or both and is aimed at preventing fixed contractures and a painful shoulder-hand syndrome. It also prevents muscle deconditioning, strengthens the uninvolved side, promotes venous circulation, and provides the patient with self-help activity. A foot board should be provided, prolonged flexion postures should be avoided, a bandage-roll may be kept in the paralyzed hand to prevent finger flexion, and a flaccid arm should be supported in a sling to prevent shoulder displacement.

It is important to position the bed so that the patient with a hemianopia does not have his intact visual field facing a blank wall, and all visitors and staff should approach the patient from the intact side. The bedstand with the patient's personal belongings, telephone, urinal, nurses' call-button and television control should all be within reach of the nonparalyzed hand. The patient should be encouraged to feed, bathe, dress, and groom himself as much as possible. This will diminish the patient's dependence on the staff and the feelings of helplessness and worthlessness that are common to a person who is suddenly rendered hemiplegic.

Convalescent Phase Management

As soon as the patient's general medical condition is stable and he is alert and eating, the patient should be evaluated by a physiatrist or physical therapist. A treatment plan should be outlined that encourages the patient and provides the opportunity to achieve maximum independence, even partial or complete restoration to the previous life situation.

Mobilization. In addition to the usual orthostatic hypotension that accompanies attempted sitting and ambulation following a period of bed rest, the hemiplegic is especially prone to falls. Close supervision is mandatory when sitting the patient on the edge of the bed with legs dangling, when attempting transfer to a chair or commode, or when attempting standing or walking. Ambulation can be carefully attempted when the patient can lift the paretic leg 45 degrees off the bed. Blood pressure must be monitored and the patient must not be left unattended. The patient's ability to ambulate should be evaluated by the physical therapist and a program should be recommended that provides a secure progression from parallel bars to a walker and to a cane. Ankle bracing may be desirable to provide a dorsiflexion assist and avoid toe dragging, tripping, and falls. An experienced orthotist can provide valuable assistance in good bracing.

Spasticity of the paretic extremities may be associated with spontaneous clonus and muscle spasm that is disruptive and painful. Diazepam (Valium), dantrolene sodium (Dantrium), or baclofen (Lioresal) may provide some relief.

Activities of Daily Living. Physical and occupational therapists can teach the patient how to dress, how to modify a bed and utilize an overhead trapeze, how to transfer from bed to a wheelchair or chair and from a chair to a toilet, and how to equip a bathroom, a shower and a stairway for optimal support. Special eating utensils, furniture and other environmental modifications can be devised to assist the patient and those caring for him to achieve maximum independence.

Language Function. Speech therapy is of limited value to the aphasic patient. A speech therapist can make an accurate assessment of the patient's language function (particularly the ability to comprehend) and educate those dealing with the patient about the amount of deficit and its meaning. Speech therapy for aphasics may provide valuable supportive psychotherapy.

Psychological Function. Feelings of helplessness, fear, and sometimes worthlessness may overwhelm the hemiplegic patient and his family and may be a major obstacle to rehabilitation. Aphasia or alterations of intellect or affect may produce additional frustrations. Financial burdens and decisions about extended care, home care, or nursing home placement must be anticipated by the physician and appropriate emotional support and agency referral should be provided.

The almost inevitable depression that develops in the newly hemiplegic patient is usually best handled by providing understanding, education about realistic expectations for the degree of recovery, and reassurance. While this kind of reactive depression is not generally responsive to antidepressant medication, selected patients, especially those with associated insomnia, may benefit from amitriptyline (Elavil), 50 mg. orally taken at bedtime. The dosage may be increased to 100 to 150 mg. daily and is best given all at bedtime.

The long-term rehabilitation of the patient with hemiplegia is aimed at helping him achieve optimal recovery of function and modifying his activities and immediate environment to best accommodate his residual neurologic deficit. The majority of recovery from the motor deficit will have occurred in 2 to 3 months (though aphasia may continue to recover over many months). However, the patient may continue to learn compensatory actions with the unaffected hand and leg and environmental modification can result in improved functional adaptation that continues for many months.

EPILEPSY IN ADOLESCENTS AND ADULTS

method of
JONATHAN H. PINCUS, M.D.
New Haven, Connecticut

Epilepsy traditionally has been divided into two broad etiologic categories: symptomatic and idiopathic. The term symptomatic epilepsy is applied to seizure disorders with an identifiable cause, such as encephalitis, tumor, trauma, or known metabolic disease. In these conditions, seizures are considered to be a symptom of another disease. The term "idiopathic" epilepsy literally means seizure disorders that arise spontaneously and exist in the absence of other diseases of the nervous system. This term is too broadly used when applied to all convulsive disorders in which no cause has yet been identified irrespective of the age or family history of the patient. "Idiopathic" epilepsy as such usually begins in childhood or adolescence, and a positive family history is most helpful in making a reliable diagnosis when there may be a genetic predisposition. In older patients with negative family histories, epilepsy "of unknown cause" should be labeled as such, and the incomplete causative diagnosis left for further evaluation.

It must be recognized also that the concept of idiopathic epilepsy actually is artificial. Epilepsy is surely the result of a physiologic dysfunction, but the actual biochemical or neuroanatomic locus of the abnormality is not specifically known. In this sense, idiopathic epilepsy is "symptomatic," that is, symptomatic of an unknown abnormality. A high proportion of relatives of patients with idiopathic epilepsy, even focal, have abnormal eletroencephalograms (EEGs), yet most of these persons never have clinical seizures. Some patients who have idiopathic epilepsy also show other symptoms of brain dysfunction and have a history of events known to be associated with brain damage. Acquired brain damage may promote expression of the genetic trait and to the extent that it does, the resulting seizures are "symptomatic" of brain damage. It is also true that even in symptomatic epilepsy the mechanism by which identifiable lesions cause seizures is not well understood. Not every patient with a brain tumor, for example, has seizures. In all epileptic patients, whether they have idiopathic or symptomatic epilepsy, seizures are not constant, even though the lesion may be constantly present and the electroencephalogram (EEG) consistently abnormal. It seems likely that other factors must prevent seizures from occurring all the time in such cases, as well as certain factors being precipitating.

Clinical Classification

The classification of epilepsy is important in the choice of therapy. *Grand mal* seizures are characterized by total loss of consciousness and stereotyped motor activity. Initially there is a tonic stage, during which the body stiffens and breathing stops. This is followed by a clonic phase characterized by rhythmic shaking of the extremities and trunk. This sequence may last for a minute or two and sometimes repeats. After the convulsions stop there is a postictal depression of consciousness, including drowsiness, confusion, headache, and somnolence, which may last from a few minutes up to a day or two. About 50 per cent of patients experience some sort of aura, which usually precedes the attack. An aura is an integral part of the seizure. In fact, an aura must be considered to be a seizure even when it is not followed by a grand mal attack. Usually it is an ill-defined sensation of not feeling well; sometimes it is essentially a brief psychomotor seizure. Patients with focal lesions in the cortex are apt to have an aura (visceral or sensory) that can be related to the damaged area. Usually auras are of several seconds' duration, but grand mal seizures may be preceded by prodromal periods of several hours' or even days' duration, during which the patient does not feel well, is confused, or may be elated or depressed.

The tonic phase of a grand mal seizure coincides with generalized synchronous spikes on the EEG. The clonic stage is characterized by grouped spikes separated by slow waves. During the postictal phase, low voltage slow waves are seen. In about half the cases of grand mal seizures, the interictal waking EEG is normal. In the remainder, paroxysmal features including spikes, sharp activity, and slow wave bursts may be seen. If EEGs are recorded during sleep, abnormalities not seen in the waking EEG may be recorded, but 25 to 30 per cent will still remain normal. Grand mal seizures may occur in the absence of any structural defect but may also be seen in patients with generalized or focal cerebral disease.

Petit mal (centrencephalic, absence) seizures are characterized by a loss of awareness, during which there is no motor activity other than blinking or rolling up of the eyes. The episodes are brief, usually lasting less than 10 seconds. Patients do not fall to the ground, and there is no postictal depression. These seizures occur in childhood and early adolescence and are rarely seen in anyone over 20 years old. Fifty to 75 per cent of patients with petit mal epilepsy do not have other types of seizures. The electroencephalographic pattern associated with petit mal seizures (in over 80 per cent of cases) is the 3 cycles per second spike-wave discharge. The EEG is seldom normal in the interictal state, and it is especially sensitive to overbreathing. The term petit mal is often mistakenly applied to other forms of seizures, particularly psychomotor seizures, when some automatisms are present.

Focal seizures (partial simple) may be motor, sensory, or both. In patients over the age of 10 years they usually indicate focal disease in the side of the brain opposite the affected side of the body. Focal seizures may occur in the so-called "jacksonian march," starting in the distal parts of one extremity and moving proximally. The seizures are not necessarily associated with unconsciousness, but generally when they advance to both sides of the body, consciousness is lost. Very often in the postictal phase a phenomenon known as "Todd's paralysis" occurs. This is a transient paralysis of the affected part of the body that indicates that there probably is a structural abnormality in the opposite side of the cerebrum. Todd's paralysis may also follow grand mal seizures and it then might have the same focal significance. Certain metabolic abnormalities may give rise to focal seizures in the absence of any structural abnormality. Among these disturbances are hypoglycemia and hypocalcemia.

Minor motor seizures are a category of epilepsy in which motor activity may be less dramatic and less prolonged than in other types, but the disorder of the central nervous system associated with them is not necessarily minor. Minor motor seizures may be divided into several kinds: In an *akinetic seizure* the patient appears to fall to the floor passively without warning. His antigravity muscles seem to have relaxed. These spells may be of very short duration and after 2 or 3 seconds he may get up quickly without any postictal depression. Akinetic seizures, however, are probably not actually akinetic but rather myoclonic; they often result from active flexion of the neck and hips. The fall forward in the standing or sitting position may result in injury to the head and face. Until such seizures can be controlled with medication, these patients must sometimes wear protective helmets to protect the face and head. Akinetic spells usually first occur in the juvenile period but may be seen in adolescence and early adulthood. While these seizures may be seen in association with petit mal epilepsy and as a manifestation of idiopathic epilepsy, in most patients they are associated with brain damage and have a poor prognosis for normal intellectual development. They may thus be seen as a counterpart of infantile spasms in an older age group.

Akinetic seizures are often associated with an EEG pattern of spike and wave discharge that differs in frequency and form from the typical petit mal type. Hence, it is referred to as "atypical" spike wave.

Myoclonic jerks involving smaller muscle groups or the flexors or both and extensors of the hips may occur alone or as a prodrome to grand mal seizures. In either case, they may also be a part of a mild idiopathic seizure disorder and are not necessarily an ominous sign. Myoclonic jerks occasionally occur in healthy persons as they are falling asleep. This is called sleep myoclonus, and it is a normal phenomenon. Myoclonic jerks are not always associated with nonprogressive disorders, however. They occur in degenerative, infectious, and progressive diseases such as myoclonus epilepsy of Unverricht, subacute sclerosing panencephalitis (Dawson's encephalitis), in storage diseases, and in certain metabolic disorders (e.g., uremia).

The terms *psychomotor seizures* (partial-complex seizures) and *temporal lobe epilepsy* are often used synonymously. Like many oversimplifications, this is largely correct: discharges that produce psychomotor seizures usually, but not always, originate in deep, medially placed nuclei in the temporal lobe, which consists of the amygdala, uncus, and hippocampus. They may also arise from virtually any other part of the limbic system, not all of which is located in the temporal lobe. In addition, other areas of the nervous system may be the source of the discharges causing psychomotor seizures. These discharges may arise from subcortical, frontal, diencephalic, or upper brainstem regions and then spread through one or both temporal lobes. In most patients, however, electrical activity spreads to the temporal lobes so that the characteristic electroencephalographic abnormality is temporal spiking unilaterally or bilaterally. Nonetheless, there are no pathognomonic electroencephalographic configurations that make a diagnosis of psychomotor seizures absolutely certain, and the resting EEG is often normal. However, during continuous EEG monitoring in sleep or following sleep deprivation characteristic abnormalities may occur.

The manifestations of psychomotor seizures fall usually into four categories: (1) subjective experiences, (2) automatisms, (3) postural changes, and (4) autonomic changes. The *subjective feelings* including forced, repetitive and disturbing thoughts, alterations of mood, sensations of impending disaster and anxiety, as well as inappropriate familiarity or unfamiliarity (déjà vu, jamais vu). Some patients have episodes of depersonalization, dreamlike states, or sensations like those of alcoholic intoxication. Visual distortions such as macropsia and micropsia, auditory distortions, olfactory and gustatory hallucinations, and abdominal pain, are some of the most common sensory experiences. Abdominal pains associated with psychomotor seizures may be so severe as to simulate an acute abdominal emergency and in some cases exploratory laparotomies have been performed.

The *automatisms* of psychomotor seizures are much more difficult to recognize as ictal events than the tonic-clonic stages of a grand mal seizure. They tend to be repetitive and often are oral activities such as lip smacking, chewing, gagging, retching, or swallowing. Some patients may perform a variety of complicated acts that seem to blend with normal behavior. However, the behavior usually is inappropriate. The repetition of a phrase over and over again and the buttoning and unbuttoning of clothing are common. A few patients may assume bizarre *postures* resembling those of catatonic schizophrenia. These positions are held for variable periods of time. Some patients have fugue states. Fortunately, outbursts of directed, aggressive behavior are extremely rare during seizures. *Autonomic changes* include salivation, pupillary dilatation, increased gastrointestinal motility and perspiration.

In some patients with psychomotor epilepsy there may be prolonged episodes of abnormal behavior lasting for hours or days. Although epilepsy is very rarely manifested solely as a prolonged behavioral disturbance,

the clinician should include some form of associated seizure disorder in his differential diagnosis when considering episodic, and especially patterned, behavioral abnormalities even when they are prolonged.

The Principles of Therapy

The major principles of therapy for epilepsy are simple: (1) An appropriate primary drug should be chosen. (2) It should be used alone at a moderate dosage. (3) The dosage should be increased until either seizures are controlled or toxic symptoms appear. (4) Serum drug levels should be monitored to assure compliance, absorption, and to help assess subjective complaints that may be incorrectly attributed to the drug by the patient. (5) If it is not possible completely to control seizures at nontoxic doses, the dose should be lowered and a second drug should be added. (6) If complete control is reached, some consideration should be given to tapering and discontinuing the first drug. (7) If a drug is totally ineffective in controlling seizures, it should be discontinued.

The usual symptoms of overdosage are shared by most of the major anticonvulsants. These are: (1) sedation, (2) nystagmus, (3) mild mood changes, and (4) ataxia. In addition, when serum levels of the drug are above the usual therapeutic range, various psychiatric symptoms such as disorientation, memory loss, depression, and psychosis can develop. In some instances of phenytoin intoxication, seizures even increase. Milder behavioral symptoms that are commonly described by patients with high anticonvulsant blood levels include feelings of lower energy levels and initiative, and decreased sociability and ability to concentrate. Unfortunately, some patients experience these symptoms when blood levels are well below the "toxic" range. Phenobarbital and primidone are especially likely to cause this.

Complete seizure control may not be possible without some degree of toxicity. In such cases the functional capacity of the patient should determine what is an acceptable degree of seizure control. In general, among adult and adolescent epileptics, grand mal seizures are easiest to control and psychomotor seizures are the most difficult.

Choice of Drug

For grand mal, focal motor and sensory, and psychomotor seizures, the primary drugs are: phenytoin (Dilantin), barbiturates (phenobarbital, primidone [Mysoline]) and carbamazepine (Tegretol). There are at present no data indicating which of these is the most effective, but generally phenytoin has been preferred as it is less sedating than the barbiturates and has been in use longer than carbamazepine.

For petit mal, the drug of choice is ethosuximide (Zarontin) followed closely by a drug recently introduced to the American pharmacopeia, valproic acid, (Depakene). Acetazolamide (Diamox) and trimethadione are rarely used today but are also effective. Acetazolamide is especially useful in female patients whose seizures flurry around the time of menses, and it can be administered intermittently for several days before and during the period.

For minor motor seizures, phenobarbital is often the first drug tried. Though it is often ineffective in controlling minor motor seizures, it may help in some patients. However, phenobarbital controls the grand mal and psychomotor seizures, which are often associated. Valproic acid may be particularly effective in minor motor as well as absence spells. Acetazolamide, ethosuximide, clonazepam, and diazepam are others that have been used effectively. The number of drugs that have been tried is a reflection of the limited usefulness of each, although both valproic acid and clonazepam have been recent welcome additions to the therapeutic armamentarium. The ketogenic diet may be useful in difficult cases. Used mainly in children with minor motor or absence seizures, it may also be effective in these clinical seizure forms in adults and adolescents and even can control psychomotor and grand mal seizures. It has usually been considered too unpalatable and complicated for use in adolescents and adults but an apparently tolerable diet which induces ketosis ("Atkin's" diet) has been devised mainly for purposes of losing weight that we have found to be effective in controlling seizures in an occasional patient who, for one reason or other, refuses or cannot take medications or in whom medications have proved ineffective.

Surgery in Epilepsy

There are very few seizure disorders that will not respond to some medical measures, but a small number of unfortunate patients suffer from severe seizures that cannot be controlled by medical therapy. For such patients, there are three major surgical approaches, and they all seem to be effective in certain cases:

1. The most widely used approach involves the actual *removal of brain tissue,* within which is an epileptogenic focus. When there is focal onset of seizures, the removal of tissue in the involved area can provide seizure control when other measures fail. When seizures are multifocal, this approach is unlikely to benefit patients.

2. *Commissurotomy* is another approach. Here, the corpus callosum and sometimes other tracts that connect the right and left hemispheres are severed. In general, the best results have been obtained in patients with infantile hemiplegia, with a shrunken, scarred hemisphere that serves no function other than to cause generalized seizures. When such patients fail to respond to anticonvulsant therapy, removal of the damaged hemisphere (hemispherectomy) can effectively control seizures, but commissurotomy is the more conservative surgical procedure, as it prevents seizure activity from spreading from the damaged to the normal hemisphere.

3. A third surgical approach to control epilepsy involves *cerebellar stimulation* via implanted electrodes. Considerable experimental work has been done on the effect of cerebellar stimulation on seizures, but the data are conflicting and difficult to interpret. Suffice it to say that some investigators have shown termination of seizures in association with cerebellar stimulation, others have shown enhancement of seizures, and some have shown both. Although extremely interesting, this mode of therapy must still be regarded as of unproved value. For a brief summary of the indications for uses of antiepileptic drugs, see Table 1.

Major Drugs Used

Phenytoin (Diphenylhydantoin, Dilantin, DPH). Phenytoin is the drug of choice for grand mal, focal, and psychomotor seizures. The usual initial adult dose of phenytoin is 300 mg. per day, and it can be given in a single dose, ordinarily. The therapeutic blood level is between 10 and 20 micrograms per ml. In most patients blood levels in this range are not associated with sedation but sometimes they may be. When patients are started on the standard daily dosage, it requires approximately a week for phenytoin levels to rise to a plateau in or near the therapeutic range. This standard dosage of phenytoin is often too low. Often 400 mg. per day is necessary and in rare patients, 500 mg. may be necessary. In two patients we have seen, 700 mg. were necessary to produce serum levels of 10 to 20 micrograms per ml. In some instances, 300 mg. per day produces levels below 10 micrograms per ml. but 400 mg. per day produces levels above 20 micrograms per ml. along with unpleasant side effects. In such patients, it may be wise to make use of the 50 mg. tablet which can bring the total dose to 350 mg. per day.

Recent reports indicate that during pregnancy decreased gastrointestinal absorption of phenytoin may affect seizure control adversely. Some patients have required more than three times their maintenance dose of phenytoin to maintain serum levels in the therapeutic range during pregnancy. Drugs can adversely affect anticonvulsant blood levels. Isoniazid, chloramphenicol, dicumerol,

TABLE 1. **Clinical Pharmacology of Commonly Used Anticonvulsants**

DRUG	USUAL DAILY ADULT DOSE	THERAPEUTIC SERUM LEVEL	SERUM HALF-LIFE (HOURS)	TIME TO ACHIEVE STEADY STATE WITHOUT PRIMING DOSE	MAJOR INDICATIONS
Phenytoin	300–400 mg.	10–20 μg./ml.	24–48	5–10 days	Grand mal, focal psychomotor
Phenobarbital	90–120 mg.	15–40 μg./ml.	96	3 weeks	Same
Primidone*	750–1000 mg.	5–15 μg./ml.	6–9	1–2 days	Same
Carbamazepine	600–1200 mg.	4–10 μg./ml.	8	2 days	Same
Ethosuximide	750–1000 mg.	40–100 μg./ml.	60	2 weeks	Petit mal, minor motor, myoclonic
Clonazepam	1–3† mg.	20–70 ng./ml.	24–48	5–10 days	Same
Valproic acid	1000–1250 mg.	undetermined	6–8	1–2 days	Same

*Primidone is used primarily for control of psychomotor seizures. Its major metabolite is phenobarbital.

†Up to 20 mg. may be needed to achieve therapeutic levels.

disulfiram, or sulthiame can markedly increase phenytoin levels by inhibiting the enzyme that degrades phenytoin. There is some evidence that anticonvulsant agents such as carbamazepine and dipropylacetate can lower phenytoin serum levels, though there is some question as to whether this lowering changes the amount of "free phenytoin" in the serum.

The therapeutic effect of phenytoin can be related to "free" as opposed to albumin-bound phenytoin. The free fraction ordinarily comprises 10 to 20 per cent of the total serum phenytoin. In conditions associated with hypoalbuminemia such as uremia, phenytoin levels may be strikingly low, even though the amount of "free" phenytoin is unchanged. If phenytoin blood levels in such patients are raised to the usual therapeutic range, patients experience toxicity. A direct estimate of free phenytoin concentrations can be made in saliva or spinal fluid.

It has been the practice of most physicians to prescribe anticonvulsants in divided doses, and patients have been advised to take their medication three and even four times a day. Pharmacokinetic analysis based on blood levels indicates that this is usually an unnecessary way of prescribing medication and often works to the detriment of seizure control, since patients are more likely to forget their medication when it must be taken so frequently. The half-life of an anticonvulsant is the time it takes for the serum level to drop to half its steady state level after the drug has been discontinued. Drugs with half-lives of more than 24 hours seldom need be given more than once a day.

To achieve appropriate phenytoin blood levels fully and rapidly in a patient, it is possible to administer 1.0 to 1.5 grams within a 24 hour period. This can be accomplished orally by giving 500 mg. in three doses 12 hours apart, following with the usual daily maintenance dose. This also

can be achieved even more rapidly by the intravenous administration of phenytoin, which can be infused at a rate not exceeding 50 mg. per minute. No more than 500 mg. should be given in a single dosage in this manner as cardiotoxic reactions from too rapid administration have been documented in elderly patients or in those with underlying cardiac disease. The treatment can be repeated 2 to 6 hours later with relative safety, and in this manner phenytoin can be used to treat status epilepticus. Intramuscular administration of the drug should be avoided because absorption is unpredictable from muscle, and muscle necrosis can be caused by the injection.

Phenytoin is available in 100 mg. capsules, 50 mg. tablets, and a liquid suspension that contains 25 mg. per ml. (roughly 125 mg. per teaspoonful). The suspension is not recommended because it is difficult to mix well and minor errors in filling the teaspoon can result in major alterations in the dose. There is excellent correlation between blood level and therapeutic response for phenytoin and blood levels should be obtained when it is expected that the therapeutic range has been reached. If the level is low and if there is definite evidence of good compliance, the dosage should be raised to therapeutic levels. In the face of persistently low blood levels, it may be wise to admit the patient to the hospital and directly supervise the administration of the drug. Daily blood levels should be obtained and if they rise, direct evidence of poor compliance will have been obtained. Confronting the patient with this usually has a salutory effect upon his future compliance.

Adverse effects of phenytoin can be divided into four groups: (1) acute or chronic intoxication, (2) allergic hypersensitivity reactions, (3) rare metabolic side effects, and (4) common metabolic side effects.

Intoxication with phenytoin closely correlates with elevated blood levels. Most adults will show nystagmus, ataxia, and coordination difficulties at blood levels exceeding 20 to 30 micrograms per ml. Chronic phenytoin intoxication can be confused with dementia. Choreoathetosis and seizures have been reported in patients with toxic levels. A mild peripheral neuropathy that is usually clinically insignificant has been reported in patients who have been on phenytoin for more than 10 years. Myasthenic syndromes have been reported that respond to lowering the dose.

Allergic manifestations include a diffuse, morbilliform rash, which usually begins during the second week on phenytoin therapy. The Stevens-Johnson syndrome and exfoliative dermatitis are rare. Lymphadenopathy occurs in less than 1 per cent of patients and a full-blown picture of serum sickness has been reported. A Hodgkin's-like reaction and lupus erythematosus syndrome may rarely occur, but both are usually reversible when phenytoin is discontinued. Any allergic manifestation is an absolute contraindication to continuing phenytoin therapy. Hypocalcemia and osteomalacia have been reported occasionally in patients on anticonvulsant therapy that has included phenytoin. These have been reported mainly in institutionalized patients on poor diets who have not been exposed to adequate sunlight. Rarely, hyperglycemia has been reported in patients receiving phenytoin and clotting defects and clinical bleeding within the first few days of life have been reported in infants born to mothers on anticonvulsants, including phenytoin. Evidence suggests that phenytoin increases the incidence of congenital malformations two to fourfold. In particular, cleft palate, cleft lip, congenital heart defects, hypertelorism, failure to thrive, and psychomotor retardation have been noted.

Common side effects include gingival hyperplasia, which is seen in up to 40 per cent of patients receiving phenytoin and is more common in children than in adults. Though good dental hygiene helps to alleviate the problem, it can become serious enough to require gingivectomy. It is not seen in patients with dentures. A small percentage of patients have an increase in facial hair, which is particularly unpleasant for adolescent girls and young women. A megaloblastic anemia related to folic acid deficiency occurs occasionally. Artifactual lowering of thyroid function indices without a true alteration of thyroid function is also commonly encountered. Phenytoin may elevate the ceruloplasmin level.

There is anecdotal evidence that phenytoin can worsen petit mal and minor motor spells.

Phenobarbital. Phenobarbital and related barbiturates (such as meprobarbital [Mebaral]) are used for the control of grand mal, focal, and psychomotor seizures. Phenobarbital may also be used in minor motor and petit mal seizures, not so much for control of these as for control of possible associated grand mal and psychomotor seizures. The usual daily dose for an adult is 90 to 120 mg. daily. Therapeutic blood levels range from 15 to 40 micrograms per ml. The upper end of the therapeutic range, however, can rise with continued exposure to the drug as tolerance to its side effects develops. Some patients are able to tolerate 50 and 60 micrograms per ml. after prolonged exposure. On the other hand, phenobarbital does produce sedation in many patients whose blood levels are at the lower end of the therapeutic range.

In the past, it has been assumed that phenobarbital levels were quickly achieved when a person started on the daily maintenance dose, but this is not the case. It often takes almost 3 weeks to achieve steady state levels in the therapeutic range when a patient is started on 90 to 120 mg. per day. When double the ordinary dose is given for 4 days, the time required to achieve therapeutic levels is reduced to 4 days. To achieve therapeutic levels acutely, phenobarbital must be administered intravenously at a rate of 50 mg. per minute. The total dose should equal 7 to 10 mg. per kg. of body weight. This will result in blood levels of 15 to 25 micrograms per ml. Given this way, phenobarbital is effective in controlling seizures within 15 minutes.

The half-life of phenobarbital is very long, approximately 96 hours. An orally administered dose leads to a peak blood level approximately 18 hours after administration. For this reason, it is not reasonable to ask patients to take phenobarbital in divided doses. Phenobarbital is not bound to protein as is phenytoin, and blood levels in uremic states and in other conditions associated with hypoalbuminemia are accurate. Phenobarbital can be given orally, and the dose is available in 15, 30, 60, and 90 mg. tablets. When it is needed for the rapid control of seizures, medication should be given intravenously. Intramuscular administration should be reserved for those rare situations in which a patient requires maintenance daily doses and for one reason or another does not have an intravenous line and cannot take medication orally. A liquid form of phenobarbital is available that contains 4 mg. per ml. It has its major use in the pediatric age range.

Dose-related toxicity includes sedation, nystagmus, ataxia, and difficulties with learning and memory. The "paradoxical" reaction seen in minimally brain-damaged children and some brain-damaged older persons of hyperkinetic and disorganized behavior is sometimes encountered. Allergic reactions, as with other medications, include drug rashes. A state of relative folic acid deficiency with megaloblastic anemia can be seen unusually, and the drug may induce a higher rate of congenital malformations when it is administered to pregnant women. There is some evidence that it can damage the developing immature nervous system.

Primidone (Mysoline). Primidone is effective for treating grand mal, focal, and psychomotor seizures. Its major side effect is sedation. Patients who have not previously taken a barbiturate, who are started on primidone directly, can find small doses extremely sedating. Patients who have had prior experience with barbiturates have much less of a problem. Primidone (Mysoline) is available in scored 50 mg. and scored 250 mg. tablets. In patients who have received prior barbiturates, primidone may be substituted directly for phenobarbital. Two hundred and fifty (250) mg. of primidone is roughly the equivalent of 30 mg. of phenobarbital.

In measuring the blood level of primidone, one should evaluate not only the primidone level but also the phenobarbital level, as primidone is metabolized to phenobarbital. The kinetics of phenobarbital have been discussed above. Primidone has a much shorter half-life (6 to 9 hours), and it reaches a peak blood level approximately 3.5 hours after the medication is administered. Therapeutic levels of primidone are considered to range between 5 and 15 micrograms per ml. Although primidone itself probably has some anticonvulsant action, its major metabolites, mainly phenobarbital, are the main anticonvulsants. Primidone is generally given in divided doses.

The side effects and toxicity of primidone are essentially the same as those of phenobarbital and phenytoin. As the drug is available only as an oral preparation, it cannot be used in the acute treatment of epilepsy. If there is intercurrent illness or surgery that prevents the oral administration of the medication, parenteral phenobarbital must be substituted temporarily.

Carbamazepine (Tegretol). Carbamazepine is a major drug for psychomotor epilepsy, and in Europe it is considered the drug of choice in that condition. It can also be used for grand mal and focal seizures. The recommended dose for seizures is to begin at 1 tablet (200 mg.) per day. Usually, therapeutic levels are achieved at 600 to 1200 mg. per day in divided doses. Drug levels do correlate with clinical control and the therapeutic range is from 4 to 10 micrograms per ml. There is a rather short half-life of approximately 8 hours, so the drug must be given in divided doses. One or two tablets every 8 hours is an effective way of administering the drug.

Toxicity includes fatigue, nystagmus, dizziness, and slurred speech. It is not uncommon for the white blood cell count to drop below 5000 per cu. mm. in patients taking this drug. Unless the count drops below 3000 per cu. mm., there should be no reason to discontinue the medication. Six cases of aplastic anemia, five of which terminated fatally, were reported during the 1960s in patients who were receiving carbamazepine. For this reason, patients receiving the drug should have white blood cell counts before the drug is started and then on a weekly basis for a month and on a monthly basis for 6 months, following which a blood count every 3 months is advisable. However, agranulocytosis is exceedingly rare in association with the use of this medication, and some have even questioned a causal relationship. Other rare reactions include hepatic dysfunction and allergic rashes. The possible teratogenicity of carbamazepine has not been fully investigated. Although it is an extremely effective drug, and it may become the drug of choice in the treatment of psychomotor epilepsy in this country as it already has in Europe, it is not now used in this manner because of concern about hepatic dysfunction, bone marrow depression, and possible teratogenicity.

Ethosuximide (Zarontin). The major indications for the use of ethosuximide are petit mal seizures and minor motor/myoclonic seizures. Because this form of seizure is more common in children than adults, it is used primarily in the pediatric age range. The usual daily adult dose is 750 to 1000 mg. The therapeutic blood level ranges from 40 to 100 micrograms per ml., and it takes 5 to 6 days to achieve the steady state if the patient is begun on maintenance doses. The serum half-life is rather long (about 60 hours), and peak blood levels are achieved roughly 6 hours after oral administration. It is supplied in capsules of 250 mg. and as a syrup in which 1 teaspoon is the equivalent of 250 mg. The side effects include sedation and ataxia. Particularly in adults, signs of central nervous system (CNS) stimulation may be noticed. These have included euphoria, hyperactivity, night terrors and psychotic episodes (which are virtually indistinguishable from paranoid schizophrenia), and increased libido. Depressive states with suicidal tendencies have also been reported. Most of these disturbing central nervous system effects have been reported in adults. This is all the more striking for the drug is used almost exclusively in children and is rarely used in adults. The actual incidence of these side effects is not known, but it may be rather high. The only evidences that the drug causes CNS stimulation in children are anecdotal reports that have linked ethosuximide with an increased frequency of grand mal seizures in patients in whom the drug was used alone. Allergic reactions include skin rashes and a lupus erythematosus syndrome that responds to discontinuation of the medication.

Clonazepam (Clonopin). Clonazepam is used primarily for minor motor seizures (akinetic-myoclonic seizures) and in patients with absence (petit mal) seizures who have failed to respond to ethosuximide. European data indicate that it may be effective in psychomotor seizures. The usual daily adult dose is 1 to 3 mg. per day, but up to 20 mg. may be necessary to achieve therapeutic blood levels (20 to 70 nanograms per ml.). It takes 5 to 10 days to achieve a steady state level on maintenance doses, and the blood half-life varies from 18 to 50 hours. The side effects are essentially the same as the other benzodiazepines and include sedation and ataxia as well as rare hypersensitivity reactions.

Valproic Acid (Depakene). Valproic acid is indicated for use in patients with absence seizures primarily. It also may be helpful in other seizure types. The drug is administered orally and is available in a 250 mg. capsule as well as a syrup containing 250 mg. per teaspoon. The recommended starting dose is 15 mg. per kg. per day with increments of 5 to 10 mg. per kg. per day made at 1 week intervals until seizures are controlled or side effects occur. The serum half-life is rather short (4 to 6 hours), and for this reason it must be given in divided doses. Gastrointestinal side effects are common and include diarrhea, cramps, nausea, and vomiting. Toxic reactions include sedation and ataxia. Hemapoietic depression, hepatic dysfunction, and allergic rashes have rarely been noted. Valproic acid has important interactions with other drugs. It may potentiate the CNS depressant activity of alcohol, and there is evidence that the drug reduces the total phenytoin concentration, presumably by competing with phenytoin at serum protein binding sites; yet, it appears not to cause a reduction in unbound (free) phenytoin serum concentrations. The use of valproic acid with clonazepam may worsen petit mal seizures.

Status Epilepticus

Repetitive seizures with incomplete recovery of the baseline neurologic function between seizures is defined as status epilepticus. In general, it is not wise to spend too much time in heuristic arguments concerning whether a particular patient is in status epilepticus or is having frequent seizures just short of status. The only major problem facing the clinician is: "Should the seizures be treated acutely?" If the answer is no, oral administration of medication is advisable; if the answer is yes, the patient should be treated as though he had status epilepticus.

The treatment of status epilepticus requires the insertion of an oral airway and possibly an endotracheal tube, and placement of an intravenous line. Every effort should be made to limit the total amount of fluid administered in order to minimize cerebral edema.

The drug of choice is phenobarbital which should be administered at a rate of 50 mg. per minute intravenously until a total dose of 7 mg. per kg. of body weight has been given. If seizures continue 30 minutes after the administration of phenobarbital, another 3 mg. per kg. should be administered. Doses of this magnitude are essential to achieve blood levels within the therapeutic range (15 to 30 micrograms per ml.).

The second drug to use if adequate doses of intravenously administered phenobarbital fail to control seizures is phenytoin. With concomitant monitoring of blood pressure and electrocardiogram, phenytoin should be administered intravenously at a rate not exceeding 50 mg. per minute to a total dose of 1 gram. If circumstances allow, this total dose of phenytoin should be administered in two portions, 2 or 3 hours apart in order to avoid cardiac depression.

If these measures fail, intravenous diazepam should be tried. Usually 10 mg. is needed in the adult to stop the seizures. In many centers, diazepam is considered the treatment of choice; however, we do not agree. Although diazepam may stop seizures acutely, its anticonvulsant action is short-lived and does not last more than 30 minutes; for this reason, the drug cannot be used for maintenance therapy. While diazepam can be administered two or three times with 20 minute intervals in between, if seizures continue, another drug must be tried.

Although the anticonvulsant action of diazepam is short-lived, its effect as a respiratory depressant is not and it may be dangerous to use adequate doses of phenobarbital after diazepam has failed because these drugs are synergistic in depressing respiration. Thus, we prefer to use drugs that will not only act rapidly but will also provide sustained anticonvulsant coverage.

Other adjuncts to the treatment of repetitive seizures are: paraldehyde and lidocaine. Paraldehyde should be administered as a 4 per cent solution in isotonic saline solution given by intravenous drip. Lidocaine should be given as an intravenous bolus of 1 mg. per kg. followed by an infusion of 10 to 30 micrograms per kg. per minute. The half-life of lidocaine is rather short (about 2 hours). (This use of lidocaine is not listed in the manufacturer's official directive.) Widespread use of this drug in the management of cardiac arrhythmia has led to the development of methods to measure lidocaine levels in the blood so that close monitoring can be achieved. Therapeutic levels of 2 to 5 micrograms per ml. are the goal. There is some evidence that phenobarbital augments the anticonvulsant effects of lidocaine and protects against the neurotoxicity of the drug itself so that the use of lidocaine following the unsuccessful use of phenobarbital and phenytoin is a reasonable recourse for the control of persistent and repetitive seizures. Infusion can be maintained for 12 to 48 hours and then discontinued. By this time, the conditions that provoked the episode of seizures may have resolved.

Alcohol Withdrawal Seizures

Alcohol withdrawal seizures may be unassociated with underlying brain damage or may be associated with it. In the former case, the seizures are characteristically single, brief, and generalized though occasionally, two or even a flurry of brief seizures may occur in a relatively short period of time. Seizures generally occur within 2 or 3 days following withdrawal from alcohol. The neurologic examination and electroencephalogram (EEG) are within normal limits though increased sensitivity to photic stimulation may be noted. It is generally not advisable to treat such patients with anticonvulsant maintenance therapy. Further abstention from alcohol would effectively prevent future problems of alcohol withdrawal, but if, as is usually the case, the patient should continue to drink, it is not likely that he would take his anticonvulsant medication. Prolonged or focal seizures indicate brain damage, and such patients should be fully investigated and probably treated for epilepsy even if alcohol withdrawal has precipitated a seizure.

Epilepsy in Pregnant Women

The incidence of congenital malformations is somewhat increased in children born to epileptic women and in most cases this has been ascribed to anticonvulsant therapy. Phenytoin has been identified as the major offender. Approximately half the women with idiopathic epilepsy experience an increase in the frequency of seizures during pregnancy. While there can be many theoretically plausible causes for this, a recent study of pregnant women who were receiving phenytoin or phenobarbital or both showed that serum anticonvulsant levels dropped during the pregnancy. If this is a common occurrence in pregnant women, it would explain the tendency for seizures to increase in frequency during pregnancy. Many authorities now recommend that serum anticonvulsant levels be monitored and adjusted carefully during pregnancy to avoid increased seizures. While it is quite reasonable, this course of action carries with it the risk of an increased incidence of congenital malformations caused by the anticonvulsants. In the absence of definitive information, it would probably be wise to continue the medication that the patient was receiving before she became pregnant, whatever the blood level, increasing the dosage only if seizures develop.

During pregnancy, a woman should receive vitamins with supplementary folic acid as most of the major anticonvulsants, especially phenytoin, can induce folic acid deficiency.

Infants born to mothers receiving anticonvulsants, especially phenytoin, can experience bleeding in the neonatal period that is related to a decrease in vitamin K–dependent clotting factors. Pregnant women receiving anticonvulsants should be given water-soluble vitamin K, 5 mg. by mouth, at least once a week during the final month of pregnancy.

Discontinuance of Medication

There is very little from data concerning the safety of discontinuing medication with regard to the chances of seizure recurrence. Some studies in children have indicated that after complete seizure control for 4 years if anticonvulsant medication is discontinued, approximately 25 per cent of patients will have recurrences over the next 5 years, most of which occur in the first 6 months following withdrawal. In general, the results for post-traumatic epilepsy are better. A recurrence rate following medication withdrawal in adults has been quoted as being as high as 80 per cent, even if the seizure remission on medication had lasted for 2 years. In general, we have encouraged most patient to continue their anticonvulsant medication indefinitely. If they are extremely anxious to discontinue medication and they have been seizure-free for 4 years or more and if the EEG is normal or only mildly abnormal, we have agreed to gradually taper and discontinue medication over a 2 to 3 month period.

EPILEPSY IN CHILDREN

method of
MARY LOUISE SCHOLL, M.D.
San Diego, California

Epilepsy, characterized by recurrent seizures, is a symptom of abnormal neuronal activity within the central nervous system. Seizures vary greatly in their clinical manifestations. Approximately 60 per cent of patients with epilepsy have one type of spell; the remaining 40 per cent have two or more types. In order to facilitate treatment, seizures may be classified in the following categories: major motor, minor motor, petit mal, psychomotor, seizure equivalents, mixed seizures, and febrile seizures.

Although seizures usually appear during infancy or childhood in the majority of epileptics, all children who have seizures are not labeled epileptics. There are a few patients who have one seizure during a period of physical or emotional stress, whose electroencephalograms display abnormalities suggesting a lowered seizure threshold, but who do not continue to have recurrent spells. The repetition of the attacks is an important factor in the diagnosis.

The underlying cause of epilepsy should be elucidated if at all possible before treatment is instituted. Seizures may be the first clinical manifestations of a cerebral tumor or of other types of acute or progressive central nervous system disease. A thorough evaluation of the patient is imperative. This should include a detailed medical history, general physical and neurologic examinations, an electroencephalogram made during waking, drowsing, and sleeping states, and, if indicated, computed axial tomography (EMI scan), x-ray films of the skull, a lumbar puncture, and other spinal procedures and blood tests.

Febrile Seizures

Seizures associated with fever occur frequently in children. They account for half of all seizures experienced by children under 5 years of age. Although these spells may recur, they do not necessarily imply that the child is, or will be, an epileptic. The majority of young children who have seizures during the febrile state only are usually not potential epileptics. Febrile seizures are divided into two groups: (1) *primary* or benign, those in which the fever is the essential contributing factor, and (2) *secondary* or epileptic, those in which the fever acts only as a precipitating factor.

Primary febrile seizures usually occur in children 3 months to 6 years of age who are intellectually and neurologically normal. The seizures are always generalized and short in duration (15 minutes or less). The child's electroencephalogram, made during the afebrile state, is always normal. There is frequently a positive family history of febrile convulsions. Two to 3 per cent of these children subsequently develop epilepsy.

More than 50 per cent of children with secondary febrile seizures will eventually develop a convulsive disorder. These children frequently display electroencephalographic abnormalities during the afebrile state. The onset of the disorder may occur very early in life or after the age of 6 years. Their seizures may be prolonged or focal. Evidence of delayed intellectual development or discernible neurologic abnormalities prior to the first febrile convulsion is not uncommon. A family history of epilepsy or a history of significant brain insult or head trauma is frequently obtained.

Treatment of Febrile Seizures. Occasionally febrile seizures may be prevented in some patients by the administration of phenobarbital and acetylsalicylic acid every 4 hours during periods of fever. This sporadic therapy is usually not successful in children who develop high fevers rapidly. These patients may have a seizure before the parent is aware of the illness or before the drugs, taken by mouth, can be assimilated. Daily anticonvulsant therapy should be prescribed for this group of patients, for any child having had two or more primary febrile convulsions, and for all children who have any of the following: (a) onset of a febrile seizure under the age of 1 year, (b) a prolonged or focal seizure with fever, (c) multiple febrile seizures within a 24 hour period, or (d) a previous history of neurologic deficits or mental retardation. These children are more at risk of developing neurologic sequelae as a result of febrile seizures. The drugs of choice are phenobarbital, 30 to 60 mg. (½ to 1 grain), or mephobarbital (Mebaral), 50 to 100 mg. once daily at bedtime. During periods of illness with fever the maintenance dose is repeated every 8 to 12 hours. If these drugs are not tolerated, as indicated by persistent lethargy, hyperactive behavior, irritability, or rash, phenytoin sodium (Dilantin) may be used, although it is less effective in preventing recurrent febrile seizures. Treatment should be continued until age 6.

Treatment of Status Epilepticus

Prolonged seizures are a threat to life. The mortality rate in status epilepticus is 10 per cent. *Status epilepticus is a medical emergency.* The patient should be given the same type of treatment as other patients in coma. An adequate airway must be maintained, the seizures must be controlled as quickly as possible, and the patient must be attended at all times.

Anticonvulsant drugs may be given intravenously, intramuscularly, or by rectum. Drugs for rectal administration should be maintained in the homes of patients who have a history of previous status epilepticus. Therapy is administered promptly at the onset of the seizure. The patient can then be transported to the hospital for additional care.

Drugs administered *intravenously* exert their effects promptly and the dosage can be readily controlled. If this route is selected, the drugs must be given *slowly* over a 2 to 3 minute period *in order to avoid apnea.* If the status ceases before the suggested dosage has been administered, the injection should be discontinued. It can be repeated at a later time if there is a recurrence of the seizures. The following drugs are commonly used *intravenously:*

Sodium phenobarbital, 4.4 to 6.6 mg. per kg. (2 to 3 mg. per pound) of body weight.

Amobarbital (Amytal Sodium) 6.6 to 8.8 mg. per kg. (3 to 4 mg. per pound) of body weight.

Phenytoin (Dilantin), 4.4 mg. per kg. (2 mg. per pound) of body weight; newborns and very young infants require much higher doses, 13.2 to 17.6 mg. per kg. (6 to 8 mg. per pound) of body weight.

Acetazolamide (Diamox), 5.5 mg. per kg. (2.5 mg. per pound) of body weight.

Diazepam (Valium), 5 to 10 mg. total dosage irrespective of body weight. This drug acts very promptly. It is effective in all types of status epilepticus (see package insert).

Chlordiazepoxide (Librium), 50 to 100 mg. total dosage irrespective of body weight (see package insert).

Paraldehyde,* 0.33 ml. per kg. (0.15 ml. per pound) of body weight; each milliliter of paraldehyde should be diluted in 10 ml. of isotonic saline solution or 10 ml. of 5 per cent glucose in water. A combination of the two, namely, 3.5 ml. of isotonic saline and 6.5 ml. of 5 per cent glucose in water, can be used as an alternative. This is given by intravenous drip which enables the physician to regulate the rate of flow to the patient's need.

Lidocaine (Xylocaine), 4 mg. per kg. per hour in a continuous intravenous glucose infusion, may be given to young infants and children with status that are resistant to *reasonable* amounts of other drugs (investigational for this use).

Sodium phenobarbital, amobarbital (Amytal Sodium), diazepam (Valium), and chlordiazepoxide (Librium) can be given repeatedly every 20 to 60 minutes. However, when large doses are required to terminate seizures one must be alert to cardiopulmonary arrest, and supportive equipment should be readily available at all times. Blood levels of drugs should be monitored frequently.

If the *intramuscular* route is used the recommended dosages are as follows:

Sodium phenobarbital, 4.4 to 6.6 mg. per kg. (2 to 3 mg. per pound) of body weight.

Amobarbital (Amytal Sodium), 6.6 to 8.8 mg. per kg. (3 to 4 mg. per pound) of body weight.

Phenytoin (Dilantin), 4.4 mg. per kg. (2 mg. per pound) of body weight.

Acetazolamide (Diamox), 5.5 mg. per kg. (2.5 mg. per pound) of body weight.

Diazepam (Valium), 5 to 10 mg. total dosage irrespective of body weight.

Chlordiazepoxide (Librium), 50 to 100 mg. total dosage irrespective of body weight.

Paraldehyde,* 0.33 ml. per kg. (0.15 ml. per pound) of body weight with a maximum of 10 ml.; not more than 5 ml. should be injected at any one site.

Phenytoin, acetazolamide, and diazepam or chlordiazepoxide may be given in addition to either paraldehyde or one of the barbiturates, since the action of these drugs is synergistic, not accumulative. The initial dose may be repeated in 30 to 60 minutes if necessary. Caution should be used in giving large amounts of barbiturate since respirations may be compromised.

The following drugs may be given by *rectum:*

Secobarbital (Seconal), 8.8 to 11 mg. per kg. (4 to 5 mg. per pound) of body weight.

Chloral hydrate, 44 to 55 mg. per kg. (20 to 25 mg. per pound) of body weight; the total dose should not exceed 2 grams.

Paraldehyde,* 0.66 ml. per kg. (0.3 ml. per pound) mixed with 1.32 ml. per kg. (0.6 ml. per pound) of vegetable oil. This is given as a retention enema.

Ether and thiopental sodium (Pentothal) have been found to be effective in the control of status epilepticus. These general anesthetics should be administered by an *anesthesiologist.*

A state of prolonged confusion is characteristic of petit mal status and psychomotor status. These states may be differentiated by electroencephalography. Two and one half to 3 per second spike-wave discharges are present in petit mal status. These can be readily distinguished from other types of cerebral dysrhythmia. Although petit mal status is generally self-limiting, it occasionally may be prolonged or may terminate in a grand mal seizure. Diazepam (Valium) given intravenously in a dosage of 5 to 10 mg. will generally terminate petit mal status abruptly. Other drugs that may be used are acetazolamide (Diamox), sodium phenobarbital, and paraldehyde. The same drugs may be effective in psychomotor status.

THE EPILEPTIC CHILD

Aims of Treatment

1. It is of prime importance to prevent the recurrence of seizures by the use of anticonvulsant drugs. With the medications presently available, about 75 per cent of children will obtain complete seizure control. Another 15 to 20 per cent will show moderate improvement, and 5 to 10 per cent will be unimproved or will appear to have their spells aggravated by medication.

---

*Fresh paraldehyde should always be used. In contact with air this drug slowly oxidizes to acetic acid. Paraldehyde should be stored in a well-filled, tight, light-resistant container at a temperature of 30°F.

*Fresh paraldehyde should always be used. In contact with air this drug slowly oxidizes to acetic acid. Paraldehyde should be stored in a well-filled, tight, light-resistant container at a temperature of 30°F.

2. It is imperative that the child understand his illness in order that he may learn to live comfortably with it and will ultimately assume the responsibility of his own medication. Every child should be given an explanation of his illness. The complexity of the explanation should be adapted to the child's age and his ability to comprehend. He should be given an opportunity to express his feelings and ask questions about his disorder each time he visits his physician.

3. Parents of the epileptic child tend to be anxious, to be overprotective, to impose excessive restrictions, and to be lax with discipline. Alleviating parental fears and guiding and supporting parents in their relationships with sick children is a major contribution to therapy.

4. The cooperation of school personnel, friends, and others in frequent contact with the patient is important if he is to adjust socially and psychologically. The physician must take an active role in soliciting this cooperation.

Principles of Drug Therapy

1. Treatment should be started with one drug. The initial daily dosage is generally about a third of the anticipated average daily dose. The drug is then gradually increased every 5 to 7 days until seizure control is established or symptoms of overdosage appear. One should not hesitate to increase a drug as long as there is no evidence of toxicity. If symptoms of overdosage appear, the daily dosage should be reduced to the maximal level of tolerance. Toxic symptoms such as lethargy, drowsiness, or slowed mentation are often more of a handicap to the child than recurrent seizures. In fact, there are some patients whose seizures will become remarkably more frequent if they are maintained in a drowsy state. The goal of therapy is not only to control the seizures but also to have an alert, normally functioning patient.

2. If the original drug is not effective in controlling the seizures it may be gradually replaced by a second drug or the drugs may be combined. Two new drugs should never be added simultaneously to the patient's regimen. Each drug should be evaluated separately. No course of treatment can assure immediate control for any one patient. Numerous trials of therapy may be required. Persistence is the key to successful control. When one drug or a combination of drugs fails, another should be tried.

3. If the seizures occur frequently, the success of the drug can be determined in several weeks or months. However, if the attacks are infrequent, many months may be required to establish the efficacy of a specific medication. Patients or members of the patient's family should keep an accurate record of the number, duration and severity of the seizures. A simple method for accomplishing this is to list the seizures on a calendar.

4. In order to maintain a relatively constant blood level, the drugs should be taken regularly each day in single or divided doses.

In order to assure that the child receives medication regularly, the number of doses should be curtailed to a minimum, as compliance is generally proportional to the number of doses prescribed daily.

5. The patient and his family should be cautioned about withdrawing medication abruptly, since status epilepticus may result. If, for some reason, the patient is unable either to take or to retain the drugs by mouth, they may be given, in the majority of patients by subcutaneous, intramuscular, or intravenous injection.

6. Many children who have no specific evidence of structural brain pathology outgrow their seizures before or at puberty. Anticonvulsant therapy should be continued until the patient has remained free of seizures for 1½ to 3 years. The medication may then be *gradually* withdrawn over a 6 to 12 month period. There is no reliable method for determining in advance whether a patient will remain seizure-free after medication is eliminated. This can be established only by giving the patient a trial without drugs. If discontinuation of drugs is not accomplished before puberty it should not be attempted during this period.

7. Patients taking anticonvulsant drugs should have physical examinations at regular intervals. Those patients taking medications known occasionally to produce harmful effects on the hemopoietic, hepatic, or urinary systems should have appropriate blood or urine studies frequently at the onset of therapy and at more prolonged intervals when tolerance has been established.

Specific Drug Therapy*

Table 1 lists the most commonly used medications.

It is well known that anticonvulsant drugs are more beneficial in one type of seizure than in another. Thus, the drugs chosen should be specific for the type or types of seizures being treated. In order to make a wise choice of drugs the physician must be familiar with the details of the patient's preictal, ictal, and postictal states, as well as with his electroencephalographic abnormalities. A brief description of the various types of seizures and the recommended drug therapy follows:

---

*The physician should be familiar with the information in the manufacturers' official directives before using these agents.

TABLE 1. **Anticonvulsant Drugs Used for Children with Epilepsy***

| DRUG | | | | | TYPE OF SEIZURE BENEFITED | | | |
Generic Name	*Proprietary Name*	AVERAGE DAILY DOSE	FORM	SIDE EFFECTS	*Major Motor*	*Minor Motor*	*Petit Mal*	*Psycho-motor*
Chloroquine (investigational)	Aralen	125–500 mg.	125–250 mg. tablet	Blurring of vision; anorexia; bleaching of hair	−	−	+	−
Quinacrine hydrochloride (investigational)	Atabrine	100–200 mg.	50–100 mg. tablet	Yellow discoloration of skin; nausea; diarrhea	−	−	+	−
Bromides, triple		1–4 grams	500 mg. per tablet; elixir, 1 gram/teaspoonful	Drowsiness; rash	+	+	−	−
Methsuximide	Celontin	600 mg. to 1.2 grams	300 mg. capsule	Drowsiness; headache; anorexia; rash	−	+	+	+
Clonazepam	Clonopin	0.5–6 mg.	0.5, 1, 2 mg. tablet	Drowsiness; ataxia; behavioral problems; confusion; depression; excessive salivation	−	+	+	−
Valproic acid (Sodium Valproate)	Depakene	250 mg. to 1.25 grams	250 mg. tablet; syrup, 250 mg. 1 teaspoon	Nausea; vomiting; drowsiness; loss of hair	+	+	+	−
Methamphetamine hydrochloride	Desoxyn	2.5–5 mg.	2.5 mg. tablet	Anorexia; irritability; insomnia	+	+	+	+
Dextroamphetamine sulfate	Dexedrine	5–15 mg.	5 mg. tablet; elixir, 5 mg./teaspoonful; 5, 10, 15 mg. capsule	Anorexia; irritability; insomnia	+	+	+	+
Acetazolamide	Diamox	250–750 mg.	250 mg. tablet	Anorexia; numbness of extremities	+	+	+	+
Phenytoin (diphenylhydantoin)	Dilantin	30–400 mg.	30, 100 mg. capsule; 50 mg. Infantab; 100 mg./teaspoonful; suspension (delayed action), 100 mg. capsule	Gingival hypertrophy; nystagmus; ataxia; diplopia; hirsutism; tremor; rash; nausea; vomiting	+	+	−	+
Metharbital	Gemonil	100–400 mg.	100 mg. tablet	Drowsiness; irritability	+	+	−	+
Chlordiazepoxide	Librium	30–60 mg.	5, 10, 15 mg. capsules	Drowsiness; ataxia; syncope	+	−	+	+
Mephobarbital	Mebaral	100–400 mg.	30, 50, 100, 200 mg. tablets	Drowsiness; irritability	+	+	−	+
Mephobarbital and diphenylhydantoin	Mebroin	2–4 tablets	1 tablet contains 90 mg. of mephobarbital and 60 mg. of diphenylhydantoin	As for diphenylhydantoin and mephobarbital	+	−	−	+
Meprobamate		400 mg. to 1.2 grams	200, 400 mg. tablet; 200 ml./teaspoonful suspension	Drowsiness	−	−	+	−
Methylphenylethylhydantoin	Mesantoin	100–400 mg.	100 mg. pink tablet	Ataxia; tremor; drowsiness; rash; blood dyscrasias	+	−	−	+
Phensuximide	Milontin	1.5 grams/day	500 mg. capsule; 250 mg./teaspoonful suspension	Drowsiness; headache	−	+	+	−

*The doses mentioned in this table are average doses. For specific dose recommendations, precautions, and other information see the official manufacturer's brochure for each drug before using.

Table continued on the following page

TABLE 1. Anticonvulsant Drugs Used for Children with Epilepsy (*Continued*)

Generic Name	Proprietary Name	Average Daily Dose	Form	Side Effects	Major Motor	Minor Motor	Petit Mal	Psycho-motor
Primidone	Mysoline	250–750 mg.	250 mg. scored tablet; 250 mg./teaspoonful suspension	Drowsiness; ataxia; anorexia; irritability; personality changes	+	+	−	+
Paramethadione	Paradione	600 mg. to 1.8 grams	300 mg. capsule; 300 mg./ml. solution (drops)	Photophobia; hiccups; anorexia; blood dyscrasias	−	+	+	−
Ethotoin	Peganone	750 mg. to 1.5 grams	250, 500 mg. tablet	Drowsiness; ataxia; diplopia; tremor; rash	+	+	−	+
Phenobarbital		100 mg.	15, 30, 60, 100 mg. tablet; elixir, 15 mg./teaspoonful	Drowsiness; irritability	+	+	−	+
Diphenylhydantoin, phenobarbital, and desoxyephedrine	Phelantin	2–4 capsules	1 capsule contains 100 mg. of diphenylhydantoin, 30 mg. of phenobarbital, and 2.5 mg. of desoxyephedrine	Anorexia most common; other side effects as for diphenylhydantoin and phenobarbital	+	+	−	+
Phenacemide	Phenurone	1–2 grams	500 mg. tablet; 300 mg. enteric-coated tablet	Rash; anorexia; nausea; vomiting; hepatitis; personality changes; blood dyscrasias	+	+	−	+
Methylphenidate hydrochloride†	Ritalin	10–60 mg.	5, 10, 20 mg. tablet	Nervousness; anorexia; nausea	+	+	+	+
Carbamazepine	Tegretol	200 mg. to 1 gram	200 mg. tablet	Dizziness; drowsiness; diplopia; blurred vision; rash; aplastic anemia	+	−	−	+
Imipramine hydrochloride†	Tofranil	10–40 mg.	10, 25, 50 mg. tablet	Restlessness; agitation; dry mouth; rash; blood dyscrasias	−	−	+	−
Trimethadione	Tridione	900 mg. to 1.8 grams	300 mg. capsule; 150 mg. dulcet; 150 mg./teaspoonful solution	Photophobia; hiccups; anorexia; blood dyscrasias	−	+	+	−
Diazepam	Valium	5–30 mg.	2, 5, 10 mg. tablet	Ataxia; drowsiness; nausea; dizziness	+	+	+	+
Ethosuximide	Zarontin	750 mg. to 1.5 grams	250 mg. capsule; syrup, 250 mg./teaspoonful	Gastric distress; nausea; dizziness; drowsiness	−	+	+	−

†This use of this agent is not listed in the manufacturer's official directive.

Major Motor Seizures.   Major motor seizures may be generalized or partial (focal) in nature. A warning symptom (aura) may be experienced by the patient before the seizure ensues. The type of aura varies considerably from one patient to another. If generalized (grand mal), the spells start with loss of consciousness followed by a sudden collapse of posture. A tonic phase followed by clonic movements is the usual sequence of events. Cyanosis may or may not appear as the result of a brief cessation of respirations. Saliva frequently exudes from the mouth. Incontinence of bowel and bladder occurs frequently. If the seizure is prolonged, it is generally followed by a deep sleep lasting minutes or hours. If short in duration, a period of confusion and irritability may be noted before the patient becomes fully aware. The presence and duration of tonic or clonic movements differ from patient to patient. The atonic attack, which frequently resembles a simple syncopal attack, is the most frequently undiagnosed or inaccurately classified spell. It can be differentiated from the latter in that the period of unconsciousness usually exceeds 2 minutes, there may be incontinence during the attack, and confusion, lethargy, and sleep frequently follow this type of seizure.

Focal (partial) seizures may or may not be associated with loss of consciousness. The duration of unconsciousness is usually directly proportionate to the severity of the spell. These attacks may be tonic, clonic, tonic-clonic, or atonic in type. Sensory changes are frequently present in the affected parts. A temporary paresis or paralysis (Todd's paralysis) of the involved extremity, or extremities, may follow a focal motor seizure.

The cost as well as the efficacy of a drug must be considered when prolonged therapy is anticipated. Phenobarbital is inexpensive and highly effective in controlling major attacks. It is the first drug of choice except for children who are slow learners in school. Phenytoin (Dilantin) is frequently required to obtain control of seizures.

Mephobarbital (Mebaral) generally produces less sedation than many of the other barbiturates. Because of this, it is frequently used in children. The therapeutic dose is about twice that of phenobarbital.

Primidone (Mysoline) when used alone or in combination with a hydantoin such as phenytoin (Dilantin), methylphenylethylhydantoin (Mesantoin), or ethotoin (Peganone), is an excellent anticonvulsant. Irrespective of the age of the patient, this drug must be started in a relatively small dose (one sixth of a tablet, or 40 mg.) and then gradually increased every 3 days if side effects of drowsiness and ataxia are to be avoided. If the child becomes markedly irritable or hyperactive as a consequence of taking barbiturates or primidone, the medication should be discontinued. These symptoms interfere with academic progress and the development of good social relationships. These are more handicapping on long term than inadequate seizure control.

When ataxia, hirsutism, or gingival hypertrophy limits the use of phenytoin (Dilantin), methylphenylethylhydantoin (Mesantoin), ethotoin (Peganone), or carbamazepine (Tegretol) may be substituted. Patients generally tolerate these drugs better, as they infrequently produce side effects. Aplastic anemia has occurred rarely in patients taking methylphenylethylhydantoin (Mesantoin) and very rarely in patients receiving carbamazepine (Tegretol). Nevertheless, this side effect is such a serious one that it is imperative for all patients receiving these drugs to have monthly blood tests.

Acetazolamide (Diamox), chlordiazepoxide (Librium), diazepam (Valium), clonazepam (Clonopin), and valproic acid (Depakene) are useful adjuncts to the previously mentioned anticonvulsant drugs, but, when given alone, these drugs have not been very successful in controlling major seizures. When valproic acid (Depakene) is used with phenobarbital, phenobarbital blood levels are increased; when used with phenytoin (Dilantin), blood levels of phenytoin decrease. Diazepam (Valium), clonazepam (Clonopin), and valproic acid are particularly beneficial to patients whose seizures are activated by a flashing light (strobe sensitive).

Phenacemide (Phenurone) is the most toxic of all the drugs. It may be used with caution for patients who are resistant to other types of therapy. Anorexia is usually the heralding symptom of toxicity. The drug should be stopped immediately if this symptom appears. All patients receiving this drug should have monthly blood counts.

Compounded drugs, such as Phelantin, containing phenytoin, phenobarbital, and desoxyephedrine, and Mebroin, containing phenytoin and mephobarbital, are useful in treating patients who require several drugs. They simplify the daily regimen of medication. Phelantin is essentially beneficial for patients who become drowsy on a combination of phenobarbital and phenytoin and for patients who have nocturnal seizures during deep sleep. The desoxyephedrine will lighten the sleep. In this state the patient is less susceptible to spells.

Dextroamphetamine sulfate (Dexedrine), methamphetamine hydrochloride (Desoxyn), and methylphenidate hydrochloride (Ritalin) are frequently used to combat lethargy and drowsiness induced by other anticonvulsants. An alert, active child is less prone to have seizures. In children who experience only nocturnal seizures a long-activating dextroamphetamine sulfate (Dexedrine spansule) given just as the child is getting into bed will not interfere with the onset of sleep but may control the spells by eliminating the very deep sleep during which these seizures usually occur. If this given alone does not control the seizure, it can be combined with phenytoin (Dilantin).

Minor Motor Seizures. Minor motor seizures, which are frequently associated with organic brain disease, include akinetic and myoclonic attacks. Akinetic attacks, usually associated with a momentary loss of consciousness, consist of a precipitous, brief loss of postural control that may be clinically manifested by an abrupt fall, a forward flexion of the trunk (salaam spell), or a sudden nodding of the head. Normal posture is regained almost immediately. The seizures may recur many times during the day. Because of the rapidity of the change in posture, injuries are frequently sustained. A hockey helmet or other protective type of headgear may be required to shield the child from serious injury.

Myoclonic seizures, which consist of brief muscle contractions, may be generalized (massive) or restricted to several muscle groups (isolated). The muscle contractions may produce sudden flexion or extension. There is no loss of consciousness with the attack. They may recur many times during the day, but are especially frequent when the patient is either falling asleep or awakening. They are often triggered by emotional stress, tactile stimulation, or abrupt sound.

These seizures are generally resistant to treatment. Combined drug therapy is usually required. Diazepam (Valium), clonazepam (Clonopin), and valproic acid (Depakene) are the drugs of choice. Each of these drugs should be started in a small dose and gradually increased in order to avoid somnolence, fatigue, and other unpleasant side effects. Clonazepam (Clonopin) and valproic acid (Depakene) should not be given together, as there is a danger of absence status. Mephobarbital (Mebaral) and acetazolamide (Diamox) combined with either ethosuximide (Zarontin), trimethadion (Tridione), or imipramine hydrochloride (Tofranil)* may be efficacious. Other drugs such as metharbital (Gemonil), paramethadione (Paradione), phenytoin (Dilantin), and primidine (Mysoline) may be beneficial.

Infants with massive myoclonic jerks associated with the hypsarrhythmic pattern on the electroencephalogram have a poor prognosis in regard to mental development and neurologic maturation. If these seizures occur within the first 3 months of life, they are usually associated with severe, irreversible, and often progressive brain disease. They are very resistant to any type of drug therapy. On the other hand, the idiopathic group, with onset of seizures usually after 4 months of age, respond well to ACTH gel. This is given once daily by intramuscular injection in the dose of 30 to 40 units. The dose is decreased weekly by 5 units until a daily dose of 5 units is reached. The ACTH is then discontinued, and the patient is placed on oral hydrocortisone cypionate (Cortef Fluid), 10 mg. three times daily. The dose of this is gradually reduced and ultimately removed over the ensuing 6 to 8 months. If the seizures recur during the hydrocortisone treatment, the ACTH gel treatment may be repeated. The prognosis for this group is much more optimistic than for those having an early onset of seizures.

Petit Mal Seizures. This classification includes only patients who have simple staring spells, associated with loss of awareness for 5 to 30 seconds, and whose electroencephalograms display the typical 2½ to 3 per second spike and wave pattern. Frequently, there is some minimal rhythmic twitching of the eyelids or eyebrows at a rate of about 3 per second. The patient usually stops his activity, including speech, but will not fall. There is no confusion after the attack. The child is immediately aware of his surroundings. He is not cognizant of the spell. The seizures may be infrequent or may recur several hundred times a day. The spells can generally be precipitated if the patient is made to hyperventilate. This type of seizure is rarely seen after puberty. The prognosis for these patients is excellent.

Ethosuximide (Zarontin) is the drug of choice in the treatment of petit mal because of its efficacy and its sparsity of side effects. It is started in the dosage of 1 capsule (250 mg.) per day and increased 1 capsule every 3 days until seizure control is established. The maximal dose used is generally 8 capsules per day. Phensuximide (Milontin) and methsuximide (Celontin) may be used but they are usually not as effective as ethosuximide (Zarontin). Diazepam (Valium), clonazepam (Clonopin), and valproic acid (Depakene) are very efficacious drugs in petit mal. These drugs are introduced slowly and increased gradually until control of seizure is obtained. Trimethadione (Tridione) may successfully control attacks in children who have been resistant to other drugs. Rarely, it is necessary to combine it with another of the mentioned drugs. If trimethadione (Tridione) is used, it should be given simultaneously with a barbiturate or phenytoin (Dilantin) since alone it may produce grand mal attacks in some susceptible patients. Other drugs that can be used either alone or combined with the previously mentioned medications are paramethadione (Paradione), acetazolamide (Diamox), imipramine hydrochloride (Tofranil), (investigational) dextroamphetamine sulfate (Dexedrine), methamphetamine hydrochloride (Desoxyn), quinacrine hydrochloride (Atabrine) (investigational), or chloroquine (Aralen) (investigational).

Photophobia is a frequent side effect of the "diones." Patients may be more comfortable if they wear dark glasses on sunny days. All patients taking trimethadione (Tridione), paramethadione (Paradione), ethosuximide (Zarontin), and quinacrine hydrochloride (Atabrine) should have monthly blood examinations, as rare cases of aplastic anemia have been reported in patients taking these drugs. If the total neutrophil count drops below 1500 the medication should be stopped promptly. Nephrosis is an extremely rare complication of trimethadione therapy. Nausea and anorexia, the main side effects of ethosuximide, may usually be avoided if the medication is given after

---

*This use of imipramine is not listed in the manufacturer's official directive.

meals. As mentioned previously, clonazepam (Clonopin) and valproic acid (Depakene) should not be given simultaneously, as petit mal may occur.

Psychomotor Seizures. Because of the unusual behavioral changes that occur during psychomotor attacks these spells may be misinterpreted as bouts of mental derangement. They are characterized by a clouding of awareness and the performance of inappropriate, disorganized motor acts. These vary from simple grasping or searching movements of the hands to acts of roaming about the room, moving objects, or dressing and undressing. These children always have a vague or frightened facial expression, there may be pallor or flushing of the skin, there may be chewing and smacking movements of the lips, and the patient may mumble or repeat bizarre, irrelevant phrases. If approached during an attack these children may become combative. The attacks vary from seconds to several minutes in duration and are usually followed by confusion, drowsiness, or fatigue. These seizures tend to occur in flurries, several in one day or daily for several consecutive days, followed by days or weeks without symptoms. Auras, such as déjà vu, vertigo, gastric discomfort, "funny feeling" in the head, fear, tinnitus, micropsia, or macropsia often precede these attacks.

Phenytoin (Dilantin), phenobarbital, mephobarbital (Mebaral), primidone (Mysoline), and carbamazepine (Tegretol) are the drugs of choice in the treatment of these spells. At times methylphenylethylhydantoin (Mesantoin) may be more efficacious than phenytoin (Dilantin). Ethotoin (Peganone), acetazolamide (Diamox), diazepam (Valium), chlordiazepoxide (Librium), and phenacemide (Phenurone) are useful in this disorder. Combined therapy is generally necessary to control psychomotor attacks.

Seizure Equivalents. Seizure equivalents may occur without convulsions or loss of consciousness. These are very common in children and are the most subtle and most difficult to detect. They include recurrent symptoms such as abdominal pain, headache, nausea, cyclic vomiting, nightmares, sleepwalking, night and day terrors, disorders of behavior, enuresis, hyperthermia, and hypothermia. These may appear singly or several of them may be combined in the same patient. The diagnosis is established by history, electroencephalographic findings, exclusion of other causative factors, and response to anticonvulsant therapy. There are times when it is impossible to differentiate seizure equivalents from symptoms secondary to other conditions. Phenytoin (Dilantin) is the drug of choice since it is specific for epilepsy. Other medications may be employed if this is not beneficial. If the patient improves on therapy and one wishes to establish a relationship between cessation of symptoms and anticonvulsant therapy, a placebo can be substituted. There will be a recurrence of symptoms if it is a true seizure equivalent.

Mixed Seizures. Children frequently have more than one type of seizure. This is usually immediately apparent in most patients. Rarely, some patients may give a history of having only major motor attacks (grand mal) but are resistant to anticonvulsant drugs, which are generally efficacious for this type of attack. The details of the history and a reevaluation of the electroencephalogram should always be made when children do not respond to drug therapy, since any minor seizure may trigger a major convulsion if conditions are optimum. If therapy is not directed toward the minor attack, the major episode cannot be avoided. Therapeutic failures may be due to a mixed seizure disorder being unrecognized and inadequately treated. Combined drug therapy is usually required to control patients with more than one type of seizure.

Surgical Treatment

Surgery is very rarely considered in the treatment of seizure disorders in children. It would be contemplated only for the following reasons: (1) if the seizures continued unabated in spite of intensive drug therapy and the child were significantly disabled because of his attacks, or (2) if there were evidence of a progressive brain lesion that would be amenable to extirpation. Children displaying spike foci on the electroencephalogram without demonstrable cerebral lesions should not be explored surgically. Spike foci migrate in children and ultimately disappear in the majority of patients. A spike focus that persists in the anterior temporal region after the patient has reached the late teens or early 20s may require surgery.

HEADACHE

method of
MICHAEL ANTHONY, M.D.
Sydney, Australia

The vast majority of patients presenting themselves to the physician complaining of headache are suffering from chronic headache. Acute and subacute headaches are very commonly accompanied by other equally prominent symptoms (and frequently signs) referable to the nervous or other systems, that are difficult to overlook. In view of the above, this article shall only deal with the management of chronic headache and in particular with the management of migraine and tension ("muscle contraction") headache.

MIGRAINE

Introduction

The effective treatment of migraine presupposes a correct diagnosis. While this article does not deal with the clinical aspects of the disorder, it should be emphasized that migrainous headaches are episodic in nature with intervals of variable duration of headache freedom between attacks. Headaches that are supposedly migrainous but occur daily over weeks or months, should be regarded with suspicion, unless they are the result of excessive use of ergotamine preparations. In the vast majority of patients a careful history will clearly establish the pattern of the headache. In a few, where doubt remains, the patient should be investigated further or referred to the specialist for an opinion.

Pathophysiologic Considerations

A rational approach to the treatment of migraine also presupposes some knowledge of the main physiologic and humoral changes that accompany the attack. These are:

Changes in Cranial Vessels. The initial phase of the migraine attack is one of reduced cerebral perfusion, and this is generally thought to be responsible for the neurologic prodromal symptoms, e.g., aphasia, hemiparesis, fortification spectra, photopsia, whereas the headache is caused by dilatation and edema of the extracranial arteries.

Biochemical Changes. 1. A fall in plasma serotonin during the attack, which aids vasodilatation due to the withdrawal of the normal vasotonic influence of the amine. This has been observed in 81 per cent of patients studied.

2. Platelet monoamine oxidase activity has been found to be reduced during migraine, and this may be relevant to the serotonin loss mentioned above, as it is this enzyme which is responsible for the final breakdown of serotonin.

3. Certain free fatty acids (FFA), particularly stearic, palmitic, and oleic, are known to be potent releasers of platelet serotonin in vitro, and it is relevant that two groups of workers have recently reported significant increases in total plasma FFA levels during migraine. They could possibly act as serotonin releasers and in that case this may explain the susceptibility of certain patients to develop migraine following a fatty meal.

4. In women, migraine can occur in or about the time of menstruation. It has been shown that during the premenstrual period there is rapid fall in plasma levels of estradiol and that preventing this fall by regular injections of the substance can postpone the arrival of migraine. The regular administration of progesterone under similar circumstances has no effect on the headache. This finding explains, at least partly, the common clinical observation that administration of the contraceptive pill produces or aggravates migraine in some women.

Clinical Considerations

The first approach to the treatment of migraine should be an attempt by the medical practitioner to get as much insight as possible into the patient's problems, personality make-up, and reactions to various stresses in the environment. Psychologic treatment is rarely effective, but an understanding attitude goes a long way in sustaining the patient.

The role of precipitating or trigger factors is undecided, but if certain foods, e.g., fatty foods, chocolates, oranges, or certain wines, or some physical factor such as bright, hot sun bring on an attack, these should be avoided. However, it appears unnecessary that all migrainous patients should avoid certain foods or physical factors, unless these are definitely known to precipitate attacks.

Aggravating factors should be looked for, identified, and treated, where possible. These include arterial hypertension, cervical spondylosis, oral contraceptive or estrogen medication, mental depression, or excessive use of ergotamine.

Several other measures have been suggested and tried in the treatment of migraine — histamine desensitization, prevention of salt and water retention, surgical division of cranial autonomic pathways, ligation of extracranial vessels, and neck manipulation — all without effect on the course of the disorder. Drug treatment, however, seems to be the most satisfactory means of controlling the attacks. In the light of the physiologic and biochemical changes during migraine, the aim of treatment is to prevent vasodilatation, particularly in the external carotid bed, and therefore drugs used in the control of migraine fall into the following groups:

1. Those drugs producing vasoconstriction, e.g., ergotamine tartrate, dihydroergotamine, serotonin, and noradrenaline (including other sympathomimetic amines); the latter only for experimental purposes.

2. Those drugs acting as competitive serotonin inhibitors, by simulating the action of serotonin on receptor sites, e.g., methysergide, pizotifen (not available in the United States), cyproheptadine.

3. Those drugs blocking β-adrenergic receptor sites on blood vessels and thereby diminishing vasodilator responses, e.g., propranolol, pindolol (may not be available in the United States).

4. Drugs that inactivate monoamine oxidase and prevent the metabolic breakdown of vasoactive monoamines, e.g., serotonin and noradrenaline. These include phenelzine and tranylcypromine.

Treatment of the Acute Attack

Simple Analgesics. Many patients have migraine of such mild degree that no medical attention is necessary, and simple analgesics such as aspirin, acetaminophen (paracetamol), or codeine phosphate, either alone or in combination, give excellent relief. It is only when attacks cannot be controlled by such remedies that specific therapy will be required.

Ergotamine Therapy. Ergotamine tartrate in one form or another is the cornerstone of treatment of the migraine attack. It is effective in relieving attacks in about 80 per cent of patients. Its use, however, is bedevilled by an exaggerated fear of potentially harmful side effects. In fact, vasoconstrictive phenomena are rare with therapeutic doses, providing the patient does not suffer from vascular disease (arterial or venous), hypertension, impaired renal or liver function, or sepsis. Ergotamine is best avoided in pregnancy, although it can be used with caution if really indicated, as it has little oxytocic effect.

Ergotamine Habituation. The daily use of the drug may lead to habituation, a state characterized by daily rebound headache when the effect of the drug ceases a few hours after it is taken. This leads to further medication, producing a vicious circle, which can only be broken by a careful supervised withdrawal, best carried out in a hospital. During the "weaning-off" period which may last 2 to 4 weeks, headaches should be treated by analgesics such as pentazocine, 30 to 45 mg. intramuscularly, or codeine phosphate, 30 to 45 mg. orally, to be repeated in 4 hours if necessary, Narcotic analgesics such as meperidine (pethidine) or morphine should be avoided in view of the chronicity of the disorder and the possibility of dependence. Antiemetics such as prochlorperazine or thiethylperazine could be used to relieve nausea and vomiting, either parenterally or as suppositories. Once the daily use of ergotamine has ceased, the patient should be given preventive therapy, if he experiences two or more headaches per month.

Selection and Use of an Ergotamine Preparation. There is a large number of preparations containing ergotamine tartrate, either alone or in combination with other therapeutic agents, but not all are suitable for every patient. A trial and error method has to be used until individual patients find the most suitable one for themselves. To be fully effective, ergotamine tartrate should be given early in the attack and in proper doses. Unfortunately, with doses of more than 2 to 3 mg. ergotamine tartrate taken at once, many patients complain of side effects such as nausea, aching muscles, or signs of peripheral ischemia. In order to forestall such side effects it is probably reason-

able to ask patients to take 2 mg. ergotamine tartrate at the onset of the attack, and to repeat this in 30 to 60 minutes if no improvement is noted in that time. Rest in darkness seems to enhance the action of the drug. Ergotamine tartrate is available in a variety of dosage forms and dosage regimens.

Adjunctive Drug Treatment. Other treatment, such as sedatives or hypnotics, might be quite helpful in combination with ergotamine tartrate in relieving the acute attack. It is surprising how many patients have found that "sleeping off" an attack is a successful way of gaining relief. In such a patient, 100 to 200 mg. of sodium pentobarbital (pentobarbitone) or 5 to 10 mg. nitrazepam (not available in the United States) could be useful. If vomiting is severe, prochlorperazine or thiethylperazine could be used to control it, either as suppositories or parenterally administered.

Prevention of Frequent Attacks

Continuous medication for the prevention of frequent attacks of migraine should be considered in any patient who experiences two or more attacks per month. The aim of treatment is to prevent the headache completely, or materially reduce its severity. Many drugs are used for this purpose and the most important are described below.

Phenobarbital (Phenobarbitone), Belladonna, and Ergotamine. A combination of phenobarbital, 20 mg., belladonna, 0.1 mg., and ergotamine tartrate, 0.3 mg. The dose is 1 tablet two or three times daily. It is useful mainly in children and in some adult patients in whom the rate of improvement is about 35 per cent.

Pizotifen (Not Available in the United States). At present, this is the drug of choice for the adult who is given preventive treatment for the first time. It has both antiserotonin and antihistaminic effects. Initial treatment is 1 tablet (0.5 mg.) three times daily, which is increased a week later to 2 tablets three times daily. At the latter dosage improvement rate is about 50 per cent. Its two most common, and possibly the only significant, side effects are drowsiness and weight gain due to increased appetite. Drowsiness can be prevented by introducing the drug slowly, as suggested above. The effectiveness of the drug should be assessed at the end of a month, preferably two months. A change to another drug can be made at the end of that period if there has been less than 50 per cent reduction in the frequency of the attacks.

Cyproheptadine. The mode of action, its structure, and side effects are similar to those of pizotifen. The initial dose is 1 tablet (4 mg.) three times daily, increasing to 8 mg. three to four times daily in a few days. The rate of improvement is about 45 per cent. It may be used in some patients where pizotifen is not available or has failed.

β-Adrenergic Antagonists. Propranolol has been studied extensively in the prevention of migraine. (This use is not listed in the manufacturer's official directive.) The rate of reduction of headache frequency by 50 per cent or more in the 7 clinical trials published so far varies from 55 to 81 per cent. The dose used was 60 to 160 mg. daily and the drug can be given on a twice daily dosage. Side effects are usually mild and no patient had to abandon treatment because of them. The most common are insomnia and fatigue. In two small trials using pindolol (may not be available in the United States), a drug with an indole ring nucleus but a typical β-blocking side chain, the drug was no more effective than placebo in the prevention of headaches. However, in a recent trial using pindolol and comprising a larger number of patients (79), it was found that 52 per cent of patients improved by experiencing less than half the number of headaches. The dose of pindolol used was 2.5 mg. (half a 5 mg. tablet) initially and gradually reaching 2.5 mg. four times daily, over a period of 1 week. The common side effects were nausea, ataxia, continuous headache, or cramps in legs or buttocks. These occurred in 15 patients, but only 8 abandoned treatment because of them. The incidence of side effects can be appreciably reduced by introducing the drug slowly, as suggested earlier. Of course, it is to be understood that the drugs are not prescribed when contraindications exist, particularly a history of asthma or bronchial constriction or decompensated cardiac failure.

Methysergide. The drug acts by simulating the action of serotonin on receptor sites. As a result, it increases vascular tone and therefore, vasoconstrictive phenomena at the periphery is one of its more important side effects. The similarity of its action to serotonin is also reflected by another potentially serious but fortunately very rare complication, i.e., fibrotic reactions in the retroperitoneal space or the heart valves. It has been noted that valvular fibrosis due to methysergide and those seen in the carcinoid syndrome are very similar.

Despite these potential complications, methysergide is by far the most useful effective drug in the treatment of migraine and, provided it is used carefully, there is no need to fear serious complications. A test dose of 0.5 mg. (half a tablet) should be given initially to exclude idiosyncrasy, followed by 1 mg. daily and gradually increased to 1 mg. four times daily or 2 mg. two times daily, over a period of 1 week. The drug is best given after meals to reduce the risk of gastric irritation.

Withdraw the drug for 1 month in every 6 in order to forestall the development of retroperitoneal fibrosis. In any case, patients on methysergide should be kept under regular medical supervision for side effects (peripheral vasoconstriction, intermittent claudication, pallor of extremities, angina, indigestion, epigastric pain, exacerbation of preexisting peptic ulcer, retroperitoneal fibrosis). Therefore, contraindications to methysergide treatment (most of them relative) include ischemic heart disease, peripheral vascular disease, hypertension, peptic ulceration, thrombophlebitis, and pregnancy. Eight to 10 per cent of patients are unable to tolerate methysergide, chiefly because of vasoconstrictive side effects, while 30 to 40 per cent experience temporary side effects, mainly muscle cramps or abdominal discomfort which, however, disappear within a few days or weeks. About a quarter of patients become almost headache-free with regular medication, while another 40 per cent improve substantially.

Monoamine Oxidase (MAO) Inhibitors. These drugs prevent the breakdown of serotonin and other vasoactive amines, and therefore lead to their accumulation in the body. Their disadvantage is the potentially serious side effects of paroxysmal hypertension following ingestion of foodstuffs containing tyramine and dopamine, e.g., cheese, vegetable or meat extracts, red wines, broad beans, etc. They also modify the action of a number of drugs and should never be used with meperidine (pethidine), morphine, reserpine, or other hypotensive agents.

MAO inhibitors are effective in preventing migraine in about 80 per cent of patients, even in those who fail to respond to other forms of preventive therapy. The drugs commonly used are phenelzine, 15 mg. three times daily, or tranylcypromine, 10 mg. three to four times daily. (This use of phenelzine and tranylcypromine is not listed in the manufacturers' official directives.) The use of MAO inhibitors for the prevention of migraine should be reserved for those patients with headaches resistant to other forms of medication. They should never be prescribed without a clear understanding of their mode of action, their side effects, and the exact dietary and drug restrictions that the patient has to observe carefully.

Clonidine. This hypotensive agent, which depresses both constrictor and dilator responses, has been found useful in the control of migraine. (This use of clonidine is not listed in the manufacturer's official directive) The dose used is much smaller than that recommended for hypertension. The usual dose is 25 to 50 micrograms, three times daily. Rates of improvement vary from those similar to placebo up to 53 per cent and side effects are uncommon and insignificant.

TENSION ("MUSCLE CONTRACTION") HEADACHE

The mechanism of tension headache remains an enigma. In view of recent research work, the contribution of muscle contraction is now highly questionable.

This form of headache is most unlike migraine. It is generally diffuse, poorly localized, of daily occurrence, low-grade in intensity, has a dull aching quality and rarely is it accompanied by other symptoms. Like migraine, 75 per cent of sufferers are women. Tension headache has its onset mostly during early adult life and persists most severely during the most productive years of one's life.

Treatment

1. Reassure the patient that there is no serious underlying cause. Sympathetic listening to the patient's problems and a full physical examination are mandatory. Skull x-rays and a brain scan are not unreasonable simple investigations, if they had not been performed before.

2. Psychologic treatment is very rarely effective. Simple, common-sense advice regarding various aspects of the patient's life may be more rewarding.

3. Relaxation, mental or physical or both, may be helpful and should be tried in every patient as a matter of course.

4. Pharmacotherapy still appears to be the mainstay of treatment.

Anxiolytic drugs, particularly diazepam, 2 to 5 mg., three times daily are quite helpful. If the patient responds, continue for about 6 months, then gradually wean him over a subsequent 2 months.

Antidepressants, particularly amitriptyline or imipramine, should be used, if the patient appears to be depressed rather than anxious. Begin with 25 mg. at night and increase the dose gradually until the patient is significantly improved or side effects appear. If the patient responds, attempt weaning after 6 months.

5. Local measures, such as heat to the neck (applied by the patient or given by a physiotherapist), neck traction, or injection of tender spots with local anaesthetic, are rarely effective.

Generally, the treatment of tension headache does not produce the same response rate as that of migraine. Our poor understanding of the mechanism of tension headache and the equally poor results of our treatment are, in fact, a great monument to our medical ignorance of the subject.

EPISODIC VERTIGO

method of
B. TODD TROOST, M.D.
Pittsburgh, Pennsylvania

Vertigo, strictly defined, refers to the *illusory* sensation of unidirectional movement. The patient may experience an illusion of environmental spin or of self-rotation. Unfortunately, most patients do not present solely with "true" vertigo as defined. The most common complaint is one of "dizziness," representing a host of symptoms. The physician must elicit, through careful history taking, the set of symptoms actually experienced by the individual patient. Some common symptoms reported are listed in Table 1.

It is clear that episodic sensations of vertigo, unsteadiness, or presyncope are produced by an exhaustive variety of causes. Rational therapy should be directed to the actual cause if it can be determined by history taking, physical examination, and laboratory evaluation. It should be acknowledged that despite all these, a significant number of patients cannot be easily diagnosed as having (1) peripheral vestibular, (2) central neurologic, or (3) systemic disorders as a cause for their complaints. In the absence of a definitive diagnosis, the physician may resort to empiric therapy directed at a set of symptoms and periodic reevaluation of the patient.

Peripheral Causes of Vertigo

"Peripheral" causes result from dysfunction of the vestibular end organ (semicircular canals, utricle and saccule; see Table 2).

Peripheral vestibulopathy is a category including nonspecific terms such as "labyrinthitis" that imply unproved inflammatory mechanisms.

TABLE 1. **Descriptions of Episodic Vertigo or "Dizziness"**

Vertigo	Bouncing
Unsteadiness	Falling
Imbalance	Swimming
Spinning	Staggering
Fainting	Moving
Lightheadedness	Passing out
Swaying	Tilting
Twisting	Listing
Blurring vision	Rocking
Disorientation	Oscillating
Poor equilibrium	Rolling

TABLE 2.   **Peripheral Causes of Vertigo**

1. Peripheral vestibulopathy
   (includes: labyrinthitis, vestibular neuronitis, acute and recurrent peripheral vestibulopathy
2. "Benign" positional vertigo
   (includes: benign positional nystagmus, benign paroxysmal vertigo)
3. Post-traumatic vertigo
4. Vestibulotoxic drug-induced vertigo
5. Meniere's syndrome
6. Other focal peripheral disease
   (includes: local infection, degeneration, genetic anomalies, tumor, otosclerosis, fistula and rarely focal ischemia and others)

It has been defined as single or recurrent episodes of sudden vertigo lasting from hours to a few days. The patient may experience a single or recurrent episodes of relatively severe vertigo with nausea or vomiting, especially evoked by movement but often not by a particular head position. A small number of such patients are eventually found to have more specific causes of their symptoms.

"Benign" positional vertigo refers to a symptom complex classically described as indicative of benign and peripheral (end organ) disease. These symptoms, differentiated from central neurologic symptoms, are outlined in Table 3.

The signs and symptoms of "benign" positional vertigo are transient (rarely longer than 60 seconds) and occur when the patient assumes a certain position, such as lying down and turning in bed or turning the head while driving. It has been correctly pointed out that such symptoms occur only upon change of position. Other causes of vertigo may be intensified by position change, but also occur spontaneously.

Post-traumatic vertigo may immediately follow head trauma with the implication of end organ damage (in the absence of other central or peripheral nervous system signs). The time to onset of symptoms is usually hours or days, but can be many weeks. The symptoms are those of peripheral vestibulopathy or benign positional vertigo.

Vestibulotoxic drug-induced vertigo is a category including those agents presumed or documented to have caused persistent injury to the peripheral end organ. Among such agents are streptomycin and gentamicin. Symptoms from bilateral end organ injury may persist despite immediate discontinuation of the drug. A distinction is made from the large group of agents that may cause any of the symptoms of vertigo (Table 1). Cessation of such drugs (grouped in systemic causes; see Table 4) usually results in diminution of symptoms as the drug is metabolized and excreted.

Meniere's syndrome is reviewed elsewhere in this volume. It includes attacks of severe vertigo and vomiting, tinnitus, fluctuating hearing loss, ill-described aural sensations of fullness and pressure, and spontaneous recovery in hours to days. The symptoms may be mimicked by other end organ disorders.

A wide variety of other focal diseases is included in the final category, including acute otitis media, chronic ear infection, heritable degenerative disorders of the end organ and local tumors. While focal ischemia or "stroke" of the end organ is often cited as a specific cause of vertigo, such isolated involvement is difficult to document. Vascular disease producing ischemia or infarction is usually accompanied by additional neurologic signs and symptoms and is therefore included in central or systemic categories depending upon actual cause.

TABLE 3.   **Characteristics of Peripheral vs. Central Vertigo**

SYMPTOM OR SIGN	PERIPHERAL	CENTRAL
Latency (time to onset of vertigo or nystagmus)	~ 3 to 45 seconds	No latency Begins immediately
Fatigability (signs and symptoms decrease after onset)	Yes	Persists
Adaptation (habituation) (lessening signs and symptoms with repetition of provocative maneuver)	Yes	No
Nystagmus direction	Direction fixed	Direction changing
Intensity of signs and symptoms	Severe vertigo, marked nystagmus, systemic symptoms such as nausea	Usually mild vertigo, less intense nystagmus, rare nausea
Reproducibility	Inconstant	More consistent

Central Causes of Vertigo

Central neurologic causes result from dysfunction of the vestibular portion of the eighth nerve and the vestibular nuclei within the brainstem and their central connections (Table 4).

Neural connections with the central vestibular nuclei include interaction with the vestibular portions of the cerebellum (primarily cerebellar flocculus), the visual sensory system, and afferent connections from muscle, joint, and tactile receptors.

Generally, central causes of vertigo are less common than peripheral or "systemic" causes. The symptoms are usually less prominent. Other neurologic involvement is recognized by the presence of additional objective neurologic signs on examination. Such signs include other cranial nerve abnormalities such as papilledema, facial weakness or numbness, ataxia, weakness, and hyperreflexia or sensory loss.

Brainstem ischemia (transient ischemic attack [TIA]) should be accompanied by symptoms in addition to vertigo or dizziness before such a diagnosis may be entertained. Among such symptoms are *transient* loss of vision, diplopia, perioral numbness, unilateral ataxia, and drop attack. If actual brainstem infarction occurs, neurologic signs should be present on examination such as those mentioned above.

Demyelinating disease should be diagnosed only following documentation of disseminated central nervous system lesions such as optic neuritis, transverse myelitis, internuclear ophthalmoplegia or other brainstem signs not due to other causes.

Cerebellopontine angle tumors uncommonly present solely with episodic vertigo. Special neurodiagnostic investigations are always needed to confirm this diagnosis (see laboratory investigations).

Multiple or isolated cranial neuropathies may be caused by focal or systemic involvement, due to a variety of causes including vasculitis, granulomatous disease, and meningeal carcinomatosis, but often elude precise diagnosis. Evidence of systemic involvement is elicited by history, physical examination, and laboratory evaluation.

Posterior fossa lesions in a variety of locations are unusual causes of isolated vertigo. The symptoms are usually mild and possess the central characteristics outlined (Table 2). Diagnosis and therapy directed to the underlying cause follow the appearance of new signs and symptoms. It is appropriate to note that newer high resolution rapid computed tomography has had a major impact in early diagnosis of monosymptomatic posterior fossa disease.

Seizure disorders, especially temporal lobe or psychomotor epilepsy, are rare causes of dizziness or vertigo. The patient's history almost always reveals additional symptoms such as loss of awareness, automatic behavior, or generalized seizure activity following an aura of vertigo. However, many patients with psychomotor seizures, documented by additional history and electroencephalography, occasionally have isolated auras, which include many of the symptoms listed in Table 1. Treatment of seizure disorders is discussed elsewhere in this volume.

Systemic Causes of Vertigo

"Systemic" causes have been given a separate category to include more widespread conditions that can secondarily effect peripheral and central vestibular structures to produce vertigo (Table 5).

Side effects of drug ingestion are frequently a cause of many of the symptoms in Table 1. Those listed (Table 5) are among the most common offending agents. It is imperative that every attempt be made to determine the type and quantity of medication being taken by the dizzy patient. Frequently, the elimination or reduction of medication such as mild "tranquilizers" will produce a clear-cut improvement.

The multiple causes of presyncope or postural hypotension are often responsible for complaints of vertigo or dizziness. Again, careful

TABLE 4. **Central Neurologic Causes of Vertigo**

1. Brainstem ischemia and infarction
2. Demyelinating disease: multiple sclerosis
3. Cerebellopontine angle tumor; acoustic neuroma, meningioma, cholesteatoma, etc.
4. Cranial neuropathy; focal involvement of eighth nerve or in association with systemic disorders
5. Intrinsic brainstem lesions (tumor, arteriovenous malformation, etc.), rare
6. Other posterior fossa lesions (primarily other intrinsic or extra-axial masses of the posterior fossa such as hematoma, metastatic tumor and cerebellar infarction)
7. Seizure disorders (rare)

TABLE 5. **Systemic Causes of Vertigo and Dizziness**

1. Drugs (including anticonvulsants, hypnotics, antihypertensives, alcohol, analgesics, tranquilizers, etc.)
2. Hypotension, presyncope (including primary cardiac causes and postural hypotension from a wide variety of causes)
3. Infectious disease (including syphilis, viral and other bacterial meningitides, and systemic infection)
4. Endocrine disease (including diabetes and hypothyroidism particularly)
5. Vasculitis (including collagen-vascular disease, giant cell arteritis and drug-induced vasculitis)
6. Other systemic conditions (including hematologic disorders [polycythemia, anemia, dysproteinemia], sarcoidosis, granulomatous disease, and systemic toxins)

historical review and documentation of physical findings such as cardiac arrhythmia or postural hypotension may direct further investigation and therapy.

Among the endocrinopathies that can cause disorders of equilibration are diabetes and hypothyroidism. Diabetes, with effects upon systemic vasculature and the nervous system, should be carefully ruled out. While much less common as a specific cause, hypothyroidism should be considered in patients with undiagnosed symptoms of vertigo. The remaining systemic conditions rarely present with isolated vertigo, but are included as additional primary or secondary causes that may produce such symptomatology.

The vestibular system functions to provide man with (1) spatial orientation, whether still or experiencing acceleration; (2) visual fixation during head or body movement or both (vestibulo-ocular reflex); and (3) feedback control of muscle tone to maintain posture. These functions and their control mechanisms are complexly interconnected. Thus the symptoms of episodic vertigo may reflect disturbances in more than one system. For example, the combination of "multiple sensory deficits" producing disorientation or dysequilibration may occur when vision as well as peripheral sensory structures are impaired.

An intact person may easily confuse afferent sensory information. This is exemplified by the sensation of spin or true vertigo experienced during full field optokinetic stimulation. Almost every person, while quietly seated, will still experience a compelling illusion of rotation while viewing a moving environment of optokinetic stripes (the circular-vection illusion). It is therefore not surprising to find patients with subtle abnormalities of peripheral or central vestibular mechanisms who experience definite momentary periods of disorientation while viewing a moving patterned environment. Some patients experience episodic vertigo during vehicular travel while observing repetitive visual patterns.

Most younger patients can easily compensate for unilateral peripheral vestibular damage. Frequently, older patients cannot, indicating either *bilateral* peripheral vestibular dysfunction or a separate central abnormality that decreases their ability to compensate. Episodic vertigo often can not be grouped into a specific category of peripheral, central, or systemic causes. The symptom complex may well represent a combination of abnormalities including incomplete adaptation.

Diagnostic Procedures

Specific quantitative tests of vestibular function may document the degree of dysfunction, provide insight into the actual mechanisms, and serve as a guide to therapy. A brief review of some quantitative tests of vestibular function and neuroradiologic procedures is given.

Electronystagmography (ENG). Most ENGs are performed in semiquantitative fashion, without (1) absolute values of eye movement position or velocity, (2) individual eye movement records, (3) reliable normal values and (4) subsequent correlation with specific pathology. Such tests are best utilized to define clear-cut peripheral disease (e.g., canal paresis). The documentation of "central" pathology is less reliably defined. ENG, nonetheless, provides a written documentation of vestibular function. With improved methodology and ongoing clinicopathologic correlation, quantitative eye movement recordings will yield useful information.

Quantitative Posturography. Quantitative analysis of the Romberg test provides a technique for evaluation of more widespread disorders of equilibration. Cerebellar, peripheral neuromuscular, vestibular nerve, and peripheral labyrinthine disturbances will become better differentiated as this procedure becomes documented and data are accumulated.

Quantitative Rotational Testing. A more physiologic assessment of peripheral vestibular function than caloric irrigation is provided by measurement of ocular movement during actual rotation (vestibulo-ocular reflex [VOR]). Such tests are performed in relatively few laboratories at present, but have the potential of providing reliable VOR data that will be useful in conjunction with other tests of vestibular function in defining diagnostic categories.

Computed Tomography (CT). Rapid, high resolution CT scanning has had a major impact on neurologic as well as neuro-otologic diagnosis. Newer techniques include intrathecal contrast enhancement. This technique in addition to hypocycloidal polytomography and stereoscopic posterior fossa positive contrast procedures will provide even earlier diagnosis of central and peripheral lesions.

Therapy

Therapy is outlined for *symptomatic* treatment of episodic vertigo. When definitive diagnosis such as acoustic neuroma, hematologic disorder, or systemic vasculitis has been made, the therapy must be directed to the underlying disorder.

Therapy for Vertigo and Associated Symptoms

A. Antihistamines
1. Meclizine (Antivert, Bonine), 25 mg. orally every 4 to 6 hours
2. Cyclizine (Marezine), 50 mg. orally every 4 to 6 hours; 100 mg. suppository, rectally every 6 to 8 hours; injectable form cyclizine

lactate, 1 ml. (50 mg.) intramuscular every 4 to 6 hours
3. Dimenhydrinate (Dramamine), 50 to 100 mg. orally every 4 to 6 hours; 100 mg. suppository, rectally every 12 to 24 hours; injectable form, 1 ml. (50 mg.) intramuscular every 4 to 6 hours; for intravenous therapy each ml. is diluted in 10 ml. of sodium chloride injection U.S.P. and injected over a period of two minutes

B. Anticholinergics
1. Scopolamine, 0.6 mg. orally every 4 to 6 hours
2. Atropine, 0.2 mg. orally every 4 to 6 hours; atropine tablets (injectable form), 0.4 mg. may be given sublingually

C. Sympathomimetics—ephedrine, 25 mg. to 50 mg. orally every 4 to 6 hours

D. Combination preparations
1. Donphen tablets. Composition: phenobarbital, 15 mg.; hyoscyamine sulfate, 0.1 mg.; atropine sulfate, 0.02 mg.; scopolamine hydrobromide, 6 micrograms. One or two tablets orally every 6 to 8 hours
2. Scopolamine, 0.6 mg., with ephedrine 25 to 50 mg., orally every 4 to 6 hours
3. Scopolamine, 0.6 mg., with promethazine, 25 to 50 mg., orally every 4 to 6 hours

E. Tranquilizers
1. Promethazine (Phenergan), 25 to 50 mg. orally every 4 to 6 hours; suppositories, 25 or 50 mg. rectally every 4 to 6 hours; injectable form, 25 to 50 mg. intramuscular every 4 to 6 hours
2. Chlorpromazine (Thorazine), 10 to 25 mg. orally every 4 to 6 hours; injectable form, 25 mg. intramuscular every 6 hours
3. Diazepam (Valium), 5 to 10 mg. orally every 4 to 6 hours

F. Antiemetics
1. Trimethobenzamide (Tigan), 250 mg. orally every 6 to 8 hours; suppository, 25 mg. rectally every 4 to 6 hours
2. Prochlorperazine (Compazine), 5 to 10 mg. orally every 6 to 8 hours; suppository, 25 mg. rectally every 12 hours

G. Others
1. Haloperidol (Haldol), 0.5 to 1.0 mg. every 8 to 12 hours
2. Bucladin. Composition: buclizine hydrochloride, 50 mg.; 50 to 100 mg. orally every 24 hours
3. Innovar. Composition: fentanyl, 0.05 mg.; droperidol, 2.5 mg.; this combination agent for parenteral intramuscular injection has been recommended for severe episodes of vertigo even though it is not listed as one of the indications for the drug in the manufacturer's prescribing information. Experimental protocols for its intravenous use in acute and recurrent severe vertigo show promising results. However, it must be regarded as experimental at this time.

MENIERE'S DISEASE

method of
RALPH A. NELSON, M.D.
Los Angeles, California

A diagnosis of classical Meniere's disease is based on a triad of (1) sensorineural hearing loss, (2) severe vertigo with nausea and vomiting, (3) tinnitus in the affected ear.

The attacks occur in episodic fashion, rarely lasting more than a few hours. Hearing tends to fluctuate between periods of exacerbation and remission, and the ear generally exhibits a sensation of fullness. Tinnitus is usually a "roaring," corresponding to those lower frequencies principally involved in the hearing loss.

In early stages of the disease, episodes are often severe and may be atypical, with symptoms confined to only vertigo or hearing loss. Over a period of time however, one will normally be able to elicit all the symptoms necessary to complete the triad. Diagnostic evaluation during this interval should include, in addition to the history and physical examination, those radiologic, audiometric, and serum studies necessary to eliminate other entities from the differential diagnosis. Later stages of the disease involve greater frequency but generally decreased severity of vertiginous episodes, while a progressive loss of hearing occurs.

Management

Meniere's disease may be managed in a stepwise fashion, depending on severity of symptoms and response to treatment. Elimination of disabling vertigo is the principal aim, but preservation of hearing is strongly desired. Both goals may be attained through medical regimens. However, surgical procedures are available in the event of medical failure.

Treatment of the Acute Attack. A patient with an acute episode of Meniere's presents as a disabled person with nausea, vomiting, inability to maintain balance, and uncomfortably loud tinnitus. Motion aggravates the symptoms and the patient will normally resist being moved about. Nystagmus is present.

Initial evaluation should seek to exclude (1) infectious, (2) traumatic, or (3) vascular causes for the neurologic symptoms. Vital signs, otoscopy, funduscopy, and a brief neurologic examination are performed.

An intravenous catheter is used to establish a route for medication and to correct any dehydration. Atropine, 0.4 to 0.6 mg. given subcutaneously, has been a standard emergency treatment. More recently, intravenous diazepam (Valium) has been used very successfully to stabilize acute episodes. I usually start with 5 mg. and will use as much as 20 mg. if necessary to control vertigo. Constant supervision of the patient is mandatory when administering intravenous diazepam.

Other medications such as intramuscular diphenhydramine (Benadryl), 50 mg., or dimenhydrinate (Dramamine) may be used as may suppositories. Oral medications may be effective in controlling symptoms over the next 24 hours. Intravenous histamine, 2.75 mg. over 1½ hours in 250 ml. of fluid, is also used each day for 3 days and may be followed with daily intramuscular histamine.

Long-Term Management. Long-term management must be based on: (1) definitive diagnosis as arrived at through a complete neuro-otologic evaluation; (2) medical therapeutic success in prevention of further vertiginous attacks and the progressive hearing loss that accompanies them; and (3) surgical intervention if medical measures fail to control the disease.

Medical Management

The precise cause of Meniere's disease is unknown, and for that reason types of medical therapy have been empiric. The methods include (1) the "Furstenberg" approach, using a salt-free diet and diuretics to reduce endolymphatic pressure and (2) the "House" approach, directed at each of the several possible etiologic sources of Meniere's.

I prefer the multiple drug approach, which includes (1) niacin in flushing doses of 50 to 200 mg. orally twice daily; (2) propantheline bromide (Pro-Banthine), 15 mg. twice daily; (3) bioflavonoid twice daily; (4) sublingual histamine 1:10,000, 2 drops twice daily; (5) diphenhydramine (Benadryl), 50 mg. at bedtime; and (6) dimenhydrinate (Dramamine) or meclizine (Antivert), 50 mg. three times daily as needed for control of mild vertiginous symptoms.

Medical management must also be directed at eliminating metabolic disorders such as thyroid disease, pituitary-adrenal disease, hypoglycemia, hyperlipoproteinemia, and diabetes mellitus, all of which have been associated with Meniere's disease.

Surgical Management

Surgical intervention is reserved for the patient in whom medical therapy is unable to prevent disabling vertigo or progressive hearing loss. It can be separated into procedures that preserve hearing and those that destroy it.

Procedures to preserve hearing include, in order of preference: (1) endolymphatic sac–subarachnoid shunt operation; (2) middle fossa vestibular nerve section; and (3) Cody tack operation. Sac operations provide the least morbidity to hearing, whereas middle fossa nerve section and Cody tack operations have a higher incidence of hearing loss. Overall results with the sac operation show elimination of vertigo with stabilized hearing in 60 per cent of patients. Another 20 per cent are improved considerably.

Meniere's patients who have lost useful hearing but still suffer from the disabling effects of vertigo should have a destructive procedure. Labyrinthectomy with destruction of the semicircular canals and cochlea is 85 per cent successful in eliminating vertigo. The most complete procedure is a vestibular nerve section through the translabyrinthine approach when Scarpa's ganglion is excised.

Prognosis

Most patients are managed successfully by medicines. However, progression of disease with expectation of medical rescue may compromise surgical attempts to stabilize hearing. Success with sac operations for eliminating vertigo and stabilizing hearing has been very encouraging and has led to earlier surgical intervention.

An entire spectrum of treatment is now available for Meniere's disease and a logical long-term management plan can be formulated, progressing to traditional destructive procedures only after exhausting several low morbidity approaches.

VIRAL MENINGOENCEPHALITIS

method of
DONALD GILDEN, M.D.
Philadelphia, Pennsylvania

Virus infection of the nervous system may be conveniently classified into four general types, each with different clinical features and outcomes. The most common form is *viral meningitis* or "aseptic meningitis," which is characterized by fever, headache, and stiff neck and occasionally accompanied by nausea, vomiting, irritability, lethargy, photophobia, vertigo, and pain in the back, neck, or abdomen. Physical examination reveals only fever and signs of meningeal irritation and rarely an associated rash. The most common causative agents are mumps virus, the enteroviruses (Coxsackie virus and Echo virus), California encephalitis virus, and the virus of lymphocytic choriomeningitis, in that order.

The second most common form of viral infection of the nervous system is *virus encephalitis,* the clinical symptoms of which are the result of viral invasion of the cerebral parenchyma. In addition to the above described features, there may be alterations in the patient's state of consciousness, focal and generalized seizures, hemiplegia, hemisensory loss, hemianopia, and cranial nerve palsies. The most common cause of serious viral encephalitis in the United States today is herpes simplex virus. The arthropod-borne viruses (St. Louis encephalitis virus, Western equine encephalitis virus, and Eastern equine encephalitis virus) may also cause an acute, devastating neurologic catastrophe, leaving in its wake serious residua characterized by mental changes, ataxia, hemiplegia, and often death. The third type of viral encephalitis consists of the *post-* or *parainfectious encephalopathies* associated with the exanthematous childhood diseases, such as measles and chickenpox The neurologic features are identical to those that may follow vaccination with live or inactivated virus. Pertinent symptoms and signs include headache, fever, mental changes, and focal neurologic deficit, which often occur 7 to 14 days after virus infection, although they may also occur at the time of rash. The fourth type of viral meningoencephalitis includes *chronic forms of encephalitis of proven viral cause.* Examples are subacute sclerosing panencephalitis (SSPE) and progressive multifocal leukoencephalopathy. These disorders are characterized by slowly progressive neurologic deterioration occurring over a period of many months or years. Mental changes occur early. Focal neurologic deficits are common, and myoclonic seizures are frequent in the later stages of SSPE.

Spinal fluid findings in the first two types of viral meningoencephalitis include normal or increased cerebrospinal fluid (CSF) pressure. CSF is clear or slightly opalescent and may contain 10 to 2000 cells per cubic mm., the average cellular response being in the range of 30 to 300 cells. Mononuclear cells usually outnumber polymorphonuclear leukocytes (PMN), although PMN may be seen within the first 24 to 48 hours after infection. The level of CSF protein is slightly elevated but does not usually exceed 100 mg. per dl. (100 ml.). CSF glucose is usually normal (except in some instances of mumps and lymphocytic choriomeningitis), and no microorganisms are seen on Gram stain, acid fast stain, or India ink preparations of the CSF sediment. The spinal fluid is always sterile on culture with conventional bacteriologic and mycologic media.

Management

The greatest hazard in management of patients with viral encephalitis is misdiagnosis and failure to detect a nonviral infection of the central nervous system (CNS) that requires definitive treatment. Therefore, as part of the "treatment" of virus infection of the nervous system, all disorders that may simulate viral meningoencephalitis should be excluded. This includes inadequately or partially treated bacterial meningitis, CNS vasculitis, granulomatous meningitis (tuberculosis, sarcoidosis, fungal infections, toxoplasmosis, CNS syphilis), and brain abscess with or without subdural empyema. As it may be extremely difficult to distinguish between inadequately treated bacterial meningitis and viral meningoencephalitis, if doubt exists about the presence of bacterial infection, it may be best to commit the patient to an antibiotic regimen for bacterial meningitis of unknown cause. Borderline depression of the CSF glucose, marked elevation of the CSF protein, or persistence of PMN in the CSF may suggest the presence of a disease other than viral meningoencephalitis. When the diagnosis is in doubt, repeated CSF examination is indicated.

The primary treatment of viral encephalitis consists of the management of the patient who has an altered state of consciousness, convulsions, metabolic derangements, and increased intracranial pressure. The efficacy of specific antiviral agents is still unproved.

Supportive Measures. Bed rest is advisable. Isolation may be preferred until the nature of the responsible agent can be reasonably well established. Isolation may be particularly necessary in patients who have an associated pneumonitis with cough and in patients returning from other countries with aseptic meningitis or encephalitis. Precautions should be observed in handling clothes and materials from patients, especially stools. Headache may generally be relieved with aspirin, acetaminophen, or codeine; rarely meperidine, 50 mg. every 4 to 6 hours, may be necessary. Fever may be treated with aspirin. Most viruses are thermolabile and modest temperature elevation may serve as a natural defense mechanism.

The patient should be assured of an adequate airway. Repeated suctioning may be necessary to prevent airway obstruction. Endotracheal intubation and sometimes tracheostomy are necessary. Vital signs (blood pressure, pulse, the reaction of the pupils to light, and the state of consciousness) should be recorded every 1 to 2 hours. Oral feedings should be given only to conscious patients with intact brain stem function and normal bowel sounds. Patients in coma may develop urinary retention, often necessitating a condom catheter for males or repeated aseptic catheterization. Patients should be placed on an alternating pressure air mattress and turned at least every 2 hours. If the patient is unable to move, passive limb movement should be performed frequently. Styrofoam boots or tennis shoes to keep the feet dorsiflexed may be necessary. Extreme hyperthermia may have an adverse effect on the encephalitis, in which case a cooling blanket may be necessary to keep temperature below 37°C. (98.6°F.). Patients with encephalitis may develop an inappropriate secretion of antidiuretic hormone and become water intoxicated, leading to deepening coma and possibly seizures. Close monitoring of serum electrolytes and urinary output is essential, and fluid restriction may be necessary. In rare instances hypertonic saline solution will have to be given to restore fluid and electrolyte balance.

Specific Therapy

Seizures. Initial seizures, particularly status epilepticus, may be treated with diazepam, 10 mg. intravenously, given slowly with continuous monitoring for respiratory depression. Anticonvulsant therapy should follow this initial treatment. A loading dose of phenytoin, 1.0 to 1.5 grams, given intravenously not to exceed 50 mg. per minute, or phenobarbital, 100 to 200 mg. intravenously not to exceed 25 mg. per minute should be given. Maintenance doses of phenytoin are 300 to 400 mg. per day in divided doses and phenobarbital 100 to 200 mg. per day in divided doses. Phenytoin should not be given intramuscularly. Blood anticonvulsant levels can be monitored as a useful aid to effective therapy. It is probably advisable to continue anticonvulsant medication for several months after recovery from the acute illness.

Cerebral Edema. Cerebral edema constitutes a major threat and may be the most frequent cause of death due to herpes simplex virus encephalitis. Incipient herniation syndromes can be temporarily managed with osmotic diuretics. Adults should be given approximately 500 ml. of a 20 per cent mannitol solution administered for a half to 1 hour (approximately 7.5 to 10 ml. per kg.). The repeated use of osmotic diuretics is decreasingly effective, and rebound increases in intracranial pressure may occur. Osmotic diuresis may be used in conjunction with insertion of an endotracheal tube and forced hyperventilation by an Ambu bag. When cerebral edema must be treated more definitively, dexamethasone should be administered intravenously at an initial dose of 10 mg. followed by 4 to 8 mg. every 4 to 6 hours for the first 24 hours. The possible benefit derived from corticosteroids for treatment of incipient herniation is probably greater than the risk that steroids will potentiate virus infection.

Antiviral Agents. Various antiviral agents have been tried in the treatment of virus encephalitis, particularly for herpes simplex type 1 encephalitis. Initially, promising reports for idoxuridine (IUDR) and cytosine arabinoside (Ara-C) have not been confirmed. Moreover, both drugs have considerable toxicity and Ara-C has immunosuppressive properties. Ara-C has been reported to be more effective than placebo in a controlled study of disseminated herpes zoster infection.

Adenine arabinoside (Ara-A, Vidarabine) is less toxic, and initial reports indicate its usefulness in herpes simplex virus type 1 encephalitis (investigational for this use). The dose is 15 mg. per kg. per day given intravenously over a 12 hour period for 5 to 10 days. Reduction of significant neurologic sequelae, however, requires early institution of drug therapy. Initial reports of the success of this drug need to be confirmed.

The use of interferon inducers (poly I:C; statolon) for treatment of viral infections remains to be tested in man. Interferon inducers do not reduce morbidity or mortality after experimental virus infection of rodents unless given before or at the time of infection.

Laboratory Data. Attempts should be made to identify the agent responsible for the virus infection. Acute and convalescent sera (4 to 6 weeks later) should be sent to the State Health Department for serologic testing. The throat, stool, blood, and CSF should be cultured. Repeated CSF examination may be necessary, especially to rule out CNS tuberculosis or fungus infection. Computed tomography brain scanning is a useful adjunct for monitoring of cerebral edema, detecting the onset of hydrocephalus, or helping to rule out cerebral abscess.

MULTIPLE SCLEROSIS
method of
GERALD F. WINKLER, M.D.
Boston, Massachusetts

Multiple sclerosis is a disease of the central nervous system characterized pathologically by foci of myelin destruction with relative sparing of axons, nerve cell bodies, and the other elements of nervous tissue. It is characterized clinically by episodic focal disorders of the spinal cord and brain that remit and recur, usually over a period of 2 to 3 decades. Typically, the attacks and lesions are disseminated in time and space within the central nervous system, although there are certain sites of predilection.

Treatment

The extremely variable and unpredictable course of multiple sclerosis makes it most difficult to evaluate any therapeutic regimen. No specific therapy exists. Management must therefore consist of symptomatic and supportive measures.

Treatment of the Acute Exacerbation

Rest is still considered a very important aspect of the management of the acute attack. For severe exacerbations, complete bed rest with bathroom privileges is fully justified. Where this cannot be achieved in the home setting, hospitalization is warranted. For exacerbations of lesser magnitude, diminished activity proportional to the diminished endurance and easy fatiguability, which so often characterizes such exacerbations, is called for. In this circumstance patients are advised to pay close attention to the priorities of what they must do and to conserve their energy for the accomplishment of only the high priority tasks.

ACTH and Corticosteroids. Two controlled studies (Miller et al.: Lancet, 2:1120, 1961; Rose et al.: Neurology, 20, No. 5, Part II, May, 1970) indicated that there was some value to ACTH treatment. The principal conclusion of the American Cooperative Study was that short-term, high-dosage use of ACTH hastened the evidences of improvement of symptoms and signs, but it could not be stated that the ultimate extent of improvement was greater than that attained by placebo. The study further concluded that their results provided no basis for recommending long-term use of ACTH in the treatment of multiple sclerosis. Currently, however, hospitalization for ACTH administration to treat acute exacerbations of multiple sclerosis is not reimbursable by Medicare, Medicaid, or private third-party payers because the Food and Drug Administration (FDA) has not found evidence of its substantial efficacy in treating multiple sclerosis. This determination has been made by panels established by the FDA to review drugs placed on the market before passage of the 1962 Kefauver Amendment, which required substantial evidence of efficacy. At present, this matter is under intensive review. The FDA Neurologic Drugs Advisory Committee, chaired by Guy McKhann of Johns Hopkins University, has recommended that ACTH be approved for use in acute exacerbations of multiple sclerosis. Furthermore, this committee found no evidence that the action of ACTH differs from that of corticosteroids in the treatment of multiple sclerosis.

These medications are capable of causing lysis of lymphocytes, reducing cerebral edema, stabilizing lysosomal membranes, and increasing the conductivity of nerve fibers. Thus steroids can work via mechanisms other than immunosuppression. It has been reported (Aita: Arch. Neurol., 35:183, 1978) that MS lesions detected by contrast enhancement on CT scanning may resolve with the use of corticosteroid therapy.

It is considered that the use of ACTH or corticosteroids is particularly suitable for a patient with acute optic neuritis, an acute first attack of multiple sclerosis or rapid worsening of the multiple sclerosis.

Since most acute exacerbations of multiple sclerosis begin to recover within a 2 week period,

the use of these medications is generally not started unless the patient has gone at least 2 weeks following an acute exacerbation without recovery. However, in circumstances where the exacerbation is particularly severe and disabling, and in the case of optic neuritis, it would be appropriate to begin the medications earlier. In patients with chronic MS who are having gradual deterioration, there is some justification for giving the patient a trial of this course of treatment.

An example of a dosage schedule for ACTH is as follows:

Aqueous ACTH, (20 units per ml.) 80 units intravenously for 6 to 8 hours in 500 ml. of 5 per cent dextrose and water for three days.

ACTH gel (40 units per ml.) intramuscularly in a dose of 40 units every 12 hours for a period of 7 days. The dose is then reduced by 10 units every 3 days as follows: 35 units twice daily for 3 days; 30 units twice daily for 3 days; 50 units once daily for 3 days; 40 units once daily for 3 days; 30 units once daily for 3 days; 20 units once daily for 3 days; 20 units every other day for 3 doses.

If prednisone is to be used, the following schedule would be suitable: 80 mg. daily for 7 to 10 days; 60 mg. daily for 5 days; 40 mg. daily for 5 days; 30 mg. daily for 5 days; 20 mg. daily for 5 days; 10 mg. daily for 5 days to complete a 4 to 6 week course.

For both ACTH and prednisone the precise dosage schedules are arbitrary and are set forth here only as examples.

The following measures are advocated in an attempt to prevent side effects:

Potassium supplements to prevent hypokalemia. Liquid potassium is advocated because the tablets have been known to cause perforation of the small bowel. Potassium chloride, 1 to 3 grams daily, is administered. Serum electrolytes are monitored at least twice a week.

Mental stimulation and sometimes psychosis can occur on these medications. A mild tranquilizer such as chlordiazepoxide, 10 mg. three or four times a day, is often helpful. Sleeping medication is also frequently needed when patients complain that they are unable to sleep because their minds are racing. Euphoria or depression may, however, become so severe that it becomes necessary to terminate the medication.

Gastrointestinal bleeding should be watched for carefully by the monitoring of the hematocrit and the stools. An antacid is given between meals and at bedtime, prophylactically.

Sodium retention can cause peripheral edema. The patient should be weighed regularly, salt intake restricted, and, if necessary, an oral diuretic can be prescribed.

Hirsutism and acne occur during the course of treatment but disappear when the medication is stopped. Some women complain of loss of hair after ACTH is stopped, but this phenomenon is generally moderate and self-limited.

ACTH and corticosteroids can activate tuberculosis. Therefore, a chest x-ray should be taken before therapy is begun. For those who have a previous history of tuberculosis, a prophylactic course of antituberculous therapy is worthy of consideration.

Paradoxically, there are occasions in which the use of the medication may impair the patient's ability to walk because it reduces the spasticity of the lower extremities which the patient was using as a crutch.

There are occasional patients who report that they require long-term alternate day steroid therapy in order to maintain the improvement they derived from the acute course of treatment. There is no statistical validation for this schedule of treatment. When the characteristics of the individual patient are particularly persuasive regarding the value of long-term treatment, the advantages of such a course of action must be carefully weighed against the well-recognized disadvantages of long-term steroid therapy (osteoporosis, aseptic necrosis of the femur, cataracts, hypertension, increased susceptibility to infection, etc.).

Indications for Hospitalization. Hospitalization of multiple sclerosis patients is commonly necessary at first to obtain studies to assist in the diagnosis and to exclude other forms of neurologic disease. In-hospital treatment is often required during acute exacerbations of visual disturbances, incoordination, paralysis, sensory defect, and other symptoms and signs of the disease. In-hospital treatment may also be required for management of long-term consequences of multiple sclerosis, such as urinary tract and other intercurrent infections, decubitus ulcers, severe spasticity, contractures, respiratory failure, and for illnesses suffered in common with the population as a whole. The symptoms of multiple sclerosis may worsen and the patient may require hospital care in response to an acute febrile or systemic illness that would be of little consequence to other people. In such instances, the stay may, of necessity, be prolonged. Rehabilitation programs for multiple sclerosis patients should have clearly identified feasible goals as well as measurements of achievement. (Patient Management Committee, Medical Advisory Board, National Multiple Sclerosis Society, 1974).

Management Between Exacerbations

Immunosuppressive Therapy. The idea that multiple sclerosis may possibly be caused by an immune phenomenon has led quite naturally to a consideration of immunosuppressive therapy. At present, there is no statistical evidence to indicate that this therapy is effective. The real and theoretical risks of such treatment (infection, neoplasia) make it necessary to consider this form of treatment to be purely investigational. The same comments apply to antilymphocytic globulin, which is capable of causing serious side effects including fever, rashes, thrombocytopenic purpura, and a Coombs' positive anemia (MacFadyen et al.: Neurology, *23*:592, 1973).

Dietary Treatment. As with many diseases lacking a specific therapy, attempts at finding beneficial dietary modifications have been legion. The best known has been the low-fat diet advocated by Swank. In a review of 20 years of the use of this low-fat diet in patients with multiple sclerosis (Swank, R. L.: Arch. Neurol., *23*:460, 1970), Swank concluded that the course of the disease in these patients was less rapidly progressive than in untreated patients available in the literature for comparison. Swank acknowledges that such a comparison is not as satisfactory as a randomized control. There is even less evidence to support the efficacy of sunflower oil, vitamin E, and megavitamins. At present, the consensus is that no diet has been scientifically shown to modify the natural course in multiple sclerosis. It would seem best to advocate only a varied, well-balanced diet. Reduction of the animal fat content of such diets can be justified on the basis that it may reduce the likelihood of development of atherosclerosis but not on the basis that it will benefit multiple sclerosis.

Pregnancy. Uncomplicated multiple sclerosis has almost no effect upon pregnancy. If a neurogenic bladder exists, a gravid uterus will interfere with bladder and bowel function. Urinary tract infection will be more frequent. Studies differ in their estimates of the effect of pregnancy on the relapse rates of multiple sclerosis. It does appear that there may be some heightened risk of relapse, particularly during the first 3 months postpartum. One factor may be exhaustion from the chores of caring for a newborn infant. In counseling patients one must take into consideration the current size of the family, the severity of disability already sustained by the patient, and the means available to provide the mother with additional help during the postpartum period so that she will not be subject to exhaustion. The need for help in the care of the children must be stressed. (Donaldson, R. O.: *Neurology of Pregnancy,* Saunders, 1978).

Immunizations. Because of the suspicion that disordered immune mechanisms may play a role in the pathogenesis of multiple sclerosis and because of the relationship between some immunizations and the occurrence of acute monophasic demyelinative disorders of the central and peripheral nervous system, some clinicians have been understandably reluctant to have their MS patients receive immunizations. This concern was heightened by the reported association between swine flu vaccination and the Landry-Guillain-Barré syndrome. However, Bamford et al. (Arch. Neurol., *35*:242, 1978) reported that in a series of 127 patients, equally divided between those who received the swine flu vaccination and those who did not, there was no significant difference in the incidence of exacerbations of multiple sclerosis or toxic reactions to the vaccine. Brooks et al. (Neurology, *28*:393, 1978) consider that, at this time, split product vaccines are the immunogen of choice in influenza virus prophylaxis for MS patients because, both in MS patients and in controls, this vaccine had a lower incidence of immediate side effects than did the whole virus immunogen.

House Pets.   Recently, attention has been directed to a suspected association between house pets and multiple sclerosis. In particular, Cook and Dowling (Lancet, *1*:980, 1977) reported that exposure to small indoor pets (cats or dogs) was significantly higher in their MS group than in their control group. In response, Poskanzer et al. (Lancet, *1*:1204, 1977, stated that they found no significant differences in degree of contact among MS patients and controls to over a dozen domestic farm animals and house pets. This matter is still sub judice. Therefore, there does not appear to be sufficient evidence to justify advising the wholesale elimination of household pets. Even assuming the existence of a true causal relationship, it is doubtful that elimination of such contact after the disease has become manifest would be of any value to the patient. Kurland and Brian (Ann. Neurol., *3*:97, 1978) comment, "It is certain that for the present, a skeptical perspective must be maintained and cautious judgment employed in the evaluation of this newest lead in the search for the cause of MS."

Management of Chronic Problems

Treatment of Spasticity.   Spasticity is a general term that covers a variety of physiologic phenomena. For patients afflicted with painful flexor spasms of the lower extremities, baclofen (Lioresal) has proved highly effective and is now approved for general marketing. Although dosages should be titrated on an individual basis, an advisable starting dose for most patients is 5 mg. every 3 days until a therapeutic response or a maximum dosage of 20 mg. four times a day is reached. Thus far, laboratory tests have shown no drug-related abnormalities and significant effects on blood pressure and pulse rates have not been

observed. Drowsiness can occur. Baclofen acts to block excitatory synapses on spinal motoneurons, especially those in the primary afferent pathway.

Dantrolene acts to produce a purely peripheral effect on excitation-contraction coupling in muscle fibers and produces reduction in spasticity by actual weakening of the muscles. This, combined with the side effect of hepatotoxicity has dissuaded me from using this medication.

Diazepam (Valium) has the capacity to lessen muscle tone in spastic patients. It is worth trying, but one should be alert for the side effects of drowsiness and depression.

For those patients who are bedridden with total loss of lower extremity and bladder function, severe sustained flexor tone that impedes proper nursing can be dealt with by surgical rhizotomy or intrathecal injections of phenol. These measures are not advocated for those patients who retain some lower extremity or bladder function because the procedure itself may abolish such function.

Bladder Dysfunction.   The management of bladder dysfunction in multiple sclerosis was discussed in a most comprehensive manner by John Sullivan in Current Therapy 1977. The discussion which follows has been abstracted and modified from Dr. Sullivan's 1977 Current Therapy article by Elliott Marcus for Current Therapy 1978.

Bladder dysfunction may create intolerable embarrassment and discomfort. Most importantly, it may lead to early debility and death of the patient from recurrent infection and by promoting the development of decubitus ulcers.

It is our custom to inquire about bladder function early in the course of the disease. Often, the patient is unaware of subtle changes that have occurred. Urgency and incontinence are noted, of course, by the patient, but decreased bladder sensation, diminished force of the stream, and a lengthening of the intervals between voiding may have gone unnoticed.

Formerly, we tended to oversimplify and to think in terms of upper and lower motor neuron types of bladder disturbance. Thus urgency, frequency, and uninhibited incontinence implied a suprasegmental lesion, a spastic bladder. Conversely, a large capacity, disturbance of bladder sensation, difficulty in initiating voiding, and finally frequency, dribbling urination, and overflow incontinence equaled a segmental lesion and an atonic insensitive bladder. Animal experimentation, study of spinal cord injury patients, cystometry, and electromyography have provided more detailed and accurate information. However, multiple sclerosis does not provide a complete, static, and permanent lesion as in spinal cord injury. All varieties of neurogenic bladder may be seen in patients with multiple sclerosis, and a patient may show evidence of incomplete lesions at more than one level in the nervous system. Cerebral, brainstem, cerebellar, cord, and conus medullaris lesions may influence bladder function in varying degrees in the same patient.

UNINHIBITED NEUROGENIC BLADDER. Lesions that interrupt the pathways from the frontal cortex to the pontomesencephalic reticular formation may result in the uninhibited neurogenic bladder. Since this system receives input from the cerebellum, basal ganglia, thalamus, and hypothalamus, the potential for plaques to partially interrupt this system can be readily understood. Inhibition of the micturition reflex may be defective. The patient has a decreased bladder capacity, but no residual urine. Infection, therefore, is not a problem. The uninhibited contractions may be modified by anticholinergic medication such as oxyphencyclimine (Daricon). (This use of oxyphencyclimine is not listed in the manufacturer's official directive.) Therapy is begun at 5 mg. twice daily and the dose titrated as necessary. The patient is instructed concerning excessive effects resulting in urinary retention. Propantheline bromide (Pro-Banthine), 15 mg. two or three times a day, may be employed instead of Daricon. (This use of propantheline is not listed in the manufacturer's official directive.)

REFLEX NEUROGENIC BLADDER. Lesions of the spinal cord above the conus medullaris produce this type of disorder, i.e., a spastic bladder. In multiple sclerosis, the total picture may be present or various fragments may be encountered, depending upon the degree of damage to the spinal cord. Voluntary initiation of urination may be lost. There are uninhibited contractions and a reduced bladder capacity, and there may be residual urine. The latter is due to outlet obstruction, often caused by increased tone of the periurethral musculature. Some degree of bladder sensation may be retained, particularly if the lesions are located above the midthoracic spinal cord.

Early recognition and treatment of fragmentary and minor degrees of reflex neurogenic bladder are essential, because infection and interstitial cystitis may lead to a small contracted bladder, ureteral reflux, and pyelonephritis. The patient is trained from the beginning to regulate fluid intake in evenly measured amounts throughout the day, and to void "by the clock," ideally at 2½ to 3 hour intervals. Uninhibited contractions may be alleviated by anticholinergic drugs, as in the uninhibited neurogenic bladder. In severe degrees of reflex neurogenic bladder in males, it may be necessary to reduce resistance to outflow by doing a sphincterotomy and collecting urine with a condom and leg bag. In females, there is no satisfactory external collection system, and we may be forced to use a balloon plastic catheter. The largest

size should be used to reduce intravesical pressure and to minimize the danger of plugging of the catheter by accretions. A plugged catheter must be cleared immediately. The incidence of bacteriuria rises sharply with an inlying catheter; if clinical signs of infection occur, short-term treatment with antibiotics is indicated. The selection of the antibiotic should be based on the results of sensitivity studies. We have found the combination of trimethoprim and sulfamethoxazole (Bactrim) to have a wide-range effect and to be convenient in dosage and relatively free of side effects.

AUTONOMOUS NEUROGENIC BLADDER. In multiple sclerosis, the autonomous neurogenic bladder represents involvement of the conus medullaris and interruption of the vesical reflex arc. As there are varying degrees of sensory and motor-paralytic bladder, clinically it may be confused with spastic urgency, because if sensation is partially retained, there may be a sense of urgency with frequency and overflow incontinence. Urologic evaluation reveals a loss of voluntary micturition, voiding by the Credé method and abdominal straining, a large residual, and impaired bladder sensation. There may be local signs, a change in sacral sensation, and a loss of the anal reflex. In patients with minor degrees of sensory and motor paralysis the use of bethanechol (Urecholine) four times daily will be beneficial. The patient must develop methods of initiating voiding by coughing, contracting abdominal muscles, and compressing the lower abdomen. More severe degrees of dysfunction may require removing any obstruction to outflow (bladder neck resection) and a condom and collection bag in the male. Females may be taught sterile catheter technique for intermittent self-catheterization four times daily. In multiple sclerosis patients, fine hand control may be lost, and members of the family may have to assist the patient.

BLADDER SHOCK. An acute exacerbation causing damage to the spinal cord may cause bladder shock in multiple sclerosis patients. Infection or other trauma may also induce this in a patient who has previously had a reflex neurogenic spastic bladder. The shock bladder may persist for days or months and is characterized by inability to void, loss of bladder tone, and absence of bladder contractions. This will present a changing and often confusing picture, and repeated urologic monitoring will be necessary to recognize returning function. In the meantime, bladder drainage will be necessary, preferably by intermittent sterile catheter technique. If this is not available, a plastic tube suprapubic drainage or balloon catheter may be necessary.

Patients who are unable to completely empty the bladder and those who have an indwelling catheter will develop bacteriuria. If there are no clinical signs of infection, this is not terribly important, although patients may complain of the odor of the urine. Acidifying the urine by the use of ascorbic acid and methenamine mandelate (Mandelamine) should inhibit bacterial growth of both gram-positive and gram-negative organisms, but it is least effective for Proteus and Pseudomonas organisms. In general, it is not a good practice to use antibiotics prophylactically.

Where all conservative measures have failed and urinary incontinence has necessitated an indwelling catheter with consequent chronic urinary tract infection that threatens renal function, construction of an ileal loop bladder is indicated.

Bowel Management. Constipation and fecal impaction are particularly prone to occur in inactive incapacitated patients. Frequent small diarrheal movements may be an indication of impaction. Stool softeners, suppositories and enemas are sometimes necessary on a regular basis. Sudden bowel urgency and incontinence occur in rare patients. They can only be dealt with by prophylactic evacuation of the bowel with the aid of a suppository an hour or two in advance of special occasions.

Trigeminal Neuralgia. Trigeminal neuralgia, characterized by lancinating pains in the face, sometimes associated with trigger points, is often a symptom of multiple sclerosis when it occurs in younger patients. In MS patients the trigeminal neuralgia is caused by a placque of demyelination at the root-entry zone of the trigeminal nerve. Treatment of this symptom is the same as for idiopathic trigeminal neuralgia. Phenytoin (Dilantin) is the medication of first choice, in doses adequate to produce a therapeutic level of 10 to 20 micrograms per ml. (This use of phenytoin is not listed in the manufacturer's official directive.) If phenytoin fails to give relief, carbamazepine (Tegretol), a somewhat more effective medication but one that has a small yet definite propensity to produce marrow suppression, can be tried beginning with doses of 100 mg. twice daily and increasing if necessary to doses of 800 to 1200 mg. per day. The therapeutic range is 4 to 13 micrograms per ml. The drug should be taken with meals. After control of pain is achieved, a maintenance dosage of 400 to 800 mg. per day is usually adequate. At least once every 3 months an attempt should be made to discontinue the medication. Carbamazepine may produce dangerous and alarming side effects, primarily consisting of hematopoietic, cardiovascular, hepatic, and renal disturbances. Complete blood counts including platelet and possibly reticulocyte counts and serum iron determinations should be performed before initiating therapy. In addition, the tests should be repeated, possibly weekly, during the first three months of therapy and at monthly intervals thereafter for at least 2 to 3 years. The medication should be discontinued if there is confirmed evidence of bone marrow depression (erythrocyte count less than 4 million per cu. mm., hematocrit less than 32 per cent, hemoglobin less than 11 grams per dl. (100 ml.), white blood count (WBC) less than 4000 per cubic ml., platelet count less than 20,000 per cubic ml., and/or iron greater than 150 micrograms per dl.

When control of the trigeminal neuralgia by medication is inadequate, a selective thermal rhizotomy (radio frequency lesion of the trigeminal ganglion) stands an excellent chance of producing relief of pain with preservation of touch sensation.

Dorsal Column Stimulation. In the early 1970s there was a flurry of interest in the implantation of dorsal column spinal cord stimulators for the purpose of achieving improvement in voluntary motor control and sensory appreciation. It does not appear that this method of treatment has lived up to its early expectations and it cannot be recommended as an established therapy for these purposes.

The Spastic or Ataxic Gait. It is of course desirable that the patient remain ambulatory as long as possible. However, this may not be done at the expense of exposing the patient to injury from falls. Some patients express extreme reluctance to adopt the use of a cane or walker because they regard it as "giving in" or because they feel that it will have an adverse effect on how they are regarded by others.

When the gait is unstable and the patient is prone to fall, the patient should be encouraged to consult a physical therapy department where he can be instructed in the adoption of a broad-based gait to improve balance and where the various aids to walking, such as a crutch or walker, can be tried and the patient instructed in their use.

The services of the physical therapist are also of value in instructing the patient and the family in the performance of active and passive range of motion exercises for the purpose of maintaining full mobility of spastic limbs.

Exercises. For patients who are bedridden, full range of motion exercises become even more important in the prevention of contractures. In addition, proper care of the skin to prevent decubiti becomes of extreme importance. In such patients urinary incontinence must be dealt with effectively because prolonged contact of the skin with urine-soaked bedding enhances the rate of skin breakdown. Since many bedridden patients have sensory loss, they are all the more prone to development of decubiti, and changes of position every two hours, skin inspection, adequate padding to pressure points, and the use of a water or air mattress are important preventive measures.

Alterations in Affect.　Depression is actually more common than euphoria in multiple sclerosis. Of course, it is not a symptom specific to this disorder. When it occurs in severity sufficient materially to impair the patients' ability to cope, antidepressant medications or psychiatric consultation are indicated.

Seizures.　Seizures occur in about 5 per cent of MS patients. The source is usually a placque at the junction of cerebral white matter and gray matter. The treatment is the same as that of epilepsy.

Intention Tremor.　Intention tremor is commonly seen in multiple sclerosis patients due to the frequent involvement of the cerebellar peduncles. To the extent that this cerebellar ataxia of the extremities is aggravated by emotional tension, the use of a minor tranquilizer may be helpful, provided that the side effects of drowsiness and depression do not outweigh any benefits achieved. Some ataxic patients derive improvement in their limb coordination by wearing weighted wrist and ankle bands that serve to dampen the amplitude of the intention tremor. An occasional patient will exhibit extremely severe intention tremor. On rare occasions it may be justifiable to consider stereotaxic ventrolateral thalamotomy, an effective measure for abolition of this particular movement disorder. It is best to do this procedure on only one side in order to avoid an increased incidence of complications.

Prognosis

The study by Percy et al. (Arch. Neurol., 25:195, 1971) surveyed all the cases of multiple sclerosis diagnosed in Rochester, Minnesota at the Mayo Clinic and seen 25 years later. They found that 74 per cent of the patients were still living at the end of 25 years, compared with an expected figure of 86 per cent for the general population. Furthermore, two thirds of the 25 year survivors were still ambulatory. The average life expectancy following the diagnosis of multiple sclerosis is 25 years and the normal life expectancy is reduced by no more than 15 per cent.

The public perception of multiple sclerosis is that of a disease with a far worse prognosis. Many patients, when they first learn of their diagnosis, become very concerned that they are doomed to a wheelchair existence. In fact, for every patient who is confined to a wheelchair, there are four or five who are ambulatory and who would not be recognized by a casual observer as having the disease at all.

Because of the widely held pessimistic view of the outlook for multiple sclerosis patients, many physicians have been hesitant to inform patients of their diagnosis. For those patients who are merely suspected of having multiple sclerosis but in whom there is insufficient evidence to arrive at that conclusion with reasonable confidence, it is best not to suggest the diagnosis to the patient or stress it in the medical record because, if it later turns out that the patient does not have multiple sclerosis, there will have been caused unnecessary anxiety, and the premature entry of a diagnosis of multiple sclerosis into the medical record tends to inhibit the consideration of alternative diagnoses by any physicians who may subsequently have occasion to treat the patient.

For those in whom the diagnosis of multiple sclerosis is considered to be reasonably well established, it is desirable, in the vast majority of cases, to inform the patient of the diagnosis. This should be coupled with a realistic explanation of the statistical prognosis. It is advantageous to make the patient aware of the existence of the National Multiple Sclerosis Society and to encourage the patient to contact and join the local chapter of the organization. Such membership will provide access to updated information about the disease. The Society chapters can, in addition, be of substantial help to patients in coping with a variety of social, psychologic, and paramedical problems that may arise. In this age of widespread medical enlightenment in the community, it is no longer feasible or desirable to attempt to conceal the diagnosis. When relatives ask that the diagnosis be withheld from the patient, it should be pointed out that such an attempt would be doomed to failure and would only result in the ultimate undermining of the patient's trust and confidence.

MYASTHENIA GRAVIS
method of
CHRISTIAN HERRMANN, JR., M.D.
Los Angeles, California

Myasthenia gravis is a disorder of neuromuscular transmission of the striated voluntary muscles of the body. It is characterized by variable weakness and easy fatigability. After a short rest of the muscles there is partial to total recovery of strength. Extraocular, facial, and oropharyngeal muscles are commonly affected but the neuromuscular junctions for any of the voluntary striated muscles of the body may be involved. Commonly, it has onset in women before age 40 and in men after age 40. Either sex may be affected at any time, however. About 12 per cent of infants born to myasthenic mothers have a transient transmitted form of neonatal myasthenia which remits permanently in days or weeks. Pregnancy is generally not contraindicated in myasthenia.

Anticholinesterase Therapy

Anticholinesterase drugs are the usual first line of treatment for myasthenia gravis. Their action is attributed to inhibition of cholinesterase at the neuromuscular junction, permitting acetylcholine to accumulate and facilitate the remaining neuromuscular transmission. The three most frequently used are neostigmine bromide (Prostigmin), pyridostigmine bromide (Mestinon), and ambenonium chloride (Mytelase). These partially reduce the defect in neuromuscular transmission and improve strength but are not in themselves a cure.

A fourth, very short-acting anticholinesterase, edrophonium chloride (Tensilon), is used to aid in the diagnosis of myasthenia gravis and assess the effectiveness of dosage of anticholinesterase drugs mentioned. It is not used as an ongoing form of treatment. A list of commonly used anticholinesterase drugs and comparable dosage forms and routes of administration is given in Table 1.

The anticholinesterase drugs do not naturally occur in man nor are they lacking in patients with myasthenia gravis. Excessive anticholinesterase therapy may have adverse effects, increasing the weakness and provoking other unpleasant and potentially dangerous side effects. These are listed under Cholinergic Crisis in Table 2.

Anticholinesterase therapy by mouth may be cautiously started with ½ of a 15 mg. tablet of neostigmine (7.5 mg.) or ½ of a 60 mg. tablet of pyridostigmine (30 mg.) at 4 hour intervals or two to three times daily. For patients complaining of weakness in chewing and swallowing, it is best given 30 to 60 minutes before meals. Gastrointestinal effects will be less if it is taken with a small amount of milk, crackers, bread, or other bland food in the stomach. It should not be taken with coffee, fruit, or tomato juice, or carbonated or alcoholic beverages, which may increase the parasympathomimetic side effects on the gut, bladder, bronchi, and mucus glands.

The dosage may be increased gradually and the time interval shortened between doses only if these are followed by objective improvement in symptoms and signs. The physician and patient both must realize that anticholinesterase drugs usually do not restore muscle strength to more than 80 per cent of normal with optimal dosage. Weakness of extraocular muscles, oropharyngeal muscles, respiratory muscles and other muscles at times selectively or together may show little improvement in strength with anticholinesterase medication.

Neostigmine and pyridostigmine are quite similar in their action and effectiveness. Some patients note more muscarinic side effects such as abdominal cramps, diarrhea, nausea, tearing, salivation, and sweating with neostigmine than with pyridostigmine. The action of neostigmine is 30 to 45 minutes shorter than that of pyridostigmine. Weakness involving extraocular, oropharyngeal, and facial muscles may be more favorably improved with pyridostigmine. A few patients find that neostigmine provides more prompt and slightly greater improvement in muscle strength than pyridostigmine.

Additional helpful forms of pyridostigmine include the syrup containing 60 mg. in 5 ml. (approximately 1 teaspoonful). This is more palatable and easily administered and adjusted for young myasthenic children. Patients with swallowing difficulty may handle this form easier and with

TABLE 1. **Anticholinesterase Drugs Used in Diagnosis and Management of Myasthenia Gravis**

DRUG	FORM	ADULT SINGLE DOSE AND ROUTE	USUAL EFFECTIVE DURATION AND RANGE
Tensilon (edrophonium chloride)	10 mg. per ml.	2–10 mg. IV	10 minutes (2 minutes to 2 hours)
Prostigmin (neostigmine methylsulfate)	0.25, 0.5, and 1.0 mg. per ml.	1 mg. IM	2 hours (2–4 hours)
Prostigmin (neostigmine bromide)	15 mg. tablet	15 mg. oral	3 hours (2–5 hours)
Mestinon (pyridostigmine bromide)	10 mg. per 2 ml.	2 mg. IM	2 hours (2–4 hours)
Mestinon (pyridostigmine bromide)	60 mg. tablet	60 mg. oral	4 hours (3–7 hours)
Mestinon Timespan (pyridostigmine bromide)	180 mg. tablet (slow release)	90–180 mg. oral	8 hours (6–12 hours)
Mestinon Syrup (pyridostigmine bromide)	60 mg. per 5 ml. syrup	60 mg. per 5 ml. (1 tsp. oral)	4 hours (3–7 hours)
Mytelase (ambenonium chloride)	10 mg. tablet	5–10 mg. oral	6 hours (4–8 hours)

TABLE 2. **Symptoms and Signs of Myasthenic and Cholinergic Crisis**

MYASTHENIC CRISIS	CHOLINERGIC CRISIS	
	Muscarinic symptoms and signs:	*Nicotinic symptoms and signs:*
Ocular ptosis	Sweating	Muscle fasciculations
Dysarthria or anarthria	Salivation	Dysarthric speech
Dysphagia or aphagia	Lacrimation	Dysphagia
Dyspnea or apnea	Abdominal cramping	Trismus
Facial weakness	Nausea	Muscle cramps and spasms
Masticatory weakness	Vomiting	General weakness
Difficulty handling secretions	Diarrhea	
General weakness	Urinary frequency	*CNS symptoms and signs:*
	Incontinence of bowel and bladder	
	Miosis	Restlessness
	Blurred vision	Anxiety
	Bradycardia	Vertigo
	Bronchorrhea	Headache
	Substernal pressure	Confusion and stupor
	Dyspnea and wheezing	Coma
	Bronchospasm	Convulsions
	Pulmonary edema	

greater safety than with the tablets. It is also readily given by nasogastric tube. The other useful form of pyridostigmine is the Mestinon Timespan tablet containing 180 mg. of pyridostigmine. About one third of the dosage is released like regular pyridostigmine and the remainder is released over the next 6 to 12 hours. When given at bedtime it allows the moderate to severe myasthenic to sleep through the night without awakening to take regular anticholinesterase medication. It is not recommended for daytime use in the moderate or severe myasthenic requiring larger doses of anticholinesterase for whom the regular forms of the drug give more prompt and dependable release and absorption. Some mild myasthenics may find the Mestinon Timespan form of pyridostigmine satisfactory in the daytime. Usually only moderate to severe myasthenics require anticholinesterase medication during sleeping hours and the dosage may be reduced by one half to two thirds of that taken during the waking hours.

For patients temporarily unable to take their anticholinesterase drugs by mouth or unable to swallow, a parenteral form of neostigmine methylsulfate or pyridostigmine bromide may be given. The equivalent of a 15 mg. tablet of neostigmine is 1 to 1.5 mg. of neostigmine methylsulfate intramuscularly. The similar equivalent of a 60 mg. tablet of pyridostigmine bromide is 2 mg. of pyridostigmine bromide intramuscularly. Parenteral anticholinesterase therapy is seldom more effective than the oral route and is not practical for long-term care of the patient.

Ambenonium chloride (Mytelase) is a third available oral anticholinesterase drug but is used less frequently than neostigmine and pyridostigmine. Those patients failing to respond well to neostigmine or pyridostigmine may be tried carefully on ambenonium. Its effectiveness is generally less in weakness involving cranial nerve musculature than in the extremities. Its duration of action is a bit longer than that of pyridostigmine. Muscarinic toxic side effects are not prominent, but nicotinic and central nervous system symptoms and signs of toxicity may appear. These include muscle twitching and weakness for the nicotinic manifestations and headache, restlessness, and anxiety for the central nervous system. Between 5 and 7.5 mg. of ambenonium chloride is equivalent to 15 mg. of neostigmine or 60 mg. pyridostigmine tablets. When starting ambenonium treatment, begin with 5 mg. at 4 to 6 hour intervals and increase by 2.5 mg. per dose in the presence of objective improvement and absence of undesirable side effects.

It is helpful to examine patients just before their dose of anticholinesterase and approximately 45 to 60 minutes after it. Helpful points to test are ability to sustain upward gaze, looking for fatigue of the lid levators or extraocular muscles or both; continuous counting on a single breath gives a rough estimate of respiratory muscle strength; continuous counting may also detect fatigue of the speech muscles; the time the patient is able to keep the arms or legs or both elevated may be an indication of fatigability in these muscles; the number of times the patient is able to cross and uncross one thigh over the other, squat and arise, or repeatedly compress a rolled up partially inflated blood pressure cuff or hand dynamometer are simple tests of strength and fatigability of neuromuscular junctions in these areas. The ability of the patient to close his jaw tightly against resistance, protrude his tongue into each cheek against resistance, elevate the soft palate, cough, swallow, and talk is useful to assess oropharyngeal strength.

Measurement of the vital capacity is a simple assessment of respiratory muscle function and reserve. It is weakness in the oropharyngeal or respiratory muscle strength or both that constitutes the greatest single threat to the myasthenic's life. Treatment should be directed toward achieving optimal improvement in these areas.

The edrophonium chloride (Tensilon) test, which is a helpful diagnostic aid in myasthenia gravis, may also be used in an attempt to determine the adequacy of ongoing anticholinesterase treatment. One hour following the oral anticholinesterase medication, the patient's strength is measured. Then the patient is given 2 mg. (0.2 ml.) of edrophonium chloride intravenously and strength is retested after 30 seconds to 2 minutes. If the strength is significantly improved, the dosage of oral anticholinesterase medication may be increased. If the strength is unchanged or declines, the oral anticholinesterase dosage should not be raised. A control placebo injection may be helpful for comparison. If muscarinic and nicotinic effects appear after 2 mg. of edrophonium chloride, along with increased weakness, then the oral anticholinesterase dosage should be lowered.

Although certain differences are noted among neostigmine, pyridostigmine, and ambenonium, overall results are quite similiar. Of the three, pyridostigmine appears to be the most frequently used.

Crisis

The myasthenic may have increased weakness in his oropharyngeal or respiratory muscles or both, so that he is unable to maintain a patent airway or adequate respiratory exchange or both. Bilateral weakness of the vocal cord abductors may obstruct the airway or weakness of the respiratory muscles or both may prevent adequate ventilation. This is called crisis. It may be due to an increase in the myasthenia gravis itself. In this instance it is called myasthenic crisis. This is usually provoked by infections, especially upper respiratory infections. Menses, failure to take anticholinesterase medication, vigorous physical activity, certain drugs, and emotional upsets are other causes of myasthenic crisis.

Drugs having an unfavorable effect on neuromuscular transmission that may provoke crisis include most hypnotics and tranquilizers, phenothiazines, thiazides, quinine, quinidine, procainamide, ether, d-tubocurarine, pancuronium, morphine, and mycin aminoglycoside antibiotics.

Cholinergic crisis may be caused by too much anticholinesterase medication. It may develop in the course of a spontaneous remission, following thymectomy or from an over-enthusiastic use of anticholinesterase drugs by the physician or patient. Some patients become unresponsive, insensitive or resistant to anticholinesterase drugs, particularly when the dosage is gradually increased to high levels over a long period of time. The symptoms and signs of myasthenic and cholinergic crisis are listed in Table 2.

Whatever the underlying causes, the crisis usually develops rapidly with deterioration of the patient and constitutes an emergency. Prompt control of the airway and respiration is essential. Meticulous tracheobronchial toilet and treatment of infection are also important. The edrophonium chloride (Tensilon) test may be helpful to determine whether additional anticholinesterase is needed as outlined before. However, some patients may give a positive response to edrophonium chloride but fail to improve and even get weaker when more of the other anticholinesterase medication is given.

Because it is frequently impossible to determine rapidly the cause or causes of the crisis, tracheal intubation and positive pressure assisted respiration and equipment to aspirate secretions may be lifesaving. This may be followed by tracheostomy using a cuffed tracheostomy tube attached to the positive pressure respirator.

In the presence of cholinergic crisis or unresponsive and insensitive resistant state, anticholinesterases are stopped for 3 days or longer, following which the patient's strength and vital capacity may improve. This allows neuromuscular junctions that may be damaged and depolarized to recover. Fluid balance and nutrition may be maintained parenterally or by nasogastric tube. At times some patients withdrawn from anticholinesterase improve to such an extent that they may function for several days or weeks without anticholinesterase medication.

Atropine is best saved for use only sporadically or in emergency to counteract the muscarinic side effects of anticholinesterase drugs. Regular use obscures the signs of cholinergic intoxication. With atropine, oral and tracheobronchial secretions are reduced, and become thick, tenacious, and hard to aspirate. They tend to plug the bronchi and provoke atelectasis.

Sedative and tranquilizing drugs should be avoided in the anxious, apprehensive myasthenic because these symptoms and signs may be those of failing respiratory function rather than a psychologic reaction to illness. Such drugs may aggravate hypoxia and hypercapnia, setting up a vicious cycle of respiratory and cardiac depression, with vagal activity already increased by anticholinesterase medication leading to arrhythmia and asystole.

The patient in crisis should be turned frequently, given postural drainage, percussion to the chest, and careful tracheobronchial toilet. Auscultation of the chest, chest x-rays, and fiberoptic bronchoscopy may be helpful to remove mucus plugs. Smears, cultures, and sensitivities of tracheobronchial secretions and appropriate antibiotics will aid in recovery and reduction of mortality. Periodic determination of blood gases aids in the evaluation of the adequacy of mechanical ventilation and need for oxygen supplementation, adjustment of depth and rate of mechanical respiration, and so on. Automatic, periodic sighing available on some mechanical respirators may help prevent atelectasis and contractures of the chest wall from lack of full range of movement because of weakness. The lung in most myasthenics in crisis is normal once infection and atelectasis are overcome. For this reason compressed air is best used for long-term operation of the positive pressure respirator.

Thymectomy

Improvement or remission of myasthenia gravis following thymectomy has been reported in up to 80 per cent from several centers dealing with large numbers of myasthenic patients. It is most apt to occur in patients without thymoma, although thymoma, which may occur in 15 per cent of patients with myasthenia gravis, is also an indication for thymothymectomy, since up to 40 per cent of thymomas may become invasive or malignant. Thymectomy may alter autoimmune processes present in myasthenia, although exactly why improvement or remission occurs is not understood. Results cannot be predicted with certainty in any single patient. Thymectomy does not appear helpful in congenital myasthenia. It is not recommended for patients over 60 years of age in whom the thymus is usually atrophic, in debilitated patients, or those with thymoma showing evidence of malignant spread. Thymectomy is not undertaken as an emergency procedure in a patient whose myasthenia is rapidly worsening, in the presence of active pulmonary infection or pregnancy. Improvement following thymectomy may not occur for weeks or months. The operative risk is small in the hands of a competent thoracic surgeon in a facility where neurologic and medical staff are familiar with the disorder and have intensive care facilities including respiratory support available. The patient is allowed to take usual doses of anticholinesterase medication with small sips of water up to the time of surgery. Postoperatively, the anticholinesterase medication is resumed in 12 to 24 hours when weakness occurs. The dosage requirements may be less than pre-

operatively. Meperidine (Demerol) rather than morphine is used to relieve pain.

The transcervical or suprasternal approach to the thymus has been used at a few centers, but this is not usually satisfactory for removal of thymomas and may not allow removal of all thymic tissue. Most centers continue to use a median sternotomy, which avoids these problems.

Prethymectomy treatment of the myasthenic with moderate or severe oropharyngeal or respiratory muscle weakness or both, using alternate day corticosteroid therapy for weeks or months to improve strength and stabilize the patient before surgery, may be useful in a few patients of this sort. It is generally not recommended for all patients.

Corticosteroid Therapy

We no longer use intramuscular ACTH therapy but instead use oral corticosteroid therapy, usually prednisone, on an every other day schedule. While some workers have used alternate day prednisone as the first choice of treatment even in limited essentially ocular myasthenia gravis, we have generally reserved its use for those patients with more generalized weakness not responding favorably to anticholinesterases or thymectomy or both. It may be considered in older patients not suitable for thymectomy. However, both the patient and physician should be aware of the long-term commitment, side effects, risks, and complications associated with the chronic use of corticosteroids. While strength may improve greatly, the majority of patients placed on corticosteroids remain dependent upon them for their improvement and may not be withdrawn without recurrence of myasthenic weakness in subsequent weeks or months. In some the improvement may be maintained on lower doses of corticosteroid than those required to initiate the improvement.

Since there may be some paradoxical worsening of the myasthenia when first beginning corticosteroids, they are best started in a hospital setting with staff familiar with this form of treatment in myasthenia and facilities for mechanical respiratory support and intensive care should these be needed. Patients who are anergic or who have positive skin tests for tuberculosis are best given prophylactic isoniazid (INH) and pyridoxine. We recommend that patients on corticosteroids maintain a high protein, high potassium, high calcium diet moderately low in fat and carbohydrate and avoid free sugars. Supplemental 10 per cent sugar-free potassium chloride may be needed to maintain the serum potassium in upper normal levels. The blood count, serum potassium and blood sugar are checked at office visits. Liver function tests may be obtained from those on isoniazid

(INH) as well as progress chest films at 6 to 12 month intervals. Bone density may be checked radiographically annually for evidence of osteoporosis, particularly in older patients. The eyes may be watched for evidence of cataracts. We also recommend that patients taking corticosteroids take antacids or nonfat milk 1 to 2 hours after each meal and at bedtime.

We prefer to start alternate day prednisone at 20 or 25 mg. and increase this by 5 mg. every second or third dose cycle. When improvement in strength that is usually not immediate begins, the dosage may be maintained at that level. We have seldom exceeded 100 mg. on alternate days. For those patients already requiring mechanical respiratory support or tracheostomy or both, higher initial starting dose of up to 100 mg. on alternate days may be given in an attempt to reverse the severe weakness sooner.

Adjuvant, Immunosuppressive, and Other Therapy

Ephedrine sulfate, 25 mg. two or three times daily, appears to help some patients. A few appear to benefit from calcium given as the gluconate or lactate in doses of 1 to 2 grams three or four times daily. Intramuscular injections of pooled immune serum globulin have been considered helpful to a few patients with recurrent infections who are not responding to other forms of treatment. Immunosuppressive drugs, including azathioprine, cyclophosphamide, and methotrexate, have been used for long-term treatment of a few patients not responding to the more usual treatments. (This use of these agents is not listed in the manufacturers' official directives.) The improvement with these may require weeks or months of treatment and entail side effects and risks. Currently, plasmapheresis in combination with azathioprine and intramuscular injections of pooled immune globulin has been successful in reversing weakness of a few patients severely incapacitated with oropharyngeal or respiratory muscle weakness or both in a limited series of cases at special centers for clinical investigation. Since it requires special facilities and skills and presents significant risks, it warrants further evaluation at clinical research centers in selected patients. Thoracic duct drainage remains in a similar investigational category.

Drugs to Avoid or Use Cautiously

Many drugs interfere with neuromuscular transmission. Mycin or amino glycoside antibiotics may increase neuromuscular block. These include streptomycin, dihydrostreptomycin, colistin, neomycin, kanamycin, gentamicin, vancomycin, and polymycin. They should be avoided, but if the patient has an infection requiring the use of one of these, it is best given in the hospital with close supervision and facilities for mechanical airway and respiratory support available.

Ether should be avoided as an anesthetic agent. D-tubocurarine pancuronium, succinylcholine, and related muscle relaxants are best avoided since the myasthenic is markedly sensitive to the first two of these and may have an unpredictable response to the third.

Quinine, quinidine, and procainamide may also increase neuromuscular block. Magnesium sulfate is contraindicated.

Tranquilizers and sedatives are best avoided or prescribed in half the usual dose. Morphine is a respiratory depressant and is best not used in myasthenics who tolerate meperidine (Demerol) generally well. Most myasthenics tolerate small amounts of local anesthetics such as procaine or lidocaine (Xylocaine) for dental work or minor surgery well, but since a few may experience temporary worsening of their myasthenia, the dentist or surgeon is best prepared to have equipment for emergency airway and temporary mechanical respiratory support on hand if needed.

Corticosteroids and ACTH may initially aggravate myasthenic weakness and are best started if needed in the hospital. Cathartics and enemas also may aggravate myasthenia and are best avoided or used sparingly.

Care for Surgery

Myasthenics may require surgery apart from thymectomy. Preoperative enemas are avoided. The patient may take his usual anticholinesterase drug with small sips of water up to the time of surgery. If preferred, this may be converted to a parenteral dose of neostigmine or pyridostigmine. Meperidine and atropine are satisfactory preoperative medication. Muscle relaxants are avoided. Spinal anesthesia or inhalation anesthesia, other than ether, may be given. If the patient has had significant oropharyngeal or respiratory muscle weakness or both preoperatively, the endotracheal tube may be left in postoperatively until the patient is awake and demonstrates stable respiratory function, monitored by vital capacity. Anticholinesterase therapy may be resumed parenterally as weakness develops or by nasogastric tube when the patient is no longer nauseated and has normal bowel sounds. Pyridostigmine syrup may be useful at this time. Often the dosage requirements for anticholinesterase are less than preoperatively. If antibiotics are used, those listed above known to interfere with neuromuscular transmission are avoided. Meticulous care should be given to the respiratory tract to promote full expansion of the lungs using intermittent positive pressure breathing, assisted coughing, and careful tracheobronchial toilet to prevent atelectasis and pulmonary infection.

Outlook

The majority of patients with myasthenia gravis lead gainful, productive satisfying lives. Better and newer forms of treatment, including improved means for mechanical respiratory support, antibiotics to combat infections, and our understanding of the pathophysiology of neuromuscular transmission in myasthenia, have contributed to the greatly reduced mortality and increased longevity. It is important for patients to learn to pace their physical activities. Patients and their families benefit from learning the nature of myasthenia and general principles regarding management to reduce unnecessary anxiety and promote a smoother course.

TRIGEMINAL NEURALGIA
(Tic Douloureux)

method of
JOHN M. TEW, JR., M.D.
Cincinnati, Ohio

Definition

Neuralgia is paroxysmal pain in the distribution of a nerve with minimal or no demonstrable neurologic deficit. Tic douloureux or trigeminal neuralgia is unique in that it is common (0.1 to 0.2 per cent), causes excruciating pain for long periods of time, and nearly always can be relieved by medical or surgical therapy. The condition is due to a disorder of the trigeminal nerve or a lesion in the brain stem. In most instances, the specific cause is unknown. However, compression of the trigeminal nerve by blood vessels, benign tumors or demyelinating plaques have been suggested as causative factors.

The diagnostic features of tic douloureux are characteristic and the condition has been recognized for as long as 20 centuries. Nevertheless, confusion still prevails about the cause and appropriate course of therapy. Spasmodic excruciating pain of paroxysmal nature, radiating into the zone of the trigeminal nerve, elicited by cutaneous stimuli in the innervation of the fifth cranial nerve is tic douloureux.

Medical Treatment

The diagnostic criteria now include amelioration of pain by carbamazepine (Tegretol). The initial treatment of all tic douloureux must be *medical*. While myriad "remedies" have been advocated in the past, confirming Osler's famous dictum that: "Our knowledge of any disease is in inverse proportion to the number of remedies promulgated for it," there can be little doubt that carbamazepine and certain other anticonvulsant substances exert a salutary effect on tic douloureux. Patients with this condition should not be subjected to inconsequential drug therapy, for example, vitamins and vasodilators, nor should they be submitted to procedures on the mouth, teeth, sinuses, or nerves at a distance (acupuncture).

Carbamazepine (Tegretol) is available in 200 mg. tablets and is administered as one half tablet (100 mg. twice daily) with progressively increasing dosage until a therapeutic blood level (1 to 8 micrograms per ml.) or control is achieved. Effective dosage may amount to as much as 1200 to 1600 mg. per day, depending on tolerance and side effects. In my judgment the hematopoietic and hepatic effects have been overstated. However, the monthly monitoring of blood count and liver enzymes is recommended for the first 6 months. The drug should be continued until the pain is controlled or intolerable side effects develop, then slowly discontinued. If this regimen is ineffective, one may add phenytoin (Dilantin), 300 to 600 mg. per day, until therapeutic levels of 10 to 20 micrograms per ml., or clonazepam (Clonopin), 1.0 mg. twice or thrice daily. (This use of phenytoin and clonazepam is not listed in the manufacturers' official directives.)

Those who are not effectively controlled or who develop uncontrollable side effects should be offered the appropriate surgical treatment promptly.

Surgical Treatment

Partial destruction of the sensory pathway and elimination of painful input has been the major goal of surgical therapy. Injection of sclerosing agents such as alcohol or phenol, peripheral section, or avulsion of nerve trunks may provide short-term relief (3 months to 3 years) and can be performed safely under most circumstances. However, these procedures are rarely effective for recurrent pain or pain involving multiple divisions of the nerve. The goal of modern surgical therapy is long-term control, minimal neurologic deficit, and negligible surgical morbidity.

Percutaneous Trigeminal Rhizotomy

Percutaneous rhizotomy most nearly satisfies all aspects of this goal. A simple, safe procedure, when performed by an experienced surgeon, it eliminates the perception of pain and preserves the tactile sensibility and motor function of the face and mouth. In this procedure, a needle is placed under radiographic control into the trigeminal rootlets adjacent to the pons. Electrical stimulation of the nerve fibers in the awake patient permits precise localization of the needle electrode. A thermal lesion generated by radiofrequency current is monitored by temperature control and by the response of the patient to noxious stimuli. Patient satisfaction with percutaneous rhizotomy is high. Ninety-three per cent of patients rate their result as good or excellent. Side effects are few, other than occasional occurrence of temporary blurring of vision and paresthesias of the face. The latter is the major significant side effect and is the principal reason that we must continue to look for other forms of medical and surgical therapy. An occasional patient (less than 1 per cent) will find the disagreeable sensations so obtrusive that they are constantly miserable (anesthesia dolorosa).

Trigeminal Decompression—Recent Observations

Recent observations suggest that trigeminal neuralgia may be permanently controlled by decompressing the nerve as it enters the pons (root-entry zone). Impingement by arteries, veins, benign neoplasms, and dural bands has been found. The operative procedure performed by microsurgical technique is demanding and potentially hazardous, even in the healthy patient. Nevertheless, the early encouraging results indicate that the excruciating pain can be relieved while sparing the patient the risk of significant sensory loss. Further experience with this unique concept with careful patient follow-up is needed to determine what its eventual place might be in surgical therapy.

All other forms of surgical treatment such as sectioning the nerve in the middle cranial or posterior fossa appear less attractive unless techniques already described cannot be delivered for any of a number of reasons.

Glossopharyngeal Neuralgia

The pain of IX and X cranial nerve neuralgia is similar to that described in tic douloureux except the radiation of pain is directed toward the ear, posterior pharynx, and tonsillar region. Much less frequent than neuralgia of the fifth nerve, it has been known to occur concurrently with tic douloureux. It is impossible to distinguish the pain of the ninth versus the tenth nerve in most instances, thus the combined designation.

Carbamazepine and other anticonvulsants as described for tic douloureux are useful but apparently less effective.

If procaine hydrochloride (Novocain) block relieves the neuralgia, then the treatment consists of sectioning of the superior laryngeal nerve if the pain has been restricted to the throat. Section of the ninth and upper fibers of the tenth nerve adjacent to the brain stem or decompression of the nerve as suggested for trigeminal neuralgia should be considered since sensory paresthesias are not encountered and dysphonia can be avoided by partial sectioning of the tenth nerve. Direct sectioning of the nerve appears to be the more definitive procedure. The decompression procedure is of unproved value in glossopharyngeal and vagal neuralgia.

OPTIC NEURITIS

method of
JOHN O. SUSAC, M.D.
Winter Haven, Florida

"Optic neuritis" may refer to any acute dysfunction of the optic nerve, regardless of cause. In this section, however, optic neuritis refers to the usually idiopathic form of optic neuropathy unless otherwise indicated. Since multiple sclerosis is the cause in only 20 per cent of these patients, compassion should obviate mentioning this to the patient.

Clinical Features of Optic Neuritis

The patient complains of sudden visual loss in one eye that is often associated with pain on motion of the globe. The visual loss may progress over the next day or two and usually involves the central field (central scotoma). The acuity, which is often in the 20/200 range, may be as low as no light perception. A Marcus Gunn (afferent) pupil is a constant finding. In the absence of a Marcus Gunn pupil, one should consider: macular disease, bilateral optic nerve disease, functional visual loss or a chiasmal lesion. Special attention should be directed to the visual field of the opposite eye. Should a temporal field defect be discovered, a chiasmal syndrome is likely. Usually the optic nerve head appears normal on funduscopy, and a retrobulbar neuritis is said to exist. ("The patient sees nothing and the doctor sees nothing.") Occasionally, the disk may be swollen (papillitis), and cells in the vitreous may be seen with a slit lamp.

The overwhelming majority (90 per cent plus) of patients will spontaneously recover vision within a few weeks and will have essentially normal acuity in 3 months.

Although many clinicians use steroids, there are no convincing controlled studies to show that steroids significantly alter the eventual outcome of optic neuritis. Since the side effects of steroids are not inconsiderable, I remain a nontreater when it comes to unilateral optic neuritis.

"Chronic" optic neuritis or any slowly progressive loss of vision in an eye indicates a structural lesion. Computed tomography (CT) with orbit views and visualization of the sella and suprasellar region is mandatory in such patients. Tomography of the sella and optic foramina may also be indicated.

A detailed history will often reveal a nutritional (alcohol), toxic (drug), infectious (syphilis), systemic (temporal arteritis), or familial (Leber's optic neuropathy) basis for the visual loss. Laboratory studies, including a complete blood count, erythrocyte sedimentation rate, antinuclear antibody, fluorescent treponemal antibody, serum B_{12}, and blood sugar, may be informative.

Ischemic Optic Neuropathy

This is a well-defined entity that occurs in the vascular age group (45 years and older). Sudden visual loss is associated with pale swelling of the optic disk, often with small flame-shaped hemorrhages on its edge. An inferior nasal or altitudinal field defect is also commonly found. The nerve rapidly becomes pale. Although recurrences are not seen in the same eye, the opposite eye usually becomes affected months or years later. If one sees the patient at the time of involvement of the second eye (swollen disk), combined with the pale disk in the first eye, it may lead one to suspect the Foster Kennedy syndrome.

The erythrocyte sedimentation rate and temporal artery biopsy are normal in this condition, which is presumed to be due to arteriosclerotic involvement of small vessels. In younger patients, collagen vascular disease, especially systemic lupus erythematosus, should be considered.

Temporal arteritis must be remembered in patients 55 years and older. Although headache, polymyalgia rheumatica, jaw claudication, and other systemic symptoms are usually present, they may be entirely absent ("occult" form). Sedimentation rate is mandatory, temporal artery biopsy should be considered, and the patient should be treated with prednisone, 100 mg. daily, immediately. Occasionally, sedimentation rates may be spuriously low because the patient had been taking aspirin, indomethacin, etc.

Leber's Optic Neuropathy

This is fortunately a rare type of optic nerve disease that occurs almost exclusively in males—teens to late 20s. Sudden visual loss in one eye is associated with a pathognomonic fundus picture in the acute stage: (1) circumpapillary telangiec-

tatic microangiopathy, (2) pseudoedema of the nerve fiber layer around the disk, and (3) lack of staining on fluorescein angiopathy. One should ask about similar disease in a brother or maternal uncle. There is no effective treatment, and the second eye will become involved within a year's time.

Nutritional (Tobacco-Alcohol) Amblyopia

This is a bilateral optic nerve disease associated with cecocentral scotomas, which are best found with red test targets. This occurs in people who prefer drinking alcohol to eating regular meals. Although initially felt to be secondary to a toxic effect of alcohol, it has been demonstrated that a vitamin (thiamine) deficiency is the basis for the visual loss. Treatment includes stopping the alcohol, adequate diet, and thiamine and supplemental vitamins. Hydroxycobalamin (Neo-Betalin 12), 1000 micrograms per ml. by injection, 1 ml. weekly for ten weeks, has been advocated by Smith.

Other Causes of Optic Nerve Disease

There are many forms of unusual optic neuropathies that include carcinomatous, *Toxocara canis*, etc., that are beyond the scope of this article. The reader is referred to J. Lawton Smith's Neuroophthalmology Symposium (Vol. V, Huffman Publishing Co., 1970) and Walsh and Hoyt's Clinical Neuroophthalmology (Williams and Wilkins, 1969).

ACUTE PERIPHERAL FACIAL PARALYSIS
(Bell's Palsy)

method of
KEDAR K. ADOUR, M.D.
Oakland, California

Clinical, epidemiologic, and laboratory data have shown that Bell's palsy is an acute, benign cranial polyneuritis that is probably caused by reactivation of the herpes simplex virus. The primary disease is a sensory ganglionitis of the central nervous system with secondary motor nerve palsy. The muscle paralysis is caused by inflammation and demyelinization rather than by ischemic compression. Presenting signs and symptoms vary, depending on involvement of specific sensory and autonomic nerves. In order of frequency these are: epiphora, 70 per cent; pain, 60 per cent; ageusia (dysgeusia), 57 per cent; hypesthesia of the trigeminal and second cervical nerves, 50 per cent;

hyperacusis (dysacusis), 30 per cent; and hypesthesia of the glossopharyngeal nerve (unilateral decreased sensation of the posterior pharynx), 20 per cent. There is concomitant asymptomatic palsy of the superior laryngeal branch of the vagus nerve in 20 per cent of patients.

Acute peripheral facial paralysis does not always indicate Bell's palsy. Successful management of facial paralysis requires a confident and accurate diagnosis and a reliable estimate of prognosis. *Other diseases must be excluded before the final diagnosis of Bell's palsy is made.* After a complete and accurate history has been obtained, the evaluation for cranial neuritis should include a general neurologic examination and a thorough ear, nose, and throat examination. The nasopharyngeal and otologic examinations are mandatory. Luckily, cases of Bell's palsy are alike as peas in a pod—they are similar in history, natural course, and outcome. It is unusual to find a case of Bell's palsy that deviates from the pattern. The diagnosis of Bell's palsy may therefore be made when a facial paralysis is peripheral in origin, no evidence of systemic disease is present, the history is one of acute onset, and concomitant sensory cranial polyneuritis is present.

Prognosis and Complications

Classically, the clinical course of Bell's palsy is discussed in terms of two groups: those patients with complete and those patients with incomplete paralysis. Whereas the diagnosis of complete clinical paralysis requires a relatively finite observation, incomplete paralysis covers a wide range of severity. The most valuable tools for determining prognosis in individual patients are therefore careful observation of the progression (or lack of progression) of the paralysis and the use of electrodiagnostic tests to determine the rate and degree of nerve degeneration ("denervation" in common usage).

Electrical tests to determine denervation include percutaneous nerve excitability tests, electromyography, and facial nerve conduction velocity (facial nerve latency). No matter which electrical test is used, decreased response cannot be measured until 48 to 72 hours after the pathologic events, and severity of damage may not be apparent until days after denervation has occurred. Nevertheless, we advise percutaneous nerve excitability testing as an accurate, simple method of determining denervation. Electromyographic and facial nerve latency tests are used in fewer than 10 per cent of our patients.

As early as possible after onset of the paralysis, percutaneous nerve excitability testing is performed as a baseline for determining prognosis as well as an indication for continuation of treatment. The studies should be repeated at intervals of 5 days for 2 weeks. When a nerve branch is maximally stimulated, denervation is determined by the tester's subjective impression of the "quality" and "quantity" of the muscle motion and is therefore relative rather than absolute.

Abnormal nerve excitability remains abnormal, even when volitional facial muscle action has returned. Nerve excitability is useful only during the first weeks of the disease. There is no "critical difference" value between the affected and unaffected side to indicate impending denervation.

If the maximal nerve excitability test indicates equal muscle response on both sides of the face, the patient can be expected to have complete return of facial functions in 3 to 6 weeks, without complications of faulty nerve regeneration. The most common complications of faulty nerve regeneration are: (1) contracture, (2) synkinesis (associated facial motion), and (3) facial tics (spasms). These complications do not develop until 3 months and become pronounced at 4 months after onset of paralysis. Contracture, synkinesis, and facial spasm will not develop unless regeneration occurs. Crocodile (gustatory) tearing, the last late complication to develop, does not develop until 4 or 5 months after onset of Bell's palsy.

If the maximal nerve excitability test has shown decreased muscle response on the affected side, the complete return of facial function without complication *cannot* be expected. Some residual paralysis or a degree of contracture or synkinesis remains. The degree of contracture and synkinesis can be predicted by the degree of degeneration. The patient with only minimal or moderate denervation of the facial muscles can develop 75 to 100 per cent return of all facial function, with mild to moderate contracture and synkinesis apparent to a trained observer only. The patient can expect to have excellent return of volitional facial muscle motion between 4 to 8 weeks after onset of paralysis. In patients with severe denervation, the percentage of return of volitional facial function is decreased: contracture, synkinesis, and facial spasms are usually severe. Usually, 6 to 12 weeks are required for adequate return of facial function in severe denervation. When no response to maximal nerve excitability tests (complete denervation) occurs, return of facial function cannot be expected before 12 weeks, and the amount of volitional facial muscle motion is limited to 50 to 75 per cent of that present on the opposite side. The contracture and synkinesis also are much more severe.

Laboratory Tests

A Schirmer tear test is performed for all patients, since the presence of decreased tears is an indicator of poor prognosis. A screening 2-hour postprandial blood sugar test is advised only for patients older than 39 years. A 3-hour glucose tolerance test is performed for patients with recurrent or bilateral Bell's palsy. Unless specifically indicated, x-ray films or other laboratory tests are not obtained. The stapedial reflex test (impedance audiometry) is very accurate in assessing prognosis.

Treatment

Reassurance. Discussion of the diagnosis and of prognosis should reassure most patients. Specifically, patients are told that the paralysis is not caused by a "stroke."

Eye Care. Protection of the eye is paramount. Dark glasses should be worn during the day, artificial tears instilled at the slightest suggestion of drying, and a bland eye ointment used during sleep. Taping the eye is not recommended.

Prednisone. Prednisone so dramatically relieves the pain of Bell's palsy that analgesics have not been necessary. Although surgically oriented physicians suggest that the benefit of any medical therapy is still in doubt, prednisone has become the standard treatment in the largest facial paralysis clinics throughout the world. For adult patients, the 60 mg. dosage of prednisone (or prednisolone) per day in divided doses of 30 mg. in the morning and 30 mg. in the evening is suggested. The usual caution concerning contraindications for cortisone therapy should be observed. If the paralysis remains incomplete (partial paralysis), the schedule shown in Table 1 is usually sufficient.

The patient should be seen on the fifth or sixth day after onset of paralysis for a repeat nerve excitability test. Prednisone at 60 mg. per day should be continued for 5 more days if: (1) the paralysis is or has progressed from incomplete to complete, or (2) nerve excitability indicates any denervation. A return visit is scheduled for all patients the tenth to twelfth day after onset, at which time nerve excitability is repeated to assess prognosis. For those who are still taking 60 mg. of prednisone per day, the dose is tapered to zero over the next 5 days (total of 20 days). Prednisone

TABLE 1. **Prednisone Dosage**

	A.M.	P.M.	
Day 1	30 mg.	30 mg.	
Day 2	30 mg.	30 mg.	
Day 3	30 mg.	30 mg.	
Day 4	30 mg.	30 mg.	
Day 5	30 mg.	30 mg. ⎫	
Day 6	20 mg.	20 mg. ⎬ 2nd Visit	
Day 7	15 mg.	15 mg.	
Day 8	10 mg.	10 mg.	
Day 9	5 mg.	5 mg.	
Day 10	5 mg.	0	

should never be stopped abruptly, as rebound inflammation could lead to further denervation.

Prednisone treatment does not reduce the number of patients developing partial denervation or contracture and synkinesis but does significantly reduce the number with complete denervation, thereby making the disease less severe. Considering patients with one episode only of Bell's palsy, 24 per cent of those treated or untreated have some evidence of denervation, but only 7 per cent of those receiving prednisone have an unsatisfactory end result.

Caution: Of all Bell's palsy patients, 4 per cent develop herpes zoster vesicles 2 to 4 days after onset of the paralysis, and 30 per cent of these patients develop mildly to moderately disseminated vesicles 4 to 8 days after onset. These are natural manifestations of the disease and even if they occur while the patient is taking prednisone, the dosage should still be continued at the 60 mg. level for 14 days and then tapered over the next 5 days.

Muscle Stimulation. Faradic or galvanic stimulation is not necessary, may be detrimental to recovery, and therefore is not advised.

Surgical Treatment. Early enthusiasm for facial nerve decompression waned when several studies showed this procedure was not beneficial and might be harmful.

PARKINSON'S DISEASE

method of
DONALD B. CALNE, M.D.
Bethesda, Maryland
and HAROLD L. KLAWANS, M.D.
Chicago, Illinois

Introduction

The first effective treatment to be introduced for parkinsonism was the use of belladonna alkaloids by Charcot. These drugs were known to cause dryness of the mouth, and Charcot initiated their administration to patients with parkinsonism in an attempt to alleviate the drooling of saliva commonly encountered in such patients. It was soon recognized that the belladonna alkaloids had an unexpected beneficial effect on the rigidity and tremor of parkinsonism. Unfortunately the least obvious but most disabling clinical feature of parkinsonism—the slowness and clumsiness of movement termed hypokinesia—did not improve to any significant extent.

The succeeding years were notable for the absence of any therapeutic advance. The sterility of the pharmacologic setting is illustrated by the redundant arguments on the relative efficacy of belladonna derived from different sources, the Bulgarian preparation somehow achieving a particular vogue.

Following the Second World War, synthetic congeners of the belladonna alkaloids were introduced and virtually replaced the traditional natural products. The major advantage of the new drugs was an apparent improvement in therapeutic index so that the same beneficial results were obtained with fewer adverse reactions.

Over the last decade, a spectacular change in neurologic therapeutics has occurred with the development of levodopa as a treatment of parkinsonism. Levodopa represents a totally rational approach to treatment. Its use in parkinsonism is based upon firm biochemical observations which lead to accurate predictions of clinical efficacy. Levodopa is of crucial practical significance, because shortly after its introduction it was recognized as by far the most potent therapeutic agent available for parkinsonism. Unfortunately the efficacy of levodopa is limited by rather prominent (albeit dose-related and reversible) adverse effects.

Amantadine, the next important drug to enter the therapeutic arena for parkinsonism, differed in every respect from levodopa. Its beneficial action was discovered by a chance observation; critical studies showed that its antiparkinson efficacy was much less than that of levodopa; nevertheless, it is extremely well tolerated.

Anticholinergic Drugs

All effective drugs used in the treatment of parkinsonism prior to the advent of levodopa had central anticholinergic properties. In 1967 Duvoisin conducted an elegant series of experiments which demonstrated that these anticholinergic agents ameliorate parkinsonism by blocking muscarinic receptors at cholinergic synapses within the central nervous system. He drew this conclusion from the following observations:

1. Physostigmine is an anticholinesterase agent which inhibits the destruction of acetylcholine in both the central nervous system and the periphery. Administration of physostigmine to patients with parkinsonism exacerbates the clinical features of the disease.

2. Edrophonium is another anticholinesterase drug, but unlike physostigmine it does not readily cross the blood-brain barrier, so its actions are limited to the periphery. Edrophonium does not exacerbate parkinsonism.

3. Scopolamine and benztropine are antimuscarinic agents which cross the blood-brain barrier. Both these drugs ameliorate parkinsonism and protect patients from the deleterious effects of physostigmine.

4. Methylscopolamine and propantheline are antimuscarinic agents which do not gain ready access to the central nervous system. Neither of these drugs is capable of inhibiting the exacerbation of parkinsonism induced by physostigmine.

Although muscarinic blockade is clearly a major factor contributing to the therapeutic action of anticholinergic agents, another mechanism which may play a role is inhibition of active reuptake of dopamine. Normally, the major process responsible for the inactivation of dopamine released into striatal synapses is reuptake by the presynaptic dopaminergic nerve terminal. This active reuptake mechanism is inhibited by many of the anticholinergic agents which are employed to treat parkinsonism. Blockade of this reuptake system allows the transmitter to remain in the synaptic cleft where it can continue to act upon postsynaptic receptors. These effects reverse the decreased dopaminergic transmission in the striatum, which is the chemical basis of parkinsonism.

Anticholinergic agents achieve a worthwhile therapeutic action on tremor and rigidity, but hypokinesia (the most disabling clinical feature of parkinsonism) and loss of postural reflexes do not usually respond well.

There is no satisfactory evidence that any one anticholinergic drug is specifically effective for any one particular parkinsonian deficit, although patients often report a preference among the various alternative agents which they are commonly given. Sometimes a combination of two anticholinergic agents seems better than one, but it is seldom advantageous to give more than two anticholinergics at the same time. The initial therapeutic response to anticholinergic drugs is sometimes poorly sustained, suggesting the development of tolerance.

Antihistaminic drugs are often prescribed for parkinsonism. All the antihistaminic agents that have been found to be of value in parkinsonism have central antimuscarinic properties. It is probably the ability of these drugs to antagonize the activity of acetylcholine within the brain that accounts for their therapeutic action. Dosages of each of these agents must be adjusted individually. It is usual to start patients on a low intake, which is gradually increased until a satisfactory response is obtained or unwanted effects are encountered. Minor side effects such as dryness of the mouth and slight blurring of vision are common and may have to be tolerated in order to have an antiparkinsonian effect. Older patients appear to be more sensitive to the central side effects of these agents, and great care must be exercised in increasing these agents in the elderly. Some patients are remarkably sensitive to the central side effects and experience hallucinations in very low doses.

The most common adverse reactions to anticholinergic drugs are produced by blockade of muscarinic synapses of the parasympathetic system. They include dryness of the mouth, defective ocular accommodation, mydriasis which can precipitate glaucoma, constipation, and retention of urine. This last problem can lead to acute retention in patients with prostatic hypertrophy. Unwanted effects can also be induced through effects upon the central nervous system and include a toxic confusional psychosis and hallucinations.

Amantadine

The therapeutic effect of amantadine in parkinsonism was discovered by serendipity, and its mechanism of action remains unknown. However, in studies employing much higher tissue concentrations than those encountered in routine therapy, a number of properties have been reported which may be relevant. These include (1) increasing the synthesis of dopamine, (2) augmenting the release of dopamine, and (3) inhibiting the active reuptake process responsible for inactivating dopamine.

Amantadine has one unusual pharmacokinetic property—it is scarcely metabolized. Some 86 per cent of an administered dose is excreted unchanged in the urine.

Amantadine is of similar therapeutic potency to anticholinergic drugs, but in contrast it also alleviates hypokinesia and loss of postural reflexes. Because of its efficacy against these manifestations of parkinsonism it is particularly useful in the management of patients who respond poorly to levodopa. About 50 per cent of patients derive worthwhile benefit from amantadine; there have been conflicting reports on whether the response is sustained.

Amantadine is generally given in an initial dose of 100 mg. daily, which is doubled after a week if, as is usual, there are no adverse reactions. Since one of the more common unwanted effects is restlessness, the second dose of amantadine should not be taken late in the day.

In addition to restlessness, amantadine can cause dizziness, confusion, hallucinations, mood changes, nausea, abdominal discomfort, headache, edema, pruritus, and rarely cardiac arrhythmias. All these unwanted effects are reversible by stopping treatment. Overdosage can precipitate convulsions, so amantadine is not usually given to patients with a history of seizures. There

have been reports of livedo reticularis, a condition in which there is edema and shininess of the shins, with livedo above or below the knee or on the dorsum of the foot.

Levodopa

The therapeutic efficacy of levodopa in the treatment of parkinsonism was first demonstrated in the early 1960's. Using intravenous levodopa, Birkmayer and Hornykiewicz demonstrated a decrease in akinesia in 20 parkinsonian patients. At the same time, Barbeau independently reported improvement in parkinsonism following oral doses of levodopa. The overall impression of the usefulness of levodopa remained unclear until the efficacy of long-term oral therapy was demonstrated by Cotzias et al. These workers first used large oral doses of DL-dopa for long periods of time and were able to produce dramatic and sustained improvement. Because of the toxic nature of the racemic mixture, they substituted levodopa for DL-dopa. Using the single isomer, they produced marked beneficial effects in parkinsonian patients without the same serious toxicity. A number of investigators have substantiated these results in large series of patients, including some studies which were done as double blind trials.

Levodopa has been shown to be effective in ameliorating rigidity, hypokinesia, loss of postural reflexes, and tremor. Although it is often said that levodopa has less effect on tremor than it has on rigidity and akinesia, it has a significant antitremor effect and is clearly the most potent agent now available for the treatment of parkinsonian tremor.

Although levodopa is the most effective drug for the treatment of parkinsonism, its use is frequently associated with a variety of side effects which often limit its beneficial action. When properly managed, both the incidence and severity of these side effects can be reduced, resulting in greater therapeutic efficacy. Success of long-term use of levodopa depends to a large extent on the understanding and management of these side effects.

The major adverse reactions to levodopa can be divided into three classes. The first of these are the centrally mediated side effects which are thought to result from activity of amines formed from levodopa within the central nervous system. The second are the peripherally mediated side effects which are thought to result from the formation of active amines outside the central nervous system. The last are the mixed central and peripheral side effects. Both central and peripherally formed amines are considered to be of physiologic significance in the pathophysiology of these side effects.

The centrally mediated side effects include dyskinesias, myoclonus, and psychiatric effects.

The appearance of choreoathetoid involuntary movement, or dyskinesias, is one of the most frequent and troublesome side effects of levodopa therapy. The occurrence of the movements during chronic oral dopa therapy was first reported by Cotzias et al. in their initial study of the efficacy of long-term high dosage DL-dopa and levodopa in parkinsonism. The incidence reported during chronic therapy ranges from a low of 39 per cent to as high as 80 per cent.

The dyskinetic movements induced by levodopa are remarkably diverse. Lingual-facial-buccal movements, such as grimacing, gnawing, yawning, and choreoathetoid movements of the tongue, are the most commonly observed manifestations. Choreoathetoid movements of extremities, neck, and trunk are also common.

Barbeau et al. have made the most extensive study of these movements and have proposed an extensive classification of these dyskinesias, which includes some 47 different types of levodopa-induced abnormal movements. Their classification includes eye movements such as blepharospasms and lateral eye deviations, as well as numerous types of lingual-facial-buccal, cervical, truncal, and upper or lower extremity movements. Although the diversity of these movements is remarkable, their effect on the long-term efficacy of levodopa is much more significant.

The prevalence of these movements is definitely *related to the duration of high dosage levodopa therapy*. Very little else about these movements is clearly understood. Although there is a direct relationship between levodopa and dyskinesias, there is no absolute relationship between the onset of such movements and the daily dosage of levodopa. In many patients dyskinesias have occurred with daily doses of less than 2 grams per day of levodopa. Other patients can be on 6 or more grams per day for up to 5 years without manifesting such movements. Once the dyskinetic movements appear, their severity is related to the daily dose of levodopa. Decreasing the daily dosage of levodopa invariably reduces the dyskinesias, and increasing the daily dosage makes them worse. Unfortunately the beneficial effects of therapy may be diminished when the dose of levodopa is decreased.

Many observers have found that reducing the daily dose of levodopa by 0.5 or 1.0 gram frequently eliminates the dyskinesias or at least reduces them to an acceptable level. For many patients the most effective dose for controlling the parkinsonian symptoms is at or just below that dosage which produces the dyskinetic movements. Because of this many patients have to compromise between partial control of parkinsonian symptoms and disabling levodopa-induced choreoathetosis.

The exact mechanism by which these involuntary movements are produced is unknown. The observation that the average daily dosage of levodopa is the same in patients with and in patients without levodopa-induced dyskinesias suggests that some variable, possibly histopathologic or biochemical, may be related to the occurrence of these movements. There is evidence that levodopa produces dyskinetic movements by an effect within the central nervous system rather than peripherally. Peripheral inhibition of dopa decarboxylase decreases the various peripheral side effects of levodopa but does not reduce the incidence or severity of the movements.

It is thought that these dyskinesias are related to an abnormal response to dopamine and that the mechanism underlying such an alteration of neuronal response to dopamine is the development of denervation hypersensitivity of the dopamine receptors caused by degeneration of the dopaminergic nigrostriatal pathway. Because of this denervation these receptors may become hypersensitive to dopamine. Levodopa may elicit dyskinesias as a result of dopamine activation of these hypersensitive receptors.

If levodopa-induced abnormal movements are related to the action of dopamine at dopaminergic receptor sites, then it should be possible to alter the neuronal response to dopamine and the subsequent movements in several ways. The most direct way would be to decrease the amount of dopamine reaching the receptors, which should improve the movements. Decreasing the dosage of levodopa would effectively decrease the amount of dopamine reaching the dopamine receptors. As noted above, this does reduce the severity of levodopa-induced dyskinesias. Unfortunately, however, the beneficial effects of levodopa on parkinsonian symptoms of these same patients are usually diminished at the same time. As a result of this, levodopa-induced dyskinesias often limit both the dosage of levodopa a patient can tolerate and the therapeutic response.

Barbeau initially reported that neuroleptic phenothiazines were of value in ameliorating levodopa-induced dyskinesias. Later Postma claimed that haloperidol could relieve the dyskinesias without worsening parkinsonism. It is our firm belief that neuroleptics will improve dyskinesias only at the expense of increased parkinsonism. We therefore do not advocate the use of neuroleptic agents for the treatment of levodopa-induced dyskinesias.

Jameson has reported that pyridoxine (vitamin B$_6$) reduces levodopa-induced dyskinesias without causing a loss of the levodopa effect. In our experience pyridoxine reduces dyskinesias *only* at the cost of a very significant increase in parkinsonian deficit.

In many patients, anticholinergic agents appear to worsen levodopa-induced dyskinesias. We have found that decreasing the level of anticholinergic medication in parkinsonian patients with dyskinesias decreases levodopa-induced dyskinesias in about one third of patients. This improvement in dyskinesias is unassociated with any detectable increase in parkinsonian signs and symptoms in about half of these patients.

It has recently been suggested that deanol may be useful in ameliorating levodopa-induced dyskinesias. Miller used deanol in 11 patients with severe dyskinesias and reported remarkable improvement in these abnormal movements in 8 patients without any worsening of parkinsonism. This effect of deanol was attributed to the central cholinergic activity of this agent. It is hard to understand how a centrally acting cholinergic agent could decrease dyskinesia without any increase in parkinsonism, as physostigmine (see above) significantly increased parkinsonism. We have studied deanol in 20 patients with well established levodopa-induced dyskinesias and found it to be of little if any value.

In some patients these movements appear to be increased by amantadine. If they occur in patients already on amantadine, decreasing or withdrawing amantadine may reduce the severity of the dyskinesias.

The most reliable means of decreasing levodopa-induced dyskinesias is to decrease the level of antiparkinsonian medication, either anticholinergic or dopaminergic. Alteration in daily dosages should be done as soon as dyskinesias become prominent; since any alteration may be associated with an increase in parkinsonism, it is probably best to decrease dosages slowly and to decrease only one medication at a time.

Levodopa-induced myoclonus consists of brief, rapid, usually symmetrical muscle jerks which frequently occur during light sleep. Decreasing the daily dosage of levodopa invariably eliminates myoclonus, but in some instances this is associated with some increase in parkinsonism. Decreasing the last dose before bedtime has the greatest effect on these nocturnal movements. Anticholinergic agents appear to have no influence on levodopa-induced myoclonus.

Untreated idiopathic parkinsonism is now well recognized to be frequently associated with psychiatric symptoms. Dementia is seen in up to 40 per cent of patients with idiopathic parkinsonism, and diffuse cortical atrophy is a common finding in these patients. Patients with postencephalitic parkinsonism often show behavioral and psychologic abnormalities of many types which are felt to reflect the diffuse pathology of their primary disease. The incidence of significant depression in patients with parkinsonism of any cause is high, nearly 40 per cent in one series.

Modifying intracerebral levels of amines by the administration of oral levodopa has also been found to cause significant psychiatric side effects in parkinsonian patients. These have been reported to include agitation, confusion, depression, delirium, hypomania, delusions, paranoia, hallucinations, lethargy, vivid dreams, hypersexual behavior, and overt psychosis. These side effects may occur days to months following the initiation of levodopa therapy.

In our experience it has been useful to divide the psychiatric side effects of levodopa therapy into several types. Some patients develop a full-blown psychotic response to levodopa. These patients have hallucinations, usually of a frightening character. Reality becomes tenuous, and the patients often have paranoid delusions. Levodopa has to be decreased and often discontinued in these patients. Patients with a past history of schizophrenic reaction or paranoid psychosis appear to be particularly susceptible to such reactions. Because of this, past history of such psychiatric problems is a strong contraindication to the use of levodopa. A toxic psychosis can also occur and requires reduction or discontinuation of levodopa.

A third type of psychiatric side effect is less serious. The patients report nocturnal visual hallucinations which occur most frequently after sudden exposure to light following light deprivation, as when the patient gets up in the middle of the night to go to the bathroom. When a light is turned on, the patient may see bugs or small animals running about the room, but there are no threatening hallucinations and no clouding of the sensorium. The patient is aware that these are hallucinations and usually learns to "live with them" without difficulty. It is usually not necessary to stop levodopa therapy in such cases. Many patients reject reduction of levodopa which increases their parkinsonism, because they feel that this side effect is more tolerable than their parkinsonian motor disability.

The occurrence of all psychiatric side effects of levodopa therapy has been reported as ranging from 10 to 50 per cent, depending on the interest and acumen of the investigators and the patient population. The average incidence is about 20 per cent, making mental symptoms the third most common reaction to levodopa therapy (after gastrointestinal disturbances and dyskinesias).

The pathophysiology of levodopa-induced mental changes is unknown. As one would expect, they are a result of amine formation in the central nervous system, because the administration of a peripheral dopa decarboxylase inhibitor does not prevent them. The question has been raised of possible involvement of serotonin in the pathogenesis of these psychiatric side effects. Levodopa is known to cause a decrease in brain serotonin. Two investigators have claimed success in treating levodopa-induced psychosis with the serotonin precursor L-tryptophan.

Severe psychiatric side effects of levodopa are usually treated by reduction or discontinuation of levodopa. Neuroleptics themselves exacerbate the symptoms of parkinsonism, so that a reduction in levodopa is a more direct and physiologically reasonable choice of therapy. Patients with severe psychotic reactions may nevertheless require temporary neuroleptic therapy. Depression in parkinsonian patients on levodopa often responds to treatment with tricyclics. Conventional monamine oxidase inhibitors should not be used in patients receiving levodopa because of the possibility of hypertensive crises.

Another side effect thought to be mediated in the central nervous system is emesis. The symptom complex of anorexia, nausea, and vomiting is perhaps the most common reaction to levodopa administration. These are also among the first side effects to appear in initiating levodopa therapy and often limit both the starting dose and subsequent increments of levodopa therapy. Symptoms of nausea and revulsion from food usually occur within a half hour of taking levodopa. Nausea is usually most marked in the mornings, particularly if the levodopa is taken on an empty stomach. Nausea and subsequent vomiting are dose related in that a large initial dose or a sudden increase in dosage often initiates or exacerbates them. There is also, however, a tendency to develop tachyphylaxis to these side effects. It is our impression that there may be somewhat less tolerance to the feeling of anorexia or loss of appetite.

Treating levodopa-induced nausea by administering standard phenothiazine antiemetics is of no value. These neuroleptics reduce the patient's nausea and vomiting but also worsen his parkinsonism. As in the case of the levodopa-induced dyskinesias and psychosis, neuroleptics reduce side effects only at the cost of increased parkinsonism. Duvoisin reported successful treatment of levodopa-induced nausea and vomiting with diphenidol, a trihexyphenidyl analogue with no known antiparkinsonian effect. He used diphenidol because it had been shown to antagonize the effect of apomorphine (a dopamine

agonist) on the emetic center. Duvoisin reported that diphenidol relieved symptoms of nausea and vomiting in 17 out of 25 patients who had been unable to tolerate levodopa because of these side effects. Diphenidol had no effect on parkinsonism.

The most reasonable approach to emesis is a preventive one. Levodopa should be started in very small doses, in combination with an extracerebral decarboxylase inhibitor (see below).

Cardiac arrhythmias and myocardial infarction have been reported in patients receiving levodopa. The significance of such reports is unclear, as these problems are relatively common in the parkinsonian age group. It is difficult to judge the exact contribution of levodopa therapy to the appearance of cardiac arrhythmias, and its contribution, if any, to the occurrence of myocardial infarction seems even more uncertain.

Levodopa-related arrhythmias are considered to be due to the effect of peripherally formed catecholamines on the beta adrenoceptors of the myocardium. Their incidence should be decreased by concurrent administration of a dopa decarboxylase inhibitor or by the use of a beta-adrenergic antagonist such as propranolol.

The only clinically significant side effect of levodopa in which amines formed in the periphery and in the brain are both felt to play a role is hypotension. Calne found that the resting systolic and diastolic pressures are decreased by about 10 mm. in supine parkinsonian patients taking levodopa. Since this same decrease occurred when patients were given a peripheral decarboxylase inhibitor, they proposed that this effect of levodopa on the set of the blood pressure was due to an effect on the central nervous system.

Peripheral baroreceptor reflexes are also modified by levodopa therapy. The ability of patients to sustain an adequate blood pressure on assumption of the upright posture is impaired by levodopa. This postural hypotension is mediated at least in part by peripheral mechanisms and is decreased by dopa decarboxylase inhibitors. Patients receiving levodopa often complain of lightheadedness, dizziness, or even syncope when rising from a bed or a chair. Hypotension has been seen in about a third of patients taking levodopa, and can be a serious problem in the patient with an already compromised cerebral or myocardial circulation. Fortunately, tachyphylaxis is common and most patients show no evidence of postural hypotension after 2 or 3 months on levodopa. If hypotension is a problem, it usually responds to decreasing the daily dosage of levodopa.

There are other side effects of levodopa therapy which are less common and usually of much less clinical significance. These include gout, distortions and hallucinations of taste, darkening of urine, polyuria, mydriasis, and glaucoma.

The most common problem encountered in patients who have been taking levodopa over several years is abrupt fluctuation between exacerbations of parkinsonism and dyskinesia. The cause of these "on-off" phenomena remains obscure, but many factors might contribute. At present there is no satisfactory way of alleviating "on-off" phenomena, although several manipulations of therapy have been advocated. These include (1) stopping levodopa temporarily and restarting at considerably lower dosage; (2) slight reduction of levodopa intake; (3) more frequent administration of levodopa without altering the total daily dose; (4) concomitant administration of extracerebral decarboxylase inhibitors (with reduced dosage of levodopa); and (5) administration of a dopaminergic agonist such as bromocriptine.

Extracerebral Decarboxylase Inhibitors

In 1967 Bartholini et al. suggested that the therapeutic action of levodopa might be improved by concomitant administration of an extracerebral inhibitor of L-aromatic amino acid decarboxylase, the enzyme required for converting levodopa to dopamine. Two such inhibitors have been introduced into routine therapy, carbidopa (in the United States and Europe) and benserazide (in Europe). These drugs block the conversion of levodopa to dopamine at the periphery and thus prevent certain toxic reactions such as cardiac arrhythmias. Since the inhibitors cannot cross the blood-brain barrier, levodopa can still be converted to dopamine in the striatum, where it is needed. It is probable that carbidopa and benserazide penetrate the area postrema (close to the "emetic center" in animals), because both drugs reduce the nausea induced by levodopa, which is thought to be of central origin.

Carbidopa and benserazide are both formulated in combination with levodopa, the former in a 1:10 ratio (Sinemet) and the latter in a 1:4 ratio (Madopar). A recent carefully controlled double blind cross-over study failed to reveal any significant difference in the therapeutic or adverse effects of Sinemet and Madopar.

From the previous discussion it is evident that the major advantage of using extracerebral decarboxylase inhibitors is reduction of nausea and decreased risk of cardiac toxicity. In addition, it is usually possible to build patients up to maximum tolerated dosage more rapidly when they are taking peripheral decarboxylase inhibitors. It is usual to start frail patients on Sinemet 100 or Madopar 125 thrice daily, increasing according to tolerance. In more robust patients Sinemet 250 or Madopar 250 may be used, with similar increments adjusted for each patient individually.

Which Drug for Which Patient?

Since an appreciable number of patients develop serious adverse reactions to levodopa after several years of therapy (in particular, "on-off" phenomena), most neurologists are growing more cautious with the use of this drug. It is probable that "on-off" reactions are related to the cumulative dose of levodopa. Therefore, instead of treating patients as soon as possible with as much as possible, there is a tendency to save levodopa therapy until the patient really needs it, and then to administer the minimal dose that will achieve adequate functional improvement. Each patient must be considered individually. For many mild new cases of parkinsonism, it is appropriate to monitor the patient's progress without giving any medication. Anticholinergics or amantadine should be tried in those whose deficits are more advanced, or whose income or psychologic well-being is threatened by their disease. When anticholinergics and amantadine prove inadequate, levodopa may be given in combination with a decarboxylase inhibitor; since the build-up of levodopa dosage is facilitated by blockade of L-aromatic amino acid decarboxylase, there is no longer any place for starting patients on levodopa alone.

Surgery

James Parkinson reported that tremor improved after a stroke, his account providing the basis for an attempt to help patients by producing selective lesions of the nervous system. Early surgical procedures involved deafferentation by posterior rhizotomy of the spinal segments concerned with the most florid involuntary movements. The results were inconclusive, and there followed an era in which it was fashionable to inflict lesions to the corticospinal pathways. Excision of the motor area of the cerebral cortex, ablation of the anterior limb of the internal capsule, section of the lateral segment of the cerebral peduncle, and division of the spinal pyramidal tract were all pursued with more enthusiasm among neurosurgeons than their patients. In the words of Mackay: "The surgical relief of extrapyramidal hyperkinesias seems to boil down to the artificial production of paralysis."

A more rewarding period resulted from surgical attacks on the basal ganglia. In 1954, Cooper noted that occlusion of the anterior choroidal artery led to improvement in parkinsonian tremor, and following an extensive evaluation of the relative merits of destructive lesions in various structures supplied by this vessel, the ventrolateral nucleus of the thalamus emerged the target area of choice.

Many thousands of parkinsonian patients had their tremor reduced by stereotactic procedures aimed at the ventrolateral thalamic nucleus, but the most disabling clinical feature, akinesia, was not alleviated. Attempts to correlate the postmortem findings after operation with the therapeutic outcome revealed extensive regions, including the globus pallidus, internal capsule, lateral ventricular mass of the thalamus, and the field of Forel, within which both large and small lesions can achieve satisfactory results, regardless of their precise localization.

The rationale behind surgical approaches to parkinsonism stemmed from the view that abnormal motor activity could be decreased by interfering with pathologic activity at one of the several links in the chain of events in the central nervous system which culminate in tremor and rigidity. The risk of damaging essential pathways in the course of stereotactic procedures was recognized, but it was not until the long-term results were analyzed that the major limitations of all this surgical endeavor were recognized. In 1969, Hoehn and Yahr published figures which demanded a serious reappraisal of the indications for surgery, and this revelation coincided in time with the widespread availability of powerful new pharmacotherapy in the form of levodopa. In consequence, stereotactic operations for parkinsonism have declined. Neither of the present authors has referred a parkinsonian patient for surgery in the last 5 years.

New Approaches to Treatment

Developments in the management of parkinsonism are likely to arise from new approaches designed to increase the therapeutic index of treatment—the ratio of toxic to therapeutic dosage. Now that peripherally induced adverse reactions have been decreased by the introduction of extracerebral decarboxylase inhibitors, future efforts will be made to reduce unwanted effects generated in the central nervous system. In this context, the most common problems in current therapy are dyskinesia, psychiatric disturbances, and "on-off" phenomena. Although progress has been limited in attempting to ameliorate these difficulties, there have been important conceptual advances toward increasing the selectivity of response, and some practical progress has been made in managing "on-off" phenomena. Three new approaches are of sufficient interest to justify consideration here:

Dopaminergic Agonists. Agonists which act directly on the postsynaptic receptor may theoretically be predicted to have greater specificity than levodopa if there are different categories of dopamine receptor in the central nervous system. Accumulating evidence suggests that there are, indeed, several types of dopaminergic receptors in the brain, so there is likely to be a real possibility of developing agonists which selectively activate receptors at those striatal synapses that are abnormal in parkinsonism. It is also reasonable to anticipate that agonists will emerge which have fewer effects than levodopa on noradrenergic synapses, thus generating a further level of specificity. Another useful property which can probably be achieved is a longer biologic half-life than that of levodopa. Since the enzyme responsible for converting levodopa to dopamine (L-aromatic amino acid decarboxylase) is depleted in parkinsonism, it can also be predicted that agonists, which bypass this enzymic transformation, will have a more consistent therapeutic action.

Two types of agonists have yielded encouraging clinical results:

APOMORPHINES. Cotzias et al. have shown that apomorphine has a therapeutic effect in parkinsonism, but chronic high oral dosage leads to azotemia. A more satisfactory response has been achieved with N-propyl-noraporphine.

ERGOLINES. Two ergolines have yielded good results in the treatment of parkinsonism: bromocriptine (2 brom-α-ergocryptine) and lergotrile.

In our experience, bromocriptine is at least as effective as levodopa (with or without an extracerebral decarboxylase inhibitor). We have found that some patients derive more benefit from bromocriptine than any other therapy, particularly if previous treatment with levodopa has led to prominent "on-off" reactions. Optimal treatment has often been achieved with a combination of bromocriptine and levodopa.

Adverse reactions to bromocriptine are qualitatively similar to those of levodopa, but in addition we have encountered erythema, tenderness, and edema of the ankles, which are dose dependent and reversible. Occasionally bromocriptine may induce peripheral vasospasm when the extremities are cold.

Lergotrile has been studied less extensively than bromocriptine, but Lieberman's initial report was encouraging, and we have confirmed that this drug elicits a therapeutic response. More evidence is necessary before the efficacy and toxicity of lergotrile can be compared with those of other medications.

Selective Monamine Oxidase (MAO) Inhibitors. Collins et al. have shown that two forms of MAO exist in the rat, termed MAO_A and MAO_B. MAO_A oxidizes norepinephrine (NE), serotonin

(5HT), and dopamine, whereas MAO_B destroys dopamine but not NE or 5HT. Hence a specific inhibitor of MAO_B can be expected to lead to elevation of brain dopamine, without concomitant effects on NE or 5HT. Deprenil, a selective inhibitor of MAO_B, has recently been investigated by Birkmayer et al. in parkinsonism. These workers have reported striking potentiation of the therapeutic response to levodopa (in combination with an extracerebral decarboxylase inhibitor) when deprenil is administered intravenously, intramuscularly, or orally. Further studies are needed to define optimal dose regimens and evaluate deprenil in a more prolonged therapeutic setting.

The Role of Peptide Transmitters. The concept of "peptidergic" transmission in the brain is now becoming accepted, and Barbeau has recently reported substantial potentiation of the therapeutic action of levodopa following intravenous injection of MIF (MSH release–inhibitory hormone). Confirmation and extension of these observations would be of considerable interest.

Acknowledgment

We wish to thank Miss Pat Gerdes and Miss Vernita Bergmeyer for typing the manuscript.

PERIPHERAL NEUROPATHY

method of
WILLIAM A. SIBLEY, M.D.
Tucson, Arizona

Nonspecific Treatment and Management of Complications in Polyneuritis

General Care. 1. Bed rest is important in severe cases. A foot board should be provided for patients with weakness of the feet to help prevent contracture at the ankles. For patients with severe pain and tenderness of the limbs, a bed cradle can prevent the discomfort produced by the pressure of the bed clothes.

2. Patients with severe weakness should be repositioned and turned frequently. This allays postural discomfort and helps prevent pulmonary infection. Also, patients remaining supine and immobile for prolonged periods may develop added foot weakness due to compression of the peroneal nerve between the head of the fibula and the mattress.

3. A well balanced diet containing basic vitamin requirements is essential. Multivitamin sup-

plementation is provided for all patients but is of special importance in those with alcoholic and nutritional neuropathies, in whom large doses are employed (see below). If difficulty in swallowing develops, a puree diet may be fed through a small plastic nasogastric tube.

4. Pain relief may usually be obtained with aspirin, 0.6 gram (10 grains), or dextropropoxyphene (Darvon), 32 to 64 mg., every four hours as required. Codeine, 32 mg. (1/2 grain) or meperidine (Demerol), 75 to 100 mg., every four hours may be necessary for more severe pain in the acute stages of illness; the latter drug should be used sparingly, however, to prevent addiction.

Management of Respiratory Failure. In the acute stages of the Guillain-Barré syndrome, diphtheritic polyneuritis, and porphyrinuric polyneuritis, weakness of respiratory muscles may develop rapidly over the course of a few hours. Successful management of respiratory failure depends upon advance planning to handle such an emergency and early recognition of the complication. Late appreciation of respiratory distress makes treatment more difficult because one may be dealing then with an exhausted or semistuporous patient. If the process is detected early in its development, orderly treatment can be undertaken and the patient can be prepared to cooperate fully. Thus, in the early progressive stages of the types of polyneuritis mentioned, the following plan is appropriate:

1. The patient must be observed frequently.

2. A mechanical respirator with which the physician is familiar should be immediately available.

3. Preparations for possible tracheotomy and bronchoscopy should be made well in advance of the need for these procedures. Tracheotomy is essential if difficulty in swallowing is associated with a weak cough. Aspiration of secretions through a bronchoscope will be necessary if signs of atelectasis appear.

4. A mechanical respirator is indicated when respiratory weakness of significant degree is present. Respiratory failure is often heralded by anxiety, restlessness, and a weak cough. Vital capacity measurements should be made frequently when there is doubt and may indicate progressive difficulty; if the vital capacity drops to 25 per cent of its normal value, a respirator will be required. Ventilatory capacity is also commonly followed by making serial observations of the patient's ability to count aloud rapidly as high as possible on one expiration, after maximum voluntary inspiration. Most patients can normally count to 20 or higher on one expiration; if the ability to count in this manner drops below 15, a respirator should be used without further delay. In general, *if one is in doubt as to whether respiratory weakness has progressed*

to the point of requiring mechanical assistance, this is an indication for using a respirator. The rapid unpredictable progression of respiratory distress seen in many patients is the reason for this policy.

The use of oxygen without ventilatory assistance is unwise for patients with respiratory weakness, since it may depress the respiratory center, thereby promoting narcosis from carbon dioxide retention.

Miscellaneous Complications. Urinary retention or incontinence may require an indwelling catheter, but these complications are exceptional in polyneuritis; when urinary symptoms occur they are usually transient phenomena. Persistent evidence of a neurogenic bladder should make one question the diagnosis of polyneuritis.

Abdominal distention due to adynamic ileus is seen in some patients, but it is usually of short duration. When severe, it should be treated by removal of fecal impactions, a small tapwater enema, and insertion of a rectal tube. The intermittent application of hot stupes to the abdomen and small doses of parasympathomimetic drugs such as bethanechol chloride (Urecholine) may also be helpful; 2.5 to 5 mg. of bethanechol may be given subcutaneously.

Physiotherapy. Physical therapy is important in all stages of illness and should usually be given at least twice daily for 15 to 20 minutes. With very ill patients who have severe muscle weakness such treatment should be confined to passive range-of-motion manipulations, which will prevent stiffening of joints and contracture of muscles and tendons. Care must be taken not to overstretch weakened muscles and tender nerve trunks, however.

As improvement in muscle strength occurs and pain subsides, mild active resistance exercises may be instituted and the time devoted to such therapy gradually increased. Vigorous exercise does not hasten the process of nerve healing and regeneration and may occasionally cause relapse in patients convalescing from some forms of polyneuritis. Electrical stimulation of muscles and nerves does not aid recovery.

Specific Measures

Alcoholic and Nutritional Deficiency Polyneuritis. Nutritional polyneuritis is usually due to complex multiple dietary deficiencies, even though a specific vitamin lack is of special importance in certain syndromes (e.g., thiamine deficiency in beriberi, nicotinamide lack in pellagra). Hence, it is important to provide comprehensive dietary therapy and vitamin supplementation in all patients. Alcoholic polyneuritis is a special problem since it is the most common form of polyneuritis in this country; although most evidence favors the view that alcoholic neuritis appears chiefly as the result of dietary inadequacy, a direct toxic effect of alcohol on the nerves may play a role.

Specific treatment of alcoholic and nutritional deficiency polyneuritis should consist of:

1. Abstinence from alcohol.

2. A high-protein, high-carbohydrate diet containing 2000 to 3000 calories per day and adequate sources of vitamins A and C.

3. Vigorous therapy with vitamins of the B group is of primary importance in these patients. To initiate therapy it is desirable to give the B vitamins parenterally to ensure adequate absorption. Thiamine, 50 mg., riboflavin, 20 mg., pyridoxine, 20 mg., nicotinamide, 200 mg., and pantothenic acid, 10 mg., are appropriate daily doses during the first 4 to 5 days of treatment. After this, oral preparations containing approximately one half these dosages should be given daily until recovery.

Diabetic Neuropathies. The symmetrical polyneuropathy that develops slowly over the course of many years in some diabetic patients, manifested chiefly by sensory disturbances in the distal portions of the lower extremities, is usually not influenced by any type of treatment; in many of these patients ischemia of nerves associated with arteriosclerosis obliterans in the lower extremities is a major contributing factor.

However, a more rapidly developing symmetrical polyneuritis, mononeuritis multiplex, or radiculitis may evolve over a period of days or weeks in some diabetic patients, and the radiculitis may closely simulate the picture produced by a herniated intervertebral disc. These patients with diabetic neuritis of subacute onset show a strong tendency to improvement over a period of several months regardless of the therapeutic regimen employed.

1. Careful control of the diabetes and prevention of persistent hyperglycemia should be attempted by means of diet, and insulin or oral antidiabetic agents, as indicated. This would appear to be important since the complication of polyneuritis, in some series, has been higher in poorly controlled subjects. Experimentally, there is a positive correlation between persistent hyperglycemia and (a) accumulation of sorbitol in nerves and (b) microvascular pathology in nerves.

2. Supplementary therapy with oral B vitamins is usually provided but is of uncertain value.

Infectious Polyneuritis (Guillain-Barré Syndrome, Polyneuritis with Facial Diplegia). Infectious polyneuritis appears in both mild and severe forms. Two decades ago there was a high mortality rate, varying from 15 to 40 per cent in most series, death usually occurring from respiratory failure and associated pneumonia. However, it should be remembered that patients surviving the acute phase of the disease usually recover completely, residual neurologic deficit being infrequent. Hence, treatment during the first few weeks of the illness must be carefully managed and should consist of the following:

1. Bed rest is important until improvement is well under way. After definite improvement is noted the patient may be gradually mobilized as indicated by the results of muscle testing. Active exercise and ambulation attempted too early may occasionally cause relapse.

2. Careful attention must be given to anticipate and treat respiratory difficulty (see above). Patients in the early stages of this disorder should be treated only in hospitals in which mechanical respiratory assistance is immediately available.

3. Adrenal steroid or corticotropin (ACTH) therapy has, in many patients, been associated with rapid improvement or cessation of progression. Such treatment may have value when given early in the course of the illness but probably has no effect after the first 2 to 3 weeks. Although this type of therapy is difficult to evaluate because of the variable course of infectious polyneuritis, sufficient suggestive evidence of benefit has accumulated to warrant at least a trial of therapy with these agents in most patients (a) in whom respiratory failure seems likely and (b) those who deteriorate rapidly while under observation. Prednisone, 40 mg. daily in divided doses, is given for the first three days; 30 mg. daily is given for a second 3 day period; after this, the dosage is gradually reduced to a lower maintenance level as permitted by the condition of the patient. In fulminant polyneuritis one may elect to use hydrocortisone intravenously during the first two days of treatment in a dose of 300 to 400 mg.; in such instances therapy is then continued with oral prednisone, as outlined. Antacid therapy is given routinely to patients who receive adrenal steroids; a low-salt diet and supplementary potassium chloride, 0.6 gram four times daily, are given to patients treated with hydrocortisone or ACTH.

If some improvement is not noted after a few days of steroid treatment, prolonged use of these agents is not justified because of the increased risk of bacterial infection and peptic ulceration. Massive doses of steroids probably should not be used since there is at least a theoretical risk of impairing the immune response to various viruses that may cause this form of neuropathy (Epstein-Barr, cytomegalic inclusion virus, hepatitis virus). However in at least one patient in whom cytomegalovirus (CMV) virus was isolated, alternate day prednisone, 100 mg., was associated with good clinical recovery (Arch. Neurol., *136*:100, 1976).

Idiopathic Relapsing Polyneuritis. This neuropathy is clinically similar to the Guillain-Barré type except for its chronic relapsing course. The benefit of chronic prednisone therapy in a large number of patients is much more clearly established. Dramatic improvement is often seen within a few days; continued well-being can frequently be shown to be highly dose-dependent with symptoms of relapse becoming evident within days or even hours when dosage is reduced below a certain critical level. Treatment is usually started with prednisone, 60 mg. daily, with antacids, and changed to alternate-day therapy as soon as possible. A diphasic response with initial worsening, followed shortly by improvement has been described also (Arch. Neurol., *33*:794, 1976).

Uremic Neuropathy. Polyneuritis often occurs in patients with renal failure. An apparent increase in the incidence of this complication in patients treated with peritoneal dialysis or hemodialysis is probably due to longer survival of these patients, and longer exposure to the unknown factors in uremia responsible for the nerve damage. Many patients have recovered from this neural damage with continued more adequate dialysis. Renal transplant is the most effective treatment.

Neuritis Due to Chemical Toxins. Arsenical polyneuritis is treated with dimercaprol. The dosage is 2.5 to 3.0 mg. per kg. of body weight, given as a 10 per cent solution in peanut oil, intramuscularly. This dose is repeated every 4 hours for the first 2 days, then twice daily for 7 to 10 days. Treatment should be begun as soon as possible after arsenical exposure. If therapy is started after the seventh day following arsenical ingestion, the use of dimercaprol does not apparently influence the course of the neuropathy.

The polyneuritis occasionally seen during treatment with isonicotinic acid hydrazide (INH) or hydralazine can be corrected by giving pyridoxine, 50 mg. three times daily.

Neuropathy occurring during treatment with nitrofuran drugs is more common in patients with renal insufficiency. This may be either a distal symmetrical polyneuropathy or one affecting primarily cranial nerves; in the latter instance ocular palsies, and weakness of facial and pharyngeal muscles may simulate myasthenia gravis. The neuropathy usually clears within a few weeks after the drug is withdrawn.

The treatment of lead poisoning with calcium disodium versenate is outlined elsewhere in this volume. Treatment of the polyneuritis caused by most other chemical toxins is supportive (consult section on Poisonings).

Neuritis Associated with Collagen Diseases. A mononeuritis multiplex commonly develops in patients with periarteritis nodosa, although, exceptionally, a symmetrical polyneuritis has been observed. Peripheral nerves may also be involved in systemic lupus erythematosus and rheumatoid arthritis, but neuropathy is much less common in these disorders. Treatment is that of the underlying disease, usually with adrenal steroids.

Neoplastic and Granulomatous Neuropathies. Symmetrical polyneuropathies seen in some patients with malignant neoplasms are usually not due to direct invasion of nerves by tumor tissue. Some of these cases may be due to nutritional deficiency, but the cause in most instances is not known. Improvement has occurred in some patients after resection of the primary tumor.

Direct invasion of the nerves by lymphomas or metastatic carcinoma may be helped by x-ray therapy, if the process is localized. Widespread direct involvement of nerves can often be alleviated by appropriate chemotherapy, especially in instances of lymphomatous or leukemic infiltration.

In cases of sarcoidosis single or multiple nerve trunks may be involved directly by the granuloma. Treatment with adrenal steroids is often effective in such patients.

Porphyria. The polyneuritis seen in acute intermittent porphyria often remits spontaneously; at present there is no specific treatment.

Treatment of porphyrinuric neuritis is chiefly supportive, with the following specific points to be remembered:

1. Barbiturates, sulfonamides, and griseofulvin must be strictly avoided, for they are capable of precipitating acute attacks.

2. Chlorpromazine, in doses of 25 to 50 mg. four times daily, seems to be the most useful drug presently available in the management of this illness. Chlorpromazine facilitates management of the severe pain experienced by these patients and beneficially influences the delirium and other mental symptoms often associated with the disease.

3. If additional sedation is required, chloral hydrate, paraldehyde, or meprobamate may be used. Meperidine (Demerol) may be necessary to control the pain of acute attacks, but should be used sparingly because porphyric patients easily become addicted.

4. Care must be taken to anticipate and detect respiratory failure as outlined elsewhere in this discussion.

Carpal Tunnel Syndrome. Compression of the median nerve as it passes through the restricted carpal tunnel at the wrist causes pain, paresthesias, and sensory loss in a median nerve distribution in the hand; there may be varying degrees of atrophy of the thenar eminence. Frequently appearing bilaterally, and most common in females, it is one of the most frequent of those neuropathies due to mechanical factors. Idiopathic cases may be related to occupational trauma, but since the syndrome has been reported as a complication of rheumatoid arthritis, acromegaly, myxedema, and multiple myeloma, attention should be given to detection and treatment of these possible underlying diseases. Regardless of cause, however, relief of symptoms is usually obtained by surgical division of the transverse carpal ligament at the wrist.

ACUTE HEAD INJURIES IN THE ADULT

method of
KENNETH R. SMITH, JR., M.D.,
and JOHN F. SHEA, M.D.
St. Louis, Missouri

Trauma is the most common cause of death and disability between the ages of 2 and 40 in the United States. Approximately two thirds of all motor vehicle injuries have craniocervical trauma, and brain injury is the most common cause of death in these patients. Perhaps nowhere else in medicine is the prompt initial evaluation and course of therapy as important as in the decisions involved in treating head injuries. A number of characteristics of the brain must be remembered in dealing with head trauma.

1. The brain is enclosed in a rigid container, the skull, and any increase in the volume of the cranial cavity is at the expense of brain, blood or spinal fluid (Monro-Kellie Doctrine).

2. The brain's respiration is 95 per cent aerobic and it can withstand only short periods of hypoxia before permanent neuronal dysfunction results.

3. There seems to be no functional regeneration of the neurons in the central nervous system and all measures must be taken to minimize damage to the surviving neurons after a head injury.

4. Quite often the initial evaluation of the head-injured patient is made by the ambulance attendant, paramedic, or nurse in the emergency room, each of whom may have varied training in dealing with head injuries. Precious minutes have elapsed before the patient is seen by a physician and therapy is instituted.

Noting these facts, it is the responsibility of neurologists and neurosurgeons to instruct those involved in the emergency care and transport of the head-injured patient in order to minimize additional damage to the brain or spinal cord. The major complications of head injury, which include hypoxia, cerebral edema, and intracranial hemorrhage, will be discussed and their treatment outlined.

Initial Evaluation at Scene of Accident

In dealing with any patient with suspected head or spinal cord trauma, an adequate airway must be the first priority. The A, B, Cs should be remembered: airway, breathing, and circulation. The upper airway must be cleared of any obstruction such as vomitus, dentures, clotted blood, and so on. If the chest is expanding normally and the patient appears to have adequate ventilation, a nasal cannula with oxygen should suffice. If the patient is not breathing, an oral pharyngeal airway should be inserted and the patient ventilated with an Ambu bag. If the attendant is experienced, an endotracheal tube may be inserted, remembering to keep the neck in a neutral position. All head injury patients should be suspected of having an associated cervical spine injury and appropriate measures to immobilize the spine should be undertaken. An attempt should be made to insert a nasogastric tube, as aspiration pneumonia is one of the most common causes of death in a head-injury patient. Instilling 60 ml. of an antacid in the nasogastric tube may also help in neutralizing the gastric acidity. An intravenous line with 16 to 18 gauge Medicut should be inserted to have ready access if anticonvulsants, steroids or mannitol are needed. The patient should then be transferred without delay to the emergency room. The paramedic should alert the emergency room so that preparations to receive the patient will have already commenced.

Physical Assessment in the Emergency Department

As soon as the patient arrives in the emergency department, the airway should again be assessed and arterial blood gases obtained. The radiology department should have already been notified and a portable lateral cervical spine radiograph should be taken and viewed by the physician for proper alignment. The vital signs and neurologic findings should be recorded on a continuous flow sheet and a record kept of all drugs given to the patient. If the patient is hypotensive due to hypovolemic shock, this is never due to a closed head injury. The abdomen should be evaluated as well as the thoracic contents as causes for the hypotension. Spinal cord injury may also cause hypotension but the pulse is slow rather than rapid as in shock. The extremities should also be evaluated for fractures, as a frac-

tured femur or pelvis may be associated with massive blood loss. Shock must be treated immediately and must take precedence in the treatment. Until whole blood is available, immediate volume replacement with a plasma expander such as 6 per cent serum albumin must commence. Crystalloid volume replacement is hazardous in a head injury, due to the 3 for 1 replacement rule. Since it has a molecular weight of less than 8000, the fluid leaks into the interstitial space in a short time. Three liters of lactated Ringer's or isotonic saline solution add approximately 450 mEq. of sodium to the serum. Dextrose in water is more dangerous than saline solution and should never be given initially. Blood should be drawn and sent to the laboratory for a type and cross match, complete blood count (CBC), blood urea nitrogen (BUN), electrolytes, and amylase, and urine analysis should be done. A Foley catheter should be inserted in order to monitor urinary output and to decompress the bladder. A comprehensive neurologic examination should then be done.

The single most important item in the initial evaluation of a head-injury patient is the ability to assess and record changes in the level of consciousness. Consciousness is usually maintained by the reticular activating system in the brain stem and since the brain stem is firmly anchored in the posterior fossa, it frequently bears the full brunt of an impact to the head. A temporary neuronal dysfunction results and the patient may lose consciousness. Such terms as lethargic, stuporous or obtunded should be avoided in describing the head-injury patient. A very effective coma scale has been devised by Brian Jennett and involves only three categories; eye-opening, best verbal response, and best motor response to command. A copy of this may be found in Emergency Medicine, 9:3, 1977, and should be placed in a conspicuous area in the emergency department. The pupils should be evaluated for size, reactivity, and shape. The position of the eyes should be noted as to conjugate gaze, roving movements or fixed ophthalmoplegia. Remember that the eyes look toward a destructive lesion, i.e., clot or contusion and away from an irritative lesion, i.e., seizure focus. If the cervical spine is in proper alignment, the oculocephalic reflex should be tested. Mydriatic drugs must not be used to dilate the pupils. The ears and nose should be examined for cerebrospinal fluid (CSF) leakage. Periorbital and post-auricular ecchymosis indicate basilar skull fractures and when accompanied by CSF leakage, the possibility of post-traumatic meningitis must be remembered. The scalp should be palpated for lacerations, fractures, and subgaleal hematomas. A boggy temporalis muscle may indicate an underlying pterion fracture and associated extradural hematoma. Next, the motor system should be evaluated for weakness, paralysis, and muscle tone. The tendon reflexes should also be evaluated for symmetry and presence. A sensory examination with a pin is done always comparing the two sides. If the patient is uncooperative or comatose, the response of the patient to painful stimuli is noted. The posture of the patient should be noted as to whether he is decorticate with flexed upper extremities and extended lower extremities or if he is decerebrate, showing extensor posturing in the upper and lower limbs. The superficial reflexes should be tested, including the Babinski, superficial abdominals, and cremasteric reflexes. Anal sphincter tone should be evaluated and at the same time, a rectal examination for blood, bone, prostatic pathology, etc. is done, especially if there is an associated pelvic fracture. One should also note the type of respiration, as Cheyne-Stokes respiration usually indicates a cortical lesion, central neurogenic hyperventilation indicates a midbrain lesion and an irregular or ataxic type of respiration indicates damage to the lower brain stem. A brain-injured patient should rarely be given narcotics for pain relief, as these will depress the most important evidence of brain function, the level of consciousness, and may affect pupillary size.

Diagnostic Studies

After the patient's respiration has been stabilized, the shock has been treated and the neurologic status is not deteriorating, further studies may then be indicated. Skull x-rays may be useful in identifying depressed skull fragments, fractures that cross arterial channels, air-fluid levels in the paranasal sinuses, and pneumocephalus. A brow-up lateral skull film often shows the C1-C2 cervical vertebrae well and can supplement the lateral cervical spine film. A chest x-ray and an abdominal radiologic examination may also be indicated. With the advent of computed scanning, a CT scan is probably the procedure of choice to diagnose intracranial hematoma as it has the least associated mortality and morbidity. The patient must be accompanied in the scanning room by an experienced observer, constantly watching level of consciousness and vital signs. If a computer scan is not available, cerebral angiography is the next procedure of choice to diagnose hematoma.

Intracranial pressure recording is now being done at many neurosurgical centers. The recording devices may be epidural, subarachnoid, or intraventricular in type. A continuous pressure measurement allows one to evaluate drug therapy and to plan surgical intervention. Lumbar puncture should be avoided in acute brain injuries. The knowledge of the presence of sub-arachnoid hemorrhage is of little therapeutic value and the pressure manometrics may not accurately reflect intracranial pressure. A lumbar puncture might also cause acute brainstem coning into the foramen magnum and rapid demise of the patient.

Medical Management

1. All patients with lacerations and abrasions are given tetanus prophylaxis.

2. Patients are kept in a 40° head-elevated (Fowler's position) posture in the intensive care unit bed in order to facilitate jugular venous drainage as cerebral venous pressure tends to equal intracranial pressure.

3. Fluid therapy should be kept at 1500 ml. per 24 hours and the serum and urine electrolytes and osmolality should be monitored carefully, especially if dehydrating agents are used. Inappropriate antidiuretic hormone secretion and diabetes insipidus are frequent complications of head injuries and may be the cause of the deteriorating neurologic status. Plain dextrose in water should not be used in the initial management as it may enhance brain swelling.

4. Respiratory therapy must be aimed at avoiding hypoxia and hypercarbia, as this combination will increase the amount of blood in the brain with resultant increase in intracranial pressure. A tidal volume of 10 to 12 ml. per kg. with a respiratory rate of 16 to 18 per minute and 15 sighs per hour should suffice if ventilatory assistance is needed.

5. If an endotracheal tube is still indicated after 48 to 96 hours and if the patient is still in coma, a tracheostomy is done to facilitate pulmonary toilet and removal of added dead space.

6. The use of steroids has been controversial but we still use them in hopes of reducing cerebral edema by stabilizing the blood brain barrier and recently steroids have been shown to decrease CSF formation. An initial bolus of 16 mg. of dexamethasone intravenously followed by 4 mg. intravenously is given every 6 hours and this is tapered as clinical improvement is evidenced. We have been using cimetidine to inhibit gastric acid secretion in these patients along with antacids.

7. Anticonvulsants are used prophylactically in severe brain injuries and phenytoin sodium is the drug of choice. An initial loading dose of 1 gram is given in the first 24 hours and then a maintenance dose of 300 to 400 mg. is given every 24 hours. Since intramuscular absorption is erratic, the intravenous or nasogastric tube is used. Phenobarbital is also used and 32 to 64 mg. is given intravenously every 6 hours. Diazepam is a poor anticonvulsant in the head-injured patient; it has a marked and long-lasting respiratory depressant

effect compared to its short-acting anticonvulsant action.

8. The Foley catheter is removed after the first 24 hours and intermittent catheterization is done on a routine schedule; this has lowered our incidence of urinary tract infections. The urine specific gravity should be measured every 4 to 6 hours.

9. Prophylactic antibiotics are used only if there is a dural laceration or CSF leakage and meningitic doses are used. If there is associated pulmonary or urinary tract infection broad-spectrum antibiotics are used until the culture reports are ready.

10. Temperature regulation may be impaired due to an injury to the hypothalamus and hyperthermia must be treated until normothermia returns. A cooling apparatus is quite useful but should not be placed directly on the skin of the patient. Aspirin and acetaminophen (Tylenol) may also be used.

11. If the patient is deteriorating rapidly as evidenced by focal signs such as a decrease in the level of consciousness, pupillary dilatation, or a change in vital signs such as a widening pulse pressure and bradycardia, immediate measures must be undertaken. Mannitol should be rapidly infused at a dose of 1 to 1.5 grams per kg. Mannitol buys time and commits the physician to notify the neurosurgeon in order that further diagnostic studies may be undertaken.

12. With all the sophisticated monitoring equipment available, the best method of patient care still remains repeated clinical observations and good nursing care.

Types of Injuries and Their Treatment

Scalp Lacerations. The scalp is quite vascular and copious blood loss may occur if hemostasis is not quickly attained. This is especially true in children with their small blood volume. The wound should be irrigated, palpated, and debrided of all foreign material and the wound closed in layers, including a tight closure of the galea aponeurotica.

Intracranial Hemorrhages. EPIDURAL HEMORRHAGE. This type of extradural hemorrhage is usually associated with a skull fracture, especially near the pterion. The middle meningeal vessels are torn with resultant accumulation of blood. An initial period of unconsciousness may be followed by a lucid interval of a few hours and then progressive rapid neurologic deterioration occurs. The brain may be acutely shifted with resultant compression of the brain stem against the sharp edges of the tentorium. The third nerve is compressed and a rapid sequence of paralysis, coma, and death will ensue if decompression is not speedily done. Craniotomy with removal of the blood clot and control of the bleeding meningeal vessels is the treatment of choice. The mortality rate of an acute epidural hematoma is approximately 20 per cent. This is one of the most rewarding neurosurgical procedures to be done, in that frequently the patient will make a complete recovery if the diagnosis is made rapidly.

SUBDURAL HEMATOMA. A subdural hematoma is usually caused by a shearing injury to the brain, and one of the cortical bridging veins is torn. This type of clot is usually associated with a brain laceration or contusion. There may or may not be an associated skull fracture. Subdurals may be acute, subacute, or chronic. The treatment is a wide craniotomy with removal of the clot and the dura may have to be left open and the bone flap left out to allow for brain swelling, which almost invariably is massive with a subdural hemorrhage. The mortality rate is quite high, approaching 60 to 70 per cent, due to the severity of the brain injury.

INTRACEREBRAL HEMORRHAGE. The incidence of intracerebral hemorrhage after head injury is seen more frequently than previously thought, as recently evidenced by CT scanning. Very often, the frontal lobe and the temporal lobes are contused due to the many projections and ridges on the floor of the anterior and middle cranial fossa. The contused area may then bleed into the associated lobe and cause a shift of the cerebral structures. Surgical evacuation of the clot may be necessary, especially if the clot is large and the shift is great.

Concussion. A concussion is a temporary loss of consciousness due to an alteration of the brain stem reticular formation. The patient, when first seen, will frequently have amnesia, which is usually post-traumatic but may be also pretraumatic. A concussion is usually only temporary and there are no permanent neurologic sequelae. Criterion for admission to the hospital for active observation include the following: unconsciousness lasting more than 30 minutes; pre- or post-traumatic amnesia; skull fracture, especially if it crosses suture lines or vascular channels; severe headaches and vomiting; post-traumatic seizures; lethargy or behavior change; and associated focal neurologic deficit.

Contusion. A contusion is a bruising of the brain, usually caused by rotational forces. There are areas of superficial damage to the brain found at the crests of the gyri with streaks of hemorrhage at right angles to the cortical surface of the temporal lobe and inferior surface of the frontal lobe. They are also found under fractures and under the area of impact. A contusion may also be seen on the side of the brain contralateral to the impact, and this is a contre-coup lesion. These lesions usually heal in a few weeks, but the associated edema may cause massive brain swelling and controlled hyperventilation; osmotic diuretics and steroids may be necessary to control edema.

Follow-up Care for Head-Injury Patients

Postconcussion Injuries. This syndrome is often seen and consists of headaches, extreme fatigue, psychiatric problems, muscle spasm, etc. This is best treated by aspirin and emotional support.

Post-traumatic Epilepsy. Prophylactic anticonvulsants are routinely given to any patient with a documented seizure, dural laceration, depressed skull fracture, or a severe head injury. We continue these anticonvulsants until the patient is seizure free for at least 12 to 24 months. Blood levels of the anticonvulsants may be checked to see if a therapeutic level of the drug has been achieved.

Physical Therapy. This is extremely valuable for the head or spinal cord injured patient and may have to continue for a period of many months in order that the patient may achieve the maximum return of function.

Accident Prevention. This is the single most important aspect in dealing with head or spinal cord injuries. Physicians and allied medical personnel should support highway safety laws, wearing of shoulder and lap belts, strict enforcement of the drinking-while-driving laws, and education of the general public in accident prevention.

HEAD INJURIES IN CHILDREN

method of
LUIS SCHUT, M.D.,
and D. A. BRUCE, M.D.
Philadelphia, Pennsylvania

As many as one third of all patients in a pediatric surgical service are admitted because of trauma and 50 per cent of these have experienced head trauma. One child in 10 will suffer a significant head injury with disturbed level of consciousness during the school years. One third of these, or 3 per cent of all children, will be hospitalized during the school years for head injury.

The mortality from head injury in the pediatric age group is 1 to 2 per cent, or approximately 4000 children per year. The mortality rate from more specialized neurosurgical units is considerably higher—10 to 13 per cent. In severe head injury with coma, the mortality remains at 50 per cent.

The postconcussion syndrome, mental and personality changes, and other evidence of mild to severe brain damage have been described frequently in head-injured children. However, the incidence of post-traumatic sequelae is gratifyingly low—3 to 4 per cent of all head injuries. Following severe head trauma, the incidence of severe and prolonged neurologic, intellectual, or personality problems is high. If coma exceeds 24 hours following injury, significant sequelae can be expected in 10 to 50 per cent of patients. Nonetheless, many patients make a remarkable recovery and are able to return to school and become self-supporting despite neurologic deficit. Two to 5 per cent of patients with severe head injury will remain permanently and severely handicapped.

Several important technologic innovations in the last 2 years have enabled us to increase our knowledge of the pathophysiology significantly. The application of axial transmission computed tomography (CT scanning) and emission computed tomography for measurements of local cerebral blood volume (LCBV) have added a new chapter to our knowledge of the anatomic and physiologic changes occurring in the injured brain. The use of continuous intracranial pressure (ICP) monitoring has allowed us to define exactly the time course and magnitude of the intracranial pressure changes and measure the effectiveness and duration of therapeutic drugs. Finally, the realization that only a small percentage of even the more severe injuries can be benefited by surgery encourages the development of a team approach to the problem of head injury. This includes the anesthesiologist, pediatrician, and neurosurgeon as a minimum.

Initial Management

Nothing can be done to reverse the immediate effects of the primary head injury. The cellular death and disruption that occur at the time of impact are not yet amenable to therapy. The secondary events (brain swelling, brain edema, hypoxia and shock) are all amenable to correction. Therefore, it is to this secondary head injury that all our efforts are directed.

It has been shown that 50 per cent of children dying from head injury are awake at the time of admission to hospital, yet 70 per cent of deaths occur within the first 48 hours. These figures emphasize that the mortality is due to rapid progression of some secondary events, since coma and death did not result at the moment of impact.

This secondary injury is due to alterations in the arterial gases secondary to respiratory difficulties, alterations in systemic blood pressure, and alterations in the intracranial pressure. Any obstruction of the airway, common in the unconscious patient, will result in arterial CO_2 tension or decrease in the oxygen tension. CO_2 is a potent cerebrovascular vasodilator. Hypercarbia leads to an increase in cerebral blood volume, causing secondary increase in intracranial pressure, increase in end-capillary pressure leading to increased fluid infiltration into the tissue and edema. Hypoxemia will lead to further decrease in tissue

Po_2 in areas of the brain already limited in oxygen availability by edema or elevated intracranial pressure and systemic shock will lead to ischemic hypoxia of the brain if the arterial pressure is low enough. Delayed formation of an intracranial mass lesion (epidural, subdural, or intracerebral hematoma) will lead to an increase in intracranial pressure and a decrease in cerebral blood flow and further ischemic damage.

Only 7 per cent of head trauma patients admitted to our service require surgery, stressing that head injury is not a surgical disease but rather has a complex pathology best treated in an intensive care unit by team effort.

The time from injury to arrival in the hospital is a period of great risk. An improperly positioned child may develop airway obstruction and suffer his or her secondary injury before arriving at the hospital. To avoid this, good ambulance facilities and, in particular, well-trained ambulance personnel are vital. When the injury has occurred to the freely mobile head, concern for cervical spine injury should always be entertained. This necessitates careful transport, probably best performed if the patient is unconscious in the lateral position with the cervical spine straight and supported.

Upon arrival in the hospital immediate clearing of the airway manually and assisted ventilation with a mask and oral airway are usually adequate to maintain low CO_2 and normal Pao_2. Lateral spine films can then be obtained to ensure the absence of cervical fracture or dislocation or both. In patients grade III and IV our policy is to insert a nasotracheal or oral tracheal tube for further transport of the patient (Table 1). This requires the early and full involvement of an anesthesiologist. All diagnostic studies are then performed under light general anesthesia with thiopental (Pentothal), nitrous oxide and oxygen, and pancuronium if required. See Figures 1 and 2 for treatment steps.

Table 1. Clinical Grading of Head-Injured Patients

Ia.	Normal consciousness *without* focal signs
Ib.	Normal consciousness *with* focal signs
IIa.	Lethargic *without* focal signs
IIb.	Lethargic *with* focal signs
IIIa.	Confused or stuporous *without* focal signs
IIIb.	Confused or stuporous *with* focal signs
IVa.	Coma (pain response or less) *without* focal signs
IVb.	Coma (pain response or less) *with* focal signs

The importance of the team approach is immediately apparent. While the anesthesiologist is controlling the airway the pediatrician is establishing an intravenous line, drawing routine blood studies, and doing a full systemic examination to identify injuries other than to the cerebrum. At the same time, the neurosurgeon can evaluate the neurologic status of the patient. The early presence of all members of the team allows each one to evaluate the patient before any drugs have been given. If no CT scan is available and no arteriography immediately planned in a patient who is not comatose, then endotracheal intubation may be too traumatic and attempts may lead to further problems. Thus, control with an oral airway and frequent suctioning with the patient in a semiprone position is probably the best way to protect the airway and maintain normal blood gas tensions.

Skull x-rays should always be obtained in the severely injured child. In cases of minor trauma with an alert patient, x-rays should be obtained in children under 1 year of age. Twenty-one per cent of all head-injured patients admitted to our service have a skull fracture. Forty-six per cent of patients aged less than 1 year have sustained a fracture. Injury, particularly falls, in the first year of life is frequently associated with a skull fracture but no

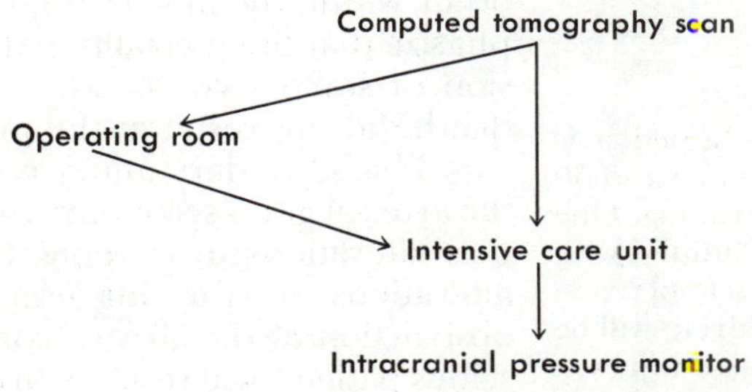

Figure 1.

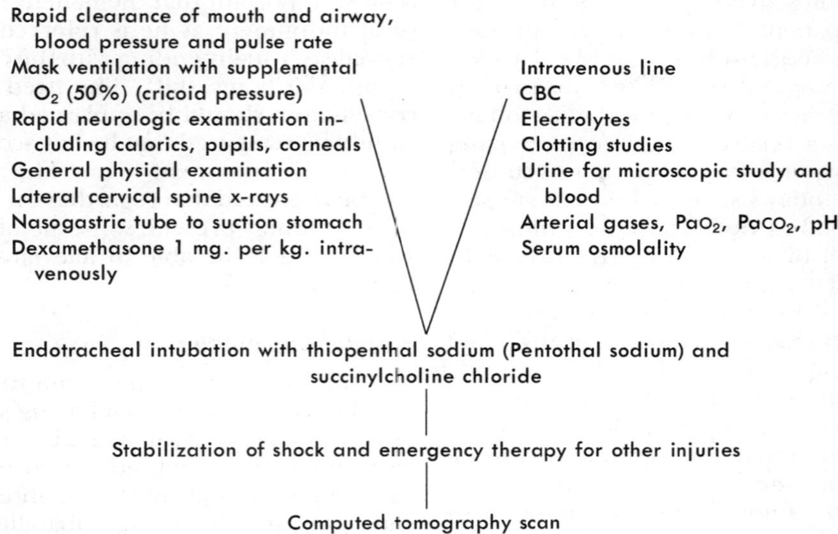

Figure 2. Head injury treatment protocol for patients with severe head injury [i.e., no spontaneous eye opening, no verbal response (speech or crying), no spontaneous purposeful movements].

alteration of consciousness. X-rays of the cervical spine and chest are routinely obtained in the severely injured patient. Routine blood studies including complete blood count (CBC) and differential, electrolytes, blood urea nitrogen, creatinine, sickle cell preparation, prothrombin time, partial thromboplastin time, and blood type are routinely obtained. Urine is obtained for evidence of blood. When a CT scan is available, this is unquestionably the best special study. If no CT scan is available, then repeated careful neurologic evaluations are the key to further investigation. *Any* deterioration in neurologic status should be an indication for arteriography. This is almost always preferable to exploratory burr holes. The patient in deep coma should be studied early with arteriography since there is no way to know whether the coma is a result of primary diffuse injury or due to secondary injury (i.e., swelling or intracranial hematoma). Infrequently, both conditions exist. As many children require therapy for elevated intracranial pressure (10 per cent) as require surgery.

We obtain an immediate CT scan on all grade III and IV patients. If a surgical lesion is seen then the appropriate operation is performed and the patient returned to the intensive care unit (ICU) following surgery with an intracranial pressure monitor in place. If no mass lesion is seen, the patient is returned to the ICU where an intracranial pressure monitor is inserted. If the patient is irritated by the nasotracheal tube and the intracranial pressure is normal, the tube is frequently removed. If the intracranial pressure is high or the patient tolerates the endotracheal tube well, it is

left in place for at least 24 hours. Patients who require an endotracheal tube for airway maintenance but who are restless are usually treated with either small doses of morphine intravenously or with pancuronium and controlled ventilation.

Seizures are usually treated with phenytoin (Dilantin) in older children. If phenobarbital is used for the younger children, good airway maintenance is extremely important. Occasionally, because of apparent rapid deterioration, mannitol 0.5 to 1 gram per kg. in 20 per cent solution is given. Following mannitol it is important to complete an intracranial study to rule out a mass lesion which may now be masked as a result of the hyperosmolar therapy. The role of steroids remains controversial in head injury, but we have generally used them. Recent evidence suggests that a significant effect is obtained by using doses of 1 to 1.5 mg. per kg. of dexamethasone for a period of 9 days.

BRAIN TUMORS

method of
GLENN A. MEYER, M.D.,
and LARRY E. KUN, M.D.
Milwaukee, Wisconsin

Introduction

In his recently published autobiography, *No Man Alone,* the late Wilder Penfield describes his early operative experience in New York prior to moving to Montreal. During a memorable week, he performed long arduous craniotomies for tumor on three patients with three prompt postoperative deaths. In the subsequent five decades, neurosurgical capabilities have improved sufficiently that death or major morbidity following craniotomy is a relatively rare event evoking prolonged discussion at the complications conference. Obviously, today's surgeons do not surpass Dr. Penfield in skill or dedication. The improvement is the result of much more effective tools, techniques, and medications, both for the neurosurgeon and his colleagues in neuroradiology, neuroanesthesia, radiation therapy, and neurologic nursing.

The diagnostic work-up of patients with brain tumors with specialized angiography and second generation CT (computed tomographic) scanning (often supplemented with multidirectional tomography and radionucleide scanning) provides the surgeon with a detailed map of the spatial and vascular characteristics of the tumor and occasionally an accurate prediction of the histology. Thus, the surgeon can accurately focus his efforts, via the least traumatic route, on the tumor mass, whether located on the surface or deep within the brain. The need for blind biopsies has been eliminated.

Nonoperative Methods of Treatment

Treatment with synthetic steroids often provides many weeks or months of comfortable life. One must accept, and if necessary prepare the patient for, the discomfort of hyperadrenalism, but this should not deter the use of steroids when necessary for control of tumor morbidity. The dose must be titrated against the patient's signs and symptoms and may vary from 0.5 to 100 mg. per day of dexamethasone or its equivalent. The medication is given in divided doses three or four times daily accompanied by antacid therapy.

The use of osmotic diuretics can be lifesaving and may provide time for diagnosis and elective surgery. Their use may be indicated both in the hospital during acute exacerbations of intracranial hypertension (mannitol, 0.25 to 1.0 gram per kg. intravenously every 3 to 6 hours) or more chronically (glyceryl, 0.8 to 1.2 ml. per kg. orally every 4 to 8 hours). Some means of intracranial pressure measurement may aid materially in guiding steroid and osmotic therapy both acutely and chronically.

The ability to follow safely and accurately tumor size with CT scans has encouraged neurosurgeons to observe the biologic behavior of small benign tumors in the elderly. Occasionally, such patients with very indolent lesions can be spared the necessity for craniotomy.

In treating patients with incurable tumors, it is most important that the patient not feel a sense of abandonment as he is referred to a series of specialists, usually ending with the chemotherapist or nursing home staff. The need for additional consultation should be explained and the patient should be reassured that he has access to all members of the treatment team. The patient should also be reassured that regardless of what problems the tumor may present, some member of the team will invariably be able to alleviate the pain and suffering.

Hospital Capabilities

It is our opinion that brain tumor treatment should occur in a hospital having sufficient numbers of neurosurgical patients to allow the development of specialized neurosurgical nursing care. Such a unit ideally has an intensive care area with patient monitoring capabilities. This does materially increase the chance for morbidity-free surgical treatment. The nonphysician staff must be trained in both neurologic diagnostic techniques and the use of monitoring instrumentation. The training must be followed by a sufficient case load to maintain staff skills.

Another crucial hospital capability is immediate access to a CT scanner, staffed 24 hours a day and in close proximity to the postoperative ward. The scanner can be lifesaving in diagnosing and localizing postoperative hematomas that are not necessarily at the site of tumor resection.

Operative Considerations

It is important to begin daily bacteriostatic shampoos as soon as craniotomy is scheduled. Prophylactic intravenous antibiotics (e.g., nafcillin, 1 gram every 4 hours) begun just before surgery are recommended in patients with increased risk of infection such as those involving a shunt for cerebrospinal fluid.

Coordination with a neuroanesthesiologist is crucial, especially where techniques such as intraoperative hypotension are required.

With markedly vascular lesions, the immediate preoperative embolization of major feeding arteries, usually by a neuroradiologist using catheter techniques, may be crucial to the success of an operation.

In our opinion, elective craniotomies should be done in operating rooms equipped to handle the full gamut of complicated neurosurgery. Included are an operative microscope and microneurosurgical instruments including those required for vascular lesions. Instrumentation for constant monitoring of blood pressure and blood gases as well as for air embolism is essential.

TABLE 1. **Treatment of Brain Tumors**

| TUMOR | SURGERY | | RADIATION THERAPY | | | CHEMO-THERAPY | | RANGE OF MALIG-NANCY 0–4 | AGE PREDILECTION | | LOCATION PREDILECTION Tentorium | | |
	Pallia-tive	Cura-tive	Local	Total Brain	Total CNS	Sys-temic	Intra-thecal		Older	Younger	Above	Below	Other Specific
Malignant glioma grades III–IV glioblastoma	+	−	−	+	±	+	−	3–4	+	−	+	±	−
Glioma grades I–II	+	±	±	±	−	−	−	1–2	−	+	±	+	−
Meningiomas	±	+	±	−	−	−	−	0–2	+	−	±	±	−
Metastatic	±	−	±	+	−	±	−	2–4	+	−	+	±	−
Oligodendro-gliomas	+	−	+	±	−	±	−	2–3	+	−	+	−	−
(Neurinomas) Schwannomas	±	+	±	−	−	−	−	0–1	+	−	−	+	+
Pituitary adenomas	±	+	+	−	−	−	−	0–1	+	−	+	−	+
Cranio-pharyngioma	±	±	+	−	−	−	−	0	−	+	+	−	+
Medullo-blastoma	±	−	−	−	+	+	+	4	−	+	−	+	−
Ependymoma	+	±	+	−	±	±	±	1–4	±	±	±	±	−
Hemangioblastoma	±	+	±	−	−	±	−	0–3	+	−	±	+	−
Pinealoma	±	−	±	+	±	+	±	1–4	±	+	−	−	+
Optic glioma	±	±	+	±	−	±	−	0–3	−	+	−	−	+
(Pontine) brain stem glioma	±	−	+	−	−	±	−	1–4	−	+	−	−	+

Key: + yes or usually; − no or never (almost never); ± maybe or occasionally

Intraoperative recording of cortical evoked potentials can be crucial for preservation of neurologic function, particularly with intrinsic lesions of the brainstem and with those involving the primary visual pathways.

Craniotomy

Details of operative techniques are not relevant, but Table 1 gives an overview of what the neurosurgeon can expect to accomplish with individual tumors. The general principle of obtaining a tissue diagnosis, in almost every patient if at all possible, is followed. This principle is also applied to such lesions as pineal area tumors, since the risk of exposure of deep basal and midline tumors is now sufficiently reduced. Thus, the patient with a rare benign tumor in these less readily accessible areas may be spared the potential morbidity of radiation therapy. The authors do not practice "biopsy only" technique with malignant gliomas, since tumor debulking and internal decompression are

important to achieve maximum benefit from radiation and chemotherapy.

Anterior basal routes of exposure may be required for successful treatment of lesions expanding the sella turcica or eroding the clivus; transsphenoidal and transpharyngeal approaches are used, respectively. The lateral cervical approach to the clivus has little if any application.

A preoperative cerebrospinal fluid shunt may markedly improve the operative results in patients showing deterioration from hydrocephalus. This commonly occurs with posterior fossa tumors such as medulloblastomas.

Continuing neurosurgical follow-up should be provided for all brain tumor patients with performance of repeat CT scanning at appropriate intervals and when there is an abrupt change in neurologic condition. Occasionally a change in the biologic behavior of the tumor such as development of a cyst or localized tumor mass may dictate the need for craniotomy late in the course of an incurable tumor. This is more likely to occur in tumors treated by radiation therapy without prior craniotomy, i.e., optic gliomas and brainstem gliomas.

Radiation Therapy

General Considerations. Irradiation is utilized in the management of most patients with brain tumors. The indications for radiation therapy and the techniques of treatment depend upon the patient's age and functional status, the tumor location and histology, and the surgical resectability. Successful treatment depends upon understanding the natural history of brain tumors with maximal exploitation of the differential responsiveness to irradiation of normal brain tissue and neoplastic tissue. In many instances radiation therapy can be shown to improve neurologic function, prolong survival, and improve the quality of survival.

Modern radiotherapy employs megavoltage equipment and patient localization techniques that permit relatively high doses of radiation to precisely defined volumes. CT scanning increases the accuracy and safety of such treatment by enhancing our knowledge of tumor behavior and the precision of field definition. While wide-field irradiation of the entire cranium or the entire neuraxis (brain and spinal cord) is indicated for many patients with central nervous system neoplasms, limiting the volume of irradiation to localized, relatively noninvasive tumors is a distinct advantage in controlling the later lesions.

With the exception of the peculiarly radiosensitive pineal germinomas, irradiation of most primary brain tumors requires doses approaching the tolerance of normal brain. Treatment fractionation with low daily doses (150 to 180 rad), total doses below 5500 rad in 6 to 8 weeks, and reduction of field size when feasible minimize the occurrence of postirradiation complications. One must balance the potential benefits of treatment against the risks of damage to normal brain structures.

Normal Tissue Reactions. During treatment one may occasionally see nausea, appetite suppression, or lassitude; however, most patients experience no immediate reaction except alopecia and cutaneous erythema. With megavoltage irradiation, patients will usually have regrowth of hair within six months.

An important and poorly understood reaction to radiation therapy is the development of headache, lassitude, low grade fever, or enhanced local neurologic symptoms and signs 4 to 8 weeks after the completion of treatment. This syndrome has been attributed to a transient, partial demyelinization within the treated volume. Symptoms and signs are diminished by corticosteroids, with spontaneous resolution in 5 to 30 days. Knowledge of this is particularly important, since it mimics tumor progression.

Late complications months to years following irradiation are fortunately rare, but instances of brain necrosis and major vascular occlusion have been reported. In most patients, these relate to excessive doses (rarely seen below 7000 rad), rapid treatment regimens, repeat courses of irradiation, or field techniques allowing excessive inhomogeneity.

Treatment of Specific Tumors

Malignant Gliomas. Postoperative irradiation improves both the quality and length of survival in patients with grade IV lesions. In addition, a small number of patients with grade III lesions achieve disease-free survival in excess of 5 years.

Metastatic Tumors. Cranial irradiation provides effective palliation for patients with metastatic brain tumors. Most patients experience significant improvement in neurologic symptoms following treatment, although long-term, disease-free survival in any patient with documented brain metastasis is rare. Rapid fractionation schemes (3000 to 3600 rad in 2 to 2.5 weeks) have been well tolerated and effective in this group of patients, in which median survival following documentation of metastasis is measured in months.

Pituitary Adenomas. Small field sellar irradiation is indicated in the primary or postoperative management of many patients with pituitary neoplasms. Significant suprasellar extension reduces the likelihood of irradiation control, and large or rapidly developing visual field defects are indications for more prompt decompression via a neurosurgical approach, usually followed by postoperative irradiation. Reduction of tumor size and hormonal production (e.g., growth hormone in eosinophilic adenomas) is gradual following irradiation, with favorable changes usually demonstrable over several months to a few years post treatment. The transsphenoidal surgical approach to small functioning adenomas is an alternative form of initial therapy and may be curative, although there is need for longer follow-up with this relatively new treatment modality.

Medulloblastoma. Medulloblastoma is a moderately radiosensitive lesion that can be cured in approximately 50 per cent of the patients radically treated to the entire neuraxis (craniospinal irradiation). Such techniques are laborious and require exquisite immobilization and attention to treatment details but result in a gratifyingly long, disease-free survival without serious treatment-related sequelae.

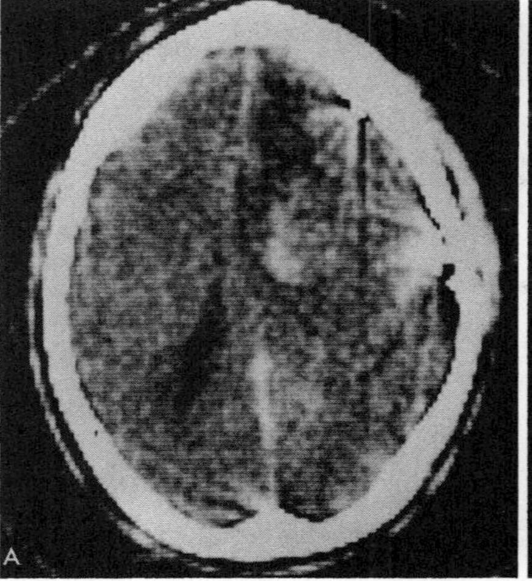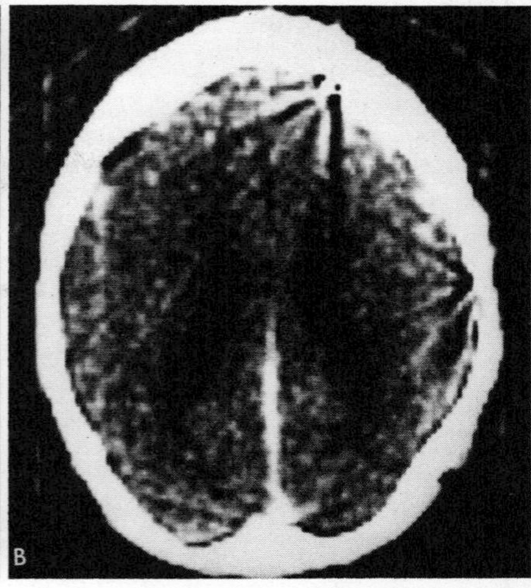

Figure 1. This patient, now age 15, was treated by the authors beginning with craniotomy for tumor debulking of his grade III glioma on 10/19/76, followed by completion of 6000 rads whole brain radiation on 12/29/76 and CCNU-procarbazine therapy beginning 2/3/77. Only traces of the contrast-enhanced tumor shown in *A* were present in *B* at follow-up on 2/7/78.

Other Tumors. Local radiation is often used with incompletely resected low-grade gliomas, meningiomas, and craniopharyngiomas. Localized treatment without prior surgery is also commonly given to pinealomas, optic gliomas, and brainstem gliomas. The treatment decision in such lesions requires multidisciplinary input.

Chemotherapy

Chemotherapeutic agents have demonstrated effectiveness in certain brain neoplasms. Transient responses of up to several months or a few years are reported in malignant gliomas, brainstem neoplasms, medulloblastomas, and ependymomas. The adjunctive use of antineoplastic agents with surgery, with or without irradiation, has marginally improved survival time in patients with malignant gliomas. Tumor-free survival of significant duration, however, has been only infrequently noted following the use of such agents.

Most responses have occurred with the use of nitroureas (BCNU, CCNU, MeCCNU), procarbazine, high dose methotrexate, and vincristine. Sporadic responses have been noted with alkylating agents (cyclophosphamide, thiotepa), imidazole carboxamides (DTIC), and the newer epipodophyllotoxin (VM-26). Although the blood brain barrier is not intact within the center of the tumor mass, normal vessels retarding drug transport across this pharmacologic barrier exist around the periphery of the tumor where infiltrative growth is present. Indeed, most responses in malignant gliomas and brainstem neoplasms have been limited to the lipid-soluble nitroureas and procarbazine. Some medulloblastomas respond markedly but transiently to the addition of vincristine, cyclophosphamide, and methotrexate. Systematic combination chemotherapy has yet to increase either disease-free or total survival time with medulloblastomas. Very occasionally an unexpectedly good result can be achieved (see Figure 1).

The chapter provides guidelines only. For further neurosurgical details concerning specific tumors, the reader is referred to Youman, J. R.: *Neurological Surgery*, Volume III, Saunders, 1973. For further information concerning radiation therapy see Bouchard, J.: *Radiation Therapy of Tumors and Diseases of the Nervous System*, Lea & Febiger, 1966.

RHEUMATOID ARTHRITIS

method of
ROY FLEISCHMANN, M.D.,
and J. DONALD SMILEY, M.D.
Dallas, Texas

Rheumatoid arthritis (RA) is a systemic disease that has a variable onset and course in which about 35 per cent of patients have acute onset of disease that spontaneously resolves within 6 to 12 months. About half have disease characterized by exacerbations and remissions. The remaining 15 per cent of patients have progressive, destructive arthritis and may also have involvement of organs other than the musculoskeletal system. When first seen, it may be difficult to determine to which category the patient belongs, yet this classification will determine the therapeutic modalities required. The physician must also determine whether the patient's pain is caused by active inflammation or by old, destructive changes. This decision is determined by the medical history, physical examination, x-rays, and laboratory tests. The presence of active disease is characterized by joint inflammation, which includes synovial proliferation, effusions, tenderness to palpation, warmth, and redness. Significant morning stiffness lasting more than one hour and easy fatigability are also signs of active disease. The presence of crepitance and instability without synovial proliferation, effusions, warmth, redness, or tenderness reflect irreversible destruction of cartilage and supporting joint capsular tissue.

The therapy of rheumatoid arthritis consists of the judicious selection of anti-inflammatory agents, physical therapy, and surgical procedures. Each must be tailored to the individual patient. Thus, a patient with mild disease should be treated with anti-inflammatory drugs in an orderly progression with careful assessment of each drug. The physician should start with the least toxic agent, and only when this fails to suppress inflammation should the next potentially more toxic drug be used.

A general program that includes adequate rest and sleep and a nutritious diet should be outlined for patients with active disease.

Although physical therapy is of value for most patients, vigorous exercise of involved joints accelerates damage. Mild range of motion exercises should be designed to prevent contractures. Patients without active inflammation may do more vigorous muscle strengthening and active range of motion exercises. Initially, a trained physical therapist should instruct the patient to protect inflamed and weakened joint structures, and an occupational therapist should teach other ways to perform daily activities when damaged joints interfere.

Drug therapy may be divided into nonsteroidal anti-inflammatory drugs, steroids, and cytotoxic drugs. Non-narcotic analgesic agents are used concomitantly to treat pain along with anti-inflammatory drugs but are rarely used alone. Aspirin is the first drug used to treat RA because it is anti-inflammatory, analgesic, and has a long, successful history of effectiveness and low toxicity. It is also the least expensive drug useful for RA. Adult patients are given 3.9 grams (12 tablets) daily with meals and this dosage may be increased to as much as 5.85 grams (18 tablets) in divided doses. Nonresponsive patients or, occasionally, those receiving very large doses should be monitored by serum salicylate levels, which should be between 18 and 32 mg. per dl. (100 ml.). Tinnitus is also an excellent sign of hypersalicylism. About 45 per cent of patients with RA respond satisfactorily to aspirin therapy. About 5 per cent of patients develop gastrointestinal symptoms, which may be treated with antacids or by the use of alternative forms of salicylate. Several salicylate preparations are now available that may be better tolerated than aspirin (Magan, Trilisate, Mobidin). Timed-release aspirin is absorbed in the small intestine and may be also associated with less gastrointestinal symptomatology. Aspirin in a dosage of 12 to 18 tablets daily can cause significant constipation. The laxative effect of magnesium-containing antacids, when combined with aspirin (Ascriptin, Bufferin) or used concomitantly, may be their principal advantage to the patient with RA. Toxic hepatitis is a recently emphasized side effect of aspirin. Slight elevation of the liver enzymes are not thought to be cause for aspirin withdrawal. Most patients with RA will have some relief with aspirin and can tolerate salicylates in one form or another. Aspirin rarely causes complete remission of RA, although it may help to control inflammation.

Patients who cannot tolerate aspirin or have an incomplete response after a 4 week trial are candidates for other nonsteroidal anti-inflammatory drugs. These agents are similar to aspirin in their anti-inflammatory effects. There are three proprionic acid derivatives, ibuprofen (Motrin), naproxen (Naprosyn), and fenoprofen (Nalfon). All are given in relatively high dosage to be effective in active RA. Aspirin should not be given with these drugs because it interferes with their absorption and accelerates their renal excretion. The daily dose of ibuprofen necessary varies between 1600 and 3200 mg. given in four divided doses. (This dose is higher than that listed in the manufacturer's official directive.) Naproxen can be given as 250 to 375 mg. twice daily, an advantage to most patients. Fenoprofen is given as 1200 to 2400 mg. daily in four divided doses.

Indomethacin (Indocin), 75 to 200 mg. daily in three to four divided doses, and tolmetin (Tolectin), 1200 to 1600 mg. daily given in three to four divided doses, are both anti-inflammatory and analgesic and may be given with aspirin. Both drugs are more likely to produce gastrointestinal side effects than the proprionic acid derivatives.

Phenylbutazone (Butazolidin), 300 to 400 mg. daily in three or four divided doses, is an effective anti-inflammatory agent, but, because of its potential bone marrow toxicity after prolonged use, it should be reserved for acute, short-term treatment or after trials of the above drugs have shown them to be ineffective.

In patients with early or mild disease, each of these drugs should be evaluated for a 2 week period. Even though one drug fails to help, another drug of the same class may be helpful.

If the patient continues to have inflammation for 6 months and a systematic trial of the above drugs has not been effective, then a course of gold therapy should be instituted. Numerous controlled studies have shown that gold is effective in 60 to 65 per cent of patients with severe RA in reducing inflammation and slowing progression of the disease. The patient should be told it will require 3 to 5 months before it can be determined whether or not the arthritis will respond to gold.

Before each succeeding gold injection, the patient should have a white blood count (WBC), platelet count or platelets on smear, and a urinalysis for protein. A significant drop in the WBC, platelet count, or the development of 2+ or greater proteinuria should delay the next gold injection until the abnormality is resolved. At that time, gold injections can be resumed with small test doses (5 mg. per week, etc.). If the abnormalities return then gold therapy should be abandoned. In addition to the above, the patient should be questioned and examined for skin rash, petechiae, or stomatitis, and if these are present, gold should be halted until the symptoms are resolved.

Gold therapy is initiated with 10 mg. gold thiomalate (Myochrysine) or gold thioglucose (Solganal) given intramuscularly. The following week the patient receives 25 mg. and then 50 mg. in subsequent weeks. A clinical response is usually seen between 400 to 800 mg. If no response is obtained by 1 gram, then it may be assumed that gold is not effective. When the patient reaches 1 gram of gold, and has shown a good response, the frequency of injections may be reduced to every 2 weeks for 2 months. If still doing well, then injections may be reduced to every 3 weeks for another 2 months. If still doing well, injections can be given once a month indefinitely. WBC, platelet count, and urine protein determinations should still be obtained before each gold injection.

D-penicillamine (Cuprimine) has been shown to be useful in the treatment of RA even in patients in whom gold was not effective. (This use of D-penicillamine is not listed in the manufacturer's official directive.) During therapy with penicillamine the same clinical and laboratory measurements are assessed as with gold. WBC, platelet count, and urine for protein should be done every 2 weeks for the first 3 months and then monthly thereafter. Treatment is initiated with 250 mg. 30 minutes before breakfast for three months. If no adverse side effect develops, then the dose is increased to 500 mg. daily, which may be given before breakfast and lunch if gastrointestinal symptoms develop. After an additional three months, if no adverse side effects have developed, the dosage may be raised to 250 mg. before each meal (750 mg. daily) beginning with the seventh month. The frequency of side effects rises dramatically with dosages of 1 gram or more daily, but in some patients higher doses may be required to achieve efficacy. The side effects most frequently seen with penicillamine are skin rash, leukopenia, thrombocytopenia, proteinuria, and loss of taste or smell.

Some rheumatologists use hydroxychloroquine (Plaquenil) in a dose of 250 to 500 mg. daily in those patients who have not responded to other nonsteroidal anti-inflammatory drugs. Hydroxychloroquine has been shown to have a modest anti-inflammatory effect on RA during short-term use. Its long-term benefits are questionable, however, and the unpredictable occurrence of retinitis has caused us not to use the drug in patients with RA.

Cytotoxic agents such as cyclophosphamide (Cytoxan), chlorambucil (Leukeran), methotrexate, azathioprine (Imuran), or 6-mercaptopurine (Purinethol) have all been used effectively in unusually severe RA. They each have serious side effects, including increased frequency of the development of malignancies. They should, therefore, be reserved for only those patients with life-threatening disease not controlled by any of the above drugs and should be administered only by experienced rheumatologists with meticulous supervision. None of the cytotoxic drugs are officially approved for use in RA by the Food and Drug Administration.

Glucocorticoids given in sufficient doses are potent anti-inflammatory agents that dramatically improve RA in most patients. Unfortunately, they do not halt progression of the disease and most patients develop signs of hypercortisonism. In many, the side effects with prolonged use are worse than the original disease. Postmenopausal females and physically inactive patients are especially at risk to develop osteoporosis and compression fractures of the spine. Every effort should be made not to use glucocorticoids in the treatment of rheumatoid arthritis. However, certain situations, such as bleeding peptic ulcer or eye or systemic vascular involvement, may require their use. In most patients with RA given glucocorticoids, the dosage should not be more than the equivalent of 7.5 mg. of prednisone daily.

Surgical treatment of rheumatoid arthritis may be considered in two categories of patients: those with active inflammation and those who are inactive but with residual joint damage. In most patients with active disease, surgery is contraindicated because the surgically corrected joint may be destroyed by continued inflammation. Synovectomy of the knee joint may produce pain relief for up to two years after the procedure, but there is no difference in the long-term destruction between surgically synovectomized joints and unoperated control joints 5 years later.

In patients with inactive disease who have major joint deformity, joint replacement has become a well-recognized and successful form of therapy. There are now prostheses available for the hip, knee, shoulder, elbow, wrist and ankle, and small joints of the hands and feet. Total hip replacement and perhaps knee joint procedures give reasonable expectation of success. Other joint replacements should be recommended with greater caution.

Proper use of the therapeutic modalities now available should provide major relief for most patients and will slow or halt progression of the disease in many. The judicious use of physical therapy and surgical repair can often restore some degree of functional ability in those with inactive disease.

JUVENILE RHEUMATOID ARTHRITIS

method of
JAMES T. CASSIDY, M.D.
Ann Arbor, Michigan

Before a physician can begin treatment of juvenile rheumatoid arthritis (JRA), he must be sure that the diagnosis is firmly established, as it is often one of exclusion. By definition, JRA begins before the age of 16 years. Objective arthritis must be distinguished from arthralgia, pain in the joints. Arthritis is defined as swelling in one or more joints, or by the presence of two or more of the following signs: limitation of range of motion, tenderness or pain on motion, and increased heat. Arthritis must persist for a minimum of 6 weeks in at least one joint in order for the clinician to be reasonably sure that the diagnosis is JRA. Last, the clinician should be confident that other forms of chronic inflammatory joint disease have been excluded, especially the other connective tissue diseases and infection.

The diagnosis of JRA has been materially aided by recognition of three distinct types of onset of disease. These are defined by a constellation of clinical signs and symptoms during the first 6 months of disease. With *polyarticular onset,* arthritis begins in five or more joints, usually the knees, ankles, and wrists. *Oligoarthritis* is defined as onset of disease in four or fewer joints. Quite often only a single joint is involved, often the knee. *Systemic onset* of disease is characterized by daily spiking fevers to greater than 39°C. (102.4°F.) and the appearance of a characteristic erythematous nonpruritic rash; there is usually prominent involvement of viscera, including marked lymphadenopathy, hepatosplenomegaly, pericarditis, and leukocytosis.

Treatment

As in adults with rheumatoid arthritis, therapy in children with JRA is supportive and not curative. Management of this disease strives toward control of the clinical manifestations and prevention of deformity. As JRA is characterized by chronic or recurrent inflammation of the joints and supporting tissues, treatment in many patients must be prolonged. It is this length of therapy that often determines its ultimate acceptability to the child and his family and judgment as to its safety by the physician. Acute articular inflammation results in transient disability, swelling, and pain. Chronic inflammation, on the other hand, may result in permanent deformity and erosion of cartilage and bone. Although the eventual prognosis in the majority of children with JRA is excellent, at onset of the disease the physician has no absolutely reliable indices to predict eventual recovery or disability. Treatment in all patients must therefore be directed toward suppression of articular inflammation, prevention if possible of secondary deformities and contractures, and medical control of systemic disease.

The philosophy of management of JRA should be to start with the simplest, most conservative measures. If these forms of treatment prove ineffectual or inadequate, the physician can move on to other therapeutic modalities in an orderly fashion. The more potent or toxic therapeutic agents such as the immunosuppressive drugs should only be used in life-threatening disease with full recognition of their calculated risks and only in accepted experimental protocols.

Aspirin. Aspirin is the only pharmacologic agent of indispensable value in the treatment of children with JRA. It is effective in suppressing the signs of inflammation and fever in the majority of children with JRA. In addition, aspirin has a demonstrated record of safety. Administration should be divided into 4 or 5 doses given with meals or with food at bedtime. Administration of aspirin during the night is generally not necessary in view of the prolonged excretion of salicylate by the kidneys after therapeutic levels are achieved. Treatment with aspirin may be begun at 75 to 100 mg. per kg. per day. The higher doses are tolerated best in children under 25 kg. of body weight. Serum salicylate levels are sometimes helpful as an aid to correct dosage because of the lack of verbally communicated signs of toxicity such as tinnitus in the very young child. The appropriate level varies from child to child but is usually between 15 to 25 mg. per dl. (100 ml.) measured 2 hours after the morning dose. It may be difficult to reach serum levels of this magnitude in children with systemic disease, but increasing the daily amount of aspirin beyond 130 mg. per kg. often results in toxicity. Aspirin in the young child must be used cautiously as salicylism can occur rapidly. Some children will experience abdominal pain or vomiting while on aspirin therapy. This can usually be controlled by taking the salicylate with food or by administration of antacids, or it may be overcome by changing temporarily to a liquid preparation (choline salicylate). Enteric-coated aspirin is generally not recommended unless the coating will reliably dissolve in the duodenum (Ecotrin). In our experience, peptic ulcer disease or significant gastrointestinal bleeding in children on aspirin therapy is rare.

Some children develop a nonspecific hepatitis related to salicylate therapy. This occurs most frequently when the serum salicylate levels are in the toxic range (>35 mg. per dl.). The transaminase enzymes may be elevated in as many as 50 per cent of children on therapeutic levels of aspirin. Transient elevation of these enzymes in a child who is otherwise not showing signs of salicylate toxicity is not in itself an indication for stopping the drug. If they remain elevated, or the levels are high, aspirin may be temporarily stopped, if feasible, or the dosage decreased by at least 20 per cent. If the transaminase enzymes remain elevated, the aspirin should be discontinued until they return to normal. Treatment may be reinstituted at that time at a lower dose, which can be gradually and cautiously increased.

Satisfactory control of inflammation will be achieved in approximately 70 per cent of children with aspirin alone. For children who do not respond to this regimen or who respond inadequately after a 6 month trial period, other drugs must be considered.

Other Nonsteroidal Anti-inflammatory Agents. Most of the nonsteroidal anti-inflammatory agents have not been authorized for use in children. They would be used for control of pain, stiffness, and inflammation in selected children who have been unresponsive to aspirin. Tolmetin,* 200 to 300 mg. four times a day or 25 mg. per kg. per day, has been demonstrated to be effective in children. For patients over 14 years of age, other agents may be tried such as naproxen,* ≤ 750 mg. daily, or ibuprofen,* ≤ 2400 mg. a day. Indomethacin,* in a dose of 25 mg. two to four times a day, may be particularly effective for control of fever in the older patient with JRA. Phenylbutazone* is seldom used in pediatric rheumatology.

The failure of one anti-inflammatory agent does not preclude the possibility of successful treatment of a patient with another drug. Therefore, more that one drug may be used in the resistant case for trial periods of approximately 4 to 8 weeks. It is usually not considered advisable to

---

*See manufacturer's official directive. The safety and effectiveness of this agent have not been established for use in children.

administer any of these agents in combination with aspirin.

Acetaminophen, in doses of 325 to 650 mg. two to three times a day, may be particularly helpful in the control of the temperature spikes that are seen in the systemically ill child. This medication has no anti-inflammatory action, however, and should not be used for basic management of the disease. Likewise propoxyphene may be used occasionally for relief of pain but not as an anti-inflammatory agent.

Gold Salts. Gold salts have been found as effective in the treatment of children with JRA as in adults with rheumatoid arthritis. Preparations in general use are gold sodium thiomalate and aurothioglucose. They are indicated in children whose polyarthritis has been unresponsive after 4 to 6 months of a conservative program of management. Administration of gold salts should be under the direction of a rheumatologist. Before these drugs are begun, the child's hematologic, renal, and hepatic functions must be evaluated. A test dose of approximately 5 mg. should be given intramuscularly on the initial visit. Weekly doses thereafter are gradually increased until approximately 0.75 mg. per kg. per week is given ($\leq$ 50 mg.). Weekly treatment is continued for approximately 20 weeks to a total dose of 15 mg. per kg. ($\leq$ 1000 mg.). If satisfactory improvement or remission has been achieved, maintenance therapy is continued every 2 weeks for 3 months and then every 3 weeks for 3 months. At that point, if objective signs of improvement continue, the child may be placed on monthly gold injections. A complete blood count and urinalysis must be obtained each week before administration of gold salts and assessment of the child for any toxicity, especially dermatitis, bone marrow depression, hematuria or proteinuria, or mucosal ulcerations should be done. Decrease of the white blood cell count below 5000 per cu. mm., a fall in the absolute neutrophil count by 50 per cent, proteinuria, hematuria, or clinical signs of gold toxicity are indications for at least a temporary cessation of therapy. In selected cases therapy may be cautiously resumed at a lower dose after the child's condition returns to normal. However, severe leukopenia, neutropenia, or proteinuria, or an exfoliative rash are absolute contraindications to a reinstitution of therapy. It is generally estimated that approximately 25 per cent of children started on gold salts will not be able to complete a course of treatment because of toxicity, usually hematuria or dermatitis. Approximately 25 per cent will not experience substantial relief of their articular inflammation while on gold, and the remaining 50 per cent will have beneficial results or a complete remission.

Antimalarial Drugs. Hydroxychloroquine is a useful adjunctive agent in the treatment of JRA. Its use has been greatly restricted in recent years because of concern over the development of retinitis. The initial dose of hydroxychloroquine is 5 to 8 mg. per kg. per day ($\leq$ 600 mg.). After 6 to 8 weeks this dose should be reduced and total treatment should probably not be prolonged beyond one year. An ophthalmologic examination should be performed before therapy and every 3 to 6 months thereafter. Although it would be unusual for retinal toxicity to occur at this dose, any suspicion of retinitis would mandate that the agent be discontinued permanently because the drug is cumulative. Corneal deposition may occur and is not an indication in itself for permanently discontinuing the drug. It should be noted that the use of hydroxychloroquine in juvenile rheumatoid arthritis is not indicated in the drug insert (the manufacturer's official directive).

Corticosteroid Agents. The corticosteroid drugs are useful in the treatment of three aspects of JRA. They may be used orally in life-threatening disease or in lower dosage for the treatment of chronic uveitis. An ophthalmic steroid is prescribed for the treatment of chronic uveitis. Intra-articular steroids are of limited use for treatment of a single joint that continues to be inflamed in a child who has otherwise responded well to conservative therapy or as adjunctive aid for physical therapy to one or more joints in order to achieve a carefully outlined objective. Intra-articular injection should not be used more than 2 or 3 times in a single joint during a restricted interval of time.

Chronic uveitis in children with JRA is usually insidious in onset. Early detection will only occur if periodic slit lamp examinations are done by an ophthalmologist of all children with JRA. Currently, it is recommended that examinations be obtained every 3 months for the first 2 years of disease in children with oligoarthritis, and every 6 months thereafter for a period of 7 to 10 years. In other children with JRA, chronic uveitis is less common and slit lamp examinations should be done at 6 month intervals for the first 5 years of disease. Uveitis is most likely to occur in the very young girl with oligoarthritis and positive antinuclear antibody tests. Primary treatment of chronic uveitis must be under the supervision of an ophthalmologist and usually consists of corticosteroid eye drops and an atropine-like drug to dilate the pupil and prevent posterior synechiae.

Prednisone is the steroid analog usually chosen for use systemically. For severe uncontrolled systemic disease with marked cachexia or disability, prednisone may be started in a dose of 0.5 to 1 mg. per kg. per day ($\leq$ 40 mg.) as a single dose in the morning or in divided doses. Once satisfactory control of the disease is achieved or the physician determines that satisfactory control is not going to occur, the medication should be gradually decreased and eventually discontinued. It is important that both the child, if possible, and his parents realize that total control of the signs and symptoms of JRA may not be possible and that it may be necessary to accept some manifestations of activity in exchange for a reduction in corticosteroid toxicity. In some children with severe unresponsive polyarthritis, alternate day prednisone may be useful but we have not found this to be generally true.

Growth retardation is the most significant aspect of steroid toxicity in children. JRA in itself retards development and growth. A child may regain some of the loss in linear growth in time, be it the result either of his disease or steroid therapy, but it is our experience that this does not happen very often or it is not complete in terms of resumption of the previous isodevelopmental channel. The other side effects of corticosteroid medications are an increased susceptibility to infections, addisonian crisis, Cushing's syndrome, cataracts, and glaucoma.

It needs to be emphasized that there is no place in the treatment of a child with oligoarthritis for systemically administered corticosteroids. These children are almost never systemically ill. At the very most, persistent marked inflammation in one or more joints would best be treated by a limited course of corticosteroid injections (prednisolone tertiary-butylacetate).

D-penicillamine. D-penicillamine has not been approved for use in JRA but is being tried in experimental protocols. Current data suggest that it may be as effective as gold salts and no more toxic. The maximum dose is 10 mg. per kg. per day ($\leq$ 750 mg. per day). This maximum dose is reached after three increments of 12 weeks each. A complete blood count, platelet count, and urinalysis are done each week. Important toxicities of D-penicillamine are drug-induced lupus, dermatitis, and immune-complex nephritis.

Immunosuppressive Agents. Immunosuppressive agents should be used in JRA only in experimental protocols and only for life-threatening exacerbations of disease. The drugs most commonly considered are azathioprine and cyclophosphamide. Leukopenia or bone marrow aplasia may result from either of these agents. The potential for development of malignancy is the most important consideration in the use of these drugs. Sterility has been associated with all of the immunosuppressive agents, particularly those of the alkylating variety. A unique indication for the use of immunosuppressive drugs in JRA may be the development of amyloidosis.

Physical and Occupational Therapy. Maintenance of function and prevention of deformity by physical therapy and splinting cannot be overemphasized. This is especially true for children who may be confined to bed or wheel chair because of the activity of their disease or pain. During periods of acute inflammation of the joints physical therapy might best consist of supervised rest and range of motion in a Hubbard tank. However, atrophy of the extensor muscles and later of the flexors begins early and a program should be developed to strengthen these muscle groups. As weight bearing is sometimes impossible because of pain or contractures, passive and then active motion of selected muscles must be prescribed. Swimming and tricycle riding are particularly helpful because they avoid placing weight on the joints. Cock-up night splints for the wrist and posterior splints for the knees are useful for preventing malpositioning of these joints. If the hips are involved, a prone lying board will help to prevent hip flexion contractures. For severe contractures serial casting with active exercises each time the cast is removed may be effective; forced extension at these changes should be avoided. Maintenance of reduced contractures often requires passive exercises and gentle stretching by the parents and the use of resting splints. Cervical spine malpositioning may be avoided by use of a soft collar and a writing table with a tilt top on which the child can do his homework.

Orthopedic Surgery. Synovectomy does not significantly affect the long-term course of the arthritis but may be useful in carefully selected children for relief of mechanical impairment of joint motion related to synovial hypertrophy, as in the knees. Tenosynovectomy may be considered to decrease the risk of tendon rupture over the dorsum of the wrist. A well thought out plan of reconstructive surgery can be of great importance in the few children who enter the late teenage period or adulthood with marked disability. Total joint replacement, particularly of the hip, might be indicated at that time when bone growth has ceased.

Education and Counseling of Family and Patient. As the prognosis for the majority of children with JRA is excellent, it is extremely important that parents and child, if possible, understand the concept of the disease and its management. A considerable amount of effort must be expended in explaining to them the nature of JRA, expectations during the period of initial therapy, and the course of the disease. This counseling should be initiated by the physician and reviewed by the clinic nurse and social worker. These educational efforts must be constantly reinforced and it is often useful to ask each person to write down questions about problems and bring them to the clinic interviews. More than 50 per cent of the families of children with JRA manifest psychiatrically important and often severe emotional disturbances. A major goal of the management of the child with JRA is to help in the formation of as nearly a normal psychologic and social development as possible. Continued attendance at school is encouraged whenever possible; at the least, home instruction is indicated for all but the very ill patient.

The child's nutrition is an important factor in the long-term management of JRA. Generalized growth retardation almost invariably occurs during active periods of the disease. This may be exacerbated by corticosteroid therapy or relative malnutrition. Vitamin supplementation is often indicated.

Prognosis

As a general rule 70 to 90 per cent of children with JRA make a satisfactory recovery from their disease without serious disability. A certain smaller percentage of children who recover will have a recurrence of arthritis in adulthood. The final outcome of JRA in any child is associated, in general, with the type of onset of disease. Children with systemic onset are the most prone to develop life-threatening and sometimes fatal complications. The functional result in children with persistent polyarthritis is less favorable than in the other groups. The child who has oligoarthritis does best from the standpoint of joint disease but may suffer from the complications of uveitis.

Approximately 1 of 10 children with JRA enters adulthood with severe functional disability. The child most likely to do poorly is the one with a later age of onset, early involvement of the small joints of the hands or feet, early appearance of bone erosions, unremitting disease, prominent systemic features, positive rheumatoid factor tests, and subcutaneous nodules. The prognosis for sight in children with chronic uveitis is probably improving related to early detection and better management; however, blindness occurred in approximately 70 per cent of the children with this complication.

A child's potential for growth is an important factor working in favor of the physician and his program. To a great extent it is this potential for further physical and psychologic growth that enables so much to be accomplished in the child with JRA.

ANKYLOSING SPONDYLITIS

method of
SURAWUT PRICHANOND, M.D.
and JOHN L. SKOSEY, M.D., Ph.D.
Chicago, Illinois

Ankylosing spondylitis is an inflammatory disease that affects primarily the axial skeleton and large peripheral joints. Inflammation may also occur in other organs, for example, the eyes, aorta, lungs, urethra, and intestinal tract. Although the cause of ankylosing spondylitis is unknown, it has a definite genetic predisposition (HLA B27). Certain types of infections are believed to trigger the process in the susceptible host. The natural course of the disease is unpredictable, characterized by recurrent exacerbations with variable systemic features, but in many patients it leads to a chronic crippling disorder. The onset of ankylosing spondylitis is usually during early adult life. Nine times more men are affected than women. Although the spine is usually the first area affected, initial symptoms may occur peripherally in hips, shoulders, knees, or heels or, rarely, as the result of an extra-articular manifestation (e.g., iritis, aortic insufficiency). Early systemic features may include fever, anorexia, weight loss, fatigue, and anemia. Successful therapy depends upon early diagnosis and treatment with regular follow-ups.

Education

To obtain early cooperation of the patient, the physician should inform him of the nature of his disease, the rewarding outcome to be expected from total management, and of the potential disasters that could occur as a result of the patient's ignoring his responsibilities. An optimally successful management program requires a well-motivated patient willing to adhere to the guidelines established for him. The physician must explain clearly the goals of therapy, provide detailed information about medications, and stress the importance of physical therapy.

Goals

The primary goals of therapy are suppression of inflammation and pain, maintenance of functional ability, and prevention of deformity through maintenance of range of motion of both axial and peripheral joints, of muscle strength, and of posture. Additionally, extra-articular complications that may occur during the patient's course must be detected early and treated promptly, and ankylosing spondylitis must be differentiated from other closely related diseases such as Reiter's disease and psoriatic arthritis.

Medications

Although there is no specific therapy for ankylosing spondylitis, many things can be done to achieve the goals. The rewards of total management of this disease instituted early are quite gratifying. The aims of medication are to suppress inflammation, stiffness, and pain and thus to enable not only relief of symptoms but also effective physical therapy. Agents that have proved beneficial in ankylosing spondylitis include phenylbutazone, indomethacin, aspirin, and other nonsteroidal, anti-inflammatory agents. Although some physicians consider aspirin the drug of first choice, it is usually insufficient when there is moderate or severe involvement of the spine, shoulders, or hips. Provided that there is no contraindication (e.g., cardiac, renal, hepatic, or peptic ulcer disease), phenylbutazone is the drug of choice in patients with moderate disease with restriction of motion and evidence of calcification. This drug has a remarkable specificity for symptomatic relief in ankylosing spondylitis and has been shown to retard the ossification of the lumbar vertebrae which occurs in this disease. Initially, phenylbutazone should be given in divided doses, 200 to 300 mg. daily. It is advisable to reduce this to the smallest maintenance dose possible after symptoms have improved and the erythrocyte sedimentation rate has decreased. Once control has been established, a maintenance dosage of 100 mg. daily is often sufficient.

Approximately 25 per cent of patients receiving phenylbutazone experience side effects, which include various skin eruptions, peptic ulcer, fluid retention, vertigo, insomnia, visual disturbance, nephrotoxicity, and bone marrow suppression (agranulocytosis or aplastic anemia). The fact that these adverse reactions are usually related to dosage represent another reason for using only the minimal amount required to control symptoms. Periodically, the drug may be withdrawn completely to determine if it is still needed. Such withdrawal attempts are recommended only after the first 6 months of therapy and only in totally asymptomatic patients. Patients receiving phenylbutazone must be followed periodically in a systematic fashion. Thrombocytopenia and aplastic anemia are rare; nevertheless, patients must be evaluated regularly for these potentially serious complications.

Indomethacin, a drug that has also been shown to be effective in the suppression of articular symptoms of ankylosing spondylitis, may be used as an alternative to phenylbutazone. The initial dose should be 25 to 50 mg. four times daily; the average daily maintenance dosage of indomethacin, required for suppression of articular manifestations, is 100 mg. More than this amount may be needed in patients with active disease of the hips or other peripheral joints or with marked spinal involvement. With even low maintenance doses of indomethacin, certain susceptible individuals may develop side effects such as dizziness, headache, or peptic ulceration. If the patient cannot tolerate phenylbutazone or indomethacin, other nonsteroidal, anti-inflammatory agents such as naproxen (Naprosyn), ibuprofen (Motrin), fenoprofen (Nalfon), or tolmetin (Tolectin) may be tried. These medications should be given with meals, with the exception of fenoprofen, the absorption of which may be retarded by food. Concomitant antacid therapy may also be required.

Gold salts and antimalarial drugs (chloroquine and hydroxychloroquine) are of no significant value in the treatment of ankylosing spondylitis. Muscle relaxants (carisoprodol and mephenesin) have also been shown to be of no value. Because of the efficacy of indomethacin and phenylbutazone, not only as anti-inflammatory agents but also in the suppression of pain, analgesics are rarely needed in ankylosing spondylitis. Corticosteroid drugs are less effective than phenylbutazone and indomethacin and have more long-term side effects than these drugs. However, in severe progressive disease uncontrolled by other measures, prednisone in a dosage up to 10 mg. per day may be tried. The use of systemic corticosteroids in the management of aortitis accompanying ankylosing spondylitis has yet to be evaluated. Corticosteroid treatment is mandatory in uveitis associated with ankylosing spondylitis (see below). Inflammation of peripheral joints may be treated with intra-articular injections of appropriate corticosteroid drugs. Contraindications such as joint instability, local infection, or septicemia must be observed, and the patient must be restrained from undue joint stress (e.g., weight bearing) during the period of steroid action. Intravenous iron dextran has been shown to aggravate symptoms of patients with ankylosing spondylitis.

Physical Measures

The aims of physical therapy are to maintain range of motion and muscle strength and to prevent deformities. Physical therapy in ankylosing spondylitis includes many therapeutic exercises and postural corrections. The physical therapist should demonstrate to the patient the techniques of execution of the exercises. Appropriate exercises may be divided into three groups: (1) range of motion, (2) extensor muscle strengthening exercises, and (3) other special exercises. These exercises can be done in an optimally effective manner only after the inflammatory process has been brought under full control. The exercise program may be facilitated by first applying heat to affected areas in order to take advantage of its analgesic effect and to relax muscles and other soft tissues. Range of motion exercises of the neck, shoulders, hips, and dorsal spine should be done regularly. Static muscle contraction exercises, especially of the quadriceps and abdominal muscles, are very important. Extension exercises of the spine are among the most important. Costovertebral joint involvement may eventually lead to restriction of chest expansion. Thus, breathing exercises are very important to maintain existing motion and to increase the effectiveness of diaphragmatic breathing. Swimming is an excellent form of general exercise for all muscle groups, especially the thoracic, hip, and spinal muscles. Diving should be prohibited because of the risk of atlantoaxial subluxation and fracture of the cervical vertebrae. The exercise program must be performed daily and must be reevaluated periodically as part of the regular follow-up. The patient must incorporate the prescribed exercise program into his daily life. He should be advised to use a firm mattress and preferably no pillow or the lowest pillow tolerated. He should be instructed to lie prone on the floor or bed intermittently in order to prevent kyphosis and neck and hip flexion. While standing, it is helpful for patients to place their backs against a straight wall. A firm, straight backed chair with headrest should be used. Bowling and golfing are unsuitable and must be avoided. Sexual intercourse may be difficult for patients who have severe back and hip involvement, and the physician should give practical advice to these patients. Patients with severe hip flexion contractures may be able to accomplish intercourse by lying side by side with or by a rear approach to their sexual partners. Intercourse may be accomplished more easily by some couples with the man lying flat in the supine position.

Radiation Therapy

We feel that there is no role for radiation therapy in the modern treatment of ankylosing spondylitis, as the risk of complications far outweighs the potential benefits. The risk of developing leukemia after radiotherapy is ten times greater than that of nonirradiated patients or of the general population. Other risks include bone marrow depression, transverse myelitis, and radiation sickness. Furthermore, phenylbutazone is more effective than radiotherapy in providing symptomatic relief and functional improvement.

Surgery

Hip flexion deformities unresponsive to medical and physical therapy should be treated by surgery. After total hip surgery full medical and physical management must be continued in order to prevent reankylosis. Posterior spinal osteotomy must be seriously considered should severe fixed flexion deformity of the spine develop. It is generally agreed that spinal osteotomy should be done only by very skilled and experienced surgeons because of the high risk of this procedure.

Management of Associated Conditions

Anterior uveitis must be treated promptly in order to prevent blindness and other complications. Atropine and corticosteroids administered locally are usually sufficient to control ocular inflammation, but systemic administration of corticosteroids may be necessary in some cases. Cardiac complications, which include aortic insufficiency, heart block, and congestive failure, are managed utilizing conventional therapies for such conditions. Pulmonary infections are managed by prompt identification of the infectious agent, specific therapy directed toward the infectious agent, and chest physical therapy to maintain maximum lung expansion and to promote bronchopulmonary toilet. The neurologic complications of ankylosing spondylitis are particularly recalcitrant to therapy. Corticosteroids and surgery fail to improve the cauda equina syndrome. Prolonged immobilization of cervical spine and even cervical fusion may be necessary, should atlantoaxial subluxation result in cord compression. Associated inflammatory bowel disease is treated in the conventional manner. Indomethacin is contraindicated in inflammatory bowel disease.

Follow-up

Periodic visits to the physician are important to ensure that the entire medical and rehabilitation programs are being properly carried out. In order to follow the course of the patient, the physician should make objective measurements such as Shober's index and other measurements of spinal motion, chest expansion, and occiput to wall and finger to floor distances. Periodically, the patient should be asked to demonstrate his daily exercise program so that the physician, with the aid of the physical therapist, can be certain that it is being performed properly. Complete blood counts, including platelet count, should be done monthly while patients are receiving phenylbutazone. Electrocardiogram, chest x-ray, and spinal and peripheral joint x-rays may be done periodically to assess the progression of disease. The physician should be alert to the possibility of extra-articular complications. Medications and physical therapy programs should be adjusted appropriately during these follow-up visits.

BURSITIS AND CALCIFIC TENDINITIS

method of
A. DEAN STEELE, M.D.
Temple, Texas

The numerous bursae situated between musculoskeletal structures to allow relatively friction-free motion are subject to inflammation from various causes. Bursal inflammation may occur as part of a systemic rheumatic disease, such as rheumatoid arthritis and other collagen diseases, or as part of the crystal deposition diseases—gout and pseudogout—and rarely may be caused by bacterial infection. Most attacks of bursitis are nonspecific and often presumed to be related to degenerative changes that may be aggravated by activity and trauma. The subdeltoid, olecranon, trochanteric, prepatellar, and anserine bursae are among those most often involved.

Tendinitis also may occur as part of a collagen disease, but it is usually nonspecific in origin or associated with calcification visible on x-ray. Calcification is commonly seen with tendinitis in the rotator cuff of the shoulder.

The treatment of bursitis and tendinitis is aimed at relief of pain, suppression and elimination of the underlying inflammatory or causal pathologic process, and restoration of normal function of involved structures. When specific diseases are identified as the etiologic problem, treatment is aimed at their control.

In the acute stage, pain may be so severe that narcotics are necessary for adequate relief until the inflammatory process can be controlled. Meperidine, 50 to 100 mg. every 4 hours, or hydromorphone (Dilaudid), 2 to 4 mg. every 4 hours orally, may be given. Codeine, 60 mg. every 4 hours, may suffice. The involved structure should be immobilized: the upper extremities by using a sling and/or splints and the lower extremities by using a splint or crutches. Moist heat or cold applications may be used several times daily for 20 to 30 minute periods.

Initial efforts to suppress inflammation may include local injection of corticosteroids in the insoluble forms such as prednisolone tertiary butylacetate or triamcinolone hexacetonide. Doses equivalent to 20 to 40 mg. of prednisone may be administered in combination with 1 to 2 ml. of lidocaine. At the same time oral anti-inflammatory agents may be started; indomethacin, 100 mg. as an initial dose, 25 to 50 mg. four times daily for 5 to 7 days with tapering of the dose as response permits over the next week. Common side effects from indomethacin include gastric irritation, occipital headaches, and light-headedness. Phenylbutazone, 200 mg. three times daily for 2 days, then 100 mg. four times daily for 1 to 2 weeks may also be used. Possible side effects include gastrointestinal irritation, sodium and fluid retention, skin rash, and bone marrow depression. The efficacy of newer nonsteroidal agents in these conditions remains to be demonstrated.

When sizeable amorphous deposits of calcium in the involved area are seen on x-ray, local injection of lidocaine and aspiration of calcareous material may be tried.

As the acute process evolves into a subacute stage, lesser analgesics such as propoxyphene or continued use of codeine may suffice. Rest and use of moist heat or cold applications should be continued.

As decreased pain and inflammation permit, the patient should begin range of motion exercises of the affected part, with gradual increase in use and general activity as tolerated. Specific muscle strengthening exercises should be prescribed on a slowly progressive basis if weakness has developed.

If chronicity ensues, the use of analgesics, moist heat or cold applications, and exercises may be continued. Repeated corticosteroid and local anesthetic injections may be used. Calcific deposits may require surgical removal, at which time reconstructive surgical procedures may be performed as deemed appropriate.

OSTEOARTHRITIS

method of
LAWRENCE J. KAGEN, M.D.
New York, New York

Osteoarthritis, or degenerative joint disease, is marked by pain, stiffness, limitation of motion, and bony deformity of involved joints. Anatomic examination demonstrates deterioration of articular cartilage, with areas of abrasion, softening, flaking, and fibrillation, and in severe cases, denudation of underlying subchondral bone, cystic areas of bone rarefaction, and zones of sclerosis with new bone growth and remodeling. New bone formation manifested by osteophyte production occurs at the margins of the articular cartilage. The progress of degenerative joint disease is generally slow, and inflammatory signs are absent. There are, however, occasional situations in which rapid change or mild inflammation or both may be present. Degenerative joint disease is the most common form of "arthritis"; x-ray evidence of its presence will be found in most older persons, often in the absence of symptoms.

The cause of degenerative joint disease is not known, although trauma, abnormalities of joint alignment, or support, as well as familial factors, are recognized as predisposing conditions.

Treatment

Explanation and Patient Discussion. Because symptomatic osteoarthritis is usually a chronically recurring problem, an understanding and cooperative patient is an important part of the treatment program. In discussions with the patient, two areas may require explanation. First, the progress of degenerative joint disease is usually slow, not generalized, and symptoms are often episodic. Severe involvement in one area does not imply a poor outlook in other joints. Moreover, symptomatic improvement may be expected in the absence of extensive joint destruction. In most patients, all this points to a favorable prognosis.

The second area, on the other hand, deals with the fact that the pathogenesis and cure for degenerative joint disease are not known. In certain situations cartilage and bone change may progress, resulting in painful loss of joint function, even though the patient has tried to adhere to the therapeutic program offered. In these rare, severe cases, treatment may have to be more extensive and include mechanical aids, physical retraining, or surgery.

Reassurance. Psychologic support based on a candid understanding of the clinical situation is helpful. Most patients with osteoarthritis, although limited at times by pain and stiffness, will not become seriously crippled, or disabled. The presence of bony enlargements such as Heberden's nodes does not imply an unfavorable prognosis and should not be the cause of unnecessary fear.

Rest and Reduction of Stress. In symptomatic patients, periods of rest or relaxation during the working day are useful, particularly if the history indicates a relation of stress or activity to production of symptoms. When weight-bearing joints are involved, constant standing should be avoided. Proper methods of lifting and of work should be encouraged. In some cases, supports such as crutches or canes may be used to reduce stress on involved joints during walking. Use of the cane in the hand on the side opposite to the symptomatic joint of the lower extremity generally achieves the best support during walking. Properly prescribed shoes that support normal foot alignment and weight bearing and reduce inequality of leg length, if present, are important parts of the treatment program.

Exercise. The goals of exercise are to maintain: (a) muscle strength in support of involved joints, (b) proper posture and joint position, and (c) range of joint motion.

Overuse of the joints may increase stress and worsen the condition. Exercises that lead to joint pain and stiffness are to be discouraged. Vigorous use of involved joints, such as in programs of running or jogging, may aggravate symptoms and joint damage. Gentle range of motion exercises, isometric exercise, and programs designed to build muscles around joints without undue joint stress, for example, straight leg raising in the case of the knee, are most useful.

Heat. Heat delivered locally, by electric pad, moist hot pack, or paraffin bath (for the hands), or generally, in a warm tub or shower, may relieve muscle spasm and pain. Heat can be used with good effect during episodes of pain and muscle spasm associated with osteoarthritis of the spine. Modalities such as diathermy that provide deep heat should be used with caution by trained persons to avoid excessive heat absorption.

Drug Therapy. The objective of medication is to minimize symptoms. The concurrent use of physical measures mentioned here may allow a reduction in doses needed. The doses given here may be modified according to the response and need of the individual patient. Three classes of agents are employed: (a) analgesics, (b) anti-inflammatory drugs, and (c) muscle relaxants.

ANALGESICS. Aspirin, 650 to 975 mg. (10 to 15 grains) every 4 to 6 hours. This agent, which also possesses anti-inflammatory properties, is extremely useful in the therapy of degenerative joint disease. Common side effects include tinnitus, which usually disappears with reduction of maintenance dose, and gastrointestinal distress. Antacids are useful in the control of the latter symptom.

Acetaminophen, 325 to 650 mg. every 4 to 6 hours. This analgesic is useful in patients sensitive to, or unable to use, salicylates. It seems most suitable for short-term relief of mild pain.

Propoxyphene hydrochloride, 65 mg. three or four times daily; propoxyphene napsylate, 100 mg. three or four times daily. These agents are generally well tolerated without gastrointestinal side effects. Propoxyphene is often used in combination with salicylate or other anti-inflammatory measures.

In general these three agents will be helpful in controlling symptoms of pain in most patients. In some patients other agents have been used, including pentazocine hydrochloride, 50 mg. every six hours, and ethoheptazine, 75 mg. every four to six hours. Addicting agents should be avoided, if possible, in chronic treatment.

ANTI-INFLAMMATORY AGENTS. Although inflammation is not usually regarded as prominent in the pathogenesis of degenerative joint disease, several agents with anti-inflammatory effects may produce excellent treatment results.

Aspirin (see above).

Indomethacin, 25 mg. four times daily. Gastrointestinal intolerance, headaches, and occasional changes in mental function are probably the most commonly encountered side effects.

Ibuprofen, 300 to 400 mg. three or four times daily. Gastrointestinal intolerance and dizziness are the most commonly noted side effects.

Fenoprofen, 300 to 600 mg. four times daily. Gastrointestinal intolerance, somnolence, and tinnitus are reported side effects.

Phenylbutazone and oxyphenbutazone, 100 mg. three or four times daily. These agents are very effective and may be used in an acute flare or episode of disease. Because of the danger of serious side effects such as agranulocytosis, interference with production of bone marrow elements, and gastrointestinal ulceration they are generally not used for periods longer than 1 week.

Intra-articular injection of corticosteroids may provide temporary relief of pain in joints with evidence of acute flare or inflammation. However, these agents may have deleterious effects on cartilage and further add to joint deterioration. Injections, therefore, should be performed infrequently, and patients should be cautioned against overuse or stress of joints during the period of symptomatic improvement.

MUSCLE RELAXANTS. If muscle spasm contributes to symptoms, diazepam, 2 to 10 mg. three times daily, may provide relief. As somnolence may be a side effect, higher doses should be reserved for acute treatment where bed rest is needed, as with lumbar spine pain.

Other Modalities of Treatment. For local disease certain other modalities may be of use.

CERVICAL SPINE. A supportive collar can be used for acute situations. Traction may also be employed but should be avoided if there are signs of spinal cord compression or vascular embarrassment.

LUMBAR SPINE. A firm mattress provides most comfortable support. Bed rest and pelvic traction may be used during acute episodes.

WEIGHT REDUCTION. Weight reduction is usually advised to reduce stress on weight-bearing joints in overweight patients.

SURGERY. Orthopedic surgery may be recommended when a comprehensive program of medication along with physical measures has failed, and when findings indicate operative intervention can correct anatomic abnormality. Procedures available, at present, include osteotomy with realignment (e.g., for the knee), implantation of prosthetic joints (e.g., for the knee or hip), joint debridement, and joint fusion. The last procedure relieves pain but may lead to increased stress and degeneration of other nearby joints.

Obstetrics and Gynecology

ANTEPARTUM CARE

method of
CHARLES S. MAHAN, M.D.
Gainesville, Florida

Importance

To the time honored goals of good prenatal care (healthy mother—healthy baby), we have recently added the broader concern, healthy family. Studies showing relationships of positive bonding and attachment phenomena during and after pregnancy with decreased incidence of "failure to thrive" and child abuse have gained wide-spread attention and acceptance.

With most American families limiting their number of children to two or three, it is no surprise that patients and health care personnel alike are more concerned than ever about a "top quality" product of each pregnancy. Modern prenatal care, as outlined here, can help achieve that result in at least 90 to 95 per cent of pregnancies that carry beyond the first trimester.

General Objectives of Modern Prenatal Care

1. The prevention of emotional and physical problems that would adversely affect pregnancy outcome.

2. Detection and treatment of health problems that would endanger the mother or fetus or both.

3. Education of the mother and the family regarding good emotional and physical health care during pregnancy and for the rest of her life.

Prepregnancy Visit

This visit provides a chance for a review of the woman's health status with an eye toward concep-
tion in the near future. A rubella titer can be checked, smoking and drugs stopped. Oral contraceptives should be stopped at least 3 months before conception, due to increased chances of anomalies and abortion if taken during that period of time. Intrauterine devices should be removed at least one full cycle before conception occurs. Emphasis should be placed on good nutrition at the time of conception and in early pregnancy. The idea of the prepregnancy visit is rapidly catching on with women in the United States and should be strongly encouraged.

Confirmation of Pregnancy

Pregnancy tests should be made easily available to women, as confirmation is an important step in ultimate acceptance of the pregnancy. Many good office tests are currently available for the detection of HCG (human chorionic gonadotropin) and are usually positive (with 98 per cent accuracy) by 40 days after the last menstrual period. A positive pregnancy test is a crisis for many women and they need counseling at this point about their choices: continuation or termination of the pregnancy.

First Prenatal Visit

History. General information should be obtained at this time, including the patient's occupation, her age, parity, and the extent of her knowledge about pregnancy and health.

MENSTRUAL HISTORY. 1. Usual pattern of menses.

2. Last normal menstrual period.

3. Recent contraception use—may help to determine time of conception in confusing situations.

4. Calculation of the estimated date of confinement (EDC), often best left until after completion of the physical examination to confirm uterine size. The EDC is calculated by Naegele's

rule: Subtract 3 months from the day of the last normal menstrual period and add 7 days.

PAST OBSTETRIC HISTORY. 1. Determining parity (FPAL): F = full-term (or over 2500 grams), P = premature (or under 2500 grams), A = abortions (or under 500 grams), L = number of living children. Thus a para 2-1-1-3 has had two full-term children, one premature, one abortion and now has three living children.

2. Careful attention should be paid to all details and complications of previous pregnancies such as : when, where, gestational age at delivery, prenatal complications, length of labor, type of delivery, hemorrhage, hypertension, infection, Rh immune globulin, blood transfusion, size of baby, Apgar scores, child's development since birth, child's name, and sex.

A history of bad outcomes with previous pregnancies (such as a stillbirth) places the woman in a high risk group for the current pregnancy.

FAMILY HISTORY. Other than genetic diseases such as Tay-Sachs or Huntington's chorea, positive family histories for such illnesses as diabetes, hypertension, or heart disease have interest only as regards the woman's future health status. Family history has little effect on the course of pregnancy; however, family illnesses should be recorded so that a complete data base for future reference and primary care can be obtained.

PAST MEDICAL HISTORY. 1. Overall statement of general health.

2. Hypertension.

3. Diabetes.

4. Heart disease including history of rheumatic fever or scarlet fever.

5. Venereal diseases.

6. Urinary tract infections.

7. Anemia.

8. Allergies.

9. Endocrine diseases.

10. Infertility.

11. Surgery, especially gynecologic surgery.

12. Blood transfusions.

13. Psychiatric disorders.

14. Alcohol and nicotine intake (amount).

15. Drug use and abuse.

HISTORY OF PRESENT PREGNANCY. 1. Bleeding since last menstrual period.

2. Pelvic pain.

3. Quickening or perception of fetal movement.

4. Tiredness.

5. Breast soreness and enlargement.

6. Nausea and vomiting.

7. Weight gain or weight loss.

8. Headache.

9. Bowel symptoms.

10. Urinary symptoms.

11. Drugs ingested.

Physical Examination. A thorough, top to bottom, physical examination should be done at the first prenatal visit to determine health status and detect preexisting health problems. For many a young woman this may be the first complete physical examination she has had for many years, if ever. Special attention should be paid to the following:

1. Weight and height.

2. Pulse and blood pressure.

3. Fundoscopic examination of the eye, as a baseline in case of future development of high blood pressure in pregnancy.

4. Teeth—severe caries will sometimes be an indication that the patient might not be able to take in adequate amounts of protein due to difficulty in chewing.

5. Thyroid.

6. Heart—murmurs, irregularities, rate. Flow murmurs and premature beats are common during normal pregnancy.

7. Breasts—breast self-examination should be encouraged and taught at that visit if not already being done.

8. Abdomen—scars, tumors, uterine size, fetal heart tones.

9. Neurologic examination, with special attention to any abnormalities in deep tendon reflexes or evidence of congenital clonus. These findings would be important later if the patient developed preeclampsia.

10. Varicosities.

11. Pelvic examination: external genitalia—any unusual lesions or inflammation. Vagina and vault—if there is evidence of vaginitis, wet mounts with saline and potassium hydroxide should be done at this time. Cervix—scarring from old tears or previous surgery, any evidence of premature dilatation or effacement, any bleeding lesions on the cervix that need to be treated in early pregnancy. At this time a Pap smear and gonorrhea culture should be done from the cervix. Uterus—size (in weeks), shape, consistency. Signs of uterine myomas or uterine anomalies. Adnexa masses or tumors. Rectovaginal examination.

12. Pelvic measurements: intertuberous diameter in centimeters. Pubic arch in degrees. Diagonal conjugate in centimeters. A description of the depth of the sacral curve. The size and placement of the ischial spines. The width of the sacrospinous ligament in finger-breadths. Following the pelvic measurements, a general description of the pelvis should be made and a comment concerning the adequacy of the pelvis for the vaginal delivery of a fetus presenting by the vertex.

Routine Laboratory Tests in Pregnancy. 1. Hematocrit, done at first visit and every 2 months thereafter (normal is 31 per cent or above in pregnancy).

2. Blood type and Rh determination, done at first visit.

3. Atypical blood antigen screen, repeat at 26 and 32 weeks in Rh negative patients.

4. VDRL, done at first visit and 32 weeks.

5. Gonorrhea of cervix, done at first visit and 36 weeks.

6. Urinary infections screen, done at first visit and 28 weeks (cheaper methods such as Bacturcult and Uroglox have been developed and are available for office use).

7. Pap smear, first visit.

8. Rubella titer, first visit. In most laboratories a titer of over 1:10 indicates immunity.

9. Sickle cell screen (black patients), hemoglobin electrophoresis must be done if this test is positive to determine the kinds and amounts of abnormal hemoglobin present.

10. Fasting and 1 hour after 50 gram glucose load blood sugar test, done only at 28 weeks unless there is a history of a close family member with insulin-dependent diabetes or a history of a previous baby weighing over 9 pounds. If this history is present, the tests are done at the first prenatal visit as well as at 28 weeks.

11. Urine, dip stick for glucose, protein, and ketones. This is done at each visit.

Subsequent Visits

Frequency. Depends on risk factor assessment after the history, physical examination, and laboratory testing are done at the first visit. The risk factors are best recorded in problem-oriented fashion. The ACOG-approved prenatal forms sold by the Hollister Co. are ideal for this.

HIGH RISK. Poor obstetrical history, hypertension, diabetes, heart disease, venereal disease, urinary tract infection, malnutrition, Rh sensitization, previous cesarean section, infertility, age over 37 or under 16, depression, or other. See woman at least every two weeks until 32 weeks, then weekly or twice weekly.

LOW RISK. No health hazards to pregnancy found. See every 4 to 5 weeks until 32 weeks; every other week until 36 weeks; then every week.

Procedures. 1. Weight.

2. Laboratory tests (see First Prenatal Visit).

3. Blood pressure.

4. History—fetal movement, headache, visual disturbances, edema, vaginal bleeding, nausea and vomiting, other complaints and problems.

5. Physical examination—the height of the uterine fundus is measured in centimeters with a measuring tape. The tape is placed from the top of the symphysis pubis to the top of the uterine fundus. After the twentieth week of pregnancy the measurement in centimeters should almost equal the number of weeks of pregnancy; palpation of fetal position; fetal heart tone auscultation with fetal stethoscope or the doppler instrument or both; estimated fetal size after 28 weeks; descent and engagement of the presenting parts; vaginal examination near term; examine extremities for edema.

6. Roll-over test. Done at 28 to 34 weeks to predict which mothers may develop pregnancy-induced hypertension. Blood pressure first taken in the left lateral recumbent position and the normal pressure in that position is recorded. Patient is then turned to the supine position and the blood pressure is taken within 2 minutes of being turned. If there is a diastolic elevation of over 15 mm. Hg, there is a 75 per cent chance that the patient will develop hypertension before the end of the pregnancy.

7. Answer questions.

Counseling. Most physicians and clinics have found it very helpful to have a printed list or pamphlet that lists routine advice and instructions to patients for the more usual health problems and discomforts of pregnancy. Some new thinking in certain of these areas will be listed here:

WORKING. Most low risk women can continue their occupations until near term, providing they can have adequate rest periods when needed. Each person's case must be considered individually, remembering that most housework is more energy-consuming than many jobs women have out of the home.

SEXUAL INTERCOURSE. Recent studies have shown that many women switch from vaginal to oral intercourse during pregnancy as a matter of choice, mostly because it is more comfortable for them. However, there is no contraindication to vaginal intercourse in most pregnancies. Women with a history of premature labor in past pregnancies are advised to abstain from vaginal intercourse in the last 2 to 3 months of pregnancy. If this is unrealistic in certain cases, they are advised to use condoms to catch the semen. There is a concern that the prostaglandins in semen may help stimulate premature labor.

SPORTS. It has been shown that regular sports activity and exercise decreases many of the usual pregnancy discomforts in participating women. Women are advised to use common sense in this regard. Sports that would cause back injury or other severe bodily injury are to be avoided, especially after the twentieth week of pregnancy. Examples of such sports would be snow and water skiing and horseback riding. Tennis, running, and bicycling are popular sports that the low-risk mother can participate in without incident if she uses good judgment. All of these sports keep the pelvic and back muscles in good shape for labor.

Swimming is probably one of the best sports for the pregnant woman as it is refreshing, exercises most muscles, and is very safe right up until term.

TRAVEL. Travel is not restricted in the low-risk woman until 3 weeks before term and this is only to prevent the possibility of being caught "away from home base" in labor. If people *must* travel (death of a parent, etc.), a copy of the prenatal record should be carried with the patient as well as the name of a competent doctor in the area she is visiting.

DRUGS. Only three commonly used drugs have been studied and found to be safe in pregnancy:

1. Prenatal vitamins with folic acid.
2. Oral iron preparations.
3. Dicyclomine (Bendectin) for nausea and vomiting. The patient should understand that nearly all other drugs are suspect and their use has to be balanced against possible ill effects on the fetus. Patients should be advised to call the physician before medicating themselves with any drug, whether "over the counter" or prescription. Diuretics are indicated *only* for congestive heart failure.

Alcohol is a drug. More than 2 to 3 ounces (60 to 90 ml.) per day on a regular basis during pregnancy has been shown to be teratogenic.

Nicotine is also a drug. Any amount of smoking has been related to reduced fetal potential but the severity is directly related to the amount smoked. Patients should be strongly and repeatedly advised to stop smoking while pregnant and to stay off nicotine after delivery since room air smoke is also detrimental to newborns.

The most commonly prescribed drug in the United States is diazepam (Valium), which has been shown to be related to fetal teratogenesis in humans if taken during pregnancy. (See manufacturer's official directive—use in pregnancy.) Women taking this drug should be advised to stop before getting pregnant.

Childbirth Preparation. Parents are advised to read widely on pregnancy physiology and birth and to ask questions. The father and any children over 5 years of age are invited to accompany the mother on any or all office visits so that they may share in the positive aspects of pregnancy, such as hearing the fetal heart tones with the doppler instrument.

Excellent prenatal education groups exist in most communities (International Childbirth Education Association, LaLeche League, American Society for Psychoprophylaxis in Obstetrics), and these groups provide support and role models to couples, especially those that may have moved away from their extended family. Prenatal and postpartum parenting classes are also valuable for most families.

Couples should be strongly advised to participate in any community, clinic, office, or hospital classes since it is shown that childbirth preparation greatly reduces pain and anxiety in labor and reduces the need for drugs and anesthetics.

All of these elements are crucial to the establishment of strong bonding, a unique relationship between mother and child that lasts forever and which has strong effects on the ultimate caretaking of the child by the parents.

Nutrition. Nutrition research in the last 10 years has revolutionized the way we advise pregnant mothers. Malnutrition to some extent underlies many of our most serious problems in pregnancy: toxemia, intrauterine growth retardation, abruption of the placenta, severe anemias, and possibly premature labor.

The pregnant woman of average height should eat a high-calorie, high-protein diet in enough quantity to gain 25 to 30 pounds during the pregnancy. Most of that weight should be gained in the second half of pregnancy. Edema is normal in most pregnant women and not due to salt excess, so women are now advised to salt their food to taste.

Obese women should gain the same 25 to 30 pounds as the woman of normal weight. Women who were underweight for their height before the pregnancy began should be advised to gain *more* than 30 pounds during the pregnancy.

Pregnant women under age 16 will need special nutritional help, since they are growing rapidly, and will need to take in more protein and calories than the average woman to gain the 25 to 30 pounds.

Food supplement programs for poor mothers (such as WIC) have been very successful in producing healthier and larger babies and are now available in most parts of the United States.

Iron and folic acid are considered the only necessary supplements if food intake is adequate.

Breast-feeding. Most evidence now available shows that undoubtedly "breast is best," and advises obstetricians and pediatricians to try to sell breast-feeding to mothers. Many women are becoming aware of this and, as a result, the incidence of mothers who choose breast-feeding has rapidly escalated the past 5 years.

It is important to stress nipple preparation, starting about the fifth month of pregnancy. LaLeche League manuals and "The Complete Book of Breastfeeding" are very helpful guides to the primigravida. Lanolin is helpful in nipple preparation and care.

Dental Care. Dental hygiene is important, as dental caries increase during pregnancy. This is not due to lack of calcium but rather to an increase in caries-producing bacteria due to a favorable environment for bacterial growth in the mouth caused by the increased estrogen production in pregnancy. The gums become more hyperemic and friable around the second month of pregnancy, increasing the frequency of bleeding gums. Regular brushing of the teeth and massage of the gums with the finger may help prevent this.

Dental x-rays may be taken any time during pregnancy, but the abdomen should be shielded by a lead apron. Routine dental work should be reserved for the second trimester, but emergency work can usually be done with relative safety if the dentist and physician will consult each other about anesthetic and antibiotic use.

"Stretch Marks." Striae of pregnancy on the breast and abdomen can be successfully prevented or lessened by the routine application of cocoa butter to these areas starting in early pregnancy.

Varicose Veins. Each pregnancy can make lower extremity varicose veins worse, especially if the woman has a genetic predisposition to them. Most women cannot afford to be off their feet long enough to make a difference and so gradient-pressure pregnancy leotards can be a good investment in preventing further vein damage and increased comfort.

Bowels. Constipation is a common problem and usually can be relieved by adjusting the dietary intake. Increased fluids, fruits, and bran cereals all help (and are good dietary components even in the absence of constipation or pregnancy). Mild laxatives (such as milk of magnesia) taken infrequently in low dosages appear to be safe, but dietary adjustment should be the first priority.

Hemorrhoids. If not already present these may appear early in the second trimester as the uterus gets big enough to put pressure on the hemorrhoidal vein system. A dietary program to soften stools (see Bowels above) is important. Applications of local anesthetic ointments and sitz baths also are helpful. In severe cases suppositories (such as Wyanoids) need to be used but delivery of the baby often provides the only real relief.

Colds. Mild upper respiratory infections in pregnancy should be managed with bed rest and fluids. If drugs are needed for fever or muscle aches, use acetoaminophen by mouth every four hours; for coryza, use pediatric phenylephrine (Neo-Synephrine) nose drops or spray; for cough, use honey or molasses by mouth.

Edema. This occurs normally in most pregnant women and is not thought to be a reliable sign of developing pathologic processes. If ankle edema becomes so severe as to be uncomfortable, bed rest on the left side will help mobilize the fluid, increase urination, and decrease the edema.

Pediatrician. The family having their first child will usually ask for help in selecting someone to care for the child if the physician providing prenatal care does not take care of children. It is important to know the practice of the pediatricians or family physicians in your community, especially if the mother plans to breast-feed. The breast-feeding mother needs very supportive physicians and family members.

Many physicians providing infant care are now arranging to see the first-time parents in their offices before delivery to meet them and to outline suggested preparations for the baby and for baby care after delivery.

Labor and Delivery. The woman and her "coach" need to discuss labor and delivery with the physician at least 3 to 4 weeks before the expected date of confinement (EDC).

Their Lamaze or prenatal classes may have raised concerns about hospital policies, but such anxieties are decreasing now that more hospitals have family-centered care.

Concerns that surface at this time often involve the possibility of cesarean section, fetal monitoring, circumcision, length of hospital stay, and anesthesia. Time should be allotted to answer these concerns with oral or written information.

Many physicians are advising low-risk women who have been to Lamaze classes to stay at home until labor is quite advanced (if membranes are intact) to decrease the anxiety of hospitalization and its effects on labor.

It is important at this time to be sure that a complete set of the patient's prenatal records have been transferred from the office or the clinic to the hospital.

Prevention and Treatment of Pregnancy Complications

Genetic Disorders. Of the thousands of genetic problems that affect the fetus, the most common is mongolism or Down's syndrome, occurring most frequently in the offspring of women over 37 years of age. These women (and others with possible genetic problems) should be referred to a center that does genetic amniocentesis and cell culture. The best time for this to be done is between 14 and 16 weeks after the last menstrual period.

Abnormal Uterine Growth. After 20 weeks, in the nonobese woman, the uterus should grow at such a rate that the height of the uterus in centimeters is close to the number of weeks gestation (such as 28 cm. at 28 weeks). If this does not happen, suspicion should be aroused concerning:

Multiple Pregnancies. 1. The uterine growth is ahead of the dates.

2. Diagnosis by ultrasound examination.

3. Treatment is to stop work; modified bed rest from 28 to 36 weeks with only mild activity; stop vaginal intercourse.

4. Follow the growth of both fetuses with ultrasound.

5. High calorie and protein intake to anticipate a 40 to 50 pound weight gain.

Fetal Anomalies. 1. Poor uterine growth, size less than dates.

2. Ultrasound or x-ray (may fail to show soft tissue anomalies).

3. Suspicion of anomaly often difficult to confirm.

4. Sometimes excessive uterine growth—polyhydramnios.

Intrauterine Growth Retardation. 1. Uterine size less than dates.

2. Diagnosis: serial ultrasound examinations show fetal skull size (biparietal diameter) that falls below the standard for the gestational age.

3. Therapy: increased dietary intake, bed rest on left side to aid fetal growth and to decrease hypertension.

4. Assess fetal age with lecithin-sphingomyelin ratio by amniocentesis. Deliver as soon as mature.

Breech Presentation. If this presentation persists after 36 weeks:

1. X-ray pelvimetry to assess pelvic measurements.

2. Flat plate x-ray of abdomen to rule out fetal anomalies or an extended fetal head.

3. Ultrasound to assess fetal size by measuring biparietal diameter (BPD) of fetal skull. If BPD is greater than 10 cm. a very large baby is present.

4. If any of these tests are not normal or if a footling breech or large baby is present, discuss the definite possibility of cesarean section with parents.

Anemia. 1. Definition: hematocrit less than 30 per cent or hemoglobin less than 10 mg. per dl. (100 ml.).

2. Iron deficiency is the cause of 95 per cent of anemias in pregnant American women.

3. Work-up: A serum iron level below 40 micrograms per dl. confirms iron deficiency as the cause of the anemia. A therapeutic response to iron treatment can also be used as confirmation.

4. Replace iron orally as the sulfate or gluconate salt two to three times daily. The therapeutic goal is to increase the hematocrit or to keep the hematocrit from dropping any lower. An average of 2 weeks of iron therapy is needed before a response is seen. Oral iron is as effective as any other route of administration and should be used unless the patient cannot or will not take it.

5. Review the patient's diet to be sure her nutrition is adequate and to rule out pica (ingestion of laundry starch, ice, clay).

6. Folic acid deficiency is rare since folic acid is usually present in prenatal vitamin supplements in much more than the minimum daily requirement.

Diabetes. 1. In gestational diabetes the glucose tolerance is abnormal only when the patient is pregnant. This can be managed with dietary control alone but must be carefully done since adequate calories and proteins are needed for optimal fetal growth. The help of a certified nutritionist is a necessity here.

2. In the insulin-dependent diabetic (IDD) the most important goal of therapy is to adjust the pregnant woman's insulin to keep her blood sugars in the normal range, preferably below 100 mg. per dl., at all times throughout pregnancy.

3. Insulin levels should be controlled on an ambulatory basis rather than in the hospital. This is done by frequent visits for blood sugar determinations daily until they are brought under control. Fasting and postprandial blood sugar values are usually used to manage insulin levels.

4. An individualized diet must be tailored for the patient considering all aspects of her diabetes and her pregnancy. Again, this is best done by a qualified nutritionist.

5. The insulin-dependent diabetic patient should be followed with tests for fetal well-being (see below).

6. Plan the delivery of the insulin-dependent diabetic patient when the lecithin-sphingomyelin (L/S) ratio and ultrasound confirm fetal maturity, usually 37 to 38 weeks.

7. Plan the delivery to occur in a perinatal center since there is a high chance of cesarean section and necessity for neonatal intensive care.

8. Babies of the insulin-dependent diabetic mother should have the same perinatal mortality and morbidity rates (excluding the increased number of fetal anomalies in the diabetic mother) as the low risk mother if excellent perinatal care is given.

Infections in Pregnancy. Urinary Tract Infections. 1. All pregnant women should be screened for urinary tract infections at the first prenatal visit with an inexpensive bacteriologic or chemical method (Bacturcult, Uroglox, etc.).

2. Seventy to 75 per cent of urinary tract infections in pregnancy are due to *Escherichia coli*. This organism is colonized in vaginal introitus from the bowel and later pushed into the urethra during intercourse.

3. Treatment: This is important even in asymptomatic women as 20 per cent of those with asymptomatic bacteriuria in pregnancy will later develop pyelonephritis if untreated. Treatment is with sulfisoxazole, 2 grams at once and 1 gram four times a day for 10 days until 32 weeks of pregnancy or ampicillin 500 mg. four times a day for 10 days at any time of pregnancy.

4. Follow-up treated women with monthly cultures.

RUBELLA.   1. A titer of less than 1:10 in most laboratories indicates *no* immunity to rubella.

2. If exposed to rubella, the titer should be repeated in 3 to 4 weeks after exposure. If there is a greater than three-fold rise in titer, acute infection has occurred.

3. If rubella infection is proved in the first 3 to 4 months of pregnancy, there is a high risk of congenital anomalies in the fetus. The patient should be counseled and made aware of this risk so that she may elect a therapeutic abortion if desired.

4. If rubella infection is proved in the last half of pregnancy, the baby may be born with active rubella infection and therefore may be shedding the live virus. These babies are a danger to nonimmune women in labor and delivery areas and nursery workers.

5. All women of child-bearing age working in a hospital or clinic or office should obtain rubella titers and should receive immunizations if the titer is low.

6. It should be noted on the prenatal chart if the mother has a titer of less than 1:10 that she should be offered vaccination in the immediate postpartum period before her hospital discharge. This is safe in nursing as well as non-nursing mothers, as long as they are advised to protect themselves from pregnancy for the first 3 months after immunization.

GONORRHEA.   1. Present in 5 per cent of pregnant mothers.

2. Diagnosis: culture on modified Thayer-Martin culture medium at first prenatal visit and at 32 to 34 weeks.

3. Treatment: aqueous procaine penicillin G intramuscularly or oral erythromycin in the same dose that is used for nonpregnant women.

4. A test of cure culture is important.

5. The sexual partner should be treated and condoms should be used for the rest of the pregnancy.

6. Gonococcal arthritis is more common in pregnant women and responds well to outpatient treatment with standard doses of penicillin.

SYPHILIS.   1. VDRL is false positive in as high as 5 per cent of pregnant women. Syphilis can be ruled out by performing an FTA-ABS test on the blood.

2. Secondary syphilis is the most common form seen in pregnant women. The typical skin rash and condyloma lata are the most common symptoms.

3. Treatment is intramuscular benzathine penicillin in the same dosage as for the nonpregnant woman. Erythromycin in the same dosage but for double the period of time as for the nonpregnant woman.

4. Follow-up VDRL's should be done a month later to be sure that the titers are declining toward a normal level.

5. The sexual partner should be contacted and treated and condoms should be used for the rest of the pregnancy.

HERPES GENITALIS.   1. Diagnose by a history of vesicles that turn into ulcers usually on the vulvar area. More accurate diagnosis can be obtained by scraping the ulcer and doing a Pap smear of the scrapings. If herpes is present, inclusion bodies are seen in the squamous cells.

2. Apply povidone-iodine (Betadine) solution liberally to lesions until healed to avoid bacterial superinfection and to speed healing.

3. Advise the use of condoms if coitus is planned after the lesions heal to avoid the chance of reinfection by the partner.

4. If active lesions recur or are still present near term, the family should be advised of the possibility of cesarean section as the method of choice for delivery. It is important to stress the necessity of immediate transport to the hospital if the membranes rupture with lesions present, as the cesarean section should be done within 4 hours after membranes rupture.

GROUP B STREPTOCOCCAL INFECTIONS.   1. A growing problem causing serious new-born infections and death.

2. Diagnosis: Streptococcal cultures during pregnancy in women with a past history of group B Strep. neonatal infection.

3. Treatment: None known yet. Penicillin prophylaxis of the mother is not effective and is of questionable value in infants whose mothers have had a positive culture.

Intrauterine Assessment of Fetus

Ultrasound.   1. B mode scans can be used to check for anomalies, twins, location of the placenta, and biparietal diameter of the fetal skull as an index of gestational age, fetal size, and fetal growth.

2. Biparietal diameters are more accurate if a series of measurements can be done monthly before 32 weeks.

3. Presently, ultrasound is too expensive to use as a routine examination for all mothers.

X-ray.   Currently the only major indication for this procedure in evaluation of the fetus is to attempt to discover bony congenital anomalies or a deflexed fetal head in breech presentations.

Amniocentesis.   This should be done only with the aid of ultrasound to prevent fetal or placental damage by the needle.

1. Lecithin-sphingomyelin (L/S) ratio: If greater than 2, this test usually means that there is enough surfactant present in the fetal lung to pre-

vent respiratory distress after the fetus is delivered. This is one of the most significant advances of modern obstetrics.

Testing the L/S ratio should be considered if there is a question of the estimated confinement being correct in women in whom repeat classical cesarean section is needed. If a repeat low segment cesarean section is necessary, awaiting labor in women with questionable due dates is safer than amniocentesis.

2. Creatinine: The creatinine level increases in amniotic fluid as pregnancy advances. If the level is greater than 2 mg. per dl., the fetus is usually mature. This is not quite as valid as the L/S ratio.

3. Bilirubin levels: These can be measured in Rh-sensitized mothers starting at 25 weeks of pregnancy. These are more accurate than blood antibody titers. Rh sensitization is becoming rare due to the availability of immune globulin and women with sensitization should receive care in regional perinatal centers.

Hormone Assays. These tests are seldom used alone but are most often used in conjunction with other fetal assessment tests. Both estriols and human placental lactogens (HPL) are usually valid only if serial results are obtained and trends can be assessed. For both tests, a downward trend that eventually falls below the normal level can be taken as a sign of serious fetal jeopardy in certain diseases of pregnancy. Both tests may have to be done daily near term, to catch deterioration of the pregnancy quickly enough to act in time.

1. Urinary estriol: Estriol measurements are an index of the well-being of the fetal-placental unit. Twenty-four hour urine specimens are necessary and are usually followed serially starting at 30 to 32 weeks of pregnancy.

Estriol measurements are especially helpful in following diabetes in pregnancy, intrauterine growth retardation, and hypertensive disorders in pregnancy. Normal estriol values are between 12 to 30 mg. per 24 hours near term.

2. Serum Human Placental Lactogen (HPL) is primarily an index of the well-being of the placenta. Single blood samples can be drawn and are usually followed serially after 32 weeks. This test is especially good for following hypertensive diseases in pregnancy and intrauterine growth retardation but not especially good for following diabetes in pregnancy. The mean value of HPL from 32 to 36 weeks is 7.5 micrograms per ml.

Tests with the External Fetal Monitor. 1. The nonstress test: This test can be done in the clinic or office on high-risk patients if a monitor is available. In the healthy fetus, fetal movements result in sudden slight increases in the fetal heart rate. If the monitor records no increase in fetal heart rate during movements, the fetus may be ill.

2. The stress test: This is usually done in the hospital. Uterine contractions (if not occurring spontaneously) are induced by low dose intravenous oxytocin infusion until three contractions of 40 to 60 seconds duration occur in a 10 minute period.

A test is read as negative if no late decelerations are present in relation to uterine contractions. A positive test is read when late decelerations occur with more than half of the contractions. If the test is negative, it needs to be repeated only every 7 days.

Conclusion

Using the above outline of modern antepartum care and by providing careful interconceptional care of the woman, with an eye toward a possible future pregnancy, we can today expect an excellent pregnancy outcome for the mother, baby, and family.

An interested, humanitarian physician or midwife applying these concepts in an atmosphere of warm interest in family development can help make pregnancy and birth an important, happy growth experience rather than one of life's major crises.

ABORTION

method of
PAUL F. BRENNER, M.D.,
and DANIEL R. MISHELL, M.D.
Los Angeles, California

Introduction

The medical management of an abortion (termination of a pregnancy prior to a gestational age compatible with fetal viability) depends upon several factors.

1. Whether the abortion is commenced spontaneously or is to be induced.

2. The gestational age to which the spontaneous abortion proceeded: threatened, inevitable, incomplete, complete abortion.

3. Have two or more consecutive abortions immediately preceded the present spontaneous abortion: habitual abortion.

4. Has the fetus succumbed without a spontaneous attempt to evacuate the uterus: missed abortion.

5. Has the present abortion been complicated by sepsis: septic abortion.

6. To what gestational age has the pregnancy advanced prior to the elective induction of abortion: first trimester, second trimester?

General Considerations

1. All women undergoing a spontaneous or an induced abortion should receive family planning counseling.

2. Certain other complications of pregnancy such as ectopic pregnancy, trophoblastic disease, and multiple pregnancy should be considered.

3. Whenever the uterine cavity is invaded with either suction or sharp curettage, the operator must accurately determine beforehand the size and position of the uterus and must know the methodology and risks of the equipment he has chosen to use.

4. Upon completion of the spontaneous or an induced abortion, immune globulin, human (RhoGAM), should be administered within 72 hours to Rh negative patients who were not previously immunized.

5. If fetal tissue (chorionic villi) is not seen when the specimen is examined histologically, the presence of an ectopic pregnancy should be suspected.

Spontaneous Abortion

Spontaneous abortion is the involuntary termination of a pregnancy prior to a gestational age compatible with fetal viability. The medical management of spontaneous abortion depends upon the extent to which the evacuation of the products of conception has proceeded.

Threatened Abortion. A threatened abortion is manifested clinically by uterine bleeding occurring prior to 20 weeks' gestation, which may or may not be accompanied by uterine cramping and which does not result in cervical dilatation.

1. Eliminate cervical and vaginal causes of bleeding by inspection.

2. Evaluate uterine size.

3. Bed rest: 48 hours.

4. Abstinence from coitus and douching for 14 days.

5. Gestagen therapy is not advocated. The use of synthetic gestagens or progesterone has not been proved to have a beneficial effect in preventing abortion and may have a deleterious effect on the fetus when administered during pregnancy.

Inevitable Abortion. An inevitable abortion is manifested clinically by uterine bleeding and pain occurring prior to 20 weeks' gestation and accompanied by cervical dilatation.

1. Do not delay in an effort to save the pregnancy.

2. Hospitalize the patient and evacuate the products of conception from the uterus (see incomplete abortion).

Incomplete Abortion. An incomplete abortion is manifested clinically by uterine bleeding and pain occurring prior to 20 weeks' gestation and accompanied by the incomplete evacuation of the products of conception from the uterus.

1. Hospitalize the patient.

2. Nothing by mouth.

3. Evaluate uterine size.

4. Blood type and Rh, complete blood count.

5. Blood to be saved for cross match.

6. Initiate an intravenous infusion of 1000 ml. 5 per cent dextrose with lactated Ringer's solution containing 30 units of oxytocin.

7. Local anesthesia (paracervical block) or general anesthesia.

8. Uterus is less than 12 weeks size: evacuate the products of conception from the uterus by dilatation if necessary and either suction or sharp curettage.

9. Uterus is greater than 12 weeks size: initiate labor with intravenous oxytocin using gradually increasing concentrations.

10. Oxytocin administered with solutions not augmented with electrolytes may cause water intoxication.

11. Transfuse the patient when either her vital signs or her hemoglobin concentration or both indicate the need for blood replacement.

12. Save all tissue evacuated from the uterus and send for gross and microscopic examination.

13. Monitor the patient's vital signs at sufficiently frequent intervals as indicated.

14. Observe the patient until her overall condition is judged satisfactory.

Complete Abortion. A complete abortion is manifested clinically by the evacuation of all the products of conception from the uterus.

1. If all the products of conception appear to have been passed intact, the uterus is well contracted, and there is minimal bleeding, administer methylergonovine maleate (Methergine), 0.2 mg. orally every 4 hours for six doses.

Missed Abortion. A missed abortion is the involuntary failure to expel the products of conception 8 or more weeks after fetal demise and less than 20 weeks.

1. Serial determination of uterine size. Uterus stops growing and may decrease in size.

2. Serum fibrinogen and platelet count once a week.

3. After documenting fetal death by falling or negative human chorionic gonadotropin (HCG) levels, evacuate the products of conception.

4. Uterus is less than 12 week size: see incomplete abortion.

5. Uterus is greater than 12 weeks and less than 20 weeks size: initiate labor with a suppository containing prostaglandin E_2 placed intravaginally or with intravenous oxytocin if there is a contraindication to prostaglandin E_2 therapy.

Habitual Abortion. Habitual abortion is the involuntary termination of three or more consecutive pregnancies prior to a gestational age compatible with fetal viability.

1. The medical management of the abortion is the same as detailed for spontaneous abortion.

2. In addition, an investigation as to the possible cause of the recurrent pregnancy loss should be undertaken.

Hysteroscopy or hysterosalpingogram: Uterine causes which might lead to habitual abortion include congenital anomalies, submucus leiomyomata, intrauterine synechiae, and incompetent cervical os.

Karyotype of both partners: the incidence of chromosomal abnormalities decreases as the gestational age increases.

Serum thyroid-stimulating hormone (TSH). There is disagreement concerning the role of hypothyroidism, if any, with habitual abortion, but this diagnosis may be excluded by a normal serum TSH.

Endometrial biopsy late in the luteal phase, day 26. The inadequate luteal phase is demonstrated when the histologic dating of the endometrium is two or more days out of phase with the dating of the menstrual cycle based on the time of presumed ovulation basal body temperature (BBT) in at least 2 cycles. There is disagreement concerning the role of the inadequate luteal phase, if any, with habitual abortion, but this diagnosis may be excluded when the dating of the endometrium is in agreement with the cycle date based on the onset of the menses after the biopsy.

3. After a second trimester abortion an investigation in search of a uterine cause should be initiated. A high probability exists that a uterine defect is present, and a delay until further pregnancy wastage occurs is not warranted.

4. The patient with an incompetent cervix should have a cervical cerclage (McDonald procedure) at 14 weeks' gestation in the next pregnancy.

5. Submucus myomas associated with a second trimester abortion or multiple first trimester losses should be removed (myomectomy).

6. Uterine synechiae may be lysed under direct observation via the hysteroscope.

7. If either partner is found to have a chromosomal defect, genetic counseling should be provided to the couple.

8. Progesterone administered as a 25 mg. rectal suppository twice a day or as 12.5 mg. daily injections is used as replacement therapy for the inadequate luteal phase.

Septic Abortion. A septic abortion is an abortion, spontaneous or induced, that is associated with sepsis, which may or may not be limited to the uterus.

1. Hospitalize the patient.

2. Nothing by mouth.

3. Blood type and Rh; complete blood count.

4. Two units of blood cross matched for transfusion.

5. Serum fibrinogen; total platelet count.

6. Serum chemistries: prothrombin time, glucose, bicarbonate, urea nitrogen, sodium, potassium, chloride, calcium, inorganic phosphate, creatinine, uric acid, and alkaline phosphatase.

7. Culture the cervix.

8. Blood cultures, aerobic and anaerobic.

9. Gonorrhea culture of the cervix.

10. Supine and upright roentgenograms of the abdomen; examine for intraperitoneal gas and myometrial gas.

11. Monitor the patient's vital signs at sufficiently frequent intervals as indicated.

12. Insert a Foley catheter.

13. Record intake and output.

14. Initiate an intravenous infusion of 1000 ml. 5 per cent dextrose with lactated Ringer's solution.

15. Initiate antibiotic therapy, including penicillin and an aminoglycoside.

Aqueous penicillin G, 5 million units intravenously administered over 30 minutes every 6 hours. Once the patient is afebrile for 24 hours the antibiotic can be changed to ampicillin, 0.5 gram orally four times a day. The total course of antibiotics is 10 days.

Gentamicin, 60 to 80 mg. intravenously administered over 30 minutes every six hours for five days, or kanamycin, 7.5 mg. per kg. of body weight intramuscularly every 12 hours for five days (total daily dose 15 mg. per kg.).

16. A third antibiotic should be added to the regimen if there is evidence of septic shock, pelvic abscess, or the septic abortion is associated with an intrauterine device.

Clindamycin, 60 mg. intravenously administered over 30 minutes every six hours, unless diarrhea occurs, then select chloramphenicol (Chloromycetin), 1.0 gram intravenously administered over 30 minutes every six hours.

17. If the septic abortion is associated with the use of an intrauterine device (IUD), remove the IUD only after therapeutic levels of antibiotics are attained.

18. Evacuate the products of conception from

the uterus by dilation if necessary and either suction or sharp curettage only after therapeutic levels of antibiotics (2 hours) are attained. Removal of the focus of infection is the primary treatment.

19. Exploration of the abdominal cavity and possible hysterectomy should be considered in:

The septic patient whose abortion occurred under uncertain circumstances and there is peritoneal gas on the upright abdominal film.

The septic patient whose myometrium is extensively occupied with gas.

The septic patient with gas in the myometrium and intravascular hemolysis.

The septic patient with gas in the myometrium and renal failure.

The septic patient who fails to respond to antibiotic therapy and curettage.

20. Save all tissue evacuated from the uterus and send for gross and microscopic examination.

Voluntary Abortion

The elective induction of abortion is the voluntary termination of a pregnancy prior to a gestational age compatible with fetal viability.

Mini-Abortion. A mini-abortion is the voluntary termination of a pregnancy prior to 7 weeks' gestation.

1. Positive pregnancy test. The radioreceptor assay (RRA) and radioimmunoassay of the beta subunit of HCG are highly sensitive assays that can be used to diagnose early pregnancy.

2. Menstrual extractions should not be performed on nonpregnant women whose menses are delayed.

3. Blood type and Rh; complete blood count.

4. Local anesthesia: paracervical block.

5. Evaluate uterine size.

6. Evacuate the products of conception from the uterus. Minimal cervical dilatation (4 to 6 mm.) may be required. Use a flexible plastic cannula attached to a suction apparatus. Carefully inserting and withdrawing the cannula in all planes of the uterine cavity aspirate until no further tissue can be obtained.

7. Save all tissue evacuated from the uterus and send for gross and microscopic examination.

8. Monitor the patient's vital signs at sufficiently frequent intervals as indicated.

9. Observe the patient until her overall condition is judged satisfactory.

First Trimester Elective Induction of Abortion. A first trimester elective induction of abortion is the voluntary termination of a pregnancy prior to 12 weeks' gestation.

1. Positive pregnancy test.

2. Evaluate uterine size. The uterus must be 12 weeks' gestational size or less.

3. Nothing by mouth.

4. Blood type and Rh; complete blood count.

5. Blood to be saved for cross match.

6. Local anesthesia (paracervical block) or general anesthesia.

7. Initiate an intravenous infusion of 1000 ml. of 5 per cent dextrose with lactated Ringer's solution containing 30 units of oxytocin.

8. Evacuate the products of conception from the uterus. The length of the uterine cavity is determined with a sound. No instrument is placed in the uterus at a distance greater than the length of the cavity. The cervix is dilated as necessary with dilators of progressively increasing diameter. Using a rigid cannula attached to suction of 55 to 70 cm. Hg, the instrument is carefully inserted and withdrawn in all planes of the uterine cavity until no further tissue can be aspirated.

9. The uterine cavity is explored with a sharp curette.

10. Save all tissue evacuated from the uterus and send for gross and microscopic examination.

11. Monitor the patient's vital signs at sufficiently frequent intervals as indicated.

12. Observe the patient until her overall condition is judged satisfactory.

Second Trimester Elective Induction of Abortion. A second trimester elective induction of abortion is the voluntary termination of a pregnancy which has advanced beyond 12 weeks' gestational age but not to 24 weeks'.

1. Positive signs of pregnancy. Fetal heart, fetal movements, roentgenographic or ultrasound evidence of the fetus.

2. Evaluate uterine size.

3. Hospitalize the patient.

4. Nothing by mouth.

5. Blood type and Rh; complete blood count.

6. Blood to be saved for cross match.

7. Initiate an intravenous infusion of 1000 ml. of 5 per cent dextrose with lactated Ringer's solution unless hypertonic saline is to be used.

8. If the abortion is to be induced with hypertonic saline it is best to use a solution containing a reduced electrolyte concentration such as a 5 per cent dextrose with 0.5 isotonic saline solution for intravenous infusion. Since oxytocin is a frequently used adjunct with hypertonic saline, the administration of a solution containing some electrolytes will reduce the possibility of water intoxication.

9. Evacuate the products of conception from the uterus. The intra-amniotic placement of abortifacient should not be attempted prior to the sixteenth week of gestation.

Remove 200 (50 to 250) ml. of amniotic fluid and replace it with an equal volume of 20 per cent sodium chloride solution. The intravascular placement of hypertonic saline may lead to serious circulatory or central nervous system reactions.

Disseminated intravascular coagulopathy is another serious side effect. Cardiac and renal diseases are contraindications to the use of the saline solution.

The intra-amniotic placement of a single dose of 40 mg. prostaglandin F2 alpha is an alternative abortifacient for second trimester pregnancies. Gastrointestinal side effects, pyrexia, cervical lacerations, live births, and asthmatic attacks (bronchospasm) are complications associated with this method. The use of prostaglandin is contraindicated in patients with asthma, hypertension, and cardiac disease.

10. If an abortion is not successfully induced in 48 hours, initiate intravenous oxytocin.

11. If an abortion is not successfully induced in 72 hours after the initial intra-amniotic placement of the abortifacient (24 hours after the addition of oxytocin), administer a second dose of the abortifacient.

12. If the placenta is not expelled within 2 hours following the passage of the fetus, it should be delivered by surgical intervention.

13. All women undergoing second trimester elective induction of abortion following the passage of the products of conception should have a sharp curettage to ascertain that no further products of conception are present in the uterus.

14. Save all tissue evacuated from the uterus and send for gross and microscopic examination.

15. Monitor the patient's vital signs at sufficiently frequent intervals as indicated.

16. Obtain a complete blood count 2 hours after delivery of the placenta. Initiate antibiotic therapy if infection is present.

17. Observe the patient until her overall condition is judged satisfactory.

18. A hysterotomy may be performed to evacuate the products of conception from the uterus if the patient has had a previous cesarean section or leiomyomata uteri.

19. Serum chemistries: liver and renal function screen. These tests should be obtained on all patients who are to have a hysterotomy, hysterectomy, or general anesthesia.

20. A hysterectomy may be performed to terminate the pregnancy if there is pelvic disease associated with the desire to terminate the unwanted pregnancy.

Perforation of the Uterus

1. Carefully observe the patient.
2. Laparotomy is indicated for:
Lateral uterine perforation.
Perforation with the suction apparatus.
Omentum or bowel injury or both with a sharp curette.
Hemorrhage.

RESUSCITATION OF THE NEWBORN

method of
JOHN R. RAYE, M.D.
Farmington, Connecticut

Resuscitation is required for any newborn who, in the first minutes of life, cannot establish adequate ventilation to meet his needs for oxygenation and carbon dioxide excretion or whose cardiac output is inadequate to supply essential organs. The goal of an effective resuscitation is intact survival. The attainment of this goal requires the availability of adequate equipment and supplies, the anticipation and rapid assessment of the needs of the individual patient, appropriate therapy, and attention to postresuscitation care.

Equipment and Supplies

Equipment and supply needs are listed in Table 1. These items must be present in the delivery room and their availability confirmed at the start of each nursing shift. All personnel responsible for neonatal resuscitation must be fully acquainted with the equipment, its use, and location. Wall charts of drug dosages and sizes of airway management equipment are helpful in the delivery room.

Anticipation

An effective resuscitation requires advance planning. Planning should identify the persons responsible for resuscitation and their specific roles. Three people are required when ventilation, external cardiac compression, and drug therapy are necessary for the severely depressed patient. Practice resuscitation using available models

TABLE 1. **Resuscitation Equipment and Supplies**

Radiant warmer
Air and oxygen sources with variable concentration blender and flow regulator
Suction source with regulator
Suction catheters: 5, 6, 8, 10 Fr.
Bulb syringe
Oral airways: 000, 00, 0
Resuscitation bag capable of supplying >80% oxygen with in-line pressure manometer
Face masks: 0, 1
Endotracheal tubes and stylets: straight, 2.5, 3.0, 3.5, 4.0 mm.
Laryngoscope with straight blades: 0, 1
Stethoscope
ECG monitor with oscilloscope and clothespin or needle leads
Umbilical catheter tray including 3.5, 5 Fr. umbilical catheters and 3-way stopcocks
Syringes, needles, tape, tincture of benzoin
Heparin solution

(dolls, ketamine-sedated kittens) should be performed on a recurring basis to ensure the development of adequate skills.

With modern obstetrical management the need for resuscitation should be predicted in most situations. Skilled persons must be available at the time of delivery. Previous obstetrical problems, abnormalities of fetal growth, maternal hypertensive diseases, evidence of prepartum asphyxia judged by fetal heart rate alterations, and, most importantly, premature delivery can be used as high-risk indications in preparing for resuscitation. Any infant whose special needs can be identified in advance should be delivered in an environment best suited to meet these needs. This may require transport of the high-risk mother to a regional perinatal center for delivery.

Assessment

An effective resuscitation requires constant evaluation of airway patency and adequacy of ventilation and cardiac output. The evaluation of neuromuscular tone may be a helpful adjunct observation; a flaccid infant usually requires more vigorous and prolonged support. The Apgar score has been widely used as an indicator of the need for resuscitative support. It is not appropriate, however, to be entirely directed by a scoring system or to wait for the 1 minute score prior to initiating resuscitation. Absent or ineffective respirations require ventilatory support and a low cardiac output requires correction regardless of "score."

As soon as the infant is delivered he should be toweled dry while being placed under the radiant warmer. The infant must be left naked both for assessment of vital signs and to allow direct exposure for radiant warming. Following positioning to promote drainage of secretions and airway patency the initial assessment of ventilation and heart rate is made. Resuscitation is begun if there is evidence of compromise of airway patency, ventilation, or cardiac output. A general treatment procedure is shown in Figure 1.

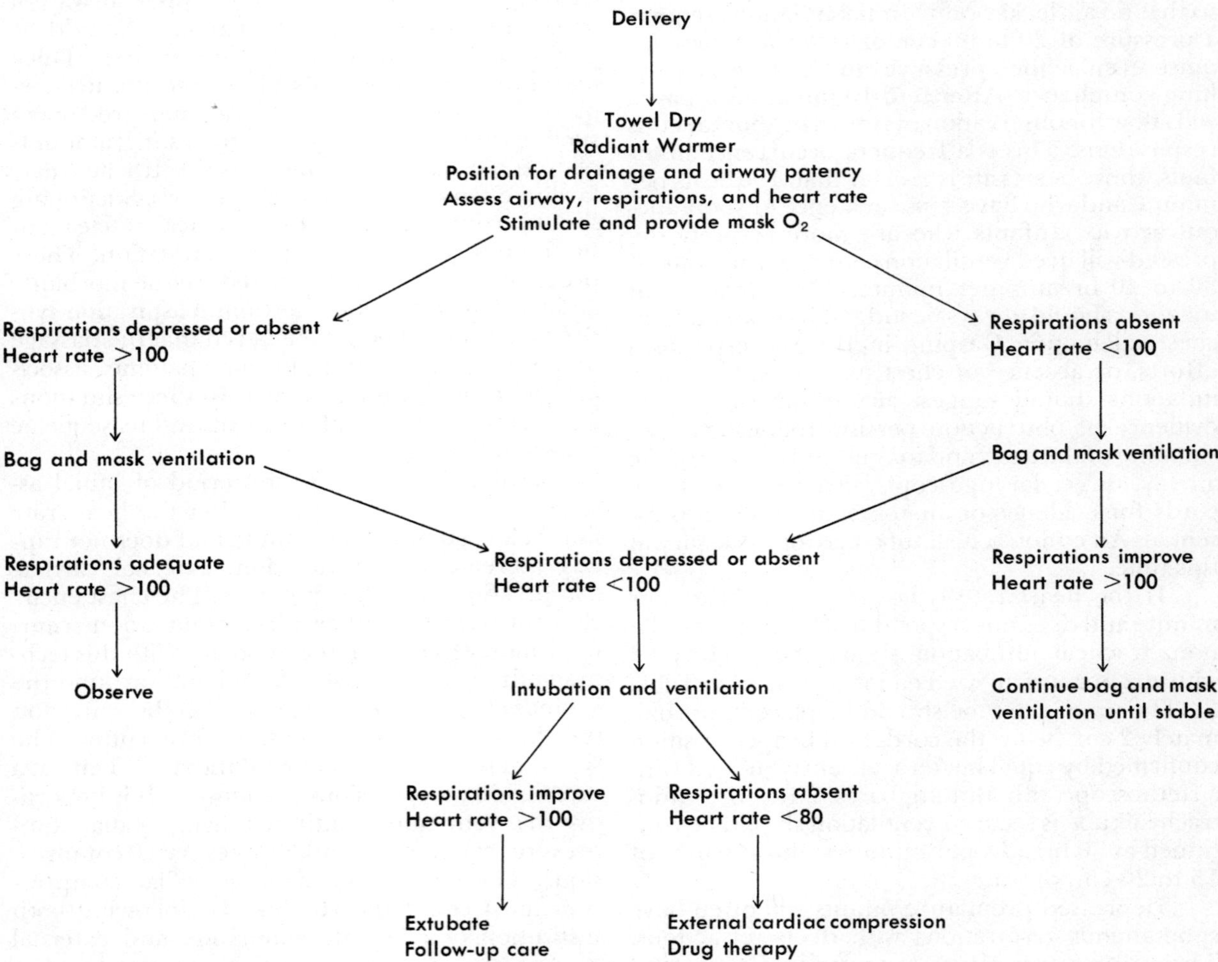

Figure 1. Simplified resuscitation plan.

Treatment

Airway. A lateral Trendelenberg position facilitates drainage of secretions and prevents the tongue from moving posteriorly, resulting in airway obstruction. Suction of the nares and mouth with a bulb syringe will clear most remaining fluid. Deep hypopharyngeal suctioning may stimulate vasovagal reflex episodes which interfere with effective resuscitation. In most infants the stimulation from drying and suctioning will result in the initiation of effective spontaneous respirations. Mask oxygen may facilitate recovery.

Breathing. Infants who have not initiated spontaneous respirations at the completion of the previous actions will now require bag and mask ventilation with oxygen. Many self-inflating bags are unable to deliver oxygen at a concentration of greater than 40 per cent and should be adapted to deliver at least 80 per cent oxygen. The infant is placed with slight extension of the head (sniffing position) to enhance airway patency. An oral airway will maintain the forward position of the tongue. The mask is applied very tightly to the face so that no air leaks occur. Initial inflations require a pressure of 20 to 30 cm. of water and may require even higher pressures in the face of poor lung compliance. After 5 to 10 inflations a pause will allow for observation of return of spontaneous respirations. This is a frequent occurrence in infants whose heart rate is greater than 100 beats per minute and who have some evidence of spontaneous activity. Infants who are more severely depressed will need ventilation continued at a rate of 30 to 40 breaths per minute. The adequacy of inflation should always be judged by evaluation of chest wall motion. Gasping, ineffective respiratory efforts, or absence of chest motion with normal inflations should suggest airway obstruction. If evidence of obstruction persists following repositioning of the head and tongue and suction of the airway, direct laryngoscopic visualization of the cords for evidence of anatomic obstruction is essential. An endotracheal tube may be necessary at this time.

If the heart rate is less than 100 beats per minute and does not respond to initial bag ventilation, tracheal intubation should be performed with an appropriate sized endotracheal tube (Table 2). The tip of the tube should be placed approximately 2 cm. below the cords and proper position confirmed by equal bilateral air entry judged with a stethoscope at both lung bases. After the endotracheal tube is secured ventilation should be continued at 30 breaths per minute with pressures of 15 to 20 cm. of water.

Depressed premature infants will often have spontaneous respirations with deep retractions. These respiratory efforts are often ineffective and require that the infant receive vigorous support, including early endotracheal intubation.

TABLE 2. **Guidelines for Selection of Airway Equipment**

WEIGHT	ORAL AIRWAY	ENDOTRACHEAL TUBE	SUCTION CATHETER FOR ENDOTRACHEAL TUBE (FR)
<1250	000	2.5	5
1250–2500	00	3.0	6
>2500	0	3.5	8

Infants born in an environment of amniotic fluid contaminated with thick, particulate meconium require special attention, with major modifications in resuscitation protocol. This does not apply to thin watery meconium-stained fluid. As tracheal aspiration of meconium appears to be entirely a postnatal event, meconium-stained infants should have thorough hypopharyngeal suctioning as soon as the head is delivered even before delivery of the chest. If this is impossible, thorough hypopharyngeal suctioning should take place immediately after delivery. If gasping occurs prior to clearing the hypopharynx and upper airway of meconium, direct tracheal suctioning should be performed to remove particulate matter. Thick meconium, because of its high viscosity, may require the use of the endotracheal tube directly as a suction catheter. The installation of small amounts of isotonic saline solution into the trachea may facilitate removal of particulate debris. Suctioning should continue until the trachea is clear of meconium prior to continued ventilation. These procedures will significantly reduce the morbidity and the mortality from meconium aspiration syndrome. It should be remembered that the passage of meconium in utero is, in some patients, associated with significant asphyxia. In these situations aggressive treatment of asphyxia and its sequelae is also indicated.

Cardiac. If during the period of initial assessment or at any time thereafter the heart rate falls below 80 beats per minute and does not rapidly increase with ventilation, external cardiac compression should be initiated. The chest encirclement technique of cardiac compression seems to be most effective in the neonate. With this technique the operator places both hands around the infant's chest with the finger tips on the spine and the thumbs together over the midsternum. The sternum is compressed toward the spine 1 cm. at a rate of 100 compressions per minute. It is imperative that ventilation continue during cardiac compression at a rate of 2 inflations every 10 compressions. The person performing cardiac compression must count the rhythm. If, following both institution of adequate ventilation and external cardiac compression, the heart rate remains low drug therapy should be utilized.

Drugs. The drugs listed in Table 3 must be

TABLE 3.   **Drugs for Newborn Resuscitation**

Glucose	5 ml. per kg. of 10% solution over 1 minute
Sodium Bicarbonate	2 mEq. per kg. of 7.5% solution diluted at least 1:1 over 2 minutes
Epinephrine	0.1 ml. per kg. of 1:10,000 solution
Atropine	0.03 mg. per kg.
Naloxone (Neonatal Narcan)	0.01 mg. per kg.
Albumin	15 ml. per kg. of 5% solution over 2 minutes
	4 ml. per kg. of 25% solution over 5 minutes
Calcium	100 mg. per kg. of 10% calcium gluconate or 30 mg. per kg. of 10% calcium chloride over 2 minutes
Ringer's Lactate	15 ml. per kg. over 2 minutes

available. It is helpful to have a wall chart giving the usual doses of each drug in the resuscitation area so that errors are not made in the emergency setting.

As soon as it is apparent that severe asphyxia is present and that the infant will require prolonged resuscitation, a central line should be placed. Placement of an umbilical arterial line provides both an intravascular access route as well as a means for monitoring blood gas and acid-base status and blood pressure. For the less experienced, an umbilical venous catheter may be more easily introduced and may suffice for interpretation of acid-base status and drug infusion. Ideally, the venous line should lie in the inferior vena cava but may be used in the emergency setting when located within the portal sinus. It is imperative that free return of blood be documented prior to the infusion of drugs into a catheter.

Infants who are asphyxiated will rapidly exhaust glycogen stores and will benefit from an exogenous glucose supply during resuscitation. Glucose is given as an infusion of 10 per cent dextrose in water at a dose of 5 ml. per kg. over 1 minute. This dose may be repeated at 15 minute intervals during the resuscitation period.

Although there is considerable controversy regarding the use of sodium bicarbonate infusions in neonates, it still appears appropriate to use this buffer during resuscitation when ventilation is adequate to excrete the added CO_2 load. Older data do suggest that early buffering may both delay the onset of central nervous system (CNS) damage and prolong the period during which an effective resuscitation can be performed. It does appear, however, that rapid changes in osmolality related to rapid infusions of concentrated bicarbonate solutions may be dangerous. For this reason the standard 7.5 per cent bicarbonate solution should be diluted at least 1:1 with either 10 per cent glucose solution or water. Bicarbonate is given at a dose of 2 mEq. per kg. over 2 minutes by

the clock. Subsequent doses of bicarbonate are indicated on the basis of significant metabolic acidosis demonstrated on blood acid-base measurements.

If the heart rate remains low following ventilation and external cardiac compression, epinephrine, 0.1 ml. per kg. of 1:10,000 dilution, should be given through the central line. In addition, atropine, 0.03 mg. per kg., may be given, particularly if reflex vagal episodes have been noted. Calcium infusions are used by some to improve myocardial contractility (5 to 10 mg. per kg. of elemental calcium; 0.3 ml. per kg. of 10 per cent calcium chloride or 1 ml. per kg. of 10 per cent calcium gluconate).

The use of naloxone hydrochloride (Narcan) should be considered in any depressed neonate born to a mother who has received narcotic analgesia. The dose of 0.01 mg. per kg. may be given intravenously or intramuscularly if there is adequate peripheral perfusion. Narcotic effects may outlast the effect of the antagonist and require additional naloxone doses every 30 to 60 minutes.

Infants who do not respond to basic resuscitative measures or who have evidence of hypovolemia including hypotension, poor peripheral perfusion, and weak pulses following oxygenation, or who have progressive acidosis often benefit from volume expansion. Hypovolemia should be considered, particularly following a history of vaginal bleeding, partial cord compression, or severe intrauterine asphyxia. Although blood is the ideal volume expander, technical problems associated with the use of placental blood are major and limit its usefulness. O-negative blood cross matched to the mother prior to delivery may be used. An acceptable alternative is the use of albumin solutions, 15 ml. per kg. of 5 per cent or 4 ml. per kg. of 25 per cent solutions. If signs of improved perfusion are noted following the initial dose, the infusion may be repeated. If neither blood nor albumin solutions are available, 15 ml. per kg. of Ringer's lactate will provide temporary volume expansion.

Follow-up.   Care following active resuscitation is extremely important. Attention should be paid to the maintenance of a neutral thermal environment. Intravenous glucose solutions should be continued when significant asphyxia has been present and blood glucose concentrations monitored by Dextrostix. Acid-base status should be followed with attention directed to the roles of persistent hypothermia or hypovolemia as causes for metabolic acidosis. If acidosis persists following control of these variables, subsequent additional slow infusions of buffer may be necessary. Blood carbon dioxide measurements will help assess adequacy of spontaneous ventilation and persistent hypercarbia ($Paco_2 > 65$ mm. Hg) may signal the need for prolonged ventilatory support. The oxygen needs of patients following resuscitation change very rapidly and ambient O_2 concentrations must be regulated to prevent both hypoxia and hyperoxia, keeping the infant's Pao_2 between 50 and 80 mm. Hg.

Severe asphyxia may result in postresuscitation sequelae such as seizures, acute renal tubular necrosis, disseminated intravascular coagulation, hepatic necrosis, and myocardial or brain damage. Hypoglycemia and electrolyte abnormalities are common. The anticipation of these problems may require transfer of the infant to an intensive care facility.

ECTOPIC PREGNANCY

method of
FREDERICK J. FLEURY, M.D.,
and RANDOLPH WM. ROLLER, M.D.
Springfield, Illinois

Ectopic pregnancy refers to implantation of the zygote in a site other than the uterine cavity. Approximately 95 per cent of such pregnancies are located in the uterine tube, while implantations in the abdominal cavity, uterine cornua, ovary, and cervix occur in decreasing order of frequency. A coassociation between ectopic pregnancy and residues of pelvic inflammatory disease can be found in as many as 50 per cent of patients, but any factor that can prevent or slow transport of the fertilized ovum down the tube may predispose to ectopic implantation.

The ratio of ectopic to normal intrauterine pregnancies varies from 1:300 to as high as 1:125. Approximately 10 per cent of those having an ectopic pregnancy will have more than one ectopic pregnancy. Current maternal mortality studies indicate that more than 100 women die annually in the United States from this condition, or 1 death per 800 ectopic pregnancies. Prompt diagnosis and immediate proper treatment are essential to prevent maternal death.

The most important element in the diagnosis of ectopic pregnancy is a high index of suspicion. Any patient presenting with the triad of abdominal pain, vaginal bleeding, and a history of irregular menses must be considered to have an ectopic pregnancy until proved otherwise. A careful clinical history and physical examination are the first diagnostic tools. Characteristically, these patients present with amenorrhea, with or without abnormal vaginal bleeding, the sudden onset of pelviabdominal pain, and a tender adnexal mass. They are typically 2 to 4 or more weeks late for their menstrual period and often have a history of pelvic inflammatory disease, infertility, or both. When tubal rupture has occurred, the patient presents in severe shock secondary to massive intraperitoneal hemorrhage. This represents a surgical emergency of the highest degree. For the patient in this situation, there is no time or need for further diagnostic procedures and rapid vascular volume expansion and operative therapy are indicated.

In the group of patients with appropriate history and physical findings but stable vital signs, time is available for further investigation to establish the proper diagnosis. Culdocentesis may be performed in an attempt to discover free-flowing, nonclotting blood in the cul-de-sac. Paracentesis, when positive, is equally helpful. The latter procedure may be somewhat less painful for the unanesthetized patient than culdocentesis, but if paracentesis is negative, culdocentesis should be performed. These procedures are not indicated for the patient if the decision for surgical intervention has already been made.

Another group of patients may be diagnosed as having "possible" ectopic pregnancy because of atypical signs and symptoms. These patients must be very carefully examined and studied to prevent both unnecessary delay and unnecessary surgery. In the stable patient with mild to moderate discomfort, a standard pregnancy test may be helpful, as it is positive in 50 per cent of patients with ectopics. The rapid slide test for the beta subunit of human chorionic gonadotropin (HCG), a more sensitive indicator of possible pregnancy, may prove helpful in some situations. Culdocentesis may also be positive in this group. However, positive results can occur from the ruptured corpus luteum cyst and from retrograde flow of blood from the uterine cavity at the time of menses or spontaneous abortion. Diagnostic laparoscopy has proved helpful in this group of patients and has the special advantage of possibly eliminating unnecessary laparotomy. Other disease states such as pelvic inflammatory disease, adnexal accidents, and appendicitis may then be ruled out. Laparoscopy in the face of a definite need for laparotomy is contraindicated.

A final and yet very important consideration

is that a few young patients will present with a classic picture of ectopic pregnancy with the exception of a stable blood pressure and a normal pulse. These young patients can paradoxically maintain a pulse below 90 per minute in spite of their pain and massive intraperitoneal bleeding. The blood pressure begins to fall in these patients as a late sign of intraperitoneal hemorrhage. This must be remembered to prevent undue delay in therapy.

With severe intraperitoneal hemorrhage, one or two intravenous lines should be established immediately using an 18 or larger gauge needle. Immediate intravascular replacement with lactated Ringer's or low molecular weight dextran is imperative. Transfusion with whole blood is recommended in the face of severe hypotension. In nearly all patients the intravenous solutions will maintain adequate blood pressure until there is sufficient time to type and cross match the patient's blood. In the extreme case, however, it may be necessary to use noncross-matched O-negative or type-specific blood. In a few patients, one may have to intervene surgically to control the hemorrhage without waiting for a return of normal vital signs. In less extreme circumstances, when surgical intervention is indicated but with less emergency, the patient can be adequately transfused and stabilized as she is prepared for operation.

The procedure of choice for the tubal ectopic pregnancy is salpingectomy with cornual resection to prevent future ectopic implantation at this site. A Pfannenstiel incision should be used. It must be remembered, however, that the midline approach is the fastest route with the best exposure and always should be used when any delay might endanger the patient. Once the involved tube has been identified, it should be immediately clamped to prevent further blood loss. The ovary on the involved side is not removed unless its blood supply has been compromised.

The surgeon may attempt to repair a minimally damaged uterine tube when the contralateral tube is surgically absent or diseased. Salpingotomy is associated with a reported incidence of 16 per cent recurrence compared to the 10 per cent recurrence of ectopic pregnancy in the uninvolved tube after salpingectomy. Patients should be informed of the distinct possibility of repeat ectopic gestation in the repaired tube. Fortunately, in this group of patients with minimally damaged tubes, there is usually enough time before operation to discuss this conservative approach and have the patient share in the decision making process.

If the present ectopic pregnancy involves the patient's only remaining tube and conservation is not possible, salpingectomy only should be done. It is often stated that the uterus becomes a "useless" organ after removal of the second tube and should therefore be removed. It is our opinion that the uterus should not be removed unless there is specific gynecologic indication and the patient's condition is stable.

The less common forms of ectopic pregnancy are also treated surgically. Abdominal pregnancy poses a serious problem. Laparotomy with removal of the fetus should be accomplished once the diagnosis is made, regardless of gestational age. The placenta and fetal membranes should be left in situ as placental separation usually results in massive uncontrollable bleeding. These patients must be followed carefully because of a high incidence of complications.

As a rule, cornual pregnancies present following rupture and extensive hemorrhage. As a result, these patients are in grave condition, and hysterectomy is often required. Cornual resection can be considered in the less severely compromised patient who desires further child-bearing potential and whose uterus is not too severely damaged.

Ovarian pregnancy is clinically indistinguishable from tubal gestation and therefore is not diagnosed until laparoscopy or laparotomy. This condition can be treated with wedge resection rather than oophorectomy except when the entire ovary is involved or destroyed.

Cervical pregnancies are very uncommon and often present as painless vaginal bleeding. The vaginal approach to evacuation of the cervical gestation often results in severe bleeding and success with this method is infrequent. On occasion, ligation of the cervical branches of the uterine arteries may be attempted, but hysterectomy may be the best method of treatment.

An ectopic gestation is a potential cause of Rh isoimmunization. It is therefore important to identify the Rh negative patient and provide her with prophylactic Rh immunoglobulin if indicated.

In summary, the management of ectopic pregnancy depends upon the severity of the patient's pain or hypotension. Rapid circulatory volume replacement, transfusion, and operation are imperative for the critically ill patient. For the comfortable and stable patient, more time exists for further diagnostic procedures. Once the decision to operate has been made, further testing is unnecessary and surgery should be accomplished as rapidly as possible.

HEMORRHAGE IN LATE PREGNANCY

method of
EMANUEL A. FRIEDMAN, M.D.
Boston, Massachusetts

Vaginal bleeding in the third trimester of pregnancy continues to pose a serious threat to the life and well-being of both the gravida and her offspring. It continues to be a leading cause of maternal mortality and perinatal wastage. There has been a gratifying trend in recent years toward improvement for the mother as a consequence of more readily available means for counteracting shock, replacing blood loss, administering anesthesia, expeditiously emptying the uterus surgically, recognizing and correcting coagulopathies, and stemming otherwise uncontrollable blood loss by operative vascular ligations. Improved outcomes for the fetus are primarily related to measures aimed at conservatism and delay, where possible, in effecting delivery; moreover, major advances in neonatal care for the premature infant have considerably enhanced survival. The basic principle in managing patients with hemorrhage in late pregnancy involves weighing the benefits of aggressive intervention for purposes of terminating the pregnancy in the interests of the mother against the risks of delay with the objective of improving fetal salvage by allowing the fetus to mature in utero.

Preliminary Evaluation

An immediate assessment of patient status is essential. If there is heavy vaginal bleeding with evidence of cardiovascular instability, aggressive intervention will be necessary. Although such patients are in the minority, they demand prompt, expert, and aggressive management. For the remainder, well in the majority, more careful evaluation and deliberate diagnosis and treatment are in order.

The patient should be hospitalized and given bed rest. Her vital signs should be monitored. An intravenous infusion should be instituted with a large-bore needle to permit immediate access to a vein, should it become necessary for purposes of rapid blood replacement. Suitably cross matched blood must be made available. Aside from blood typing, laboratory examinations should include hematocrit, urine analysis, and coagulation studies. The latter minimally include bleeding and clotting times and observation of a clot for lysis; if available, determination of fibrinogen, prothrombin time, fibrin split products, and platelet count are useful. Use of a central venous pressure catheter may also be useful, especially for the patient with active bleeding or cardiovascular instability or both.

For diagnosis of the underlying cause of the bleeding, only the most cursory attempts need to be made for the patient with catastrophic hemorrhage. Here, it is far more critical to mobilize all efforts toward preventing or correcting hypovolemic shock. No more than a superficial vaginal examination by speculum is necessary in order to ascertain that the bleeding originates from within the uterus and is not instead coming from a polyp, varix, laceration, erosion, or neoplasm on the cervix, vagina, vulva, or perineum. If it can be established that the bleeding is coming from within the uterus under these exigent circumstances, prompt intervention should follow.

When bleeding is less active or actually abating, more extensive evaluation should be undertaken. In addition to the speculum examination of the vagina, the condition of the abdomen should be noted, particularly with reference to focalization of the pain, guarding, tenderness, and rebound. Uterine size, contour, irritability, and relaxation should be determined. Assessment of the fetus should include its size, presentation, and heart tones, the last being best evaluated by continuous beat-to-beat electronic fetal heart rate monitoring. A line drawn with marking pencil on the abdominal wall will denote the upper border of the uterus and serve to signal any subsequent uterine enlargement due to concealed retroplacental bleeding. Objective placental localization by means of ultrasonography, when available, has almost totally replaced all other techniques because of improved safety unaccompanied by sacrifice in accuracy.

Ultrasonography can also provide an indirect measure of fetal maturity by giving the biparietal diameter of the fetal head. A more critical assessment of functional fetal maturity is available in the lecithin-sphingomyelin ratio of amniotic fluid; when this ratio is greater than 2:1, pulmonary maturity is reasonably assured so that respiratory distress will be unlikely to occur in the neonatal period. Ultrasound imaging techniques also permit visualization of retroplacental clot formation to aid in the diagnosis of abruptio placentae. It should be stressed that a placenta previa identified early in the third trimester may later in pregnancy be found to have "migrated" to a higher site within the uterus, thereby reducing or eliminating further risk of hemorrhage.

The source of vaginal bleeding may rarely be a fetal umbilical vessel. This occurs with a velamentous insertion of the cord, a condition in which the umbilical vessels course between the chorion and amnion before entering the main body of the placenta. In vasa previa, one or more of these vessels crosses the internal cervical os and may there be subjected to damage, particularly at the time the membranes rupture. If suspected, the diagnosis can be made by examining the blood for fetal erythrocytes or fetal hemoglobin. When vasa previa is diagnosed, cesarean section should be undertaken at once if the fetus is alive and sufficiently mature to be likely to survive after delivery.

Management of Placenta Previa

Whenever possible, the patient with placenta previa should be treated expectantly. It is rare for the first episode of bleeding to end fatally (although possible, of course). If bleeding is massive or unremitting, intervention by cesarean section should be undertaken at once. If not, an expectant management program can be instituted. The patient is observed for progression or recurrence of bleeding. No pelvic or rectal examinations are permitted. Abstinence from intercourse or other intravaginal manipulations is mandated. Blood is replaced as lost. The fetal condition is periodically monitored. Use of glucocorticoids for purposes of accelerating fetal lung maturity is instituted if less than 34 weeks' gestational age. Dexamethasone can be given either orally or intramuscularly in 4 mg. doses every 8 hours for 48 hours.

Such a program of observation and support allows the fetus to mature, while awaiting either the onset of another episode of hemorrhage or of spontaneous labor. Proceeding directly to definitive diagnosis by intravaginal transcervical digital examination will invariably precipitate hemorrhage by disrupting the placental site overlying the internal os. Hemorrhage will force premature intervention. The possible advantages of delay, particularly in allowing the fetus to mature further and perhaps in migration of the placenta away from the internal os, will thus not be attainable. Therefore, one should try to maximize opportunities for expectancy if at all feasible and practicable.

Patients with documented total or central placenta previa must ultimately be delivered by cesarean section. Only rarely is it acceptable to permit a patient with partial or marginal placenta previa to undergo labor with the presenting fetal part tamponading the bleeding maternal uterine vessels. This approach should be reserved for the occasional multipara in active labor with little or no vaginal bleeding. Definitive digital exploration within the cervix for the purpose of clarifying the diagnosis should be undertaken immediately prior to cesarean section. However, it must not be done unless everything is in readiness for either abdominal surgery or pelvic delivery (the so-called "double set-up"), including anesthesia, blood, instruments, and personnel. Once the characteristic spongy or gritty placenta is palpated, one must proceed immediately to perform the indicated cesarean section. Delay will result in excessive blood loss.

The choice of cesarean section technique is arguable. Transverse incision through the lower uterine segment tends to increase both fetal and maternal blood loss from the placental site, although it does provide good access to the placental site for purposes of providing surgical hemostasis. Generally, the classical (vertical upper uterine) incision is preferable, particularly since the lower segment tends to be poorly thinned out, very vascular, and easily traumatized; moreover, the fetus is relatively inaccessible through a lower segment incision.

Management of Abruptio Placentae

Differentiation between placenta previa and abruptio placentae is generally based on differences in clinical presentation, the latter being characterized by uterine contractility, irritability, and pain. Clear-cut distinction, however, is not always achievable. Therefore, one should entertain the possibility of placenta previa in any patient who presents with significant bleeding in the third trimester. Although abruptio placentae is often a catastrophic complication of pregnancy, it can be relatively innocuous, subsiding without adverse effect. The more severe variety subjects the patient to the hazards of profuse hemorrhage, not always entirely apparent because large amounts of bleeding may be concealed within the uterus. Furthermore, this condition superimposes the hazards of coagulopathy as well, probably on the basis of absorption of thromboplastin from the retroplacental site.

Patients with abruptio placentae deserve to be delivered as quickly and as atraumatically as possible, except for those with the mildest clinical manifestations. The latter include those with stable cardiovascular status, normal coagulation parameters, and no fetal distress. Any gravida with uterine tetany, shock, evidence of fetal compromise, or coagulopathy warrants intervention. This also applies to those with a progressive clinical picture. It should be recognized that the longer the delay before delivery, the greater the likelihood of hemorrhage, disseminated intravascular coagulation, and fetal death.

Blood should be administered to replace loss. If the fetus is alive, continuous monitoring should be undertaken; if less than 34 weeks' gestational age and some delay in delivery is anticipated, glucocorticoids can be given.

The choice of mode of delivery depends on the patient's condition, specifically the amount of blood she has lost and the rate of continued bleeding, and how favorable the cervix is for induction of labor. If appropriate, amniotomy can be done and oxytocin infusion administered for purposes of inducing or stimulating labor and effecting vaginal delivery. In general, about 4 hours (and no more than 8 hours) of such stimulation is given. If the clinical manifestations worsen or if labor is not progressing well, cesarean section may be invoked to terminate the pregnancy. Alternatively, cesarean section should be done if conditions are particularly unfavorable for vaginal delivery or the initial presenting picture interdicts any delay in evacuating the uterus.

Rarely with abruptio placentae, the myometrium may be so inspissated with blood that it cannot contract. This condition, called Couvelaire uterus, results in uncontrollable bleeding from the atonic uterus at the placental site. Bleeding from this site can only be stanched if the uterus can be made to contract with uterotonic agents. Failing this, hysterectomy may be necessary. For the woman who may wish to retain her reproductive potential, bilateral hypogastric artery ligation may be tried; if this is ineffectual, one could proceed with ligation of the ovarian arteries in the infundibulopelvic ligaments or, more preferably, at their point of anastomosis with the ascending branches of the uterine arteries in the utero-ovarian ligaments. This usually reduces the blood flow sufficiently to the uterus to stop the bleeding. The uterus will not become totally ischemic, however, because there will still be adequate circulation by way of anastomoses with the descending branches of the uterine arteries.

Although the underlying inciting factors for the development of disseminated intravascular coagulation terminate abruptly as soon as the uterus is emptied, coagulation parameters must be carefully monitored. The appearance of widespread hemorrhagic tendencies with bleeding from various sites requires intensive treatment, particularly aimed at restoring depleted clotting factors. The best approach is the use of fresh whole blood. Specifically replacing fibrinogen may also be useful. Details of management of this complication are dealt with elsewhere. Heparin as a means for blocking the intravascular coagulation process does not appear to have a place in the management of the coagulopathy resulting from abruptio placentae.

TOXEMIA OF PREGNANCY
method of
E. J. QUILLIGAN, M.D.
Los Angeles, California

Toxemia of pregnancy, known by a host of other names such as preeclampsia-eclampsia, pregnancy-induced hypertension, hypertension in pregnancy, is really one of a combination of two or more of three basic diseases, preeclampsia-eclampsia, essential hypertension, or renal disease. The disease develops in the second or third trimester of pregnancy. It is characterized by hypertension, a systolic pressure greater than 140 mm. Hg, or which increases more than 30 mm. Hg above previously recorded levels or a diastolic pressure greater than 90 mm. Hg or which increases more than 15 mm. Hg above the baseline levels. There may also be proteinuria, 1+ or greater on two successive specimens collected 6 hours apart and uncontaminated by vaginal secretions, or edema of the hands, face, or body. More severe disease will be manifested by higher blood pressure levels (greater than 160/100), significant albuminuria (greater than 1 gram per day), or convulsions. Symptoms that may alert the physician that more severe disease is developing include severe headaches, scotoma, and epigastric pain.

The ultimate therapy for toxemia of pregnancy is delivery; however, the physician's thinking must always be tempered by the severity of the maternal processes and its effect on her as well as the effect of the disease or therapy on the fetus and newborn. Mild forms of the disease and, occasionally, even the more severe forms may improve dramatically with bed rest alone, so this is the first therapy for all patients. In general, this is best done in the hospital, as the patient, removed from her home environment, really rests. While in the hospital the patient should receive a diet with a reasonable protein content (at least 1 gram per kg. of body weight), and a normal sodium chloride content. Diuretics are contraindicated even though the patient may be edematous. Bed rest alone is sufficient to initiate a diuresis in most patients. In the past patients were given phenobarbital to encourage them to rest more. This is usually not necessary. While in the hospital the patient should be weighed daily, have her blood pressure taken four times per day, and have a urine sample examined for albumin once daily. Occasionally, in the very mild forms of the disease one may prescribe bed rest at home. If this is to be done, the patient must be told of the symptoms of rapidly developing disease, e.g., scotoma, headache, and epigastric pain, and seen very frequently, i.e., every 2 to 3 days. If the patient does not improve or any of the signs become worse, she must be admitted to the hospital immediately.

The duration of this keystone of therapy, bed rest, in toxemia of pregnancy depends upon the stage of pregnancy in which the disease develops, the severity of the disease and the response to bed rest, and, finally, the effect of the disease on the fetus. For example, a patient developing a mild form of the disease at 40 weeks' gestation would simply be delivered by induction of labor after a few hours' rest in bed. On the other hand, patients frequently develop the disease early in the third trimester when it would be a distinct disadvantage to the fetus to be delivered. In such instances, the maternal progression of the disease and the effect of the disease on the fetus will determine whether the pregnancy should be terminated.

Fetal evaluation is best performed by both biophysical and biochemical methods. The biophysical tests include the response of the fetal heart rate to fetal movement and to maternal uterine contractions. A fetus who shows at least two accelerations of the fetal heart rate of 15 beats per minute or greater associated with fetal activity in a 20 minute period is normal. Since the fetus normally has periods of inactivity, it may be necessary to record for 40 minutes or longer to detect fetal activity. Also a fetus who does not show any late decelerations of the fetal heart rate when the mother is having uterine contractions with a frequency of three contractions per 10 minutes is normal. Since the reverse is not necessarily true, i.e., no cardiac accelerations or late decelerations with contractions, indicating an abnormal fetus, caution must be used in delivering the premature fetus on the basis of these tests. If the fetus is premature we require, in addition to the above, an abnormal estriol (urine or plasma) value in the mother to interrupt pregnancy.

As stated above, just as maternal progression of the disease may indicate therapy in addition to bed rest, so too may the stage of the disease on first observation indicate further therapy. Should the patient develop eclampsia (most severe form of the disease), every effort should be made to prevent convulsions. This is best done with magnesium sulfate. Magnesium sulfate is indicated whenever there is a significant possibility of convulsions developing as evidenced by increased deep tendon reflexes, a rising blood pressure, previous convulsions, premonitory symptoms (headache,

scotoma, epigastric pain) or finally a patient in labor even with mild disease. The initial dose of magnesium sulfate is 3 to 4 grams in a 20 per cent solution given slowly (over 5 to 10 minutes) intravenously. This may be followed by either intravenous or intramuscular magnesium sulfate. If given intravenously the dose should be 1 to 2 grams per hour and if intramuscularly, 10 grams of a 50 per cent solution given as 5 grams injected deeply in each buttock with 1 ml. of procaine in each syringe and 5 grams of a 50 per cent solution deep intramuscularly every 4 hours. The dose intravenously or intramuscularly must be reduced if the deep tendon reflexes are absent, the respiratory rate is reduced (<12 per minute), or the urinary output is less than 25 ml. per hour. Magnesium sulfate if given during delivery should be continued for 12 to 24 hours after delivery because while delivery is the ultimate therapy of the disease the patient is still at risk of convulsing for the next 24 to 48 hours. Whenever magnesium sulfate is administered, there should be a syringe of calcium gluconate (5 to 10 ml. of 25 per cent solution) available to counteract magnesium toxicity.

Occasionally, the patient with toxemia of pregnancy will have oliguria or even anuria. In this situation fluids should be given sparingly, to replace loss, or preferably with the assistance of central venous or wedge pressure. Fluid overload can occur with oliguria rather easily and pulmonary or cerebral edema is still one of the three principal causes of maternal death in toxemia, the other two being cerebrovascular accident and convulsive anoxia. If pulmonary edema does develop, furosemide, 40 mg. intravenously, should be given. This is the only indication for the use of diuretics in this disease. If fluids are to be used we prefer Ringer's lactate; however, the type of fluid to be used must take into account prior therapy. If diuretics have been used extensively, the patient may need more sodium chloride.

One complication that may result in maternal death is cerebrovascular accident. In order to prevent this, one may use a hypotensive agent. Hypotensive agents are not routinely used because reduction in maternal blood pressure may reduce uterine blood flow and thus imperil the fetus. However, if there is a significantly increased risk to the mother as judged by a diastolic blood pressure of 110 mm. Hg or higher, hypotensive agents should be used. The preferred agent is hydralazine because it may relieve renal vascular constriction. We prefer to give 2 mg. pulses every 2 to 5 minutes until the diastolic pressure reaches 100 mm. Hg. When the pressure starts to rise, additional doses should be given. When the patient is postpartum and the fetus need not be considered, a lower diastolic pressure, i.e., 100 mm. Hg, should trigger the use of hydralazine.

Toxemia of pregnancy is a serious disease; however, early diagnosis and prompt and conservative therapy can give excellent results for both mother and fetus.

OBSTETRIC ANALGESIA AND ANESTHESIA

method of
MIGUEL COLÓN-MORALES, M.D.
San Juan, Puerto Rico

Morton's demonstration of ether anesthesia, in 1846, initiated what soon made possible the separation of pain and surgery. Unfortunately, and in spite of all efforts, similar complete separation of pain and childbirth has not yet been achieved.

There are fundamental considerations responsible for the difficulties encountered with the relief of pain during labor and delivery. They must be well understood prior to any attempt to provide analgesia or anesthesia for the obstetric patient, lest more harm than good result.

The change in emphasis from mother to fetus during recent years and the concern for the long-term effects of depressant drugs on the newborn, together with the manpower shortage in well trained obstetric anesthesia personnel, have complicated the present situation even more.

Recently there have been favorable changes in the practice of obstetric anesthesia and analgesia. The introduction of new drugs and techniques, the increased knowledge concerning the alterations in physiology of the pregnant woman, the more accurate assessment of the fetus through monitoring and the increasing availability of well trained and experienced personnel to provide analgesia and/or anesthesia to the obstetric patient have modified to a certain extent our attitudes toward the problem of pain relief during childbirth and its potential hazards. There is at present no ideal anesthetic agent or technique for childbirth. All known analgesics or anesthetic drugs pass through the placental barrier to the fetus with its immature organs and in its state of intermittent hypoxia and acidosis during labor and delivery.

There is, however, enough evidence to suggest that *properly* administered analgesia and/or anesthesia reduces mortality and morbidity of the newborn. This represents a challenge to all physicians concerned, especially to obstetricians, anesthesiologists, and pediatricians.

Basic fundamental knowledge and special skills are essential for the proper management of pain during labor and delivery and should be part of the armamentarium of every physician who assumes the responsibility for participating in the care of the obstetric patient during childbirth.

Fundamental Considerations

Pregnancy causes physiologic alterations of great importance in the respiratory and cardiovascular systems. Such alterations must be kept in mind in order to provide safe obstetric anesthesia or analgesia.

Respiratory System Alterations. During the later part of pregnancy, respiratory rate and depth are increased to cope with the rise in O_2 requirements. The dyspneic-like effect is the result of the pressure of the enlarging uterus on the diaphragm. When the fetal head engages in the pelvis—"the lightening"—around the thirty-sixth week of gestation, the condition improves. Because of the increased O_2 requirement, any respiratory depression resulting from increased dosages of sedatives, analgesics, or anesthetics may lead to maternal hypoxia and its hazards to the already hypoxic fetus during labor and delivery (see Figure 1).

Cardiovascular System Alterations. Increase in blood volume occurs early in pregnancy. There is a greater rise in the plasma than in red blood cells. The result is the anemia of pregnancy, which must be corrected by means of iron. The increase in volume will serve to compensate for the loss of blood during delivery. There is also a gradual rise in cardiac output and pulse rate. These facts must be kept in mind in patients with heart disease because of the greater burden imposed on the heart.

During the last trimester of pregnancy, pregnant women lying in the supine position may suffer from hypotension caused by a decrease in venous return resulting from the pressure of the gravid uterus on the inferior vena cava and pelvic veins. This is called the Inferior Vena Cava syndrome. Although compression of the inferior vena cava occurs in 85 per cent of pregnant women, during the last trimester, when in the supine position, severe symptoms are manifested in only 8 to 10 per cent; this is due to compensation by an increase in heart rate and by diversion of the blood through the paravertebral veins and into the azygous vein. A rise in vasomotor tone and peripheral resistance compensates and often prevents a fall in maternal blood pressure but does not necessarily correct an impairment with uteroplacental perfusion. Regional anesthesia with resul-

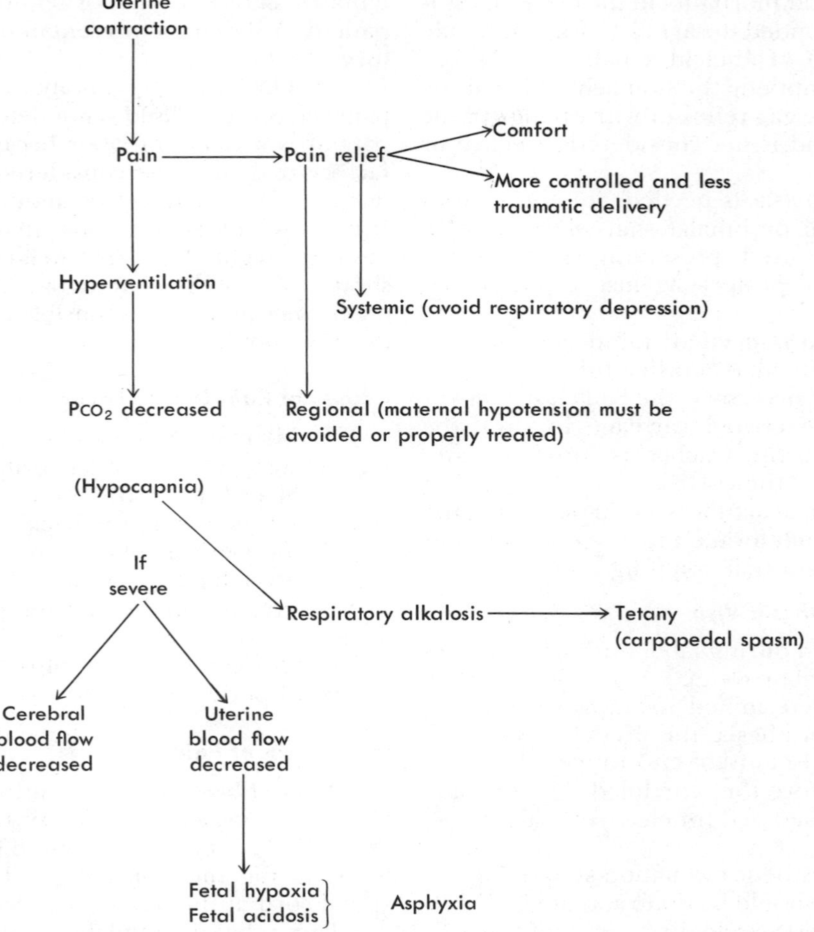

Figure 1.   Effects of pain and hyperventilation on mother and fetus.

tant peripheral vasodilation may prevent adequate compensation to maintain maternal blood pressure. Compression of the aorta (Poseiro effect) may maintain maternal blood pressure in the upper extremities but may result in a drop in blood pressure of the uterine arteries.

The Placenta

The placenta serves as the lungs, liver, and kidney of the fetus during pregnancy and parturition. Anything interfering with normal placental circulation will affect the growth and development of the fetus and its adaptation to the external independent environment after birth. All drugs used for obstetric analgesia and anesthesia will cross the placental barrier—with the one exception of the muscle relaxants, when used in small doses.

Obstetric Maternal Deaths

Causes: (1) Hemorrhage, (2) infection, (3) toxemia, (4) heart disease, and (5) anesthesia.

Obstetric Anesthesia Deaths

Causes: (1) Aspiration of vomitus (most common), (2) hypotension, and (3) respiratory failure.

Aspiration of Vomitus

1. "Prepare for the worst and it will seldom happen."

2. All parturients must be considered to have full stomachs. The onset of labor slows emptying of the stomach, and continued gastric secretions accumulate in the stomach during labor.

3. Fifty per cent of the obstetric deaths caused by anesthesia are attributable to the aspiration of vomitus.

4. Prevention—"an ounce of prevention is worth a pound of cure." During her prenatal visits, both the obstetrician and the anesthesiologist should warn the patient against taking solids or liquids by mouth once labor has started. During labor, the use of antacids is recommended to serve the specific purpose of neutralizing acidity of the gastric secretions. A pH above 2.5 is a must to re-

duce mortality and morbidity in the event of aspiration. Recommended dosage is 15 to 30 ml. (one half to 1 ounce) of antacid a half hour before delivery time. Emptying the stomach artificially by stimulation of the gag reflex or with apomorphine is rarely used and is not considered effective or practical.

When anesthesia is needed, for the sake of safety a regional or inhalational *analgesia* technique should be used, preserving tracheolaryngeal reflexes to protect against aspiration if vomiting occurs.

If anesthesia is needed, rapid endotracheal intubation is essential. A "crash intubation" is performed, using, if necessary, the Sellich maneuver (pressure on the cricoid cartilage to close the esophagus) while the trachea is intubated and sealed by inflating the cuff.

The endotracheal tube is left in place until the patient is completely awake and able to protect her airway in the event that vomiting occurs.

Predelivery Anesthesia Visit

Relief of pain during labor and delivery does not start in the labor room.

If we are determined to improve obstetric analgesia and anesthesia, the predelivery visit to the anesthesiologist must be encouraged. It should be done well before the scheduled delivery date (EDC) or date scheduled for elective cesarean section.

1. A preanesthetic evaluation adapted to the obstetric patient should be done at that visit, preferably by the anesthesiologist.

2. The different types of analgesia and anesthesia available for delivery, as well as the psychologic methods, should be discussed and a tentative choice or plan of action described to the patient. A slide-type presentation may be satisfactory.

3. The final decision about what method of pain relief will be used is not determined until the patient is actually in labor because of the many factors that must be considered in making this decision. Such an interview should help remove all fears and misconceptions that the expectant mother might have. A well-informed patient should be a well-behaved patient through more confidence in those responsible for her pain relief during labor and delivery.

Causes of Pain During Labor

1. Myometrial anoxia—contraction of muscle during a period of relative anoxia causes pain.

2. Stretching of the cervix—a painful sensation is felt, mainly in the back.

3. Traction on tubes, ovaries, or peritoneum.

4. Stretching of supporting ligaments.

5. Pressure in the urethra, bladder, and rectum.

6. Distention of the muscles of the pelvic floor and perineum.

Mechanism of Pain

Nerve fibers carrying painful sensations during the *first stage* of labor enter the spinal cord at the T10, T11, and T12 levels. The painful sensations during the *second stage* of labor enter the spinal cord at the S2, S3, and S4 levels.

Pain relief during labor and delivery may be accomplished through (1) psychologic methods, (2) pharmacologic methods, or (3) a combination of both.

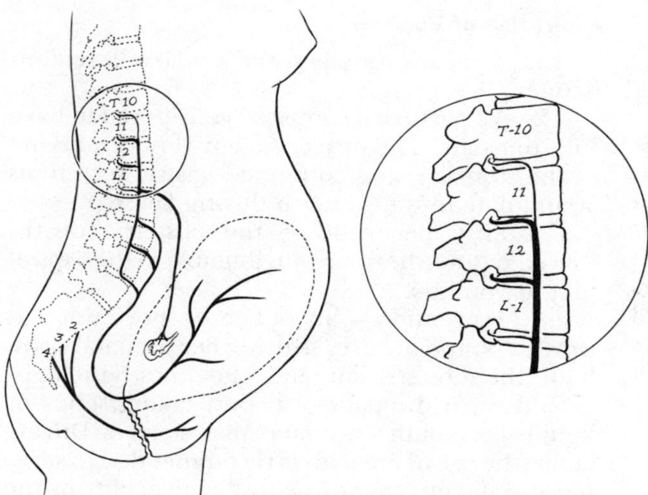

Figure 2. Parturition pain pathways The uterus, including the cervix, is supplied by sensory (pain) fibers which pass from the uterus to the spinal cord by accompanying sympathetic nerves in the following sequence: uterine, cervical and pelvic plexuses, the hypogastric nerve, the superior hypogastric plexus, the lumbar and lower thoracic sympathetic chain, and thence through white rami communicantes and posterior roots. The primary pathways (shown as thick lines in the inset) enter the eleventh and twelfth spinal segments, whereas the secondary auxiliary pathways enter at T10 and L1. The pathways from the perineum pass to the sacral spinal cord via the pudendal nerves. (Modified from Bonica, J. J.: Principles and Practice of Obstetric Analgesia and Anesthesia. Philadelphia, F. A. Davis Company, 1967).

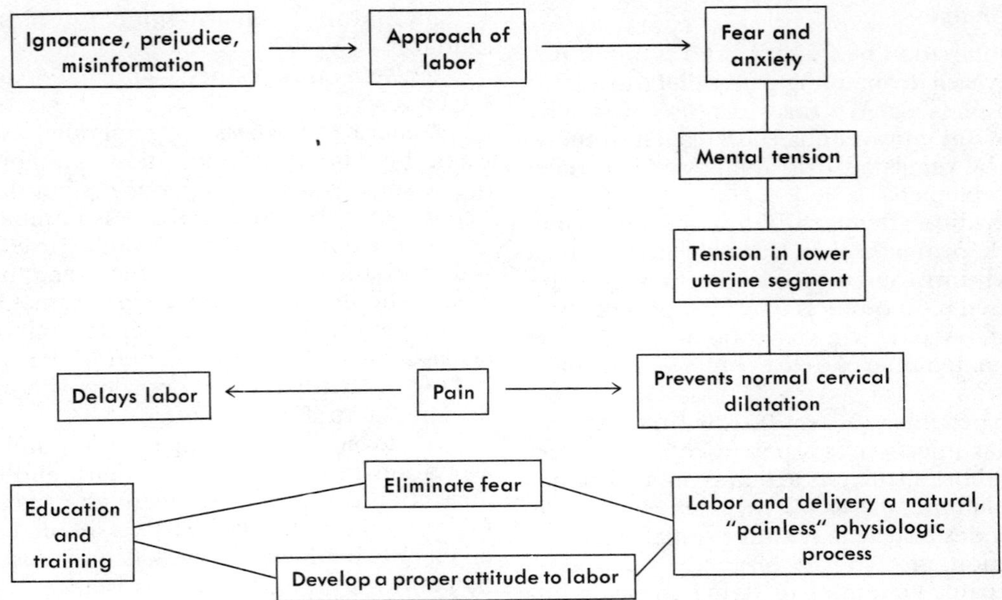

Figure 3. Natural childbirth (Dick Read method).

Psychologic Methods of Pain Relief

These include (1) natural childbirth (childbirth without fear, Dick Read method), (2) psychoprophylactic method (Lamaze, Vellay), and (3) hypnosis.

Unfortunately psychologic methods for pain relief during labor and delivery are not suitable for everyone. The decision to use natural childbirth should be made several months before the estimated date of confinement. It takes time to learn the special exercises and to condition the mind in order for this method to be most effective. The ultimate objective should be to minimize the use of pharmacologic analgesia and/or anesthesia.

Preparation for Natural Childbirth. 1. Eight lectures in the basic anatomy and physiology of pregnancy.

2. A program of exercises and relaxation to be practiced throughout pregnancy.

Unfortunately great emphasis is placed on *conscious* and *spontaneous* delivery, and this can lead to severe psychologic trauma to patients who require operative delivery.

Psychoprophylaxis. Psychoprophylaxis was started in Russia, but was later developed in France by Lamaze and Vellay. It is based on the pavlovian concept of conditioned reflex training. Since women associate childbirth with pain, psychoprophylaxis aims to decondition the patient and then create new positive reflexes.

Method: The patient receives a series of illustrated lectures on the conditioned reflex and the physiology of normal labor. Then she is taught a series of exercises, which she practices during pregnancy. These include different breathing patterns and pain-reducing procedures—e.g., massage of the lower abdomen; and pressure on the anterior superior iliac crest when contraction increases in intensity. This is a form of distraction therapy.

In contrast to the method of natural childbirth, the patient in a psychoprophylaxis program is made aware that labor may be abnormally painful and that other forms of analgesia may be necessary. In the event she asks for pharmacologic pain relief or requires operative delivery, she does not feel that she has failed.

Hypnosis. Hypnosis is defined as a state of altered consciousness characterized by heightened suggestibility. Its exact mode of action is not known. Fifteen to 20 per cent of patients cannot be hypnotized. Only about 30 per cent of those who have been trained in the method achieve a relatively pain-free labor. The technique is very time consuming. Some patients may learn self-hypnosis. The majority require the presence of the hypnotist at the onset of labor and during the second stage.

Hypnosis should not be used in psychiatrically disturbed patients.

To summarize: Each one of these psychologic methods has its enthusiastic followers. At present, perhaps an individualized application of these techniques, alone or as an adjunct to the judicious use of the pharmacologic methods, might come closest to the ideal goals we are searching for in the management of pain relief during childbirth.

Systemic Analgesia

A combination of narcotics and tranquilizers serves very well in obtaining pain relief during the first stage of labor. We favor the use of smaller dosages by the intravenous route, given in increments or by regulated drip until adequate relief of pain is obtained.

Meperidine (Demerol), 25 to 50 mg., combined with promethazine (Phenergan), 25 mg., given slowly intravenously or by the intramuscular route, is used most often. It may be repeated every 3 to 4 hours. Avoid giving narcotics within 2 hours of the estimated time of delivery to avoid neonatal depression.

Alphaprodine (Nisentil), 20 mg. by intramuscular injection, is a potent respiratory depressant. Short lasting, its action is about 1 hour.

Scopolamine, 0.2 to 0.3 mg., may be used if amnesia is desired. It may cause restlessness and disorientation.

Diazepam (Valium), 5 to 10 mg. intravenously, may be very effective in allaying apprehension.

Promethazine (Phenergan), 25 mg. intravenously, an antihistaminic tranquilizer and antinauseant, will potentiate the effects of meperidine (Demerol).

In the event that narcotic depression is observed in the parturient prior to delivery, naloxone hydrochloride (Narcan) may be used intravenously in increments of 0.1 to 0.2 mg. at 2 to 3 minute intervals to the desired degree of reversal. This may help reduce the depressant effects of narcotics in the newborn.

Inhalational Analgesia

A low concentration of anesthetic agents may be administered for short periods to provide pain relief during labor and even delivery. The mother remains conscious and maintains her airway, and her protective reflexes are active. The progress of labor is not affected. There is no effect on the fetus because of low concentration. The effect of these agents may be reinforced during the second stage of labor by using a pudendal block or by local infiltration of the perineum.

The agents used are N_2O and O_2 in a 50-50 mixture. Methoxyflurane (Penthrane), 0.3 to 0.5 per cent, may be added for more profound analgesia. These agents may be self-administered under close supervision by a nurse or physician. By using the Penthrane Analgyzer adequate analgesia may be obtained during contractions.

Types of Anesthesia

1. Local infiltration of the episiotomy site.
2. Pudendal block.
3. Paracervical block.
4. Low spinal or saddle block.
5. Epidural block—lumbar epidural or caudal.
6. General anesthesia—inhalational or intravenous.

General anesthesia is generally used only when there is a contraindication to regional anesthesia such as central nervous system disease or hypovolemia, or when delivery is imminent.

The least potent agent should be used to avoid a depressant effect on the fetus and newborn. There should be at least 25 per cent O_2 in the anesthetic mixture. Recommended mixtures are (1) N_2O and O_2 in a proportion of 3:1, or (2) an N_2O-O_2 mixture in 1:1 proportion with methoxyflurane 0.3 to 0.5 per cent.

To avoid the consequences of vomiting and aspiration in the obstetric patient, endotracheal intubation is highly recommended once a patient is given general anesthesia. This should be undertaken only by those highly skilled in crash intubation and with the necessary assistance. It must be kept in mind that the lighter and shorter the anesthesia, the less depressant drugs will reach the infant before birth.

Pudendal Nerve Block. The pudendal nerve is the main supply of the perineum. It arises from the second, third, and fourth sacral nerves. The nerve is blocked most easily where it lies close to the tip of the ischial spine.

Pudendal nerve block should be performed in primigravidas when the cervix is fully dilated and the presenting part is at station $+2$, and in multiparas when the cervix has reached 7 to 8 cm. of dilatation.

Pudendal block provides satisfactory anesthesia for spontaneous delivery, low forceps extraction, breech delivery, and episiotomy repair or repair of laceration.

Transvaginal Technique. With the tip of the index finger inside the vagina, locate the ischial spine and palpate the sacrospinous ligament. A 10 ml. syringe, with a long No. 20 spinal needle guided by the index finger, is used. Three ml. of anesthetic solution is injected into the sacrospinal ligament. The needle is pushed deeper; as it enters the loose tissue behind the ligament, aspiration is attempted to avoid intravascular injection, and then 7 ml. of the anesthetic solution is injected. The procedure is then repeated in the opposite side.

Transperineal Technique. A skin wheal is raised with local anesthetic midway between the anus and the ischial spine. With the index finger in the vagina as a guide, the needle is directed toward the posterior surface of the ischial spine's inferior tip and into the pudendal canal. If no blood is aspirated, inject 3 ml. of solution beneath the inferior tip of the spine; another 3 ml. is injected

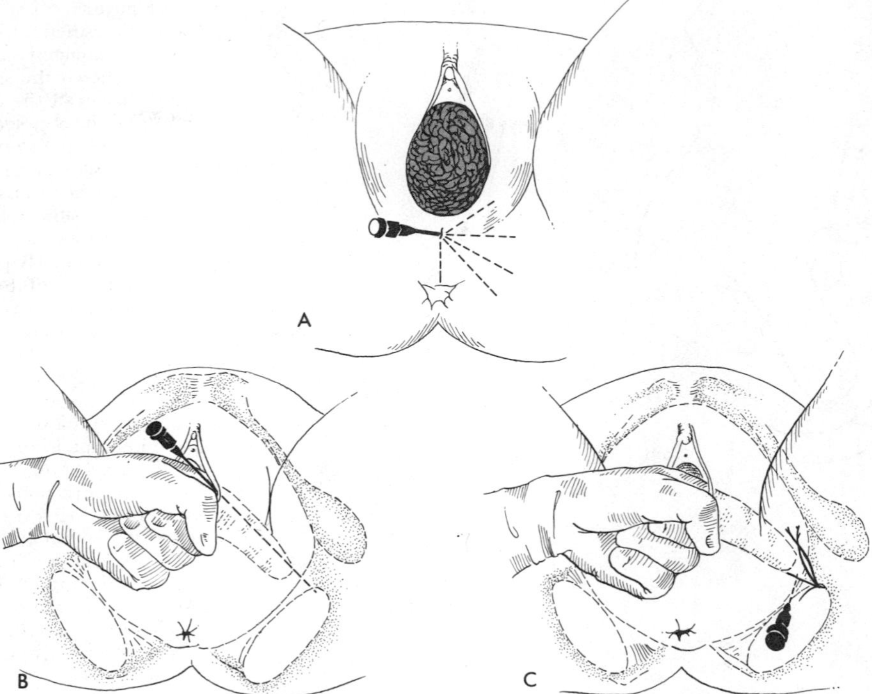

Figure 4. *A,* Local anesthesia: direct infiltration. *B,* Pudendal nerve block: transvaginal route. *C,* Pudendal nerve block: percutaneous transperitoneal approach. (Redrawn from Oxorn, H., and Foote, W. R.: Human Labor and Birth. 2nd ed. © 1968 by Meredith Corporation, Appleton-Century-Crofts, New York.)

after relocating the tip of the needle under the superior tip of the ischial spine. The needle is then inserted a little beyond the spine into the greater sciatic notch and 4 ml. of solution is injected. The procedure is then repeated in the opposite side.

Satisfactory anesthesia should take place in 15 minutes.

Paracervical Block.　　Paracervical block is used to relieve uterine and cervical pain. The local anesthetic of choice is injected within the lateral fornices at 4 and 8 o'clock 1 cm. deep. Precautions are taken to avoid intravenous injection by frequent aspiration. The injection is done once labor is established and a cervical dilatation of 4 cm. is reached. Duration of anesthesia is 1 hour. Paracervical block is used for the relief of first stage labor pains. It has no effect on areas innervated by the pudendal nerve (vagina, perineum, and vulva). Continuous paracervical block may be used by placing plastic catheters in the paracervical areas. At present no helpful instruments are available to facilitate this technique.

Fetal bradycardia sometimes follows paracervical block (incidence, 10 to 85 per cent). It may be followed by neonatal depression and even death.

Toxicity of Local Anesthetics. Local anesthetics are rapidly transferred across the placenta into the fetus. Once in the fetus there is rapid uptake by the heart, the brain, and the liver. Susceptibility of the fetal heart to local anesthetics

administered to the mother may be explained by the relatively high concentrations of the local anesthetic in the fetal heart, similar to that in the mother.

Myocardial toxicity of local anesthetics is enhanced by *hypoxia* and *acidosis.* Therefore drug levels well tolerated by the mother may be responsible for severe myocardial depression observed in the partially asphyxiated fetus. Similarly, local anesthetics may accumulate in the fetal brain and later result in respiratory depression at birth.

Factors of importance in toxicity include the dose and the rate of drug absorption from the site of injection.

In paracervical block the drug is injected in a highly vascular area and may result in transiently elevated drug levels in fetal blood associated with fetal *bradycardia* and *acidosis.*

To reduce the hazards of toxicity to the fetus and newborn:

1. Use less toxic drugs.

2. Reduce maternal and fetal blood levels of anesthetic by (a) using the smallest dose that will provide adequate analgesia, (b) using rapidly metabolized drugs (e.g., chloroprocaine), and (c) using long-acting drugs (e.g., bupivacaine), which will require less frequent reinjection.

Toxic Reactions to Local Anesthetic Drugs.　　True hypersensitivity to the local anesthetic drug, causing sudden death after injection

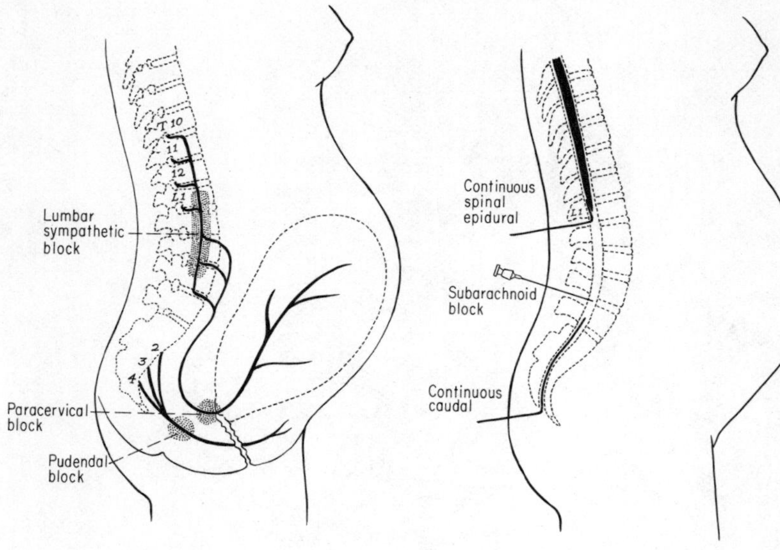

Figure 5. The most common regional anesthetic techniques used for obstetric analgesia-anesthesia. On the left are shown the site of injection and the diffusion of the local anesthetic (depicted by the stippled area) for "minor" blocks. Both paracervical block and pudendal block can be achieved by inserting a needle transvaginally, whereas lumbar sympathetic block is achieved by the paravertebral technique which entails insertion of a 3 to 4 inch needle 4 cm. lateral to the tip of the spinous process of the second lumbar vertebra and advancing it so that its point comes to lie on the anterolateral surface of the vertebra anterior to the attachment of fascia or iliopsoas muscle. Injection of a maximum of 10 ml. of solution on each side will interrupt labor pain pathways and produce relief of pain associated with uterine contractions. Bilateral paracervical block achieves the same effect, whereas bilateral pudendal block will relieve perineal pain caused by distention of the perineum by the presenting part. (Modified from Bonica, J. J.: Atlas of mechanisms of pathways of pain and labor. What's New, 1960, pp. 216–217.)

of a small dose, is extremely rare. Allergy occasionally develops in dentists or pharmacists after repeated contact.

Toxic reactions usually result from (1) overdose from too large volume or too high concentration, (2) inadvertent intravascular injection, or (3) very rapid absorption. They may also occur when the rate of absorption of the drug exceeds the rate at which it is neutralized.

Signs and symptoms: Central nervous system (CNS) stimulation, as manifested by restlessness, dizziness, fine muscular twitching (e.g., facial muscle), or generalized convulsions; leading to hypoxia, loss of consciousness, obstruction of airway, vomiting, aspiration, further obstruction, further hypoxia, depression of vital centers in medulla, and at last respiratory and circulatory failure.

It must be remembered that most local anesthetics are rapidly detoxified by the liver and that blood concentration soon falls below toxic levels.

Treatment consists of the following measures:

1. Maintain an airway.

2. For apnea, give artificial respiration, either mouth-to-mouth or by bag and mask.

3. For pulselessness: artificial circulation, external cardiac compression, epinephrine (Adrenalin), sodium bicarbonate, calcium gluconate or chloride.

4. Hypoxia must be treated promptly by giving O_2 by mask.

5. Convulsions may be controlled by diazepam (Valium), 5 to 10 mg. intravenously, or by thiopental (Pentothal), 50 to 100 mg. intravenously. If immediate intubation is available, a short-acting muscle relaxant may be used to stop convulsions and allow ventilation and adequate oxygenation promptly.

6. Consider the possibility of a reaction or sensitivity to epinephrine (Adrenalin) in the anesthetic solution. This should be short lasting if treated promptly with oxygen, reassurance, and adequate ventilation.

Low Spinal Anesthesia (Saddle Block Anesthesia). After adequate preparation of the back, with the patient in the sitting position, the subarachnoid space is entered with a No. 26 or 25 spinal needle.

A hyperbaric mixture of equal volumes of tetracaine (Pontocaine) 1 per cent solution and dextrose 10 per cent solution is injected: tetracaine (Pontocaine), 4 mg. (0.4 ml.); dextrose, 40 mg. (0.4 ml.). The patient remains in the sitting position for at least 5 minutes after injection.

The injection should not be made during a contraction to avoid a higher level of the anesthetic.

This anesthetic technique is used when the cervix is fully dilated and when low forceps can be used easily to extract the head.

Lumbar Epidural Analgesia and Anesthesia. The pain of the first stage of labor may be very effectively relieved by blocking the afferent impulses from the uterus to the eleventh and twelfth thoracic segments via sympathetic pathways. Blocking the sacral roots at this stage is unnecessary and also undesirable. Relaxation of the pelvic floor muscles will affect proper flexion and rotation of the baby's head as it passes through the birth canal.

Lumbar epidural anesthesia may be given by single injection or by continuous technique. The latter is used more frequently, as it provides analgesia for the greater part of the labor. The optimal time to use it is when labor is well established and the cervix is dilated 4 to 6 cm. in primigravidas and 3 to 4 cm. in multiparas.

The *technique* for this procedure is as follows:

1. The patient lies on her side or sits up.

2. Her back is prepared with povidone-iodine (Betadine) or pHisoHex.

3. A No. 17 Tuohy needle is inserted in the second or third lumbar interspace with the bevel pointing cephalad.

4. Epidural puncture is made by the loss of resistance technique.

5. A test dose of 5 ml. of the solution of the local anesthetic of choice is injected into the epidural space.

6. After a 2 minute interval, if there is no evidence of intrathecal injection, a vinyl plastic tube is inserted through the needle for a distance of about 3.75 cm. (1½ inches). The needle is removed over the catheter. The catheter should never be pulled back lest it be severed by the sharp tip of the needle.

7. Antibiotic ointment is applied around the tubing and skin and properly covered, using gauze and tape so as to avoid kinking of the vinyl plastic tubing.

8. A needle and syringe filled with the local anesthetic of choice is connected to the distal end of the plastic tubing.

9. The patient lies on her back, and a second dose of anesthetic, 10 to 15 ml., is injected to avoid unilateral analgesia.

10. During labor the patient should lie on her side to avoid inferior vena cava compression.

11. When labor pain returns, more of the local anesthetic agent is injected through the catheter.

12. When the patient starts feeling pelvic pain and is fully dilated, the perineal dose, 10 to 15 ml., is given while she is in the sitting position. The patient remains sitting for about 5 minutes to allow the anesthetic solution to descend by gravity toward the sacral roots.

Anesthesia for Cesarean Section. There is no "ideal" anesthetic for cesarean section. There is a risk to the mother and fetus inherent in all known techniques. The final decision will depend on the needs of the patient and the skill of the anesthesiologist or obstetrician.

ELECTIVE CESAREAN SECTION. Regional anesthesia is strongly recommended—local, lumbar or sacral epidural, or spinal anesthesia. Our preference is *spinal anesthesia.*

Technique: Intravenous infusion is started with a 16 gauge indwelling catheter. Initial blood pressure and pulse are taken and recorded. Five hundred to 1000 ml. Ringer's lactate solution is given rapidly. Spinal anesthesia is administered with the patient sitting or on her side. The drug used is tetracaine 1 per cent solution diluted in 10 per cent dextrose, 50 : 50 mixture. The dosage is 6 to 10 mg., depending on the position used (sitting up, lateral decubitus) and the height of the patient. The patient is then placed in a supine, 10 degree Trendelenburg position for approximately 30 seconds. The Colón-Morales (C-M) uterine displacer is applied, displacing the uterus to the left. Blood pressure and pulse are taken repeatedly. The displacer is readjusted if necessary. If there is a drop in blood pressure below 100 mm. Hg systolic, the uterine displacer is readjusted. If the blood pressure drops below 90 mm. Hg systolic in spite of the intravenous fluids and uterine displacement, 12.5 to 25 mg. of ephedrine is given intravenously.

EMERGENCY CESAREAN SECTION. Spinal or general anesthesia is used, depending on the cause for the emergency situation.

In hypotensive states or in fetal distress, regional anesthesia may not be applicable. In such an urgent situation, general anesthesia may be favored.

The *technique* for emergency cesarean section is as follows:

1. The patient is placed in the supine position.

2. The uterine displacer is applied, displacing the uterus to the left.

3. Blood pressure and pulse are taken.

4. The patient is draped.

5. When the obstetrician is ready to start surgery, a sleeping dose of thiopental (Pentothal) is given intravenously (150 to 250 mg.); an $N_2O–O_2$ analgesic mixture (50:50) is started, and 40 to 60 mg. of succinylcholine is given intravenously, followed by endotracheal intubation. After delivery of the infant, 0.3 to 0.5 per cent methoxyflurane (Penthrane) is added to the analgesic mixture, or meperidine (Demerol) in small repeated doses is given intravenously to provide analgesia.

Postspinal Headache. Postspinal headache is due to leakage of cerebrospinal fluid through the puncture hole; it usually starts on the second or third day after administration of spinal anesthesia. The patient feels relief from the headache when recumbent, but the headache gets worse when she is sitting up or standing. It may be short- or long-lasting, mild or severe. The incidence is markedly reduced if 24 to 26 gauge spinal needles are used for the puncture.

Treatment encompasses the following measures:

1. The patient should be kept flat in bed for 12 to 24 hours.

2. The foot of the bed may be raised slightly to reduce cerebrospinal fluid (CSF) hydrostatic pressure at the site of the puncture hole.

3. One thousand ml. of intravenous fluid (isotonic saline or Ringer's lactated) is given, and the patient is asked to drink plenty of fluids.

4. Vasopressin (Pitressin) may be given in a dosage of 0.5 to 1.0 ml. intramuscularly to speed up rehydration.

5. Analgesics and tranquilizers should be given—codeine, 30 mg. (½ grain), or diazepam (Valium), 5 to 10 mg. intravenously, intramuscularly, or orally.

6. If headache persists in spite of the aforementioned treatment, an injection of isotonic saline solution into the caudal or epidural space should be tried.

7. A blood patch in the epidural space has also been advocated and has been claimed to be very effective.

Caudal Anesthesia. Blocking the sacral nerves provides complete analgesia of the lower uterine segment as well as the vulva and perineum.

Technique: The patient is placed in the knee-chest position or in the lateral position with her bottom leg straight and top leg flexed.

Landmarks include the sacral cornua, tip of coccyx, and sacral hiatus.

The area is prepared, leaving a plug with antiseptic over the anus. With the middle finger and thumb, identify the sacral cornua. Then identify the tip of the coccyx with the index finger. Slide the finger cephalad, identifying the sacral hiatus. Inject a local anesthetic into the skin over this area.

For a single caudal injection, insert a No. 20 or No. 18 gauge needle into the sacrococcygeal membrane at an angle of 45 degrees, recognizing the sacral canal by the loss of resistance. Depress the tip of the needle toward the intergluteal cleft until it lies almost parallel to the dorsum of the sacrum and advance the needle 2 cm. along the sacral canal. Aspirate to check for blood or cerebrospinal fluid; if negative, inject air or saline, with fingertips over the sacral area feeling for swelling or crepitus. If present, reinsert the needle until no crepitus is felt or no blood is aspirated. If spinal fluid is aspirated, abandon the procedure. When the needle is in the correct position, inject the local anesthetic solution slowly after a preliminary test dose of 3 ml. has been used to make sure the dura

has not been entered. Wait 5 minutes after the test dose injection and check for weakness of the legs. If the test dose is negative, inject the local anesthetic—e.g., lidocaine (Xylocaine) 1.5 per cent, 20 to 25 ml. with repeated aspiration, or bupivacaine 0.5 per cent, 20 to 25 ml.

For the continuous technique, use a Tuohy No. 18 needle and thread a vinyl catheter into the caudal canal.

Intravenous Anesthesia. Ketamine has been used for pain relief in vaginal delivery. Dosage is 12.5 to 25 mg. administered intravenously at crowning. This dosage may be repeated if indicated to a maximum dosage of 100 mg. If necessary, local anesthesia may be used for the removal of the placenta or repair of episiotomy. With the aforementioned dosage schedule, Akamatsu reports that "No untoward effect was encountered in mother or infant."

The Colón-Morales (C-M) Uterine Displacer—"The Third Hand"

The administration of spinal and/or epidural anesthesia prior to cesarean section relaxes abdominal muscles, causing the pregnant uterus to fall to the right, resulting in compression of the inferior vena cava. Cardiac output is decreased owing to inadequate venous return, and the uteroplacental perfusion may be impaired.

The C-M uterine displacer (left uterine displacement device) was specifically designed for the physiologic management of the supine hypotension syndrome reducing the need for use of intravenous fluids or vasopressors. Properly adjusted, the C-M uterine displacer will reposition the uterus, relieving pressure on the inferior vena cava, thus increasing venous return, central venous pressure, cardiac output, mean arterial pressure, and systemic vascular resistance. Maternal normotension and uteroplacental perfusion are restored.

Initial Care of the Newborn After Vaginal or Abdominal Delivery

In every cesarean section a physician highly skilled in newborn resuscitation should be present with the necessary equipment to provide the best possible care during those important first few minutes of life.

An *accurate* Apgar scoring of every newborn at 1 and 5 minutes of life should be done by the physician in charge of the initial care of the newborn or by a nurse who has been taught how to score an infant accurately. The Apgar Score Timing Unit (Fig. 6) has made such temporal accuracy possible.

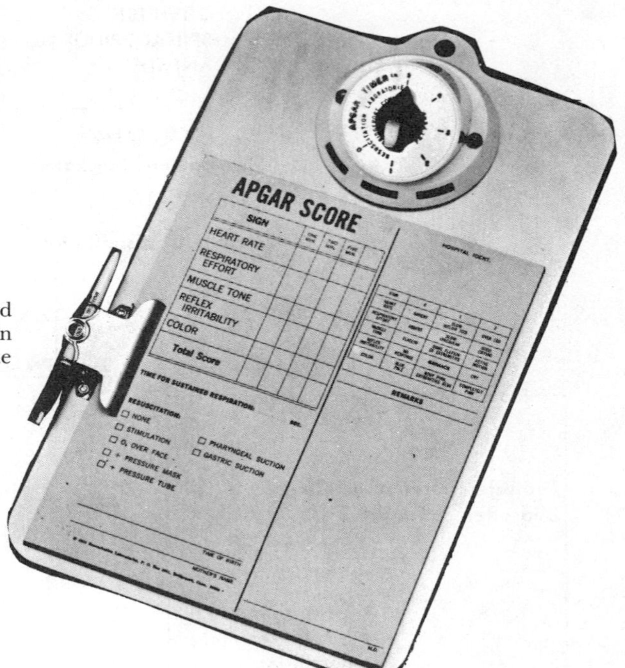

Figure 6. The Apgar Score Timing Unit was developed by the department of Anesthesiology of Teachers Hospital in Puerto Rico to provide a simple technique for more accurate recording of the newborn score.

Technique for Scoring. 1. Observations are made exactly at 1 and 5 minutes after delivery of the entire infant.

2. The modalities listed are obtained according to Table 1 and appropriate values assigned.

3. In order to be consistent, and to gain the full advantage of proper treatment and prognosis, it is imperative that scores be recorded in their proper sequence.

Significance of the Apgar Score. As in other pathologic conditions, treatment of newborn depression rests upon accurate diagnosis. The various physical signs are conveniently summarized by the Apgar score. This has little relation to oxygenation but does reflect the degree of acidosis. A score from 7 to 10 generally applies to a "vigorous" infant, 4 to 6 to a "depressed" infant, and 0 to 3 to a "markedly depressed" infant.

In addition to the predictive value for survival, there is a relationship between the score and the development of neuromuscular deficits in childhood.

In the words of Dr. Virginia Apgar, "Nine months' observation of the mother surely warrants one minute's observation of the baby!"

Analgesia and Anesthesia in Special Obstetric Situations

Multiple Delivery. Be very careful with the administration of sedatives, analgesics, or tranquilizers because of the effect on the fetuses and the progress of labor.

Avoid the supine position at all times to prevent the hazards of aortocaval compression.

The possibility of prematurity must be kept in mind.

Regional anesthesia—saddle block or pudendal block—is given after the cervix is fully dilated and the presenting part is at least at the +2 station.

If intrauterine manipulation is necessary, halothane or ether anesthesia may be necessary to relax the uterus.

Breech Delivery. Avoid overdosage with systemic analgesic drugs during the first stage of labor.

Regional anesthesia—saddle block or pudendal block—is given when the cervix is fully dilated and the presenting part is at the +2 station.

If the aftercoming head becomes trapped, be ready to relax the uterus with deep halothane anesthesia.

Prematurity. Avoid analgesics. Regional anesthesia—lumbar epidural or spinal—is safe,

TABLE 1. **Apgar Scoring Chart**

SIGN	0	1	2
Heart rate	Absent	Slow (below 100)	Over 100
Respiratory effort	Absent	Slow irregular	Good crying
Muscle tone	Flaccid	Some flexion of extremities	Active motion
Reflex irritability	No response	Grimace	Cry
Color	Blue pale	Body pink extremities blue	Completely pink

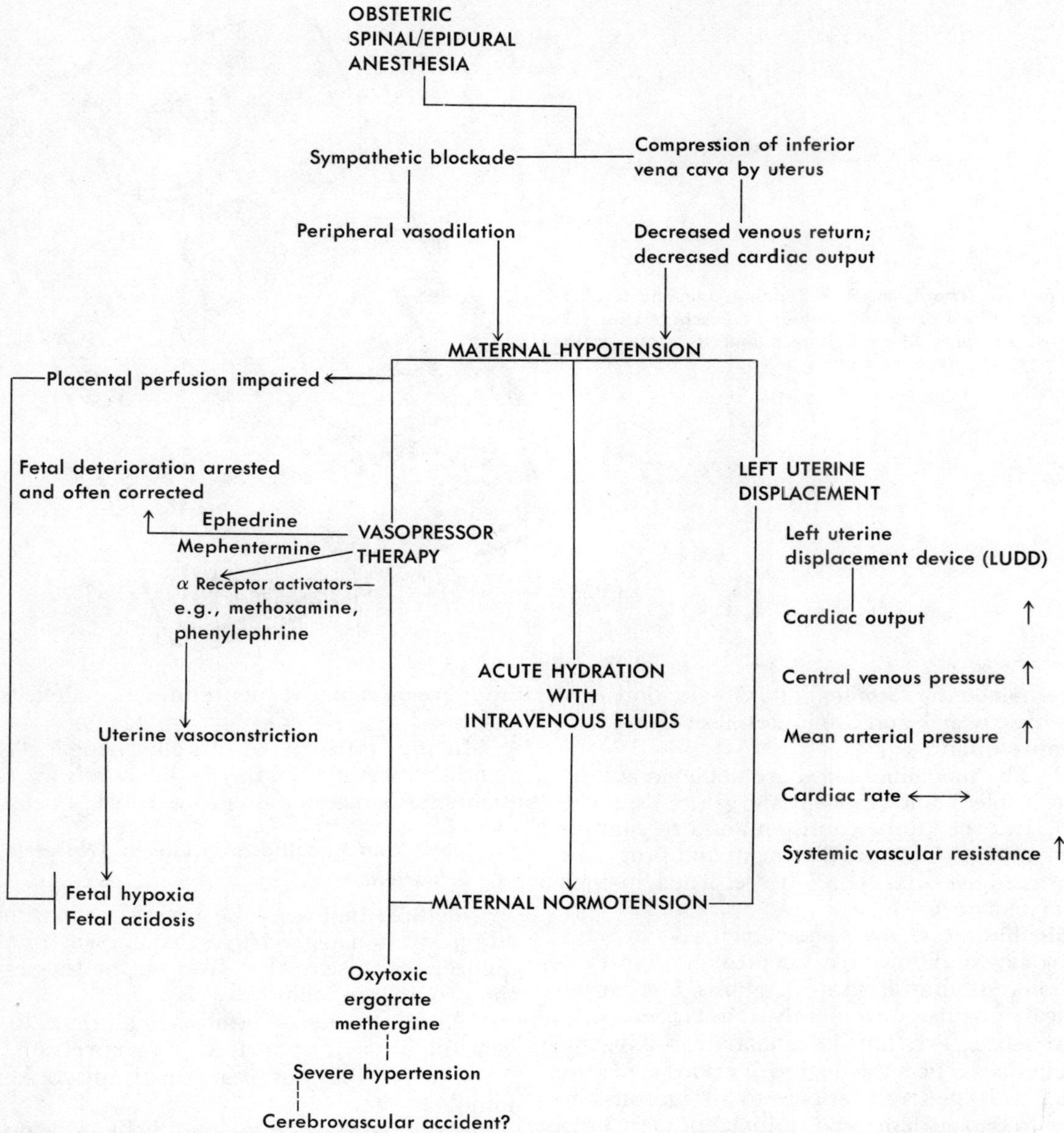

Figure 7. (From scientific exhibit of supine hypotensive syndrome, physiologic versus pharmacologic management. Presented by Miguel Colón-Morales, M.D., during annual meetings of American Medical Association and American Society of Anesthesiologists.)

but avoid maternal hypotension by uterine displacement or hydration or with ephedrine, 12.5 mg. intravenously, if needed. General anesthesia should be avoided. Paracervical block is too risky. Pudendal block is used for delivery.

Preeclampsia. The presence of uteroplacental insufficiency should caution one against any techniques causing hypotension.

Care must be taken with vasopressor drugs. There is increased sensitivity in these patients.

Diabetes. In all forms of diabetes the fetus should be considered at risk. Regional anesthesia is preferred for cesarean section. Paracervical block should be avoided.

Rheumatic Heart Disease. Avoid any increase in oxygen consumption—e.g., tachycardia or myocardial depression. Provide some analgesia. In the first stage, segmental epidural block or paracervical block may be used. In the second stage, pudendal block, saddle block, or caudal block is used for terminal delivery.

Mandatory Safety Measures in Obstetric Analgesia and Anesthesia

1. Well secured indwelling intravenous cannula.

2. Ready availability of blood. (a) Type and cross-match every obstetric patient when admitted

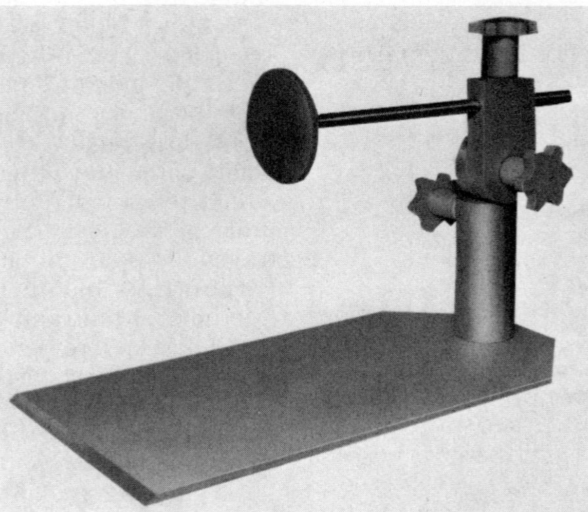

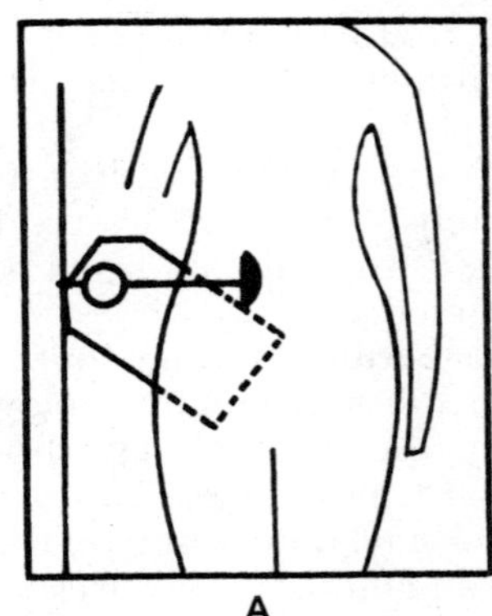

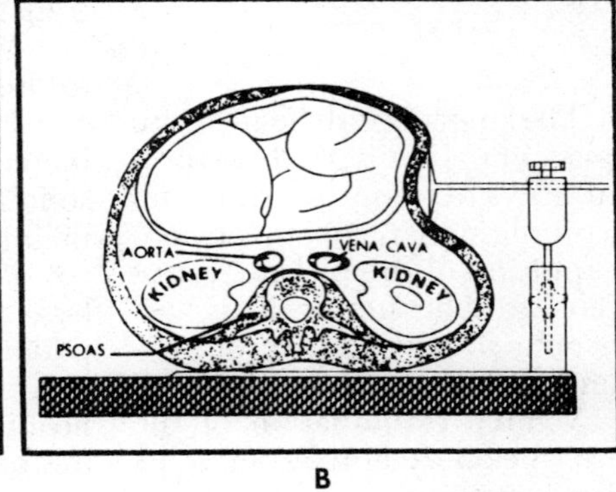

Figure 8. The C-M uterine displacer. Instructions for use: After regional anesthesia is administered, place patient in supine position. Raise patient's right side enough to allow for placement of plate under right lumbosacral region (or mattress), positioning the vertical post cephalad to minimize interference with the surgeon *(A)*. Displace the uterus manually to the left and adjust pressure pad so as to gently maintain the uterus in the desired position *(B)*. As soon as the peritoneal cavity is opened, the horizontal rod may be released so as not to interfere with intra-abdominal manipulation by the surgeon. (Developed by Miguel Colón-Morales, M.D.)

in labor. (b) Have 500 ml. of type O Rh-negative blood available in the delivery room at all times.

3. Suction equipment in good working condition.

4. A rapid-tilting delivery table.

5. Strict observance, through patient education, of nothing by mouth (solid or liquid) with onset of labor contractions, with the one exception of recommended alkali oral therapy.

6. Administration of antacids throughout labor and about 1 hour prior to scheduled cesarean section, to neutralize acidity of stomach contents.

7. Presence of an anesthesiologist or anesthetist capable of performing a rapid endotracheal intubation under difficult conditions and of treating the complications of local anesthetics and regional techniques.

Conclusion

The fact that, in spite of all efforts, childbirth and pain have not yet been divorced is good evidence of the serious difficulties encountered so far in solving this problem.

Great progress has been made, especially during the last 2 decades, but such progress must be considered partial solutions to a very difficult problem.

Let us all hope and work for a breakthrough in the not too distant future. In the meantime let us make the best possible use of all the knowledge, the skills, and the manpower available, to do the best we can with what we have to protect the mother, the fetus, and the newborn. We will be protecting future generations and perhaps even mankind.

POSTPARTUM CARE

method of
TAKEY CRIST, M.D., F.A.C.O.G.,
F.A.C.S.
Jacksonville, North Carolina

Introduction

The term puerperium or postpartum period includes the period elapsing between the end of the third stage of labor and the return of the genital tract to its normal nonpregnant state.

Management of the patient during this time span can be divided into three phases: (1) hospital care, including the delivery room, recovery room, and postpartum unit; (2) home care; and (3) the postpartum office visit.

Hospital

Delivery Room. The puerperium begins with the delivery of the placenta. This period requires careful management and attention to ensure an uneventful and uncomplicated recovery period. Immediately after expulsion of the placenta, care should be taken to ensure that the uterus is well contracted. The placenta should be carefully inspected to determine that membranes and placenta are intact. Manual examination of the uterus is carried out to rule out retained fragments as well as uterine abnormalities.

The fundus is gently but firmly massaged to help express clots and to ascertain that it remains firmly contracted.

If intravenous infusion is used, oxytocin may be administered by this route in the amount of 20 units per 1000 ml. of 5 per cent dextrose in water.

The cervix is inspected for lacerations and repaired if indicated. Further inspection is made of the vaginal vault for lacerations or hematoma formation.

The episiotomy is repaired with 2–0 chromic interrupted and running sutures. An estimate of blood loss is made, and, along with blood pressure, pulse and respirations are recorded before transfer from the delivery room.

Testosterone enanthate and estradiol valerate (Deladumone OB) is administered intramuscularly to suppress lactation in the mother who wishes to bottle-feed. It may be administered with the delivery of the infant's head or immediately before transfer from the delivery room.

Recovery Room. Ideally, postpartum recovery should take place in a separate recovery area. Regardless of areas of recovery, the procedure should remain the same. For patients who have no complications, this intensive care period should be carried on for at least 2 to 4 hours. Care should include a sterile perineal pad with T-binder. The pulse, blood pressure, and respirations are recorded every 15 minutes. Careful attention should be given to uterine firmness. The fundus must be gently massaged every 15 minutes and blood loss recorded. Excessive bleeding or inability of the uterus to remain firm should result in administration of intravenous fluids, along with 20 units of oxytocin (Pitocin) per 1000 ml. of intravenous solution and/or ergonovine maleate (Ergotrate) or methylergonovine maleate, (Methergine) intramuscularly.

The bladder region should be palpated frequently to detect distention. Bladder distention must be prevented, by catheterization if necessary, to avoid prolonging the time required for recovery of normal bladder tone and function.

Following spinal or epidural anesthesia, the patient must be able to move her legs before she is transferred to the postpartum unit.

Visitors in the recovery area should be limited to the child's father.

If the patient desires to breast-feed immediately following delivery, this may be allowed so long as the baby's normal body temperature is maintained.

Postpartum Nursing Unit. It is felt that for both the physical and psychologic well-being of the patient, the hospital stay should be at least 72 hours. In most cases, 3 to 5 days is the normal hospital stay, depending on the condition of both infant and mother and the establishment of a satisfactory feeding routine. The routine orders that must be included are as follows:

1. Routine vital signs, including temperature, pulse, respirations, and blood pressure, are recorded at least four times a day.

2. A regular diet is given unless contraindicated.

3. Early ambulation is encouraged.

4. The patient may shower on the second postpartum day.

5. Catheterization is advised every 6 to 8 hours if the patient is unable to void.

6. Instruction should be given as to proper perineal care.

7. A heat lamp is provided three times daily for 15 minutes beginning the first postpartum day. If the patient desires, sitz baths twice daily may be used.

8. Complete blood count (CBC) is taken the morning after delivery.

9. Urine culture is also taken the morning after delivery.

10. Empirin compound with codeine, 30 mg. (Empirin No. 3) can be given every 3 to 4 hours as desired for pain. If the patient is allergic to codeine, propoxyphene (Darvon), 65 mg. every 3 to 4 hours as necessary, may be substituted.

11. Dioctyl calcium sulfosuccinate and danthron (Doxidan), 2 capsules, can be given at bedtime beginning the day of delivery as a laxative.

12. Secobarbital sodium (Seconal), 100 mg., may be given at bedtime for sleep.

13. Unless contraindicated, methylergonovine maleate (Methergine), 0.2 mg. three times daily, can be given.

14. Breast-feeding mothers are instructed to wear good supportive brassieres, preferably a nursing brassiere. Emollient cream (Massé Cream) may be applied to the nipples and areolae three times daily.

15. Bottle-feeding mothers are instructed to wear snug-fitting supportive brassieres. If engorgement becomes uncomfortable, ice packs may be applied.

16. If indicated in Rh-negative mothers, a RhoGAM work-up is done and immune globulin (human) RhoGAM is given intramuscularly after satisfactory laboratory cross-match.

It is important that the patient be observed for any postpartum complications. The most important of these are hemorrhage, puerperal infection, thrombophlebitis, mastitis, and cystitis and pyelitis. Careful attention to the temperature is important at this time. A temperature of 100.4°F. (38°C.) on two consecutive occasions should result in further thorough investigation as to the cause, followed by the appropriate treatment.

Excessive bleeding should be immediately investigated and appropriate action taken, which usually includes administration of intravenous therapy and, if necessary, whole blood replacement.

Home Care

The 4 to 6 week period after discharge is a continuation of the patient's transition to her normal nonpregnant state. It is important that she be given specific instructions before discharge as to how to care for herself. Before being sent home, an examination should be done, including inspection of the breasts and nipples and examination of the perineum for healing, the uterus for involution, and the abdominal wall for relaxation.

Discharge instructions should be discussed and written instruction sheets given to the patient. Activity may be gradually increased, beginning with light activity and 1 to 2 hour rest periods per day for the first 10 to 14 days, and gradually increasing to full normal duties at 6 weeks. Light exercises may begin in 2 weeks and these, also, gradually increased. Continuation of prenatal vitamins and iron for approximately 6 weeks is advised for bottle-feeding mothers and as long as nursing continues in breast-feeding mothers.

Sexual intercourse may be resumed at the discretion of the couple, making sure that the patient and her partner have been instructed in the use of birth control. No restrictions as to shower or tub baths are given. The patient is advised to maintain a well balanced diet. Contraception is discussed with the patient. If the nonbreast feeder desires oral contraceptives, she is instructed to begin pills. If she is not breast feeding and engorgement occurs, she is instructed to wear a good light supportive brassiere day and night. Any stimulation to the breast is to be avoided. Ice packs and acetaminophen (Tylenol) are given for discomfort. She is told to report at once any increase of pain in her episiotomy, localized pain or reddened areas in the breasts, excessive bleeding, abnormal pain, or fever. An appointment for a return visit to the office in 6 weeks is mandatory.

Postpartum Office Visit

The postpartum visit is necessary to determine the rate of return to a normal nonpregnant state, and to be sure there has been a healthy adjustment between mother, baby, and the family unit. Family planning measures are discussed.

During this visit, weight, blood pressure, temperature, pulse, respiration, urine sugar, and protein are recorded. An evaluation of breast, abdomen, and lower extremities is made.

A pelvic examination is done, giving special attention to healing of the perineum, vagina, and cervix. A careful bimanual examination is done to determine uterine involution and absence of any adnexal disease. A Papanicolaou smear is also done at this time.

Resumption of menstruation should be discussed and the breast-feeding mother instructed that menstruation may not occur while she is lactating, but may occur at irregular intervals. It should be emphasized to her that breast feeding is not a form of birth control.

The bottle-feeding mother should be reassured that normally periods will not resume for 8 to 10 weeks.

Contraception is discussed at this visit. If oral contraception has already begun, instructions are reinforced. If the patient is breast feeding, oral contraception is not used until the baby is weaned. If a diaphragm is chosen, proper fitting and instruction for proper use are carried out. If the patient chooses an intrauterine device (IUD), it can be inserted at this time. If nonprescription contraception is desired, she is encouraged to use foam and condoms.

A pelvic examination is usually repeated after 6 months and 1 year. Adequate postpartum care over a year may prevent or even cure conditions that would otherwise cause trouble in later years.

CARE OF THE LOW-BIRTH-WEIGHT INFANT

method of
RICHARD S. BAUM, M.D.
Indianapolis, Indiana

Babies Born Too Small or Too Soon

1. Low-birth-weight (LBW) infants still represent the single largest contributor to infant mortality in the United States, and are disproportionately represented among the developmentally handicapped. In recent years, however, many innovations have slashed LBW mortality by more than 50 per cent and nearly eliminated once common spastic diplegia. A new technology has demonstrated that survival depends upon more than "a will to live." Perhaps more important have been recognition of the necessity for a heightened sense of anticipation, the establishment of special referral centers (with infant transport teams), and a willingness to refer mothers and babies for special care.

2. These factors have created a medical-legal climate that presently compels consultation or referral for many of the problems of this vulnerable group of patients.

3. The following guidelines are offered for use when backup resources are limited by time or distance, or when the infant's stability appears to make referral unnecessary.

Before Delivery

1. Unless the mother is in driving labor, do not accept delivery of the LBW baby as inevitable. Encourage bed rest, and seek consultation in reference to cerclage or other means of buying time for additional fetal growth. Consider transferring the mother to a referral center if she is likely to produce an infant who is assured of transfer.

2. In the event that labor cannot be halted, attempt to provide at delivery a person whose sole responsibility is the skillful resuscitation of the baby. Ideally, these skills should include the ability to pass an endotracheal tube. Warm the environmental temperature of the delivery room, and alert the referral center if transfer is anticipated.

The First Minutes

1. Continue efforts to minimize heat loss by toweling the baby dry immediately. Only efforts critical to normal cardiorespiratory function should be made; postpone eye care and bathing.

2. Recognize that in very low birth weight infants (usually less than 1500 grams) the Apgar score is an imprecise predictor of survival—*do not* withdraw support from the LBW patient solely on the basis of low Apgars. *Do* let resuscitative efforts be guided by the baby's color and pulse.

3. If, with gentle suctioning of the oropharynx, toweling, and oxygen the pulse is not greater than 100 beats per minute, begin inflation of the lungs by bag and mask (preferably fitted with a 100 per cent O_2 adapter). If positive pressure bagging fails to reverse bradycardia within an additional 30 to 60 seconds, intubate (try 3.0 mm. tube when the baby weighs less than 1500 grams, 3.5 mm. when weight is greater than 1500 grams) and continue ventilation with O_2. Check breath sounds in both axillae to ensure proper placement: diminished air entry on left could mean a tube too far down on right. Later, confirm the tube position with x-ray and adjust the tip to the interclavicular midpoint. If an endotracheal tube is left in place in a gestationally immature baby, bag the infant with just enough pressure to produce "normal" chest expansion (start at 20 to 25 cm. H_2O); if the infant can ventilate itself and continuous positive airway pressure can be applied, first offer at 4 to 6 cm. H_2O.

4. For marked bradycardia (less than 40 per minute) apply external cardiac massage in midsternum, using pressure from two fingers at 80 to 100 times per minute.

5. Reduce abdominal distension with nasogastric tube. Place gently to avoid precipitating apnea or bradycardia.

6. If bicarbonate or glucose is pushed intravenously (peripheral or umbilical vein—never artery!), do not exceed 1 mEq. $NaHCO_3$ or 1 ml. dextrose in water ($D_{25}W$) per minute.

7. When the cord is clamped, leave at least 2 cm. for possible umbilical catheterization. In addition to a screening examination of the baby, have the placenta examined for sites of blood loss: vascular anastomoses with twin gestation, retroplacental clot, vessel tears, etc.

8. If meconium is present in the amniotic fluid, suck out oropharynx, then nostrils, with DeLee catheter before the shoulders are delivered and the first breaths taken; if, after immediately moving the baby to the warmer, meconium can be observed in oropharynx, pass a DeLee tip or endotracheal tube (no more than 2 cm.) below the cords and suction meconium that may still be in the trachea.

The First Hours

1. Adjust environmental temperature to achieve a neutral thermal zone and reduce energy requirements. (Try incubator 93 to 95°F. [33.9 to 35°C.] for infant below 1500 grams, 91 to 93°F. [32.8 to 33.9°C.] above 1500 grams.) Heat losses can be reduced by wrapping extremities lightly with plastic film or gauze. Check temperatures frequently to avoid overheating.

2. Administer 0.5 mg. vitamin K intramuscularly.

3. Obtain baseline hematocrit immediately and ascertain the adequacy of peripheral perfusion by capillary filling time (fingertip pressure on skin) or, if available, by blood pressure (prefer *mean* BP greater than 35 mm. Hg for small premature, greater than 40 mm. Hg for a larger premature). In the face of acute illness, attempt to keep central (deep vessel) hematocrits in the 40 per cent range with whole blood or packed cells; if red blood cells are unavailable, try to improve perfusion with plasma suspension, e.g., plasma protein fraction, human (Plasmanate) at 10 ml. per kg.

4. High heelstick hematocrits warrant check of central hematocrit (deep vessel) and for distressed LBW infant with marked polycythemia (defined arbitrarily as *central* hematocrit greater than 65 per cent) hemodilution by partial exchange transfusion should be considered (safer than phlebotomy).

5. Check Dextrostix on admission and hourly thereafter until normoglycemia is assured (most hypoglycemia manifests in first four hours). Try to keep above 40 mg. per dl. (100 ml.) and below 120 mg. per dl. Correct symptomatic hypoglycemia with 1 ml. per kg. dextrose in water ($D_{25}W$) pushed slowly by intravenous route. At least partial protection from low blood sugar is afforded by $D_{10}W$ at a baseline rate of 60 to 70 ml. per kg. per day. If unable to place intravenously, judicious use of $D_{10}W$ by nasogastric tube may hold off low glucose levels. Periodically, check true plasma glucose (remember, Dextrostix are simply a screening device).

6. When respiratory distress is present:

Obtain anteroposterior and cross-table lateral chest x-rays (rule out pneumothorax, tap significant extrapleural air).

Obtain blood or tracheal cultures or both, and initiate parenteral penicillin 150,000 to 200,000 units per kg. per day). (Group B streptococcal sepsis is often clinically indistinguishable from hyaline membrane disease.) If the possibility of gram-negative infection exists, add gentamicin (5 mg. per kg. per day) or kanamycin (15 mg. per kg. per day).

Oxygen should be raised only to that level sufficient to abolish cyanosis. Continuation of oxygen therapy must be according to a strict protocol with specific written orders and serial blood gas measurement to avoid hypo- or hyperoxygenation or both (danger of retrolental fibroplasia and the high likelihood of successful litigation if the baby is blinded through inappropriate oxygen use). Attempt to maintain arterial PaO_2 between 50 and 70 mm. Hg: radial, temporal, or umbilical catheter with tip at T_8 or L_3-L_4 preferred sites. If arterial gas is unattainable, "arterialized" heelstick or fingertip samples are acceptable, but capillary PaO_2 exceeding 40 to 50 mm. Hg is unacceptable. Initially, arterial oxygen tensions should be sampled at least every 2 hours; later obtain whenever there are significant changes in clinical status or inspired oxygen concentration is raised or lowered.

Progressive expiratory grunt coupled with a rising oxygen requirement may necessitate continuous positive airway pressure (CPAP); a sharply rising $PaCO_2$ or a PaO_2 that cannot be maintained above 50 mm. Hg suggests a need for intermittent positive pressure, preferably intermittent mandatory ventilation (IMV). Most respiratory failure in LBW infants is reversible with these modalities.

7. In the absence of respiratory distress, feeding by the gastrointestinal route may be begun within 4 hours. Progression of feeds is contingent upon successful meconium passage, absence of abnormal distention, and absence of vomiting or increased gastric residuals.

The First Days

1. Nipple feeds should be confined to the stable baby of at least 33 to 34 weeks' gestation. The less mature, but stable, infant is fed best by indwelling nasogastric tube (intermittent bolus started every 2 hours) or (in experienced hands) by continuous nasogastric or transpyloric feeds.

2. If the first feeding of sterile water is accepted, the use of breast milk can be encouraged (freshly collected or refrigerated is preferable to frozen). If unavailable, a hypo-osmolar, nonlactose-containing formula such as Isomil 20 may be accepted better than more standard cow's milk based formulas. Whatever is used, one fourth to one half strength feedings initially may be tolerated better than 20 calories per ounce (30 ml.) feeds. The goal is advancement to growth promoting daily intake of about 120 calories per kg.; occasionally 150 to 180 calories per kg. may be required. This may take more than a week to achieve, even in a stable premature. During these first days, adequacy of hydration takes precedence over calories.

3. Baseline fluid requirements are increased to 80 to 90 ml. per kg. on day 2, and at least 100 ml. per kg. per day thereafter. Daily weights and at least every 8 hours urine specific gravities are useful for monitoring adequacy of intake (urine can be collected in cotton balls taped to perineum).

4. Monitor serum levels of sodium, potassium and calcium. After day 1, most babies require 3 mEq. per kg. per day of sodium and 2 mEq. per kg. per day of potassium. Hypocalcemia is common in LBW infants; seizures or extreme irritability might warrant slowly given intravenous calcium gluconate, but generally hypocalcemia is

treated more safely by the gastrointestinal route. (Calcium gluconate, 400 mg. per kg. per day, probably is tolerated well; more may be needed, but give cautiously.)

5. Anticipate hyperbilirubinemia, especially when both extensive bruising and marked immaturity are present. The physician may start phototherapy for jaundice if noted within the first 24 hours, but concommitant checks must be made for sensitization (blood group, Rh, Coombs') and abnormal RBC morphology, and do *not* continue phototherapy when indirect bilirubin values remain far below exchange levels, or when direct bilirubin is greater than 2 mg. per dl. For the very small premature, exchange transfusions may be warranted at bilirubin levels as low as 10 mg. per dl. If phototherapy is used, insensible water losses will be increased and fluid intake will need to be adjusted upward.

Considerations in Continuing Care

1. After the initial weight loss, postnatal growth patterns should approximate fetal growth at the same postconceptual age. Deviations that would warrant special concern include flattening of the weight curve ("late metabolic acidosis" correctable with bicarbonate), failure of head growth (nutritional inadequacy? chronic perinatal infection?), or too rapid head growth (hydrocephalus?).

2. Critical, life-threatening medical illnesses such as septicemia or meningitis often express themselves first through remarkably "soft" signs, such as lethargy or slight hypothermia. Sepsis must be considered whenever there is any deviation from previous stability. Suspicions of infection would warrant cultures of blood, cerebrospinal fluid (CSF) and urine, and a chest film (rule out pneumonia.) Parenteral ampicillin (100 mg. per kg. per day) and gentamicin (5 mg. per kg. per day) could be an appropriate antibiotic combination, pending culture results.

3. Recurrent apnea or progressive respiratory distress or both may appear after days or weeks of comparative stability. Consider especially measures for pneumonitis and sepsis, congestive heart failure, anemia, and metabolic disturbances such as hypocalcemia or "late metabolic acidosis," or referral for continuous positive airway pressure (CPAP), intermittent mandatory ventilation (IMV), or special medications.

4. Surveillance for surgical problems also must be maintained. Beware especially of abdominal distention or hematest positive stools or both, which may herald necrotizing enterocolitis. (When in doubt, nothing by mouth is the safest course, especially if intravenous hydration can be maintained.) Inguinal hernias are very common in LBW infants, and should be repaired before discharge *if* appropriate surgical care and anesthesia can be arranged. There are no valid medical indications for routine circumcision of these infants.

5. "All prematurely born infants treated with oxygen" should have examinations for retinopathy of prematurity (recommendation of Committee on Fetus and Newborn, American Academy of Pediatrics).

6. Drops in the hematocrit are to be expected, but still require at least weekly monitoring, if not actual transfusion. The use of packed cell transfusion to boost hematocrit into the 40s should be considered especially in the face of apneic episodes, acute illness, or when baseline pulses rise well beyond 160 without corresponding rises in reticulocyte count.

7. A multivitamin preparation containing vitamin C and 400 I.U. vitamin D should be given to LBW infants, whether on breast milk or formula. Other recommended supplements for premature infants include vitamin E (25 I.U. per day) and folate (50 micrograms per day for well infants and 100 micrograms per day for sick infants).

8. An iron-fortified formula is preferable to formula without iron for the preterm infant. Although breast milk contains a significant amount of iron that is well-utilized by term infants, utilization is less certain in the preterm infant, and 2 mg. per kg. per day of ferrous sulfate drops may be helpful.

Parents and Prognoses

1. Psychologic support of parents can be as important as physical care of the baby in shaping its later development. Most LBW infants survive and the majority will do well: an optimistic view, therefore, stands a good chance of being the most honest view; conversely, undue pessimism is likely to provoke detachment between parents and baby, or lifelong parental overprotectiveness (vulnerable child syndrome).

2. Frequent and close physical contact between parents and baby not only is helpful but essential if the parents eventually are to cope with their offspring with skill and serenity.

3. The fathers' anxieties often are as high as the mothers', although less likely to be expressed. It is fairer to the family if efforts are made to communicate with both parents at the same time, rather than have one interpret the physician's words to the other.

4. Although the outlook for most LBW survivors is good, realistically some will be developmentally abnormal. In the first months of life, however, it is difficult to distinguish this group with certainty. Landmarks are likely to be delayed at least by the number of weeks the baby was born ahead of schedule.

5. If a baby does die, the physician's job is not at an end. Tiny babies do not necessarily generate tiny grief, and one or two visits with a sympathetic doctor may be quite helpful in easing parents through the many months of the grieving process.

NORMAL INFANT FEEDING

method of
H. S. HARRISON, M.D.,
and P. J. JAKUBEC, M.D.
Morgantown, West Virginia

Birth. Breast feeding if at all possible and as soon as possible. Proprietary formula in the hospital and proprietary formula with iron on discharge. Soy formula for those with a strong family history of allergy.

Two Week Check. Check on weight gain, urine output, tolerance to formula. Discourage early introduction of solids.

Four Months. Advise mothers that they *may* now start offering cereal diluted with formula or breast milk. Waiting until 6 months is encouraged. Rice cereal, vegetables, fruits.

Four to Six Months. Egg yolk may be added.

Six Months. Meats are added. Lamb or veal is suggested as the first meat. Continue with breast milk or proprietary formula.

Nine Months. Egg white is added.

One Year. Whole milk is now given. A hematocrit is obtained at this time. Weaning from the bottle should start now. There is more leeway regarding the time of weaning from the breast.

Family practitioners and pediatricians spend a great deal of time counseling parents regarding the proper nutrition of their children. There is a voluminous daily literature regarding nutrition in children and it is difficult for the practicing physician to sort out the true experts from the food faddists, so it is no surprise that parents are somewhat confused.

The growing infant needs relatively more nutrients than does the adult. In addition to added nutrients for growth, he needs additional amounts for the higher metabolic rate and more rapid turnover. Also, bone growth imposes special nutritive requirements. In contrast to these handicaps, there are certain nutrients in which he is favored because he received a surplus during fetal life. These include iron, copper, and vitamin A.

Breast-feeding

Breast-feeding should be encouraged by obstetricians, family practitioners and pediatricians. Breast milk contains less casein, more alpha-lactalbumin, and practically no beta-lactalbumin. The two main characteristics of the amino acid composition of human breast milk are the methionine-cysteine ratio and the relatively low content of phenylalanine and tyrosine. This fits very well with the metabolic capacity of amino acid metabolism in the newborn and premature. The breast milk is more easily digested. Breast milk contains IgA, which imparts local immunity at the gastrointestinal level, and also maternal macrophages, which impart some local immunity. Breast milk also causes hyperplasia of the absorptive cells of the gastrointestinal tract. Some water-soluble vitamin D is also given to the infant in breast milk. The most common food allergy is to cow's milk, and this is averted by breast-feeding. Hypernatremia and the high solute load coming from cow's milk formulas, as well as the disastrous consequences resulting from errors in formula mixing with hyperosmolality, are avoided with breast-feeding.

Young mothers beginning to breast-feed in the hospital are told on the first day that they should alternate breasts and that the infant should nurse both breasts at each feeding. The mother is taught to break the suction with her finger to release the infant from the breast. We tell mothers to nurse five minutes at each breast per feeding the first day, ten the second and fifteen the third to avoid excess trauma to the nipple. Some infants may want to nurse every one to two hours and others will be fairly regular at three hours. Most infants can be fed on demand, but an occasional infant wants to nurse constantly and the mother may need some advice about scheduling. Mothers are advised that the infant will periodically outgrow the milk supply and be fussy for a day or two and that more frequent nursing quickly increases the supply. Supplementary bottles are discouraged, as they interfere with the natural supply and demand. Mothers are told that on occasion a supplementary bottle can be used and soy formula is used to avoid cow's milk protein. Babies are given to the breast as soon as possible after birth and on the delivery table if possible. Breast-fed babies do not have to have water or Karo supplementations and should not be introduced to a rubber nipple at all.

Bottle-fed Babies

The first feeding is started within 4 to 6 hours and sooner in very large infants, infants of diabetic mothers, or in those at risk for hypoglycemia. The first feeding is sterile water and is used to test for tracheoesophageal fistula. This is followed by 1 or 2 sugar water feedings and then a cow's milk formula is used. We use a proprietary formula and in the normal infant we use iron in the formula from the time he leaves the hospital to avoid confusion from changes. Babies are fed every 3 to 4 hours on a demand schedule unless the infant is having trouble with nursing too frequently or too infrequently. Babies on proprietary formulas are offered water once or twice a day and the mothers are told to let the infant's thirst determine how much water he takes. Weight is checked in 2 weeks and mothers are made aware of the need to watch the number of diapers being wet in a day as a method of determining the adequacy of food intake.

Beikost (Any Food Other Than Milk)

Cereal. Rice is usually the first cereal offered and it is started at 4 months. It is given primarily as a vehicle for iron. Also, it is used because of the ease of altering its consistency. Mothers are told that as solid food is added the infant will cut back slightly on the amount of milk consumed. Cereal does not make the baby sleep through the night.

Fruits. Home-prepared fruits or baby food are used. Apples and pears are the first to be introduced and pineapple is one of the last. Prunes are used on occasion for constipation. Home-prepared fresh fruits are good but home canned fruits may contain more sugar than commercial baby food. Because fruit juices are less well tolerated and cause some infants to spit up and others to develop diarrhea, they are initially diluted. Rashes around the lips are often due to ingested fruits and juices. Since fruits have a higher caloric density they should be introduced in small amounts.

Vegetables. Some pediatricians feel that vegetables should be offered before fruits so that the infant will not develop a sweet tooth and, therefore, have a lifetime craving for excess carbohydrate. This has not been proved, however. Beets are not given the young infant because they produce a magenta colored urine and this causes great parental and physician concern. Corn is very allergenic and is introduced much later. Infants should never be forced to eat a food they do not like. If a food is consistently refused, it should be removed from the diet and reintroduced several weeks later. Carrots are well tolerated as the first vegetable and green beans or peas are also usually well tolerated.

Meats. Meats are introduced at 5 to 6 months. Veal is often the first meat, although the infant may have lamb, beef, or chicken. Mothers who wish to prepare their own fresh food for the baby are warned that meats spoil very easily and should always be refrigerated and kept only for 48 hours. It is preferable to prepare the meat at each meal and either grind it in a blender or use a hand food mill at the plate. The use of fried foods and gravies is discouraged.

Desserts. Mothers are told to avoid puddings, custards, and other desserts.

Eggs. Egg yolks are added at 5 to 6 months and egg whites not until 9 months because of the allergenicity of egg whites; this allows the kidney to be more mature for handling this protein load.

Skim Milk. Skim milk should not be used before one year of age. The young infant has to drink too large a quantity to get enough calories for growth and this markedly increases the protein and solute load his kidneys must handle. Also, some fat is required and especially linoleic acid.

Calories

Energy requirements vary with each age and from one infant to another. The requirement for activity is surprisingly great, particularly in small infants; crying alone has been shown to double the metabolic rate. A placid infant may survive on as little as 70 calories per kg., whereas one who cries a great deal may require 130 calories or more. Usually the infant needs 100 to 120 kcal. per kg. per day for the first 6 months and 90 to 100 kcal. per kg. per day the second 6 months.

Protein

Average nitrogen requirement varies from 300 mg. per kg. per day at birth to 100 mg. per kg. per day as an adult. Breast milk provides between 2.0 and 2.5 grams per kg. of protein. Newer infant formulas are similar. The widely used rule that 15 per cent of the total calories should consist of protein appears to provide more than the minimum requirements in infancy. Older children are usually given 25 per cent and an additional allowance is made for children on vegetarian diets due to the quality of the protein.

Amino Acids

The true needs of amino acids are impossible to obtain and no artificial pattern has been obtained which is superior to that of whole egg or human milk.

Fat

In feeding normal infants it appears desirable to include a certain amount of fat in the diet, but there is no strong case for feeding particular fats, for the differences are small. Some linoleic acid seems necessary for healthy skin.

Carbohydrates

Although infants have been fed on carbohydrate-free diets for many months, this is not a practical procedure. The development of ketosis is difficult to avoid. As a rule, roughly half of an infant's caloric requirement is supplied as carbohydrate.

Water

The need for water is often overlooked in the infant. The healthy infant in the temperate climate needs 75 ml. per kg., and 150 ml. per kg. gives an adequate margin of safety. In subtropical conditions, 175 ml. per kg. may be needed.

Minerals

Mineral requirements are, for the most part, not accurately defined. With the exception of iron, the breast-fed infant appears to be adequately supplied, and it may be assumed that the quantities ingested are well above his minimum requirements. Both cow's milk and breast milk provide insufficient iron and after the stores present at birth become depleted, iron deficiency develops unless a supplement is given. Under exceptional circumstances, when a milk-free diet must be used, fortification of the diet with calcium may be advised. An intake of 200 to 300 mg. per day appears to be adequate.

The requirements for the trace elements copper, manganese, cobalt, zinc and selenium are not known with accuracy at the present time.

Fluoride

An excess of fluoride leads to discoloration and mottling with increased brittleness of the dental enamel, whereas a deficiency predisposes to dental caries. In our area, well water contains no fluoride, so those who do not have fluoridated water and those who are breast fed are given supplements beginning at three months.

Vitamins

The following requirements must be met:
Vitamin A: 1,500 I.U. per day is definitely protective
Vitamin C: 25 to 35 mg. per day is needed.
Vitamin D: 400 I.U. per day is protective
Thiamine: 0.2 mg. per day
Riboflavin: 0.5 mg. per day
Pyridoxine: 0.5 mg. per day
Nicotinic acid is manufactured from tryptophan and must be supplied when protein intake is marginal. Choline, likewise, is similarly related to the intake of methionine. Vitamin B_{12} and folic acid require no consideration, providing the diet contains an adequate supply of vitamin C and provided antibiotics are not being given. Vitamin

C and vitamin D need to be supplied to infants on breast milk or unfortified cow's milk. Vitamin C is lost during pasteurization or boiling and must be supplemented. Vitamin A deficiency is seen only in special circumstances such as when skim milk has been employed for feeding for a prolonged period of time. Vitamin E is said to be sometimes deficient in premature infants. The consistent opinion of the Committee on Nutrition of the American Academy of Pediatrics has been that normal children receiving a normal diet do not need vitamin supplementation over and above recommended daily allowance (RDA) levels. Megavitamin therapy as a treatment for learning disabilities and psychoses in children, including autism, is not justified on the basis of documented clinical results.

Artificial Feeding

1. Estimate the caloric requirements from the weight.
    0–3 months: 120 kcal./kg.
    3–6 months: 115 kcal./kg.
    6–9 months: 110 kcal./kg.
    9–12 months: 105 kcal./kg.
2. Estimate the daily quantity of the formula needed from the knowledge of the number of calories provided from the formula. Most formulas contain 20 calories per ounce (30 ml.). Check to see that an adequate protein allowance (2.5 mg. per kg.) and water allowance (150 ml. per kg.) are provided.
3. Divide this into the number of feedings needed.

Obesity

Most breast fed babies become quite chubby by 8 months of age. Foman, however, found that the breast-fed baby who had been fed solid food later was the least likely to be obese at 2 years of age. In treating obesity in the infant, one must keep in mind that marked weight reduction is not desirable. Enough calories and protein for brain growth must be available at all times. A moderate reduction in the number of calories consumed, along with encouragement of activity, will allow the child to grow into his weight. Adding some water to whole cow's milk or infant formula to slightly reduce calories may be indicated along with the avoidance of highly sweet foods. Fomon noted that infants on skim milk took more volume than those on whole milk. He fears that if excessive gastric filling becomes recognized by the infant as the signal to discontinue feeding, the infant may then become obese when introduced to foods of higher caloric density. Breast-fed infants consume more cholesterol than cow's milk fed babies, yet apparently do not develop more atherosclerosis and do not have higher cholesterol levels later. At our present level of knowledge, I would not recommend diets that markedly restrict cholesterol other than generally to encourage American families to eat less butter and meat and to try to use chicken and fish in the diet.

Vegetarianism

At the present time in our culture, a number of dietary cults have arisen, and as physicians we must deal with these as many of our patients adhere to such diets with religious zeal. If a semivegetarian diet is followed, excluding only the eating of meat, little difficulty is experienced in achieving adequate intakes of most nutrients. If nearly all animal products are avoided and restrictions are simultaneously placed on the intake of other foods (such as grains, legumes, or fruits), as is the case with some vegans and other very restrictive vegetarians, achieving an adequate intake of nutrients becomes more difficult. The diet may be inadequate in protein, vitamin B_{12}, vitamin D, calcium, or iron. It is our practice to take a careful dietary history; those vegetarians who are also consuming milk and eggs are felt to be giving their children an adequate diet. All vegetarians are advised that vegetable protein is not a complete protein because it does not contain all amino acids and, therefore, an adequate mixture of cereals and legumes of various kinds is very necessary in order that amino acid deficiency does not develop.

DISEASES OF THE BREAST

method of
JAMES H. THOMAS, M.D.
Kansas City, Kansas

Introduction

The treatment of breast disease begins with a well-informed patient. The extensive publicity concerning breast carcinoma and the desire of many patients to participate in the decision-making process provides the physician the unusual opportunity to educate a willing patient population. Additionally, the availability of centers for detection of breast diseases allows for thorough education of patients as to the necessity of frequent self-examination and examination by a physician. Patients should be advised as to their risk for the development of breast carcinoma and those deemed to be at "high risk" should be encouraged to establish a program for frequent reevaluation.

Anomalies

Amastia. Complete absence of one or both breasts is one of the rarest breast anomalies. There are usually associated underdeveloped or absence of structures of the shoulder girdle, chest or arm on the side of the rudimentary breast. There is some evidence for a familial tendency. Implantation of a breast prosthesis is advisable in these persons.

Accessory Breast Tissue. Accessory breasts and nipples occur frequently in orientals, and are twice as frequent in females as in males. These structures are usually situated along the milk line between the axilla and groin, and are most frequent in the axilla. In half of the cases these anomalies are bilateral. Most accessory breasts consist of a very small areola and nipple that have no physiologic function and are not subject to disease. Accessory breasts containing glandular structures are subject to all diseases that afflict the normal breast. When a cosmetic problem, accessory breasts and nipples should be excised.

Precocious Development. Breast enlargement before age 8 or 9 years is abnormal. Abnormalities in ovarian, adrenal, or central nervous system function should be sought.

Failure of Development of the Female Breast. When the breast fails to develop, ovarian agenesis must be considered. Turner's syndrome is characterized by sexual infantilism, short stature, and web neck. In these patients estrogen therapy will usually result in breast development.

Adolescent Hypertrophy. Marked hypertrophy in females may require reduction mammaplasty. This should be done only after all anticipated pregnancies have been completed. Hypertrophic breasts in male patients, gynecomastia, should be removed both for cosmetic benefit to the patient and for excluding the possibility of carcinoma. In selected patients with obvious cause, for example, cirrhosis, estrogen therapy, or hypertrophy-producing drug therapy, conservative management may be selected.

Breast Abnormalities of Physiologic Origin

Abnormal Lactation. Lactation not associated with pregnancy or continuing long after breast feeding has been terminated may be due to a variety of causes: (1) the stimulus of suckling or manual manipulation of the breast or nipples, (2) trauma to the chest wall or any type of surgical procedure involving the chest wall, (3) pituitary necrosis resulting from severe obstetrical hemorrhage, "Sheehan's syndrome," (4) pituitary adenomas as well as other pituitary neoplasms may disturb the hypothalamic pituitary relationship, (5) section of the pituitary stalk performed for diabetic retinopathy, (6) hypothyroidism in both adolescent girls and adult women.

Galactocele. In women in whom lactation has been established and suppressed by terminating nursing more or less abruptly the inspissated milk may produce a lactocele, a cyst containing thick, creamy milk. On physical examination this lesion has all the characteristics of a benign neoplasm, being rounded, well delineated, and moveable within the mammary tissue. It is usually situated over the central breast area. Aspiration in a patient who has a history consistent with this anomaly is diagnostic. No further treatment is required if the characteristic milky fluid is removed.

Infections in the Breast

Lactational Mastitis. A common complication of nursing is the development within the breast of a localized area of inflammation. Often a slight elevation of temperature is present. Treatment should include: (1) cessation of nursing, (2) administration of antibiotic, preferably erythromycin, 250 mg. four times a day, and (3) the application of warm moist heat. Such therapy will usually result in resolution of the infection.

Lactational Breast Abscess. Occasionally, mastitis devolves into an obvious abscess. Fluctuation is extremely uncommon. The presence of a tender mass lesion and clinical evidence of infection require immediate therapy. Treatment consists of antibiotic therapy directed toward *Staphylococcus aureus* coagulase-positive, and immediate incision and drainage. Awaiting development of fluctuation often will lead to extensive breast damage.

Recurring Subareolar Abscess. This is a special type of recurring low-grade infection of the subareolar region. It has no relationship to lactation and is characterized by spontaneous rupture and development of sinus tracts, often at the base of the nipple. Abscesses should be drained following initiation of antibiotic therapy. After the inflammation has subsided, the sinus tract should be surgically excised.

Miscellaneous Breast Disorders

Nipple Discharge. Premenopausal milky discharges are associated with breast function and require no therapy. Any bloody discharge must be explained. Most bleeding lesions are within 2 cm. of the nipple and can be found by palpation with expression of blood through the nipple. The appropriate duct should be totally excised by a formal quadrant excision. Most bleeding is caused by intraductal papillomas, 85 per cent of which are benign.

Nipple Erosion. Paget's disease should be suspected. Biopsy of the nipple and areolar area is definitive. With Paget's disease there is always an associated deep malignancy, and therefore all patients with Paget's disease should be treated for breast carcinoma.

When nipple erosion develops in a nursing patient, breast-feeding should be discontinued and the skin lesion treated with a topical antibiotic-steroid ointment.

Nipple Retraction. Inversion is most often normal. A history of recent development, however, arouses suspicion of new disease and indicates the necessity for retroareolar biopsy.

Traumatic Fat Necrosis. Many patients with this lesion are unable to recall the injury. Characteristically there is ecchymosis, redness of the skin with skin retraction, and often a tumor at the site of skin retraction. Additionally, enlarged axillary nodes may be present. Differentiation from a primary adenocarcinoma of the breast is mandatory. The nature of the lesion can only be determined by excisional biopsy and microscopic examination.

Mondor's Disease. A thrombophlebitis of the superficial veins of the breast; this lesion masquerades as disease of the breast and thus comes to the attention of surgeons. Characteristically, patients develop acute pain in the breast followed by development of a tender cordlike structure in the region of the thoracoepigastric vein. No treatment is required other than reassurance of the patient by the physician.

Neoplasms of the Breast

These lesions most often present as dominant breast masses and require thorough evaluation. Physical examination remains the major method of assessing breast masses although mammography and computerized axial tomography of the breast have contributed to early diagnosis and management. Mammography should be reserved for those patients at high risk for the development of breast carcinoma, and preferably utilized in patients 45 years of age or older. When a suspicious lesion is identified by mammography and is not palpable on physical examination, this area may be localized, excised, and the specimen subjected to mammography to confirm that the lesion is included in the biopsy. All dominant masses regardless of the patient's age require biopsy. If, on physical examination, the mass is cystic in nature, aspiration with a 20 gauge needle is indicated. Complete disappearance of the cyst must occur. Fluid should be sent for cytology. If the lesion does not completely disappear with the aspiration or recurs, excisional biopsy should be undertaken.

Cystic Disease. Cystic disease is the most frequent lesion requiring breast biopsy. Once cystic disease has begun, new cysts can be expected to develop at regular intervals until the patient is postmenopausal. Cystic disease, because it is bilateral and related to menses, is in some way an expression of abnormal ovarian function. The patient may give a history of rapid development of a lesion of considerable size. On examination, these lesions are firm, often painful, and relatively moveable. When a dominant mass is identified, biopsy of the mass is indicated. This may be preceded by aspiration in a patient who has previous biopsy proof of cystic disease. These patients should be followed closely, especially those with "florid" disease, as the risk of breast carcinoma is increased when compared to the normal population.

Adenofibroma or Fibroadenoma. Characteristically these are lesions of youth, and may be in some way associated with estrogen stimulation of the breast during the pubescent period. Adenofibromas are the third most common tumor of the breast in American females. They are exceeded in frequency only by carcinoma and cystic disease. These lesions are often small painless tumors discovered accidentally by the patient. On physical examination they are most often rubbery and freely moveable within the breast tissue. Surgical excision is curative. In patients under 25 years of age the lesion may be followed for a relatively short period of time, not to exceed 3 months. If the tumor recurs in a patient following an excision, reexcision is indicated. If the tumor is larger than 5 cm. or has a history of rapid growth, it is wise after exposure of the lesion to remove a small wedge for frozen section to rule out the possibility of cystosarcoma phylloides.

Cystosarcoma Phylloides. This tumor is often derived from a fibroadenoma or adenofibroma. The diagnosis is based on microscopic appearance and not clinical characteristics. It contains both fibroepithelial and very cellular stromal components. These lesions are unpredictable, but are most often benign. This determination can only be made by clinical follow-up. Wide excision, along with a zone of surrounding breast tissue is recommended. For this reason any tumor that is large (5 cm.) and has the clinical characteristics of a fibroadenoma should be exposed for a frozen section prior to excision. If cystosarcoma phylloides is present, removal of the tumor with a rim of surrounding breast tissue will prevent the likelihood of recurrence.

Intraductal Papilloma. These papillary neoplasms characteristically result in a bloody or serosanguineous nipple discharge. On occasion there is an associated tumor. Examination can define the quadrant responsible for the discharge. Appropriate therapy is surgical excision of the responsible quadrant. A frozen section will determine the character of the lesion. If an intraductal

carcinoma is present, an appropriate mastectomy should be performed.

Breast Carcinoma. PREOPERATIVE EVALUATION. A chest x-ray and routine laboratory work-up are the only tests ordered. Isotope scans are indicated only when clinical symptoms are present. Careful examination of the supraclavicular fossa should be performed. Metastasis to nodes in this location contraindicate surgery for cure.

PRIMARY CARCINOMA, OPERABLE FOR CURE. If there is minimal breast carcinoma (lesions less than 0.5 cm.) a modified radical mastectomy, including complete axillary dissection with removal of the deltopectoral fascia overlying the pectoralis major and minor muscles, is indicated. Lesions greater than 0.5 cm. should be treated with radical mastectomy. Inner quadrant or subareolar lesions should be treated with an Urban type internal mammary node dissection with complete repair of the chest wall using anterior rectus abdominis fascia. Inflammatory carcinoma of the breast (defined as greater than one third of the breast involved with peau d'orange and proven subdermal lymphatic involvement with carcinoma) is treated with radiation therapy. All primary breast carcinomas should be evaluated at the time of surgery for the presence of estrogen receptors for subsequent management of the patient if recurrences develop.

ADJUVANT THERAPY. Adjuvant chemotherapy utilizing cyclophosphamide (Cytoxan), methotrexate, and 5-fluorouracil may be indicated in those premenopausal patients with regional node involvement. Likewise, adjuvant therapy should be considered in special situations such as inflammatory carcinoma and breast carcinoma developing during pregnancy. The role of adjuvant ablative therapy in the management of patients with inflammatory carcinoma and those who develop carcinoma during pregnancy is at present undetermined.

RECURRENT CARCINOMA. Biopsy is indicated in all patients with recurrent carcinoma where tumor is accessible. Approximately 1 gram of tumor placed in liquid nitrogen is utilized for determination for the presence or absence of estrogen receptors. Those premenopausal patients with positive estrogen receptors are subjected to oophorectomy followed by adrenalectomy when relapse occurs. Chemotherapy consisting of cyclophosphamide, 50 mg. daily by mouth, methotrexate, 25 mg. intravenously each week, and 5-fluorouracil, 500 mg. intravenously every week and continued for 8 weeks with a 4 week rest period, is indicated in those patients whose tumors are not positive for estrogen receptors and those patients in whom tumors recur folllowing successful ablative therapy. X-ray therapy may be utilized to control local bony and recurrent chest wall disease. The postmenopausal patient with recurrent disease (that is, greater than 5 years postmenopausal) who has positive estrogen receptors is best treated by diethylstilbestrol, 15 mg. a day in divided doses. Responders to hormone manipulation should be considered for adrenalectomy. Adrenalectomy should be performed transabdominally if the ovaries are present to allow for concomitant bilateral oophorectomy. A posterior approach, removing the twelfth rib, is preferred if previous oophorectomy was performed. Replacement therapy of 50 mg. of cortisone acetate daily, 37.5 mg. in the morning and 12.5 mg. in the afternoon, is favored. Chemotherapy should be employed after all hormone manipulative therapy has failed and in those patients who do not have significant levels of estrogen receptors.

Special Problems with Recurring Carcinoma

Lymphangitic Pulmonary Spread with Shortness of Breath. Prednisone, 60 mg. by mouth daily.

Hypercalcemia. Prednisone, 60 mg. daily infusion, or mithramycin.

Pleural Effusion. If little disease exists elsewhere, open thoracotomy and pleurectomy are preferred. Instillation of nitrogen mustard through a chest tube, using systemic therapy dose levels, can be utilized to lessen effusion. Intrathoracic quinacrine hydrochloride (Atabrine), 200 mg. a day for 5 days, can also be tried. (This use of quinacrine is not listed in the manufacturer's official directive.) Great caution should be exercised in treating patients with intracavity nitrogen mustard who are also on systemic chemotherapy.

Isolated Bone Lesions. Radiation therapy.

Cerebral Metastasis. Neurosurgical excision or radiation therapy if multiple lesions are present.

Cortical Destruction of Weight-bearing Bone. Orthopedic intervention with internal fixation if possible.

ENDOMETRIOSIS

method of
TIFFANY J. WILLIAMS, M.D.
Rochester, Minnesota

Endometriosis is the presence of endometrial glands and stroma outside their usual location in the uterine cavity. The condition refers specifically to "external" endometriosis and not to "internal" endometriosis or adenomyosis. Mild and asymptomatic endometriosis may require no therapy. Conservative surgery is indicated when infertility is associated with endometriosis, after completion of fertility evaluation. Definitive surgery is indicated for older women and for those with extensive and symptomatic endometriosis. The relationship of endometriosis to malignancy exists but has been documented only infrequently. Endometrioid carcinoma of the ovary is always a possibility but possibility alone is not an indication for surgery in the absence of an ovarian tumor when diagnosis is mandatory.

Therapy

Accurate diagnosis is needed before initiation of any therapy, whether medical or surgical. Testosterone, estrogens, progesterones, and currently danazol have been utilized with varied degrees of success. Not all endometriosis is responsive, not all responses persist, and not all patients tolerate the side effects of the medications.

Steroidal agents have been used as part of preoperative preparation. Their use seems unnecessarily time-consuming, as well as expensive. In addition, success in treating intestinal lesions and ovarian masses with these agents has been limited. With ovarian lesions, malignancy must be excluded, which generally precludes any hormonal temporization. In young women with associated infertility, hormonal therapy will be contraceptive and may waste valuable time—time that is better spent in trying to become pregnant after surgery.

Surgery

Surgical management is divided into two broad categories: diagnostic and therapeutic. The most common diagnostic category is that of the adnexal mass. Women may have extensive endometriosis and be asymptomatic. In such women, the presence of an ovarian neoplasm must be ruled out.

The surgical therapy may be further subdivided also into two categories: conservative and definitive. Conservative surgery refers to any procedure that allows the patient to retain her childbearing potential. Definitive surgery refers to complete surgery, that is, hysterectomy and bilateral salpingo-oophorectomy with excision or destruction of the endometriosis.

The patient with endometriosis may present in two ways: with infertility and with secondary symptoms. Infertility is noted in nearly 30 per cent of women and may be the primary problem, and secondary symptoms, such as dysmenorrhea, dyspareunia, and pain, are found in nearly 30 per cent of women undergoing exploration.

Accordingly, patients with endometriosis may be considered in two related groups: (1) those who are young or whose family has not been completed or both and (2) those who are older or who have completed their family or both. Because of these possibilities, preoperative discussion is necessary so the surgeon will know the patient's wishes and can act in her best interests.

Conservative Surgery. Conservative surgery with preservation of the uterus, tubes, and ovaries is indicated in the young and infertile woman. Examination under anesthesia, dilatation and curettage, exploratory celiotomy, lysis and excision of adhesions, mobilization of uterus, and resection or fulguration of endometriosis with accurate peritonization are indicated. Uterine suspension is indicated to prevent prolapse and adhesions into the cul-de-sac and may be associated with plication of the uterosacral ligaments. The adnexa likewise may require suspension in order to prevent prolapse and scarring into the pelvis. Tuboplasty and myomectomy are indicated if infertility is associated with tubal occlusion or myomas. When pain or dysmenorrhea is part of the symptom complex, presacral neurectomy is appropriate. Thorough lavage of the pelvis and incision should be done to minimize implantation or spread of the endometriosis. Warm isotonic saline is a satisfactory solution to use.

Patients undergoing such conservative therapy have about a 40 per cent chance of a successful pregnancy, success usually being achieved within the first 2 years; however, symptoms recur at a similar rate, and additional surgery because of endometriosis is required in 16 per cent of these patients.

Definitive Surgery. Definitive surgery involves a castrating hysterectomy with excision or destruction of the endometriosis. It is always indicated in women with extensive disease who are near menopause and even in younger women with extensive disease. The source of the endometriosis, as well as the hormonal stimulant, is removed. The younger woman who has undergone definitive surgery, however, may tolerate cyclic hormone replacement without recurrence of symptomatic endometriosis. Even if symptoms recur, the use of the medication can be stopped.

Ovarian function could be preserved by surgery consisting of hysterectomy only. About 10 per cent of patients so managed have recurrence or persistence of dysmenorrhea, dyspareunia, or pain, and 6 per cent require additional surgery for endometriosis. Thirty per cent of women require hormones within 5 years. Therefore, ovarian preservation should not be considered in the perimenopausal female. Ovarian tissue may be conserved in the younger patient, with a calculated risk that symptoms may recur and additional surgery may be needed.

DYSFUNCTIONAL UTERINE BLEEDING
method of
H. OLIVER WILLIAMSON, M.D.,
and CHARLES C. TSAI, M.D.
Charleston, South Carolina

Dysfunctional uterine bleeding (DUB) is abnormal, anovulatory, and not due to genital tract pathology or systemic disease. Often preceded by infrequent menses or even amenorrhea, it is the prolonged or excessive bleeding that usually requires the therapy described here. DUB is more common in the postmenarchal and premenopausal epochs but can occur during any of the reproductive years. It is presumed due to disturbances in the central nervous system (CNS)-hypothalamic-pituitary axis. Evaluation and therapy depend upon the extent of the bleeding and the age of the patient, which in turn influence the type of lesions necessary to be excluded to arrive at the diagnosis.

Abnormal Bleeding

Normal cycles occur within 21 to 35 days, last 3 to 7 days and do not exceed 100 ml. in amount. Cycles 21 days or shorter and bleeding lasting longer than 10 days or causing anemia, shock, or significant clotting is abnormal. A fall of several points in the hematocrit should be considered indicative of excessive blood loss; however, vacillations associated with premenstrual edema may make such interpretations difficult.

Anovulation

Failure to ovulate frequently allows continued estrogenic stimulation to the endometrium, setting the stage for abnormalities of bleeding. The simultaneous decline in estrogen and progesterone is associated with predictable withdrawal bleeding. In its absence, a variety of endometrial changes may occur that can be associated with irregular bleeding. These may proceed into hyperplastic states and there is an increased incidence of endometrial carcinoma developing in such patients. Accordingly, the disorder should be appropriately treated. The reproductive outlook for these patients when studied in prior years has not been good. This state may now be improved with the availability of better methods of inducing ovulation such as with clomiphene citrate (Clomid).

Basal body temperature charting, endometrial biopsy or dilation and curettage (D and C) may be helpful in determining whether a given cycle is ovulatory or not. However, for an endometrial sample to be meaningful, it would have to be obtained just before or during the first day of bleeding to indicate if ovulation had occurred. Accordingly, one may assume that bleeding is anovulatory if the cycle is shorter than 21 days. Also, if bleeding is excessively prolonged, then one seldom is justified in awaiting the onset of another bleeding episode to confirm the ovulatory status. Hence, it does not seem imperative to prove that the current cycle is anovulatory before instituting therapy.

Exclusion of Organic Lesions

Although many advances have been made in testing hypothalamic-pituitary-ovarian function, DUB usually presents as a summation of effects of repeated bouts of anovulation. Testing at one point in time may seldom be meaningful. Accordingly, the diagnosis still remains a presumptive one but after reasonable organic lesions have been excluded. Prompt examination is imperative and should not be deferred because the patient is bleeding. Delay of definitive therapy for genital malignancy and pregnancy aberrations such as ectopic gestation may result if such a tack is taken.

Table 1 should be considered as a guide only as to the history and physical examination. Should therapy fail, the patient should be interrogated again, reexamined, and additional studies obtained if indicated. The patient 30 years of age or older and the patient with failure of adequate hormonal therapy should be curetted (Table 1).

Therapy

Dysfunctional uterine bleeding is often self-limited. When bleeding is not excessive, expectant observation may be preferable. When repeated episodes occur, hormonal therapy is usually employed. If the hematocrit (hemoglobin) starts to drop, hematinic therapy is added, but if anemia

TABLE 1.   **Minimal Pre-therapy Evaluation**

DISEASE	HISTORY	PHYSICAL (DO NOT DEFER BECAUSE OF BLEEDING)	LABORATORY
Thyroid	Heat or cold intolerance, constipation, skin changes	Thyroid palpation, eye signs, pulse changes, reflexes	T_3 and T_4; TSH if suspect hypo; obtain prior to estrogen therapy
Liver disease	Previous hepatitis, jaundice, exposure to hepatotoxins; family history; pain	Palpable liver, jaundice	SMA 12
Blood dyscrasia	Family history, easy bruisability, bleeding from other sites	Petechiae, hepatosplenomegaly, extra-genital bleeding	CBC, PT, PTT, platelet observation (count?)
Genital trauma or foreign body	History of IUD	Full exam with anesthesia if necessary; consider IUD removal; explore endometrial cavity for possible lost IUD	Rape evaluation if suspected; culture if necessary; x-rays of abdomen if suspect lost IUD not detected on exam
Genital tract infections	Dysuria, urinary frequency, vulval or vaginal itching, cohort infection	Strip urethra, tenderness to cervical manipulation, adnexal tenderness or mass	CBC, sed rate, temperature elevation, wet and KOH smears of vaginal secretion if indicated. Urethral and cervical GC culture. Cervical biopsy of lesion (erosions)
Vaginal or cervical malignancy	Postcoital bleeding, prior abnormal cytology, history of prenatal DES exposure or poor reproductive history in mother	Full visualization of vagina and cervix, Schiller staining, and colpomicroscopy if DES history positive	Biopsy any lesions, Papanicolaou smears
Endometrial lesions	Laborlike contractions, history of previous diagnosis of uterine anomaly or myomata, dysmenorrhea, dyspareunia	Palpation for uterine bossilations, vaginal exam for prolapsed polyp or myoma, uterosacral or cul-de-sac nodularity with tenderness, ovarian cyst with endometriosis	Office endometrial biopsy (curettage) if post adolescent. Full D&C with cavity exploration with forceps if adenomatous hyperplasia or more severe lesion found or failure of therapy. Hysteroscopy, hysterography or laparoscopy if indicated

Table continued on the following page

TABLE 1.　**Minimal Pre-therapy Evaluation** (*Continued*)

DISEASE	HISTORY	PHYSICAL (DO NOT DEFER BECAUSE OF BLEEDING)	LABORATORY
Fallopian tube carcinoma	Bloody hydrorrhea	Palpable adnexal mass	Exploration if failure of therapy and suspect mass significant
Ovarian tumor or polycystic ovary syndrome	Pelvic region heaviness, discomfort or pain. Antecedent amenorrhea	Palpable adnexal mass, hirsutism, obesity	Endometrial biopsy (hyperplasia with functioning tumors and PCO). Plasma estrogens (for functioning tumors), FSH, LH, steroid assessment (for PCO) prior to hormonal therapy. UCG for rare primary choriocarcinoma. Ultrasonography if indicated
Ovulational and pregnancy aberrations: Ovulational bleeding	Mid cycle	Minimal bleeding	Correlate with basal body temperature and menstrual history
Implantational	Occurring approximately day 24 of 28 day cycles	Defer endometrial assessment with first slight episode of bleeding	Basal body temperature chart
Threatened abortion	History of pregnancy symptoms	Defer endometrial assessment with first slight episode of bleeding	UCG, ultrasonography if indicated
Incomplete abortion	Tissue passage, clotting, pain	Cervix dilated	UCG, ultrasonography if indicated
Ectopic	Tearing abdominal or shoulder pain, dyspnea, thirst	Bulging cul-de-sac, tenderness to cervical manipulation, afebrile, shock signs	Culdocentesis, UCG, ultrasonography if indicated
Trophoblastic disease	Antecedent pregnancy	Enlarged uterus (?)	UCG, D&C (suction?)
Exogenous hormones or drugs	History of skipping or discontinuing oral contraceptives, therapy for endometriosis (including oral preparations, injections or pellets), acne, hirsutism and psychotherapeutics	Condition under history; do not assume drug cause of bleeding	

develops, transfusion should be employed if indicated and uterine curettment done.

Hormonal Therapy

Table 2 presents in outline form the more generally accepted regimens of hormonal therapy of DUB. It is suggested that one should become thoroughly familiar with one regimen according to the manufacturers' recommendations and then employ others only if side effects develop or there are specific indications for changing (Table 2).

Combination estrogen and progestogen therapy has simplicity to recommend it, for the patient has to deal with only one type of medication. However, it is important to stress to the patient that she should not miss tablets and that she should take them approximately at the same time each day. Skipping tablets may precipitate bleeding. When multiple tablets are necessary, they should be spaced throughout the day. Nausea may be possibly averted by taking them with food. Should a history of disorders contraindicating estrogen-containing medications be obtained, e.g., migraine headaches, vascular disease such as thrombophlebitis, pulmonary embolus, or hypertension, then these medications should be avoided. Desirable as it would seem to control or prevent bleeding in immobilized patients, the frequency of thromboembolic phenomenon under such circumstances would seem to contraindicate their use.

If the patient responds to hormonal therapy, some degree of assurance can be had that an endometrial lesion is not present. Should recurrence of abnormal bleeding ensue on discontinuance of therapy, it has been the practice in past years to reinstitute therapy and continue it for longer periods of time, e.g., 6 months to one year. However, serious questions are now being raised regarding the use of such potent progestogens in patients with menstrual disorders, for they are the very ones apt to develop postpill amenorrhea. Although clomiphene citrate can be utilized to correct such conditions in most women wishing to achieve ovulatory cycles for reproduction, its use in DUB is not generally advocated. (This use of clomiphene citrate is not listed in the manufacturer's official directive.) Accordingly, one must consider the ramifications of long-term use of combination contraceptive preparations before embarking on their use.

Combination therapy does not produce a normal appearing endometrium, in that it is rapidly converted to a secretory phase and may show a rich decidual response. Should the patient subsequently undergo D and C, the pathologist should be notified of the therapy for he may cogitate unnecessarily over the diagnosis of an ectopic pregnancy.

Sequential Hormonal Therapy. The sequential use of estrogen then estrogen and a progestogen for the treatment of patients with disorders of menstruation has been followed for many years and found to be effective, generally well tolerated, and productive of a relatively normal appearing endometrium. Therapy is divided into an estrogenic hemostatic phase followed by estrogen and then estrogen plus progestogen to mimic the normal cycle (substitutional phase). If bleeding is of insufficient magnitude to warrant D and C, hemostasis is achieved by administering oral estrogens. One usually starts at a lower dose and if bleeding does not slow or cease, the dose is escalated episodically every few days until hemostasis is achieved. If bleeding is relatively brisk, but insufficient to warrant immediate D and C, parenteral equine estrogens may be added to the oral preparation. Usually 25 mg. are injected intravenously though it may be given intramuscularly. This may be repeated in 6 to 12 hours if necessary. However, if bleeding is still brisk at the end of this, D and C should be reconsidered. The parenteral preparation is said to cause polymerization of mucopolysaccharides in the ground substance of small blood vessels, causing them to be more resistant to bleeding, though questions are being raised regarding the effectiveness of such therapy. The oral preparation should be simultaneously continued with the parenteral preparation, as it is relied upon for endometrial proliferation.

Once hemostasis is achieved, the oral estrogen is continued at the same dose level for 20 additional days. A progestogen is given for the last 10 of these 20 days. On discontinuance of such therapy, withdrawal bleeding usually occurs within 10 days. A second cycle of therapy is then instituted 5 days after the onset of bleeding. The estrogen dose is usually reduced to more physiologic levels if pharmacologic doses were necessary to achieve hemostasis.

Should breakthrough bleeding occur after hemostasis is achieved but while the patient is still on the estrogen portion alone, the estrogen may be increased. However, if bleeding persists, then the patient should be considered for curettage. If bleeding occurs while the individual is on the estrogen and progestogen, therapy should generally be discontinued for 5 days and a new cycle started, including the hemostatic phase if necessary. It should be stressed that the medication should be taken regularly, for skipping doses may induce abnormal uterine bleeding. After three such cycles, something on the order of 80 per cent of patients will have return of normal ovulatory cycling. If they do not, they should be reevaluated, reconsidered for D and C, and if this is not indicated, may be recycled for longer periods.

Conjugated or esterified equine estrogens have the advantage over synthetic estrogens of being well tolerated orally (less nausea), but the disadvantage of being relatively expensive. However, hormonal therapy is far cheaper than a D and C. One should not utilize long acting estrogens such as chlorotrianisene (Tace), for this will not allow a rapid drop in plasma levels, which in turn are necessary for rapid changes in the endometrium and consequent clean-cut withdrawal bleeding.

Should dydrogesterone (Duphaston or Gynorest) be utilized as the progestogen, it is best given in divided doses because of its rapid metabolism (short action).

Because of its complexity, patients employing the sequential regimen should be provided with a written schedule for the medication with the suggestion that they check off each dose as taken and also record any bleeding.

Injection Therapy. When one suspects that the patient cannot or will not take oral medications satisfactorily, then injectable therapy may be preferable. As with oral sequential therapy, hemostasis is achieved by the administration of estrogen. This is based upon the fact that ordinarily the proliferating endometrium in the absence of an endometrial lesion does not bleed. Although having an activity when given by injection of approximately 2 weeks, 17 hydroxyprogesterone caproate is a relatively weak progestogen and may not consistently give a normal appearing endometrium. However, it is usually of sufficient potency to provide satisfactory cycling in the majority of patients.

Progestogen or Progesterone Therapy. Patients with dysfunctional uterine bleeding are anovulatory, yet usually exhibit manifestations

TABLE 2. **Hormonal Therapy of Dysfunctional Uterine Bleeding**

TYPE OF THERAPY	HEMOSTATIC PHASE (DOSES GIVEN DIVIDED UNTIL BLEEDING CEASES AND PROCEED TO SUBSTITUTIONAL PHASE)		SUBSTITUTIONAL PHASE	CYCLING (2 OR MORE CYCLES)	COMMENT
	Drug	*Dosage*			
Combination	Enovid and Ortho Novum	10–40 mg.	10 mg. for 20 days then to cycling	10 mg. daily starting on day 5 for 20 days	Escalate dose to maximum of 40 mg./day for breakthrough bleeding and maintain same dose in substitutional phase
	Ovulen and Ovral	2–6 tablets	2 tablets daily for 20 or 21 days then to cycling	1 or 2 tablets daily for 20 or 21 days starting on day 5	Escalate dose to maximum of 6/day for breakthrough bleeding and maintain same dose for substitutional phase
Sequential	Conjugated equine est.	3.75–10 mg.	Continue same estrogen dose necessary for 20 additional days. Add progestogen for the last 10 days of estrogen therapy. Proceed to cycling. Progestogens (some with added estrogen): Provera, 10 mg. Norlutin, 10 mg.	Minimum dose of estrogen daily for 20 days starting on day 5. Add full dose of progestogen last 10 of the 20 days of estrogen therapy	If breakthrough bleeding on estrogenic phase, escalate to maximum dose for hemostasis and continue same dose in substitutional phase; if on progestogen and estrogen phase, discontinue and restart hemostatic phase in 5 days
	Esterified estrogens	3.75–10 mg.			
	Ethinyl estradiol	0.15–0.5 mg.			
	Ethinyl estradiol 3 methyl ether	0.15–0.5 mg.			
	Diethylstilbestrol	2–5 mg.			

Injection	Estradiol valerate	20 mg. on day one or when 1st seen; 14 days later start substitutional phase	Norlutate, 5 mg. Enovid, 5 or 10 mg. Ovulen Ovral Ortho Novum, 10 mg. Duphaston, 15 mg. in divided doses Gynorest, 15 mg. in divided doses Estradiol valerate 50 mg. and 17 hydroxy progesterone caproate 250 mg. (Delalutin). Proceed to cycling phase	On day 28 repeat hemostatic dose and 14 days later substitutional doses	May give 375 mg. of 17 hydroxy progesterone caproate on day four if bleeding or on day 21 if not should rapid conversion of endometrium to secretory phase be desired
Progesterone or progestogen only therapy	Progesterone in oil Oral Provera Norlutin Norlutate Gynorest or Duphaston			25–50 mg. IM every 28 days 10 mg./day for 5–10 days every 28 days 10 mg. per day for 5–10 days every 28 days 5 mg./day for 5–10 days every 28 days 5 mg. t.i.d. for 5–10 days every 28 days	Hemostasis achieved slowly

of estrogen activity including endometrial prolif-eration or even hyperplasia. Assuming that the estrogen is adequate, the use of progesterone alone has been advocated. However, progesterone is not a hemostatic drug. If a patient is bleeding on institution of therapy, bleeding will not be con-trolled possibly for a week or longer after the injection. Aqueous preparations of progesterone are to be avoided because of a propensity to cause painful sterile abscesses. The oral progestogens can be used in a similar fashion, being given daily for 5 to 10 days. An objection to the progesterone only therapy is that one cannot rely upon the es-trogen being constantly present; i.e., levels may vacillate (this is usually what provokes the bleeding for which the patient is complaining); hence, this may lead to irregular bleeding during the interval off progesterone or progestogen. Also, profuse bleeding usually follows the withdrawal of therapy. This added blood loss in a patient who has already possibly depleted her iron stores may lead to anemia where it did not previously exist. Cyclic withdrawal bleeding using progesterone or a progestogen is thought prophylactic in preventing endometrial hyperplasia and possibly endometrial carcinoma in those predisposed such as in the polycystic ovary syndrome. Here it is given every 30 to 90 days. Ideally, the patient should remain off therapy for several months each year to ascer-tain if remission has occurred.

Failure of Hormonal Therapy.   If bleeding per-sists after hormonal therapy at maximum doses, it is unlikely that the patient has dysfunctional uterine bleeding. The patient should be totally reassessed, including repeat physical examination. Consideration should be given to additional diag-nostic procedures. Hysterography or hysteros-copy may be necessary to detect a polyp or myoma that might have been missed at D and C. Explora-tion for a functional ovarian tumor is no longer generally necessary, for one can obtain plasma estrogen levels that are generally quite high when such tumors are present. Pregnancy tests may be helpful in the missed diagnosis of incomplete abortion, ectopic pregnancy, or even in the rare primary ovarian choriocarcinoma or trophoblastic disease. Further hematologic evaluation and con-sultation may be in order.

Dilatation and Curettage

Evacuation of the endometrium is still to be considered in patients with DUB, particularly when it is of hemorrhagic proportions. This is the most rapid method of achieving hemostasis. Not only is it usually therapeutic, it is often diagnostic. However, it is generally not the first mode of ther-apy in the adolescent. When hormonal therapy has failed, D and C should be considered, for frequently one will find an old incomplete abor-tion, polyp, or other organic lesion that has been overlooked. Curettage should not be overly vigor-ous, for totally denuding the endometrium can lead to endometrial sclerosis with the attendant possibility of amenorrhea and infertility. Also, an incompetent cervical os can result from traumatic cervical dilatation. Suction curettage is considered less traumatic and more thorough than sharp curettage. It can often be carried out as an office procedure under sedation and local anesthesia using small flexible curet tips. Cervical dilatation with laminaria may be a useful adjunct. One may miss an endometrial lesion or even a fibrotic in-complete abortion by this technique. If the patient is overly anxious, then general anesthesia may be employed. Should suction curettage fail to achieve hemostasis, the reassessment including sharp curettage may be in order.

Hysterectomy

If a woman has completed her childbearing, and particularly if she has been subjected to multi-ple curettages or difficulty is had in matching blood, then this procedure may be preferable to repeated D and C and attempts at medical control. However, it is generally viewed as a failure at diag-nosis and should be considered as a last resort and then only after thorough evaluation. One would not wish to remove a cancerous uterus without proper assessment and appropriate preoperative therapy if indicated.

Therapy Not Recommended

One author has stated "the use of ergonovine or pituitary preparations that control acute bleed-ing, androgens to check bleeding and restore the cycle or irradiation (x-ray or radium) to re-establish or eliminate cyclic menstruation are use-less, needless or hazardous." To this is added de-pomedroxyprogesterone, which may actually pro-duce dysfunctional uterine bleeding. The use of endometrial cryosurgery in resistant dysfunction-al uterine bleeding may lead to permanent infer-tility and amenorrhea. Clomiphene citrate theo-retically would appear desirable since it will normalize hypothalamic-pituitary function in most anovulatory patients with endogenous estro-gen production. However, it is such a potent drug, its use should be reserved for patients in their re-productive years wishing to achieve pregnancy. The empiric use of thyroid is not generally advo-cated. However, investigation employing thyroid-stimulating hormone releasing factor and measurement of thyroid-stimulating (TSH) re-sponses appear to delineate potential hypothyroid patients before alterations in baseline TSH or con-ventional thyroid hormonal assays as T_3 or T_4 are manifest. Accordingly, a reversal in opinion of those opposing empiric thyroid therapy for DUB may be in the offing. Usefulness of luteinizing hormone and its superactive analogues in this disorder has not yet been delineated.

Adjunctive Therapy

Psychiatric support of these patients should not be overlooked. On probing, most such patients will be found to have attendant psychologic disturbances and indeed some authorities feel that it is probably the principal cause of DUB. Accordingly, many of these patients may respond to psychiatric support.

Since blood loss is a component of most of these patients' problems, satisfactory hematinics should be prescribed concomitant with other therapy. If there is a question of dietary adequacy, multivitamins might be added; however, seldom are nutritional deficiences the cause of abnormal uterine bleeding in the United States.

Bleeding Associated with Ovulatory Cycles

Bleeding at the time of ovulation (Kleine Regel) has been attributed to the rapid fall in estrogen after the preovulatory surge. Usually, this is of such small proportion that it is of no concern to the patient. Its timing in relation to ovulation or mittelschmerz is highly suggestive of the diagnosis. Curettage is said to frequently cure the problem, but if it does, then it is more likely that a polyp was present. Irregular endometrial shedding or inadequate corpus luteum function as a recurrent problem involves probably much less than 1 per cent of the patients presenting with bleeding disorders. Accordingly, it is seldom of clinical importance but will usually respond to progestogen or progesterone therapy in the latter half of the cycle.

AMENORRHEA

method of
PAUL GABOS, M.D.
Pittsburgh, Pennsylvania

Amenorrhea, the absence of menstruation, is a *symptom* associated with a host of endocrine and nonendocrine disorders. For the sake of classification and treatment, amenorrhea may be either *primary* or *secondary*. Primary amenorrhea may be defined as an absence of spontaneous periods by age 18. If, however, normal growth and secondary sex characteristics such as breast and hair development have not occurred by age 16

TABLE 1. **Classification of Causes of Primary Amenorrhea**

I. Gonadal Abnormalities
   A. Gonadal dysgenesis: Turner's syndrome (XO) or mosaicism (XO/XX, XO/XY etc.)
   B. Testicular feminization
   C. "Resistant Ovary" syndrome
   D. "Pure" gonadal dysgenesis: XY karyotype
   E. Mixed gonadal dysgenesis, true hermaphroditism, male pseudohermaphroditism: XY karyotype

II. Extragonadal Abnormalities
   A. Hypothalamic-pituitary dysfunction
      1. Physiologic delayed menarche
      2. Psychogenic
      3. Chronic illness: gastrointestinal disorders, diabetes, lymphoma, renal disease
      4. Hypogonadotrophic hypogonadism: Kallman's syndrome and variants
      5. Stein-Leventhal syndrome
   B. Mullerian dysplasia or urogenital sinus dysplasia: absence of vagina, uterus and imperforate hymen
   C. Central nervous system tumor, trauma or infection: chromophobe adenoma, craniopharyngioma, encephalitis
   D. Other endocrine disorders: thyroid dysfunction, congenital adrenogenital syndrome
   E. Genital tract infections: tuberculosis
   F. Feminizing ovarian tumors
   G. Unresponsive endometrium

along with amenorrhea, a pathophysiologic state must be considered. A classification of causes of primary amenorrhea is included in Table 1. Secondary amenorrhea may be defined as occurring in a female who has had spontaneous periods and some or normal secondary sex characteristics and then stops menstruating for a period of 6 to 12 months. Severe secondary oligoamenorrhea with periods occurring three to four to five times yearly may be as significant and caused by those disease states causing secondary amenorrhea. Along with secondary amenorrhea, other signs or symptoms such as virilization and galactorrhea may be present and enable one to further classify the causes. Classification of causes of secondary amenorrhea is included in Table 2. Menopause is considered a physiologic state and is discussed elsewhere in this text.

It should be emphasized that amenorrhea, either primary or secondary, is merely a symptom of an underlying disorder. The therapeutic use of hormones (e.g., estrogen, birth control pills) should be withheld until the underlying cause is identified. The use of such hormones could mask or aggravate the underlying disorder.

Appropriate studies to determine the underlying cause may *selectively* include: (1) history and physical examination, (2) vaginal smear for maturation index, (3) buccal smear for Barr bodies, (4) quinacrine staining of peripheral blood smears for Y chromosome, (5) karyotype, (6) sella tomography, (7) bone age, (8) neurologic evaluation and visual fields, (9) thyroid evaluation, (10) radioimmunoassay for FSH, LH, prolactin, testosterone

TABLE 2. **Classification of Causes of Secondary Amenorrhea**

I. Normal Ovarian Function—Acquired
  A. Asherman's syndrome
  B. Endometrial destruction (tuberculosis, irradiation)
  C. Hysterectomy
II. Decreased Ovarian Function
  A. High gonadotrophins
    1. Premature ovarian failure
    2. Surgical castration
    3. Radiation castration
  B. Low or normal gonadotrophins
    1. Hypothalamic-pituitary dysfunction
      a. Psychogenic
      b. Nutritional (anorexia nervosa)
      c. Nongonadal endocrine disorders (thyroid, adrenal)
      d. Systemic infections and chronic diseases
      e. Pharmacologic (psychotrophic drugs, "post pill")
      f. Idiopathic
    2. Organic central nervous system disease
      a. Sheehan's syndrome
      b. Tumor
      c. Trauma
III. Increased Ovarian Androgen Secretion
  A. Gonadotrophins variable
    1. Polycystic ovary syndrome
    2. Ovarian hyperthecosis, ovarian stromal hyperplasia
    3. Masculinizing ovarian tumors

and 17 hydroxyprogesterone, (11) 24 hour urine for 17 ketosteroids, 17 hydroxycorticoids, and cortisol, (12) endoscopy to visualize the gonads, (13) appropriate hormone stimulation and suppression test, and (14) biopsy of gonads.

PRIMARY AMENORRHEA

Gonadal Abnormalities

Gonadal Dysgenesis. 1. Substitutional therapy is indicated from the time of "assumed" normal menarche (ages 12 to 16) to "assumed" menopause (age 45 to 50). Starting the first day of the month, conjugated estrogens (Premarin), 1.25 mg. daily for 25 days, monthly. Medroxyprogesterone acetate (Provera), 10 mg. daily day 21 to day 25 of Premarin therapy, monthly. Withdrawal "periods" will occur. Premarin, 2.5 mg. daily or twice daily, may be initially used in girls with very poor secondary sex characteristics. Estradiol (Estrace), 1.0 mg., or diethylstilbestrol, 0.5 mg., may be substituted for Premarin therapy.

2. Anabolic agents have been used without much success to stimulate growth.

3. Endometrial aspiration, biopsy, or dilation and curettage (D and C). The use of medroxyprogesterone to oppose the action of estrogen on the uterine endometrium and breast should protect against the possible occurrence of endometrial adenomatous hyperplasia or breast carcinoma in the predisposed woman. However, periodic endometrial aspiration, biopsy or D and C should be considered. An exact time interval for the performance of these procedures has not been established.

4. Although a few spontaneous pregnancies have occurred, sterility should be explained to these young women with gentleness and empathy.

Testicular Feminization. Because of the increased incidence of gonadal tumors, once *development* of the secondary sex characteristics has occurred, gonadectomy should be performed. Substitutional estrogen and progesterone therapy as outlined with ovarian dysgenesis is then initiated to "assumed" menopause. These patients are normal from a psychologic, social, and sexual standpoint. They should never be told of the histologic diagnosis of the gonads. An increased incidence of suicide has been reported.

Resistant Ovary Syndrome. This should be treated as outlined for ovarian dysgenesis. Unusually high doses of human menopausal gonadotrophin (Pergonal) have been successfully used to induce ovulations in occasional instances.

"Pure" Gonadal Dysgenesis. Patients with dysgenetic gonads and XY karyotype (except for testicular feminization) should have bilateral gonadectomy once the diagnosis *has been established*. There is an increased incidence of gonadal tumors (gonadoblastoma and dysgerminoma) and virilization in these patients.

Extragonadal Abnormalities

Hypothalamic Pituitary Dysfunction. PHYSIOLOGIC DELAYED MENARCHE. These patients are best treated with observation and reassurance and followed with maturation indices at 6 month intervals until menses have been established. The use of hormones should be avoided.

PSYCHOGENIC. This is a very rare occurrence. Appropriate psychotherapy is indicated.

CHRONIC DEBILITATING ILLNESS. This includes diseases such as colitis, diabetes, lymphoma, renal disease. Treatment of the underlying disorder and management as outlined with physiologic delayed menarche are indicated.

HYPOGONADOTROPHIC HYPOGONADISM (KALLMANN'S SYNDROME). Substitutional estrogen-progesterone therapy as outlined with ovarian dysgenesis. Once pregnancy is desired, human menopausal gonadotrophin (Pergonal) in higher than usual doses and human chorionic gonadotrophin (HCG) will induce ovulation. Clomiphene citrate (Clomid) is of no help. Gonadotrophin-releasing hormone is not yet available for clinical therapeutic induction of ovulation.

STEIN-LEVENTHAL SYNDROME. Treat as outlined in the discussion of secondary amenorrhea.

Müllerian Aplasia or Dysplasia and Urogenital Sinus Dysplasia. Imperforate hymen is best treated with hymenotomy or hymenectomy done under anesthesia. If hematocolpos or hematometria has occurred then D and C, postural drainage, and coverage with ampicillin or cephalexin (Keflex), 250 mg. four times daily for 7 to 10 days, is indicated. An absent vagina may be initially treated by daily, progressive perineal dilation with vaginal dilators (after Frank). If unsuccessful, vaginal reconstruction according to Wharton or McIndoe may be considered. Perhaps these vaginal reconstructive plastic procedures are still best done prior to anticipated marriage or anticipated sexual relations. These patients should have an intravenous pyelogram to rule out renal anomalies.

Central Nervous System Tumors. Treat as discussed under secondary amenorrhea.

Other Endocrine Disorders. Treatment of thyroid and adrenal disorders is outlined in the section on endocrine disorders.

Genital Tract Infection. An excellent discussion of the treatment of genital tuberculosis can be found in another section of this text. Tuberculosis endometritis may be treated for a period of 18 months to 2 years with the following regimen: (1) isoniazid (INH), 300 mg. per day by mouth; (2) ethambutol, 15 mg. per kg. of body weight once per day by mouth; (3) cycloserine, 250 mg. twice daily by mouth; (4) pyridoxine (vitamin B_6), 100 mg. daily by mouth. Observation for side effects involving the central nervous system and liver is necessary.

Feminizing Ovarian Tumors. These tumors are rare. Unilateral excision and possibly unilateral radiation depending on the histology of the tumor may be the treatment of choice. If bilateral oophorectomy and hysterectomy are performed, substitutional estrogen and progesterone therapy as outlined under ovarian dysgenesis should be used.

Unresponsive Endometrium. These patients have normal hypothalamic-pituitary-ovarian physiology with ovulation but fail to menstruate. No treatment is necessary. A normal pregnancy can occur spontaneously.

SECONDARY AMENORRHEA

Normal Ovarian Function

Asherman's Syndrome. Treatment consists of (1) D and C, (2) intrauterine device (IUD) insertion at the time of the D and C to prevent the reapproximation of the uterine walls, (3) immediate high dose estrogen therapy for 2 to 3 months to stimulate endometrial proliferation. Conjugated estrogens (Premarin), 1.25 to 2.5 mg. twice daily (or three times daily as tolerated) for 25 days, with medroxyprogesterone acetate (Provera), 10 to 20 mg. daily day 21 to day 25 of Premarin therapy.

Endometritis-Tuberculosis. Pelvic inflammatory disease secondary to tuberculosis is treated as outlined under primary amenorrhea.

Hysterectomy. With conservation of the ovaries during the reproductive years, naturally, no substitutional therapy is necessary.

Decreased Ovarian Function

High Gonadotrophins. PREMATURE OVARIAN FAILURE. Premature ovarian failure causing secondary amenorrhea may be due to congenital or acquired hypoplasia, "resistant ovary" syndrome, autoimmune reaction akin to thyroiditis and premature menopause of unknown cause. The prognosis for return of spontaneous ovulatory periods is very poor. Substitutional estrogen and progesterone therapy as outlined for ovarian dysgenesis is indicated until assumed "normal" menopause. These patients, too, should be treated with understanding and emotional support. Resistant ovary syndrome and autoimmune reaction ovaries have occasionally responded to very high doses of human menopausal gonadotrophins to induce ovulation and pregnancy.

SURGICAL AND RADIATION CASTRATION. Treatment is as outlined for ovarian dysgenesis.

Low or Normal Gonadotrophins. HYPOTHALAMIC-PITUITARY DYSFUNCTION. *Psychogenic.* When all other causes of secondary amenorrhea are ruled out, then a diagnosis of psychogenic amenorrhea is permissible. Nonetheless, it remains the most common cause of secondary amenorrhea. Although the gonadotrophins are low or normal in this most interesting aspect of reproductive physiology, they may also be elevated. An extreme example of this may be the Stein-Leventhal syndrome. Treatment includes: (1) proper evaluation which allows reassurance to be readily accepted; (2) oral contraceptive agents to induce periods should be avoided since they may further alter the hypothalamic-pituitary axis; (3) clomiphene citrate (Clomid) (100 mg. daily* for 5 days) to prove the presence of an intact hypothalamic-pituitary ovarian axis may be tried but its continued use to try to stimulate the return of normal function is usually unsuccessful and unwarranted; (4) periodic 6 month follow up to reassess the amenorrhea and to reassure the patient of her excellent prognosis for future spontaneous periods and pregnancy is advisable; (5) if necessary, the temporary use of a mechanical method of contraception is advisable.

---

*This dose may be higher than that listed in the manufacturer's official directive.

Nutritional Weight Gain or Weight Loss.
Weight gain or loss, especially if rapid, may cause
secondary amenorrhea. Diet should be planned
with this in mind. The extreme nutritional (really
psychogenic) problem associated with
amenorrhea is naturally anorexia nervosa.
Treatment progresses in the following manner:
(1) correct the starvation (hyperalimentation may
be necessary to prevent death), (2) psychotherapy,
(3) independent diet selection, and (4) continued
close follow-up and support. This is certainly a
serious disorder, which is difficult to treat, and
expert help is required. Although the weight loss
may be regained amenorrhea may persist for
months or years.

Nongonadal Endocrine Disorders. These are
not common causes of secondary amenorrhea. An
excellent review of nongonadal treatment including adrenal and thyroid glands is found in the
endocrine section.

Chronic Diseases. Treatment of the chronic
disease will eventually lead to spontaneous return
to ovulatory cycles. The patient may be compe-
tently treated as outlined under psychogenic
amenorrhea.

Pharmacologic. Amenorrhea following the
use of oral contraceptive agents (post-pill) occurs 1
to 2 per cent of the time or less. Organic causes for
amenorrhea must be considered if spontaneous
periods have not returned within one year after
stopping the pill and *especially* if menstrual dysfunction was present prior to the use of the pill.
This problem is best managed by observation. If
pregnancy is desired clomiphene citrate (Clomid),
50 to 150 mg.* daily for 5 days for 4 to 6 months
with or without human chorionic gonadotrophin
(HCG), may be of help.

ORGANIC CENTRAL NERVOUS SYSTEM DIS-
EASE. *Sheehan's Syndrome.* Replacement treatment for panhypopituitarism includes (1) cortisone acetate, 37.5 mg. daily (increase with
metabolic stress), (2) sodium levothyroxine
(Synthroid), 0.2 to 0.3 mg. daily, (3) conjugated
estrogens (Premarin), 1.25 mg. daily for 25 days of
the month with medroxyprogesterone acetate
(Provera), 10 mg. daily on day 21 to day 25 of
Premarin therapy, (4) ovulation induction for
pregnancy is possible with menotropins (Pergonal) plus human chorionic gonadotrophin
(HCG).

Tumors. Transsphenoidal surgery using the
microscope has become a popular and effective
method of treatment of pituitary adenomas. With
incomplete excision, postoperative radiation is indicated. Other brain tumors involving the

hypothalamic area are treated by appropriate
neurosurgical intervention.

Chromophobe adenomas, eventually, most
often present with amenorrhea, galactorrhea,
and hyperprolactinemia. The patient with
amenorrhea and inappropriate lactation should
be followed with prolactin radioimmunoassay
done at 6 month intervals and yearly sella tomography. Other causes of amenorrhea and galactorrhea such as pregnancy, on a psychogenic basis,
use of drugs (birth control pills and tranquilizers)
and hypothyroidism must be considered. Galactorrhea and amenorrhea unassociated with central nervous system tumors may be treated medically. However, the patient must be continuously
observed for tumors. Levodopa and clomiphene
citrate are usually not successful in inducing
ovulatory periods. Ergot derivatives, such as
bromocryptine (Parlodel), are now available for
the treatment of patients with hyperprolactinemia
and amenorrhea without an associated central
nervous system tumor, such as a chromophobe
adenoma. Parlodel is a dopamine agonist. The
recommended dosage of Parlodel is 2.5 mg. two or
three times daily, with meals, and the duration of
treatment should not exceed 6 months.

Trauma. Hypothalamic insufficiency secondary to trauma is treated as outlined under
Sheehan's syndrome. Induction of ovulation for
conception is treated with menotropins plus HCG.
Gonadotrophin releasing hormone is an alternate
method of ovulation induction that may obviate the
hyperstimulation syndrome. It is, however, not
clinically available at the present time.

Feminizing Ovarian Tumors

Treatment of true functioning tumors of the
ovaries must take into consideration the histologic
nature of the tumor, the patient's age, and her
reproductive desires or intentions. If surgical or
radiation castration results, then appropriate
estrogen replacement is indicated.

Increased Ovarian Androgen Secretion

Stein-Leventhal Syndrome. About 5 to 10 per
cent of these patients may present with primary
amenorrhea. However, the presence of severe
secondary oligoamenorrhea or amenorrhea is
most common. Because of the hyperestrogenic
state, adenomatous hyperplasia or carcinoma of
the endometrium in predisposed persons may
occur at an early age. Treatment consists of the
following: (1) medroxyprogesterone acetate, 10 to
20 mg. daily for 5 days every 6 to 8 weeks may be
used to oppose estrogen action and induce
periods; (2) to arrest hair growth, and especially if
contraception is desired, a combination oral contraceptive agent such as norethindrone-mestranol

---

*This dose is higher than that listed in the manufacturer's
official directive. See official directive before use.

(Ortho Novum 1/50-21) or ethynodiol-mestranol (Ovulen 21) may be used; (3) if pregnancy is desired, clomiphene, 50 to 100 mg. daily for 5 days for 4 to 6 months with or without HCG, may be tried; (4) wedge resection of the ovaries in selected patients and with clomiphene citrate failure can be considered; (5) if clomiphene citrate fails, then menotropins in selected patients and with caution may be used for infertility by a physician experienced in the use of this drug.

Ovarian Hyperthecosis and Stromal Hyperplasia. These present clinically not unlike the patient with Stein-Leventhal syndrome. The diagnosis is made histologically from sections of the ovary usually treated with wedge resection for "Stein-Leventhal syndrome." Virilization may be more pronounced. These two conditions may occur late in the patient's reproductive life. Bilateral oophorectomy may then be performed to arrest the virilization and better study the ovaries for a masculinizing ovarian tumor. Principally, treatment is as outlined for Stein-Leventhal syndrome.

Masculinizing Tumor. The comment for feminizing tumors applies to masculinizing ovarian tumors occurring during the reproductive years.

Conclusion

In concluding this discussion regarding amenorrhea perhaps a few additional comments should be made regarding ovulation induction. In the United States there are two principal drugs available for ovulation induction for patients wishing to get pregnant. Clomiphene citrate (Clomid) is an oral tablet used for anovulatory or oligo-ovulatory patients with an intact hypothalamic-pituitary-ovarian axis. The manufacturer of the drug suggests that adequate trial with Clomid should consist of one or two tablets daily (50 to 100 mg. daily) starting day 5 of the cycle for 5 days and three treatment cycles. The patient should be followed monthly for ovarian cyst formation, which is a major side effect. However, physicians experienced in the use of this drug not uncommonly may increase the dosage to as high as 150 to 200 mg. a day* for 5 to 7 days for longer periods of time. HCG, 5000 to 10,000 international units, is at times also added 5 to 7 days after discontinuing the Clomid. It should be noted that the pregnancy success rate with these higher doses and use for a longer period of time is quite low, however. The drug should be used with caution with patients with proven pelvic endometriosis.

Human menopausal gonadotrophin (Pergonal) is the second drug used, by injection, to induce ovulation for pregnancy, especially in patients in whom Clomid has failed. The dosage is controlled by the amount of total estrogen being secreted by the ovaries, determined either by blood estrogen or 24 hour urine estrogen determinations. The patient may have to be followed in the office at daily intervals. The drug is quite expensive and the side effects, although uncommon, can be more serious and for this reason should be used only by a physician experienced in the use of this drug. The incidence of multiple pregnancies with Clomid is about 1 in 20 or 5 per cent and twin pregnancies are most often seen, whereas the incidence of multiple births with Pergonal is 1 in 5 or 20 per cent. Of this 20 per cent, approximately 75 per cent are twins and about 25 per cent are triplets or other multiples. A severe side effect with Pergonal is the hyperstimulation syndrome, in which massive ovarian cysts, ascites, and pleural effusion may occur along with hypotension and oliguria or anuria. Several cases of arterial thrombosis have been reported. This, obviously, is not an innocuous drug and should be used with caution and only by physicians experienced in its use.

DYSMENORRHEA

method of
ANN B. BARNES, M.D.
Boston, Massachusetts

Dysmenorrhea is crampy lower abdominal pain associated with menstruation. The pain may radiate to the back, groin, and lower thighs following the cutaneous distribution of the sensory nerve roots shared with the reproductive organs. Malaise, nausea, less often vomiting, diarrhea, syncope, and flushing may be associated complaints. Dysmenorrhea is a complex of symptoms, not a disease.

Primary dysmenorrhea occurs during intermittent uterine contractions, which cause increased intrauterine pressure, diminished blood flow, and overall increased uterine tonus. Repeated consultations and physical examinations are needed to exclude associated pelvic pathology.

Secondary or acquired dysmenorrhea is painful menstruation associated with pelvic pathology, including uterine anomalies, imperforate hymen, endometriosis, leiomyoma uteri, particularly submucous fibroids, endometrial polyps, passage of fragments of menstrual endometrium (membranous dysmenorrhea), endometritis, cervical stenosis, adenomyosis, pelvic inflammatory disease (acute and chronic), an intrauterine device (IUD), and psychosocial reactions.

---

*This dose of clomiphene is higher than that listed in the manufacturer's official directive.

Dysmenorrhea should be distinguished by history and physical examination from gastrointestinal complaints, including constipation, colitis, regional ileitis, lactose intolerance, appendicitis, or rare disorders such as episodic Mediterranean fever. Urinary tract disease should be ruled out. Confounding reproductive tract pathology such as torsion of ovaries, tubes, or their cysts may require exclusion by laparoscopy.

The incidence of primary dysmenorrhea of sufficient severity to interfere with work performance or school attendance in the menstruating population at risk is estimated as 5 to 30 per cent. Most previous studies emphasize an onset 2 years following the menarche and a disproportionate number of teenagers. However, recent studies from Scandinavia include women in their 20s and 30s and into their 40s, suggesting that a reconsideration of the distribution problem must be considered. The individual suffering, her recurring financial and social losses, as well as the impact on society's productivity makes the treatment of dysmenorrhea of great consequence. For instance, if we recall that the female population between ages 13 and 45 in the United States is 49 million and assume 10 per cent have significant dysmenorrhea for 3 days each month, a total of over 170 million days per year are in some measure compromised by symptoms or by incapacity or both. The sales of over the counter remedies of varying effectiveness burgeon proportionately.

Knowledge of the cause of dysmenorrhea is fragmentary but advancing rapidly. Increased intrauterine pressure by a balloon, induced uterine contractions with intravenous prostaglandin F-2 alpha, and intermittent diminished uterine blood flow may each reproduce the pain of dysmenorrhea. Significantly, other women may undergo the same provocative tests without complaint. The uterine blood vessels and muscle bundles are innervated by autonomic nerves arising from the sacral nerves and hypogastric plexus. These course along the blood vessels. Additional sympathetic ganglia are found adjoining the uterus. Adrenergic, cholinergic, and dopaminergic nerves have been identified. This work on the interaction of the nervous system with the uterine contractions is an area of current research on dysmenorrhea.

Estrogen experimentally potentiates the alpha adrenergic response of short frequent uterine contractions. Progesterone experimentally following estrogen treatment reduces the number of alpha adrenergic receptor binding sites with no change in binding affinity. Consequently, uterine contractions are less frequent but of longer duration. A diurnal variation in uterine contractions may be depressed by depletion of adrenal catecholamines with reserpine or alpha adrenergic blockade such as phentolamine.

Beta-2 adrenergic agonists such as terbutaline, isoxsuprine, and fentoteral hydrobromide diminish the frequency and intensity of uterine contractions as well as relaxing uterine blood vessels.

Prostaglandins are also involved in uterine contractions and may induce dysmenorrhea-type pain. Prostaglandin F-2 alpha appears to induce contractions whereas E-2 decreases contractions; thus, not only their local presence in endometrium and myometrium is important but also their relative ratios. Prostaglandin F-2 alpha and E-2 are found increased in late secretory endometrial stages and in menstruation over levels in the proliferative and early secretory stages. However to date, imbalances in dysmenorrheic as opposed to normal women have not been substantiated. Beta-2 adrenergic stimulation appears to inhibit the contracting action of prostaglandins, indicating the complex interactions of local prostaglandin and the state of the sympathetic nervous system. Birth control pills diminish synthesis of prostaglandin.

Treatment of Primary Dysmenorrhea

As in the treatment of all symptoms, a placebo effect may be expected in as much as one third of patients. The physician's attentiveness, empathy, and attitude towards the patient and her complaint will substantially facilitate relief. Simply ruling out pelvic pathology or defining a benign cause may be sufficient encouragement to permit the patient to accept some discomfort without resorting to a chronic regimen of costly medication. Alternately, local heat in the form of heating pads or baths may provide relief.

Hot tea, coffee, or cocoa with or without ethanol-containing beverages and nonprescription remedies such as Vanquish or Midol may contain sufficient caffeine, theobromine and theophylline, which are vasodilators, diuretics, and smooth muscle relaxants through their beta sympathomimetic action, to bring adequate relief. In general, the side effects of nonprescription remedies are sufficiently less than those of prescribed drugs and are preferred.

Beta Sympathomimetic Agents. Terbutaline and isoxsuprine and fentoterol hydrobromide have been shown to relieve dysmenorrhea but are unacceptable to patients because they induce tremor and palpitations; they have not been officially approved for this use.

Progesterone, either as medroxyprogesterone acetate (Provera), 10 mg. by mouth daily on days 21 through 26 of the menstrual cycle, or as dydrogesterone (Duphaston), 10 to 20 mg. in divided doses daily from day 15 through 25 of the cycle, may bring relief to many patients without effect on ovulation (this use of these two agents is not listed in the manufacturers' official directives). Progesterone's action is probably on a pharmacologic as well as a placebo basis. For patients suffering migraine as well as for those with a familial predisposition to diabetes mellitus, hypertension, coagulation defects, and history of genital tract cancer, progesterone alone may be preferable to the birth control pill.

Birth control pills provide the most frequent, prompt, and prolonged relief. No particular combination or brand has been shown to be superior over any other. Their effect on teenage growth and development is not understood. Older patients who smoke a package of cigarettes daily will be placed at markedly increased risks for cardiovascular complications.

Analgesics, often combined with aspirin, are frequently offered to patients; however, they may interfere as much with the patient's work, studying, or driving as the symptoms themselves.

Anti-inflammatory agents such as aspirin and indomethacin, which interfere with the synthesis of prostaglandin, help some patients. Aspirin is taken as 600 mg. every four hours for 1 to 2 days. Indomethacin (Indocin), 25 mg. by mouth four times a day, is most effective if started 3 to 8 days prior to menses and continued through the second day of menstruation (this use of indomethacin is not listed in the manufacturer's official directive). Epigastric distress frequently makes either agent unacceptable. Most gastrointestinal diseases are specific contraindications.

Flufenamate inhibits prostaglandin synthesis and its binding to cells. It has been shown to be effective in clinical trials in Europe but is not presently available in the United States.

Acupuncture may provide relief for some patients, although double blind trials proving its efficacy are not available.

Surgical. Presacral neurectomy and uterine suspensions have no proven efficacy beyond that of a placebo. Their risk and cost cannot justify their use.

Psychotherapy per se has no substantiated effect; however, some patients complain of dysmenorrhea in association with familial conflicts such as parental adolescent interchange. Counseling at a variety of levels by a social worker, psychologist, or psychiatrist, may relieve the overall situations sufficiently as to diminish the specific complaint.

Treatment of Secondary Dysmenorrhea

Secondary dysmenorrhea generally responds to appropriate treatment of the underlying pathology. This holds true for dysmenorrhea of psychosocial origin, as stated earlier. Attempting to identify underlying causes and supporting the patient's efforts to minimize them may be helpful. When treatment of underlying pathology is not feasible, such as when an indicated hysterectomy is refused by a patient wishing to retain her childbearing potential, treatment regimens for primary dysmenorrhea may be selected, with due consideration of its effect on the underlying disease. Lesser operations, such as the removal of endometriomas or release of pelvic adhesions, may be combined with the treatment of primary dysmenorrhea to provide relief as well.

MENOPAUSE

method of
JOHN G. DALEY, M.D.
Wilmington, North Carolina

The human female enters menstrual life with a limited number of ova contained in her ovaries. Eventually, the number of developing graafian follicles diminishes to a number incapable of secreting sufficient estrogen to generate endometrial proliferation. The resulting cessation of menstrual life is referred to as the menopause. The ovaries continue to secrete estrogen, or androgen, which may be converted to estrogen in peripheral tissues, for some time after menstrual cessation.

The menopause problem is a phenomenon peculiar to this century and is, in part, iatrogenic, as the influence of medical science through the years has resulted in increasing life expectancy, and women now live long enough to experience not only the menopause, but also its most serious complications of osteoporosis and bone fractures. The menopause results from a hormonal deficiency and, like other endocrine deficiencies, should be treated with replacement.

The use of estrogen for menopausal patients has recently become a matter of controversy. Great concern has been generated by recent reports suggesting a possible relationship between estrogen therapy for the menopausal patient and endometrial carcinoma. These data have had a profound effect on attitudes about estrogen replacement. Patients have been frightened by conclusions drawn in the lay literature. Even those patients who require estrogen for their metabolic needs are reluctant to use it. Some gynecologists have abandoned estrogen therapy, while others have liberalized their indications for hysterectomy as a preventative measure in premenopausal patients. These kinds of decisions seem unjustified. The data thus far presented are inconclusive and only confirm the concept that prolonged, excessive use of unopposed estrogen may lead to endometrial hyperplasia, and, in predisposed women, to adenocarcinoma. Inappropriate use of the estrogen is to be condemned, but estrogen still has a place in the care of the menopausal female.

Multiple psychosocial events often occur in the lives of middle-aged women, causing emotional reactions that may confuse and compound the menopausal syndrome. Unfortunately, many menstruating women have estrogen prescribed unnecessarily in an attempt to alleviate these symptoms. Other women, at this stage of life, become very concerned with their body image and undertake restrictive diets. Consequent symptoms of hypoglycemia are frequently misinterpreted as the menopausal onset, despite continuing regular menses. Hypertension, hypothyroidism, and side reactions from certain drugs are other conditions frequently misdiagnosed as early menopause. Although it is true that the gonadotropins, particularly the follicle-stimulating hormone (FSH), begin to rise prior to the cessation of menses, persistent menstruation attests to the fact that there remains sufficient endogenous estrogen to stimulate endometrial growth. Estrogen replacement therapy should be reserved strictly for deficiency states. To determine deficiency, the female vagina offers several opportunities to "bioassay" the endogenous estrogen level. The condition of the vaginal epithelium, the clarity and amount of cervical mucus, and the percentage of superficial cells in a hormone cytology smear are useful methods of evaluating estrogen levels.

The menopausal syndrome is well tolerated by most women, but others are incapacitated by hot flashes, night sweats, or dyspareunia. Although other drugs are available or are under investigation for control of these symptoms, estrogen replacement for this deficiency syndrome is the best method of therapy currently available. Even women who require little support for their symptomatology may require estrogen for their metabolic needs. As the life expectancy of women lengthens, larger numbers of patients are experiencing osteoporosis and serious bone fractures in their later life. Some of these women will die from complications of their fracture and most others will live as invalids the remainder of their lives. Estrogen therapy can prevent this sequence of events. Postmenopausal females whose vaginal analysis indicates an estrogen deficiency should be on small doses of estrogen to maintain these metabolic needs. The dose of estrogen must be individualized for each patient, and should be the smallest dose necessary to meet her need.

Therapy

Climacteric (Perimenopause). Despite increasing availability of health education material, most women are ignorant of the nature and significance of the menopause. With education, reassurance, and some psychotherapeutic support, this period of life can be endured by most women with little difficulty. During this phase there is usually sufficient endogenous estrogen and replacement is rarely necessary. However, some patients with prolonged intervals between menses may need estrogen support for their menopausal symptoms. In this case, 0.625 mg. of estrone sulfate (ES) each day for 21 days will usually suffice. During the last 7 days of the 21-day therapeutic period, medroxyprogesterone acetate (MPA), 10 mg., is added to the estrogen regimen so that the effect of both hormones ends simultaneously. The progestogen is added to assure complete and concise menstrual withdrawal. Following a week of no therapy, during which time menses begins, the patient resumes the estrogen-progestogen cyclic therapy. Eventually, with the decreasing endogenous source of estrogen, there will be insufficient stimulus for endometrial growth and the patient will become menopausal (see menopause below). In some patients prolonged intervals can be followed by very heavy menses. Endometrial biopsies in some patients may demonstrate endometrial hyperplasia. Patients without this diagnosis can be managed by medroxyprogesterone acetate, 10 mg. each day for the first 7 days of each month. After 3 months, the drug is stopped. If hypermenorrhea resumes, the drug is reinstituted and continued until the patient no longer experiences withdrawal menses. Should the medroxyprogesterone acetate fail to result in normal withdrawal menstrual flow, the patient should be evaluated with an examination under anesthesia and a dilatation and curettage.

Another disturbing manifestation of this period of menstrual life is the frequent, prolonged, and occasionally heavy menses. This bleeding pattern may not be entirely an endocrine abnormality. Hypertension, uterine descensus, bleeding diathesis, or uterine pathology may be contributing causes. In this age group uterine carcinoma may be manifesting with frequent and irregular bleeding. Thus, colposcopy-directed biopsies, fractional curettage or evaluation for these other conditions would be in order. If the recurrent bleeding pattern persists after the dilatation and curettage (D and C), the patient should be treated with estrone sulfate, 2.5 mg. each day for 21 days, with medroxyprogesterone acetate, 10 mg., added during the last 7 days of the 21-day cycle so that both hormones end simultaneously. After a 1-week interval, during which the patient should have a normal withdrawal menses, the estrone sulfate–medroxyprogesterone cyclic therapy is repeated. The rather large dose of estrone sulfate is used to eliminate possible breakthrough bleeding. These cycles are continued for 5 months. The results of therapy can be evaluated by assessing the character of the spontaneous menses during the sixth month. If, after the first course of therapy, the frequent, hypermenorrheic pattern continues, the therapy is reestablished for another 5 months. Eventually, the patient's endogenous source of estrogen will diminish and she will become amenorrheic, at which time therapy is discontinued.

Menopause. Patients suffering from symptoms directly related to the menopause, i.e., hot flashes and flushes, sweats, and dyspareunia, will require estrogen replacement. The goal of estrogen therapy is to find the dose that will relieve the symptoms without stimulating endometrial growth, an achievable goal in most patients. The vagina, serving as a "bioassay," is the key for diagnosing estrogen deficiency and for monitoring estrogen replacement. The patient is started on 0.3 or 0.625 mg. of estrone sulfate each day except the first 5 days of the month. Some patients will require higher doses of estrogen to control symptoms, and menstrual withdrawal will be necessary (see below). However, with time the dosage may be reduced. Monthly interruption of estrogen therapy has traditionally been done on the assumption that bleeding will occur if the endometrium is being stimulated. However, the technique is unreliable. Patients who do break through during this nontherapeutic interval may already have developed endometrial hyperplasia through preceding cycles. The vaginal hormonal cytology smear is useful in these patients. If the karyopyknotic index can be maintained below 15 per cent, there is little likelihood of endometrial growth. As a crosscheck, the patient is asked to take medroxyprogesterone acetate, 10 mg., along with the estrone sulfate during the last 7 days of the month every 4 months, so that the effect of both hormones ends simultaneously. If no endometrium has developed, no withdrawal flow will take place. If menses does occur following the medroxyprogesterone acetate therapy, the dose of estrogen should be reduced if possible (see below). After 2 or 3 years of therapy, the estrogen may be discontinued as a trial to determine if the patient's menopausal symptoms without therapy have reduced to a tolerable level. A clue that an improved symptom tolerance has been achieved is the absence of symptoms during the first of the month when the patient is without estrogen therapy. If, after the discontinuation of estrogen, unbearable symptoms recur, the therapy is resumed and discontinued in trial fashion yearly thereafter. Some women will require estrogen supplement for severe symptoms throughout life.

Once estrogen is discontinued and menopause symptoms are minimal, the condition of the vagina must be observed continually for evidence of vaginal atrophy. Some women will continue to have sufficient endogenous estrogen for their metabolic needs, but the majority will have to resume low-dose estrogen therapy to maintain proper protein metabolism and to prevent calcium loss. These patients should also receive semiannual progestational therapy as a test for endometrial build-up.

Occasionally, even the smallest dose of estrogen necessary to control symptoms will stimulate endometrial growth. In these patients, medroxyprogesterone acetate must be added to the cyclic regimen the last 7 days of each month. With time, these patients may also be removed from their estrogen therapy, as their symptomatology becomes less severe. Unfortunately, some may require continued low dose therapy for their metabolic needs. Combined estrogen-androgen therapy may be beneficial in this situation. However, in some patients, the choice is between discontinuing therapy and risking future bone fracture with all of its attendant complications or continued menstrual withdrawal into later years. For these patients, any change in the character of the withdrawal flow or any bleeding between menses must be investigated.

Although other estrogen substances of comparable dose can be used in place of estrone sulfate, this estrogen is preferred because it is well tolerated, readily enters into enterohepatic circulation, has a physiologic half life, has less effect on clotting mechanisms, and is promptly cleared by the kidneys. A 21 carbon progestogen is preferred because it does not manifest an antiestrogen effect on liver protein synthesis. Oral contraceptives should be avoided because of their potential hazard for patients in this age group.

VULVOVAGINITIS

method of
EDUARD G. FRIEDRICH, JR., M.D.
Milwaukee, Wisconsin

The term vulvovaginitis implies a combined infection of the vulva and vagina by a single causative agent. However, except for candidiasis and herpes infections, this is an unusual occurrence. Most instances of combined inflammation represent primary infections of the vagina with secondary irritation of the vulvar tissues by the vaginal discharge. This latter condition is more appropriately termed "reactive vulvitis" and may be seen with a variety of vaginal infections. The proper management of the vaginal condition results in disappearance of the vulvar irritation. Topical corticosteroid preparations applied to the introitus and lower labia will accelerate this response. Hydrocortisone 1 per cent with iodochlorhydroxyquin (Vioform) 3 per cent

TABLE 1. **Vulvovaginitis**

	CANDIDA	TRICHOMONAS	ATROPHY	HEMOPHILUS
Complaint	Pruritus	Discharge	Bleeding	Odor
pH	4 to 5	5 to 7	6 to 7	5 to 6
Discharge	Thick, cheesy	Thin, copious	Scanty, purulent	Gray, creamy
Wet smear	Hyphae (KOH)	Motile protozoa	WBC, parabasals	Clue cells

From Friedrich, E. G. Jr.: *Vulvar Disease*. W. B. Saunders Co., 1976.

cream is particularly effective for this purpose when applied to the vulva twice daily for 10 days.

It is the primary vaginal infection to which specific diagnostic and therapeutic steps must be applied. The exact nature of the vaginitis must be determined prior to any attempt at therapy. Most cases of "stubborn" or "resistant" infections are simply instances of misdiagnosis or result from the lack of any diagnostic attempt. Every case of vaginitis has a specific cause, and most can be quickly categorized by observation of the patient's complaint, the character of the discharge, analysis of the vaginal pH with a strip of indicator paper, and the wet smear findings (Table 1).

Once the causative agent is determined, therapy can then be specifically directed. In order of their frequency, the common primary vaginal infections include those due to *Candida, Trichomonas,* atrophic conditions, *Hemophilus,* and herpes simplex virus.

Candida

When the pH is in the low physiologic range and budding hyphae are seen on the KOH smear, the diagnosis of candidiasis is made. The vaginal walls are inflamed and a three-dimensional cheesy discharge is often present. If the vulva is involved, it is similarly reddened and covered with a fine gray sheen. This infection represents the most common form of vaginitis. The primary treatment of *Candida* infections of the vagina consists in:

1. Removal of as much of the pasty white discharge as possible.

2. Thorough painting of the entire vaginal surface with a 1 per cent aqueous solution of gentian violet. If the external vulvar tissues are also involved, these are painted in a similar fashion. Care is taken to absorb any excess dye and the hazards of fabric staining are explained to the patient.

3. Coitus is prohibited.

4. A fungicidal cream, one applicator full, is deposited in the vagina at bedtime. Miconazole nitrate (Monistat) and clotrimazole (Lotrimin) both seem to give excellent results. The patient is seen again after 1 week, and if the infection remains, the same treatment is repeated. Rarely are more than 2 such courses of treatment necessary.

Recurrent *Candida* infections require further investigation. Patients with subclinical diabetes mellitus may often present initially with vulvovaginal candidiasis and such patients should have a glucose tolerance test done. Poor hygiene habits, especially wiping the anus from the back to front after defecation, transfer organisms from the anal canal to the vagina and are responsible for many candidal infections. The population of *Candida* in the intestinal tract can be decreased by the use of oral nystatin tablets, 500,000 units three times daily for two weeks. The coital partner may sometimes harbor the same fungus on the penile skin. Five per cent boric acid in lanolin (Borofax) is an excellent topical candidicide for use on the penis in such cases. Finally, many patients relate that their recurrences coincide with a specific time in the menstrual cycle or are related to coital activity. To diminish the frequency of such recurrences, a 1-pint retention douche of 3 per cent potassium sorbate N.F., after intercourse or nightly for 1 week during the cycle phase in which they find the infection is most likely to recur, can be extremely effective.

Trichomonas

Trichomonads thrive in a basic pH and produce a copious, often foamy discharge. The Papanicolaou smear alone is an unreliable indicator of infection but the finding of motile protozoa on a saline wet smear is diagnostic. Treatment consists of:

1. Metronidazole, given orally to both partners, 250 mg. three times daily for seven consecutive days. Because of an Antabuse-like effect noted in some patients, alcohol ingestion should be warned against and for this same reason, patient compliance with a 7-day schedule involving a weekend, is often less than ideal. Alternate regimens shown to have equal effectiveness include 500 mg. twice daily for five days or a single dose of 2 grams. These latter schedules however lack current Food and Drug Administration approval.

2. Metronidazole is contraindicated in the first trimester of pregnancy and during lactation, and at these times trichomonas infections may be successfully treated with hypertonic saline douches (1 cup of table salt to 4 cups of water),

twice daily for five days. The douche pressure should be controlled by having the bag no higher than shoulder height when in a sitting position. Positive pressure douche apparatus should not be used for this purpose.

Trichomonas infections are considered to be sexually transmitted, and when the initial diagnosis is made, an endocervical culture should be taken to rule out concomitant gonorrhea.

Atrophic Conditions

Whenever the maturation of vaginal squamous epithelium is compromised because of the relative lack of estrogen, there will be a concomitant decrease in available glycogen substrate for normal flora. In these situations, pathogenic bacteria may gain control and result in bacterial vaginitis. Such conditions exist in premenarchal children, in women on oral contraceptives, during pregnancy and lactation, and also in the postmenopausal decades. Oral estrogen replacement does not always prevent the development of atrophic vaginitis. The saline wet smear of the scanty purulent discharge will often show copious white blood cells mixed with parabasal vaginal epithelial cells. The key to therapy for such cases consists in topical estrogen application:

1. During the first 2 weeks, a sulfa-containing estrogen cream should be used. AVC with dienestrol (AVC/Dienestrol) offers these two drugs in combination.

2. Thereafter, a weekly application of an estrogen-only preparation will prevent a recurrence of the condition.

In children, however, it is not necessary to continue prophylactic estrogen. Fragments of toilet paper contaminated with feces and other bits of foreign matter that gain entrance to the vagina are usually the inciting cause in the pediatric age group, and hygienic education is the best form of prevention.

Hemophilus

Hemophilus vaginalis vaginitis is a distinct entity, although the causative bacteria has yet to be taxonomically classified. Vaginal infection by the organism is usually a sexually-transmitted disease, resulting in a creamy gray-white discharge, which is often malodorous. Vaginal squames with adherent surface organisms, "clue cells," are frequently noted in the wet smear, and the vaginal pH is usually between 5 and 6. Ideally, both partners should be treated. The approaches to therapy available are:

1. Cephradine, 500 mg. four times daily for 6 days.

2. Alternatively, metronidazole 500 mg. twice daily for 7 days has been shown to be highly effective but lacks current Food and Drug Administration approval.

3. Although not as effective as the above choices, ampicillin, 500 mg. four times daily for 5 days, may be of benefit to some patients.

Herpes Simplex

The type II variety of herpes simplex virus is the cause of an increasingly common sexually-transmitted disease than often results in combined vulvovaginitis. The primary infection is characterized by diffuse painful coalescent ulcerations of the vulva with fever, lymphadenopathy, and malaise. The vagina may appear grossly normal or else show some reddening accompanied by a seropurulent discharge. Papanicolaou's smear of the vagina and contact cytosmear of the vulvar ulcerations will demonstrate the cytopathic effect of the virus and confirm the clinical diagnosis. If viral cultures are available these should be performed instead. Recurrent attacks may develop in some patients, but these lack constitutional symptoms and are generally confined to small areas of the vulvar skin.

The treatment of herpes infections is directed toward:

1. Relief of pain with oral analgesics.

2. Prevention of surface viral spread and secondary bacterial infection with topical applications of 10 per cent povidone-iodine solution (Betadine).

3. Promotion of healing with wet compresses of 1:40 Burow's solution; or three times daily applications of 1 per cent hydrocortisone with 3 per cent iodochlorhydroxyquin (Vioform) cream for 1 week.

Vaginal and cervical involvement can be treated with povidone-iodine (Betadine) douches twice daily and nightly applications of povidone-iodine (Betadine) vaginal gel.

Primary infection may last beyond 10 days, but recurrent episodes are generally gone within 1 week. No therapy has been successful in preventing recurrences. If the infection is noted during pregnancy, then frequent Papanicolaou's smears or viral cultures of the vagina and cervix are indicated to monitor the presence of continued virus. If obvious lesions or positive cytologic smears or cultures are present at the time of delivery, cesarean section is indicated, provided the membranes have not been ruptured for over 4 hours, to prevent transmission of the virus to the newborn with the resultant risks of morbidity and mortality.

Other Causes

Less frequent causes of vaginitis include foreign body infections, i.e., the forgotten tampon, salivary and allergic vaginitis, and the unusual desquamative vaginitis in which the epithelium is sloughed despite an apparently normal hormonal milieu. Anaerobic colonization of a forgotton tampon usually results in a malodorous purulent discharge. Removal of the tampon followed by a rinse of the vagina with a one half strength hydrogen peroxide solution is curative. The patient with salivary vulvovaginitis may have to decrease or discontinue oral-genital sexual practices, while those who have become allergic to semen will benefit from the use of a condom. If fertility is desired, such patients may obtain some relief from diphenhydramine hydrochloride (Benadryl), 50 mg., prior to intercourse. Desquamative vaginitis will often respond to the treatment recommended for atrophic conditions. Even though the hormonal pattern appears normal, topical estrogen preparations with or without sulfa drugs can be of distinct benefit in this condition if continued on a daily basis for 2 to 3 weeks.

Finally, there remains a group of patients with distinct complaints of burning and dyspareunia, discharge, and malodor, who, on physical examination, show no evidence of vaginal infection. Such patients may be suffering from psychosomatic vulvovaginitis, and their symptoms may represent an unconscious defense mechanism used to avoid coitus. In such patients, any form of therapy simply reinforces the patient's problem and delays successful therapy, which consists in sympathetic psychiatric counseling.

Every patient with vulvovaginitis deserves a thorough and thoughtful diagnostic evaluation. Only then can specific and effective therapy be instituted.

PELVIC INFLAMMATORY DISEASE

method of
PHILIP B. MEAD, M.D.
Burlington, Vermont

Inflammation of the female pelvic viscera may result from venereal (exogenous) infections, and may follow intrauterine device (IUD) insertion, obstetrical delivery, abortion, or gynecologic surgery (endogenous infections). Such infections can be manifested pathologically as salpingitis, tubo-ovarian abscess, pelvic abscess, pelvic cellulitis, endomyometritis, or septic pelvic thrombophlebitis. Bacteriologically, these infections are caused by *Neisseria gonorrhea*, group A beta hemolytic streptococci (community-acquired infections); or by organisms present in the normal cervical-vaginal flora (gram-negative enteric bacilli, enterococci, and anaerobes including *Bacteroides fragilis*) acting as primary or secondary invaders.

Uncomplicated (Lower Tract) Gonorrhea

1. Diagnosis of endocervical gonorrhea is made by Thayer-Martin cultures. Gram stained smears are unreliable in females. Although as many as 80 per cent of women with positive endocervical cultures for gonorrhea will have symptoms referrable to this infection, these symptoms are usually too nonspecific to be of aid in the diagnosis.

2. Patients with positive cultures should be treated with aqueous procaine penicillin G, 4.8 million units intramuscularly, divided into two doses and injected at different sites during one visit, together with 1 gram of probenecid by mouth just before the injections. Alternative regimens (not as effective), include ampicillin, 3.5 grams, and probenecid, 1 gram by mouth, given at the same time; or tetracycline hydrochloride, 1.5 grams by mouth followed by 0.5 grams by mouth four times per day for 4 days, for a total dose of 9.5 grams.

3. Penicillin-allergic patients with lower tract gonorrhea can be treated with tetracycline, or with spectinomycin, 2 grams intramuscularly in one injection. Pregnant, penicillin-allergic patients should be treated with erythromycin, 1.5 grams by mouth followed by 0.5 grams four times daily for 4 days since tetracycline is contraindicated in pregnancy and spectinomycin has not been proved safe. This regimen is only about 75 per cent effective.

4. Follow-up endocervical and other appropriate cultures should be obtained from women 3 to 14 days after completion of treatment.

5. Treatment failures usually represent reinfections, but are occasionally due to antibiotic resistance. Penicillinase-producing strains of *Neisseria gonorrhea* are rarely found in the United States, but are being isolated in increasing number from other countries. Patients shown to have penicillinase-producing strains of *Neisseria gonorrhea,* or those who fail on an initial regimen of either procaine penicillin G, tetracycline, or ampicillin should be retreated with spectinomycin intramuscularly in a single dose of 2 grams.

6. Women with known recent exposure to gonorrhea should receive the same treatment as those with gonorrhea, regardless of culture results. The sexual partners of all patients with culture-proved gonorrhea should be traced and appropriate cultures obtained.

7. A reagin test for syphilis should be performed at the time of treatment for lower tract

gonorrhea and if therapy other than procaine penicillin was used, it should be repeated in 3 months.

Acute Salpingitis

Salpingitis will develop in 10 to 17 per cent of patients with untreated endocervical gonorrhea. Acute salpingitis can also occur coincident with intrauterine device (IUD) usage and as a reexacerbation of a previous gonorrheal salpingitis. Approximately 50 per cent of acute salpingitis is gonorrheal, and the remainder (nongonococcal salpingitis) is a polymicrobial infection caused by gram-negative enteric bacilli, anaerobes, Chlamydia and enterococci.

1. Endocervical cultures for *Neisseria gonorrhea* should be obtained from all patients presenting with acute salpingitis.

2. Hospitalization should be strongly considered for women with an adnexal mass suggestive of an abscess, temperature greater than 38°C. (100.5°F.), patients unable to take oral medications, in the presence of upper abdominal peritoneal signs, when diagnosis is uncertain, in those who fail to respond to outpatient therapy, and for the rare pregnant patient. Some authorities believe that all patients with acute salpingitis should be hospitalized.

3. The following regimens have been found to be adequate for gonococcal salpingitis in outpatients: 1.5 grams of tetracycline hydrochloride given as a single oral dose followed by 500 mg. orally four times daily for 10 days.

Aqueous procaine penicillin G, 4.8 million units intramuscularly divided into at least two doses and injected at different sites at one visit, or 3.5 grams of oral ampicillin. One gram of oral probenecid is given along with either penicillin or ampicillin, and both are followed by 500 mg. of ampicillin, taken orally, four times a day for 10 days.

4. For hospitalized patients: aqueous crystalline penicillin G, 20 million units intravenously daily, or ampicillin, 1 to 2 grams intravenously every 4 hours, until clear-cut improvement occurs, followed by 500 mg. ampicillin taken orally four times a day to complete 10 days of therapy. Since it is not possible to distinguish gonococcal from nongonococcal salpingitis clinically, many physicians add an aminoglycoside (gentamicin 3 to 5 mg. per kg. intramuscularly daily in three divided doses), or antibiotics effective against *Bacteroides fragilis* (clindamycin, chloramphenicol or carbenicillin).

For penicillin-allergic patients use doxycycline, 200 mg. by intravenous Soluset immediately followed by 100 mg. intravenously every 12 hours until improvement occurs, then the patient can be changed to oral doxycycline, 100 mg. twice daily (this regimen should not be used in pregnancy).

5. Patients treated for acute salpingitis should receive a follow-up culture for *Neisseria gonorrhea*, as well as a follow-up serologic test for syphilis if therapy other than penicillin was used.

Pelvic Abscess

Pelvic abscess may arise as the sequela of gonorrheal or nongonorrheal tubal infection, after puerperal infections, secondary to disease of other pelvic organs (appendiceal abscess or diverticular abscess), as a complication of pelvic surgery or in association with infections related to the intrauterine device. Again, gram-negative enteric bacilli, enterococci, and anaerobes are the causative organisms, with anaerobes (particularly *Bacteroides fragilis*) the most common isolates.

1. If there is uncertainty as to the diagnosis or a suspicion of rupture, the patient should immediately undergo exploratory laparotomy. Other patients can be managed expectantly.

2. Along with general supportive and diagnostic measures, antibiotic therapy should include coverage for gram-negative enteric bacilli and anaerobic organisms. We prefer a regimen of clindamycin, 600 mg. intravenously by Soluset every 6 hours, and gentamicin, 3 to 5 mg. per kg. per day in three divided doses, injected intramuscularly. Alternative regimens include penicillin, 20 to 30 million units per day, or ampicillin, 1 to 2 grams intravenously every 4 hours, together with chloramphenicol, 1 gram intravenously every 6 hours; or carbenicillin, 24 to 30 grams intravenously, daily, given in four or six divided doses.

3. For patients being managed expectantly, colpotomy drainage is performed when technically feasible. Absolute prerequisites include that the mass be fluctuant, that it adhere to the pelvic peritoneum and that it dissect into the midline of the upper one third of the rectovaginal septum.

4. If the patient remains refractory to medical management, as evidenced by persistence of fever or an increase in the size of the abscess during the first 48 to 72 hours, then surgery is performed. If there is a favorable response during the waiting period, no change in therapy is judged to be indicated.

5. For the patient for whom surgery is indicated, a total abdominal hysterectomy, bilateral salpingo-oophorectomy, and careful exploration of the peritoneal cavity to locate and break up any purulent collections are advocated.

Intrauterine Device–Associated Infection

Patients using an intrauterine contraceptive device (IUD) have approximately a four-fold increased risk of developing pelvic inflammatory disease. Young women, nulliparous women, and patients with multiple sexual partners seem to be more likely to develop such infections. An endomyometritis is the most common infection, but all degrees of pelvic sepsis, including pelvic abscess, may be encountered.

1. Patients using IUDs should be aware of the prodromata of IUD-associated pelvic infection: dyspareunia, foul vaginal discharge, and metrorrhagia.

2. Patients suspected of having a mild endometritis can be treated on an outpatient basis with tetracycline hydrochloride, 500 mg. four times a day for 10 days, or ampicillin, 500 mg. orally four times a day for 10 days. The intrauterine device should be removed on the second day of therapy.

3. Follow-up pelvic examination is important to prove adequacy of response.

4. More severe forms of IUD-associated pelvic infection should be dealt with as described under Acute Salpingitis and Pelvic Abscess.

Pelvic Infection Following Gynecologic Surgery

Management of the febrile postoperative patient with a suspected pelvic infection is carried out as follows:

1. The presence of a fluctuant pelvic mass at the top of the vaginal vault suggests a cuff abscess. Transvaginal drainage is performed with aerobic and anaerobic cultures taken from this pus. Systemic antibiotics (ampicillin alone, ampicillin plus an aminoglycoside, or clindamycin plus gentamicin) are prescribed.

2. If pelvic examination reveals diffuse induration without a fluctuant mass, a diagnosis of pelvic cellulitis is made. Aerobic and anaerobic blood cultures are obtained, but in this situation vaginal cultures are of no value, since one is unable to obtain a meaningful and adequate specimen. Treatment consists of systemic antibiotics as described earlier.

3. In the patient with suspected pelvic cellulitis who fails to respond to appropriate antibiotic therapy, one must exclude the presence of an undrained abscess (either wound or operative site), or the development of septic pelvic thrombophlebitis. Use of ultrasonography, pelvic examination, and even examination under anesthesia will aid in the diagnosis of an undrained abscess. Appropriate surgical drainage is indicated.

4. If the patient with suspected pelvic cellulitis remains febrile despite appropriate antibiotic therapy, and an abscess cannot be demonstrated, one must be concerned as to the existence of septic pelvic thrombophlebitis. Such patients will often appear quite well despite the persistence of a hectic fever curve. A plateaulike tachycardia,

signs or symptoms of pulmonary embolization, and the presence of an ileus are additional suggestive clues. These patients should be treated with full heparinization (approximately 100 units per kg. intravenously every 4 hours or continuous infusion of approximately 1000 units per hour); if defervescence does not occur within 48 to 72 hours a diagnosis of septic pelvic thrombophlebitis is unlikely. If rapid defervescence does occur one can be sure in the diagnosis and should continue heparinization for 7 to 10 days. If pulmonary embolization has not been documented, it is probably unnecessary to maintain these patients on long-term oral anticoagulants.

UTERINE MYOMAS
method of
WALTER G. SAUNDERS, M.D.
Sheridan, Wyoming

Uterine myomas (also called fibroids) are benign smooth muscle neoplasia occurring predominantly in the uterine corpus. They are present in somewhat more than 20 per cent of women past age 35. Most are asymptomatic. Their malignancy potential is extremely low (less than 1 per cent). Myomas may grow rapidly and achieve astounding size. Frequently, they involute in menopause. Even the most skilled examiner may be confused in differentiating between adnexal disease and subserous myomas.

Complications and Management

As noted, most myomas are small (uterine size less than 12 weeks) and asymptomatic. Regardless of age, these patients should be followed more frequently, the size and interval growth of the myomas accurately documented and the patient informed as to (1) their presence, (2) size or change in size, and (3) benign condition. This provides the patient with an informed base, protects her from the overzealous surgeon, and is helpful when seeing a patient for the first time should she have attained this information from a previous physician. Patients should be screened for coexisting cervical, endometrial, or ovarian disease, which should be eliminated prior to definitive surgical therapy for myomas.

Abnormal bleeding (usually in the form of menorrhagia) is one of the most common complications of myomas. Submucous myomas are frequently the cause. They may be diagnosed by hysteroscopy or hysterography, but are best documented during fractional curettage, which has the added advantage of determining malignant disease of the endometrium and endocervix. Submucous myomas rarely respond to surgical or medical therapy short of hysterectomy. Abnormal bleeding in a myomatous uterus without submucous myomas may respond favorably to curettage or medical manipulation of the endometrium to produce more regular and less voluminous shedding.

Infarction or *torsion* are other complications associated with uterine myomas. Infarctions of intramural myomas may usually be handled conservatively, with analgesics, bed rest, and possibly antibiotics. Torsion of pedunculated myomas, though rare, may require celiotomy and myomectomy.

Pedunculated submucous myomas sometimes *prolapse* through the cervix. These complicated cases present with anemia from the menometrorrhagia, pain, and endometritis. It is preferred to stage the therapy if possible by:

1. Removing the myoma (by twisting or snaring) if possible.

2. A thorough curettage of the base and endometrial cavity.

3. Treating the attendant endometritis with broad-spectrum antibiotics (ampicillin or cephalosporins) and continuing the treatment for 5 to 10 days following curettage.

4. Medroxyprogesterone acetate (Depo-Provera) (150 to 200 mg. intramuscularly) may inhibit uterine bleeding for 4 to 6 weeks until hysterectomy can be performed at a less morbid time for the patient.

5. The magnitude of anemia sometimes necessitates transfusion.

Obstruction of nongenital structures occurs rarely until myomas are at least 14 to 16 weeks size. Ureters may be displaced in any direction and must be carefully sought during surgery. A preoperative intravenous pyelogram (IVP) is advised. Myomas attaining a size beyond 12 weeks are best treated by hysterectomy.

Myomatous complications of pregnancy range from conservatively treated infarction to pelvic dystocias from large cervical myomas to dysfunctional labors. These uncommon but dramatic complications may lead to operative delivery. *Myomectomy at cesarean section is not advised* because of the attendant hemorrhage. Myomectomies are occasionally performed in the infertile patient. If the surgery is extensive or the endometrial cavity is violated or both during myomectomy, subsequent pregnancies should best be handled by section.

Iatrogenic complications of uterine myomas are those produced by the injudicious usage of contraceptive steroids or exogenous estrogen. Myomas frequently grow when nurtured by estrogen. Such growth may produce any of the previously mentioned complications. It is suggested that alternate forms of contraception or treatment for menopausal symptoms be instituted in the patient with documented myomas.

Surgery. Surgery in the form of hysterectomy is definitive therapy for most complications of uterine myomas. It is *not* indicated for the asymptomatic patient with a small uterus. Prior to hysterectomy a recent cervical cytology is mandatory. Assessment of the endometrium is likewise necessary in the face of altered bleeding coincident with or secondary to myomas. An intravenous pyelogram (IVP) or barium enema may be extremely helpful in eliminating nongynecologic pelvic disease prior to surgery. Surgery is likewise *mandatory* if (1) the differentiation between any sized myoma and an enlarged ovary cannot be made, (2) previously quiescent myomas seem to be growing, (3) these criteria, while important at any age, *apply especially to postmenopausal women.* The choice of sugical approach depends upon the size of the myomas and particular skills of the surgeon. Large uterii are best removed abdominally and simultaneous plastic procedures can then be performed from below if indicated by physical examination.

UTERINE CANCER

method of
HENRY C. McDUFF, M.D.,
and ALAN D. STEINFELD, M.D.
Providence, Rhode Island

Uterine cancers present a continuing challenge to the physician on many fronts.

Cervical carcinoma can be easily and reliably diagnosed in its earliest stages through the use of the Papanicolaou smear, but there remains some reluctance on the part of many women to submit to this fast and safe screening test. The patient and physician thereby lose valuable time and an opportunity to diagnose and treat this disease in a highly curable stage. At the other end of the spectrum are advanced cancers of the uterus, which are all too easily identified, but too often resist the best efforts to control what frequently remains a local disease. Even the patient whose tumor is controlled may have problems stemming from the physical or emotional impact of her disease or its treatment or both.

There are several key factors in the optimal care of patients with uterine cancer. A thorough pretreatment evaluation is of fundamental importance. The basis of the clinical staging systems used for both cervical and endometrial carcinoma is the pelvic examination. This should be performed under anesthesia as a joint venture by the gynecologic and radiation oncologist. Cervical biopsies and a fractional curettage should be done; this is also a convenient time to perform cystoscopic examination. Visualization of the bladder mucosa permits assessment of possible tumor involvement. A sigmoidoscopy can also be done at the same time in patients who have bowel symptoms or in the asymptomatic patient with a large central tumor. Following the examination, a consensus opinion should be reached regarding the clinical findings and the patient definitively staged. Once this staging is agreed upon, it must never be changed.

The evaluation of the patient should also include a complete history and physical examination with particular attention paid to previous abdominal surgery or radiation, hormone ingestion, and family history of malignancy. Laboratory studies should also include a complete blood count, urinalysis, and liver function tests. A chest x-ray and metastatic series are routinely ordered. An intravenous pyelogram (IVP) should be obtained. The IVP demonstrates renal function and also identifies the position of the ureters and the kidneys. Deviation of the ureters may suggest metastatic tumor or retroperitoneal lymph nodes, and knowledge of kidney location is important in regard to radiation therapy planning. In certain patients, considering tumor size and location, a barium enema is suggested.

The role of the bipedal lymphangiogram in evaluating a patient with uterine cancer is still in question. The test does visualize many of the lymph nodes at risk for tumor involvement, but the true positive rate even in an expert's hands is only about 75 per cent. These pelvic lymph nodes, as will be seen later, receive maximum tolerable treatment by current techniques. There is no evidence at the present time that treatment of radiographically abnormal para-aortic nodes can increase survival. It yet remains to be demonstrated that information supplied by the lymphangiogram can improve survival rates, modify conventional techniques or decrease treatment associated morbidity.

The availability of adequately trained personnel and proper equipment is of paramount importance in the treatment of women with uterine cancer. A few general principles can be stated, but the details of the radiotherapeutic and surgical techniques will be discussed in later sections. Radiation must be delivered with equipment operating in the megavoltage range. The volume of tumor to be radiated must be carefully specified and steps taken to ensure daily reproducibility of each treatment. The radiation oncologist must carefully monitor the treatment, noting tumor response and effect on normal tissues. Therapists should be prepared to alter the plan of treatment if warranted by the clinical course during radiation. Similarly, the surgeon and the hospital must be able to deal with the patient in need of radical pelvic surgery. Support should be available to handle urologic or intestinal complications.

The patient is not adequately or totally cared for unless provision for long-term follow-up is available. Only in this way can the side effects of treatment be monitored and recurrent disease discovered early. Selective retreatment may include pelvic exenterative procedures, or reirradiation in hopes of long-term control or cure. Palliative radiation and chemotherapy may also be considered. Standard surveillance of a patient with uterine cancer requires follow-up examinations every 3 months for 2 years, every 6 months for 3 years and once a year after 5 years.

Cancer of the Uterine Cervix

Incidence and Etiology.   The incidence of invasive cervical cancer is decreasing in the United States due to improved surveillance, attention to risk factors, and the improving cooperation of the female population. The results of treatment show better 5 year survivals due to sophistication of radiation therapy, better use of selective radical surgery, and a continuing tendency to regionalize care in centers equipped to manage all facets of the disease.

Another factor responsible for the decreased incidence of invasive cervical cancer is a direct result of earlier cytologic sampling by physicians and family planning centers. This has resulted in a proliferation of patients demonstrating CIN (intraepithelial cervical neoplasia), CIS (intraepithelial cervical carcinoma), and VAIN (intraepithelial vaginal neoplasia).

Staging.   The treatment of cervical cancer in all major institutions is based on the clinical stage of the disease and the FIGO (International Federation of Obstetricians and Gynecologists) classification is now universally accepted (Table 1).

Treatment.   CARCINOMA IN SITU OF THE CERVIX.   We believe there to be four types of carcinoma in situ of the cervix: (1) pure, (2) carcinoma in situ with glandular invasion, (3) carcinoma in situ with lymphatic invasion, (4) carcinoma in situ with vascular invasion.

Treatment here involves some patient input in reference to age and the possibility of desired

TABLE 1. **Clinical Staging for Cancer of the Cervix**

Stage 0: Carcinoma in situ, intraepithelial carcinoma.

Stage I: Carcinoma confined to the cervix (extension to the corpus should be disregarded).

    Stage Ia: Microinvasive carcinoma (early stromal invasion).

    Stage Ib: All other cases of Stage I. Occult cancer should be marked "occ."

Stage II: The carcinoma extends beyond the cervix but has not extended to the pelvic wall. The carcinoma involves the vagina, but not the lower third.

    Stage IIa: No obvious parametrial involvement.

    Stage IIb: Obvious parametrial involvement.

Stage III: The carcinoma has extended to the pelvic wall. On rectal examination there is no cancer-free space between the tumor and the pelvic wall. The tumor involves the lower third of the vagina. All cases with hydronephrosis or nonfunctioning kidney.

    Stage IIIa: No extension to the pelvic wall.

    Stage IIIb: Extension to the pelvic wall and/or hydronephrosis or nonfunctioning kidney.

Stage IV: The carcinoma has extended beyond the true pelvis or has clinically involved the mucosa of the bladder or rectum. A bullous edema does not classify as Stage IV.

    Stage IVa: Spread of the growth to adjacent organs.

    Stage IVb: Spread to distant organs.

---

pregnancy. (1) Pure carcinoma in situ and carcinoma in situ with glandular invasion may be treated by therapeutic cone, cryocauterization, or electrocauterization if patient desires pregnancy. Careful and frequent follow-up examinations are mandatory and colposcopic surveillance is essential. If this conservative treatment is selected, hysterectomy is recommended after the age of 35 or after two successful pregnancies. It should further be mentioned that this conservative treatment is allowable as long as the identified lesion occupies no more than one quarter or 25 per cent of the exocervix. (2) When pregnancy is not a desired consideration, pure carcinoma in situ and carcinoma in situ with glandular invasion should be treated by vaginal or abdominal hysterectomy with ovarian preservation below the age of 45 and with ovarian sacrifice beyond the age of 45.

Carcinoma in situ with vascular invasion or lymphatic invasion should be treated by radical hysterectomy without node dissection and with ovarian preservation, age respected.

There is virtually no place for the use of radiation in the management of carcinoma in situ of the cervix, but the team approach is still very important; here, the consulting team member is the pathologist, because only he can properly differentiate these four types of carcinoma in situ of the cervix.

INVASIVE CARCINOMA OF THE CERVIX. General guidelines for the care of patients with various stage carcinomas of the cervix can be given. The radiation and gynecologic oncologists at the Rhode Island Hospital consider each patient's care individually and advise a treatment plan to suit the disease and the patient. Factors taken into account are the patient's general physical condition, emotional status, and social situation. For example, a patient may be suitable for a course of external radiation, but because of transportation difficulty may not be able to come for the treatment. The social worker and the oncology nurse greatly aid in solving such problems.

There is little question that invasive cervical cancer in all stages is best treated by radiation, but there are disease stages and individual considerations where surgery is recommended either as primary treatment or as an adjuvant to radiation.

Primary radical hysterectomy and node dissection is preferred in sexually active patients with Stage Ia, Ib, and in certain patients with favorably Stage IIa disease. Age, height-weight ratio, and metabolic stability are basic for surgical selection, and ovarian preservation is to be encouraged. This type of surgery also allows for persistence of a pliable and functional, though temporally shortened, vagina.

Stage Ia microinvasive carcinoma (early stromal invasion). We prefer to identify this disease stage as representing less than 2 mm. of stromal involvement. There are two different types of Stage Ia, the confluent pattern and the peg pattern. Patients with cervical cancer, Stage Ia, peg pattern, may be appropriately treated by extrafascial vaginal or abdominal hysterectomy, and Stage Ia, confluent pattern, should be managed by radical hysterectomy, but pelvic node dissection is probably not necessary.

Stage Ib. All other cases of Stage I including occult carcinoma, in which disease is totally limited to the cervix; the suggested treatment here is radical hysterectomy and bilateral node dissection with ovarian preservation, depending upon age guidelines. Older patients with Stage Ib or IIa disease and all patients with IIb and Stage III disease are treated by radiation therapy. Our policy is to begin with a course of external radiation to the whole pelvis. The pelvic volume is defined in the anteroposterior (AP) projection, superiorly by the L-5, S-1 interspace, inferiorly by a line midway through the obturator foramen, and laterally by a line 1 cm. lateral to the walls of the bony pelvis. Lateral fields are also used unless the patient is quite thin (AP diameter less than 20 cm.). The posterior limit of this field is usually the S-1, S-2 interspace, while the anterior limit extends 1 to 2 cm. in front of the anterior limit of the fifth lumbar vertebrae. These lateral fields are generally 8 to 9 cm. wide. We deliver 4500 rads maximum tumor dose to the tumor volume in 25 treatments using 10 MeV photons from a linear accelerator.

All fields are treated each day. Planning the fields is simplified by the insertion of a decayed radon seed or other suitable marker into the cervix at the time of initial examination in the Radiation Oncology Department. This is, by convention, placed at the 12 o' clock position. If there is a large amount of central disease, the whole pelvic dose may be raised to 5000 rads in 28 fractions. It must be carefully understood that this is a maximun dose, defined at the 100 per cent isodose line.

In Stage I or very early Stage II disease this course of external radiation is followed by a single intracavitary cesium insertion. We prefer the Fletcher-Suit tandem and ovoids, but patients with a narrow vaginal vault are treated by the Henschke tandem and ovoids or a protruding tandem.

There has been much discussion regarding the method of dosimetry used when both external and intracavitary radiation (brachytherapy) are employed. One attempt at solution has been to state the number of "milligram hours" delivered by brachytherapy and add the external dose in rads, thus describing the total treatment. This method ignores the rapid change in dose rate inherent in all intracavity therapy.

Another approach to the dosimetry problem has been to define doses at Points A and B. Point A is located 2 cm. superior and 2 cm. lateral to the external cervical os. This marks the place where the ureter crosses the uterine artery and is the lateral limit of the paracervical tissue. Point B is 3 cm. lateral to Point A and is said to locate the pelvic lymph nodes. Clearly, human structure is sufficiently variable so as to make the anatomic correlation of these points different in each patient. At the Rhode Island Hospital we define a tumor volume in each patient and deliver 7500 to 8000 rads to the area of the primary cervical disease. If 4500 rads is given with external radiation, intracavitary radiation must then supply an additional 3500 to 4000 rads. The total dose delivered to the pevic nodes with this system is 5500 to 6000 rads. Should the patient's anatomy preclude insertion of ovoids, the dose to the paracervical and parametrial areas can be boosted with additional external radiation.

Patients with more advanced Stage IIa, Stage IIb, or Stage III disease receive additional parametrial radiation following the intracavitary therapy. A boost of 500 to 1500 rads is given, depending upon the amount of original disease and the dose delivered by the brachytherapy.

Treatment of Stage IV disease is highly individualized. Stage IVa carcinoma of the cervix, spread of growth to adjacent organs; treatment begins with external radiation to the pelvis. The clinical situation is reassessed at 4000 rads. If there has been excellent tumor regression, surgery is attempted. This may require anterior, posterior, or total pelvic exenteration. If at 4000 rads surgery is not possible or if the patient is not surgically acceptable, external radiation is continued. The whole pelvis is treated to 5000 rads at 180 rads per treatment. The anterior and posterior fields are then reduced to approximately 10 by 10 cm. and an additional 1000 rads is given. At 6000 rads, the field is again reduced and an additional 1000 rads is delivered. It is difficult and hazardous to administer such doses of irradiation to the pelvis, but the disease threat to the patient warrants the risk. Stage IVb disease indicates spread to distant organs, and, as mentioned above, this disease entity requires carefully individualized treatment in the nature of pelvic radiation for control of local disease and chemotherapy in attempt to manage the extrapelvic spread.

Cancer of the cervix is a curable disease. With careful execution of the treatment policies outlined here, the following 5 year survival rates can be anticipated: Stage I, 80 to 90 per cent; Stage II, 60 to 70 per cent; Stage III, 20 to 30 per cent; Stage IV, 5 to 10 per cent.

SPECIAL CONSIDERATIONS. Invasive cervical cancer with a large bulky endocervical component is referred to as a "barrel-shaped lesion." This is usually a Stage IIb lesion and generally the amount of parametrial involvement is gentle.

The central disease bulk however is so large that control by radiation alone is rarely possible. These patients should be treated with external radiation, 4500 rads, followed by a modified Wertheim procedure, and then reevaluated after careful review of the microscopic findings at surgery. An additional 500 to 1500 rads is often suggested.

Recurrent cervical cancer primarily treated with radiation is best managed by surgery, and recurrent cervical cancer primarily treated by surgery is best retreated by radiation.

Treatment of invasive cancer of the cervical stump is managed stage for stage, similar to disease occurring in an intact uterus. The present emphasis on total hysterectomy for benign disease will eventually render carcinoma of the cervical stump to an historical category. Even now it is being seen but rarely, and in its place a new entity has surfaced, invasive cervical cancer inadvertently discovered in a uterus removed by conventional hysterectomy for benign disease. Treatment of this condition is again stage related and it is usually Stage Ib, occult. Radiation control is very effective but some patients again can be best managed by radical vaginectomy and bilateral pelvic node dissection.

CARCINOMA OF THE CERVIX IN PREGNANCY. Another important entity requiring therapeutic concern is cancer of the cervix occurring during pregnancy. Most of these patients are under the care of a physician and Papanicolaou smears are an integral part of the initial antepartum visit. Abnormal bleeding or discharge is a threatening symptom to a pregnant patient and, consequently, they seek advice early For this reason mainly, invasive cervical cancer in pregnancy is a low stage disease, Ib, occult, or IIa.

Carcinoma in situ of the cervix occurring during pregnancy requires the standard surveillance alluded to previously, although cone biopsy confirmation is very cautiously recommended. Treatment of this disease during pregnancy is confined to very careful surveillance and reevaluation of the lesion following delivery. Vaginal delivery is permissible; cesarean section should be done only for obstetrical indications.

Invasive cervical cancer occurring during pregnancy is managed stage for stage as if no pregnancy existed with one notable exception, termination of the pregnancy.

In the first trimester, pregnancy termination may be accomplished by external radiation and the central lesion later treated in a routine fashion. In the second trimester, pregnancy termination is best achieved by hysterotomy and then the radiation treatment is pursued. In the third trimester, cesarean section at the time chosen to recover a "good baby" is followed again by the standard radiation techniques.

Wertheim hysterectomy and node dissection is very acceptable for cancer of the cervix in pregnancy, and the decision for surgery is based on stage of disease and physical health of the mother. This procedure is very easy to perform in pregnancy after the uterus has been evacuated. The coexisting pregnancy does not accelerate the growth pattern of the disease and the disease if treated in the third trimester of pregnancy does not challenge the health of the baby if appropriate maturity studies are done prior to cesarean section.

CHEMOTHERAPY. This treatment modality in cervical cancer is not totally refined. At the Rhode Island Hospital we are pursuing a fairly aggressive protocol in the management of advanced disease: high dose methotrexate, bleomycin, and DDP (Platinum).

Carcinoma of the Endometrium

Incidence and Etiology. Adenocarcinoma of the endometrium is being seen with increasing frequency. It is now the third most common major organ malignancy in women, the incidence now exceeding that of cervix, and the ratio increasing year by year. The profile of a patient with this disease would reflect a high incidence of diabetes, hypertension, and obesity. She would be about 62 years of age, could possibly be childless or the mother of a very small family. She might give a history of an aggressive menopause or perhaps long-term estrogen usage, and she would present with postmenopausal vaginal bleeding. Her history might also reflect a previous major organ malignancy, usually breast or colon (15 to 20 per cent).

Staging. The treatment of endometrial adenocarcinoma is predicated on the clinical stage of the disease and the pathologic grade of the tumor. In 1971, the FIGO (International Federation of Gynecologists and Obstetricians) classification, embracing both stage and grade considerations, was adopted and is now also universally accepted (Table 2).

A staging examination under anesthesia is just as important here as in cervical cancer, although two examiners are not necessary. The depth of the uterine cavity is carefully recorded and a fractional D and C is imperative. The tissue recovered is presented for (1) cell type, (2) pathologic grade, (3) endocervical involvement, and (4) estrogen and progesterone receptor sites.

Treatment. Cancer of the cervix is a disease best treated with radiation, and surgery is reserved for special considerations. In carcinoma of the endometrium, the situation is reversed. This dis-

TABLE 2. **Clinical Staging for Cancer of the Endometrium**

Stage 0:	Carcinoma in situ. Histologic findings suggestive of malignancy. Stage 0 should not be included in the therapeutic statistics.
Stage I:	The carcinoma is confined to the corpus.
	Stage Ia: The cancer is present in a uterus measuring up to 8 cm. in length from the external os to the upper limits of the uterine cavity.
	Stage Ib: The carcinoma is present in a uterus measuring more than 8 cm. in length from the external os to the upper limits of the uterine cavity.
G1:	Highly differentiated adenomatous carcinomas.
G2:	Differentiated adenomatous carcinomas with partly solid areas.
G3:	Predominantly solid or entirely undifferentiated carcinomas.
Stage II:	The carcinoma has involved the corpus and the cervix (simultaneous presence of normal cervical glands and cancer in the same field will give the final diagnosis).
Stage III:	The carcinoma has spread outside the uterus but not outside the pelvis.
Stage IV:	The carcinoma has extended outside the true pelvis or has seriously involved the mucosa of the rectum and/or bladder. A bullous edema as such does not permit allotment of a case to Stage IV.

ease is best managed by surgery and radiation plays a supporting or adjunctive role.

Carcinoma in situ of the endometrium/severe adenomatous dysplasia: This condition may in rare instances be managed by oral or parenteral progestogens with careful follow-up and frequent office tissue sampling. I would suggest medroxyprogesterone acetate (Provera), 20 mg. for 2 weeks of every menstrual month. This obviously would apply to the very rare patient who wants to become pregnant. This uterus, however, will forever remain suspect.

Stage I adenocarcinoma of the endometrium is subdivided into A and B categories, according to cavity size, and further subdivided into pathologic grade of tumor I, II, III, according to the degree of cellular dedifferentiation.

Throughout the country there is wide flexibility concerning management of Stage I endometrial carcinoma. The following emphasizes the method pursued at the Rhode Island Hospital:

Stage Ia, GI. Small uterus, well-differentiated tumor, treated by extrafascial hysterectomy and bilateral salpingo-oophorectomy. If the pathology section shows any evidence of deep myometrial invasion, postoperative external radiation therapy is given to a dose of 4500 rads full pelvis.

Stage Ia, GII and GIII. These patients are managed by external radiation therapy to a dose of 4500 rads followed in 3 to 4 weeks by an extrafascial abdominal hysterectomy and bilateral salpingo-oophorectomy.

Stage Ib, GI. The uterine cavity enlarged beyond 8 cm. and a well differentiated tumor. These patients are managed by external radiation therapy to dose of 4500 rads full pelvis, followed in three to four weeks by extrafascial hysterectomy and bilateral salpingo-oophorectomy.

Stage Ib, GII and *Stage Ib, GIII* lesions are managed in the same way, namely external radiation therapy, followed by extrafascial hysterectomy.

A recent report by Creasman has identified positive pelvic lymph nodes in 3 per cent of GI lesions, 10 per cent of GII lesions, and 36 per cent of GIII lesions. This same study further identifies 11.5 per cent positive pelvic nodes associated with superficial myometrial invasion and 43 per cent positive nodes in deep myometrial invasion. These patients for the most part are a little too old, a little too obese, and a little too fragile to accept formal radical hysterectomy and node dissection, so we must here depend upon the radiation oncologist to attack these node-bearing areas.

Stage II, the disease involves the endocervix. Preoperative full pelvic irradiation, 4500 rads, is given, followed by local cesium insertion into the endocervix and upper vagina. The cesium delivers 4000 rads to the vaginal epithelium while the uterine tandem supplements the dose to the pelvic lymph nodes by delivering an additional 1000 rads. Extrafascial hysterectomy with node sampling is then performed 3 to 4 weeks following this cesium implant. Stage II endometrial carcinoma behaves like carcinoma of the cervix as well as carcinoma of the endometrium, and in rare instances where the patient's physical condition is acceptable, a Wertheim hysterectomy and node dissection can be substituted for the cesium implant and extrafascial hysterectomy. There is a high incidence of para-aortic node involvement in Stage II disease, and selective para-aortic nodes should be studied before embarking on radical surgery.

In Stage III, the carcinoma has spread beyond the uterus but is still confined within the pelvis. Treatment here involves primary external radiation therapy, 4500 rads, followed by extrafascial hysterectomy and bilateral salpingo-oophorectomy. Once again, para-aortic nodes and selective pelvic nodes should be removed for sampling. This does not infer a formal lymphadenectomy.

In Stage IV, the disease has spread to involve the adjacent bladder or rectum, or has extended beyond the true pelvis. For disease involving bladder and rectum, our treatment would be external radiation, 4500 rads, followed by cesium implantation to the cervix, uterus, and upper vagina, and later a possible attempt at cytoreductive surgery. Stage IV disease extending beyond the pelvis will be discussed under special considerations.

Special Considerations. Recurrent disease at the vaginal vault: This lesion should be seen with decreasing frequency, owing mainly to the surgical removal of the upper vagina at the time of treatment and the pre-or postoperative radiation delivered to the upper vagina. Should it occur, however, and the incidence should be much under 5 per cent, it is probably best managed by vaginal radiation if review of the previous x-ray dosages can confirm that adjacent normal tissues will not be damaged.

Adenosquamous disease: This cell pattern is no longer considered indigenous to the waters of Lake Erie. It is being reported with greater frequency in all major centers. It requires very aggressive treatment in the nature of external radiation therapy, 4500 rads, intrauterine cesium therapy, and after a 4 to 6 week interval, extrafascial hysterectomy with bilateral salpingo-oophorectomy and node sampling.

Mixed mesodermal tumors of the uterus or uterine sarcoma: These lesions also are aggressive in their growth patterns and therefore require aggressive measures for control. We suggest external radiation therapy, 4500 rads, followed by extrafascial hysterectomy, then chemotherapy with doxorubicin (Adriamycin) and dacarbazine (DTIC).

Recurrent pelvic or extrapelvic disease: The standard follow-up of patients with pelvic cancer, be it cervical or uterine in origin requires office surveillance every 3 months for 2 years, every 6 months for 3 years, and once a year after 5 years. We believe that an intravenous pyelogram performed every 3 years is important in carcinoma of the cervix follow-up and we similarly believe that a chest x-ray is important yearly in patients with adenocarcinoma of the endometrium. Should pelvic or extrapelvic recurrence appear, our present method of treatment involves the use of megestrol acetate (Megace) tablets by mouth (40 mg.), 180 to 360 mg. per day. The previously obtained hormonal receptor sites are helpful here in assessing the possible benefits of progesterone therapy. Extrapelvic Stage IV disease, or recurrent disease has been shown to respond fairly well to a combination of megestrol acetate (Megace) and doxorubicin (Adriamycin). The most favorable responders are relatively young and present with recurrence beyond 2 years of initial treatment and show low-grade tumor.

Certain patients will undergo abdominal hysterectomy for benign disease and at the time of pathology review will be found to have a coexisting endometrial carcinoma. If this is an SI, GI lesion, no further treatment is necessary. If the pathologic grading identifies GII or GIII, or if myometrial invasion is clearly identified, then full pelvic irradiation to a dose of 4500 rads should be given. If endocervical involvement is also apparent, further radiation should be delivered using cesium sources in an appropriately fitted vaginal applicator.

There is one particular type of patient with endometrial carcinoma who presents with a very dangerous metabolic profile. This is a patient with severe diabetes, a past history of vascular disease requiring constant medical surveillance, and associated extreme obesity. When these patients also harbor endometrial carcinoma, they pose a real challenge. They require very strict preoperative medical study of a formal nature, documented by physical review by a qualified internist or cardiologist or both. These very high risk patients require a different and extremely conservative, suboptimal treatment. We suggest that these patients be managed by intracavitary radium only, employing doses between 4800 and 9000 mg. hours in one or two applications, and recommending either the Heymann packing capsules or a uterine tandem and vaginal ovoids depending upon the volumetric capacity of the uterus. They

receive no surgery, they are too area bound, too obese and too medically unstable to handle external radiation. We have on occasion suggested megestrol acetate (Megace), but they receive no cytotoxic drugs.

Certain patients with early endometrial carcinoma, SIa, GI indicating early stage and a favorable pathologic grade can be electively managed by vaginal hysterectomy and bilateral salpingo-oophorectomy.

CARCINOMA OF THE VULVA
method of
PAUL B. UNDERWOOD, JR., M.D.
Charleston, South Carolina

Carcinoma of the vulva is primarily a disease of the geriatric patient and represents less than 5 per cent of the gynecologic malignancies. The majority are epidermoid carcinomas arising from the skin or mucous membranes of the vulva, although they may originate from skin appendages, Bartholin's glands, clitoris, or underlying stroma. As was not the case in the past, increasing numbers of women are seeking early medical attention for vulvar irritations and lesions. The physician should be familiar with certain premalignant conditions, even in the young female, because prevention and/or early diagnosis is the present-day answer to survival.

Premalignant Lesions

Premalignant lesions of the vulva may be classified into four categories: (1) granulomatous lesions, (2) white lesions, (3) premalignant lesions, and (4) nevi. Any vulvar irritation that does not heal with appropriate therapy must be biopsied. The accuracy of biopsy will be increased by staining the vulva with toluidine blue, which will delineate areas of epithelial hyperactivity. This technique involves the following measures: (1) wash the vulva with 1 per cent acetic acid to remove all mucus and excretions, (2) dry, (3) paint with 1 per cent toluidine blue, (4) dry, and (5) wash with 1 per cent acetic acid. Toluidine blue is a nuclear stain; hence, areas that remain blue have nuclear hyperactivity and represent areas to be sampled. Vulvar biopsy is an office procedure performed under a local anesthetic. If small, bleeding can be controlled by pressure; however, occasionally a suture of absorbable material is required for hemostasis.

The profound chronic infectious state of granuloma inguinale and longstanding condylomata acuminata with the resultant tissue reaction and scarring should be recognized as a carcinogen. Emphasis should be placed on chronicity, because in my experience, if treated early, these granulomatous lesions rarely result in carcinoma. The edematous, scarred, leather-like vulva of healed granuloma inguinale should be examined every 4 months for any ulceration. Condylomata acuminata are considered benign papillomatous lesions; however, when present for long periods of time, especially if chronically inflamed and/or ulcerated, they should be biopsied prior to the usual therapy.

The white lesion precipitates marked confusion between the terms kraurosis, lichen sclerosus et atrophicus, and atrophic and hypertrophic leukoplakia. Most authorities have recently agreed to classify these lesions as epithelial dystrophies prefixed with the words atrophic or hypertrophic. The atrophic dystrophies seldom develop malignant changes, whereas approximately 5 per cent of the hypertrophic vulvitides undergo carcinomatous changes. The management of dystrophies should be directed toward the relief of symptoms, specifically itching and dyspareunia: (1) keep the area clean and dry; (2) apply estrogen cream with 1 per cent hydrocortisone twice daily; (3) if dyspareunia is present, provide surgical relief of the introital stenosis by a midline episiotomy closed transversely; (4) with hypertrophic lesions, observe every 4 months for ulcerations or tumorfaction. Simple vulvectomies and "skinectomy" procedures should be used only when all conservative attempts fail, because in most cases a recurrence of the lesion will develop at the skin margins.

The preinvasive lesions are Bowen's disease, intraepithelial carcinoma, and Paget's disease. The eponym Bowen's disease denotes a specialized form of intraepithelial carcinoma that appears to grow more slowly; however, from the clinical standpoint, the two should be considered the same disease. These neoplastic changes usually develop in multiple areas upon the vulva, although an isolated lesion may be seen. The treatment of the solitary neoplasm should await histologic evaluation of multiple biopsies of the normal-appearing vulva. If they confirm a single abnormality, wide local excision is the treatment of choice. The typical patient with multifocal vulvar involvement can be managed either by a "skinectomy" procedure with skin graft or by a simple vulvectomy. The "skinectomy" produces excellent cosmetic results without introital stenosis. In the young female, the donor site should be from the buttocks in order to avoid embarrassing questions.

Topical 2 and 5 per cent 5-fluorouracil applied twice daily for 4 to 8 weeks has been effective in some patients. The neoplastic vulvar tissues will become ulcerated and miserable. Therefore, in my opinion, since the results are poor and the side effects high, this means of therapy should be utilized only for those patients who are believed to be medically inoperable.

Paget's disease of the vulva should not be managed by the "skinectomy" procedure, as it represents an intraepithelial spread of invasive adenocarcinoma and has a tendency to follow hair shafts. Also, truly invasive carcinoma below the epithelium can be found in approximately 10 per cent. A simple vulvectomy is therefore the treatment of choice. If invasive carcinoma is discovered after removal, a bilateral groin dissection should be performed at a later stage. The neoplastic cells involve the epithelium far beyond the gross lesion; therefore very wide margins should be obtained. If available, frozen sections of the margins for confirmation of adequacy should be obtained at the operating room table.

Five per cent of all melanomas are found on the perineum, which represents only 1 per cent of the body's skin surface. Since the majority occur after the age of 35, all vulvar nevi should be removed at the time of delivery as a worthwhile means of preventive medicine.

Invasive Carcinoma

The prognosis of a patient with invasive carcinoma is directly associated with the degree of differentiation, the size of the lesion, and its location. Most vulvar carcinomas are well differentiated; however, those arising from the clitoris are notoriously poorly differentiated. Malignancies of the clitoris or Bartholin's glands have a worse prognosis. Those occurring on the perineal body and posterior vestibule require wide labial excision, because the lymphatic drainage of the vulva swings farther lateral the more posterior the lesion. Carcinomas involving the distal urethra and lower vagina require a more radical approach. The size of the lesion is directly related to the incidence of lymph node metastasis.

The lymph drainage of the vulva is to the inguinal and femoral nodes. These nodes drain through Cloquet's nodes (a lymph node lying medial to the femoral vein and beneath the inguinal ligament) to the deep pelvic nodes. Vulvar carcinomas always involve the groin nodes before they involve the pelvic nodes, except for lesions of the clitoris in which the groin may be bypassed and the carcinoma metastasize directly to the deep pelvic nodes. Lymphatic drainage may extend to the contralateral groin, especially from the anterior vulva. The incidence of nodal metastasis varies from approximately 5 per cent for lesions less than 2 cm. in diameter to over 50 per cent for those greater than 7 cm.

With these facts in mind, therapy can be planned accordingly. The basic procedure is an en bloc radical vulvectomy and bilateral groin dissection. Cloquet's nodes should be resected separately and sent for frozen section. If positive, a deep pelvic lymphadenectomy is performed at the same sitting. If negative, the additional surgery and its complications do not warrant the pelvic lymphadenectomy. For reasons previously described, clitoral lesions are exceptions. Because of skin lymphatics, a 1 to 2 inch segment overlying the inguinal ligament and continuous with the vulva should be removed.

The technique for the groin dissection that I prefer is to undermine the abdominal skin for about 3 inches above the inguinal ligament and the skin of the thigh to the apex of the femoral triangle. All fatty and lymphatic tissue over the external oblique fascia is cleaned to the inguinal ligament. The fascia lata is incised along the sartorius muscle from the inguinal ligament to the apex of the femoral triangle, followed by its incision over the abductus longus muscle to the same apex. The saphenous vein is identified and double ligated as it exits this tissue mass. The fascia lata is incised from the inguinal ligament, beginning laterally and extending medially. By this technique, the femoral nerve, artery, and vein are cleaned of their lymphatic tissue without disturbing the more superficial lymph canals. This mass of fatty tissue is resected en bloc with the vulva. The more anterior the lesion, the more mons pubis one removes. The farther posterior, the farther lateral the labia majora are incised. If the urethra is involved, its distal one third can be excised without incontinence ensuing. All vulvar tissues external to the urogenital diaphragm are removed. The usual specimen is terminated distal to the hymen; however, the lower one third of the vagina can be excised by this approach. A finger in the rectum will permit a deeper dissection over the bowel without fear of entering it.

The technique for closure of this enormous defect is vital to prevent morbidity and complications. The sartorius muscle is excised from its origin and sutured to the inguinal ligament overlying the femoral vessels for their protection. The perineal skin and the vaginal mucosa are undermined for 2 to 3 cm. This permits closure without tension and places the suture line outside the vaginal orifice, thereby decreasing introital stenosis. A Z-plasty closure is also beneficial. Caution should be taken not to pull the urethra over the symphysis, as this may produce stress incontinence.

Suction catheters should be placed beneath the groin flaps. The groin incision should be closed with subcuticular absorbable suture to prevent folding of the skin at the suture line which may produce slough. Pressure dressings are contraindicated.

The secret to primary wound healing is immaculate wound cleanliness for 10 to 14 days. I emphasize cleaning all suture lines every 8 hours (not three times a day) with hydrogen peroxide. The patient is maintained at bed rest with feet elevated 15 degrees (to prevent thrombophlebitis) for 7 days. Suction drainage to the groins and bladder catheter is continued for a similar time. Prophylactic antibiotics are utilized. An over-the-bed cradle with a light bulb aids in maintaining dry suture lines.

If necrosis develops in the skin flaps, keep the area dry and observe as long as tensile strength of the devitalized tissue exists. This permits time for the skin flap to stick. Debridement is performed only after separation has occurred. At this point, wet soaks with one quarter strength Dakin's solution aids in wound granulation. Only rarely is skin grafting necessary.

Chronic lymphedema of the leg is another complication. For prophylaxis, elastic stockings are to be worn during awake hours for at least 3 months. Lymphangitis will contribute to permanent leg edema; therefore since most infections are streptococcal, prophylactic penicillin or erythromycin should be maintained for 1 year.

Radiation plays only a minor role in therapy of vulvar malignancies owing to its poor tolerance. Enormous lesions can be shrunk with 3000 rads delivered through a perineal port prior to radical surgery. Prophylactic irradiation to the groin and pelvis may be utilized with incomplete resection of tumor but usually produces permanent lymphedema of the leg.

Primary exenterative procedures are indicated for enormous lesions involving over one third of the urethra and vagina, or any part of the rectum. In special instances, an ileal conduit or colostomy can be utilized to permanently divert the excretory stream, permitting radical excision without the morbidity of the exenteration.

Other rare malignancies of the vulva are worthy of mention. Basal cell carcinomas do occur in the vulvar area, but usually in women over 60 years of age. Treatment is local wide resection. A low grade fibrosarcoma is occasionally seen in the subepithelial tissues. It generally metastasizes only in late stages; therefore radical local excision is adequate therapy. To the contrary, a rare, highly malignant rhabdomyosarcoma may develop in the inferior labia majora of teenagers. One should consider this diagnosis when an apparent Bartholin gland cellulitis does not heal by the usual means of therapy. A radical vulvectomy with bilateral groin and deep pelvic node dissection followed by postoperative chemotherapy with doxorubicin (Adriamycin) or VAC (vincristine, actinomycin D, and cyclophosphamide) for at least 1 year is the treatment of choice. Unfortunately, this tumor is usually beyond resection at the time of diagnosis. In such instances, local radiation plus the aforementioned chemotherapy becomes the treatment of choice. The prognosis for survival approaches zero. Another uncommon malignancy of the vulva is a melanoma. Therapy should be ultraradical excision extending to the depth of the urogenital diaphragm along with radical groin and deep pelvic node dissection.

PREOPERATIVE AND POSTOPERATIVE CARE FOR ELECTIVE GYNECOLOGIC SURGERY

method of
ROBERT E. ROGERS, M.D.,
and JAMES A. HALL, M.D.
Indianapolis, Indiana

Successful surgery demands close cooperation and communication between a qualified surgeon and the patient. Thoughtful attention to the physical and emotional requirements of the patient, meticulous attention to operative detail, and close supervision of the postoperative period are all requirements for optimal surgical care.

Preoperative Preparation

Surgical therapy must be fitted to the patient and her disease. Since variables are virtually infinite, a rigid preoperative plan is neither desirable nor possible. However, adequate preoperative preparation must include:

Patient Information and Consent. The patient and any other persons that she might desire to have informed should be thoroughly counseled as to the indications for the surgery, procedure to be performed, expected results, alternative procedures, expected convalescence, possible complications, and risk of not performing the procedure.

General Health Evaluation. A complete history and physical examination should be performed prior to admission to the hospital. Complicating factors should be dealt with prior to surgery. Good nutrition should always be stressed.

Gynecologic Evaluation. A thorough gynecologic history, along with pelvic and rectal examination, is mandatory preoperatively in all patients. Cervical cytology (Papanicolaou smear) should be performed within 3 months of surgery and any abnormalities thoroughly investigated. Hysterectomy or exploratory laparotomy should never be performed without prior endometrial biopsy or curettage to rule out the presence of carcinoma if there is a history of abnormal bleeding. Patients being operated upon for urinary stress incontinence should have other forms of incontinence ruled out by the use of intravenous pyelogram, cystoscopy, urethroscopy, cystometrogram, Bonney-Read-Marchetti test, urinalysis, and culture. Those having surgery for known or suspected cancer should be investigated for metastatic disease. The possibility of pregnancy must always be considered in a gynecology patient.

Ideally, gynecologic surgery should be scheduled during the proliferative phase of the cycle and is to be avoided during the menstrual period. If atrophic changes are present in the vagina, topical estrogen cream for up to 6 weeks prior to surgery is of great value for women undergoing vaginal reparative surgery.

Laboratory Evaluation. Indices of general health such as complete blood count, VDRL, and urinalysis should be obtained. Other medical problems may dictate further tests. Chest x-ray and electrocardiogram are generally reserved for those over 35 years of age or who have cardiopulmonary disease. Any history of abnormal coagulation should be investigated with appropriate tests.

Preoperative Orders

As there is no "routine" patient, there can be no routine orders. Areas which must be considered are:

1. Diet, including nothing by mouth for at least 8 hours prior to surgery.

2. Encouragement of maximum activity.

3. Medications, including appropriate pain and sleep preparations, as well as the patient's usual prescriptions. Low-dose heparin should be considered for those at risk for thrombosis. Patients scheduled for vaginal hysterectomy in the reproductive age group are treated prophylactically with cephalothin sodium (Keflin). Systemic bacterial endocarditis (SBE) prophylaxis should be given if there is a history of rheumatic fever or valvular disease. Preoperative medications may also be ordered by the anesthesiologist.

4. Nursing measures include daily vital signs and an initial height and weight measurement. Patients having major vaginal or abdominal surgery should have an abdominal and perineal scrub and shave. Perineal shaving is not required for minor vaginal surgery. A cleansing enema should be given. Preoperative antibacterial douching with a povidone-iodine preparation (Betadine) prior to major procedures is generally requested. Certain patients, particularly those undergoing radical cancer procedures, require more

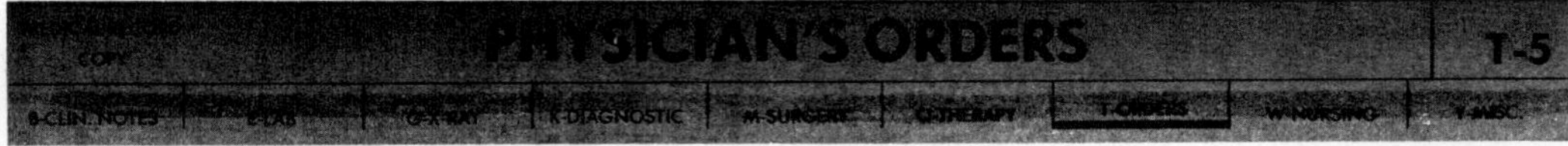

INDIANA UNIVERSITY HOSPITALS
INDIANAPOLIS, INDIANA   INSERT # 1

| Rev. 3/77 | PHYSICIAN'S ORDERS | M6552100 |

1. ADDRESSOGRAPH BEFORE PLACING IN PATIENT'S CHART ▶
2. INITIAL AND DETACH COPY EACH TIME PHYSICIAN WRITES ORDERS
3. TRANSMIT COPY TO PHARMACY

DATE	ORDERS	TRANS BY
	Diagnosis: Uterine Leiomyomata	
	Sensitivities/Drug Allergies: None known	
3/20/78		
1500 hrs:	1. Admit to Dr. Rogers for TAH-BSO in AM	
	2. Regular Diet	
	3. Up ad-lib	
	4. Tylenol 10 grains p.o. q 4 h, prn pain.	
	5. Dalmane 30 mg. p.o. q hs, prn sleep.	
	6. Routine vital signs q. shift.	
	7. CBC, VDRL	
	8. CCMS urine for U/A and C/S	
	9. T & C for 2 units whole blood.	
	10. S-S enema at bedtime.	
	11. Abdominal-perineal prep.	
	12. Betadine douche at bedtime	
	13. Chest x-ray	
	14. E.K.G.	
	15. Call for any problems	
	Dr. Rogers	
3/20/78		
1600 hrs:	1. NPO 2400 hrs.	
	2. Morphine 8 mg. I.M. on call in AM	
	3. Atropine 0.4 mg. I.M. on call in AM	
	Dr. Jones	

Do Not Write Orders If No Copies Remain; Begin New Form   Copies Remaining

PHYSICIAN'S ORDERS   T-5

Figure 1

thorough bowel preparation, and this can be accomplished by the use of oral magnesium citrate and castor oil. Psychologic preparation for this surgery is of great importance.

5. Adequate amounts of whole blood (usually 2 units) should be typed and cross matched for all major cases. Unless indicated, routine cross matching of blood for minor procedures is unnecessary.

6. An appropriate preoperative consent signed by the patient must be part of the chart prior to the procedure.

Operative Evaluation

Every patient should have a bimanual examination under anesthesia before the patient is prepped. This will allow a change in surgical ap-

INDIANA UNIVERSITY HOSPITALS
INDIANAPOLIS, INDIANA   INSERT #2

Rev. 3/77	PHYSICIAN'S ORDERS	M6552100	

1. ADDRESSOGRAPH BEFORE PLACING IN PATIENT'S CHART ▶

2. INITIAL AND DETACH COPY EACH TIME PHYSICIAN WRITES ORDERS

3. TRANSMIT COPY TO PHARMACY

DATE	ORDERS	TRANS BY
	Diagnosis: Dysfunctional Uterine Bleeding	
	Sensitivities/Drug Allergies: None Known	
3/20/78 1500 hrs:	1. Admit to Dr. Rogers D & C in AM	
	2. Regular diet	
	3. Up ad-lib	
	4. Tylenol 10 grains p.o. q 4 h prn pain	
	5. Dalmane 30 mg. p.o. q h.s. prn sleep	
	6. Routine vital signs q shift	
	7. CBC, VDRL	
	8. CCMS urine for U/A and C/S	
	9. S-S enema @ bedtime	
	10. Chest x-ray	
	11. E.K.G.	
	12. Call for any problems	
	Dr. Rogers	
	Anesthesia Pre-op	
3/20/78 1600 hrs:	1. NPO 2400 hrs.	
	2. Morphine 8 mg. I.M. on call in AM	
	3. Atropine 0.4 mg. I.M. on call in AM	
	Dr. Jones	

Do Not Write Orders If No Copies Remain; Begin New Form   Copies Remaining

PHYSICIAN'S ORDERS   T-5

MEDICAL RECORD COPY   B-CLIN. NOTES   E-LAB   G-X-RAY   K-DIAGNOSTIC   M-SURGERY   O-THERAPY   T-ORDERS   W-NURSING   Y-MISC.

Figure 2

proach if indicated with a minimum of delay. It is imperative that the bladder and bowel be empty in order to obtain an adequate examination. The quality of an examination under anesthesia is so good that it should be done even if the patient is scheduled only for minor surgery and is thought to have a normal pelvic examination. Proper positioning of the patient on the operating room table is important to avoid injury that will present itself during the postoperative period. Care must be taken to avoid contact between skin and metal if electrocautery is to be used.

Postoperative Care

It is imperative that the surgeon communicate the pertinent details of the procedure as well as the management plan during the postoperative period. This is done through clear and concise orders and a thorough written note in the chart. Postoperative orders void all prior orders and include the following areas:

1. Statement of the procedure and general condition of the patient.

2. Diet, if any.

3. Activities to include early ambulation.

4. Medications are given for pain, sleep, sedation, and nausea as needed. Antibiotics are used if indicated or continued for 48 hours if given prophylactically. If started, low-dose heparin should be continued (5000 units subcutaneously every 12 hours) until the patient is ambulatory for 48 hours. Other medications relating to general health should be ordered. Intravenous fluids should be given to maintain good fluid and electrolyte balance. Blood transfusions (packed cells) should be given to maintain the hemoglobin to near 10 grams per dl. (100 ml.). With large volume losses, whole blood rather than packed cells should be used.

5. Nursing measures include frequent vital signs, intake and output, early ambulation, pulmonary toilet, and care of drains. If infection is present, appropriate infection control measures are necessary.

6. Laboratory evaluation includes monitoring of the hemoglobin and hematocrit. Other tests are obtained as the patient's health indicates.

A brief operative note should be written in the chart. This will guide those caring for the patient until a formal dictated and typed note is returned to the chart. The written note should include the diagnosis, procedure performed, anesthesia, operative findings, blood loss, fluid replacement, presence of drains, complications, packs, and condition of the patient.

General Remarks About Postoperative Care

1. Fluid status and continued blood loss are best evaluated in the immediate postoperative period by changes in pulse, blood pressure and urinary output, not hemoglobin and hematocrit.

2. Accurate intake and output are necessary for management of fluid balance and need to reflect loss from all drains as well as insensible loss. In difficult cases, central venous pressure monitoring is of value.

3. Ambulation and pulmonary toilet should be started on the evening of surgery.

4. Return of bowel function is evidenced by spontaneous passage of flatus and diet should be withheld until this occurs. A few ice chips or water sips may be given if bowel sounds are present but no flatus has been passed.

5. Drains should be removed only when the output is minimal, not at a "routine" time.

6. A suspected ileus should be treated with nasogastric suction and by prohibiting oral intake (NPO). A bowel obstruction should be suspected if an ileus persists more than 7 postoperative days.

7. Large enemas should be avoided for bowel stimulation if an appendectomy was done.

8. Urinalysis and culture should be obtained when Foley catheter use is discontinued. Unless a catheter was anchored, culture is not necessary.

9. The usual sequence for infection is pulmonary, urinary, and wound. Less common causes for fever are thrombophlebitis, pulmonary embolus, sepsis, abscess formation, drug reaction, or phlebitis at the intravenous injection site. Antibiotics should be used to treat infection, not fever. A thorough search for the cause of the fever should always be made. Mild elevations of temperature within first 24 hours after surgery are usually caused by atelectasis and respond to improved pulmonary toilet.

Discharge Instructions

By the time of release, the patient should be fully counseled as to the diagnosis, pathologic findings, procedure performed, and complications. Full instructions regarding activity, medications, and follow-up appointment should be given to the patient and documented in the medical record.

THROMBOPHLEBITIS

method of
JOSEPH J. ROVINSKY, M.D.
New Hyde Park, New York

The disease entities of thrombophlebitis, phlebothrombosis, and pulmonary embolization constitute the triad of thromboembolic disorders.

Thrombophlebitis is initiated by an inflammatory reaction in or around a venous channel, usually peripheral but occasionally within the pelvis. Either superficial or deep veins or both may be involved. Vascular wall injury at the site of inflammation results in the development of an adherent and relatively firm thrombus. Theoretically, there should be little risk of embolization from such a thrombus; actually, the platelet thrombus may extend along the venous channel, resulting in a secondary phlebothrombosis.

In phlebothrombosis, a thrombus forms in a deep venous channel, usually in the lower extremity, initially may produce no clinical symptoms, and may extend proximally into larger venous channels. Primarily, this is a coagulation thrombus with a "white" base consisting of platelet aggregates and a "red" tail consisting of fibrin and trapped blood elements; this tail grows by apposition, undergoes retraction, and floats freely in the vein lumen. The soft, irregular thrombus readily disrupts, and frequently is the source of pulmonary emboli. The time required for such a thrombus to organize and attach to the vessel wall may be weeks, months, or even years.

Normal pregnancy creates a state of hypercoagulability and represents a period of increased thromboembolic risk. The pregnant woman physiologically manifests elevations in the concentrations of plasma procoagulants (prothrombin, proconvertin complex, accelerator globulin, and antihemophilic globulin), increased levels of fibrinogen, thrombocytosis, increased platelet reactivity, and impaired fibrinolysis—all changes observed as well after major surgical procedures. To this are added the mechanical factors of venous stasis and pelvic operative procedures. The risk of thromboembolism is 20 times greater in the puerperium than in pregnancy itself, in great part because of steroid suppression of lactation. The risk is increased three-fold by primary cesarean section as compared to vaginal delivery, increased 10-fold by repeat cesarean section, and 50-fold by cesarean section after previous major uterine surgery. A 50 per cent protective influence of blood group O has been documented, but remains unexplained.

Superficial Thrombophlebitis

This condition often develops in varicose veins during pregnancy, particularly in the third trimester and in multiparous women. The superficial varicosity becomes firm, knotty, and tender to palpation, and exhibits local symptoms of inflammation. When the disease remains localized, there is no risk of embolization.

Treatment. 1. Circulatory support with an elastic bandage or stocking extending above the area of inflammation. The patient may remain ambulatory.

2. Mild analgesics as required for comfort. Local application of heat may give some symptomatic relief.

3. Anticoagulation is not necessary and should be prescribed only if deep vein involvement is suspected.

4. Anti-inflammatory drugs such as phenylbutazone (Butazolidin), oxyphenbutazone (Tandearil), or ibuprofen (Motrin) are not necessary in what is a self-limiting process of short duration, and carry a significant risk of adverse reactions.

5. Definitive management of the varicosities should be deferred until after the puerperium.

Deep Vein Thrombophlebitis/Phlebothrombosis

The diagnosis of deep vein thrombosis is more difficult to establish, yet the hazard to the patient is much greater. The frequency of pulmonary embolization in the diagnosed but untreated patient is 2.5 per cent; each case, therefore, is potentially fatal. A clinically silent phlebothrombosis may first become evident by the appearance of a pulmonary embolism.

Diagnosis. A high index of suspicion is required, particularly in patients with a history of prior thromboembolic disease, varicose veins of unusual severity, obesity, or multiparity. Every patient with puerperal fever must be suspect. Clinical symptoms are highly variable and are well described elsewhere. When suspected clinically, the diagnosis must be confirmed by laboratory techniques.

Treatment. 1. Hospitalization and absolute bed rest. Ambulation may be permitted as soon as acute local symptoms have subsided—ordinarily about 5 to 6 days.

2. Heparin anticoagulation is the prime immediate treatment of deep vein thrombosis. In therapeutic doses, heparin inhibits the activity of tissue thromboplastin and coagulation factors VII (proconvertin) and IX (Christmas factor), combines with a plasma protein to form an antithrombin that inhibits the transformation of fibrinogen to fibrin, and impairs platelet aggregation. In the acute episode, the drug is best administered intravenously in a dilute solution (1000 units per ml.) through an indwelling catheter, either continuously (with an infusion pump) or intermittently. Intermittent injection by the intravenous route appears to be the method of choice and provides several advantages in initial therapy: It assures immediate onset of action, the duration of which is relatively predictable and dose-related. Peak prolongation of the clotting time occurs within minutes and returns to normal over a dose-related period of time. The administration of 5000 to 15,000 units of heparin produces a general duration of effect from at least 2 to as long as 6 hours; the extent and duration of clotting time prolongation for a given dose is influenced both by the patient's weight and by the presence of "heparin resistance," which usually is maximal in the early stages of thrombosis. The heparin effect may be reversed promptly by the administration of an equivalent dose of protamine sulfate.

Heparin dose requirements for the treatment of peripheral deep vein thrombosis have not been established firmly. Experimentally, it has been shown that venous thrombosis and clot propagation can be prevented when the clotting time (Lee-White) is prolonged by heparin to 1.5 to 2 times normal values. More recently, it has been demonstrated that a tripling of the control value may be necessary to prevent formation of a stasis thrombus. At these levels of clotting time prolongation, thrombus formation via the thrombin-fibrinogen pathway is prevented, and experimental venous thrombosis cannot be induced. These observations form the basis for clinical practice. A whole blood clotting time of two to three times *normal* control values (not necessarily the patient's control value, since this may be accelerated), generally requiring from 20,000 to 60,000 units of heparin every 24 hours by the intermittent intravenous route, has been found effective and safe; this corresponds to an activated partial thromboplastin time (PTT) of 1.5 to 2.5 times normal values. At this dose level, the thrombotic process is arrested in the extremities, and recanalization probably is enhanced.

3. Coumarin derivatives inhibit the synthesis of coagulation factors II (prothrombin), VII (proconvertin), IX (Christmas factor), and X (Stuart factor) by the liver, and at least 20 hours are required significantly to increase the prothrombin time. These drugs are administered orally, and the daily maintenance dose depends on an assessment of the cumulative effect of therapy by daily estimation of the prothrombin time. In the transition from heparin to an orally administered coumarin derivative, a period of overlap of the two drugs is necessary for optimal treatment, keeping in mind that coumarin derivatives fail to exert a measurable antithrombotic effect for at least 5 days. At therapeutic doses, the prothrombin time is maintained at two to three times normal levels.

4. Thrombolytic therapy. Streptokinase and urokinase are enzymes recently available for the treatment of venous thrombosis and embolism. These agents activate the innate plasminogen/plasmin system and cause the dissolution of existing thrombi. Since the enzymes induce lysis of fibrin in hemostatic plugs as well as in thromboemboli and can cause bleeding anywhere in the body, in addition to the potential side effects of fever (50 per cent of cases), allergic reactions, and renal complications, their use in peripheral deep vein thrombosis is on tenuous grounds.

5. Surgical intervention. Interruption of venous return usually is reserved for the patient who has suffered one or more pulmonary emboli despite adequate anticoagulation therapy or in whom anticoagulation therapy is contraindicated. In such patients, prompt and adequate surgical intervention may be lifesaving, protects the mother against further embolization, and involves no risk to the fetus. Ligation of the femoral veins bilaterally is not fully protective because of the frequent involvement during pregnancy of the pelvic and gluteal veins, which drain into the iliac vessels above the inguinal ligament; interruption at a higher level therefore is necessary. The inferior vena cava may be interrupted just below the level of the right renal vein either by ligation or by placement of a serrated Teflon clip. The risk of the surgical procedure in experienced hands is about 2 per cent; rarely does an enlarged uterus in pregnancy interfere with an extraperitoneal approach to the inferior vena cava. The collateral circulation in pregnancy is such that the incidence of postoperative leg swelling is minimal, and interference by the resultant hemodynamic changes with continuation of the pregnancy is extremely rare. The ovarian veins may be involved in the thrombophlebitic process, especially if sepsis is present. If a pelvic source of embolism is suspected, bilateral ovarian vein ligation also must be accomplished. After the first few weeks of gestation, there is little risk of abortion following this procedure.

6. Special considerations in pregnancy. During pregnancy, coumarin derivatives are best avoided except under most unusual circumstances; these drugs have a low molecular weight, traverse the placenta readily, and have resulted in reported cases of hemorrhagic death of the fetus, even with low dose therapy of the mother, in the absence of maternal bleeding complications, and without the trauma of labor and delivery. In addition, coumarin derivatives have a significant teratogenic potential if administered during the first trimester. Accordingly, anticoagulation should be maintained with heparin alone throughout gestation; once the required dose has been established, the patient may be taught successfully to self-administer the required three to four daily injections through an in-dwelling heparin lock. Anticoagulation should be maintained up to and through labor and delivery. Three to four days after delivery, a coumarin derivative regimen may be substituted. In puerperal thrombophlebitis, heparin should be used until subsidence of the acute, painful stage of the disease and coumarin derivatives substituted thereafter. *Anticoagulation postpartum should be maintained for 3 to 6 months* to minimize the risk of puerperal thromboembolism.

CONTRACEPTION

method of
ELIZABETH B. CONNELL, M.D.
New York, New York

Introduction

Definition. By strict definition, *contraception* is the prevention of conception, and a *contraceptive* is an agent that prevents conception. However, the

TABLE 1. **Contraceptive Effectiveness***

METHOD	THEORETICAL EFFECTIVENESS (CONSTANT USERS) (%)	USE-EFFECTIVENESS (ACTUAL USERS) (%)
Abortion	0	0
Abstinence	0	?
Chance	80	80
Coitus interruptus	15	30
Condom	5	15–25
Diaphragm	5	15–25
Douche	—	31
IUD	1–3	3–10
Oral contraceptives	0.1 to 1.0	5–25
Long-acting progestin (IM)	0.3	5–10
Rhythm	15	40
Spermicidal preparations	5	15–25
Condom and spermicidal agent	1	5
Sterilization—male	0.014	0.14+
Sterilization—female:		
Tubal ligation	0.008	0.008
Hysterectomy	0.001	0.0001

**Contraceptive Technology*—The Emory University Family Planning Program. Department of Gynecology and Obstetrics, Emory University School of Medicine, Atlanta, Georgia.

term contraception is used today in a much more general sense—control of unwanted fertility by a wide variety of preparations and techniques. In this broader sense, it is therefore appropriate to consider not only the classic methods but also the developing fields of male and female sterilization and abortion.

Theoretical vs. Use-Effectiveness vs. Extended Use-Effectiveness. The effectiveness of contraception is currently defined in three different ways. The first of these is called the theoretical or ideal effectiveness of a method. This is the effectiveness that can be obtained by the correct and consistent use of any particular preparation or method. The second is the general effectiveness of a particular method when used by large numbers of persons and includes patient errors. The third is its effectiveness when used by many people over extended periods of time. Clearly, the three measurements may have quite divergent results. This is particularly true with those methods of contraception that require repetitive performances of techniques, the success of which depends upon the long-term motivation of one or both of the sexual partners, such as the coitus-oriented methods. The second and third measurements are very important when one evaluates large-scale programs.

The theoretical and use-effectiveness rates for the most commonly used methods are shown in Table 1. It is now increasingly accepted that a method which is theoretically completely effective must also be easy to administer, inexpensive, highly acceptable, and have minimal side effects in order for its use-effectiveness to equal its theoretical effectiveness. The following evaluation of each contraceptive method will therefore include its current state of development, its effectiveness in individual and group situations, and a brief estimate of the potential of the particular method for the future.

OVUM DEVELOPMENT

Lactation

For centuries women have been aware of the fact that so long as they continued to nurse their babies, their chances of becoming pregnant were decreased. This is due to the fact that lactating women do not begin to ovulate again for some time after delivery. However, this technique is far from 100 per cent effective, because as time goes by there is an increasing likelihood that ovulation will occur while lactation is still going on. Thus, it is possible to ovulate and become pregnant without ever having a postpartum menstrual period.

One of the signs of "progress" in developing countries today is a decrease in breast feeding, stimulated by widespread advertising of infant formula products. This has been unfortunate from the health point of view, and also because it removes one of the major methods of family planning. Recognition of the importance of lactation has recently led to research on the use of hormones to stimulate lactation and keep the patient from resuming ovulation.

Oral Contraception

Development. The suppression of ovulation reached a high peak of effectiveness when it was discovered that various hormonal agents administered orally would prevent the release of eggs

TABLE 2. **Oral Contraceptives Available in the United States**

TRADE NAME	ESTROGEN	DOSE	PROGESTIN	DOSE	MANU-FACTURER
Combined					
Brevicon (21 day)	Ethinyl estradiol	0.035 mg.	Norethindrone	0.5 mg.	Syntex
Brevicon (28 day)	Ethinyl estradiol	0.035 mg.	Norethindrone	0.5 mg.	Syntex
Demulen (21 day)	Ethinyl estradiol	0.05 mg.	Ethynodiol diacetate	1.0 mg.	Searle
Demulen (28 day)	Ethinyl estradiol	0.05 mg.	Ethynodiol diacetate	1.0 mg.	Searle
Enovid-E (20 day)	Mestranol	0.10 mg.	Norethynodrel	2.5 mg.	Searle
Enovid-5 (20 day)	Mestranol	0.075 mg.	Norethynodrel	5.0 mg.	Searle
Loestrin 1.5/30 (21 day)	Ethinyl estradiol	0.030 mg.	Norethindrone acetate	1.5 mg.	Parke, Davis
Loestrin 1/20 (21 day)	Ethinyl estradiol	0.020 mg.	Norethindrone acetate	1.0 mg.	Parke, Davis
Modicon (21 day)	Ethinyl estradiol	0.035 mg.	Norethindrone	0.5 mg.	Ortho
Modicon (28 day)	Ethinyl estradiol	0.035 mg.	Norethindrone	0.5 mg.	Ortho
Norinyl-1/50 (21 day)	Mestranol	0.05 mg.	Norethindrone	1.0 mg.	Syntex
Norinyl-1/50 (28 day)	Mestranol	0.05 mg.	Norethindrone	1.0 mg.	Syntex
Norinyl-1/80 (21 day)	Mestranol	0.08 mg.	Norethindrone	1.0 mg.	Syntex
Norinyl-1/80 (28 day)	Mestranol	0.08 mg.	Norethindrone	1.0 mg.	Syntex
Norinyl-2	Mestranol	0.10 mg.	Norethindrone	2.0 mg.	Syntex
Norlestrin-1 (21 day)	Ethinyl estradiol	0.05 mg.	Norethindrone acetate	1.0 mg.	Parke, Davis
Norlestrin-1 (28 day)	Ethinyl estradiol	0.05 mg.	Norethindrone acetate	1.0 mg.	Parke, Davis
Norlestrin-1(Fe) (28 day)	Ethinyl estradiol	0.05 mg.	Norethindrone acetate	1.0 mg.	Parke, Davis
Norlestrin 2.5 (21 day)	Ethinyl estradiol	0.05 mg.	Norethindrone acetate	2.5 mg.	Parke, Davis
Norlestrin (Fe)2.5 (28 day)	Ethinyl estradiol	0.05 mg.	Norethindrone acetate	2.5 mg.	Parke, Davis
Ortho-Novum 1/50 (20 day)	Mestranol	0.05 mg.	Norethindrone	1.0 mg.	Ortho
Ortho-Novum 1/50 (21 day)	Mestranol	0.05 mg.	Norethindrone	1.0 mg.	Ortho
Ortho-Novum 1/80 (21 day)	Mestranol	0.08 mg.	Norethindrone	1.0 mg.	Ortho
Ortho-Novum-2 (20 day)	Mestranol	0.10 mg.	Norethindrone	2.0 mg.	Ortho
Ortho-Novum 10 (20 day)	Mestranol	0.06 mg.	Norethindrone	10.0 mg.	Ortho
Ovral (21 day)	Ethinyl estradiol	0.05 mg.	Norgestrel	0.5 mg.	Wyeth
Ovulen (20 day)	Mestranol	0.10 mg.	Ethynodiol diacetate	1.0 mg.	Searle
Ovulen (21 day)	Mestranol	0.10 mg.	Ethynodiol diacetate	1.0 mg.	Searle
Zorane 1/50 (21 day)	Ethinyl estradiol	0.050 mg.	Norethindrone acetate	1.0 mg.	Lederle
Zorane 1.5/30 (21 day)	Ethinyl estradiol	0.030 mg.	Norethindrone acetate	1.5 mg.	Lederle
Zorane 1/20 (21 day)	Ethinyl estradiol	0.020 mg.	Norethindrone acetate	1.0 mg.	Lederle
Minipill					
Micronor (35 day)			Norethindrone	0.35 mg.	Ortho
Nor-Q.D. (42 day)			Norethindrone	0.35 mg.	Syntex
Ovrette (28 day)			d 1-Norgestrel	0.075 mg.	Wyeth

from ovaries. Today the oral contraceptives remain the most effective method of family planning. Taken properly, they may virtually remove any fear of pregnancy. However, the use-effectiveness remains somewhat lower than the theoretical effectiveness because of the difficulty some women have in remembering to take their pills as directed. The many oral contraceptives currently available are listed in Table 2.

Side Effects. A recent survey has estimated that 9.5 to 10 million women in the United States and 30 to 40 million women in the rest of the world are now taking these preparations for conception control. Another 50 million women have used them in the past. Therefore, the evaluation of actual and potential side effects is extremely important. One of the major reasons that we do not have statistically valid answers to many of the questions being raised is seen in Table 3, which indicates the numbers of women who would have to be studied in order to answer these perplexing questions.

Many signs and symptoms, such as nausea, vomiting, breast tenderness, and breakthrough bleeding, have been correctly ascribed to the use of oral contraceptives. These symptoms were particularly common in the early years when the dosage was higher. However, with decreased dosage, the incidence of these troublesome but not serious side effects has declined markedly.

Certain other potentially serious side effects are now well documented.

THROMBOEMBOLISM. A statistically valid cause and effect relationship between use of the oral contraceptives and myocardial infarction and pulmonary and cerebral thromboembolism has been established. There appears to be a predictable risk for oral contraceptive users above and beyond the spontaneous occurrence of these disorders in untreated women. The generally accepted figure for the mortality from thromboembolic disorders caused by the use of older oral contraceptives is about 3 per 100,000 women per year. The increase in risk is presently estimated

TABLE 3. **Minimal Samples Required to Detect Differences in Disease Rates Between OC Users and Controls in Prospective Study*†**

| | | | PERSONS REQUIRED IN EACH GROUP | |
| | NO. OF YEARS AFTER ONSET OF | ANNUAL INCIDENCE RATE | *Incidence Two Times* | *Incidence Five Times* |
DISEASE	STUDY	IN CONTROLS PER 10,000	*in OC Users*	*in OC Users*
Cancer of the breast	1	2.2	85,000	11,000
Cancer of the corpus uteri	1	0.3	600,000	80,000
Cancer of the cervix	1	3.1	60,000	7500
Cancer of the breast	10	7.5	25,000	3000
Cancer of the corpus uteri	10	1.3	140,000	20,000
Cancer of the cervix	10	5.6	35,000	5000
Diabetes	1	20	9000	1200
Malformations	1	300	600	100
Thromboemboli	1	20	9000	1200

*From Seigel, D., and Corfman, P.: J.A.M.A. *203*:950, 1968. Copyright 1968, American Medical Association.

†OC = oral contraceptive. It is assumed that this is a simple random sample of "ever users" of ages between 20 and 45 years. Sample sizes for malformations are for births. The table is computed for one-tailed significance tests at 0.05 level with power equal to 0.8.

to be 4- to 11-fold. However, the more recent data suggest that as hormonal dosage is decreased, the risk also goes down proportionally.

The risk of cerebrovascular accident or stroke is currently estimated to be approximately 4 to 9.5 times greater for women taking oral contraceptives. Furthermore, newer data have shown an increased risk of myocardial infarction from use of oral contraceptives as shown in Table 4. It must be remembered that the risk of cardiovascular death must be weighed against death rates from other causes, particularly those related to pregnancy and induced abortion. The comparison is even more striking in many less developed areas of the world where the maternal mortality and morbidity are infinitely higher.

Inasmuch as there appears to be a four- to six-fold increase in the risk of thromboembolic complications following surgery in oral contraceptive (OC) users, it is recommended that the pill be stopped at least 4 weeks prior to elective major procedures and whenever a woman is going to be immobilized for a considerable period of time.

HYPERTENSION. An acute elevation in blood pressure has been reported to occur in a small number of women during the first few months of use of the oral contraceptives. In general, with the exception of this group, hypertension is not found in the first few years of use. By the fifth year, however, there is a 2.5- to 3-fold increase in the prevalence of hypertension among users as compared to nonusers. There is some suggestion that women who had an elevation in blood pressure during pregnancy are more likely to develop this complication. Blood pressures usually return to normal levels within a short time after discontinuation of the oral contraceptive.

MALIGNANCY. Three sites of the female reproductive tract are being carefully watched for possible effects of the long-term use of the oral contraceptive—breasts, endometrium, and cervix. With respect to the first two, there has been no increase to date in their incidence during those years in which there has been wider use of these preparations. In fact, it is interesting to note that recent studies suggest that the oral contraceptives may actually exert a protective effect on the anovulatory woman who has an increased risk of endometrial malignancy. In addition, it has been shown that women on the pill have a lower incidence of benign breast diseases. Since malignancies of the breast and endometrium occur primarily in women closer to the end of the child-bearing age than in the age group currently using the oral contraceptive, long-range evaluations must be carried out in order to be sure that continued safety is established.

METABOLIC CHANGES. Extensive studies of patients taking oral contraceptives have shown

TABLE 4. **Estimated Annual Mortality Rate Per 100,000 Women from Myocardial Infarction by Use of Oral Contraceptives, Smoking Habits, and Age (in Years)***

| | MYOCARDIAL INFARCTION | | | |
| | *Women Aged 30–39* | | *Women Aged 40–44* | |
SMOKING HABITS	Users	Nonusers	Users	Nonusers
All smokers	10.2	2.6	62.0	15.9
Heavy†	13.0	5.1	78.7	31.3
Light	4.7	0.9	28.6	5.7
Nonsmokers	1.8	1.2	10.7	7.4
Smokers and nonsmokers	5.4	1.9	32.8	11.7

*From Jain, A. K.: Studies in Family Planning, *8*:50, 1977.
†Heavy smoker: 15 or more cigarettes per day.

that numerous changes occur. They have a decreased glucose tolerance, elevated plasma insulin levels, and increased serum triglycerides, serum alpha 2 and beta globulins, and serum carrier proteins. Thyroxine-binding globulins are increased, leading to an increase in protein-bound iodine (PBI) and T_4 and a decrease in T_3 resin uptake, but free thyroxine remains normal. An increase in transcortin leads to an elevation of plasma cortisol and angiotensin 1; angiotensinase and plasma renin substrate are also increased. However, almost without exception, these side effects disappear shortly after discontinuance of the oral contraceptives. Therefore, the specter raised about the induction of diabetes mellitus and arteriosclerosis remains a real one, but so far sufficient data have not been obtained either to verify or to disprove such an association.

LIVER. Some patients on oral contraceptives will show a decrease in certain of the liver function tests such as the sodium sulfobromophthalein (Bromsulphalein [BSP]). In addition, serum glutamic oxaloacetic transaminase (SGOT), alkaline phosphatase, and plasma triglycerides and phospholipids may be elevated. As in other areas, the tests have returned to normal after discontinuance of the oral contraceptive. The significance of these temporary changes remains unclear. However, since estrogen is metabolized by the liver, it would appear wise not to give oral contraceptives to women who have acute or chronic liver disease.

Recently benign adenomas of the liver have been reported in women taking oral contraceptives. When these are diagnosed and treated promptly, no further trouble has occurred. However, serious hemorrhage has been reported in certain patients. It appears that the risk of developing these tumors increases after 4 or more years of oral contraceptive usage. A few women taking the pill have been found to have hepatocellular carcinoma, but no causal relationship to the pill has been demonstrated.

GALLBLADDER. Several articles have appeared recently linking the pill to an increased incidence of surgically confirmed gallbladder disease. Changes in biliary metabolism of liver pigments induced by estrogen have been suggested as the possible mechanism for the development of this complication. It is also possible that women developing gallstones might have done so in any event, but use of oral contraceptives may have accelerated the time of occurrence. The risk appears to go up after 6 or more months of use, being double after 4 or 5 years.

FETAL EFFECTS. Chromosomal changes resulting in triploidy have been reported in abortuses of women who have taken oral contraceptives. However, these changes are always lethal. There are also reports suggesting a possible association between oral contraceptive use and congenital heart disease and limb-reduction defects. For these reasons, these agents should not be used as tests for possible pregnancy.

MENSTRUAL IRREGULARITIES. Some women have breakthrough bleeding during oral contraceptive use. Others, particularly those on the higher doses of oral contraceptives, develop hypo- or amenorrhea. In most instances, this may produce anxiety but no permanent ill effects on the health of the women. It is usually rapidly reversed by stopping the medication or by changing the type of contraceptive agent. Conversely, many women who have premenstrual tension, irregular periods, heavy menses or dysmenorrhea often find that they are improved when they take oral contraceptives.

RETURN OF FERTILITY. Sufficient data have now been collected to show that most women have a prompt return of fertility after stopping the pill, the pregnancy rate 3 to 6 months post-therapy being comparable to rates obtained in noncontracepting women. A small percentage of women will not immediately begin to ovulate spontaneously, but most of them can be stimulated by the administration of clomiphene citrate or menotropins and human chorionic gonadotropin (HCG). However, a few patients have recently been reported for whom even this therapy proved ineffective and ovulation was delayed for a considerable period of time. Prolonged amenorrhea either with or without galactorrhea may result from a benign tumor of the pituitary, a chromophobe microadenoma. The diagnosis can be confirmed by performing luteinizing hormone (LH), follicle-stimulating hormone (FSH) and prolactin assays and by x-ray of the sella turcica. Successful therapy of this condition has been reported using either surgical removal or treatment with bromergocryptine (investigational).

MISCELLANEOUS SIDE EFFECTS. It is clear that certain women have additional types of responses to oral contraceptives. These responses include growth of uterine leiomyomata, fluid retention and weight gain; development of chloasma, and the accentuation of preexisting migraine and depression. As noted before, removal of the contraceptive agent will lead to the rapid relief of symptoms in almost all instances. Acne is often improved during use of the pill. Evaluation of libido changes shows no constant pattern, any alteration appearing to reflect the basic personality of the user.

Contraindications. The following are the contraindications to the use of oral contraceptives currently listed by the Food and Drug Administration: (1) thrombophlebitis or thromboembolic disorders; (2) a past history of deep vein thrombophlebitis or thromboembolic disorders; (3) cerebral vascular or coronary artery disease; (4) known or suspected carcinoma of the breast; (5) known or suspected estrogen-dependent neoplasia; (6) undiagnosed abnormal genital bleeding; (7) known or suspected pregnancy.

There are a number of conditions that might be considered as relative contraindications of greater or lesser degree in addition to those discussed before: (1) gestational diabetes or a strong family history of diabetes mellitus; (2) strong family history of breast carcinoma; (3) lactation; (4) serious psychiatric disorders, especially with a history of depression; (5) history of idiopathic jaundice of pregnancy; (6) active liver disease; (7) nulliparous women with grossly irregular menses; (8) large uterine leiomyomas; (9) gallbladder disease; (10) severe varicosities; (11) chronic cardiac disease; (12) severe hypertension; (13) severe renal disease; (14) migraine headaches; (15) obesity; (16) chloasma; (17) epilepsy; (18) sickle cell disease or trait; and (19) congenital hyperlipidemia.

CONTINUATION RATES. Continuation rates with the oral contraceptives vary tremendously from one group to another. Highly motivated patients have rates of upward of 85 per cent at the end of the first year, excluding those women who have stopped medication in order to begin a planned pregnancy. Large-scale studies in clinic settings show rates of 65 to 75 per cent at the end of 1 year, dropping to as low as 40 to 50 per cent at the end of 2 years. In general, continuation rates are somewhat higher among younger and more educated women. However, the hypothesis that women of lesser education and those in lower socioeconomic groups are not suitable candidates for the oral contraceptive is progressively being disproved. Continuing worldwide evaluation of the use of the pill as a major method of contraception supports this thesis.

LOW ESTROGEN PILLS. In efforts to decrease or eliminate the known or suspected side effects of estrogen, attempts have been made to decrease the amount of estrogen in the pill. Experience has shown that this can be done, doses as low as 20 micrograms being used. However, as the dose drops, a point is reached at which occasional pregnancies will occur and irregular bleeding patterns become a problem. Longer experience is needed to assess the gain from a lower estrogen dose against the loss of fertility and cycle control. In general, the lowest dose pill should be used that, for any given patient, provides satisfactory cycle control.

MINI-PILL. The "mini-pill" is a progestin given daily without interruption. Its mode of action remains unclear, but there is evidence to suggest that the stopping of ovulation is not of prime importance, but rather the changes in the cervical mucus, endometrium, or tubal transport.

The theoretical advantage of the "mini-pill" is that, since it does not contain estrogen, the side effects associated with the use of that hormone may be reduced or abolished. It appears that hematologic and metabolic alterations are indeed less with the "mini-pill" than with the older preparations. However, the bleeding patterns and pregnancy rates obtained with the various "mini-pill" preparations are not as satisfactory as those obtained with conventional combined therapy. Cycles tend to be irregular in about 25 per cent of patients, and some develop intermittent heavy bleeding. Pearl's Index ranges from 2 to 4 for most "mini-pills," being considerably higher in certain foreign programs in which the educational levels are lower and medical instruction of patients is less thorough than in the original domestic studies. The ultimate balance of side effects versus symptomatology remains to be clarified.

Other Routes of Hormonal Contraception

Injection. A number of preparations have been studied as injectable contraceptive agents to be administered at 1 to 3 month intervals. The potential exists for an injection that would last for 6, 12, or even a greater number of months. At present, these preparations remain in the research area, no injectable agent being as yet on the market. The product most extensively studied is medroxyprogesterone acetate (Depo-Provera), given in doses of 150 mg. every 3 months. Although this preparation is highly effective, there are still problems relative to irregular bleeding, prolonged amenorrhea, breast tumors in test beagle dogs, and delay in the return of ovulation. The United States Food and Drug Administration has recently disapproved this compound for use in the United States for these reasons.

An injectable agent has certain obvious advantages. Many patients, particularly in certain parts of the developing world, prefer injections to pill taking. Physicians working in areas where continuous medical care is lacking find injections given at frequent intervals to be especially valuable. In any area injectable contraceptive agents are ideal for patients who do not have the intellectual capability, emotional stability, or sustained motivation, or who cannot or lack the desire to use other methods.

Implants. Research is currently being carried out to evaluate continuous low dose progestins administered in Silastic capsules, rods and biodegradable microcapsules which are placed under the skin by use of a hypodermic needle. It has been suggested that such capsules could provide sustained release for as much as 5 or more years. If return of fertility is desired, the capsules are simply removed. However, certain problems still remain with this method, particularly in relation to cycle control.

Vaginal Rings. Compounds such as medroxyprogesterone acetate are being investigated, using an intravaginal Silastic ring as a carrier for hormones that are absorbed through the vaginal mucosa. The ring is left in place for approximately 3 weeks. After removal, withdrawal bleeding occurs, and a week later the same or a new ring is reinserted. This technique is still also at the investigational stage of development. It possesses the major advantage of avoiding the first pass through the liver, felt to be important in avoiding certain of the side effects produced when hormonal agents are taken by mouth and absorbed into the hepatic circulation.

Releasing Factors

Since hypothalamic releasing factors are now being isolated, the possibility of using or developing antagonists to these substances is being studied. For example, releasing factors such as the one for luteinizing hormone (LH) might be used to induce ovulation at a predictable time, during which abstinence could be practiced. Alternatively, the administration of the LH antagonist might prevent the release of LH and block ovulation. Although early results are promising, these methods will not be available in the near future.

OVUM TRANSPORT

More than a century ago it was realized that if the fallopian tubes were blocked in some way, ova could not be fertilized by sperm. From this observation have grown a wide variety of techniques for female sterilization. Most of these techniques involve the ligation, partial removal, or obstruction of the midportion of the fallopian tubes. An additional, although not quite reliable, method involves the removal of the fimbria bilaterally.

The effectiveness of most of the surgical procedures is virtually 100 per cent. Originally, they involved a hospital admission, usually being done either after delivery or abortion. More recently, increasing numbers are being carried out as elective procedures. In both instances, use of an operating room and general anesthesia have been required. Efforts have been made to find ways to carry out these procedures more quickly and easily, such as the use of the laparoscope or the culdoscope. Use of electrocautery and the application of clips, bands, and rings to the fallopian tubes have

been of help in this regard. In fact, sterilization is now the most frequently used method of family planning in both the United States and other parts of the world. Growing utilization is also being made of the simplified surgical technique known as the mini-lap.

It appears that certain of the newer methods may be carried out under local anesthesia on an out-patient basis. At the present time, these approaches are being used at many medical centers, and the applicability of these techniques in wide-scale sterilization programs, particularly where there are limited medical facilities, is being evaluated.

Research is being carried out on techniques in which materials such as silver nitrate, quinacrine, silicone polymers, and surgical adhesives are injected into the tubes, the cornual regions, or the endometrial cavity per se, in an attempt to obliterate these areas and produce permanent infertility. In addition, a great deal of work is also being devoted to attempts to find techniques that are reversible, such as temporary obstruction of the tubes by removable plastic and metal devices. The ultimate potential of these procedures for general application is not yet clear.

SPERM DEVELOPMENT

Methods closely paralleling those used by the female are currently being investigated for the control of fertility in the male. It has been known for a long time that large doses of testosterone and other androgens can prevent the maturation of sperm. However, production of azoospermia without the simultaneous production of metabolic side effects has not yet been achieved. Other hormones such as estrogens and progestins will lower the sperm count to zero, but they also concurrently decrease libido and potency. Research, therefore, continues for agents that will not allow sperm development, but that also will not interfere with any of the psychologic or physiologic functions of the male. It appears that the balanced administration of androgenic and progestogenic substances may be feasible as pills or injections. A number of hormonal agents are being placed under the skin as subdermal Silastic implants. Testicular antigens are being purified with the hope that they may be used to block spermatogenesis. Certain of these techniques look promising, but it is far too early to consider them as part of current therapy.

SPERM TRANSPORT

As in the case of the female, sterilization of the male is increasingly being used as a means of conception control. Numerous types of procedures have been and are being developed, the one most frequently employed being the conventional vasectomy in which a segment of each vas is removed. The operation is usually carried out in the physician's office under local anesthesia. It is highly effective, can be performed rapidly, and has a very low complication rate. The number of vasectomies done and clinics offering these procedures have grown steadily over the last 5 years both in this country and abroad.

A great deal of research is being conducted at present in attempts to find ways of making the vasectomy procedure consistently reversible. Clips, plugs, two-way valves, plastic threads, and many other methods are being tested in this connection. Surgical techniques obliterating the lining of the vas without destroying the surrounding muscular coat are also being evaluated in this regard. It is now clear that with minimal tissue removal it is possible later to reanastomose the vas. However, simple anatomic continuity has not yet been proved synonymous with the return of fertility. The best results obtained to date have been with the use of microsurgery, giving a return of fertility in more than three quarters of subjects.

FERTILIZATION

Natural Family Planning

Once the process of fertilization was understood, a variety of techniques were developed in order to try to prevent conception. One of the first and still widely recommended is that of rhythm, or natural family planning. This method, or course, remains the only contraceptive technique acceptable to the Roman Catholic Church. Rhythm may be carried out in two ways, one being much more effective than the other. The first is known as calendar rhythm. The days of probable ovulation are estimated by mathematical formulae based on a woman's previous menstrual history. If a woman has reasonably regular menses, this is a moderately acceptable and successful technique. However, this method prevents the woman with irregular cycles from having an active sexual life without a considerable risk of pregnancy. The second method is called the temperature rhythm technique and is quite effective. A woman takes her basal body temperature every morning and may have sexual relations only after the ovulatory rise. A more recent technique, known as the Billings Method, is based on the detection of ovulation by following the cyclic alterations in the cervical mucus and avoiding intercourse when midcycle changes appear.

All of these methods clearly require intelligence, motivation, and tremendous self-control on the part of both partners. Their popularity is understandably limited, and they are of little use in large-scale family planning programs. Furthermore, it has recently been reported that central nervous system defects, including Down's syndrome and anencephalia, occur with higher than average frequency in certain Roman Catholic populations. It has been suggested that this may be due to late fertilization occurring as the result of the failure of the natural family planning techniques.

Extravaginal Techniques

Coitus interruptus, the removal of the penis from the vagina prior to ejaculation, is probably the oldest and still one of the most widely used contraceptive techniques. When practiced by an intelligent, highly motivated male it is quite effective. However, it requires great self-control, and many men are either psychologically or physically incapable of using this method. Oral and anal intercourse and mutual masturbation are also highly successful for obvious reasons, but are of limited general application and usage.

Intravaginal Techniques

Condom. The condom, or contraceptive sheath, has been used since the eighteenth century. The original ones were made from sheep intestines. These were replaced by rubber and, most recently, by plastic. In addition to the contraceptive action of the condom, it provides a high degree of protection for both males and females against venereal disease. Faced with the rapid increase in venereal disease, public health physicians are reemphasizing the role of the condom in the contraceptive armamentarium.

When properly used, the condom is a highly effective method of contraception. It is necessary to apply the condom prior to intromission, leaving one inch free at the tip to allow room for the ejaculate. Failures occasionally result from tearing or from leakage of sperm from the open end of the condom if the penis is not removed from the vagina promptly after ejaculation.

The condom has the disadvantage of being necessarily related to the sexual act, and therefore being less acceptable to certain men and women than nonsex-related methods. In addition, certain persons find that the condom reduces the amount of stimulation during intercourse and is therefore less desirable than other techniques. Its usage is curtailed in certain areas of the world because of its long association with prostitution and venereal disease. These objections are gradually being dispelled by the development of new types of condoms, lubricated, made of thinner plastics in a wide variety of textures and colors, and also by improved patient education as to the advantages of this method.

Vaginal Diaphragm. This technique has been used since the late 1800s. Before the development of the oral contraceptive, the vaginal diaphragm was the medical technique most often used by women in the United States and in many developed areas of the world. It acts, in combination with a spermicidal cream or jelly, as a barrier to the entrance of sperm into the inner portions of the female reproductive tract. Correctly fitted and properly used on every occasion, the diaphragm is highly effective. Failures most often result from its nonuse at a time when a woman feels that she cannot become pregnant. In addition, it may be incorrectly inserted so that the cervix is not covered, or, rarely, it may be displaced during intercourse. The diaphragm must be inserted before each act of sexual intercourse, carefully checked to make sure that it is in the proper position, and left in place for 5 to 6 hours thereafter. Additional spermicide must be applied, leaving the diaphragm in situ, if coitus occurs again during this time.

Concern about the known and suspected side effects of oral contraceptives and intrauterine devices has caused many women to begin or return to the use of the diaphragm.

Douche. For centuries women have douched with water, vinegar, and a variety of herbs and chemicals after intercourse in an attempt to prevent pregnancy by killing or washing out the sperm. However, since sperm are known to be in the endocervical mucus in less than 2 minutes after ejaculation, this technique is obviously of limited or no value as a contraceptive method.

Vaginal Preparations. A wide variety of vaginal preparations have been used for contraception for thousands of years. The older methods included chemicals such as heavy metals, herb, plant, and animal preparations. Currently, a number of spermicidal agents are being employed, including jellies, creams, suppositories, tablets, and aerosol foams. In general, these techniques are not as effective as the pill and IUD. Although they are relatively easy to use and do not have to be dispensed by a physician, many women find them unacceptable because they are messy and because they prefer techniques unrelated to the time of intercourse. However, when used properly and consistently, particularly in conjuction with condoms, a high level of effectiveness may be obtained. In addition, early work suggests that certain of the vaginal agents may also exert an antivenereal disease effect, a very important fact, given our current venereal disease epidemic.

Precoital Pill

Investigation has shown that certain of the progestins and perhaps other agents administered approximately 4 hours prior to sexual relations will produce an effect on the cervical mucus that will prevent penetration by sperm. In one such study of a progestin, this effect lasted for approximately 18 hours. However, much work remains to be done on this technique before its ultimate usefulness can be determined.

IMPLANTATION

Intrauterine Devices

The latest development in this area is a new generation of intrauterine devices that contain small amounts of metals such as copper (Cu-7 and Copper T) or hormonal agents such as progesterone (Progestasert). Smaller devices were shown to produce less bleeding, but have higher expulsion and pregnancy rates. It was found that when a metal or a hormone was added to a small IUD, less cramping and bleeding resulted, and a high level of protection against pregnancy was maintained. Closed intrauterine devices should not be used since this type of device can perforate the uterus, pass into the peritoneal cavity, and trap and strangulate a segment of bowel.

Mechanism of Action. The mechanism of action of intrauterine devices has been much studied but still remains somewhat unclear. It was originally felt that the effectiveness of IUDs was dependent upon changes in tubal motility or upon infection of the endometrial tissues, but it now appears that they probably act by producing some sort of histochemical change in the endometrium. Macrophages and other leukocytes appear in the endometrical cavity in response to intrauterine devices, and in all likelihood act on the blastocyst by not permitting it to implant. The metallic IUDs probably act either on the sperm or on the blastocyst. The hormonal IUDs apparently act to change the surface of the endometrium, making it unsuitable for implantation.

Continuation Rates. The use of intrauterine contraception has increased steadily, reaching more than 15 million, 4 to 5 million of them in the United States. It currently has one of the highest continuation rates of any of the medically prescribed methods, since it requires a positive act on the part of the woman to stop using an IUD in distinction to the ease of discontinuation of the use of barrier techniques or the oral contraceptive.

Morbidity and Mortality Rates. The mortality rate for IUDs is currently estimated to be somewhere between 1 and 10 deaths per million women-years of use. Complications requiring hospitalization range from 0.3 to 1.0 per hundred women-years of use. At the present time, IUDs have a lower mortality rate but a higher morbidity rate than oral contraceptives.

While IUDs are still considered generally safe and effective, the risks, particularly of infection, perforation, bleeding, ectopic pregnancy, spontaneous abortion, septic midtrimester abortion, premature delivery, and decreased fertility, continue to pose a problem.

Clinical Management. IUD insertion should be performed during the menstrual period whenever possible. At this time there is less likelihood of carrying out an insertion in the presence of an unrecognized pregnancy, the endocervical canal is more patulous, and the bleeding incident to the insertion procedure is concurrent with the menses. An IUD of average size can be used in a uterus which sounds to a depth of 6 to 8 cm. When a uterus measures less than this, one of the smaller IUDs should be inserted. A uterine depth greater than 8 cm. may require one of the larger devices. Problems associated with the IUD may be reduced by careful insertion following a specific technique—thorough pelvic examination, cleansing of the cervical os, grasping the cervix with a tenaculum in order to straighten the canal, sounding the uterus, and the use of presterilized intrauterine devices. Syncope during insertion resulting from a vagal response secondary to anxiety or pain induced by dilatation of the cervix, may be averted by using sedatives, atropine, and a paracervical block.

The largest single advantage of the IUD is that after insertion comparatively little follow-up care and minimal patient motivation are involved. However, even the best of the uterine devices is not without side effects. Patients should be seen after the first menstrual period and at 6 to 12 month periods thereafter. Inert devices do not require removal at any specific time interval. Metal or hormone-releasing devices, however, need to be replaced at periodic intervals.

Side Effects. PREGNANCY. Currently used IUDs have a net pregnancy rate of approximately 0.0 to 5.6 per hundred women at the end of the first year. Overall protection against unwanted pregnancy may be increased by employing a barrier contraceptive method around the time of ovulation.

Pregnancy may occur after an unnoticed expulsion; it may also occur with an IUD in situ in the uterus, the tube, or the ovary. Inasmuch as the IUD is highly protective against intrauterine pregnancy, this type of gestation is statistically less likely than extrauterine pregnancy and the latter type should always be considered, especially if the symptoms are somewhat atypical. Data are now becoming available suggesting that the use of IUDs may be associated with a slightly increased risk of ectopic pregnancy. Since this complication is apparently more frequent in women who have had prior extrauterine gestations, such women should be informed about their increased risk, if they request insertion of an IUD.

In the event that an intrauterine gestation is found with the IUD in situ, it is imperative that the device be removed, if easily accessible, as soon as the diagnosis of pregnancy is made, regardless of the desired outcome. It was previously believed that removal would induce spontaneous abortion. However, it has been shown that removal not only decreases the rate of spontaneous abortion from 50 to 25 per cent but also decreases the risk of midtrimester septic abortion and premature delivery. When pregnancies have continued to term with the IUD in situ no fetal damage has been reported.

If a woman elects to continue her pregnancy and does not have her IUD removed, she must be carefully instructed when to seek medical consultation. She must be warned that the prodromal symptoms of septic midtrimester abortion are often vague and nonspecific, and the disease may run a rapidly fulminating course ending in septic shock, disseminated intravascular coagulation, and death. If symptoms of midtrimester septic abortion should occur, aggressive treatment must be instituted immediately. The uterine contents must be emptied as rapidly as possible and antibiotic therapy, effective against anaerobes, initiated. In rare instances, hysterectomy may be necessary in order to preserve the life of the patient.

CRAMPING AND BLEEDING. Cramping and bleeding are the two most frequent medical causes for removal of intrauterine devices, together accounting for more than half of all removals. These side effects appear to be directly related to the size of the device relative to the size of the uterine cavity. Removal rates for these complaints vary widely for the same device from one study to another. This undoubtedly reflects the great variation in patient motivation and acceptance, social and cultural factors, and the attitudes of the medical staff. The plastic devices (Lippes Loop, Saf-T-Coil) produce the greatest blood loss, the copper devices (Cu-7, Copper T) somewhat less, and the progesterone-bearing device (Progestasert) produces less blood loss than a normal period used as a control. Excessive bleeding of sufficient degree to require hospitalization occurs in approximately 1 per cent of women.

PERFORATION. Uterine perforation has been reported to range from 0.0 to 8.7 per 1000 insertions, and may happen either during or at some time after the insertion. Perforation through the cervix has occasionally been observed, the stem portion of the T- and 7- shaped copper devices being pushed by the contractions of the uterus through the wall of the cervix into the upper vagina. Perforation rates reflect a great many variables, including the time of insertion and the procedure used, uterine anomalies or pathology that distort the normal anatomy, the design of the IUD and its inserter, and the skill and experience of the operator.

If significant pain or bleeding are experienced during the insertion, the position of the device must be carefully checked. A perforation may, however, be "silent" and only be discovered later when the device is found to be displaced or absent, or when a pregnancy has ensued. When this happens, it is imperative to determine whether the device is still in situ and, if so, where and what associated damage, if any, has occurred. A careful investigation must be made, starting with a pelvic examination and proceeding to the use of such techniques as x-ray and ultrasonography when indicated.

If perforation of an inert linear device is found to have occurred, the situation and the minimal potential danger should be explained to the patient. Clinical judgment and patient wishes should determine whether the device is removed. These devices have often been allowed to remain in situ. However, they have been known to produce abscess formation and bowel perforation and removal is usually to be preferred. In the case of the copper-containing IUDs, removal should be effected as soon as medically feasible, since copper ions stimulate the formation of dense intraperitoneal adhesions. Closed devices should also be removed, since strangulation followed by intestinal obstruction may occur if a loop of bowel becomes incarcerated within the open portion of the device. Devices may often be removed by laparoscopy, culdoscopy, or culdotomy if they are free in the abdominal cavity. Laparotomy is necessary only when dense adhesions have been formed or when partial perforation has occurred.

EXPULSION AND THE "LOST IUD." Expulsion rates are reported to range from 0.7 to 19.3 per cent, depending on the device, when it is inserted, and the correctness of its placement high in the fundus. If the patient is not aware that the device has been expelled and if the string of the IUD cannot be seen and there are no signs of pregnancy, the presence or absence of the IUD must be determined. First, the uterus should be probed to look for a retracted string and to determine whether the IUD is still in the uterus. If the IUD is not found, ultrasonography may be used, or posteroanterior and lateral x-rays of the pelvis may be taken. The position of the uterine cavity can be indicated by the insertion of a metal uterine sound, another IUD of a different type, or by the instillation of a radio-opaque dye.

INFECTION. Contamination of the endometrial cavity with vaginal organisms inevitably occurs during insertion but usually clears spontaneously over the next month. Heretofore, intrauterine contraception has not been considered to present a danger of acute or chronic pelvic infection. However, the incidence of pelvic inflammatory disease (PID) has recently been shown to be significantly higher during the first 15 days following insertion of an IUD and a number of articles have appeared in the medical literature documenting an increased risk of pelvic infection associated with the use of IUDs.

Acute pelvic infection may occur with an IUD in place, leading to the development of tubo-ovarian abscesses or general peritonitis or both. The infection may be due to gonorrhea but also may be caused by actinomycosis, or bacteria, and in some cases it is nonspecific in nature. The signs and symptoms of pelvic inflammatory disease are the same, whether or not an IUD is present.

The most frequent presenting complaints are pelvic pain and tenderness, uterine bleeding, chills, and fever. On pelvic examination a purulent vaginal discharge, signs of peritoneal inflammation and pelvic masses are usually found. Smears and cultures for gonorrhea and for both aerobic and anaerobic bacteria should be taken from the endocervix and on occasion from the cul de sac or abdominal cavity.

Treatment should be instituted with a broad-spectrum antibiotic, which is effective against gonorrhea. The IUD may initially be left in place, but if the infection does not show a marked response to treatment within 24 to 48 hours, it should be removed.

Chronic pelvic inflammatory disease may also occur with an IUD in situ. This condition frequently has an insidious onset and is often first diagnosed by finding a small, slightly tender tubo-ovarian mass at the time of a routine follow-up visit. Early symptoms include foul-smelling leukorrhea, dyspareunia, premenstrual bloating, intermenstrual bleeding, and hypermenorrhea.

RETURN OF FERTILITY. Earlier studies concluded that IUDs did not produce any long-term effects and that the duration of use did not influence the rate of return of fertility. However, there is new evidence which suggests that intrauterine contraception is associated with a higher than normal frequency of pelvic infection and that the fertility rates following removal are lower than those in patients who had used a barrier form of contraception or no contraception at all. Furthermore, the return of fertility is slower, and the ultimate number of pregnancies are fewer as the duration of use increases.

With the advent of the new smaller medicated IUDs, this form of contraception became feasible for nulligravid women. However, because of this new information it is essential that physicians discuss the desire for future pregnancy with all women prior to the insertion of an IUD, particularly young nulligravid patients. They must be counseled that intrauterine contraception carries with it a slight but real risk of infection and temporary or prolonged infertility.

MALIGNANCY. Long experience with the use of a wide variety of IUDs has failed to reveal any evidence of an association between the use of intrauterine contraception and the subsequent development of uterine malignancy.

Removal. The three main nonmedical reasons for removing an IUD are: (1) to initiate a pregnancy, (2) to replace a drug-bearing device, and (3) personal reasons.

Medical indications for removal include: (1) pregnancy, (2) excessive cramping and bleeding, (3) pelvic and/or abdominal pain, (4) pelvic inflammatory disease, (5) displacement, (6) uterine or cervical malignancy, and (7) menopause.

Whenever feasible, removal should coincide with a menstrual period, since the endocervical canal is more patulous at that time and bleeding resulting from the removal process will be less obvious. Most devices can be readily removed from the uterus by putting traction on the strings of the device. Occasionally, it may be necessary to place a tenaculum on the cervix to straighten the cervicouterine angle. IUDs may become deeply embedded in the endometrium or actually invade the superficial layer of the myometrium. If instrumentation is required, paracervical block should be performed and a polyp forcep, an alligator clamp, or some other grasping instrument used to extract the IUD. If these efforts are unsuccessful, additional diagnostic steps should be undertaken. If partial perforation is not found, extraction should next be attempted under general anesthesia. Hysteroscopic exploration and removal under direct vision may also prove to be useful.

Contraindications. ABSOLUTE. The following are the contraindications to the use of intrauterine contraception currently listed by the Food and Drug Administration: (1) pregnancy or suspicion of pregnancy, (2) abnormality of uterus resulting in distortion of uterine cavity, (3) acute pelvic inflammatory disease or history of repeated pelvic inflammatory disease, (4) postpartum endometritis or infected abortion in the past 3 months, (5) known or suspected uterine or cervical malignancy including unresolved abnormal Papanicolaou smear, (6) genital bleeding of unknown etiology, (7) untreated acute cervicitis until infection is under control, (8) copper-containing IUDs should

not be inserted in the presence of a diagnosis of Wilson's disease, and (9) known allergy to copper (for copper-containing IUDs).

RELATIVE. The following may be considered as relative contraindications of greater or lesser degree to the use of intrauterine contraception: (1) small uterine cavity (less than 5 cm.), (2) severe cervical stenosis, (3) severe hypermenorrhea resulting in anemia, (4) severe dysmenorrhea, (5) congenital or valvular heart disease, (6) previous ectopic pregnancy, (7) anticoagulant or immunosuppressive therapy, (8) blood dyscrasias, (9) immediate puerperium, (10) benign cervical pathology, (11) nulligravidity, and (12) nulliparity.

TERMINATION OF PREGNANCY

Surgical Abortion

It is clear that the termination of pregnancy is a highly efficient means of fertility control. Abortion has been practiced for centuries and continues to be the most frequently and widely used method of fertility control. It is increasingly being legalized throughout the world because of the recognition of the high maternal mortality associated with widespread illegal abortion.

A variety of techniques for the termination of pregnancy are currently being explored. These are not considered to be strictly within the domain of this particular article and therefore will not be covered in any detail. Suffice it to say that abortion techniques used in the first trimester of pregnancy, primarily the use of suction curettage under local anesthesia in outpatient facilities, appear to be the techniques of choice at the present time. This procedure is the least disturbing to the patient, has the lowest cost, and has by far the lowest complication rates.

Prostaglandins

This interesting new group of compounds is found in almost all tissues of the body. It has been discovered that certain of the prostaglandins such as E_2 and $F_2\gamma$ have a marked effect on uterine contractility. Use has been made of this property in the induction of abortion and the stimulation of labor at term. (See manufacturers' official directive for method of use.)

GENERAL CONSIDERATIONS

It is very important that a patient actively participate in the decision-making process as to what would be the most appropriate contraceptive method for her. To do this, she must be given accurate and easily understood information re-

Figure 1.* Annual number of deaths associated with control of fertility and no control per 100,000 nonsterile women, by regimen of control and age of woman

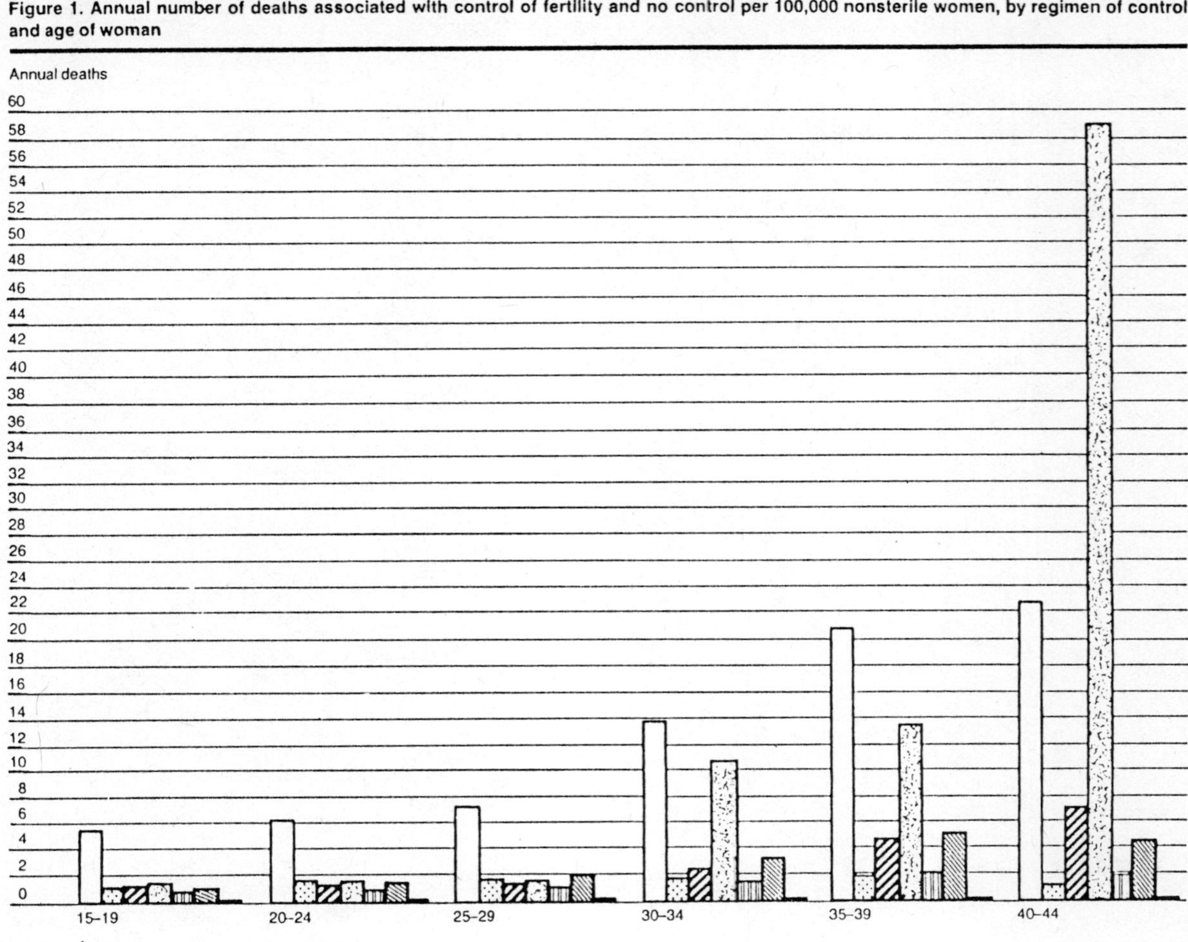

* From Tietze, C. New Estimates of Mortality Associated with Fertility Control. *Family Planning Perspectives* 9:74-76, 1977.

garding the relative safety and effectiveness of the various family planning techniques currently available (Figure 1), as well as the risk vs. benefit ratio for each individual method. If medically possible, her selection should be followed, since it is well established that tolerance of side effects and continuation rates are both better if a patient is using the method of her choice. Whether abortion is available and acceptable to a patient will influence the decision as to whether or not to use a method that is only relatively effective. Finally, it must always be made clear that if the initial selection turns out to be unsatisfactory, numerous other options exist.

ALCOHOLISM

method of
ITAMAR SALAMON, M.D.
Bronx, New York

Alcoholism has been defined by the World Health Organization as "a chronic behavioral disorder manifested by repeated drinking of alcoholic beverages in excess of the dietary and social uses of the community and to an extent that interferes with the drinker's health or his social or economic function." Abuse of alcohol to this extent indicates the presence of an underlying emotional disorder. The treatment of alcoholism, therefore, falls into two categories: treatment of the complications of excessive use of alcohol, and therapy for the underlying emotional disorder that leads to the dependence on alcohol.

Complications of Excessive Use of Alcohol

Intoxication. 1. *Mild to moderate intoxication and alcoholic stupor* are usually of short duration and, if the vital signs are normal, letting the patient "sleep it off" is all that is necessary. A mild analeptic, such as caffeine sodium benzoate, 0.5 gram intramuscularly, or a sympathomimetic amine, dextroamphetamine, 5 mg. by mouth or subcutaneously, may hasten recovery.

2. *Alcoholic coma* is a serious matter; the range between alcoholically induced surgical anesthesia and irreversible respiratory depression is very narrow. The following measures should be taken.

An adequate airway must be immediately established; an endotracheal tube may prove necessary.

Vital signs should be recorded at frequent intervals; if shock is present, appropriate therapy with fluids and vasopressors should be instituted.

A careful physical examination should be made, with particular attention to signs of trauma to the head, neck, and spinal column. If these are not apparent, the patient may be placed in a prone position with the head turned to one side to prevent aspiration in the event of vomiting. Accumulated secretions should be removed by suctioning.

Oxygen may be administered by nasal catheter or tent. A mechanical means of maintaining respiration should be available in the event of respiratory paralysis.

Gastric lavage may remove unabsorbed alcohol from the stomach and reveal the presence of hemorrhage. Care should be taken to prevent pulmonary aspiration of the return flow.

An intravenous infusion with 5 per cent dextrose in water should be started, and dehydration and electrolyte imbalances should be corrected.

Palpation and percussion of the bladder should be performed. If distention is present, it should be relieved by catheterization. If more than 500 ml. of urine is present, gradual decompression should be carried out.

In particularly severe cases of coma, dialysis may prove useful in removing alcohol from the blood.

Finally, it must be emphasized that examinations should be performed to rule out other causes of coma, to discover if other drugs have been ingested, particularly barbiturates, and to uncover any disorder to which the alcoholic is particularly vulnerable—subdural hematoma, pneumonia, meningitis, hepatic failure, and gastrointestinal bleeding.

3. *Excitement* rather than stupor may occasionally be seen because the depressant effect of alcohol removes inhibitory control mechanisms. Acute intoxication may lead to a condition characterized by nausea, vomiting, restlessness, hyperexcitability, and hyperactivity, often of an extremely violent nature. Such a state requires the use of sedatives or tranquilizers or both, and may require temporary restraint of the patient. The use of sedatives requires the caution that such drugs may further depress respiration, and the use of neuroleptics requires the caution that these compounds sometimes potentiate the effects of hypno-

tic and sedative drugs and so may also increase respiratory depression. Probably the best drug for this condition, however, is haloperidol (Haldol) in doses of 2 to 5 mg. intramuscularly every 45 to 90 minutes until agitation is relieved. The advantages of haloperidol are that it is rapidly effective, it produces only minimal or light sedation, and rarely causes hypotension. In the rare instance in which a vasopressor is necessary, 1-nor-epinephrine (Levophed) should be used. If rapid sedation is necessary, 10 mg. of intravenous diazepam (Valium), injected slowly over a period of two minutes, will usually produce dramatic results. Since there is cross tolerance between diazepam and alcohol, occasional patients will require higher doses for a therapeutic effect.

4. *Pathologic intoxication* is a syndrome of impaired consciousness and confusion, disorientation, hallucinations and delusions, violent and impulsive behavior, and profound emotional disturbances of rage, anxiety, and depression, triggered by the ingestion of small amounts of alcohol. This state is usually followed by a prolonged sleep, after which there is amnesia for the episode. Some observers feel that pathologic intoxication represents a variant of temporal lobe epilepsy in which the seizures are induced by alcohol. The acute episode may be managed in the same way as outlined under Excitement.

Withdrawal Syndrome. This syndrome is seen in patients who have been heavy drinkers for a long time, but it appears only after a period of decreased alcohol intake. There is a characteristic progression of symptoms that may terminate in a full-blown picture of delirium tremens. The syndrome usually begins a few hours after the last drink with the appearance of tremulousness, nausea, weakness, anxiety, and perspiration. There may be cramps and vomiting; hyperreflexia is prominent, and tremor becomes quite marked. Grand mal seizures may occur in the period of 24 to 48 hours after cessation of drinking ("rum fits"). Early signs of delirium (defects in attention and concentration) may become apparent, and visual hallucinations, typically of small animals (pink elephants), begin to appear. Tactile and olfactory hallucinations may also be present. As the syndrome progresses into the third day of withdrawal, the delirium becomes more manifest and the patient becomes confused, disoriented, and agitated. Finally, exhaustion, hyperthermia, and cardiovascular collapse may appear.

Management of the Withdrawal Syndrome. 1. *Tremulousness*, or "the shakes," represents the earliest and mildest stage of withdrawal. This condition can be treated on an out-patient basis if the patient is not too agitated and the

rium), 25 mg. orally four times a day until the symptoms are brought under control and then a tapered reduction over a period of 2 weeks, is effective therapy. Chloral hydrate, 0.5 to 1.0 gram at bedtime, may be used for sedation, if required.

2. Withdrawal from alcohol may precipitate *seizures* in persons who are not otherwise epileptic, although they may have a lower seizure threshold than normal persons. These seizures are frequently referred to as "rum fits"; they appear on the first or second day of abstinence, are usually generalized in nature and few in number. Therapy should consist of an initial dose of sodium phenobarbital (Luminal), 100 mg. intramuscularly, followed by phenytoin (Dilantin), 100 mg. three to four times per day by mouth. If seizures are not controlled, phenobarbital, 30 to 60 mg. three to four times a day, may be added. If an electroencephalogram shows no evidence of focal or general paroxysmal activity and there is no known underlying epilepsy, this regimen may be gradually discontinued after the patient has recovered from the withdrawal syndrome.

Seizures in the withdrawal state are particularly apt to occur in patients who have underlying epilepsy, particularly if they have stopped taking their anticonvulsant medication. Status epilepticus is a serious complication. Focal or generalized seizures may also occur on a post-traumatic basis, and these patients should receive a full neurologic work-up, with the possibility of a subdural hematoma kept strongly in mind. The management of cryptogenic epilepsy and status epilepticus is detailed in the section on Epilepsy in Adults in this text.

3. *Delirium tremens*, or incipient delirium tremens, requires hospitalization. Management of this serious condition includes the following measures:

Medication. At present the drug of choice appears to be chlordiazepoxide (Librium) because of its long duration of action, slow elimination, and cross-dependence with alcohol. Its use in alcohol withdrawal is analogous to the use of methadone in opiate withdrawal. Oral or intravenous administration is preferable to the intramuscular route as absorption of benzodiazepines from intramuscular injections is variable and unpredictable. A useful regimen is 50 to 100 mg. intravenously for immediate relief of symptoms, followed by 50 to 100 mg. orally four times a day. The precise dosage will vary according to the individual patient's tolerance, and should be adjusted to that level necessary to prevent the emergence of a withdrawal syndrome. Once the patient is stabilized, a tapered withdrawal from chlordiazepoxide (Librium) may be carried out over a 2 to 3 week period. Paraldehyde, 8 to 12 ml. orally, provides excellent nighttime sedation.

Fluids and electrolytes. These patients are usually dehydrated, and administration of fluids and correction of electrolyte abnormalities, particularly of sodium, potassium, and magnesium, are essential. Intake and output should be recorded, and a minimum of 3000 ml. of fluid should be administered daily, either by mouth or, if necessary, intravenously. A high carbohydrate, high caloric diet and multivitamins should be a standard part of the regimen, and it is imperative to begin by immediately administering a dose of 50 to 100 mg. of thiamine intramuscularly prior to the administration of glucose to avoid precipitating or aggravating a Wernicke-Korsakoff syndrome.

Restraints. The use of restraints for agitated patients should be avoided as much as possible, for they may lead to further exhaustion and injury. Severe agitation is best dealt with chemically, through the use of chlordiazepoxide (Librium) and, if necessary, intravenous diazepam (Valium). The availability of a seclusion room is desirable. General principles for the management of delirious patients apply here as well—the presence of a familiar person, constancy of surroundings, adequate lighting, both daytime and nighttime, and frequent reassurance, orientation, and explanation of procedures. These measures help allay the patient's fears and calm his agitation.

Other measures. If the patient presents with the full-blown picture of delirium tremens, vital signs should be recorded every 30 minutes. Cardiovascular collapse should be treated with fluids and vasopressors and hyperthermia combated with ice packs or a cooling mattress.

Again, it must be emphasized that the complications of alcoholism—trauma, infections, liver disease, gastrointestinal hemorrhage, and the ingestion of other drugs—must be sought and, if present, adequately treated.

Acute Alcoholic Hallucinosis. This is a less commonly seen syndrome that follows prolonged and excessive use of alcohol. It is characterized by the presence of threatening auditory hallucinations, accompanied by marked fear and occasionally delusional elaborations *in the presence of a clear sensorium*. It is not clear whether this is a psychosis directly related to the toxic effects of alcohol or whether it is a latent pathologic response made manifest by chronic alcohol usage. The management should be the same as for other acute psychotic states, utilizing a potent neuroleptic. Haloperidol (Haldol) 5 mg. intramuscularly every 2 hours until agitation is relieved, followed by oral doses of 10 to 40 mg. per day, or chlorpromazine (Thorazine),

100 to 200 mg. by mouth four times a day, are typical regimens. It is often desirable in agitated patients to increase the dosage until daytime sedation is achieved. This dosage level may be maintained for several days while improvement occurs and then is tapered to a maintenance level of 200 to 400 mg. per day. Further reduction of dosage may take place with clinical improvement. As with other alcoholic patients, the physician should carefully attend to nutritional needs.

Nutritional Disorders. Nutritional disorders arise because of the caloric and vitamin deficiencies caused by the inadequate diets of many chronic alcoholics. They include pellagra, beriberi, and polyneuropathy; treatments of these disorders are described elsewhere in this book.

1. Wernicke-Korsakoff syndrome is caused by a deficiency of thiamine and is characterized clinically by a delirious, confused state, accompanied by nystagmus or extraocular palsies and ataxia (Wernicke's syndrome). When an amnestic-confabulatory state is also present, the label of Korsakoff's syndrome is added. The mortality rate is 15 per cent, and death may be sudden and unexplained, or caused by acute congestive heart failure of the high-output type, complications of cirrhosis of the liver, or infection. Early institution of thiamine therapy may be lifesaving and may prevent a permanent deficit. Since the administration of glucose will deplete stored thiamine, thus precipitating or aggravating a Wernicke-Korsakoff syndrome in a patient with already meager stores of this vitamin, it is essential to precede any intravenous glucose drip in a chronic alcoholic with an intramuscular injection of 50 to 100 mg. of thiamine. Treatment of the Wernicke-Korsakoff syndrome consists of thiamine, 100 mg. intramuscularly for 10 days, along with oral multivitamin B complex, which is continued indefinitely. Bed rest, a nutritious diet, and early recognition and care of cardiac complications are necessary. The ocular signs will usually improve rapidly with therapy and the ataxia more gradually. Improvement in the memory deficits, however, is more variable, and slow improvement may occur over a period of a year or more. Vitamin therapy should be continued throughout this period. Depending on the state of the patient's memory deficit and his behavior, he may be able to return to his family or he may require placement in a nursing home or a psychiatric facility.

2. Amblyopia. "Tobacco-alcohol" amblyopia is thought to be due to a deficiency of multiple vitamins. Treatment includes (1) a nutritious diet, (2) multivitamin supplements, (3) thiamine, 50 mg. per day, and (4) vitamin B_{12}, 100 micrograms intramuscularly, and folic acid, 5 mg. orally once a day. Note that this treatment may mask pernicious

anemia. When the deficits appear to have cleared, the patient may be maintained on multivitamins alone.

Ingestion of Other Toxic Substances.　It should always be kept in mind that alcoholics may have ingested other toxic substances as well, and a careful history should be obtained from the patient and family. The combination of alcohol and barbiturates (or other sedative-tranquilizers) is a common one. Lead encephalopathy may follow the ingestion of home-brewed whiskey contaminated with lead from the pipes or coils of the distillation apparatus.

Methyl alcohol poisoning still occurs, particularly in "skid-row" alcoholics. Treatment consists of the intravenous infusion of 1000 ml. per hour of a 3 to 5 per cent solution of sodium bicarbonate to counteract the severe acidosis that occurs. The concomitant administration of 1 ounce of whiskey every hour for several hours is helpful in delaying the oxidation of methanol to toxic formaldehyde.

Gastrointestinal Complications.　These disorders include acute and chronic gastritis and peptic ulcer, cirrhosis of the liver and its accompanying complications of esophageal varices, ascites, and hepatic and renal failure, and pancreatitis. The management of these disorders is discussed in Section 5, The Digestive System.

The Emotional Disorder

The persistent use of alcohol to the extent that it interferes with the drinker's health, and his social and economic functioning, indicates the presence of an underlying emotional disorder. Although social and cultural patterns profoundly influence the use of alcohol, individual psychopathology is the major factor in the abuse of alcohol. This psychopathology cuts across the usual psychiatric diagnostic categories, which are of little use in indicating a propensity toward alcoholism. The personality traits which characterize the typical alcoholic are:

1. *Schizoid withdrawal:* a basic sense of estrangement or isolation from people.

2. *Depression:* feelings of hopelessness, sadness, and futility, with profoundly low self-esteem.

3. *Hostility:* a chronic rage which suffuses the personality, at times evident in all aspects of functioning, or in other cases, only becoming manifest in dreams, hallucinations, or drunken behavior.

4. *Self-destructiveness:* the combination of low self-esteem and chronic anger leading to overt self-destructive behavior, of which drunkenness is one manifestation and serious suicide attempts another.

5. *Dependency:* an infantile orientation to other persons as the providers for insatiable demands for food, love, acceptance, and comfort, and a pervadingly passive attitude toward the world.

6. *Sexual immaturity:* the lack of a firm sexual identity.

7. *Low frustration tolerance:* "I want what I want when I want it," often coupled with high aspirations, and *poor impulse control*, leading to frequent disappointments, resentments, and depression and renewed episodes of drinking and self-destructive behavior.

Treatment.　Psychotherapy. A therapeutic interaction between a person experiencing emotional distress and a therapist skilled in interpersonal relations is the preferred treatment for the chronic alcoholic. Several basic principles apply to the therapy of these patients:

1. The therapist must initially adopt a supportive, giving approach and be willing to tolerate the patient's demands, his failures, and his self-disparaging and self-destructive behavior. A moralistic attitude toward drinking on the part of the therapist is destructive to treatment.

2. Abstinence is an essential goal of treatment, and it must be total and lifelong.

3. The patient's denial of the severity of his alcoholism or the severity of his emotional problems must be dealt with as soon as possible.

4. When a spouse or other family member is involved with the patient, it is essential that he be involved in some form of counseling or therapy. There is much evidence to indicate that the alcoholic's family frequently (although unconsciously) encourage his drinking to satisfy their own unconscious needs.

Adjuncts to Treatment. *Alcoholics Anonymous* is a loosely organized, voluntary association of alcoholics that uses a variety of group techniques to help maintain abstinence. Those patients who are able and willing to participate in an AA program can receive enormous benefit and aid in rehabilitation.

Group therapy of a more formal nature may also be useful in providing support, gratification of dependency needs, dealing with denial, and comradeship with fellow sufferers.

Disulfiram (Antabuse) is a drug that alters the metabolism of alcohol so that a toxic product, acetaldehyde, is formed. The patient who has ingested alcohol while taking disulfiram (Antabuse) will experience, within minutes, a reaction that includes flushing, nausea, and vomiting, a sharp drop in blood pressure, marked palpitations, and a feeling of impending death. Dosage is from 0.25 to 0.5 gram daily, and the patient is instructed as to the serious nature of the symptoms that will develop should he drink while taking the drug. At least 4 days should elapse after a dose of disulfiram (Antabuse) before drinking may be resumed. In a motivated patient the use of this drug will often help control impulsive urges to drink.

Social agencies, where appropriate, may be utilized to help with vocational rehabilitation, job placement, living arrangements, and other aspects of the outside world with which the alcoholic must cope.

NARCOTIC POISONING

method of
JOHN ADRIANI, M.D.
New Orleans, Louisiana

Causes of Poisoning

Narcotic analgesics (strong analgesics) are the most useful drugs available for pain relief; few drugs can supplant them. Unfortunately, they are used by drug-dependent persons for nonmedical purposes. Overdosage resulting in poisoning may be due to any of the following: (1) Use of common doses in subjects with diminished tolerance (cachexia, hypothyroidism, hepatic insufficiency). (2) Accidental overdosage or overestimation of dosage. (3) Accumulation of the drug administered subcutaneously in repeated doses for pain of traumatic states in the presence of hypotension. When the blood pressure returns to normotensive levels, absorption of the unabsorbed drug results in poisoning. (4) Overestimation of dosages or exceeding of dosages in drug-dependent persons. (5) Accidental ingestion by children. (6) Deliberate overdosage for suicidal intent. (7) Additive effects with other central nervous system (CNS) depressants or potentiation as a result of drug interactions (simultaneous use of monoamine oxidase inhibitors).

Types of Narcotics

Available narcotics fall into five major chemical groups: (1) The opiates (also opoids). These are derived from opium. The derivatives in this group, all derived from phenanthrene, include morphine, diacetylmorphine (heroin), dihydromorphinone (Dilaudid), oxymorphone (Numorphan), methyldihydromorphinone (Metopon), codeine, ethylmorphine (Dionin), oxycodone (Percodan), methyl dihydrocodeinone (Dicodid), tincture of opium, camphorated tincture of opium (paregoric), hydrochlorides of opium alkaloids (Pantopon), purified opium alkaloid (Omnopon), and so on. (2) The methyl morphinan series also derived from phenanthrene, but synthetic. The important drug in this series is levorphanol (Levo-Dromoran). (3) The piperidine group. Important drugs in this group include meperidine (Demerol), anileridine (Leritine), piminodine (Alvodine), and fentanyl (Sublimaze). (4) The methadone group, which includes methadone, methadol, and propoxyphene (Darvon). (5) The benzmorphan group, which includes phenazocine (Prinadol) and pentazocine (Talwin).

A specific chemical grouping is identified in the molecular structure of the narcotics that acts at a specific receptor site on a cell and induces analgesia. The pharmacologic responses of all narcotics are qualitatively similar but quantitatively different. The signs, symptoms, management, and course of treatment of overdosage are therefore similar.

Signs and Symptoms of Narcotic Overdosage

The signs and symptoms of narcotic overdosage are marked depression of the central nervous system accompanied by sleep, stupor, or profound coma. Their severity is dose related. The skin may be clammy, pale, or cyanotic. Respiration is usually periodic, varying in rate anywhere from as low as 5 or 6 per minute. The depth in increased, but total minute volume exchange is decreased. Bradycardia and hypotension are common. The pupils are constricted to the classic pinpoint position in the early phases of overdosage with the majority of drugs. Meperidine is an exception. In the later phases, particularly in cases of severe poisoning, they may be dilated due to anoxia. The skeletal muscles are usually flaccid in some other types of coma. The body temperature is subnormal early but may rise in cases of prolonged coma resulting from infection. Most narcotics have a heterogeneous effect, i.e., they stimulate some structures and depress others. Convulsions may occur with massive dosage in infants and children, and at times in adults. These arise particularly from stimulation of subcortical centers.

Initially, the symptoms are related to the respiratory system. Later, the circulatory system is involved. If patients are untreated and inadequate ventilation persists, irreversible cerebral damage may occur. Death is usually due to anoxia in acute early phases. In prolonged, sustained intoxication death may result from cardiac failure, acute infections, renal failure, or hepatic insufficiency.

Immediate Treatment

If the cause of the depression or coma is definitely established, one is then not faced at the onset with the problem of establishing the diagnosis. It is necessary to institute the usual urgent measures necessary for treating coma from any cause. Noisy respiration always indicates obstructed respiration. However, obstructed respiration is not always noisy. The obstruction is relieved in most patients by hyperextending the head by placing the hand on the tip of the chin and extending the chin so that it points upward toward the ceiling. A pharyngeal airway usually suffices to support the tongue and the relaxed pharyngeal structures. The pharyngeal reflexes may not be completely obtunded so that there may be a tendency to eject the airway. In this case, an anesthetic ointment of 20 per cent benzocaine (Americaine) may be applied to the airway. An endotracheal cuffed catheter may be necessary if the pharyngeal airway is not tolerated.

Narcotics decrease the rate of respiration but not necessarily the depth. The exchange is described as "slow and deep." This is often a distinguishing feature between overdosages of narcotic and of non-narcotic central nervous system depressants, particularly the hypnotics, such as the barbiturates. The latter usually cause a shallow and rapid rate of respiration. Ventilation generally is inadequate, and some form of assistance must be provided with a mechanical device. Artificial respiration must be instituted promptly if apnea is present. Mouth-to-mouth breathing may be necessary at the outset until mechanical devices can be placed into operation. The bag and mask of an anesthetic apparatus serve admirably for this purpose in the operating room. Mechanical ventilators of the intermittent positive pressure breathing (IPPB) type may be used. Hand ventilators such as the Ambu likewise may be used. Apnea sometimes develops when the oxygen is commenced. This indicates that a severe depression exists and that respiration is being maintained by the aortic-carotid chemoreceptor reflexes, which are activated by the anoxic stimulus. The oxygen must be continued, however, and ventilation maintained artificially by mechanical means if this occurs. Blood gas determinations of arterial carbon dioxide and oxygen should be made periodically if available to assess the adequacy of ventilation and to avoid acidosis or alkalosis as well as anoxemia.

Circulatory Complications

The blood pressure should be determined as soon as ventilatory dysfunction is corrected or while it is being corrected by another person assisting the physician. If a hypotension is present, its severity should be assessed. A vasopressor such as ephedrine, given in increments of 15 mg. at 1 to 2 minute intervals, or phenylephrine (Neo-Synephrine), 1 mg., or methoxamine (Vasoxyl), 2 to 3 mg., may be administered intravenously. Neither phenylephrine nor methoxamine has a positive inotropic effect on the heart. Should evidence of myocardial depression be present, a drug that has a positive inotropic effect should be used, such as metaraminol (Aramine) or ephedrine. Should metaraminol be used, 10 to 20 mg. in 500 ml. of 5 per cent dextrose and distilled water may be used as a drip. Cannulation of a vein is desirable for the administration of necessary fluids as well as for the administration of drugs, blood, or plasma expanders. A slow drip of 5 per cent dextrose in distilled water may be used to maintain a patent vein if fluids are not indicated. Often the hypotension, particularly if it is mild (between 90 and 100 mm. Hg systolic), adjusts itself without therapy upon improvement of ventilation. If it does, one can assume that it was due to anoxia. Some clinicians administer lactated Ringer's or a solution of similar type to correct the hypovolemia or any existing electrolyte imbalance. Volume should be monitored when large quantities of fluid are administered to prevent cardiac overload. Hypotension caused by the combination of a narcotic and phenothiazine does not respond to sympathomimetic amines, because of the presence of an adrenergic blockade.

Pulmonary edema may result from left-sided heart failure caused by myocardial depression in cases of severe poisoning. The patient should be digitalized rapidly with 1.5 mg. of digoxin or 1.5 mg. of digitoxin or another glycoside of the physician's preference. Digoxin acts more quickly. The cardiac rhythm should be monitored with the electrocardiograph. Central venous pressure readings should be taken if possible, particularly to evaluate the effects of digitalization and fluid therapy.

Use of Antagonists

Narcotic overdosage not complicated by the presence of other drugs and factors such as anoxia, diabetic acidosis, uremia, and so on, is effectively treated by the use of antinarcotic drugs. Three drugs in this category are available— levallorphan (Lorfan), nalorphine (Nalline), and naloxone (Narcan). An allyl group replaces the methyl group on the nitrogen atom of morphine to form nalorphine, that of levorphanol to form levallorphan, and that of oxymorphone (Numorphan) to form naloxone. These drugs differ pharmacologically from the central stimulants (analeptics), which are used to antagonize depression caused by barbiturates and other hypnotics. The analeptics are stimulants and convulsants. Nalorphine, levallorphan, and naloxone are weak narcotics and do not stimulate the nervous system. Dysphoria occurs, which is unpleasant. When administered to a patient who has previously received a narcotic, these agents cause varying degrees of reversal of the depression. This reversal presumably results from competitive inhibition, that is, displacement of the narcotic from the receptors for narcotics and supplanting a strong narcotic effect with a weaker one. The most pronounced effect appears to be principally on the respiratory center. Some arousal and increase in reflex activity occur, but this is not complete. Antinarcotics are ineffective in overcoming depression caused by hypnotics, such as chloral, paraldehyde, glutethimide, and the barbiturates; they may even enhance such depression. Naloxone is the least apt to enhance the effects of other hypnotics than the other antagonists. Nalorphine, levallorphan, and naloxone given to a person dependent on the morphine-type drug who has received the usual narcotic requirement reverse the effect and precipitate withdrawal symptoms. Small doses of narcotic antagonists may precipitate severe and fatal withdrawal symptoms in drug-dependent patients. The use of antagonists is permissible in these persons, but the initial dose should be reduced to approximately one eighth or one tenth of the recommended dose for the nonhabituated patient.

Of all three drugs, naloxone is the drug of choice because it appears to lack any significant narcotic activity of its own. Levallorphan is approximately five times more potent on a milligram per milligram basis than nalorphine. Five mg. of nalorphine is approximately equal to 1 mg. of levallorphan. Naloxone is approximately 25 times more potent than nalorphine and the dosage should be scaled down accordingly. Narcotic antagonists may counteract narcotic-induced hypotension in some, but not all, patients; they may also cause sensory depression, oliguria, or nausea.

When narcotic overdosage is suspected, 0.4 mg. (1 ml.) of naloxone is given intravenously in adults. If depression is due to a narcotic, some increase in the ventilatory exchange occurs. An increase in rate and some increase in the overall minute volume exchange occur within 1 minute. Additional doses may be given at 1 to 2 minute intervals. If no response is obtained after three or four doses, one may conclude the difficulty is not due to a narcotic. The response, as a rule, is sustained for varying periods of time up to several hours depending upon the drug taken and the quantity. Should the patient lapse into the depressed state after a period of time, the incremental doses are again given. If naloxone is not available, nalorphine (Nalline) or levallorphan (Lorfan) may be used. If nalorphine is used 5 mg. is given intravenously. If levallorphan is used 1 mg. may be given. Five or 10 mg. of nalorphine or 1 or

2 mg. of levallorphan may be repeated if no response is obtained with the initial dose. If no response is obtained after using 15 mg. of nalorphine or 3 mg. of levallorphan (Lorfan), one may conclude that the difficulty is not due to a narcotic. Repeated administrations are also required if the patient lapses into a depressed phase. The use of excessive quantities of either levallorphan or nalorphine enhances the depression. Hypotension, if caused by a narcotic, is usually reversed. Nausea and vomiting, excitement, and other side effects characteristic of the narcotics are not reversed or antagonized by levallorphan. Neither nalorphine or levallorphan is suitable for antagonizing depression caused by pentazocine (Talwin). Convulsions may occur. Pentazocine is a feeble antinarcotic.

Naloxone (Narcan) is now considered to be the most useful antinarcotic for the reversal of narcotic depression induced by natural and synthetic narcotics, including pentazocine (Talwin), and for diagnosis of suspected acute overdosage of narcotics. Naloxone is essentially a pure narcotic antagonist that does not possess the agonistic properties characteristic of nalorphine or other narcotic antagonists. Naloxone possesses no pharmacologic activity in the absence of narcotics and appears to be devoid of the agonistic effects of other narcotic antagonists. It does not enhance the depression caused by barbiturates and other hypnotics and is therefore considered useful in the differential diagnosis of drug-induced coma.

Naloxone is active within 3 minutes after intravenous administration. It also may be used subcutaneously or intramuscularly. Onset of action in these instances is variable and not as rapid as after intravenous administration. It does not cause tolerance or physical or psychologic dependence. In some instances nausea and vomiting may occur as a side effect.

Doses in Infants

Depression caused by narcotics is common in infants and children, because their tolerance to the drugs is less predictable. Often codeine, used for pain relief after operations, or the tincture (paregoric) causes a morphinelike depression. This depression responds to the action of antinarcotics. The doses for infants and children should be reduced and estimated according to body weight. Generally, the initial dose of 0.01 mg. of naloxone per kg. of body weight suffices but may be repeated in increments as described for adults. The drug should be administered into the umbilical or other vein in apneic or depressed infants delivered from mothers who have received narcotics during labor. If a third fraction is ineffective, the apnea difficulty is most likely due to some other cause and not to a narcotic. In pediatric practice, as in adult practice, it is preferable to administer the doses in small fractions until the desired effect is obtained, rather than to estimate the total dose and administer it in a single injection.

Effect on Sensorium

The response with all three drugs is usually apparent within 1 to 2 minutes. Seldom are more than 2 or 3 minutes required for full establishment of respiratory stimulation. The results are never so dramatic when the drug is given intramuscularly. It is advisable, therefore, to administer the drug intravenously at all times. The oral route is not only impractical but ineffective. It is not necessary to administer a sustaining dose after the initial intravenous injection has caused reversal. No other stimulant is necessary to augment the action of nalorphine or levallorphan. In cases of mild poisoning or when arousal begins, methylphenidate may be used as a cortical stimulant to clear up the sensorium.

Other Therapeutic Measures

Gastric lavage seldom serves any useful purpose, even when drugs have been taken orally. Prior intubation with a cuffed endotracheal tube is mandatory to prevent aspiration should one feel it is indicated. It is a worthless procedure in cases of parenteral administration of the drug.

In patients with severe prolonged intoxication, a retention catheter of the Foley type should be introduced into the bladder in order to observe the urinary output, to evaluate renal function, and to prevent distension of the bladder as a result of increased smooth muscle tone of the bladder wall. Some narcotics affect the pituitary gland and release the antidiuretic hormone which frequently causes oliguria.

Treatment of Cerebral Injury Due to Anoxia

Prolonged depression of respiration may cause injury to the cerebral structures accompanied by cerebral edema. The signs, symptoms, and treatment are the same as those of brain injury that is due to anoxia for other causes. Pathologic reflexes such as positive Babinski, absent abdominal reflexes and spasticity are usually suggestive of cortical injury. The electroencephalograph may be of help in the diagnosis. Muscle twitchings and convulsions may occur owing to brain injury. Phenobarbital, 60 to 120 mg. intravenously, may control these. Various regimens have been suggested for the treatment of anoxic brain damage—hyperosmotic solutions of 20 per cent serum albumin, 50 per cent sucrose, or 25 per cent mannitol. These solutions not only allegedly remove fluid from the brain but also promote diuresis and facilitate the urinary excretion of unmetabolized narcotics and their by-products. The possibility of expansion of the blood volume and of cardiac failure must be borne in mind when these solutions are used. The value of surface cooling or deliberately induced hypothermia to prevent brain damage has never been fully assessed. Steroids are considered of benefit if administered early. Cortisone or hydrocortisone, up to 1 gram intravenously, may be used within the first few hours.

Respiratory Complications

Some narcotics release histamine. Bronchiolar constriction may be present. The presence of secretions in the tracheobronchial tree may further augment this bronchial constriction. Aminophylline, 200 to 500 mg., or 0.4 mg. of isoproterenol (Isuprel) may be administered cautiously intravenously. Some clinicians advise the use of hydrocortisone, 300 to 400 mg. slowly intravenously, or 120 to 160 mg. of methylprednisolone intravenously. Tracheal catheters may stimulate the upper airway passages and reflexly cause bronchospasm. Change in position is advised before resorting to the use of drugs.

The deeply comatose patient may develop pulmonary infections or atelectasis. Atelectasis may be of the miliary type at first and become progressive. Semiconscious patients able to respond may be encouraged to take periodic deep breaths. Comatose patients, whether breathing spontaneously or mechanically, should be passively hyperinflated periodically every 20 to 30 respirations by use of a "sigher." Comatose patients should be turned from side to side at 1 or 2 hour intervals. Diagnosis of the nature of the pulmonary infection may be made by x-ray examination. Pneumonitis and lobar pneumonia may accompany prolonged coma. This should be treated with the appropriate antibiotic or chemotherapeutic agent. Whenever possible, the organism involved should be identified from a specimen in the tracheobronchial secretions obtained under sterile conditions. Routine or prophylactic use of antibiotics is not recommended. As a general rule, penicillin or one of its variants to which the bacterial flora is susceptible is effective. The dosage, of course, should be individualized.

Fluid Balance and Electrolytes

In patients with prolonged coma, intravenous fluid therapy is indicated. The type and quantity of fluid used are guided by the aid of the hematocrit, the circulating blood volume, arterial pH, Pco_2, and Po_2 and electrolyte studies, including base deficit or excess and serum potassium, sodium, and chloride. The presence of metabolic acidosis may be corrected by intravenous infusion of sodium bicarbonate (1.4 grams per 1000 ml.).

Poisoning from narcotics heretofore did not present the serious problems encountered with hypnotics such as the barbiturates, because the general unavailability of these compounds precluded the ingestion or administration of massive doses. The illicit use of heroin and methadone and an increase in the use of propoxyphene is responsible for the increase in the number of poisonings. The increasing use of morphine in large doses by intravenous drip for cardiac surgery has also caused a greater usage of antinarcotics. Patients with prolonged periods of coma caused by the drug itself are uncommon. As a rule, most patients respond to the use of antinarcotics. Antinarcotics do not reverse the adverse effects of methotrimeprazine (Levoprome) used for analgesia. The muscle rigidity caused by fentanyl (Sublimaze) is reversed by antinarcotics.

PSYCHONEUROSIS

method of
DAVID M. HAWKINS, M.D.
Durham, North Carolina

The concept of psychoneurosis originally covered a specific group of symptom-defined psychiatric disorders felt to arise from a disturbed parent-child relationship, occurring in the patient as a conflict between his conscience (superego, parental and cultural values) and his desires, feelings, or reactions, and particularly amenable to the psychoanalytic treatment approach. It is useful to consider the elements of that concept that are retained in current psychiatric thinking as well as to identify the ways in which the concept has been broadened and changed in order to understand better the treatment and referral options available to the practicing physician.

Anxiety and the patient's mechanisms for managing it are still considered the core issues in psychoneurosis. In all of us anxiety is a useful signal that all is not well and extra attention to safety is needed. In the neurotic, anxiety is experienced in an inordinate amount or more chronically than commensurate with actual environmental danger and either (1) the experience of it is painful or disruptive in itself or (2) the mechanism of handling the anxiety, such as displacement to an object (a phobia) or an attempt to ward it off (a compulsion), is problematic or only partly success-

ful. Additionally, the chronic stance, muscle tensions, breathing patterns, and so on adopted by the person in order to respond to the environment and minimize or avoid anxiety or convert it to a more acceptable feeling (switch scare to anger, for instance) result in somatic changes and symptoms. Behavior designed to transfer anxiety or discomfort to the environment and make it "their problem, not mine" result in characterologic and personality patterns that are disruptive to personal relationships and intimacy and therefore bring symptomatic complaints from self or others. Thus, the person usually manifests a composite of disruptive or uncomfortable feelings, behaviors that are evaluated by self or others as problematic, and a characterologic pattern that is, to a greater or lesser extent, adaptive and useful or disturbing.

Psychoneurotic problems are still felt to arise from a disturbed parent-child relationship, but rather than seeing them as a defect in handling a development stage or the result of a particularly traumatic event, we now think of them in terms of how they reflect and are a part of the person's whole adaptational plan. Such a plan includes assumptions about oneself, an overall plot and outcome, the need for certain other characters to play important roles, and behaviors and habits that advance the plot and maintain attitudes which convince the protagonist that the world is as it needs to be for his story.

Each person brings into the world his own genetic strengths, weaknesses, and proclivities and encounters a unique combination of support and stresses. He is given a complex set of messages *directly* ("enjoy yourself," "don't waste time!"), *indirectly* ("Why can't you ever do anything right?" meaning that you can't or aren't expected to), *by behavior* (baby gets angry and mother may become helpful or may hold the baby nervously or angrily), and *by modeling* (father pays little attention to mother except when she acts sexy). The growing child, using his intuitive, clever, magical, inadequately informed thinking mechanism develops habits, assumes body postures, makes decisions about how the world "is" and how to survive. These become predominantly unconscious and the child proceeds with life using these various mechanisms, behaviors, and attitudes.

On the one hand, the child is dependent on parents to help define the world and teach values. This job of defining extends beyond objects and practical behavior, and the child learns certain definitions of his feelings, attitudes, and in fact himself. These may conflict with the child's spontaneously occurring feelings and wants, and to the extent that the child feels bad, guilty, afraid, inadequate, or not all right as a result of this conflict, we consider him neurotic.

On the other hand, the child is capable of independent thinking and reasoning about the world and can organize perceptions, see through faulty parental logic, figure out ways to circumvent rules, and manipulate the environment to get what he wants. Sometimes the resulting behavior is temporarily successful or gets the child immediate gratification, but does not work well for achieving long-range goals in the world. To the extent that such behavior is self- or other-defined as problematic, we consider the person character-disordered.

Most patients who come to the attention of the practicing physician for other than strictly medical reasons manifest a combination of neurotic and characterologic problems. In psychiatric parlance these are called mixed neuroses, character disorders, or character neuroses. In the remainder of this article "psychoneurotic" will refer to these mixed neurotic and characterologic problems.

Psychoneurotic Symptomatology

In order to decide on optimal treatment, the physician will need to assess beyond the symptomatic manifestation and form an impression of the adaptational plan and its supporting mechanisms, in the context of which the symptoms are occurring. When this holistic view is presented to the patient from the outset, he will likely be much more cooperative in exploring areas other than those obviously related to the chief complaint, accept consultation with specialists, or consider referral for psychologic or other treatment.

The physician's first task is to recognize that the patient is manifesting psychoneurotic symptoms. The sources for defining these symptoms are three-fold, including (1) self, (2) others, and (3) a structural concept.

Self. The patient may complain directly of the basic neurotic problem, recognizing that he has depression, low self-esteem, decreased confidence, or particular negative feelings about or assessment of self. He may complain of the effect this has on his life plan, recognizing that a particular goal (success, contentment) will not be possible unless the plan is changed (". . .unless I get help. . .unless something is done").

The patient may complain of the anxiety arising from a neurotic conflict; either the subjective feeling of anxiety or the somatic manifestation of it (palpitations, trembling, insomnia, etc.).

The patient may complain of discomfort with the mechanism by which he is partly or wholly managing the anxiety: phobia, compulsion, etc.

Others. A significant other person (spouse, parent, friend) may report discomfort with the patient's behavior directly to the physician.

The patient may report that others are uncomfortable ("my wife is concerned. . .").

The physician is also an "other." He may feel uncomfortable with the patient or the patient's behavior and should treat this as important diagnostic information.

Structural. A structural concept of psychoneurotic symptoms assumes that all of us must handle roughly similar developmental stages and issues of living and if we do not it is because we are blocked by a neurotic conflict from developing in some area. Knowledge of this manifestation of psychoneurosis requires a mediating step; that is, the patient must be compared to some organizing schema. This may be done formally, via psychodiagnostic testing, or informally as the physician assesses how the patient is dealing or has dealt with typical life issues: becoming independent of the family of origin, establishing and maintaining friendships, creating some sense of a life goal, finding self-support or value in a work situation, and dealing with major areas of behavior such as assertion, reliance on and trust in others, or establishing close relationships. If the patient has avoided or dealt poorly with some major area, this may be evidence of a psychoneurotic problem. The physician must be particularly attuned to the possibility of a structurally defined neurotic problem in those patients who present with somatic symptoms of indeterminate cause or who display exaggerated or unexpected reactions to somatic illness or to the illness of significant others.

Assessment

Having ascertained that the patient's symptoms suggest a psychoneurotic problem, the physician can consider how the person's adaptational plan is not working successfully.

The Plan Is the Problem. Some plans and the habit patterns that support them serve relatively well through a lifetime, especially if they are not too rigid and allow for change and adjustment. Some serve for part of a lifetime and then "run out," as with the professional person who works hard to finish school and become established and then becomes depressed because his plan does not cover situations in which he has time for more leisure activities and intimacy. Some plans work relatively well in the person's family of origin but do not support movement into the larger community. Finally, there are plans that were never geared to the person's best long-term interest and may have been predicated on a particularly hostile set of parental messages such as "don't exist (My troubles all started with you)" or "don't be successful (Why can't you ever do better?)." Such plans severely constrict the person's capacity for work, self-respect, and intimacy, limit his choices of action in the world, and may have a final scene that occurs in the state hospital, jail, or morgue. Problems with a faulty plan are best handled in reeducative therapy.

The Plan Needs Expanding. Many adaptational plans need augmentation when a person's life structure changes and he is faced with social and cultural changes for which he has not prepared. A young divorced woman, for instance, may find she needs to learn more assertiveness to become self-supporting. A man's driving phobia may become visible with a job change and require specific symptomatic treatment. In cases such as these, reeducative therapy may be helpful or supportive therapy, including advice, reassurance, and the recommendation to learn new skills, may be sufficient.

Temporary Breakdown of the Adaptational Pattern. Sometimes people are faced with life stresses that overwhelm their particular adaptational plans, which otherwise have sufficed. Prolonged illness, financial reverses, or family crises may precipitate psychoneurotic symptoms especially involving anxiety or depression. These patients are the best candidates for supportive therapy including psychotropic medication (anxiolytics, hypnotics, or antidepressants). It is particularly helpful to them for a physician to put their situation in perspective, calling attention to (1) usual strengths and ability to cope, (2) unusualness of the stress, and (3) the time-limited nature of the problem. This is like shining a flashlight on a dimly lit and scary object for a child. The features of the anxiety-producing situation can be seen more clearly, its size seems reduced when it is viewed in context, and the person is reassured that "overwhelmed" is a temporary phenomenon.

Treatment Options

Having spotted the symptoms and related them to the patient's adaptational plan, the physician is in a position to consider and recommend appropriate treatment. Self, other, and structurally defined symptoms are combined, the patient's resources (personal strengths, intelligence, finances, self-awareness, tolerance of discomfort, amount of environmental pressures) are considered, and a decision made to (1) provide or recommend supportive therapy, (2) recommend symptom-focused therapy, or (3) recommend reeducative therapy. It is extremely important that the patient be given as much information as possible about the decision. As long as this is done in the context of how the identified problems, especially the *self*-identified ones, are related to the patient's wishes and decisions to get along in the world, he can hear the recommendation as support rather than blame. With some patients support and an alliance with the physician must be established before further explanation and recommendation can be made.

Reeducative Therapy. When the patient has resources and motivation for investing in a major adaptational change, one of the reeducative therapies can be considered. Reeducative therapy is a combination of a therapeutic technique (psychoanalysis, transactional analysis, or gestalt therapy for example) and a commitment between patient and therapist that will see the patient through the process of (1) creating a trusting alliance; (2) revealing and delineating the patient's adaptational life plan, often identifying the forces shaping it originally; (3) formulating a new plan based on the patient's current wants, needs, and resources; and (4) learning and practicing the new behaviors that will support the new plan. One of the changes in the reeducative treatment of psychoneurosis has been a decreased emphasis on understanding the origin or genesis of the neurotic conflict and increased emphasis on how the neurotic assumptions, feelings, and behaviors are maintained and how they serve the patient in his current life. The patient is then encouraged and aided in trying on new behaviors and feelings that work better and is supported in getting used to them.

Many of the techniques or theoretical schools of therapy can be practiced in either an individual or group setting. Increasingly, group therapy is being used for the treatment of psychoneurotic problems because of (1) increased availability, (2) decreased cost, (3) ease of demonstrating to the patient the adaptational pattern and its effects on self and others, and (4) ease of generalizing support for new behavior and increased self-esteem from the therapy setting to every day life.

Symptom-Focused Therapy. Symptom-focused therapy includes pharmacologic agents aimed at alleviating symptoms connected with anxiety or depression, behavior therapy directed at changing problematic behaviors and habits, or biofeedback aimed at correcting long-standing muscle tension habits that cause somatic symptoms. There are three sets of circumstances in which symptom-focused therapy is indicated. *First*, when the symptom is seen by the patient as particularly troublesome and it is not central to the adaptational plan; for instance, a person with a driving phobia but otherwise fairly good adjustments to life might respond well to behavior modification or deconditioning, as opposed to a patient whose family relates to him almost exclusively in regard to the phobia and who has no extra-family support system. *Second*, when the patient's motivation or resources would not support reeducative therapy, symptom-focused therapy such as behavior therapy, biofeedback, or psychotropic medication may be used to ameliorate a central symptom such as a compulsion, headache, or depression. *Third*, psychotropic medication may be used to treat symptoms in a patient whose adaptational plan has broken down under temporary stress. Antidepressants, anxiolytics, or hypnotics may be called for to support the patient through the crisis; their long-term use, however, is generally a substitute for more intensive supportive or reeducative therapy and is fraught with danger. Medication may also be used during the evaluation or while a supportive relationship is being established.

In using medications supportively these points may be useful to remember: (1) The patient should be informed that the medication is supportive and temporary. This helps him keep the symptom-producing situation in context and supports his self-view as an active participant in life rather than a passive victim to be fixed or helped. Demands for increased medication often suggest that a different support or reeducative treatment is needed, facing the cause rather than trying to decrease the symptom. (2) Anxiolytics such as chlordiazepoxide or diazepam are useful and are best prescribed on a regular schedule such as 5 to 10 mg. two to four times daily for moderate anxiety; use on an as-needed (p.r.n.) basis in response to increased anxiety may reinforce anxiety-generating behavior. Barbiturates are not a good substitute for anxiolytics. (3) Antidepressants are more useful when depression is evident on mental status examination and involves biologic concomitants (sleep, appetite, concentration disturbances, etc.) than with the subjective feeling of "depression" alone. The sedative and placebo effect of small doses of antidepressants when the feeling of depression is a neurotic symptom may prevent patient and physician from seeing that more intensive intervention would be optimal.

Supportive Therapy. In supportive therapy the emphasis is not on reworking the patient's adaptational plan but in helping the patient use it more effectively, emphasizing its strengths, working around its weaknesses, and augmenting it where necessary. The agent of supportive therapy is often a physician, clergyman, teacher, or vocational counselor; or the agent may be a group, such as one of those mentioned below. What all effective supportive agents have in common is (1) authority, partly invested in them by the patient and partly established by the agent's approach, and (2) demonstrated concern for the patient's well-being and best interest. With these available the patient can experience the reassurance that he is not alone, the increased self-esteem of having his strengths and person validated, he can hear new information that may even counter information in his plan, and may feel safe enough to try on new and more effective behaviors.

A support base that is being used increasingly, either alone or in conjunction with an individual supportive relationship, is the support group. These come in many forms. Some are symptom or crisis-related, such as Mended Hearts for people who have had open heart surgery, the various ostomy groups for those who have had bowel surgery, groups for single parents, or social groups for divorced persons, Alcoholics Anonymous or Alanon for alcoholics and their families, and assertiveness training groups. Others are less specifically focused, such as men's or women's support groups, Re-Educative Counseling groups, or peer support groups for physicians. In addition to specific supportive action, these groups offer an antidote to the alienation that many persons feel in our changing society, and have partly replaced the support formerly available in close extended families.

Relating to the Patient. The physician's attitude and assumptions are generally clear to the patient, even when they are not meant to be. Seeing the patient as a person whose symptoms and presentation represent a life plan that, to various degrees, is or is not working well communicates support and allows the physician to remain flexible, to understand that there are many and changing options for intervention, and to work more *with* than *on* the patient. Finally, if referral for specific treatment is called for, it is extremely helpful for the physician to (1) contact the new therapist directly and (2) provide a follow-up visit, phone call, or letter to the patient. These steps have been shown to increase the success of treatment referral.

DELIRIUM

method of
EDWIN S. ROBBINS, M.D.,
and MARVIN STERN, M.D.
New York, New York

Delirium is an acute disorder brought about by altered cerebral function. It is quite common and should be considered whenever there is a history of drug or alcohol abuse (and withdrawal); febrile illness, especially in children; overdose of drugs, noting especially anticholinergics such as tricyclic antidepressants; cranial neoplasms or head trauma; physical trauma; postsurgical states, especially open heart surgery; cerebral anoxia often following myocardial infarction or heart failure; sensory deprivation, following eye surgery ("black patch" syndrome) or treatment in an intensive care unit; endocrine disturbances; and the administration of many drugs, particularly in crisis settings, although cumulative effects or individual idiosyncrasies must also be considered. Delirium may also be the first sign of a cerebral illness such as meningitis, but more often it follows, sometimes by several days, the appearance of the precipitating agent. It is a time-limited illness, usually resolved by the end of 5 days, though it may extend to as long as 2 weeks. Outcome of delirium is usually favorable, but prognosis is that of underlying disorder.

While some patients are not recognized to be delirious because they are quiet, minimally disorganized, and present a good social facade, most cases are characterized by sudden onset. Associated with altered states of consciousness are defects in recent memory, difficulty in learning new material, increased concern with the environment and multiple misinterpretations of events. Although attention span is short, most patients can be contacted readily and will respond to questions. Clouding of consciousness, poor judgment, and sensory misinterpretations may be manifest by the expression of lurid tales, with paranoid content. By careful questioning, it is possible to reconstruct the events leading to the distortions. Hallucinations are frequent. Visual hallucinations are most common, followed by auditory and then other somatic phenomena.

Among motor manifestations are restlessness, frequently manifested by picking at bedclothing, or tremulousness. A few patients are quiet and withdrawn. Myoclonus and grand mal seizures are uncommon. Electroencephalograms (EEGs) may be characterized by slow wave patterns, but these changes are not always present.

Treatment for delirium consists of identifying and treating the underlying illness as quickly as possible. Neurologic and psychiatric examinations are indicated. In conjunction with treating the underlying illness, specific measures are required for the delirium. These center about environmental contact, maintaining electrolyte and fluid balance, and reducing elevated temperature. Verbal contact helps diminish restlessness and panic. Use of a night light may decrease the degree of perceptual distortion. Delirious patients should not be permitted to remain in rooms by themselves or be placed in seclusion because they are noisy and disruptive. Use of restraints should be restricted as much as possible.

When the cause has been established, medicine that is not contraindicated or is a specific antidote, such as physostigmine or anticholingeric drugs, including tricyclics, should be administered.

Major tranquilizers are useful in controlling agitated, psychotic behavior. Among those which will not additionally cloud consciousness nor affect the cardiovascular system are haloperidol, perphenazine, and trifluoperazine.

AFFECTIVE DISORDERS

method of
MEL PROSEN, M.D.
Chicago, Illinois

Affective disorders, particularly depression, are the most commonly diagnosed psychiatric disorders. The lifetime expectancy of developing an affective disorder is estimated from 8 to 20 per cent, including the milder neurotic depressive disorder. This is a commonly missed diagnosis, and it is thought that only about one quarter of all the severely depressed patients who are in need of treatment actually receive it.

Definition. Affective disorders must be differentiated from those states of unhappiness and sadness that occur commonly in every human being. Furthermore, affective disorders are generally differentiated from reactive depressions, in which it is felt there is a precipitant and significant life stress, usually a loss of a loved one, so that the person has a reason to be feeling poorly. Upon resolution and working through of the problem, the person generally recovers spontaneously. Affective disorders should be confined to those persons who have a *dysphoric mood* that is pervasive and in whom there is no obvious reason or precipitating factor for the altered pathologic state. Affective disorders in which depression is the only mode of expression are termed unipolar depressions. Other affective diseases, in which there is an alteration in mood with hypomanic, agitated, pressured, excited states of function are known as the hypomanic and manic type. Persons prone to both severe depressions and one or more manic episodes are said to have bipolar affective disorders.

The term affective disorders should be reserved for the person suffering from severe dysphoric moods with pervasive loss of interest or pleasure in their surroundings. They generally tend to be sad, blue, feeling hopeless, with a lack of concern for themselves and an inability to respond to their environment in a meaningful way. Generally, their social relationships tend to suffer, including close family ties and friendships, and they are unable to work effectively and creatively. These symptoms must be prominent and persist for a long period of time. They must show significant vegetative symptoms such as severe appetite disturbances, usually weight loss: a pound a week or 10 pounds per year, or significant weight gain. There is a sleep disturbance, with either an inability to fall asleep, stay asleep, or an early morning awakening; or they tend to withdraw and sleep excessively. There is a lack of energy, easy fatigueability, chronic tiredness, or perhaps some degree of psychomotor agitation with an inability to relax or engage in activities for any meaningful period of time. There is a lack of interest in one's surroundings and usually an absence of pleasurable responsiveness in their usual activities. Libido is generally lowered, often leading to impotence. There is a feeling of self-reproach, usually of inappropriate, excessive guilt, which can almost be delusional. There is a marked diminution of intellectual function, usually indicated by an inability to think or concentrate, with lapses of recent memory. Persons with severe affective disorders usually have recurrent thoughts of death and ruminate about suicide, hoping to escape from their psychologic anguish.

Persons suffering from the manic disorder tend to be highly irritable, with expansive moods, hypertalkativeness, flight of ideas, pressured speech, an inflated self-esteem bordering on grandiosity, and a decreased need for sleep. They are easily distractable, and they tend to get involved in activities without any concern for the consequences. They tend to spend money wildly, travel impulsively, and become sexually promiscuous. There is complete lack of judgment and no inhibition. They are unable to settle down and relax on a purely voluntary basis. Most affective disorders of the depressive type are self-limiting. Acute depressive episodes generally have a good prognosis without any type of significant intervention. Spontaneous improvement definitely occurs in depression and it is hoped that the following detailed therapeutic interventions will be utilized in order to shorten and abort the depressive episode. There is a small number of patients with severe depressive illnesses who do not spontaneously remit. It is thought that about 10 to 15 per cent of the patients have significant enough depressions with a chronic course so that their level of function is never satisfactory. There is a high rate of recurrence in depressive illness, with the possibility of recurrence ranging from 40 to 50 per cent.

It is essential to interrupt a severe depressive illness in order to minimize the possibility of suicidal behavior. The suicide rate has been estimated up to 25 per cent of chronic, repeated severe depressive disorders.

The modes of therapy described here can be usually done on an out-patient basis. The criteria commonly used to indicate hospitalization are those patients with severe affective disorders who are unable to manage their lives within the presence of significant responsible family members. Patients who are self-destructive need to be admitted to the hospital and monitored very closely in an in-patient setting because their suicidal potential is not automatically diminished by being in a socalled "protective" setting. Patients who are severely depressed can lapse into what is termed a depressive stupor wherein they are unable to engage their world in a meaningful manner and are unable to care for themselves properly, so that their nutritional status and poor hygiene can lead to severe medical consequences.

The nature of the depressive illness is such that it somehow, by its nature, interferes with the various therapeutic interventions designed to curtail it. Patients with the severe affective disorder can become so hopeless and helpless that they are unable to follow the physician's recommendations properly and do not take medications as prescribed or take them in an erratic manner and do not keep appointments. They do not meaningfully participate in the physician-patient interactions so crucial in any process of intervention. Furthermore, they are prone to suicide-equivalent behavior by their lack of concern for themselves and because they generally are not able to appreciate fully the environment or interact with it in a meaningful way. They are accident prone and, if suffering from other severe medical illnesses such as diabetes, cardiovascular disorders, or severe infections, are quite likely to refuse or not remember to use their medication appropriately.

A careful evaluation of suicidal risk has to be made in every severe affective disorder. Furthermore, the agitated hypomanic states are extremely deleterious to the patients' function and often lead them to engage in detrimental activities, such as squandering their financial resources in some get-rich scheme.

Patients suffering from affective disorders present tremendous difficulties for their families and it is only natural that after a period of time, spouses and children will also be severely affected by the ravages of a patient with an untreated affective disorder. It is quite natural that close family members will become irritated and harbor resentment towards the patient; if this ambivalence becomes pathologic, the severely depressed patient might be more prone to become suicidal or feel all the more worthless and resigned to his illness. It is imperative to hospitalize patients who do not respond to interventions within 1 to 3 weeks in order to initiate more active forms of intervention and possibly to provide some type of therapy that cannot be instituted in an out-patient setting.

Suicide Risk

The patient who is a suicidal risk should be followed very closely and initially seen at least 2 to 3 times per week; the physician should make himself available by phone at all times. If a patient fails to engage early in therapy and to establish the beginnings of a relationship, the physician should hospitalize immediately.

Strong indications of *suicide risk* are found in patients over the age of 45 and patients suffering from significant traumatic events such as the loss of a loved one or disabling physical disorders that threaten their physical and economic independence. Adolescence is a tumultuous developmental stage, so that the adolescent can be especially prone to suicide.

Suicide-prone patients have usually indicated, in one form or another, some unwillingness to live and have tried to communicate their distress to the significant people in their environment. There usually is a history of prior suicide attempts and their life has indicated a prolonged self-destructive, ineffectual manner of handling stress and crises. There is usually a severe loss or threat of loss and generally an inability to respond to help. There is usually some marked inability to express openly and, quite commonly, depression has progressed to a psychotic proportion with patients who have delusions that they are rotting inside and who are terribly guilty and blame themselves for all that is not going well around them. There is usually an incidence of alcohol abuse and many suicide attempts are made under the influence of alcohol or other central nervous system depressant medications.

The patient with affective disorder requires a very close scrutiny until establishment of as good a rapport as possible with patient and family members. There should be frequent visits, and medications must be prescribed in small amounts which, if taken all at once, would not be lethal. If self-destructive behavior is evidenced, the patient should be hospitalized immediately. There should be careful monitoring of patients in the hospital, especially at the time of admission and as they begin to improve. As patients come out of severe depressive states, they might have the energy and motivation to commit suicide, which they were unable to do earlier due to apathy and severe psychomotor retardation.

It is also important to note that the hypomanic patient, because of his poor judgment, can be a severe suicidal risk. He will drive an automobile at excessive speeds and take unnecessary chances, thus increasing his vulnerability to accidents; he may also provoke violence upon himself in social situations.

Modes of Treatment

Severe affective disorders are generally managed by antidepressants, which are classified according to their structure and mode of action as tricyclic antidepressants and monoamine oxidase (MAO) inhibitors. Electroconvulsive therapy is another form of somatic therapy. Supportive psychotherapy occurs when the physician engages the patient in a professional relationship and tries to help the patient understand himself; this is an important part of all these interventions. In order to help depressed patients, it is essential to enlist their cooperation and try to promote in them some degree of optimism and willingness to collaborate in the attempt to alter their illness. This is especially important in the affective disorders in which patients tend to feel hopeless, helpless, guilty, and incapable of improving or unworthy of help. Often, as they begin to get better, they tend to undermine the various treatment modalities instrumental in their improvement.

Medication

Tricyclic Antidepressants. A tricyclic antidepressant is the treatment of choice for most depressions. About 70 per cent of patients will improve on tricyclic antidepressant medication in appropriate doses in about 4 to 6 weeks. The tricyclic antidepressants will commonly cause anticholinergic side effects initially, such as dry mouth, blurred vision, constipation, urinary retention, and palpitations. It is important to reassure the patient that these symptoms should be tolerated and that they will often dissipate in several days. As the depressed patient is prone to somatic preoccupations and concerns, it is essential to urge him to continue to take the medication at its appropriate levels with the reassurance that, in time, the side effects will diminish and the severe depression will begin to abate.

TABLE 1.   **Tricyclic Antidepressants**

GENERIC NAME	TRADE NAME	DOSE RANGE
Imipramine	Tofranil	150–300 mg./day
Desipramine	Pertofrane, Norpramin	150–200 mg./day
Amitriptyline	Elavil, Endep	75–300 mg./day
Nortriptyline	Aventyl	50–150 mg./day*
Protriptyline	Vivactil	10–60 mg./day
Doxepin	Sinequan	150–300 mg./day

*This dose may be higher than that listed in the manufacturer's official directive.

Numerous attempts have been made to determine which patients respond best to the various tricyclic antidepressants. It seems that agitated depressions respond to amitriptyline, whereas the retarded anergic depressions respond better to imipramine. There have been attempts to measure urinary metabolites of norepinephrine, methoxyhydroxyphenylglycol (MHPG). The relation between patients with high MHPG responding better to amitriptyline and patients with low MHPG responding to imipramine has been suggested.

These medications must be used in appropriate doses (see Table 1). The dose of imipramine or amitriptyline should begin at 25 mg. three times daily and should be rapidly pushed to therapeutic levels. Some patients will not absorb the tricyclic antidepressants, and in many medical centers there is an opportunity to measure steady-state plasma concentrations of the tricyclic antidepressants. Patients who do not respond well to tricyclics generally seem to have some genetically determined absorption problem that can be demonstrated in relatives with severe affective disturbances. Tricyclic antidepressants can be given at night because of their sedative effect and some of the anticholinergic discomforts can be diminished as the therapeutic effect of the tricyclic antidepressants can sustain the patient over the 24 hour period. The tricyclics should be avoided in patients who have benign prostatic hypertrophy or narrow angle glaucoma. In addition, the anticholinergic effects can be cumulative.

Severe overdoses of tricyclic medication present problems because of their cardiac toxic effects. The tricyclic antidepressants can cause palpitations, tachycardia, and severe orthostatic hypotension. On the electrocardiogram (ECG), there can be T wave depression with prolonged QT interval and an ST segment depression. With overdose, there can be severe arrhythmias with extrasystoles, atrial ventricular fibrillation, and ventricular tachycardia. In patients in whom anticholinergic effects and cardiotoxic effects should be minimized, it might be crucial to utilize a tricyclic with less anticholinergic effects such as doxepin. Allergic reactions to the tricyclics such as jaundice of the obstructive type and a hypersensitivity reaction with eosinophilia can occur. Agranulocytosis is rare (with an incidence less than 0.01 per cent). Older patients can complain of headaches, muscle cramps, and not infrequently, some pitting lower extremity edema.

Tricyclic antidepressants in bipolar depressions can precipitate a hypomanic state and also precipitate delusions and hallucinations in a patient with latent schizophrenia. Patients should be maintained on an adequate dose of tricyclics for 6 to 9 months. If there is a history of repeated, recurrent depressive disorder, the patient should be kept on the antidepressant for an indeterminate period of time with the dose gradually reduced and the medication even possibly reinstated at such times as spring and fall when recurrent depressive disorders tend to occur. It is important to remember that tricyclic drugs can interact with other medications, especially central nervous system depressants, and the patient should be judiciously advised to avoid alcohol and barbiturates. The tricyclics should be used with extreme caution and in the lowest possible doses in the elderly, who can often benefit from as small a dose of imipramine as 10 to 20 mg. per day. They should be avoided in patients prone to cardiac arrhythmias, in whom electroshock therapy, carefully monitored, would be the treatment of choice. The effect of the tricyclic antidepressant drugs in pregnancy and lactation is still unclear and they should be used with caution.

Monoamine Oxidase Inhibitors. The monoamine oxidase inhibitors (MAOI) (see Table 2) are very much less used in the treatment of severe depressive disorders. When the MAOIs were first introduced, there was concern about their causing a severe hepatotoxicity with hepatocellular degeneration and a viral-like hepatitis. There were reports of hypertensive crises when MAOIs were used by people who had eaten foods high in tyramine content. However, in the past decade, especially in the United Kingdom, MAOIs have been used, especially for refractory depressions, and, should a severe depression fail to respond to the tricyclics after 3 to 4 weeks, a trial of MAOIs is indicated.

These have been effective in severe endogenous, atypical depressions when the patients seem to have higher levels of anxiety, some paranoia, and severe obsessive compulsive symptoms with hypochondriacal ruminations. MAOI responsive patients tend to complain of extreme lassitude and the sleep disturbance tends to be one of excessive sleep; instead of a diminished appetite, they tend to eat excessively. If placed on MAOIs, patients *must* avoid foods rich in tyramine such as cheese,

TABLE 2.   **Monoamine Oxidase Inhibitors**

GENERIC NAME	TRADE NAME	DOSAGE
Hydrazine		
Isocarboxazid	Marplan	10–30 mg.
Phenelzine	Nardil	15–75 mg.
Nonhydrazine		
Tranylcypromine	Parnate	10–50 mg.*

*This dose may be higher than that listed in the manufacturer's official directive.

yeast extract, beer, wine, sour cream, cola drinks, chocolate, chicken livers, beans, figs, dates, and raisins. An extensive work-up including ECG, alkaline phosphatase, blood urea nitrogen (BUN), serum glutamic oxaloacetic transaminase (SGOT), urinalysis, and complete blood count (CBC) should be performed. Patients who have been on tricyclics should be given a washout period of 5 to 7 days before the use of MAOIs. MAIOs can cause hypotensive effects, especially orthostatic hypotension. The parenchymal hepatocellular damage can occur, and weekly determinations of liver function tests should be performed on patients taking MAOIs. Rarely, MAOIs can cause insomnia and a toxic psychosis. Acute hypertensive crisis such as convulsions, intercranial bleeding, and hyperpyrexia should be avoided by carefully indicating to patients they must avoid foods that can produce tyramines, a byproduct of bacterial fermentation. Certain other drugs must not be used in the presence of MAOIs such as amphetamines, ephedrine, phenylephrine, and various decongestant medications. MAOIs can also potentiate central nervous system depressants, and it is to be especially avoided in patients who might be abusing meperidine. The physician should be very careful not to maintain the patient on MAOIs any longer than is absolutely necessary. There should be careful monitoring of blood pressure and constant and frequent follow-ups in order to enforce the dietary restrictions required for this medication. In addition, this medication should not be given to patients who are irresponsible or erratic in following the physician's orders.

Electroshock Therapy. The most effective treatment in the management of severe affective disorders is electroshock therapy. Patients who have not responded to adequate doses of tricyclic antidepressants followed by a course of MAOIs without remission should be considered for electroshock therapy. Furthermore, the patient with a severe suicidal risk who does not respond to initial hospitalization and milieu interventions should be considered a good candidate for electroshock therapy. The patient with severe psychotic depression who is unable to respond to his environment and properly collaborate in taking antidepressant medication, resulting in malnutrition and dehydration, should be considered for electroshock therapy immediately. The overriding issue is suicidal danger, which is everpresent in every severe psychotic depression. The manic phase of manic depressive psychosis, which is often difficult to manage with phenothiazines and lithium, can be quickly brought to remission with a course of electroshock therapy. Not infrequently, severely hypomanic patients are resistant to lithium and can be nonabsorbers of phenothiazine medication,

making it essential to manage the acute phase of the illness with electroshock therapy, which will help stabilize them. Depressions of old age often respond remarkably well to a brief course of convulsive therapy, and very careful evaluation must be done, because these patients often appear to have senile dementia, and a good deal of their organic brain function will clear with the lifting of a severe retarded or agitated depression.

Certain symptoms predict *a good response* to electroshock therapy, such as anorexia, weight loss, early morning awakening, low self-esteem, feelings of worthlessness, and repetitive thoughts of self-destruction with massive feelings of guilt and somatic delusions. Paranoid, suspicious, narcissistic, depressive patients *do not respond* as well to electroshock therapy as do the severe chronic depressive character types.

Electroshock therapy can be a very safe treatment, but it does transiently raise cerebral spinal fluid pressure and is contraindicated for any condition with increased intracranial pressure such as a space-occupying lesion. A severe compensated cardiorespiratory status should alert the physician to proceed very cautiously and with sophisticated anesthetist consultation. The patient should be very carefully evaluated prior to electroshock therapy with ECG, chest x-ray, x-rays of the cervical and thoracic spines, urinalysis, and SMA-18. Patients with severe osteoporosis or healed vertebral fracture should be carefully managed with adequate succinylcholine for complete muscle relaxation, so that the seizure does not disrupt existing pathogenesis.

The patient should be adequately prepared for electroshock therapy. Most patients have terrible fears and fantasies about the implications of the treatments, and the physician should carefully review exactly what the procedure involves and deal as effectively as possible with the apprehensions of the patient, who generally tends to feel he is being punished for not getting better from other interventions. Bitemporal electroshock therapy produces both an anterograde and retrograde amnesia, and memory function should return to normal within 4 to 6 weeks and usually within 10 days after the last treatment. The patient should be carefully evaluated after each electroshock therapy session in order to keep the number of treatments to the absolute, essential minimum. Severe depressive reactions usually respond to 6 to 12 treatments. Patients should not receive anything orally after midnight, and at the time of treatment they should be given 0.6 to 0.8 mg. of atropine to block the vagal stimulating effects of the treatment. The atropine should be given intramuscularly 15 minutes before electroshock therapy or can be given intravenously along with the anesthetic. Dentures should be removed and a general anesthetic, either methohexital (Brevital), 30 to 100 mg. given intravenously, or sodium thiopental (Pentothal), can be used to put the patient to sleep. Muscle relaxation is obtained by the use of 30 to 90 mg. of succinylcholine (Anectine). Adequate preoxygenation with 95 to 100 per cent oxygen should be given prior to treatment. It is essential that the medications and general anesthesia be performed by a competent anesthetist and that there be adequate recovery facilities to monitor the patient carefully after electroshock therapy. After administration of anesthesia, the electroshock is administered by applying electrodes over the anterior portion of the temporal bone bilaterally and using a shock of 150 volts for the duration of 0.5 second.

Management of the Manic Patient

Manic patients are often very difficult to manage because of their agitated state, grandiosity, expansiveness, and because the are unable to appreciate the nature of the illness. They are unwilling or ambivalent about being controlled by people in their midst or by somatic forms of therapy. Lithium carbonate is extremely effective in the long-term management of the manic patient, but usually it is not sufficient to manage the acute phases of the illness. Phenothiazines such as chlorpromazine, 50 to 150 mg. every 3 to 4 hours, or fluphenazine hydrochloride (Prolixin), 25 mg. every 2 hours,* or haldoperidol, 5 to 10 mg. orally every 3 to 4 hours, are often necessary to help sedate the overwrought, out-of-control manic patient. These medications, of course, should be *titrated* very carefully against the severity of the patient's illness and decreased as the patient's mood begins to stabilize. In one group of affective disorders, known as rapid cycling, manic patients require very high doses of sedating phenothiazine medication in order to help them achieve some degree of control. In addition, there are some poor responders who must be managed initially with the use of phenothiazine-like medication and electroconvulsive therapy. Management of the manic episode may take from 2 to 5 days. The initial dose of lithium carbonate will vary and the patient should be started on a dose of 600 mg. the first day and increased to 900 mg. the next and gradually increased and then followed by serum blood levels scheduled on each morning. Usually the dose of lithium required to produce therapeutic blood level ranges is from 1 to 1.3 mEq. per liter. There is variation from patient to patient. The various factors that influence the lithium

blood level are age, sex, weight, and salt intake of the patient. New patients readily excrete the lithium and an increased salt intake will decrease the plasma level of lithium. The salt will compete with lithium for reabsorption in the distal tubule in the kidney. Much higher doses of lithium might be required to help stabilize the hypomanic patient, who will then be able to respond to lower doses once his hypomania is brought under control. The side effects of lithium therapy are nauseousness, mild lethargy, fatigue, and a fine tremor of the hands. Serious side effects of lithium are predominantly neurologic and can include vertigo, somnolence, hyperactive reflexes, stupor, confusion, seizures, and dizziness. Another complication of lithium is the development of a nontoxic goiter and some functional hypothyroidism. Lithium has been in use since 1949, but only in the last few years has it been used in high doses because of the accurate detection of patients suffering manic depressive disorders. The long-term effects of this medication will be evaluated over the next several years. There have been reports of a disorder resembling diabetes insipidus in some patients on long-term use of lithium. It is important to note that the thiazide diuretics can potentiate the toxic effects of lithium and, in severe intractable hypomanic situations, there are reports in the literature of thiazides being used in order to potentiate the effect of lithium.

Lithium carbonate has been the major medication to maintain and stabilize mood and should be used for an indefinite time. Careful monitoring of the patient should be done to maintain blood levels ranging from 0.5 to 1.2 mEq. per liter. Amounts required to maintain adequate blood levels generally run from 600 to 1200 mg. per day. Patients who are prone to hypomania tend to miss the episodes of elation, and may even mourn their absence, and will require particularly diligent follow-up to assure compliance with the lithium regimen to avoid deliberate precipitation of another manic episode.

There are some forms of unipolar, repeated severe depressions that can be successfully managed with lithium carbonate therapy. In patients whose response to tricyclic or MAOI therapy has been little or equivocal, a trial of lithium carbonate is in order.

Iatrogenic Causes of Affective Disorder

Reserpine is well known to cause severe psychotic depressions. L-Dopa, propranolol, methyldopa, and various steroids have been associated with depressive syndromes. Hypomanic states can be precipitated by the use of the corticosteroids. Cocaine and amphetamines can cause maniclike states, but these central nervous system

---

*This dose may be higher than that listed in the manufacturer's official directive. See official directive before using.

(CNS) stimulants are more likely to cause paranoidlike psychosis in vulnerable persons.

In summary, patients with affective disorders are a serious problem for the treating physician. They have to be taken very seriously and require immediate intervention, often hospitalization, and very close follow-up. It is important that the physician be able to provide an ambience of acceptance and understanding in order to help the severely depressed patient regain some self-esteem and feelings of worthiness and hopefulness. These severely depressed or hypomanic patients can elicit strong emotional reactions in their physicians because of their helplessness, dependence, and generalized inability to engage in a meaningful way. It is important to realize that patients who feel worthless and guilty initially are quite prone to becoming even more depressed when attempts are made to help them. This reaction has to be understood and managed carefully and alertly, so that it can then be handled effectively to help the patient benefit from a sensible combined psychologic, pharmacologic somatic intervention approach.

SCHIZOPHRENIA

method of
JARL DYRUD, M.D.,
and JOSEPH HARASZTI, M.D.
Chicago, Illinois

From earliest times the person who had "lost his mind" was not considered sick either by the community or by himself. Having become a changed person, yet sound of wind and limb, he was more to be feared than pitied.

This "changed person" was so different in behavior, affect, and thought processes from what he was before and from his fellows that in one way or another he was defined as alien to the community.

In every age the problem he presented tended to be diagnosed in terms of explanations in vogue at the time. At one time or another the majority of experts agreed that he was possessed by a spirit, that his bile was poisoning his animal spirit, that he had a diseased brain, or that he was a degenerate.

If we define treatment in its broadest sense as "how do we deal with him?, 'how does our culture define his problem?' " we can see how inseparable diagnosis and treatment really are. Any diagnostic scheme calls for or makes possible a certain range of possible responses. You cannot speak one way and think another.

We must bear in mind that madness, insanity, psychosis, and schizophrenia are all words used to describe those whose behavior is sufficiently incongruous with their circumstances, as defined by their community of fellows, so that the community defines them as outside this consensus. Whether precipitated by great emotional stress, toxic states, or a relatively mild trauma to a person of particular sensitivities, the manifest behavior may be very similar. The outcome, however, is very different. The vast majority of heavily stressed patients become nonpsychotic fairly promptly in a benign environment. The person of particular sensitivities may not. In fact, he tends to persist in a maladaptive pattern we call chronic schizophrenia as opposed to the acute reactive type.

Chronic schizophrenia, or schizophrenia proper, is a diagnostic term applied to millions of people throughout the world, yet there is no generally accepted definition of the term.

The term schizophrenia is an example of the "fallacy of misplaced singularity." Bleuler, of course, spoke of "The Group of the Schizophrenias," by which he recognized the heterogeneity of conditions subsumed under the label. The conditions include the clear-cut process schizophrenia, insidious in their onset in early adolescence and proceeding ever more malignantly into dementia; the oscillating, phasic schizophrenic conditions; the rigid, litigious paranoid schizophrenic processes that appear in the third and fourth decades of life; the acute schizophreniform psychotic episodes, from which some patients recover apparently completely and from which many more patients never reach a *restitutio ad integrum*. There are nonpsychotic conditions, too, that we label schizophrenic: the so-called latent schizophrenias, incipient schizophrenias, ambulatory schizophrenias, and even remitted schizophrenias.

Much of the research data emerging from family and genetic studies (e.g., Heston, Kety, Rosenthal, Wender and Schulsinger) point to an even broader area of schizophrenia factors than even the syndromal descriptions, and suggest a spectrum of conditions that include people with severe neurotic symptoms and even those without pathology but who show a distinctive, novel, creative outlook on reality. In some studies it has been found that subtle evidences of thought disorder can exist in settings of normal social, occupational, and family behavior. From these studies questions about etiology arise. Are the serious schizophrenias to be considered etiologically related to the neuroses? That is, if one accepts a conflict cause of neurosis such as Freud presented, can one fit the schizophrenias into such a psychoanalytic model? Or, if one accepts a thoroughgoing empirical model such as Skinner has outlined, in which all behavior is a learned outcome of its consequences, can one fit the schizophrenias into such an operant model?

The answer in our time has resolved itself into "The Schizophrenias" and has implicated a cause that may be far more complex than the conditions for which the usual psychotherapies were developed. This position does not disavow the etiologic importance of learning, family strains, and intrapersonal conflicts. Rather, with our expanding knowledge of genetic, biochemical, and quasistable personality factors we prefer to think of all of these factors as "contributory" or "necessary etiologic conditions" rather than specifically or uniquely causal. In keeping with Adolph Meyer's psychobiologic approach, we recognize that a crucial diagnostic task is the assessment of the relative contributions of familial, genetic, conflict, biochemical, psychologic, and sociocultural factors in order to be able to aim a treatment program at its proper target. For it would seem that in the severe disintegrated schizophrenic conditions, a plurality of therapeutic methods would be called for, simultaneously or sequentially, rather than reliance on one technique alone; i.e., the early treatment steps may well be focussed on reducing the ambiguity of the environment in an operant conceptual framework followed by more stress on the therapeutic relationship.

Even though we cannot neatly define schizophrenia, on any given day, 70 per cent of the long-term hospital beds in this country are occupied by people bearing this diagnosis. On this same day we would then estimate the incidence of hospitalized schizophrenic people to be roughly 160 per 100,000 population. Prevalence is a much harder figure to estimate because it includes nonpatients as well as out-patients, but a number of studies have placed it in the vicinity of 290 per 100,000 on any one day. These estimates are surprisingly uniform throughout western civilization wherever records have been kept. Thus, you can see that it is a major public health problem.

This particular sensitivity has been found to concentrate in populations in transition, i.e., adolescence to maturity, in socially disorganized populations, and in high-density populations.

David Rosenthal in the "Genain Quadruplets" summarizes three major current theoretical positions on the contribution of hereditary and environmental factors to the schizophrenias; he names these the Monogenic-biochemical, the Diathesis-stress, and the Life Experience approaches.

The Monogenic-biochemical approach holds that a single inherited mutant gene is responsible for the later appearance of schizophrenia, through the pathway of an inborn error of metabolism in a manner similar to phenylketonuria (PKU). Variability of penetrance is used to explain the fact that not all persons with the genotype demonstrate the illness. Schizophrenia is seen as a unitary phenomenon, in which environmental factors, either predisposing (in childhood) or precipitating (in adulthood), are of little import.

The Diathesis-stress approach asserts that potential schizophrenics are born with a variety of predispositions to develop a variety of the schizophrenias and that the genetic contribution is polygenic, in a manner similar to the multiple determinants of adult intelligence. Thus, normally adaptive stress-response systems in the adult may go awry.

The Life Experience approach says that some combination of unfortunate early life experience (e.g., maternal deprivation, an irrational environment) and current life stresses (e.g., adolescence, marriage, childbirth, job loss) conspire to produce the appearance of illness.

The Diathesis-stress approach seems most consistent with the heterogeneity of findings in genetic, metabolic, and psychologic studies of schizophrenia.

Bleuler's concept of "loosening of associations" is perhaps the single most characteristic feature of the illness. His "four As" of association (loose), affect (inappropriate), ambivalence, and autism are still most valuable clues to the existence of a schizophrenic process.

Heinrich Neumann, writing in 1854, stated the problem beautifully when he said it is a loosening of the patient's "togetherness" both with himself and with his community.

In our time and in our terminology schizophrenia is not a disease but a group of symptom patterns. While thought disorder has been described as the core symptom in schizophrenia by many psychologists, it has been well known among clinicians that many acute schizophrenics do not show thought disorder, even in an acute psychotic episode. In contradiction to our usual understanding of schizophrenia, which is described as an acute psychosis occurring in a clear sensorium, many acute schizophrenics appear confused, along with severe agitation, bizarre behavior, and with an affective component of excitement. It is quite possible that the approach-avoidance anxiety seen in schizophrenics is at least as important as thought disorder. The diagnosis of schizophrenia should not be made on the basis of phenomenology alone. Schizophrenia is a longitudinal illness that occurs over time with exacerbations and remissions and many other conditions can mimic the accessory symptoms of schizophrenia and the phenomenology often associated with schizophrenia. A cross-sectional approach to the diagnosis could account, at least in part, for the fact that American psychiatrists tend to overdiagnose schizophrenia. Thus, a diagnostic system should include some measure of chronicity as a diagnostic criterion. However, both these approaches, the initial one based entirely on symptomatology, one of the advocates of which is Kurt Schneider, and the other approach based on chronicity, are both narrow approaches. The second one is based more on Kraepelin's original view that schizophrenia has a deteriorating or, at least, a chronic course. A different approach would be a more flexible system based on various symptoms and signs as diagnostic criteria. This approach is seen in the newer systems, such as the Research Diagnostic Criteria. It is true that none of these sets of criteria have demonstrated clearly superior validity over others. Because of the major differences in criteria used, it is important to specify which diagnostic criteria are being used when diagnosing a patient, communicating to others, or keeping records. John Strauss, in a recent article on the treatment of out-patient schizophrenics, has outlined a multiaxial approach to diagnosis that makes sense. This approach incorporates criteria based on both symptomatology and chronicity. To become familiar with the individual dimensions of the multiaxial approach, there are several good review articles.*

We divide our approach to treatment into the treatment of the acute phase of illness and the treatment of the chronic illness in schizophrenia. During the acute phase, we first consider indica-

---

*For one dimension, Mathis, S. W., and Kidd, K. K.: Estimating the Genetic Contribution to Schizophrenia. Am. J. Psychiatry, *133*:185–191, 1976, gives a good summary of the genetic point of view. Obviously, there are a number of summaries available concerning the biochemical etiology. See Baldessarini, R.: Schizophrenia. N. Engl. J. Med., *297*:988–995, 1977. Social causes are summarized by Kahn, M. L.: The Interaction of Social Class and Other Factors in the Etiology of Schizophrenia. Am. J. Psychiatry, *133*, 177–180, 1976.

tions for hospitalization. In addition to the obvious criteria, whether or not the patient is dangerous to himself or others or whether he can take care of himself, we must point out the advantages of community psychiatric hospitals and of a time-out from stressful circumstances, both warranting short stays and obviating for many the incarceration in the chronic disease hospitals of the past. We have observed that in most patients out-patient therapy does not constitute adequate treatment for the acute phase of schizophrenia. With few exceptions, most of these patients should be hospitalized. Often they present as an acute emergency, and at that time the physician has to make a decision about the indications for antipsychotic medication. We are acutely aware of the recent popularity of rapid tranquilization in the treatment of acute schizophrenia and have observed that this treatment has not been shown to reduce the ultimate length of stay, nor does it remove schizophrenic symptoms. In fact, it masks the spontaneous recovery of the majority of schizophreniform illnesses and makes the diagnosis and appropriate medication of a schizoaffective disorder with lithium carbonate much more unlikely to happen. A week or 10 days in the hospital without medication often gives us the opportunity to identify those patients who are restored better without medication. The majority of patients who present in the emergency room in an acutely psychotic state require either no medication or only medication during their acute decompensation. In patients in whom we elect to proceed with antipsychotic medication there is a lag period before the remission of psychotic symptoms, in other words, at least 3 or 4 weeks, just as there is in the treatment of depression and affective illness. The best controlled study of this type was done by Davis, Erickson, and Haraszti at the Illinois State Psychiatric Institute, where they compared high-dose and standard-dose haloperidol in the treatment of acute schizophrenia. Their findings were that while the acute symptomatology can be controlled with rapid tranquilization, the psychotic process does not remit any more quickly than with the standard approach. Thus, there does not seem to be any clear advantage in placing a patient on chronic high-dose therapy. The best treatment would seem to be to bring the acute schizophrenia under control as rapidly as possible but then to use the lowest possible dosage of medications for subsequent treatment and also for maintenance treatment. The decision for maintenance treatment, rather than phasing out medication after the initial improvement, requires continued out-patient monitoring and dose adjustment rather than perfunctorily refilling prescriptions. In view of the danger of tardive dyskinesia, this would

appear to be the best course of action that can be recommended. During the treatment of the acute phase of schizophrenia, we would like to discourage the use of intramuscular chlorpromazine for a number of reasons. Chlorpromazine is a potent alpha-blocking agent and has been shown to have severe hypotensive effects following even a very small dosage, such as 25 mg. intramuscularly. In a controlled study of rapid tranquilization between chlorpromazine and haloperidol by Mann and Chen, they found that in 2 of 15 of their patients there was an almost fatal hypotensive reaction following chlorpromazine. This has been our experience as well. We have had at least two patients who almost died following small doses of intramuscular chlorpromazine. On the other hand, intramuscular haloperidol has been shown, in our experience, to be extremely safe. During the study at Illinois State Psychiatric Institute, intramuscular haloperidol was given to 38 patients and in no instance was hypotension found greater than 10 to 20 mm. Hg in the systolic blood pressure. It has also been shown that the acute treatment of schizophrenia requires fairly high doses of phenothiazines for effective symptom remission. Davis has shown that the average treatment dose for acute schizophrenia is about 750 mg. of chlorpromazine or its equivalent. Dosage equivalents in schizophrenia for some of the more popular antipsychotic drugs are given in Table 1.

So far, no clear superiority of any one phenothiazine has been shown over any other. Thus, preference of one phenothiazine over another should be based on side effects, rather than because some people feel there is some ad-

TABLE 1. **Drug Dosages in Schizophrenia**

GENERIC NAME	APPROXIMATE EQUIVALENT DOSE (mg.)	TRADE NAME
Chlorpromazine	100	Thorazine
Thioridazine	100	Mellaril
Mesoridazine	50	Serentil
Chlorprothixene	100	Taractan
Triflupromazine	28	Vesprin
Carphenazine	28	Proketazine
Acetophenazine	19	Tindal
Prochlorperazine	15	Compazine
Piperactezine	14	Quide
Butaperazine	13	Repoise
Perphenazine	10	Trilafon
Molindone	10	Moban
Thiothixene	3	Navane
Trifluoperazine	5	Stelazine
Haloperidol	2	Haldol
Fluphenazine	2	Prolixin

From Davis, J. M.: Arch. Gen. Psychiatry, *33*, 858, 1976.

vantage of using one drug over the other because of antipsychotic efficacy. There is little use for combined phenothiazine therapy unless one wants to mix various side effects. One possible use of a combination of two phenothiazines would be the use of a piperazine-type phenothiazine during the day to reduce the amount of sedation and the use of an aliphatic phenothiazine at bedtime, because of its increased sedative effect which helps a patient's sleep. The more recently discovered agents, such as the butyrophenones, the indol derivatives and dibenzyldiazepines, such as loxapine, have not been shown clearly superior over the other agents. Both molindone and loxapine have been shown to have comparable extrapyramidal side effects to the piperazine-type phenothiazines, and they have not been shown to have greater therapeutic efficacy than the other phenothiazines. The choice of use of any of these over the phenothiazines, therefore, should be based on whether a patient has experienced side effects to a particular phenothiazine or allergic reactions. It has been shown that a patient who might be allergic to a phenothiazine will not be allergic or there will not be a cross-reaction with butyrophenone or some of these other agents. In some treatment-refractory cases, it makes sense to try some of the newer drugs, perhaps because of different absorption or metabolic pathways that could be used to advantage. More recently, work has been done on plasma levels of psychotropic drugs, and this shows a great deal of promise in the tricyclic antidepressants. However, the advantages of using phenothiazine blood levels at this point do not show any correlation between blood level and therapeutic response. In other words, no dose response curve has been worked out for the phenothiazines in the treatment of schizophrenia. The main advantage of blood levels is to show whether or not the patient is compliant with taking his medication. Second, occasionally there are problems with the absorption of a drug because of increased metabolism in the gut wall, and blood levels can show whether or not the patient is absorbing the drug. Blood levels of neuroleptics in the treatment of schizophrenia are fraught with a number of difficulties. Some of these problems have to do with the fact that, for example, chlorpromazine has 168 different metabolites, many of which may be active metabolites, thus, measuring chlorpromazine levels alone does not give us a good idea of the effective dosage in the bloodstream. There may be a number of other metabolites that are equally effective. Blood levels may be more useful in using, for example, haloperidol, because haloperidol is metabolized by cleavage and, consequently, haloperidol levels are theoretically a better guide. However, this is tech-

nically very difficult, and very few physicians have the mass spectroscope facilities available for measuring them.

A few words of warning are in order about adverse reactions that may be encountered in the use of neuroleptics in the treatment of schizophrenia. These are the effects on the autonomic nervous system, extrapyramidal side effects, and allergic reactions that are extremely rare but can be very serious when they occur. Among these are bone marrow suppression with subsequent possible agranulocytosis and a change in the liver enzymes and cholestatic jaundice, which has been well described for chlorpromazine. Again, these tend to be hypersensitivity phenomena and usually occur early in treatment. Therefore, early in treatment it would be advisable to check the liver function and the white count with a differential periodically, perhaps every other week. This can be done easily while the patient is hospitalized. It has been our experience that a transient elevation of liver enzymes is very common; however, this is transient and does not warrant the discontinuation of medication. We would discontinue phenothiazines only if the patient starts to have a rise in bilirubin along with the liver enzymes, and if the rise in the liver enzymes is marked. A transient low elevation is not justification for discontinuing phenothiazines. Other possible effects to keep in mind are the skin and eye effects, especially with the aliphatic phenothiazines. Patients should be warned about going out into the sun, should be advised about wearing sun glasses and using effective sun screens, especially agents that contain para-aminobenzoic acid. A number of endocrine effects have been shown with the use of phenothiazines because of the tuberal and fundibular pathway of dopamine. Consequently, it has been shown that by inhibiting the prolactin inhibiting factor, there is an increase of prolactin that may account for the galactorrhea that is often seen. It is interesting that tolerance does not seem to develop for this particular side effect, whereas tolerance does develop to the extrapyramidal side effects over time. Tolerance has not been shown to develop to the antipsychotic effects of neuroleptics.

There are particular concerns about side effects in the elderly. Elderly patients generally require a lower dose of phenothiazines and the aliphatics or agents with increased autonomic side effect should be avoided in the elderly or should be used with great caution. Elderly patients can have marked reductions in blood pressure following aliphatic phenothiazines, mesoridazine, or thioridazine. Also the cardiac side effects due to phenothiazines are increased markedly in the elderly.

In a number of studies evaluating the relative merits of somatic treatment versus psychotherapy it would seem that a principal reason that nonpsychological treatment, such as drugs, consistently is superior to psychosocial measures is that the special target of each therapy has not been recognized. Drugs will reduce thought disorganization, quiet an unruly and excited patient, or mobilize a withdrawn patient. It remains for psychosocial interventions to teach and to train, to reassure and to raise self-confidence, and to help with skills for living that some patients may never have learned or learned badly. These interventions take time to become effective, but when they do there is some evidence, of which we need more to be certain, that fewer drugs are needed to maintain a patient in a stage of remission. For patients who either do not need medication or need it only in the acute phase of their illness, there is a great danger that the current fascination with antipsychotic medication will lead us away from the proper business of psychiatry, which is to teach people to live as well as they can with the neural equipment and social opportunities they have.

Physical and Chemical Injuries

BURNS

method of
DABNEY R. YARBROUGH, III, M.D.
Charleston, South Carolina

The severity of a burn injury and implied prognosis are primarily products of two factors: the depth of burn and the extent of burn. The depth of burn is ordinarily categorized as being first, second, or third degree. First degree burns are very superficial, involve the epidermis and the upper layers of the skin only, and are of little clinical importance. Sunburn is an example of a first degree burn. Second degree burns are a somewhat deeper injury and destroy the epithelium and part of the corium but spare the deeper layers of the skin from which reepithelialization can occur. Third degree burns involve the entire thickness of the skin. Spontaneous epithelialization obviously will not occur in the case of third degree burns. First and second degree burns are often referred to as partial-thickness burns and third degree burns may be referred to as full-thickness burns. Clinically, second degree burns are characterized by a reddish surface, which may or may not blanch on pressure, and blister formation. Sensitivity to light touch, pain, and pin prick is often retained, although in very deep second degree burns sensation may be minimal to absent. Third degree burns are characterized by a waxy, whitish or parchment-like appearance. There are usually no blisters and the surface of the burn is insensitive.

The extent of the burn is usually expressed in terms of the percentage of the body surface area involved by the burn. A rapid, easily remembered, and fairly accurate method of estimating the surface extent of the burn in adults is the Rule of Nines. The Rule of Nines states that the head and neck comprise approximately 9 per cent of the total body surface area; each upper extremity, 9 per cent; anterior trunk, 18 per cent; posterior trunk, 18 per cent; the lower extremities, each, 18 per cent; and the genitalia and perineum, 1 per cent. This formula is much less

TABLE 1. **Percentage Body Surface Area in Children**

AGE	HEAD AND NECK (%)	BOTH LEGS (%)
Birth–1 yr.	21	28
1–4 yr.	19	30
5–9 yr.	15	34
10–15 yr.	13	36

accurate when applied to children (Table 1). The so-called hand rule is also of some value in determining the percentage of very small or scattered burns. This rule estimates that the patient's hand is equal to approximately 1 per cent of his body surface area.

The following guidelines have been utilized in the treatment of burned patients. Patients with second degree burns of less than 15 per cent of the body surface area, or third degree burns of less than 2 per cent of the body surface area are categorized as having sustained minor burns and ordinarily can be managed satisfactorily on an out-patient basis. Patients with second degree burns of less than 30 per cent of the body surface area, or third degree burns of less than 10 per cent, with the exception of burn of the hands, face and feet are categorized as having moderate burns and usually can be treated adequately in community hospitals. Deep burns of the hands, face, and feet, more extensive burns than those categorized above, electrical burns or burns complicated by respiratory tract involvement, major soft tissue injury, or fractures are classed as critical or major burns and are best referred for treatment in a specialized burn unit or a burn center.

Treatment of Minor Burns

Only minor burns in previously healthy individuals should be managed on an out-patient basis.

Control of Pain. One of the most effective initial methods of pain management is the application of towels soaked in ice water. This technique usually results in fairly rapid initial relief of pain.

The pain will be alleviated further by application of an occlusive dressing as described later. Occasionally, it may be necessary to administer a mild narcotic such as codeine or meperidine hydrochloride.

Initial Wound Management. While the cold towels are being applied, a relatively mild narcotic, such as meperidine hydrochloride, should be administered in anticipation of sedating the patient for cleansing and debriding the wound. After the patient's pain has been relieved, the wound is cleansed and debrided. The procedure should always be done utilizing the best possible aseptic technique, including the wearing of a mask and sterile gloves. The wound is cleansed with an antibacterial emulsion such as 3 per cent hexachlorophene emulsion (pHisoHex) and sterile isotonic saline solution; all devitalized epithelium and blisters are debrided. Although wound healing will usually proceed normally beneath an intact blister, most often the blister fluid becomes contaminated and purulent, resulting in delayed healing of the underlying tissue. Consequently, it is best to debride all blisters initially.

Application of a Dressing. After the initial cleansing and debridement a sterile dressing should be applied to the injured area. The primary objectives of the dressing are protection of the wound and prevention of bacterial contamination. Secondary objectives include the relief of pain and splinting of joints. The dressing should be absorptive to soak up all burn wound exudate. An ointment-impregnated gauze should be placed next to the wound. In general, the various antibiotic ointments have not proved of value when used on minor burns. Moreover, the rate of sensitization with most locally applied ointments is quite high. Simple petrolatum gauze serves adequately. A generous amount of absorptive materials should be placed over the initial gauze layer; fluffed gauze pads accomplish this purpose adequately. The outer layer of the bandage should consist of a semielastic material such as Kling or stockinette and should be fixed in place with adhesive tape. Care must be taken to prevent undue compression of the underlying part to preclude the possibility of impeding circulation. Joints should always be dressed in the position of function.

Ordinarily, systemic antibiotics are not recommended in the management of uncomplicated minor burns. Tetanus toxoid, 0.5 ml., is given to previously immunized patients. In patients not previously immunized, 250 to 500 units of human antitetanus immune globulin is administered.

Dressing Changes. The patient is instructed to return immediately if undue pain or numbness is noted in the area of the burn or if chills or fever are experienced. Otherwise, routine dressing changes are performed at 3- to 5-day intervals, depending on the status of the wound. At the time of each dressing change it is usually wise to remove the external portions of the dressing initially, leaving any adherent dressing in place. The patient is then allowed to soak the affected part in a sterile basin containing sterile saline solution until the adherent dressing can be removed easily and without pain. If any pus is noted, a culture should be obtained. The wound should then be irrigated and washed very gently with warm, sterile, soapy saline solution. A new sterile dressing is then applied as described previously. If infection does not supervene, second degree burns should heal within 12 to 15 days. Eschar separation in third degree burns will also begin during this period. Eschar should be debrided progressively from full-thickness burns until a healthy granulating bed is obtained. If split-thickness skin grafting is required for closure of full-thickness injuries, this may be done on an out-patient basis if the area to be closed is very small. If larger grafts are required, the patient should be hospitalized.

Immediate Management of Moderate and Major Burns

The immediate measures to be taken in the management of patients with moderate and major burn injuries, listed in order of priority, include the following: (1) assurance of an adequate airway; (2) establishment of an intravenous lifeline, initiation of intravenous fluid therapy, and obtaining blood sample for laboratory analysis; (3) relief of pain; (4) catheterization of the bladder; (5) tetanus prophylaxis; and (6) estimation of extent and depth of burn.

Airway. As in any patient who has sustained major trauma, initial attention should be directed toward assuring an adequate airway. Immediate respiratory problems in the burned patient are most often related to inhalation of irritating products of combustion. Symptoms include shortness of breath, chest pain, wheezing, and coughing. Physical evidence of respiratory distress may include the use of the accessory muscles of respiration, tachypnea, and cyanosis. A history of having sustained the burn injury in a closed space or of having been involved in a chemical or electrical fire should alert one to the increased likelihood of respiratory involvement. Delayed evidence of respiratory distress developing 2 to 48 hours after injury may occur and may be caused by either upper airway obstruction as a result of edema or inhalation of irritating products of combustion. A falling arterial oxygen saturation and Po_2 may be an early warning sign.

In the face of impending or actual airway obstruction, the trachea must be intubated. The nasotracheal or peroral route of tracheal intubation are preferred. Tracheostomy should be avoided as an emergency method of tracheal intubation if at all possible, especially if the burn involves the neck. If tracheostomy becomes necessary it should be performed in the operating room with an endotracheal tube in place, if feasible. The incidence of serious pulmonary infection is greatly increased when tracheostomy must be performed through burned tissue.

Management of the smoke inhalation syndrome is a difficult and perplexing problem. Initial therapy should include placing the patient in a high-oxygen, high-humidity environment such as a croup tent, or humidified oxygen may be delivered via a face mask. Frequently, tracheal intubation or tracheostomy with positive pressure respiratory assistance will be necessary to combat the progressively falling oxygenation usually prominent in the chain of events. A mucolytic agent such as acetylcysteine should be administered by way of a nebulizer. Although there is currently great controversy regarding the usefulness of high doses of steroids in the management of the smoke inhalation syndrome, our current practice is to utilize these drugs for a 48- to 72-hour period after the diagnosis of significant smoke inhalation syndrome has been established. In addition to steroids, a broad-spectrum antibiotic is administered in an attempt to minimize secondary pulmonary infection. Additional aids to the diagnosis of this syndrome include fiberoptic bronchoscopy and ventilation-perfusion lung scans. Fluid intake should be minimized consistent with adequate resuscitation to reduce the possibility of pulmonary edema. In addition, it has been our practice to administer digitalis prophylactically under these circumstances.

Finally, some degree of carbon monoxide poisoning is not infrequent in patients with inhalation injury. Carboxyhemoglobin levels should be obtained to establish the diagnosis. If the carboxyhemoglobin level is significantly elevated the patient should be treated by the administration of oxygen.

Intravenous Fluid Therapy. After establishing an adequate airway, intravenous fluid therapy should be started. Fluids should always be administered through an indwelling, large-bore, intravenous cannula. It is preferable to perform the phlebotomy in a large vein of the upper extremity, such as the cephalic vein. It is also desirable to perform the phlebotomy through unburned tissue. Whenever possible the intravenous cannula should be placed in a position allowing use in monitoring central venous pressure. After insertion of the cannula, a blood sample should be drawn for baseline studies, including hemoglobin and hematocrit, blood typing and cross-match, blood urea nitrogen (BUN), creatinine, and routine serum electrolytes. Baseline blood pH, Po_2 and Pco_2 should also be determined if possible. Immediate blood volume replacement is then begun with lactated Ringer's solution. After fairly rapid administration of 500 ml. of the solution (in the adult), resuscitation is continued according to a calculated fluid budget.

Many methods of estimating fluid requirements for burned patients are available. The Brooke formula has proved to be quite useful. It estimates the following fluid requirements for the first 24 hours after injury:

Colloid (blood, dextran or plasma): 0.5 ml. per kg. per per cent of body surface burned.

Lactated Ringer's solution: 1.5 ml. per kg. per per cent of body surface burned.

Water requirement (dextrose and water): 2000 ml. (adults). (For water requirements in children see Table 2.)

One half the estimated fluid requirement for the first 24 hour period is given in the first 8 hours and the remaining half of the calculated amount during the succeeding 16 hour period. The fluid requirement during the second 24 hours after injury is usually approximately half that required during the first 24-hour period. In applying the formula to burns of more than 50 per cent of the body surface area, requirements should be calculated as if only 50 per cent had been burned to avoid excessive fluid administration to patients with larger burns. The Brooke formula must be regarded as an approximate guide *only*. Frequent revision of the rate of fluid administration is necessary. The adequacy of resuscitation is best judged by monitoring central venous pressure, urinary output, cardiac rate, and hematocrit. In complex cases, where the response to resuscitation is less than optimal, monitoring of pulmonary capillary wedge pressure and pulmonary arterial pressure by way of a Swan-Ganz catheter may be desirable.

TABLE 2. **Daily Water Requirements in Burned Children**

AGE	AMOUNT (ml.)
0–3 mo.	700
4–6 mo.	1000
7–23 mo.	1200
2–5 yr.	1400
6–10 yr.	1600
11–13 yr.	1800
14 yr. and above	2000

Of these various parameters, urinary output and central venous pressure are probably the most generally useful indicators. One should attempt to adjust the rate of fluid administration to maintain a urinary output of from 30 to 80 ml. per hour in an adult and a central venous pressure of 6 to 12 cm. of water. In the infant a urinary output of 15 to 20 ml. per hour probably indicates satisfactory volume replacement. Obviously, rising pulse rate and hematocrit usually indicate inadequate rates or type of fluid administration.

Relief of Pain. After insertion of an intravenous cannula, a narcotic should be administered for the relief of pain. Initially, the narcotic should always be administered intravenously to assure complete absorption. Ordinarily 15 mg. of meperidine (Demerol) are administered at 10-minute intervals until relief of pain is obtained. The total initial dose should not exceed 75 mg. in the adult and should be correspondingly less in infants, children, and the elderly.

Catheterization of the Bladder. After initiation of intravenous fluid therapy, an indwelling catheter should be inserted into the bladder. Urine within the bladder should be removed and examined for evidence of hemolysis and a routine urinalysis should be obtained. The catheter should then be attached to a closed drainage system and hourly collection and recording of urine output begun.

Tetanus Prophylaxis. All patients with major burns should receive tetanus prophylaxis. If there is a reliable history of previous immunization, 0.5 ml. of tetanus toxoid should be administered. If the patient has not been immunized previously, 250 to 500 units of human tetanus immune globulin is given. An initial immunizing dose of tetanus toxoid can be administered simultaneously in another area if desired.

After initial inspection of the burn wound and determination of the depth and extent of the burn, burned extremities should be examined carefully for evidence of circulatory impairment. The edema fluid beneath a tight, unyielding eschar may exert a tourniquet-like effect, resulting in occlusion of the circulation in an extremity. Capillary filling in unburned portions of the extremity distal to burns and in the nail beds should be examined and peripheral pulses palpated when possible. If evidence of actual or impending circulatory embarrassment is noted, incisional decompression of the burn eschar will be necessary. In decompressing the burned area, an incision is made through the full-thickness burn eschar and subcutaneous tissue to the underlying fascia. Occasionally, it may be necessary to incise the underlying muscular investing fascia as well. This should be done in a manner similar to that used in bivalv-

ing a cast applied to a fractured extremity. The procedure can ordinarily be effected with no anesthesia or with very small amounts of local anesthesia. Sterile technique should be utilized. Edema beneath burn eschars of the chest may inhibit respiratory excursions and require similar incisional decompression. Inspection of circulatory impairment should be continued at 2- to 4-hour intervals during the first 48 hours after injury.

Management of Moderate and Major Burns After the Shock Phase

At approximately 48 hours after injury, burn wound edema is maximal, loss of fluid from the vascular compartment has essentially ceased, and the danger of hypovolemic shock has passed. At this point the majority of burned persons have passed through the period of paralytic ileus and can begin to tolerate oral alimentation. The emphasis in care shifts from prevention of shock to the following three principal areas: (1) maintenance of nutrition, (2) prevention of burn wound infection, and (3) obtaining closure of the burn wound.

Maintenance of Nutrition. During the period prior to obtaining complete healing of the burn wound, the burned patient exhibits an enormous increase in daily requirements of calories and proteins. Maintenance of an optimal nutritional status is of the greatest importance during this period. In general, the objective should be to achieve a daily protein intake of 2 to 3 grams per kg. of body weight and a caloric intake of 50 to 70 calories per kg. In addition, vitamin supplements are recommended in the following amounts daily: ascorbic acid, 1500 mg.; thiamine, 50 mg.; riboflavin, 50 mg.; and nicotinamide, 500 mg. Because of the markedly increased rate of evaporative water loss through the burned skin, the patient's daily fluid intake must be followed closely. Evidence of dehydration, such as an increasing serum sodium or blood urea nitrogen (BUN), should be met by increasing the daily fluid intake. Multiple whole blood transfusions are usually required because of both diminished production and a decreased life span of red blood cells. The hematocrit should be maintained at approximately 40 per cent. Supplemental between-meal feedings are usually necessary to maintain an adequate daily intake of calories and protein.

If nutritional requirements cannot be met by enteral alimentation, intravenous alimentation must be resorted to. Even though the septic complications of total parenteral nutrition in the burned patient are significant, maintenance of nutrition is critical, and the risk of sepsis must be accepted under certain circumstances. When total parenteral nutrition is used in the burned patient, meticulous attention must be paid to sterile technique in administering the prepared fluids and the care of the central venous catheter site. Additionally, the central venous catheter must be removed and cultured at the first suspicion of sepsis. After control of catheter-related sepsis, total parenteral nutrition can usually be resumed.

Management of the Burn Wound. The two primary objectives in the management of the burn wound are the prevention of infection and early closure of the wound. In my experience these objectives have best been met by the following regimen: As soon as possible after admission, after all urgent procedures have been accomplished and resuscitation from shock is well under way, the burn wound should be washed thoroughly with a sterile detergent solution such as hexachlorophene (pHisoHex) and isotonic saline solution. Sterile precautions should be maintained during the initial cleansing and debridement of the burn wound. All loosely adherent, devitalized tissue should be removed. Fluid-filled blebs and bullae should be excised. After thorough cleansing and debridement of the burn wound, silver sulfadiazine cream (Silvadene) is applied to the wound. A light dressing is usually necessary to maintain the medication on the surface of the burn wound. Dressings and cleansing of the burn wounds are repeated daily until the patient no longer requires intravenous therapy. A daily regimen of wound cleansing and debridement in the hydrotherapy tank can then be instituted. After each daily session of cleansing and debridement, silver sulfadiazine is reapplied to the burn wound. At each session the wound is actively debrided of necrotic eschar until bleeding or pain develops. In this manner the eschar is removed as rapidly as possible. If burn wound sepsis develops despite this regimen, topical antibacterial therapy should be changed and replaced by mafenide (Sulfamylon) or topical gentamicin (Garamycin) preparations or by the subeschar administration of antibiotics selected on the basis of sensitivity studies of the offending organism.

The technique of tangential excision of the burn wound has become increasingly popular over the past few years. In this technique, the surgeon successively excises thin shavings of the burn wound with a dermatome until punctate bleeding is encountered, indicating that viable tissue has been exposed and all necrotic tissue has been excised. Although many burn surgeons utilize this technique in the management of major burns, I have felt that it is of greatest value in the treatment of deep second degree burns of the dorsum of the hand. When viable tissue has been exposed by this technique, it must be protected by immediate autografting, allografting, or xenografting.

As soon as viable granulation tissue begins to develop and necrotic eschar has been removed, wound closure by split-thickness skin grafting should be initiated. Skin grafting can usually be started approximately 3 weeks after injury.

The use of the Brown dermatome for the removal of split-thickness autografts has been found the most rapid and effective technique. Autografts are then applied to suitable granulating beds. Preferentially, no dressing is applied to the grafted wound. In areas that may be subjected to pressure or motion, however, the autografts should be immobilized by the application of a bulky occlusive dressing. When dressings are used for immobilization of the graft, they should be changed at 3-day intervals and the grafted sites inspected and cleansed gently. This procedure should be continued until satisfactory adherence of the graft to the underlying bed of tissue has been obtained.

Skin allografts and xenografts have proved extremely valuable in the management of patients with large burns. Often the patients develop clean surgical wounds but represent a poor risk for the necessary autografting procedure. Under these circumstances the application of cadaver homograft or heterograft (most commonly porcine), can be lifesaving. The homografts or heterografts should be applied in the same manner as autografts. The grafts should be removed at 3- to 5-day intervals and replaced. If the grafts are allowed to remain in place for a longer period of time, they may become so adherent to the underlying bed that they are difficult to remove. If this occurs, the patient must go through a period of rejection of the foreign grafts, thus unnecessarily prolonging the hospital course. Additionally, homografts and heterografts may serve as a useful indicator of the suitability of the recipient site for autografting.

During the period of prolonged immobilization that occurs while complete wound healing is being obtained, all efforts should be made to provide active physical therapeutic measures to the patient. The exercises administered should include active and passive exercises of as many joints as possible to maintain a full range of motion and to prevent contractures and calcification in and about the joint. The patient should be kept ambulatory as much of the time as possible.

Management of Special Types of Burns

Although the principles remain unchanged, the treatment techniques require modification for management of certain special types of burns. Included in these special types of burns are electrical burns and chemical burns.

Electrical Burns.   Electrical burns differ from the usual thermal burn primarily in the extent of injured tissue present. Electrical burns characteristically result in necrosis of a much larger volume of tissue than do thermal burns. In addition, the passage of large amounts of electrical current through certain organs and tissues may result in injuries peculiar to this entity (e.g., ventricular fibrillation and cardiac asystole). The volume of fluid required for resuscitation of victims of electrical injury is usually somewhat greater than would be estimated from the surface extent of injured tissue. It is of utmost importance to establish and maintain an adequate urine output as early as possible in the management of patients with electrical injuries. Diuretics may be required in the early stages of resuscitation to minimize the relatively high incidence of acute renal failure encountered in electrical burns. Additionally, the urine should be kept alkaline by administering sodium bicarbonate intravenously. Urine output should be maintained at a rate of 100 to 200 ml. per hour. Brisk diuresis and alkalinization of the urine should be continued until the urine is cleared of myoglobin and hemoglobin, which are frequently noted in large amounts in the urine after the extensive muscle and red cell destruction of major electrical injuries. The presence of these substances in the urine is thought to account, at least in part, for the increased incidence of acute renal failure encountered in patients with electrical injuries.

In our experience the burn wound in patients with electrical injury is best handled by early excision after initial adequate resuscitation of the patient. Consequently, the majority of patients who have sustained electrical burns should be treated in specialized institutions. These wounds will usually require several subsequent excisions in order to remove all nonviable tissue. Split-thickness skin grafting is carried out after all nonviable tissue has been removed. One exception to this method of management is the frequently seen electrical burn of the angle of the mouth in infants, sustained as a result of chewing on electrical wires. These wounds should be managed conservatively in the interest of conserving tissue and obtaining the best possible cosmetic result.

Chemical Burns.   The most common chemical burns are those resulting from contact with acid or alkali and are frequently a result of industrial accidents. Initial treatment should be directed toward copious irrigation of the affected area with water. After dilution of the acid or alkali by irrigation has been accomplished, strong acids should be neutralized with a weak base such as sodium bicarbonate. Strong bases should be neutralized with acid such as dilute acetic acid. Neutralization should not be attempted prior to dilution because of the sudden and intense increase in the exothermic chemical reaction which results. After these initial first aid measures have been performed, the burn wound should be cared for in the same manner as a simple thermal burn.

DISTURBANCES DUE TO COLD

method of
BRUCE C. PATON, M.D.
Denver, Colorado

The ill effects of cold may be *local, general,* or *both.* Localized frostbite does not result in a generalized systemic reaction, but general body hypothermia may occur without localized tissue damage. Therefore when cold injury is being treated, the possibility of wider systemic effects should be taken into account.

Chilblains (Perniones)

Acute chilblains most commonly occur in children exposed to cold and wet, as when playing unprotected in the snow. The affected parts, which are usually fingers, toes, or knees, become red, swollen, and itchy. The fingers may become stiff and the skin may split. Chronic chilblains are often found on the legs of middle-aged women and are associated with swelling, discoloration, and dermatitis. In severe and prolonged cases there may be ulceration.

Treatment.   1. The lesion can be prevented by wearing appropriate protecting clothing and avoiding exposure to cold. Patients with severe chronic pernio should be advised to consider moving to a warm climate.

2. Acute pernio can be treated with any bland ointment such as A and D or lanolin to keep the skin soft and prevent cracking.

3. Avoid local heating, which only aggravates itching and irritation.

4. Sympathectomy should be considered in extreme injuries that will not heal. The effect is not permanent, but may permit healing.

Frostbite

There are many pathologic similarities between frostbite and burns. Ultimately, both are thermal injuries to cells which, in some cases, may result in cellular death, necrosis, and loss of tissue. The pathogenesis of frostbite is still undecided.

There are two schools of thought. In the first, it is believed that the damage is due to direct cellular injury either by the cold or, secondarily, due to osmotic changes brought about by freezing of extracellular fluid. The second school believes that vascular stasis, capillary sludging, and cellular hypoxia, lead to cellular death. Since there are experimental and clinical observations to substantiate both views, it is probable that many mechanisms are involved, which should be borne in mind when deciding upon the best therapy.

The depth of injury depends upon two primary factors: (1) temperature and (2) duration of exposure. For any given temperature, the longer the exposure, the greater the injury; for any given duration of exposure, the lower the temperature, the greater the damage.

Prevention of Frostbite. In most instances frostbite can be prevented, and investigation of most cases confirms that simple principles of prevention were forgotten or violated. Contributing factors are wind, dampness, exposure to metal, and anoxemia.

Clothing should be warm, loose, windproof, and dry. Wool, furs, down, and foam make the best insulators, and several layers of loose clothing maintain heat best. Outer layers should be windproof and waterproof if exposure to wetness is likely. Boots must not be too tight, because circulation may become impaired, and socks should be loose and made preferably of wool or cotton for good absorption of moisture. Gloves should be chosen for the same properties. If metal has to be handled, inner linings or mittens should be used. Direct handling of metal without gloves should be absolutely avoided.

Dampness is an important accelerator of heat loss. If clothing becomes wet, it should be changed, and spare clothing should be carried under any circumstances in which a change of weather or a minor accident might lead to prolonged exposure.

The cooling factor of wind has been well established and worked out. The wind does not change the temperature of exposure but greatly accelerates heat loss and accordingly shortens the safe period of exposure. Whether or not frostbite or general hypothermia develops depends upon the relative rates of heat loss from, and heat production by, the body. Everything possible should be done to achieve maximal heat production, including ensuring an adequate caloric and fluid intake, while at the same time conserving heat loss by the methods outlined above.

Experimentally mineral oil has been shown to be an excellent insulator between the skin and a coolant liquid. A layer of petrolatum or other similar ointment on lips and nose tip may reduce local heat loss and the chance of minor frostbite.

Treatment. SUPERFICIAL FROSTBITE. In superficial, localized frostbite, sometimes called "frostnip," the skin becomes pale, yellowish white, and temporarily insensitive. The most common locations are the tips of fingers and nose. If left untreated, a blister may develop within 24 hours, leading to desquamation but eventual complete healing. The part should be *warmed and thawed* immediately. If possible, the patient should be brought in out of the cold. Nosetips may be covered by a warm hand, but should not be rubbed, and especially should not be rubbed with snow. Hands and feet should be either immersed in tepid to warm water or put next to the skin (in axillae, under parkas). As the part warms, it will become painful, but the discomfort will go away in 10 to 15 minutes. Excessive local heat should be avoided, because, paradoxically, cold and frozen tissue can be easily burned at temperatures which would normally be safe.

DEEP FROSTBITE. Damage to tissues deeper than the skin should be assumed in all cases in which exposure has been more than trivial. The extent of the damage may be difficult to assess. The frostbitten part is painless and anesthetic. The color may vary from white and almost waxen to purplish. Blisters do not develop for 24 to 36 hours, and blackening and mummification take 10 days or more to appear. Gangrenous tissue eventually separates spontaneously in 60 to 90 days.

FIRST AID. The first aid measures to be adopted depend upon the circumstances. If the patient is a long distance from definitive assistance or from good transportation, the part should be allowed to remain frozen, the patient's core temperature should be kept elevated, and transportation by the most effective means available should be immediately arranged. Every precaution should be taken to avoid trauma to the frozen part. But it is preferable to walk on a frozen foot rather than on one that has been thawed.

If the patient is treated at a place such as a base camp or hunting cabin beyond which there is good, rapid, and protected transportation, it may be both possible and advisable to start definitive treatment. But this should only be considered under special circumstances, and transportation by the most rapid means possible to a hospital is the preferred method of management.

HOSPITAL TREATMENT. IMMEDIATE TREATMENT. 1. Evaluate extent of injury, associated injuries, and associated conditions such as generalized hypothermia. If total body hypothermia (see below) exists, the patient's life may be in danger and treatment of hypothermia would take preference over that for frostbite.

2. Elevate the patient's body temperature with heating blankets or the like. This induces

reflex vasodilatation and improves peripheral circulation.

3. Start *intravenous infusion*. Many patients who are exposed long enough for frostbite to develop will also be dehydrated and require fluids. If the blood volume is low, peripheral vasodilatation caused by rewarming may result in a fall in blood pressure. Lactated Ringer's solution is the intravenous fluid of choice. Low molecular weight dextran (investigational for this use), 500 ml., may be used and will have an antisludging effect on the blood. A similar effect, however, can be obtained by giving slightly larger volumes of Ringer's solution, or isotonic saline.

4. *Rapid rewarming* of the frozen extremity in water at 100 to 105°F. (38 to 41°C.) can be carried out in any convenient tub. The water should be kept in motion to afford efficient heat exchange, and warm water added as necessary to keep the temperature constant. Continue rewarming until all pallor has disappeared. This usually takes about 30 minutes. Do not continue longer, because unnecessary maceration of the skin will be produced. Pain is often severe and must be treated appropriately by drugs. After thawing is complete, remove the limb from the water and dry gently by patting, not rubbing. Put lamb's wool between the digits and leave the limb exposed, resting on a sterile sheet and protected by a cage from contact with the bedclothes.

5. Antibiotics are not necessary for a clean, simple frostbite and should be used only for specific indications if infectious complications develop.

6. Tetanus booster.

LATER TREATMENT. 1. *Local care:* The part can remain exposed without dressing, covering, or ointments. Blisters should be kept intact: do not debride them, because the surfaces exposed will only become infected. At first, the limbs should rest on sterile sheets and sterile precautions should be taken when handling the part. As the part becomes dry, swelling diminishes and subcutaneous contraction and mummification begin, and cleanliness rather than sterility is all that is needed.

2. *Physiotherapy:* Whirlpool baths in water to which pHisoHex has been added should be given for 30 minutes once or twice per day. These will aid in maintaining cleanliness and in gently debriding tissue as separation begins. The limb should be scrupulously and carefully dried after each treatment.

3. *Exercise:* Active exercises shoud be started as soon as possible and the patient encouraged to move the limb and digits. Movement of fingertips, however, should not necessarily be taken as a sign of viability. Nonviable tendons activated by a viable muscle in the forearm may move digits which ultimately become gangrenous.

4. *Surgery:* There is no condition possibly requiring *amputation* in which the surgeon should be more conservative. "Frozen in January, amputate in July" may be an exaggeration but emphasizes that delay is essential until complete and final demarcation has been achieved. If this principle is followed, a surprising amount of tissue may be saved. *Skin grafting* may be necessary to cover granulating areas after desquamation of large areas of skin. Standard plastic surgical principles are followed in selecting the best type of graft. *Sympathectomy* has been advised as either an early or a later measure. If done within 24 hours of injury, there may be some improvement in skin circulation, a decrease in swelling, and diminution of pain. There is no evidence that sympathectomy reduces the ultimate extent of tissue damage. Later, causalgic pain may be incapacitating. If the pain is relieved by a test dose of 25 mg. of tolazoline hydrochloride (Priscoline) intra-arterially on the affected side, sympathectomy is indicated. *Fasciotomy* may be essential if pressure in any of the muscular compartments threatens the vascularity and viability of the distal limb. The incisions parallel to neurovascular bundles must open the fascial compartments extensively to permit release of pressure.

5. *Drugs: Antibiotics* are not necessary unless specifically indicated. *Vasodilators* such as nicotinic acid, tolazoline hydrochloride (Priscoline), and rutin have been advised. The evidence that they are beneficial is inconclusive. *Anticoagulants:* Because capillary "sludging" has been shown pathologically to be a prominent microcirculatory feature of frostbite, heparin has been advised. But this drug is not effective against this type of cellular agglutination. There is better theoretical evidence to suggest that platelet inhibitors such as aspirin, 0.6 gram (10 grains) twice daily, or dipyridamole, 100 mg. three times daily, would be of greater benefit in improving capillary flow.

6. *Rehabilitation:* A patient with severe frostbite may have to spend many weeks or months in the hospital. During much of this time active therapy is of little importance because the wait is for biological demarcation—a slow process. This is the period when occupational therapy and consideration of and preparation for future job rehabilitation may be vital in maintaining the patient's morale.

7. *Late sequelae:* Sensitivity to cold, excessive sweating, and pain are common sequelae and may persist for many years. Bone and joint changes with small areas of subarticular erosion and osteoporosis may occur. People who have been frostbitten find that they must take extra pre-

cautions to avoid exposure to cold; even then, they often have discomfort from relatively mild exposure.

Immersion Foot (Trench Foot)

Cases of both frostbite and immersion foot are encountered in their greatest numbers during wars. But neither is an exclusively military disease. Immersion foot is produced by immersion of the feet in cold or cool water for many hours to several days. Neither the ambient temperature nor the water temperature need be below the freezing point, and the condition has been seen in shipwrecked sailors forced to sit with their feet in water for many days in tropical climates.

The initial reaction is *vasoconstriction*, leading to a cold, pale, mottled limb. Upon rewarming *hyperemia* sets in and the limb becomes red, hot, painful, swollen, and edematous. This is the stage most commonly seen by physicians. Subsequently, blisters may develop and a wet, infectious gangrene may supervene, resulting in loss of the limb. Raynaud's phenomenon, hyperhidrosis, and causalgia are common late sequelae.

Treatment. PREVENTION. If conditions leading to immersion foot are anticipated, loose waterproof footwear, with several layers of loose wool socks, should be worn. Tight constrictive leggings and nonporous materials should be avoided. Dependency of the legs should also be avoided, or intermittent elevation should be used to diminish peripheral venous stasis.

THERAPY. 1. Keep limbs dry, warm, elevated, and protected from trauma. Never apply direct heat.

2. Leave blisters intact; allow broken blisters to dry by exposure.

3. *Drugs:* Pain is often severe after the initial phase of rewarming, and *narcotics* should be used if necessary. But because prolonged use of analgesics may be necessary, the danger of iatrogenic addiction must be remembered. *Antibiotics* should be used if there is moist infection and to prevent infection in a "wet" limb with broken blisters. *Heparin* should be used if there are any signs of thrombophlebitis, which is a very common complication.

4. *Nutrition:* Victims of this condition have often been without adequate food intake for a long time, and a good caloric and vitamin intake should be provided.

5. *Physiotherapy:* Active exercises without weight-bearing should be encouraged within the limits of tolerance. As convalescence proceeds, a vigorous program of rehabilitational physiotherapy should be instituted.

6. *Surgery:* As with frostbite, *amputation* should be delayed as long as possible. The likeli-hood of overwhelming gangrene is, however, much greater in this condition than after dry frostbite. Amputation of a seriously infected, life-threatening limb may be mandatory before complete demarcation has occurred. *Sympathectomy* may be of value, especially if causalgic pain is severe.

7. *Late sequelae:* Pain, sensitivity to cold, peripheral edema, and skin problems are common late sequelae. In most instances treatment is symptomatic. Pain may respond to sympatholytic agents if ordinary analgesics do not help. Advice about protection from cold may have to be given.

Generalized Hypothermia

Increasing recognition is being given to generalized hypothermia as a cause of death in people exposed to cold. Maintenance of body temperature is a balance between heat production (by metabolism) and conservation (by both physiologic and external protective mechanisms) and heat loss. When heat loss exceeds production and conservation, the body temperature will fall. The environmental circumstances under which hypothermia occurs are numerous. The cross-country skier stranded by a blizzard without proper protection, the victims of small plane crashes, or the canoeist who falls into a cold lake far from shore are all liable to die from hypothermia rather than from specific injuries. Hypothermia may occur in healthy people exposed to cold, in people with diseases that might predispose to hypothermia, or in those in whom the disease causes hypothermia. Treatment is likely to be most successful in the first category, and least successful in the third group. Recognition of the type of problem is important in deciding on treatment and in making a prognosis.

The most common causes of death in hypothermic patients are ventricular fibrillation and respiratory arrest while cold and "rewarming shock." The exact pathophysiology of rewarming shock has not been defined, but it is almost certainly circulatory failure due to hypovolemia and acidosis, accentuated by fluid shifts and metabolic changes that occur during rewarming.

As body temperature falls, oxygen consumption is reduced by 7 per cent per 1°C. Between 33 and 35°C. (91.5 and 95°F.), violent shivering starts in an attempt to raise body temperature by increasing metabolism. This effort also increases oxygen consumption. At about 30 to 32°C. (86 to 89.2°F.), consciousness lapses and respirations become very slow. Heart rate and blood pressure fall progressively until about 27 to 29°C. (81 to 84.5°F.), when atrial arrhythmias start, to be followed by ventricular arrhythmias, fibrillation, and cardiac arrest at about 25°C. (77°F.). There have been a few recorded instances of normal cardiac function in patients with rectal temperatures below 25°C., but this temperature should be regarded as a critical point below which cardiac arrest is almost certain in unanesthetized, unsupported patients.

In a person exposed to cold, wind, rain, or snow, the onset of hypothermia may be a relatively slow process with clear-cut warning signs of severe shivering, increasing exhaustion, mental hallucinations, and unreasonable stubbornness, leading to complete exhaustion and an inability to help oneself. These signs should be recognized and signal the need for starting treatment.

Body temperature may drop very rapidly in someone immersed in very cold water. There is immediate hyperventilation. Within a few minutes the muscle temperature may fall so that the victim becomes unable to move his cold limbs and drowns. Under these circumstances factors other than whole-body hypothermia must be important, because it takes approximately 30 to 45 minutes to cool to 30°C. (86°F.) an anesthetized naked patient in ice water. Reflex muscle spasm, inhibition of respiration, and possibly acute metabolic changes may also be responsible for the rapidity of onset of immobility in very cold water. It has been found that cooling is more rapid in a clothed person who is very active than in one who remains fairly still; therefore, excessive splashing is probably disadvantageous so long as the victim remains clothed, and warms a layer of water next to his skin, on the same principle as a "wet suit."

Treatment. Treatment varies, depending upon the state of consciousness of the patient.

Conscious Patient. The principles are: (1) diminish further heat loss and (2) provide additional warmth. In the field the victim should be brought into shelter, stripped of cold wet clothing, dried and surrounded by dry clothes, blankets, or a sleeping bag. Extra warmth can be provided as hot food and drink, hot water bottles, warmed blankets. If a large bivouac sac is available, two people can lie close to the victim, not so much for the extra heat as for the extra insulation. If the victim is conscious, there is seldom immediate danger of death.

It should be recognized that body temperature can continue to fall for several degrees, even after removal of the victim from the cold environment. This is particularly true after immersion hypothermia and is due to continuing heat loss from the blood into very cold skin and subcutaneous fat.

Unconscious Patient. At a core temperature of 29 to 30°C. (84.1 to 86°F.), the patient is usually unconscious. About the same temperature, the body ceases to be able to maintain its homeostasis, and body temperature slowly falls to

that of the environment. Without warmth from external sources, rewarming is physiologically impossible. If the rectal temperature is 31°C. (85.5°F.) or higher and the patient is unconscious, look for an additional cause for unconsciousness.

At first sight, the patient may be thought dead, but this should not be assumed. In the field, standard methods for resuscitation should be started, the victim should be evacuated by the most rapid method available, and every attempt be made to rewarm him.

In the hospital, body temperature should be measured by a low recording thermistor and, as rapidly as possible, the following monitoring methods should be instituted: Electrocardiogram (ECG), central venous pressure, arterial pressure, preferably by direct intra-arterial line, blood gases, drawn as above, urinary catheter for serial monitoring of urinary output, and rectal thermometer.

Mechanical manipulations—endotracheal intubation, external cardiac massage, rough handling from stretcher to table—are very likely to induce ventricular fibrillation. If ventilation is inadequate, intubation and artificial ventilation may be essential, but it should be carried out as gently as possible with constant monitoring of cardiac action. Hyperventilation with a reduction in arterial P_{CO_2} results in an increased tendency to cardiac arrhythmias and should be avoided.

If cardiac arrest occurs, external cardiac massage must be started, but the chances of restarting a cold heart without, at the same time, using very rapid rewarming are extremely slim.

In the hospital after the patient's respiration has been controlled and appropriate monitoring lines inserted, he should be warmed in a tub of warm water, 40 to 43°C. (104 to 109.5°F.). Blood gases and acid base status should be constantly monitored and bicarbonate given to counteract acidosis.

Central venous pressure is likely to be low and should be raised to 10 mm. Hg by infusions of warmed lactated Ringer's solution. Once the venous pressure has been elevated, it is safe to dilate the peripheral circulation by rewarming.

Peritoneal dialysis with warmed dialysate has been successfully used to rewarm hypothermic patients. This method has the advantage of warming the core organs before warming the periphery.

Ventilation with warmed gases increases the rate of rewarming and has the advantage of warming blood that goes first to the heart. Oxygen may be warmed by passing it through a soda lime cannister made hot by being exposed to carbon dioxide.

After the patient has rewarmed to 35°C. (95°F.), consciousness should be returning, spontaneous respiration should have been restored, and the patient should be capable of rewarming himself by normal metabolic means.

DRUGS. 1. *Cardiac drugs:* Digitalis may be necessary for very rapid atrial fibrillation with a rapid ventricular response. But atrial fibrillation usually reverts to normal spontaneously when the temperature exceeds 30°C. (86°F.). Procainamide, 200 mg. intravenously, or lidocaine, 50 to 100 mg. intravenously, is useful for controlling ventricular arrhythmias.

2. *Steroids:* Patients in the final stages of physical exhaustion and hypothermia may be suffering from acute adrenal insufficiency. Although a low serum sodium level would confirm the diagnosis, emergency administration of 200 mg. of hydrocortisone intravenously may be lifesaving, and should be given to all patients in this category.

3. Blood sugar levels may be very low. Twenty (20) ml. of 50 per cent glucose intravenously will restore blood sugar levels to normal. The level should be maintained by 5 per cent dextrose intravenously.

4. Antibiotics are not necessary unless specifically indicated.

5. Sodium bicarbonate should be used for correction of acidosis according to the formula:

$$\frac{\text{Weight in Kg.} \times \text{Base Deficit (mEq.)}}{3} =$$
$$\text{NaHCO}_3 \text{ requirement (mEq.)}$$

LATE TREATMENT. After body temperature has returned to normal, attention can be turned to associated injuries: possible respiratory complications, neurologic defects secondary to prolonged hypotension, and the like. There are no specific complications of hypothermia per se, and recovery should be rapid after rewarming.

DISTURBANCES DUE TO HEAT

method of
JOHN R. BONAME, M.D.
Birmingham, Alabama

Patients who develop problems with heat dissipation have been categorized according to symptomatology, namely: heat cramps, heat exhaustion, and heat stroke. The first two are generally mild derangements of fluid and electrolyte distribution. The third may be identical to the phenomenon now known as malignant hyperthermia and, if so, is a genetically determined condition that may be precipitated by various stimuli, including heat, stress, exercise, and a variety of drugs (notably anesthetics).

Heat Exhaustion and Heat Cramps

The patient with heat exhaustion demonstrates generalized symptoms, with weakness, hypotension, and nausea, but a cool, moist skin. In heat cramps the low salt syndrome results in localized muscle cramping. The treatment is the same in either case: (1) rest in a cool environment, and (2) hydration with salt and water orally, if tolerated, or parenterally, if not.

Heat Stroke and/or Malignant Hyperthermia

The patient usually presents with a temperature above 105°F. (40.5°C.) with hot, often dry, skin and rapid bounding pulse. Muscle rigidity may also be present. The condition may resemble acute thyrotoxicosis with storm.

As the mortality rate even with treatment still hovers above 50 per cent, prompt, aggressive attention is mandatory.

1. Administer 100 per cent oxygen and, if the patient is semi-comatose, intubate and hyperventilate to counteract the extreme metabolic and respiratory acidosis. Pa_{O_2} may remain low despite 100 per cent oxygen.

2. Start two intravenous catheters to administer fluids and draw blood. If possible, advance one catheter to measure *changes* in central venous pressure. Administer buffered electrolyte solution (preferably previously refrigerated for such emergencies) according to central venous pressure and a urinary output of 50 ml. per hour.

3. Give procainamide (Pronestyl), 15 mg. per kg. in an intravenous drip over a 20 minute period, while monitoring the electrocardiogram (ECG). This will help control arrhythmias as well as stabilize muscle calcium levels.

4. Institute aggressive external cooling by means of ice bags and fans or hypothermia blanket in conjunction with ice bags in axillae and groin. Legs should be kept slightly elevated to avoid sudden mobilization of cold blood to the heart if the patient is subsequently moved. Bony prominences must be padded or protected from excessive cooling ("burns"). Gastric lavage with cold, balanced salt solutions may be done through a double lumen tube.

5. Administer a 50 ml. ampule of 50 per cent dextrose and 10 units of regular insulin for energy consumption and to combat the initial hyperkalemia.

6. Insert a Foley catheter, chart input and output, and observe for myoglobinuria.

7. Draw blood for complete blood count (CBC), bleeding profile, plasma HCO_3^-, electrolytes, and blood gases.

8. Monitor the ECG for detection of subclinical shivering, arrhythmias, and signs of elevated serum K^+ (peaked T waves).

9. Monitor body core temperature continuously by means of nasopharyngeal or tympanic membrane probe. Because of the tendency for continued "drift," active cooling should be discontinued at a core temperature of 101°F. (38.3°C.) but reinstituted if necessary as recrudescence may occur.

10. Administer the following: (a) Methylprednisolone sodium succinate (Solu-Medrol), 30 mg. per kg. slowly intravenously, with an additional 250 mg. intravenously every 6 hours until the patient responds to overall treatment. (b) Chlorpromazine (Thorazine), 0.7 mg. per kg. slowly intravenously, in two divided doses 20 minutes apart to prevent shivering as noted on ECG. Repeat the half dose as necessary. (This use of chlorpromazine is not listed in the manufacturer's directive.) The resultant vasodilation (and heat exchange) requires more liberal fluid replacement. (c) Digitalis as necessary in those with diminished cardiac reserve or signs of failure, watching for signs of toxicity as K^+ levels fall. (d) Sodium bicarbonate ($NAHCO_3$) should be administered as long as the arterial pH is below 7.35, on the basis of 1 mEq. per kg. of body weight divided by 5 for each mEq. of venous plasma bicarbonate below 24 mEq. or for each mEq. of base deficit reported with the blood gases. (e) Mannitol (1.5 grams per kg.) if the urinary output falters or if the urine is red. (f) Heparin, 4000 to 7500 units in an intravenous drip, to run over a 6-hour period and then to be repeated if a bleeding tendency, disseminated intravascular coagulation (D.I.C.), develops.

11. The use of dantrolene sodium (Dantrium), a hydantoin derivative, used in spastic disorders, has been found experimentally useful in stabilizing intramuscular calcium in this condition. The recommended dosage is 7 to 10 mg. per kg. intravenously. To date the manufacturer, pending Food and Drug Administration approval, has not released the drug for intravenous use.

The foregoing treatment, if promptly instituted, should help prevent irreversible progression, or kidney, brain, and other organ system complications.

SPIDER BITES AND SCORPION STINGS

method of
PHILIP C. ANDERSON, M.D.
Columbia, Missouri

Arachnids

Many spiders, including imported tarantulas, trap door spiders, jumping spiders, and especially the common wolf spider in the home and the orb weavers in the garden, can bite humans, producing in the skin deep erythemas with impressive edema in superficial lymphatic chains, tumorlike reactions or ecchymoses, and even necrotic ulcerations. Some, such as the bite of Chiracanthium, the sac spider, may be mistaken by experts for the typical bite of *Loxosceles,* the brown recluse spider. Use a general plan for the treatment of all the lesser bites of arachnids; give medication for pain, suggest rest, splint the affected limb, carefully protect the area from further trauma, and apply cool packs for pain in the first 36 hours and warm packs thereafter as desired. Bacterial infection of spider bites is rare, and although precautionary warning and proper follow-up are needed, seldom are antibiotics required. If the patient's recent series of tetanus toxoid immunizations have been omitted, the corrective boosters of tetanus toxoid are necessary. Cutaneous arachnidism may be long-lasting occasionally (12 to 20 days), and the patient may not be assured of quick recovery. The most important medical concern with a biting spider is with *Loxosceles reclusa* and of second importance but of greater reputation is the black widow spider, *Latrodectus mactans.*

The Brown Recluse Spider (Loxosceles reclusa)

The range of this nocturnal, reclusive house spider has expanded naturally north and east from the Missouri-Ohio-Mississippi River valleys and artificially all across the country, being carried with household goods in moving vans. Bites may occur anywhere in the country, perhaps where one has not been seen before, and a history of recent moving of household goods from one of the central valley states would be pertinent.

In the last year, the composition of *Loxosceles* venom has been discovered. The immunology and pathology of the bite have been studied further, and controlled analyses of the therapy of bites in rabbits and guinea pigs have been extended, so some changes in therapy are noted.

The important complication of loxoscelism is hemolysis, which may induce disseminated intravascular coagulation and progress to sudden death. For all large bites (greater than 2 cm. diameter), a test for hemolysis (urine or serum) is advised about 6 hours past the bite and, again, at 12 hours or even later if the patient does not feel progressively better. Should hemolysis develop, the situation is threatening, and hospitalization may be appropriate. For large bites, usually, and for early hemolysis, I give 100 mg. prednisone (or other equivalent steroid) per day (50 mg. twice daily) for 4 days and take precautions with fluid balance and concerning inappropriate clotting (fibrinogen, fibrin split products) with the option of administering heparin. If the kidney is injured and anuria develops, we would employ dialysis promptly to maintain homeostasis. Such awesome effects of brown spider venom are extremely rare, however.

The usual case of loxoscelism is limited to the skin and may consist only of a small, painful papule or urticaria. Such mild bites, which are actually the most common type, went entirely unrecognized until a few years ago. More severe bites usually have a small necrotic center with a ring of spreading ecchymoses and blanched skin. Current work shows that no known therapy actually will prevent ulceration or shorten by much the course of healing in skin. Because local vascular damage and vasoconstriction are major components of the injury, we suggest that cold packs or injections into the lesion should be avoided. Otherwise, the therapy of cutaneous loxoscelism is the same as for lesser arachnid bites. The course of healing may be prolonged abnormally, and for the largest bites, surgical debridement and skin grafting may be needed after about 4 to 6 weeks if healing fails.

Black Widow Bites

The very young and the very elderly, especially those with hypertensive vascular disease, may have complicated reactions to the bite of *Latrodectus mactans,* but the usual bite is benign and only discomforting. The discomfort results from a release of neurotransmitters, which cause abdominal pain, cramping, muscular stiffness, and generalized aching with headache. For most patients, the benzodiazepine drugs (diazepam [Valium]) offer adequate relief. Some patients have several days of mild illness. Calcium gluconate, 10 ml. of a 10 per cent solution, given intravenously once each day for 2 or 3 days may need to be combined with diazepam (Valium) or with methocarbamol (Robaxin) for some patients. Only the most threatened patients need black widow antivenin, which, after proper skin testing for horse serum sensitivity, can be given intravenously in 50 ml. of isotonic saline solution.

Scorpions

The sting of United States native scorpions, occurring mostly in Arizona and adjoining regions, is rarely important medically, does not require treatment with antivenin, and may be managed as a trivial spider bite. Small children are the principal victims of the North American scorpion, mostly children of central Mexico. In other nations (Trinidad, Brazil, Israel, India), much more dangerous and exotic scorpions may sting adults or children, requiring immediate treatment of the wound with cold packs or ligature and prompt treatment of systemic signs with barbiturates, atropine, and the regional antivenin with the advice of regional experts.

PORTUGUESE MAN-OF-WAR STINGS

method of
IRVING G. FROHMAN, M.D.
Rockaway Beach, New York

Physalia physalis, the Portuguese man-of-war, possesses an elaborate structure for conveying and introducing potent toxin beneath the epidermal covering of contacts. This pelagic coelenterate is found seasonally in tropical and subtropical waters and may be carried to more distant zones by ocean currents. *Physalia* is actually a colony of four specialized zooids, each contributing its own function. The pneumatophore, a blue to red float, is a gasfilled bladder, kept inflated by a gas-making gland. Gastrozooid polyps enzymatically digest prey brought to them by retractile fishing tentacles. Gonodendra have the task of reproduction.

Beneath the surface of the ocean, numerous fishing tentacles, the dactylozooids, may extend as far as 100 feet from the colony. Stinging capsules, or nematocysts, line the tentacles and contain structureless fluid neurotoxin having 75 per cent of cobra venom potency. This toxin is a nondialyzable peptide, whose chief amino acid is glutamic acid. Alcohol, acetone, ether, and other organic solvents destroy crude *Physalia* toxin. Long after the death of the parent colony the toxin may remain active, requiring care in the handling of nematocyst material capable of penetrating thick surgical gloves.

Although no deaths directly attributable to the sting have been reported in the Western

Hemisphere in persons who had been in normal health, coronary exitus is on record following *Physalia* contact. Death apparently from respiratory causes has been reported following stinging by related species common to the Pacific Ocean. Linear streaking fades within 3 weeks and may leave brownish pigmentation. Slow-healing skin ulcers may follow. Systemic manifestations subside within 3 days.

Priority in treatment is directed to such manifestations as shock, respiratory arrest, cardiac complications, and skin sensitivity (consult the appropriate articles in this volume). Epinephrine, norepinephrine, atropine, antihistamines—intramuscularly and intravenously, steroids, barbiturates, morphine, and calcium gluconate have all been suggested. Local treatment that has been reported includes lathering and shaving; rubbing with wet or dry sand or a towel; applying alcohol, ether, gasoline, ammonia water, detergents, and calamine lotion; and use of steroids or procaine hydrochloride locally. Native islanders, in the absence of other agents, apply urine. Meat tenderizers, containing the hydrolytic enzyme papain from papaya sap, provide relief by toxic denaturization.

It is desirable to have a simple, effective, uniform mode of treatment available because of the possibility that a single wave can float in myriads of *Physalia* along miles of beach front. Such a catastrophe entails the need for a protocol requiring minimal personnel, supplies, and equipment that can be self-applied by those capable of helping themselves. The application of compresses moistened with aromatic spirits of ammonia to the involved area during the period of toxin activity fulfills these specifications. Attending personnel thus may be freed to care for those requiring life-support assistance.

Irreversible inactivation of *Physalia* toxin is provided by aromatic spirits of ammonia. The average composition includes 34 parts of ammonium carbonate by weight, 90 parts of ammonia water by volume, 700 parts of alcohol, water to 1000 parts. The pH is around 9.4, an alkaline medium favoring hydrolysis of the toxin.

ACUTE MISCELLANEOUS POISONING

method of
JAY M. ARENA, M.D.
Durham, North Carolina

The basic treatment for acute poisoning, whether drug or chemical, is mainly symptomatic and supportive. Overtreatment of the poisoned patient with large doses of nonspecific and questionably effective antidotes, stimulants, sedatives, and other therapeutic agents often does far more harm and damage than the poison itself. A calm attitude, with the judicious use of drugs, parenteral fluids, and electrolytes for homeostasis, and the maintenance of an adequate airway are far more effective than heroic measures, which usually are unnecessary. As a matter of fact, it is often difficult to tell whether recovery from an acute poisoning occurred because of or in spite of the treatment used. Remember: "Treat the patient, not the poison."

Severe Poisoning

1. Establish adequate airway by inserting an oropharyngeal or endotracheal tube. Often, however, extension of the head and forward displacement of the mandible are sufficient. The situation may require mouth-to-mouth breathing or mechanical respiratory equipment. Physiologic improvement of the patient's condition is often notable when tissues receive adequate oxygen.

2. Empty the stomach with a large nasogastric tube and analyze a sample of the contents. Assess the patient's general condition and obtain pertinent information.

3. Generally, legs and head are elevated to the level of the right atrium to allow venous drainage of the lower extremities and promote circulatory pooling in the head and thorax. Cardiac failure may necessitate alterations in position.

4. Elastic bandaging of the legs prevents venous stasis. Passive leg exercises are advisable if depression is extreme. The patient is turned from side to side every 2 hours to promote pulmonary drainage and reduce atelectasis.

5. Homeostasis is maintained by parenteral fluid according to blood electrolyte concentrations and urine output. An indwelling urethral catheter is placed in the bladder to permit accurate hourly measurement of output. When the kidney is not damaged, fluid therapy is aided by hourly measurement of urine specific gravity.

6. If oliguria is associated, electrocardiographic examination and frequent measurement of serum potassium are required.

7. Vital signs are recorded every 15 minutes or more frequently if values are labile or vasopressors are administered.

8. Drugs should be given only when specifically required. Rarely, such as in cyanide poisoning, is therapy with an antidote significantly urgent. Intensive supportive therapy reduces the need for medication.

9. Central nervous system stimulants should not be used to improve respiration. These drugs impart a false sense of security, and harmful reactions such as rebound depressions or convulsions

may occur. If the myocardium is hypoxic, epinephrine may induce fatal ventricular fibrillation.

10. Intravenous vasopressors such as phenylephrine, methoxamine, or other adrenergic drugs may be required if the patient has tachycardia above 110 pulse beats per minute, prolonged capillary filling time, pallor, or diaphoresis. Moderate hypotension as low as 80 mm. Hg does not necessitate vigorous therapy with vasopressors unless urinary output is depressed. Extremely potent agents, such as levarterenol bitartrate, are used for severe shock, but vasoconstrictors may significantly depress urinary output.

Oral Poisons

Attempt to remove the unabsorbed poison when the poison has been taken by mouth. Many poisons are in themselves emetics, but if vomiting does not occur spontaneously, it should be induced. However, emesis should not be attempted in caustic, corrosive, and petroleum-distillate poisoning, or if the patient is semiconscious or comatose.

In children emesis can best be induced by having them drink a glass of water or milk (never carbonated fluids), after which they should be gagged with the finger or the posterior pharynx stroked with a blunt object. Warm saline solution or mustard water as an emetic is impractical. An overdose of salt in a child could be dangerous (hypernatremia) and even fatal.

Syrup of ipecac (not the fluid extract) can be given in doses of 10 to 15 ml. and repeated in 15 to 30 minutes if emesis does not occur. For best results, 1 or 2 glasses of water (milk should not be used, as it will delay emesis) should be given after the administration of the syrup of ipecac, because emesis may not occur on an empty stomach. Activated charcoal should never be given simultaneously with ipecac, because it will absorb the ipecac and prevent its emetic effects. Recent studies indicating that induced vomiting empties the stomach of ingested poisons more effectively than does gastric lavage have produced increased enthusiasm for its use. Nevertheless, the ipecac that fails to effect vomiting either remains in the gastrointestinal tract as an irritant or is absorbed and exerts actions concomitantly with any toxins already present, and its cardiotoxic effects must be kept in mind. Syrup of ipecac or apomorphine should not be used when antiemetic drugs have been ingested, if more than an hour or two has elapsed. Gastric lavage would be safer and more effective.

If syrup of ipecac is not available, the mechanical method, gagging with fingers or spoon, is the safest and the most logical form of treatment in the home and should be tried first.

The use of table salt as a home emetic, particularly in children, should be discouraged. Fatal salt poisoning has occurred in children and adults from this obsolete method.

Apomorphine, 0.03 mg. per lb. (0.066 mg. per kg.), given subcutaneously, usually causes prompt vomiting. Since it is a respiratory depressant, it should not be given if the patient is comatose, if the respirations are slow or labored, or if the poisoning is by a respiratory depressant. Naloxone hydrochloride (Narcan) preferably, or other narcotic antagonists (see antidote chart, p. 894), will rapidly terminate the emetic effects of apomorphine and help to diminish the subsequent depression (their use, however, is not mandatory, and is often unnecessary). The combined proper use of these drugs for emptying the stomach in acute poisoning has already been shown to be effective and safe, both experimentally and clinically. The advantages are (1) rapid emesis with removal of all gastric contents, (2) no obstruction of lavage tubes, producing delays and incomplete emptying, and (3) reflux of contents (such as enteric-coated tablets) from the upper intestinal tract into the stomach.

Gastric Lavage. Gastric lavage is indicated within 3 hours after ingestion of a poison and even several hours later if large amounts of milk or food were taken beforehand or if enteric-coated or stomach emptying delaying drugs (especially the anticholinergics) have been ingested. Gastric lavage is contraindicated after the ingestion of strong corrosive agents such as alkali (concentrated ammonia water, lye) or mineral acids (considered safe here if done within 30 to 60 minutes). Strychnine poisoning, because of the danger of producing a convulsion, and the ingestion of petroleum distillates (danger of aspiration pneumonia) are also contraindications. In semi-comatose or comatose patients gastric lavage should be attempted only after an endotracheal tube with inflatable cuff has been inserted. Consult toxicology texts for specific instructions and techniques in performing a gastric lavage, especially in children.

General Rules. 1. Identify the poison.

2. Administer a specific antidote and a local antidote for residual poison not removed by evacuation of stomach contents.

3. Give an antagonist when available.

4. Administer symptomatic treatment as indicated.

5. When the nature of the poison is unknown, give activated charcoal. One to 2 tablespoonfuls to a 240 ml. (8 oz.) glass of water is suitable for oral use or lavage. The "universal antidote" is not effective and is not recommended.

6. In massive ingestions (suicidal attempts) when therapeutic results fail to reach expecta-

TABLE 1.   Therapeutic Agents*

TO NEUTRALIZE ACIDS†

1. Magnesia magma (milk of magnesia), 100 to 300 ml. (4 to 10 ounces)
2. Sodium bicarbonate (dilute solution)
3. Calcium hydroxide solution (lime water), 200 ml. (6⅔ ounces)
4. Aluminum hydroxide gel, 60 ml. (2 ounces)
5. Precipitated calcium carbonate (chalk), 100 grams (3⅓ ounces)
6. Wall plaster—crushed in water
7. Soap solution

TO NEUTRALIZE ALKALIS†

1. Vinegar (2% acetic acid), 100 to 200 ml.
2. Lemon juice, 100 to 200 ml.
3. Orange juice, 100 to 300 ml.
4. Dilute (0.5%) hydrochloric acid, 100 to 200 ml.

DEMULCENTS

1. Olive oil, 200 ml. (6⅔ ounces)
2. White of egg, 60 to 100 ml. (2 to 4 ounces)
3. Any vegetable oil, 200 ml. (6⅔ ounces)
4. Milk
5. Starch water
6. Liquid petrolatum (mineral oil)
7. Butter

EMETICS

1. Syrup of ipecac, 10 to 15 ml. repeated in 15 to 30 minutes if necessary (do not allow to remain in stomach)
2. Apomorphine, 6 mg. for adults, 1 or 2 mg. for children 1 to 2 years old, subcutaneously (0.03 mg./lb.). Respiratory depressant effect may be counteracted by Narcan, 0.01 mg./kg.
3. Household mustard or table salt used for emetic purposes should be discouraged. Fatal salt poisoning in children and adults has been documented.

STIMULANTS

1. Caffeine and sodium benzoate, 0.5 gram (7½ grains) subcutaneously
2. Nikethamide (Coramine), 5 ml. intravenously or subcutaneously
3. Pentylenetetrazol (Metrazol), 0.1 gram (1½ grains)
4. Black coffee by rectum

SEDATIVES

1. Phenobarbital, 0.03 to 0.1 gram (½ to 1½ grains)
2. Pentobarbital sodium, 0.1 gram (1½ grains)
3. Barbital sodium, 0.3 to 0.6 gram (5 to 10 grains) orally or subcutaneously
4. Chloral hydrate, 0.5 to 1 gram (7½ to 15 grains) orally
5. Sodium bromide, 0.3 to 1 gram (5 to 15 grains) orally
6. Paraldehyde, 3 to 15 ml. by mouth (double dose by rectum)

---

*From *Davison's Compleat Pediatrician*, 9th Edition, Lea and Febiger, Publisher.

†It is unlikely that serious exothermic effects will occur from the use of well diluted, mild neutralizing agents.

tions, rule out concretions in the stomach (x-ray, gastroscopy, or surgery if necessary). Give castor oil as a solvent and to hurry the material through the intestinal tract. Follow with activated charcoal.

Antidotes. Antidotes may be given to render the poison inert or to prevent its absorption by changing its physical nature (see Table 1, Therapeutic Agents).

Inhaled Poisons

Remove the victim from the gas atmosphere and apply artificial respiration if necessary.

Injected Poisons

Apply tourniquets central to the point of injection. If feasible, remove as much of the poison as possible by surgery and suction.

Absorbed Dermal Poisons

Flush skin with large quantities of water after all clothing has been removed. Shampoo the hair and soap and rinse the skin.

Chemical Burns

Flush skin with water thoroughly and repeatedly. Consult ophthalmologist for eye care as soon as possible after thorough flushing. Do not use chemical antidotes in the eye.

Supportive Measures

Adequate amounts of fluids by mouth or parenterally are important, especially if poison is excreted by the kidney. (See articles on Parenteral Fluid Therapy, pp. 435 to 438). Use of blood transfusions, exchange blood transfusions (small children), and hemodialysis if an artificial kidney is available may be helpful. Lipid dialysis is a useful technique in the treatment of poisonings by glutethimide, pentobarbital, secobarbital, phenothiazines, camphor, and other lipid-soluble substances that cannot be effectively removed by hemodialysis using an aqueous dialysate. Peritoneal dialysis with its inexpensive disposal equipment and easy technique may also be indicated and is particularly valuable for use in children.

Shock

Therapy of shock requires careful consideration of the action of the poison ingested, the administration of vasopressor agents, steroids, the replacement of fluids, and transfusion of blood when needed.

COMMON POISONS AND THERAPY

(Modified from Arena, Jay M.: *Poisoning: Toxicology, Symptoms, Treatment*, 4th Edition, Springfield, Illinois, Charles C Thomas, Publisher; and *Davison's Compleat Pediatrician*, 9th Edition, Lea and Febiger, Publisher.)

1. Acetaldehyde

See Methaldehyde.

2. Acetaminophen

This compound with a half-life of 1 to 2 hours

does not produce the gastrointestinal hemorrhagic or acid-base disturbance of acetylsalicylic acid, but it has a more subtle form of hepatic toxicity which can be serious. Treatment is symptomatic and supportive.

Oral methionine (Pedameth), 2.5 grams every 4 hours up to 10 grams, has recently been found effective in reducing the frequency and severity of acetaminophen-induced liver damage. (This use of methionine is not listed in the manufacturer's official directive.) Although this compound has few side effects and is of low toxicity, it does have the potential to aggravate a pre-existing hepatic disease, and therefore should only be given early (before 12 hours) after ingestion, before the likely acetaminophen hepatic effects take place.

N-acetylcysteine (Mucomyst), based on preliminary evaluation, appears to act as a glutathione substitute and to directly combine with the toxic acetaminophen metabolite. It is presently being recommended as the oral drug of choice (loading dose of 140 mg. per kg., followed by 70 mg. per kg. every 4 hours, for a total of 18 doses), if given within 12 hours after ingestion. (This use of N-acetylcysteine is not listed in the manufacturer's official directive.)

3. Acetanilid

Gastric lavage or emesis. Saline cathartic. Methylene blue for methemoglobinemia. Discontinue drugs in chronic poisoning or idiosyncrasies.

4. Acetic Acid (Glacial)

Magnesium oxide. Demulcents. For inhalation, treat pulmonary edema. Shock therapy.

5. Acetone

Gastric lavage or emesis. Analeptics and respiratory stimulants if necessary. Artificial respiration and oxygen.

6. Acetylsalicylic Acid (Aspirin)

See Salicylates.

7. Alkalis

Give milk and force water, followed by diluted vinegar or fruit juices by mouth. Do not use strong acids. Demulcents. Corticosteroids to prevent stricture. Esophageal dilation after fourth day. Broad-spectrum antibiotics.

8. Aminophylline

See Xanthines.

9. Ammonia (Ammonium Hydroxide)

See Alkalis. Force water.

Do not diluate with strong acids, because heat may be generated.

10. Amphetamine

Gastric lavage or emesis. Activated charcoal. Sedation or short-acting barbiturates with caution. Chlorpromazine (Thorazine), 1 to 2 mg. per kg. intramuscularly and repeat if necessary. Haloperidol (Haldol), 0.5 to 2.0 mg. three times daily, has been used effectively recently.

11. Amyl Acetate (Banana Oil, Pear Oil)

See Acetone.

12. Aniline and Derivatives (Dimethylaniline, Nitroaniline, Toluidine)

Gastric lavage or emesis. Artificial respiration and oxygen. For skin contact, thorough cleansing. Methylene blue for methemoglobinemia.

13. Antihistaminics

Gastric lavage or emesis. Activated charcoal. Saline cathartic. Do not use stimulants. Levarterenol for hypotension. Short-acting barbiturates with caution.

14. Antimony

Gastric lavage with 1 per cent sodium bicarbonate solution. Demulcents. BAL. Maintain fluid and electrolyte balance.

15. Antipyrine (Phenazone)

See Acetanilid.

16. ANTU (Alphanaphthylthiourea)

Gastric lavage or emesis. Saline cathartic. Oxygen. Avoid oils (more readily soluble).

17. Arsenic Trioxide (White Arsenic)

Gastric lavage or emesis. Thirty ml. tincture of ferric chloride and 30 grams of sodium carbonate in 120 ml. of water as antidote in lavage (remove precipitant). BAL. Shock therapy.

18. Arsine Gas

Move from environment. Exchange transfusion. BAL (ineffective). Industrial prevention with education, ventilation, etc.

19. Aspidium (Male Fern) Oleoresin

Gastric lavage or emesis. Activated charcoal. Saline cathartic. Demulcents. Short-acting barbiturates. Artificial respiration and oxygen. Avoid fats and oils.

20. Atropine

Gastric lavage with 4 per cent tannic acid solution or emesis. Pilocarpine or physostigmine (preferable) for parasympathomimetic effects. Miotic for eyes. Oxygen. Small doses of barbiturates, chloral hydrate, or paraldehyde for delirium or convulsions. Cold packs or alcohol sponging for hyperpyrexia. Indwelling catheter.

21. *Barbiturates* (Table 2)

There is no specific antidote for the barbiturates. In acute poisoning, current practices in most centers with much experience consider the immediate establishment of adequate pulmonary ventilation as well as control of shock of prime importance, whereas analeptics are considered subsidiary, if not actually contraindicated. The evidence indicates that the most favorable results are obtained by careful attention to respiratory and circulatory functions.

Forced diuresis by giving large amounts of fluids intravenously and also giving diuretics (acetazolamide [Diamox] or mercurials) reduces the need for vasopressor drugs, prevents renal complications and hyperthermia, and lessens crust formation in the respiratory tract. Contraindications are cardiac and renal disease. Pulmonary edema does not seem to be a serious hazard. Hemodialysis should be resorted to when indicated.

In addition to supportive measures, treatment for intoxication with this group of drugs should include forced diuresis with alkalinization of the urine. Dialysis need be considered only in the presence of renal function compromise. Alkalinization of the urine should be considered if intermediate or long-acting barbiturates have been ingested. The nonionized form of these drugs is highly lipid soluble and easily crosses the tubular membranes in the kidney; the ionized form is not lipid soluble and does not cross the tubular membrane. Since alkalinization of the urine increases the ionized form of the intermediate and long-acting barbiturates, tubular reabsorption is decreased, resulting in more rapid clearance of the drug. Administration of intravenous sodium bicarbonate raises the urine pH to about 8.0, a point at which the ionized form of the intermediate and long-acting barbiturates is significantly increased.

The nonbarbiturate hypnotics include glutethimide and methyprylon. The history is of paramount importance in the diagnosis of overdoses with these agents. Physical signs are not specific and may be confused with signs of overdoses of other types of CNS depressants. If lethargy, mydriasis, hypotension, flaccid paralysis, and respiratory depression are present, intoxication with these drugs should be considered. Determination of serum and urine levels may also be helpful in confirming the diagnosis. Glutethimide also produces alternating periods of coma and relative alertness; this effect is due to the periodic increases in blood levels of glutethimide resulting from its excretion via the biliary tract with reabsorption into the circulation from the gastrointestinal tract. Lethal plasma levels of glutethimide and methyprylon are not known. The approximate fatal dose of glutethimide is 10 to 12 grams and that of methyprylon is greater than 6 grams. Supportive measures, forced diuresis, and dialysis are the most effective measures for treating overdoses of these drugs. Large doses of activated charcoal have also been shown to be beneficial.

Immediate gastric lavage with a solution of saline and activated charcoal. Continue lavage

TABLE 2. **Treatment of Barbiturate Intoxication**

CONDITION	TREATMENT	GUIDES
Respiratory insufficiency	Airway, suction; endotracheal intubation, cuffed tube, lavage; humidified oxygen; mechanical ventilation, pressure- or volume-controlled ventilator	Arterial Po_2, O_2 saturation, Pco_2, pH, minute ventilation; x-ray film of chest; airway pressure
Hypovolemia	Albumin, 5% solution, 1 liter, then dextrose, 10% in sodium chloride 0.9 per cent solution; potassium chloride supplement, 40–120 mEq.	Central venous pressure, arterial pressure, urine output, and osmolality
Low urinary output	Fluid infusion: furosemide, 40 mg. I.V., or ethacrynic acid, 25 mg. I.V.	Urinary output and osmolality
Heart failure	Digoxin, 0.5 mg. I.V., followed by 1–4 doses of 0.25 mg. digoxin at 1–2 hour intervals	Central venous pressure, ECG
Pneumonia	Ampicillin sodium, 1 gram every 4 hours I.V.; methicillin sodium, 1 gram every 6 hours I.V.; chloramphenicol sodium succinate, 500 mg. every 6 hours I.V.; gentamicin sulfate, 0.75 mg./kg. every 6 hours I.M.	Sputum and blood culture, with antibiotic sensitivity; chloramphenicol after aspiration of gastric contents; gentamicin for gram-negative bacteria resistant to other antibiotics
Dialysis	Peritoneal; lipid; hemodialysis (preferred)	Barbiturate levels of 3.5 mg./100 ml. for short-acting drugs and 8–10 mg./100 ml. for long-acting agents; impaired hepatic and renal function

with isotonic saline until the return is clear. Use castor oil for instillation and withdrawal to increase solubility of sedatives and dissolve concretions. Ensure clear airway. Respiratory stimulants such as picrotoxin or pentylenetetrazol (Metrazol), administered in subconvulsive doses, are not often used in present-day therapy. Artificial respiration. Administration of 100 per cent oxygen. For circulatory depression and shock caused by depression of vasomotor center, as well as direct action on smooth muscle in blood vessel wall: pressor amines such as levarterenol (which acts directly on vascular smooth muscle). Intravenous hydrocortisone. Blood transfusions. Trendelenburg position. For water loss from skin and lungs, decrease in urine, electrolytes variable: adequate hydration with 5 to 10 per cent glucose in water to facilitate renal elimination of barbiturates. Use of electrolytes based on analysis of plasma. After the vital signs have been stabilized and adequate renal function has been ascertained, urea or Diamox-induced (forced) osmotic diuresis with alkalization of urine has proved to be effective and successful therapy in reducing mortality, severity of intoxication, and duration of treatment and hospital stay, and is now the treatment of choice in most centers. For hypostatic pneumonia resulting from hypotension and hypoventilation: prophylactic antibiotics. For depression of kidney function resulting from hypotension and central antidiuretic action of barbiturates: exchange transfusion (children). Intermittent peritoneal dialysis. Artificial kidney (lipid dialysis). For cerebral edema: mannitol or urea. (See also Narcotic Poisoning, pp. 855 to 859.)

Text continued on page 897

TABLE 3.   **Treatment of Convulsions Due to Poisoning***

DRUG	METHOD OF ADMINISTRATION AND DOSAGE	ADVANTAGES	DISADVANTAGES
Ether	Open drop	Dosage easily determined. Good minute-to-minute control. No sterile precautions	Difficult to give in presence of convulsion. Requires constant supervision by physician
Thiopental sodium (Pentothal sodium)	Give 2.5% sterile solution I.V. until convulsions are controlled. Maximum dose: 0.5 ml./kg.	Good minute-to-minute control. Can be given easily during convulsion	Doses larger than recommended may cause persistent respiratory depression. Requires sterile equipment and administration
Pentobarbital sodium (Nembutal sodium)	Give 5 mg./kg. gastric tube, rectally, or I.V. as sterile 2.5% solution at a rate not to exceed 1 ml./minute until convulsions are controlled	Good control of initial dose	No control of effects after drug has been given. Requires sterile precautions. May produce severe respiratory depression
Phenobarbital sodium	Give 1-2 mg./kg. I.M. or gastric tube and repeat as necessary at a 30 minute interval up to a maximum of 5 mg./kg.	Effects last 12–14 hours	Causes severe persistent respiratory depression in overdoses
Succinylcholine chloride	Give 10-50 mg. I.V. slowly and give artificial respiration during period of apnea. Repeat as necessary	Will control convulsions of any type. Effect lasts only 1-5 minutes. Circulation not ordinarily affected	Artificial respiration must be maintained during use. No antidote is available. Apnea may persist for several hours in some cases
Trimethadione (Tridione)	Give 1 gram I.V. slowly. Maximum dose: 5 grams	Little depression of respiration	Not effective in all types of convulsions
Tribromoethanol (Avertin)	Only by rectal instillation. 50-60 mg./kg. causes drowsiness, amnesia. 70-80 mg./kg. produces light unconsciousness and analgesia	Ease of administration and pleasant induction without mental distress and respiratory irritation	A nonvolatile anesthetic given by a route which prevents adequate control once it is administered. Contraindicated when renal or hepatic injury exists
Amobarbital sodium (Amytal)	Give 2% sterile solution. Dose range 0.4-0.8 gram	Immediate action and lasts 3-6 hours	Inhibits the cardiac action of the vagus. May produce severe respiratory depression
Diphenylhydantoin sodium (Dilantin)	Give slowly I.V. 150-250 mg. from Steri-Vial and repeat in 30 minutes with 100-150 mg. if necessary	Lack of marked hypnotic and narcotic activity	Solution is highly alkaline and perivenous infiltration may cause sloughing. Not always effective, and other anticonvulsants frequently must be used. Cardiac arrest has been reported after I.V. therapy
Paraldehyde	Give 5-15 ml. gastric tube, rectally or I.M.	Little depression of respiration. Effects last 12 hours	Harmful in presence of hepatic disease. Old and loosely stoppered solutions can break down to acetic acid and produce serious intoxication
Diazepam (Valium)	Give 2-5 mg. I.M. or I.V. Repeat in 2 hours if necessary	More effective for relieving muscle spasm associated with seizures	Hypotension and respiratory depression or muscular weakness may occur if used with barbiturates

*From *Davison's Compleat Pediatrician*, 9th edition, Lea and Febiger, Publisher.

TABLE 4. **Antidote Chart**

ANTIDOTE	DOSE	POISON	REACTION (ANTIDOTE) AND COMMENTS

Acids, weak
  Acetic acid, 1%
  Vinegar, 5% acetic acid (diluted 1:4 with water)
  Hydrochloric acid, 0.5%
	100-200 ml.	Alkali, caustic	

Activated charcoal
  Darco G (Atlas Chem.)
  Nuchar C (W. Va. Pulp & Paper; Merck)
  Norit A (Amer. Norit Co.)
	1-2 tbsp. to glass of water or a mixture of soupy consistency	Effective for virtually all poisons, organic and inorganic compounds of large and small molecules*	Broad spectrum of activity
			  No reaction except staining

Alcohol, ethyl	I.V. as 5% sol. in bicarbonate or saline sol. P.O. as 3-4 oz. of whiskey (45%) every 4 hours for 1-3 days	Methyl alcohol Ethylene glycol	Metabolizes methyl alcohol and prevents formation of toxic formic acid; glycols into oxalates

Alkali, weak
  Magnesium oxide (preferred)
  Sodium bicarbonate
	2.5% sol. (25 grams/liter)
	5% sol. (50 grams/liter)
		Acid, corrosive	Gastric distention from liberated carbon dioxide

Ammonium acetate	5 ml. in 500 ml. water	Formaldehyde (formalin)	Forms relatively harmless methenamine
Ammonium hydroxide	0.2% sol. Both are for gastric lavage		
Atropine sulfate	1-2 mg. I.M. and repeat in 30 minutes	Organic phosphate esters: Guthion, malathion, parathion, mushroom, TEPP, trithion, etc., other cholinesterase inhibitors	Atropinization

Antivenins
  Specific
    Antivenin (*Crotalidae*) Polyvalent (Wyeth)
	See circular for dosage instruction	N. and S. Amer. snakebite venoms	

Antivenin (*Latrodectus mactans*, and *curacaviensis* (Merck, Sharp, & Dohme)		Black widow spider venom	
Antivenin (*Micrurus*) (Wyeth Laboratories and C. Amaral and Cia L.T.D.A. Cloria 34, PO Box 2123, São Paulo, Brazil)		Coral snake venom	
Nonspecific		Black widow spider venom	
Adult (may be used without antivenin, *for adult only*)			
Methocarbamol (Robaxin)	On diagnosis, 1 amp. (1 gram, 10 ml.) I.V. in 15 ml. isotonic saline sol. over 5 minute period or in I.V. drip. Follow in 12 hours with 2 tab. (1500 mg.) 3 times a day for 2 days		Muscle relaxant
Orphenadrine citrate (Norflex)	On diagnosis, 1 amp. (2 ml., 60 mg.) I.V. in 5 ml. isotonic saline sol. followed in 12 hours by 1 tab. (100 mg.) 2 times a day for 2 days		Muscle relaxant
Child Antivenin	Antivenin I.V. followed in 1 hour by methocarbamol 1 tab. (500 mg.) and 1 every 12 hours for 2 days		In children the antivenin should be used; this may be supplemented with the muscle relaxant when necessary
Bromobenzene	Adult: 1 gram Child: 0.25 gram (in lavage sol.)	Selenium	
Calcium EDTA or Versene (ethylenediamine tetra-acetate) [DPTA (diethylenetriamine pentaacetic acid), more promising analogue]	25-50 mg./kg. 2% sol. 2 times a day for 5 days 50 mg./kg., 20% sol. (0.5% procaine) I.M. daily for 5-7 days Repeat these courses after 2 day rest period	Cadmium Cobalt Copper Digitalis Iron Lead (combined therapy with BAL for encephalitis) Nickel, and other metals	Nephrotoxic Increases urinary potassium excretion Use sodium salt (Na EDTA) for digitalis in place of Ca EDTA which chelates Ca ion producing hypocalcemia and reduces synergistic action of the Ca and digitalis, converting dangerous arrhythmias to sinus arrhythmias (other specific therapy preferred) Oral EDTA should not be used until all lead has been removed or absorbed from the GI tract

*Exceptions are cyanide, alcohols, boric acid, corrosives and ferrous sulfate.

ANTIDOTE	DOSE	POISON	REACTION (ANTIDOTE) AND COMMENTS
Calcium lactate	10% sol. (in lavage sol.)	Chlorinated hydrocarbons Fluoride Oxalates	
Calcium gluconate	10% sol. 5-10 ml. I.M. or I.V., may be repeated in 8-12 hours	Black widow spider and insect bites	Muscle relaxant Bradycardia Flushing Local necrosis from perivenous infiltration (methocarbamol, etc., also effective)
Chlorpromazine (Thorazine)	1-2 mg./kg. I.M.	Amphetamine*	Drowsiness Hypotension Neuromuscular (parkinsonian)
Copper sulfate	0.25–3.0 grams in glass of water	Phosphorus	Forms insoluble copper phosphide

Cyanide poison kit (Eli Lilly stock #M76)
  Amyl nitrite pearls
  Sodium nitrite
	0.2 ml. (inhalation); follow with 3.0% sol. (10 ml.) in 2-4 minutes
	and
		Cyanide	Hypotension

Sodium thiosulfate	25% sol. (50 ml.) in 10 min. through same needle and vein (repeat with ½ doses if necessary)	Iodine	Sodium thiosulfate used alone for iodine; forms harmless sodium iodide
Deferoxamine B (Desferal, Ciba) Desferal isolated from streptomyces pilosus	1-2 grams I.M. or I.V. (adults, repeat if necessary every 4-12 hours; also 5-10 grams via nasogastric tube following gastric lavage†	Iron Hemochromatosis	Diarrhea Hypotension

Dimercaprol (BAL)	*Severe intoxication*
	  Day 1: 3.0 mg./kg. every 4 hours (6 injections)
	  Day 2: Same
	  Day 3: 3.0 mg./kg. every 6 hours (4 injections)
	  Days 4-13 (or until recovery): 3.0 mg./kg. every 12 hours (2 injections)
	Mild intoxication
	  Day 1: 2.5 mg./kg. every 4 hours (6 injections)
	  Day 2: Same
	  Day 3: 2.5 mg./kg. every 12 hours
	  Days 4–13 (or until recovery): 2.5 mg./kg. daily (1 injection)
		Antimony
		Arsenic
		Bismuth
		Gold
		Mercury (acrodynia)
		Nickel
		Lead (combined therapy with EDTA for encephalitis)
		Contraindicated for iron
			Flushing
			Myalgia
			Nausea and vomiting
			Nephrotoxic
			Hypotension
			Pulmonary edema
			Salivation and lacrimation
			Temperature elevation (especially in children)

Diphenhydramine hydrochloride (Benadryl)	10-50 mg. I.V. or I.M.	Phenothiazine tranquilizers (for extrapyramidal neuromuscular manifestations)	Atropine-like effect Drowsiness
Dithizon	10 mg./kg. twice a day P.O. with 100 ml. 10% glucose sol. for 5 days	Thallium	Diabetogenic Not available for therapeutic use. May be obtained through a chemical company

Household antidotes
  Milk
  Raw eggs
  Flour
  Starches
		Arsenic
		Mercury and other heavy metals
		Same as above
		
		Iodine
			These are useful and readily available antidotes that can be used in an emergency. All have demulcent properties

Hydrogen peroxide	3% sol. (10 ml. in 100 ml. water as lavage sol.)	Potassium permanganate Oxidizing agent for many other compounds	Irritation of mucous membranes Distention of abdomen from release of gas

Iodine, tincture	15 drops in 120 ml. water	Precipitant for:
		  Lead
		  Mercury
		  Quinine
		  Silver
		  Strychnine
			Precipitants must be thoroughly removed by gastric lavage

Magnesium sulfate
Sodium sulfate
	2.5% sol. for lavage
	10% sol. I.M. and repeat in 30 minutes
	Also as catharsis for rapid elimination of toxic agent from GI tract
		Precipitant for:
		  Barium
		  Lead
		Hypervitaminosis D
		Hypercalcemia (glucocorticoid therapy preferable)	

*Recent reports have indicated that haloperidol (Haldol) is more effective in smaller doses than chlorpromazine for amphetamine intoxication.
†Some reports suggest that large oral doses of deferoxamine can be absorbed and result in systemic toxicity, and its oral use is being questioned.

Table continued on the following page

TABLE 4.   **Antidote Chart** (*Continued*)

ANTIDOTE	DOSE	POISON	REACTION (ANTIDOTE) AND COMMENTS
Methylene blue	I.V.: 1% sol. given slowly (2 mg./kg.) and repeat in 1 hour if necessary P.O.: 3-5 mg./kg. (action much slower)	Methemoglobinemia produced by over 100 drugs and chemicals: Acetanilid Aniline derivatives Chlorates Dinitrophenol Nitrites Pyridium, etc.	Perivenous infiltration can produce severe necrosis
Monoacetin (glyceryl monoacetate)	0.5 ml./kg. I.M. or in saline sol. I.V. Repeat as necessary	Sodium fluoroacetate "1080"	Not available commercially. If parenteral therapy not feasible, can give 100 ml. of monoacetin in water
Nalorphine (Nalline) or Levallorphan (Lorfan) or Naloxone (Narcan)	Adult: 5-10 mg. I.M. or I.V. and repeat in ½ hour Child: 0.1-0.2 mg./kg. I.M. or I.V. and repeat in ½ hour. Adult: 0.5-1.0 mg. I.M. or I.V. Child: 0.02 mg. per kg. I.M. or I.V. 0. 01 mg. per kg. I.V., I.M., or S.C.	Codeine Demerol Dionin Heroin Methadone Morphine Pantopon (For respiratory and cardiovascular depression)	Withdrawal symptoms Depression effects in other than narcotic compounds Produces no respiratory depression, psychotomimetic effects, circulatory changes, or miosis
Penicillamine and its derivatives (Cuprimine)	1-5 grams P.O.	Mercury and other heavy metals	Fever Stupor Nausea and vomiting Myalgia Leukopenia, thrombocytopenia Nephrosis, reversible Optic axial neuritis, reversible Ineffective when severe vomiting is prominent
Petrolatum, liquid (mineral oil)			Solvent Demulcent
Physostigmine salicylate (Antilirium)	1–2 mg. I.M. or I.V.*	Atropine and related alkaloids; anticholinergic compounds; particularly effective for the cardiac arrhythmias and CNS toxic effects of the tricyclic antidepressant drugs Atropine and related alkaloids	Excess can produce diarrhea, bradycardia, hypersalivation, rhinorrhea, and cholinergic crisis; Rx with propantheline bromide (Pro-Banthine) preferable to atropine
Pilocarpine (not being marketed in tablet form in U. S.)	P.O.: 2-4 mg. I.M.: 0.25-0.5 mg.		Antagonizes the parasympathetic (mydriasis and dry mouth), not central, effects of atropine
Potassium permanganate	1:5,000 and 1:10,000 sol. for gastric lavage	Nicotine Physostigmine Quinine Strychnine Oxidizing agent for many alkaloids and organic poisons	Strong irritant and should not be used in strong dilutions or with any residual particles
Pralidoxime iodine (2-PAM iodine) Pralidoxime chloride (2-PAM chloride)	Adult: 1-2 grams Child: 25-50 mg./kg. I.M. or I.V. as 5% sol.	Organic phosphate esters Cholinesterase inhibition by any agent: chemical, drug, etc.	Diplopia Dizziness Headache
Protamine sulfate	1% sol. I.V. slowly (mg./mg.) to that of heparin	Heparin	Sensitivity effects
Sodium chloride	1 tsp. salt to 1 pt. water (approximately normal saline sol.) 6-12 grams P.O. in divided doses or in isotonic saline I.V.	Silver nitrate Bromides	Forms noncorrosive silver chloride Hypernatremia
Sodium formaldehyde sulfoxalate	5% in lavage sol. (preferably combined with 5% sodium bicarbonate)	Mercury salts	BAL therapy should follow gastric lavage
Sodium thiosulfate	P.O.: 2-3 grams or I.M.: 10 or 25% sol. Repeat in 3-4 hours	Iodine Cyanide	
Starch	80 grams/1000 ml. water	Iodine	

*Not approved by FDA for intravenous use in children.

TABLE 4. Antidote Chart (Continued)

ANTIDOTE	DOSE	POISON	REACTION (ANTIDOTE) AND COMMENTS
Tannic acid	4% in lavage sol. Never use in greater concentrations	Precipitates alkaloids, certain glucosides, and many metals	Hepatotoxic Tannates formed should not be allowed to remain in the stomach Because of its hepatotoxicity, should be used cautiously and in no greater than 4% sol.
Universal antidote (activated charcoal alone preferable)	Two parts pulverized charcoal (burned toast); One part magnesium oxide (milk of magnesia); One part tannic acid (strong tea sol.)	Obsolete for any use	Over-rated and ineffective. Can actually be harmful in that it may give false sense of security to those who use it
Vitamin K_1	25-150 mg. I.V. Rate not to exceed 10 mg./min.	Coumarin derivatives: Coumarin Marcoumar Warfarin, etc.	Bleeding Focal hemorrhages

22. *Barium* (Soluble Salts)

Gastric lavage with 2 to 5 per cent solution of either magnesium or sodium sulfate. Ten ml. of 10 per cent sodium sulfate intravenously, repeated in 30 minutes for serious symptoms. Artificial respiration and oxygen. Procainamide for ventricular arrhythmias. Potassium.

23. *Benadryl* (Diphenhydramine HCl)

See Antihistaminics.

24. *Benzene* (Benzol)

Gastric lavage or emesis. Artificial respiration and oxygen. Shock therapy. Blood transfusion if necessary. Avoid fats, oils, alcohol, and epinephrine or related drugs (these induce ventricular fibrillation).

25. *Benzene Hexachloride* (BHC)

Gastric lavage or emesis. Wash skin thoroughly. Short-acting barbiturates. Avoid fats, oils, and epinephrine.

26. *Benzine* (Petroleum Ether, Naphtha)

See Kerosene.

27. *Beryllium*

Calcium disodium edetate (edathamil). Corticosteroids for chemical pneumonitis. Excision of skin granulomas and ulcers. Prevention with education of beryllium-using workers or operators.

28. *Bismuth* (Soluble Compounds)

Gastric lavage or emesis. Activated charcoal. Saline cathartic. BAL. Discontinue medication at first sign of toxicity. Methylene blue for methemoglobinemia.

29. *Boric Acid* (Boracic Acid)

Gastric lavage or emesis. Saline cathartic. Shock and convulsive therapy. Peritoneal dialysis or exchange transfusion.

30. *Botulism*

See pages 27 and 900.

31. *Bromides*

Discontinue all sources of bromides. Six to 12 grams of sodium chloride in divided doses with 4 liters of water daily for 1 to 4 weeks (adult dose). Isotonic salt solution or ammonium chloride intravenously in more serious cases. Hemodialysis with artificial kidney.

32. *Cadmium*

Gastric lavage or emesis. Move patient from exposure. Saline cathartic. Calcium disodium edetate (edathamil). BAL contraindicated (BAL and cadmium combination is nephrotoxic). Artificial respiration and oxygen. Antibiotics and corticosteroids for chemical pneumonitis and pulmonary edema.

33. *Caffeine*

See Xanthines.

34. *Camphor*

Gastric lavage or emesis. Demulcents. Short-acting barbiturates. Artificial respiration and oxygen. Shock therapy. Avoid fats, oils, alcohol, and opiates. Lipid dialysis.

35. *Cantharidin* (Spanish Fly, Russian Fly)

Gastric lavage (cautiously because of corrosive effects) or emesis. Demulcents. Therapy for shock. Short-acting barbiturates. Adequate fluids for diuresis. Avoid morphine because of respiratory depression.

36. Carbon Dioxide

Terminate exposure; move patient to fresh air. Artificial respiration and oxygen. Respiratory and blood pressure stimulants.

37. Carbon Disulfide

Gastric lavage or emesis, if ingested. Move from exposure. Artificial respiration and oxygen. Pulmonary edema and therapy for shock. Short-acting barbiturates. Prevention: maximum allowable concentration (MAC) must be observed at all times. For skin contact, wash thoroughly.

38. Carbon Monoxide

Move patient from exposure immediately. Artificial respiration and oxygen. Administration of 100 per cent oxygen in a pressure chamber, if available. Hypothermia. Blood transfusion or washed red blood cells given early. Chronic carbon monoxide poisoning and therapy are questionable.

39. Carbon Tetrachloride

Gastric lavage or emesis, if ingested. Move from source of exposure. Remove contaminated clothes. Artificial respiration and oxygen. Shock therapy with special emphasis on fluid and electrolytes in face of oliguria or anuria. Avoid fats, oils, alcohol, epinephrine, and related compounds. Prevention: use of less toxic chemicals such as methyl chloroform.

40. Chloral Hydrate

See Barbiturates.

41. Chlorates

Gastric lavage with care, or emesis. Demulcents. Shock therapy. Methylene blue for methemoglobinemia.

42. Chlordane

Gastric lavage or emesis. Short-acting barbiturates. For skin contamination, thorough washing of skin and removal of contaminated clothing. Avoid fats, oils, demulcents, and epinephrine, which should never be used in any halogenated insecticide poisoning.

43. Chlorinated Alkalis (Hypochlorites, Chlorine)

Careful gastric lavage or emesis for large amounts only. Diluted vinegar and fruit juices. Demulcents. Move from exposure and wash skin thoroughly. Antibiotics and corticosteroids for pulmonary edema and pneumonitis from chlorine inhalation. Oral magnesium oxide (paradoxical as it may sound) to prevent formation of irritating hypochlorous acid in the stomach.

44. Chloroform

Gastric lavage or emesis. Demulcents. Artificial respiration and oxygen. Respiratory and cardiac stimulants. Ten per cent calcium gluconate intravenously (slowly).

45. Chlorothiazide (Diuril)

Discontinue use of drug. Correct fluid and electrolyte imbalance.

46. Chromium (Potassium Salt, Chromic Oxide)

Gastric lavage or emesis. Demulcents. One per cent aluminum acetate wet dressings for skin contamination. Ten per cent edetate (edathamil) ointment for skin ulcers. Remove from source of exposure whether it be from inhalation or skin contact.

47. Cocaine

Gastric lavage or emesis. Remove drug from skin or mucous membranes. Short-acting barbiturates. Artificial respiration and oxygen.

48. Codeine

Gastric lavage or emesis. Saline cathartic. Nalorphine (Nalline), levallorphan (Lorfan), or preferably naloxone (Narcan). Artificial respiration and oxygen. Maintain body heat and fluid balance.

49. Colchicine

Gastric lavage or emesis. Saline cathartic. Artificial respiration and oxygen. Shock therapy. Discontinue or reduce dosages of drug at first sign of toxicity.

50. Copper

Gastric lavage or emesis if vomiting has not occurred. Demulcents. Shock therapy. Calcium disodium edetate (edathamil). Penicillamine derivatives.

51. Cosmetics

Deodorants (aluminum salts, titanium dioxide, antibacterial agents); depilatories (soluble sulfides or calcium thioglycolate): gastric lavage or emesis, if large amount ingested.

Hair tints and dyes: discontinue use if allergy develops.

52. Curare

Discontinue drug immediately. Endotracheal catheter and use a positive pressure artificial respirator with oxygen until muscle function returns.

Neostigmine or edrophonium chloride. Cold packs or alcohol sponging for temperature elevation.

53. Cyanides (Hydrogen, Potassium, Sodium)

Gastric lavage or emesis, if ingested. See antidote chart for cyanide poison kit. Kelocyanor (dicobalt tetracemate) is being used effectively in Europe but is not approved for United States use at present. Artificial respiration and oxygen. Remove contaminated clothing and wash skin thoroughly.

54. DDT (Chlorobenzene Insecticide, TDE, DFDT, DMC, Methoxychlor, Neotrane, Ovotran, Dilan, Dimite)

Gastric lavage or emesis. Saline cathartic. Short-acting barbiturates. Artificial respiration and oxygen. Remove contaminated clothing and wash skin thoroughly. Avoid fats, oils, demulcents, epinephrine, and related compounds.

55. Demerol HCl (Meperidine HCl)

See Morphine.

56. Detergents (Anionic and Nonionic Surfactants, Phosphate Salts, Sodium Sulfate and Carbonate, Fatty Acid Amides)

Unless taken in large quantities, no serious toxic symptoms other than gastrointestinal symptoms; at present causing havoc with public water supplies. Milk, eggwhites, mild soap solution by mouth.

57. Diamthazole (Asterol)*

Use as directed only or discontinue use. Should not be used in children under 6 years of age. Short-acting barbiturates.

58. Dichlorohydrin

See Carbon Tetrachloride.

59. Dichlorophenoxyacetic Acid (2,4-D; 2,4,5-T Esters or Salts)

Gastric lavage or emesis. Quinidine sulfate to relieve myotonia and suppress ventricular arrhythmias. Antipyretic for hyperpyrexia.

60. Dieldrin

See Chlordane (Indane Derivatives).

61. Diethyltoluamide (Dimethylphthalate, Indalone)

Gastric lavage or emesis. Demulcents. Short-acting barbiturates.

---

*This product was discontinued in the United States (1966), but is still available in Europe.

62. Digitalis (Purple Foxglove) (Digitoxin)

Discontinue use. Gastric lavage or emesis for accidental or suicidal ingestion. Artificial pacemaker. Potassium chloride, orally or intravenously, under electrocardiographic observation. Procainamide, quinidine, diphenylhydantoin (Dilantin), propranolol hydrochloride, lidocaine, or atropine.

63. Dilantin Sodium

See Diphenylhydantoin Sodium.

64. Dimethyl Sulfate

Move to fresh air; eyes, skin, and mucous membranes should be washed thoroughly with water. Weak alkali wet dressings for skin burns. Antibiotics and corticosteroids for pneumonitis. In contaminated areas deactivate by spraying with water or 5 per cent sodium hydroxide solution.

65. Dinitro-ortho-cresol (Dinitrophenol Derivatives)

Gastric lavage with sodium bicarbonate solution or emesis. For skin contamination wash thoroughly with weak alkaline solution. Oxygen and circulatory stimulants. Reduce temperature with cold packs or alcohol sponging. Maintain fluid and electrolyte balance.

66. Dioxane

See Acetone.

67. Diphenhydramine HCl (Benadryl HCl)

See Antihistaminics.

68. Diphenylhydantoin Sodium, Phenytoin (Dilantin Sodium)

Gastric lavage or emesis for ingestion. Discontinue use or reduce dosage.

69. Dithiocarbamate (Ferbam)

Discontinue use of spray. Avoid alcohol.

70. Doriden

See Barbiturates.

71. Emetine (Alkaloid of Ipecac)

Gastric lavage if emesis has not taken place. Maintain fluid and electrolyte balance. Cautious digitalization. Cardiac pacemaker until EKG is normal and pulse regular.

72. Ephedrine

Gastric lavage or emesis. Activated charcoal. Short-acting barbiturates. Phentolamine (Regitine) early, to block hypertensive effects.

73. *Epinephrine* (Adrenalin)

See Ephedrine.

74. *Ergot Derivatives*

Gastric lavage or emesis. Activated charcoal, 1 to 2 tbsp. in water. Saline cathartic. Atropine sulfate for abdominal pain and spasm, 10 per cent solution of calcium gluconate for myalgia, and papaverine HCl or mecholyl as vascular antispasmodic. Short-acting barbiturates and artificial respiration and oxygen, if necessary.

75. *Essential (Volatile) Oils*

One hundred milliliters of castor oil, then remove by gastric lavage. Saline cathartic. Demulcents. Short-acting barbiturates. Artificial respiration and oxygen. Maintain fluid and electrolyte balance.

76. *Ether*

Artificial respiration and oxygen. Maintain adequate airway, blood pressure, and body temperature.

77. *Ethyl Alcohol (Pure)* (Whiskey = 40 to 50 per cent Alcohol; Wines = 10 to 20 per cent Alcohol; Beers = 2 to 6 per cent Alcohol)

Gastric lavage or emesis. Sodium bicarbonate, 1 tsp. to 1 pt. water, every 1 to 2 hours to prevent acidosis. Intravenous bicarbonate for acidosis. Caffeine and sodium benzoate or strong coffee. Hypertonic glucose or urea for cerebral edema. Intravenous glucose for hypoglycemia. Avoid depressant drugs (barbiturates interfere with enzymatic action of alcohol dehydrogenase) and potent respiratory stimulants.

78. *Ethylene Chlorohydrin* (Ethylene Dichloride)

Gastric lavage or emesis. Move from exposure. Artificial respiration and oxygen. Thorough washing for skin contact. Epinephrine or levarterenol for maintaining blood pressure.

79. *Ethylene Glycol* (Diethylene Glycol, Propylene Glycol)

Gastric lavage or emesis. Artificial respiration and oxygen. Ten per cent calcium gluconate intravenously to precipitate metabolic product, oxalic acid, and oxalates. Maintain body temperature, fluids, and electrolytes. Short-acting barbiturates. Dialysis. Oral and intravenous ethyl alcohol (see Methyl Alcohol).

80. *Ferrous Sulfate* (Copperas, Green Vitriol; Approximately 20 per cent Elemental Iron)

Clearance with suction and maintenance of open airways. Control of shock with available intravenous fluids, blood, plasma, and oxygen. Gastric lavage with concentrated solution of sodium bicarbonate, 5 per cent disodium phosphate, or milk until returning fluid is clear. Critically ill patients should receive calcium disodium edetate (edathamil) intravenously; if none given orally, intravenous dose should be 70 to 80 mg. per kg. per 24 hours in dextrose or isotonic saline solution in an 0.5 to 2 per cent concentration; if used orally (and rate of its absorption through a gut wall damaged by iron is not known), only half the aforementioned dose should be used intravenously, 35 to 40 mg. per kg. per 24 hours. Guided by the clinical picture and daily iron levels in serum, and, if measurements are available, by the urinary output of edetate (edathamil) and iron, intravenous and/or oral calcium disodium edetate (edathamil) is continued in a total daily dose of no more than 70 to 80 mg. per kg.; duration of treatment with this drug should not be, and need not be, longer than 5 days. Deferoxamine (Desferal), a chelating agent, has been demonstrated to be effective in the treatment of acute iron poisoning. Dosage recommended is 5 to 10 grams by mouth or nasogastric tube* and 1 to 2 grams intravenously (slowly to avoid hypotensive effects) or intramuscularly. Parenteral therapy can be repeated if serum iron levels remain high. Follow-up liver function tests and study of gastrointestinal tract with a radiopaque medium for strictures.

81. *Fluorides* (Fluorine, Hydrogen Fluoride, Fluorosilicates [insoluble])

Gastric lavage or emesis with lime water (0.15 per cent calcium hydroxide), calcium chloride solution (1 tsp. per 1000 ml. water), or milk. Ten per cent calcium gluconate intravenously or intramuscularly. Demulcents. For inhalation move to fresh air. Artificial respiration and oxygen. Prophylactic antibiotics and corticosteroids for pulmonary irritation and edema. Wash skin immediately and thoroughly with water and apply magnesium oxide paste with 20 per cent glycerin.

82. *Fluoroacetate Sodium*

Gastric lavage or emesis. Saline cathartic. Ten per cent calcium gluconate or sodium glycerol monoacetate (Monacetin). Short-acting barbiturates. Procainamide for arrhythmia. For skin contact, wash thoroughly.

83. *Food Poisoning* (Botulism)

See also Foodborne Illness (pp. 26 to 29). Types A and B polyvalent antitoxin (in-

---

*There are some studies suggesting that large doses of deferoxamine can be absorbed and result in systemic toxicity, and its oral use is now being questioned.

adequately processed vegetables and meats) or Type E antitoxin (fish and marine products). Trivalent (A, B, E) antitoxin now available.* Maintain an airway. Parenteral fluids.

84. *Formaldehyde* (Formalin)

Gastric lavage with 0.1 per cent ammonia or 1 per cent ammonium carbonate solution. Saline cathartic. Combat shock or collapse; levarterenol if necessary.

85. *Glutethimide* (Doriden)

See Barbiturates.

86. *Gold*

Discontinue use of parenteral therapy. Dimercaprol (BAL). Antihistaminic therapy. Supportive therapy for renal and hematologic effects.

87. *Hydralazine* (Apresoline, Phthalazine Derivatives)

Gastric lavage or emesis. Discontinue use or reduce dosage. Maintain blood pressure.

88. *Hydrochloric Acid* (Muriatic Acid)

Do not use gastric lavage after 1 hour of ingestion. Neutralize acid with magnesium oxide, milk of magnesia, or lime water. Give demulcents. Maintain blood pressure, fluids, and electrolytes. Antibiotics and corticosteroids to prevent infection and strictures. Thorough washing of skin and application of magnesium oxide paste. Gastroscopy for determining corrosive injury to the stomach.

89. *Hydroquinone*

Gastric lavage or emesis. Saline cathartic. Methylene blue for methemoglobinemia.

90. *Hypochlorites* (Clorox, etc.)

See Chlorinated Alkalis.

91. *Iodine* (Iodoform, Iodides)

Give suspension of starch or flour or 1 to 5 per cent solution of sodium thiosulfate. If not available, use milk or egg whites. Follow by gastric lavage. Regulate fluids and electrolytes, depending on degree of renal involvement. Epinephrine, diphenhydramine (Benadryl), or hydrocortisone for anaphylactoid reaction.

92. *Isoniazid*

Prompt gastric lavage or emesis (symptoms appear within 30 minutes). Discontinue drug or reduce dosage. Pyridoxine, 200 to 400 mg. intravenously. Short-acting barbiturates intravenously for convulsions. Parenteral sodium bicarbonate for acidosis. Hemodialysis. Osmotic diuresis (mannitol, urea, furosemide, or ethacrynic acid) hastens excretion.

93. *Isopropyl Alcohol* (Rubbing Alcohol)

See Ethyl Alcohol.

94. *Kerosene* (Petroleum Distillates: Benzine, Gasoline, Naphtha, Mineral Seal Oil, etc.)

Prevent aspiration. Gastric lavage or emesis to be avoided. Fifty ml. of mineral or vegetable oil by mouth (if not forced). Oxygen and antibiotics. Corticosteroids for pulmonary edema and chemical or lipoid pneumonitis (particularly for mineral seal oil aspiration). Results are equivocal, yet since therapy is short range, it may benefit those with severe pulmonary distress and "shock" lung.

95. *Lead*

Gastric lavage with 1 per cent sodium sulfate solution, followed by saline cathartic for immediate ingestion. Calcium disodium edetate (edathamil) intravenously or intramuscularly for 5 days and repeat if necessary. Four per cent urea (30 per cent in severe cases) intravenously for encephalopathy with increased intracranial pressure: craniectomy may be necessary. Mannitol and/or adrenal corticosteroids are also used for this purpose and often preferred. Ten per cent solution of calcium gluconate or morphine for severe abdominal pain (colic). Early diagnosis and treatment are paramount in preventing death or serious sequelae in children. BAL combined with calcium disodium edetate (edathamil) therapy is more effective in lead encephalitis than use of edetate (edathamil) alone. Penicillamine (Cuprimine) as an oral chelating agent has recently been reported to be effective and may be used in adjunctive therapy as an investigational drug.

96. *Mace* (Anti-Riot Gas)

See Tear Gases.

97. *Manganese*

Remove from further exposure. Antibiotics and corticosteroids for pneumonitis. Calcium disodium edetate (edathamil) may be beneficial if given early. Antiparkinsonian drugs. Diphenhydramine (Benadryl), biperiden hydrochloride (Akineton), or methylphenidate hydrochloride (Ritalin).

98. *Marihuana*

Removal of drug exposure (characteristic "burnt rope" acrid odor on clothes and body).

---

*U.S. Communicable Disease Center, Atlanta, Georgia. Telephone number for day coverage is (404) 633-3753 (4, 5, 6); for night and weekends, (404) 633-2176.

There are no withdrawal symptoms except with extreme cases of habituation.

99. Meperidine HCl (Demerol HCl)

See Morphine.

100. Meprobamate (Equanil, Miltown, etc.)

Gastric lavage or emesis. Saline cathartic. Artificial respiration and oxygen. Maintain blood pressure with methoxamine hydrochloride. In massive ingestion, use castor oil (for possible concretion) as solvent and purge.

101. Menthol

See Phenol.

102. Mercury Compounds

Gastric lavage immediately with egg white solution or with 5 per cent sodium formaldehyde sulfoxylate; if unavailable, a 2 to 5 per cent solution of sodium bicarbonate may be used. Magnesium sulfate as cathartic (early only). BAL. Penicillamine derivatives (oral antidote). Maintain fluid and electrolyte balance and nutrition. Spironolactone (Aldactone) has prevented renal tubular necrosis in experimental animals (rats).

103. Metaldehyde (Changes to Acetaldehyde)

Gastric lavage or emesis. Demulcents. Short-acting barbiturates. Artificial respiration, oxygen, and antibiotics. Parenteral chlorpromazine and calcium gluconate.

104. Methadone (Dolophine)

See Morphine.

105. Methyl Alcohol

To prevent the formation of formic acid and formates, 10 ml. ethyl alcohol per hour can suppress the metabolism of methyl alcohol. In severe poisoning ethyl alcohol can be given intravenously in 5 per cent concentration in bicarbonate or saline solution and 3 to 4 oz. of whiskey (45 per cent alcohol) orally every 4 to 6 hours for 1 to 3 days. Combat acidosis. Hemodialysis is paramount in serious poisoning.

106. Methyl Bromide (Chloride, Iodide)

Move from exposure. Artificial respiration and oxygen. Epinephrine for bronchospasm; antibiotics and corticosteroids for pneumonitis. Prevention: safety dispensers for fumigant use.

107. Methyl Salicylate (Oil of Wintergreen)

See Salicylates. Gastric lavage, however, may be worthwhile, even several hours after ingestion, because methyl salicylate is poorly absorbed.

108. Metrazol

See Pentylenetetrazol.

109. Morphine (Codeine, Heroin, Propoxyphene [Darvon], Meperidine [Demerol], Dihydromorphinone [Dilaudid], Opium Alkaloids [Pantopon])

Gastric lavage (before loss of consciousness). Do not use syrup of ipecac or apomorphine. Activated charcoal. Saline cathartic. Delay absorption of intramuscular drug with tourniquet and cryotherapy. Maintain adequate airway, body temperature, fluids, and electrolytes. Give narcotic antagonists Nalline or Lorfan. Naloxone hydrochloride (Narcan) is preferable (see antidote chart, p. 894). Ephedrine for hypotension and bradycardia—methoxamine or phenylephrine if pulse is rapid. Doxapram hydrochloride (Dopram), 3 to 5 ml. intravenously, is the respiratory stimulant of choice, but it has short-lasting effects (3 to 5 minutes).

110. Muscarine (Some Mushrooms)

Artificial respiration with oxygen. Atropine, 1 to 2 mg. every hour until free of respiratory effects. PAM or Protopam chloride may be useful adjunct therapy. Gastric lavage or emesis if vomiting has not occurred. Thioctic acid, an investigational compound, has been reported to be effective in European trials.

111. Naphthalene (Mothballs, Repellents, etc., Paradichlorobenzene, Camphor)

Gastric lavage or emesis for ingestion. Give sodium bicarbonate every 4 hours to maintain alkaline urine and prevent renal blockage with acid hematin crystals. Blood transfusions as necessary. Short-acting barbiturates. Avoid use of milk, oils, or fatty meals. In prevention, these products should be kept out of hands and clothes of children (symptoms produced not only by ingestion but also by inhalation and transcutaneous absorption).

112. Naphthol

See Phenol.

113. Nickel (Nickel Carbonyl)

Remove from skin by thorough washing. Artificial respiration and oxygen. BAL. Antibiotics and corticosteroids for pneumonitis.

114. Nicotine

Gastric lavage or emesis. Activated charcoal. Short-acting barbiturates. Artificial respiration and oxygen; use of positive pressure resuscitator through period of respiratory failure may prevent death. Thorough washing of skin and removal of clothing will be necessary for skin contamination.

115. Nitrates, Nitrites

Gastric lavage or emesis. Saline cathartic. Methylene blue for methemoglobinemia. Maintain blood pressure with levarterenol. Short-acting barbiturates for convulsions.

116. Nitric Acid

Give large amounts of water. Neutralize with lime water, magnesia, etc. Gastric lavage cautiously if seen within the first half hour. Gastroscopy to detect caustic burns of the stomach. Demulcents. Morphine for pain, but avoid large doses and possible depression. Shock therapy. Corticosteroids to prevent stricture formation. For eye and skin contact wash thoroughly with water: *do not use chemical antidotes in the eye.*

117. Nitrobenzene

Gastric lavage or emesis. Artificial respiration and oxygen. Methylene blue, 1 per cent solution for methemoglobinemia. Avoid fats and oils.

118. Opium

See Morphine.

119. Oxalates

Gastric lavage with calcium lactate solution, 10 grams (2 tsp.) per 100 ml. Ten per cent calcium gluconate intravenously. Give milk and demulcents.

120. Paraldehyde

Gastric lavage or emesis. Artificial respiration and oxygen. Maintain body temperature, fluids, and electrolytes.

121. Paraquat

Induce vomiting with syrup of ipecac or perform gastric lavage if vomiting has not occurred. If lavage is performed, care must be taken, as paraquat may be corrosive to the esophagus.

Immediately following vomiting or lavage, give approximately 200 to 500 ml. of a 30 per cent aqueous suspension of an adsorbent clay (such as Robinson's bentonite U.S.P., or Robinson's fuller's earth U.S.P.) plus an effective dose of cathartic, e.g., magnesium sulfate, to remove paraquat from the entire gastrointestinal tract. Repeat as often as practical (every 2 to 4 hours for several days until paraquat can no longer be detected in blood, urine, or dialysate). If bentonite or fuller's earth is not immediately available, an adsorbent such as powdered activated charcoal should be used until

better clays are obtained. Oxygen should be used sparingly and cautiously for dyspnea or cyanosis, because it may aggravate the lung lesions. Forced diuresis should be started as soon as possible to remove paraquat from the blood. If renal function is impaired, hemodialysis or peritoneal dialysis may be of value. Use of forced diuresis and hemodialysis together may aid in hastening the removal of paraquat. Monitor the patient's blood urea nitrogen (BUN) and serum creatinine levels, as these are early indicators of systemic poisoning and are useful in determining the patient's progress. Also, obtain daily chest x-rays, arterial oxygen partial pressure, pulmonary function studies, and chest auscultation. Obtain urine, blood, and dialysate samples initially and at least daily to monitor the elimination of paraquat.

For skin contamination, clothing should be removed and the skin thoroughly washed with soap and water for several minutes. If the eyes are involved, they should be irrigated immediately for 10 to 15 minutes and then seen by an ophthalmologist.

122. Parathion (Phosphate Ester Insecticides) (Malathion, Systox, EPN, Diazinon, Guthion, Trithion, TEPP, OMPA, Co-Ral, Phosdrin)

Prompt induction of emesis or gastric lavage with 5 per cent $NaHCO_3$ for ingestion only. Decontaminate by removal of all soiled clothes and thorough washing of skin. Maintain clear airway and respirations with laryngeal intubation and artificial respiration and oxygen. Atropine, 1 to 2 mg. intramuscularly or intravenously and repeat at 20 to 30 minute intervals, as soon as cyanosis has cleared (chance of ventricular fibrillation). Continue atropine until definite improvement occurs and is maintained (sometimes 2 or more days). The total dosage required may be phenomenal (over 1000 mg.). PAM (pralidoxime chloride), a cholinesterase reactivator as 5 per cent solution intravenously. Avoid narcotics, barbiturates, epinephrine, aminophylline, ether, and phenothiazine derivatives, because they further reduce cholinesterase activity and some are respiratory depressants.

123. Pentachlorophenol

Gastric lavage or emesis. Removal of contaminated clothing and thorough washing of skin. Short-acting barbiturates.

124. Pentylenetetrazole (Metrazol)

Delay absorption of intramuscular drug with tourniquet and cryotherapy. Gastric lavage or emesis for ingestion. Short-acting barbiturate for convulsions. Cold packs and alcohol sponging for hyperthermia.

125. Permanganate, Potassium

Thorough lavage of stomach with 3 per cent hydrogen peroxide (10 ml. in 100 ml. of water). Milk or demulcents. Combat collapse and shock.

126. Phenacetin (Acetophenetidin)

See Acetanilid.

127. Phenol (Derivatives) (Creosote, Guaiacol, Resorcinol, Thymol)

Careful gastric lavage, followed by 60 ml. of castor oil which dissolves phenol and hastens its removal. Activated charcoal. Maintain body temperature, fluids, electrolytes. For skin and mucous membranes, wash thoroughly and follow by application of castor oil or 10 per cent ethyl alcohol. Short-acting barbiturates for convulsions and antibiotics as prophylaxis in pulmonary edema.

128. Phenolphthalein

Gastric lavage or emesis. Activated charcoal. Castor oil if given early to hasten the drug through the intestinal tract, but no other solvents because they increase laxative action.

129. Phenothiazine Derivatives

Discontinue drug or reduce dosage. In blood dyscrasias or jaundice do not change to another derivative. Gastric lavage for ingestion of large doses. Antiparkinsonian drugs are rarely necessary. Injectable diphenhydramine hydrochloride (Benadryl) is effective in treatment of extrapyramidal symptoms. Biperiden (Akineton) parenterally or orally. Methylphenidate (Ritalin).

130. Phenytoin

See Diphenylhydantoin Sodium.

131. Phosphoric Acid

See Table 1.

132. Phosphorus (Red [Nonabsorbed, Nontoxic], Yellow [Volatile and Highly Toxic], Phosphine)

Thorough gastric lavage with potassium permanganate (1:5000) or 3 per cent hydrogen peroxide. Copper sulfate, 0.25 gram in glass of water, forms insoluble copper phosphide. One hundred ml. of mineral oil as a solvent (to prevent absorption and hasten elimination) and repeat in 2 hours. Maintain body temperature, fluids, and electrolytes. Give glucose, vitamin K, and 10 per cent calcium gluconate, if indicated. Exposure to phosphine must be terminated at once, and use of contaminated water for drinking or bathing should be forbidden.

133. Physostigmine (Eserine) (Pilocarpine, Neostigmine, Methacholine [Mecholyl], Muscarine)

Gastric lavage or emesis. Maintain artificial respiration until antidote (propantheline [Pro-Banthine], which is preferable to atropine) can be given; 30 mg. intramuscularly every 6 hours may be necessary throughout entire crisis. Maintain airway and remove pulmonary secretion (postural drainage).

134. Picrotoxin

Gastric lavage or emesis. Slow absorption of injected drug by application of cold and/or tourniquet. Short-acting barbiturate. Cold packs or alcohol sponging for hyperthermia.

135. Procaine

See Cocaine—but much less toxic.

136. Pyrethrum (Insecticide Plant)

Gastric lavage or emesis unless kerosene is more suspected than pyrethrum. Demulcents. Short-acting barbiturates for convulsions.

137. Pyribenzamine (Tripelennamine)

See Antihistaminics.

138. Quaternary Ammonium Compounds (Cationic Detergents)

Gastric lavage with soapy water, milk or gelatin solution, or emesis. Demulcents or soapy solution. Maintain clear airway; artificial respiration and oxygen. Short-acting barbiturates for convulsions. Atropine recommended without good basis for its use. Avoid alcohol. Thoroughly wash with soap and water for excessive skin contacts.

139. Quinine and Cinchona-like Compounds (Quinidine, Synthetic Hydrocupreine Compounds [Optochin, Numoquin], Plasmochin, Chloroquine [Aralen], Quinacrine [Atabrine])

Gastric lavage or emesis. Discontinue use of drug. Activated charcoal. Levarterenol for hypotension. Artificial respiration and oxygen.

140. Radiation Syndrome

Remove external clothing and wash clothing and entire body with soap and water. Fresh blood or platelet-enriched plasma. Bone marrow replacement. Antibiotics as prophylaxis for infections.

141. Rotenone

Gastric lavage or emesis if vomiting has not already occurred. Wash thoroughly for skin contact. Short-acting barbiturates. Avoid fats and oils.

142. Ryania

See Rotenone.

143. Sabadilla (Cevadilla)

Demulcents. Activated charcoal. Gastric lavage is usually unnecessary because vomiting occurs early.

144. Salicylate

I. Immediate (emesis or gastric lavage)
  A. Evaluation of severity of intoxication (extrapolation method of Done)
  B. Appraisal of status of dehydration
  C. Determination of acid-base imbalance. Test urine with Phenistix paper and Nitrazene paper
  D. Determination of electrolyte imbalance
  E. Draw blood for the following laboratory tests:
    1. Salicylate level
    2. CO_2-combining content
    3. Plasma CO_2 content
    4. pH
    5. Serum electrolytes
II. Pending laboratory report
  A. Start intravenous fluids (5 per cent glucose in ⅓ isotonic saline)
  B. If dehydration is severe, hydrating solution should be given at the rate of 8 ml. per m.² body surface per minute for 30 to 45 minutes
  C. After that time, slow down hydrating solution to 2 ml. per m.² per minute
  D. Correct bicarbonate and potassium deficits as indicated (average requirement: 5 mEq. $NaHCO_3$ per kg. and 2 mEq. K per kg. for 12 hours)
  E. In presence of clinical acidosis and acid urine, $NaHCO_3$ should be given in initial hydrating solution
  F. Cool water body sponging for hyperpyrexia
III. In life-threatening intoxication, consider exchange transfusion in young children, peritoneal dialysis with 5 per cent albumin solution (Albumisol), or dialysis with artificial kidney
IV. Administer vitamin K and B complex, the route of administration depending on the condition of the patient
  V. Maintenance management
    A. Test each urine voided with Nitrazene paper

B. Periodic (frequent) determination of:
  1. Blood CO_2-combining power
  2. Blood CO_2 content
  3. Blood pH

145. Santonin

Gastric lavage or emesis. Saline cathartic. Short-acting barbiturates. Avoid opiates.

146. Sea Nettle (Portuguese Man-of-War)

See separate article, p. 887.

147. Selenium

Move from occupational environment. Eliminate from diet. Bromobenzene solution, 0.25 to 1 gram in lavage.

148. Silver Nitrate

Dilute with isotonic saline solution (0.9 per cent = 1 tsp. salt per 1 pt. water) and thorough lavage of stomach; a relatively insoluble and non-corrosive silver chloride is formed in this reaction. Sodium sulfate cathartic (1 oz. per cup of water). Milk or demulcents. Shock therapy. Meperidine (Demerol) or codeine for pain.

149. Solanine

Gastric lavage or emesis. Activated charcoal. Pilocarpine. Artificial respiration and circulatory stimulants as necessary.

150. Squill (Red, White)

See Digitalis. Gastric lavage or emesis. Demulcents. Quinidine sulfate. Avoid epinephrine or other stimulants.

151. Strychnine

It symptoms have begun, avoid gastric lavage or emesis. Activated charcoal, followed by gastric lavage if asymptomatic. Short-acting barbiturates. Avoid stimuli and opiates. Artificial respiration and oxygen. Muscle relaxants: diazepam (Valium) is particularly effective.

152. Sulfides (Carbon Disulfide, Soluble Sulfides, Hydrogen Sulfide)

Move from exposure. Artificial respiration and oxygen. Remove swallowed poison by gastric lavage or emesis. Wash skin thoroughly for skin contact and use burn therapy. Antibiotics prevent secondary infection.

153. Sulfonamides

Gastric lavage or emesis for overdosage. Discontinue drug. Alkali and large intake of fluid if renal function is normal. Hemodialysis in severe poisoning.

154. Sulfur Dioxide

Move to fresh air. Artificial respiration and oxygen. Antibiotics and corticosteroids for pneumonitis.

155. Sulfuric Acid

See Hydrochloric Acid.

156. Tear Gases

The most commonly used preparations are chloracetophenone, ethylbromoacetate, bromoacetone, bromobenzyl cyanide, and bromomethylethylketone. *Alpha-chloroacetophenone,* even though called a "gas," is actually a fine powder. In commercial blast-dispersion cartridges, it is mixed half and half with silica anhydride, and a standard shotgun primer is used as a propellant. The mixture is an effective lacrimator in concentrations as low as 2 ppm. of air. It can cause extreme irritation and edema of the mucous membranes of the nose and eyes if discharged into the face, and temporary blindness may result. *Mace* contains recrystallized 2-chloroacetophenone (0.9 per cent 1, 1, 1-trichloroethane), solvents and propellants— Freon, kerosene, methylchloroform, 4.0 per cent.

The eyes should be irrigated for 15 minutes with isotonic saline solution or water, followed by an anti-flammatory eye ointment. For clothing and skin contamination the clothes should be removed and a thorough shower taken.

157. Tetrachloroethane

See Carbon Tetrachloride.

158. Thallium

Gastric lavage or emesis. For skin contamination, wash thoroughly. Activated charcoal twice a day, 1 to 2 tbs., and potassium chloride, 3 to 5 grams daily for 5 to 7 days. BAL. Dithizon (no preparations marketed for therapeutic use), 10 mg. per kg. twice a day for 5 days. Maintain body temperature, blood pressure, fluids, and electrolytes. Antibiotics for pneumonitis. Artane for tremors and ataxia.

159. Thiocyanates

Inorganic: Gastric lavage or emesis. Saline cathartic. Give 2 to 4 liters of fluid daily if renal function is normal. Hemodialysis or peritoneal dialysis, if necessary.

Organic (lauryl, ethyl, and methyl thiocyanate, lethane 60): See Cyanides for treatment.

160. Thiourea

Discontinue use of drug. Antibiotics and corticosteroids for bone marrow depression.

161. Thiram (Tetramethylthiuram Disulfide)

Gastric lavage or emesis. Wash thoroughly for skin contact and remove contaminated clothing. Avoid fats, oils, lipid solvents, and especially alcohol. Artificial respiration and oxygen.

162. Toxaphene

See DDT.

163. Trichloroethylene

See Carbon Tetrachloride.

164. Tricyclic (Dibenzazepine) Compounds

When a patient has convulsions, coma, signs of atropinism, and cardiac arrhythmias, one should strongly suspect tricyclic antidepressant poisoning specifically, and intoxication by other anticholinergic drugs and chemicals in general.

Treatment of intoxication from tricyclic antidepressant tranquilizers is supportive and symptomatic, with particular attention to the correction of cardiac arrhythmias and maintenance of blood pressure and respiration. Vital signs should be monitored continuously. EKG monitoring is advisable, and severely intoxicated patients should be treated in an intensive care unit.

Cardiac arrhythmias may progress to cardiac arrest owing to ventricular fibrillation or asystole. Death may occur rapidly after a sudden drop of blood pressure and pulse rate. The use of defibrillators and internal or external pacemakers has been advocated. However, in one nonfatal case, an external DC defibrillator produced no alleviation of arrhythmias, and in a fatal case an external pacemaker was tried unsuccessfully. Although documentation is limited, some arrhythmias were controlled in individual patients by use of the parasympathomimetic drugs; physostigmine, drug of choice (readily crosses the blood-brain barrier, 1 mg. intravenously); pyridostigmine (Mestinon) and neostigmine (Prostigmin) or by the beta-adrenergic blocking agent, propranolol (Inderal). Since it is not possible to predict which patient will respond, it may be necessary to try more than one antiarrhythmic drug. Intravenous sodium diphenylhydantoin has had dramatic antiarrhythmic properties and may also be of value in preventing convulsions which occur frequently. Congestive heart failure is treated by digitalization. However, rapid digitalization should be avoided in a situation in which multiple ventricular ectopic beats are likely to occur. The administration of sodium bicarbonate* and potassium

---

*In one series sodium bicarbonate was the most clinically effective method of treatment of arrhythmias in children; experimental studies support this view.

may aid in treating the cardiovascular effects. Convulsions may cause a dangerous increase in the cardiac workload. Agitation, tremors, and convulsions have been successfully treated with parenteral barbiturates. However, use of barbiturates is questionable if drugs that inhibit monoamine oxidase have also been taken by the patient in overdosage or in recent therapy. Also, barbiturates may increase respiratory depression, particularly in children. It is advisable to have equipment available for artificial ventilation and resuscitation. Diazepam (Valium) has been used as an alternative to barbiturates for controlling convulsions, and is considered the drug of choice by some. Hypotension and shock may be treated by intravenous fluids of glucose, saline solution, or plasma, and cautious administration of vasopressor agents such as levarterenol (1-norepinephrine; Levophed), phenylephrine, or metaraminol which will increase blood pressure without increasing heart rate. Any of these sympathomimetic drugs may induce cardiac arrhythmia and must therefore be used with caution. Other sympathomimetic drugs such as epinephrine and isoproterenol which stimulate the beta receptor sites of the heart should be avoided, because they cause additional increases in the heart rate and may lead to fatal ventricular fibrillation. Respiration must be maintained. Intratracheal artificial respiration is effective and the need for it should be anticipated. Patients should be observed for possible recurrence of respiratory distress after resumption of spontaneous breathing. Various methods have been attempted to hasten excretion of these drugs. They are absorbed quickly from the gastrointestinal tract and are largely bound to plasma proteins. In addition, they are rapidly accumulated in the body tissues, so that high serum concentrations do not occur. They are excreted in the urine largely as glucuronides of the demethylated and hydroxylated metabolites. They are also reportedly secreted into the stomach after absorption. Beneficial effects have been reported from use of exchange transfusion, repeated gastric lavage, and osmotic diuresis. Although evidence is equivocal as to the effectiveness of osmotic diuresis in removing significant amounts of these drugs, it is the general belief that diuresis is beneficial. Osmotic diuresis with mannitol has been employed in the treatment of a number of cases of intoxication with tricyclic antidepressant drugs. In one adult, only 5 per cent of the ingested dose of amitriptyline was recovered in the urine (as amitryptyline and its principal metabolites) after a 10 hour period of forced diuresis with mannitol. Since these drugs also promote urinary retention, catheterization should be considered if diuresis is attempted. Care must also be used to prevent overhydration leading to increased cardiac workload. Continuous or repeated gastric lavage has also been recommended to speed excretion. Although continuous gastric lavage was effectively employed in a child intoxicated with imipramine who exhibited coma, convulsions, and cardiac disturbances, it may be unwise to attempt during convulsive stages. Hemodialysis and peritoneal dialysis are not effective in removing significant amounts of these drugs.

In children the tricyclics are especially treacherous. When a verified ingestion occurs, it probably would be wise to hospitalize the child for monitoring for at least 24 hours, even though the patient may be asymptomatic at the time of admission.

165. Tridione (Trimethadione)

Gastric lavage or emesis for unusual ingestion. Discontinue drug or reduce dosage. Antibiotics and corticosteroids for bone marrow depression.

166. Trinitrotoleune (TNT)

Gastric lavage or emesis. Saline cathartic. Methylene blue for methemoglobinemia. Remove contaminated clothing and wash skin thoroughly. Short-acting barbiturates.

167. Tri-ortho-cresyl Phosphate ("Machine Oil")

Gastric lavage or emesis. Treat as for paralytic poliomyelitis with hydrotherapy, massage, and orthopedic care. Respirators or rocking bed until sufficient recovery occurs.

168. Tripelennamine (Pyribenzamine)

See Antihistaminics.

169. Turpentine

Gastric lavage or emesis. Demulcents. Saline cathartic. Stimulants for depression. Artificial respiration and oxygen if necessary.

170. Veratrum (Hellebore)

Gastric lavage or emesis. Activated charcoal. Saline cathartic. Atropine every hour to block reflex fall of blood pressure. Phentolamine hydrochloride or other sympathetic blocking agents should be given if hypertension present.

171. Vitamins (Vitamin A, Vitamin D, Vitamin K)

Discontinue use or reduce dosage. Symptomatic and supportive therapy as indicated for hypervitaminosis.

172. Warfarin (Coumadin, Panwarfin)

Gastric lavage or emesis. Vitamin K in adequate dosage. Transfusion of fresh blood if hemorrhage is severe.

173. *Xanthines* (Aminophylline, Theophylline, Theobromine, and Caffeine)

Gastric lavage or emesis. Antacids or demulcents. If suppository, remove by enema. Short-acting barbiturates. Oxygen.

174. *Xylene* (Benzene, Toluene, Cumene, and Mesitylene)

Cautious gastric lavage. Fifty ml. of mineral oil left in stomach. Saline cathartic. Artificial respiration and oxygen. Avoid digestible fats, oils, and epinephrine. Wash thoroughly for skin contact.

175. *Zinc* (Sulfate, Oxide, Phosphide [Releases Phosphine on contact with water; See Phosphine under Phosphorus])

Gastric lavage or emesis for ingestion. Move patient from source of inhalation. Artificial respiration and oxygen. Antibiotics and corticosteroids for "metal fume fever" and pneumonitis.

SECTION 17

Appendices and Index

TABLE OF METRIC AND APOTHECARIES' SYSTEMS

(Approved *approximate* dose equivalents are enclosed in parentheses. Use *exact* equivalents in calculations.)

Conversion Factors

METRIC	APOTHECARIES'	METRIC	APOTHECARIES'
1 milligram (mg.)	1/64 grain	3.88 cubic centimeters or grams	1 dram (4 cc. or grams)
64.79 milligrams	1 grain (65 mg.)	31.103 cubic centimeters or grams	1 ounce (30 cc. or grams)
1 gram	15.43 grains (15 grains)	473.167 cubic centimeters	1 pint (500 cc.)
1 cubic centimeter (cc.)	16 minims		

WEIGHTS

METRIC	APOTHECARIES'	METRIC	APOTHECARIES'
0.0001 gram—0.1 mg.—1/640 grain (1/600 grain)		0.057 gram —57 mg.—7/8 grain	
0.0002 gram—0.2 mg.—1/320 grain (1/300 grain)		0.06 gram —60 mg.—9/10 grain (1 grain)	
0.0003 gram—0.3 mg.—1/210 grain (1/200 grain)		0.065 gram —65 mg.—1 grain (60 mg.)	
0.0004 gram—0.4 mg.—1/150 grain		0.07 gram —70 mg.—1-1/20 grains	
0.0005 gram—0.5 mg.—1/120 grain		0.08 gram —80 mg.—1-1/5 grains	
0.0006 gram—0.6 mg.—1/100 grain		0.09 gram —90 mg.—1-1/3 grains	
0.0007 gram—0.7 mg.—1/90 grain		0.097 gram —97 mg.—1-1/2 grains (0.1 gram)	
0.0008 gram—0.8 mg.—1/80 grain		0.12 gram —120 mg.—2 grains	
0.0009 gram—0.9 mg.—1/75 grain		0.2 gram —200 mg.—3 grains	
0.001 gram—1 mg.—1/64 grain (1/60 grain)		0.24 gram —240 mg.—4 grains (0.25 gram)	
0.0011 gram—1.1 mg.—1/60 grain		0.3 gram —300 mg.—4-1/2 grains	
0.0013 gram—1.3 mg.—1/50 grain (1.2 mg.)		0.33 gram —330 mg.—5 grains (0.3 gram)	
0.0014 gram—1.4 mg.—1/48 grain		0.4 gram —400 mg.—6 grains	
0.0016 gram—1.6 mg.—1/40 grain (1.5 mg.)		0.45 gram —450 mg.—7 grains	
0.0018 gram—1.8 mg.—1/36 grain		0.5 gram —500 mg.—7-1/2 grains	
0.0020 gram—2 mg.—1/32 grain (1/30 grain)		0.53 gram —530 mg.—8 grains	
0.0022 gram—2.2 mg.—1/30 grain		0.6 gram —600 mg.—9 grains	
0.0026 gram—2.6 mg.—1/25 grain		0.65 gram —650 mg.—10 grains (0.6 gram)	
0.003 gram—3 mg.—1/20 grain		0.73 gram —730 mg.—11 grains	
0.004 gram—4 mg.—1/16 grain (1/15 grain)		0.80 gram —800 mg.—12 grains (0.75 gram)	
0.005 gram—5 mg.—1/12 grain		0.86 gram —860 mg.—13 grains	
0.006 gram—6 mg.—1/10 grain		0.93 gram —930 mg.—14 grains	
0.007 gram—7 mg.—1/9 grain		1. gram —1000 mg.—15 grains	
0.008 gram—8 mg.—1/8 grain		1.06 grams—1060 mg.—16 grains	
0.009 gram—9 mg.—1/7 grain		1.13 grams—1130 mg.—17 grains	
0.01 gram—10 mg.—1/6 grain		1.18 grams—1180 mg.—18 grains	
0.013 gram—13 mg.—1/5 grain (12 mg.)		1.26 grams—1260 mg.—19 grains	
0.016 gram—16 mg.—1/4 grain (15 mg.)		1.30 grams—1300 mg.—20 grains	
0.02 gram—20 mg.—1/3 grain		1.50 grams—1500 mg.—22 grains	
0.025 gram—25 mg.—3/8 grain		2 grams—2000 mg.—30 grains (1/2 dram)	
0.03 gram—30 mg.—2/5 grain (1/2 grain)		4 grams —1 dram (60 grains)	
0.032 gram—32 mg.—1/2 grain (30 mg.)		5 grams —75 grains	
0.04 gram—40 mg.—3/5 grain (2/3 grain)		8 grams —2 drams (7.5 grams)	
0.043 gram—43 mg.—2/3 grain (40 mg.)		10 grams —2-1/2 drams	
0.05 gram—50 mg.—3/4 grain		15 grams —4 drams	
		30 grams —1 ounce	

LIQUID MEASURES*

METRIC	APOTHECARIES'	METRIC	APOTHECARIES'
0.03 cubic centimeter — 1/2 minim		8 cubic centimeters—2 fluid drams	
0.05 cubic centimeter — 3/4 minim		10 cubic centimeters—2-1/2 fluid drams	
0.06 cubic centimeter —1 minim		15 cubic centimeters—4 fluid drams	
0.1 cubic centimeter —1-1/2 minims		20 cubic centimeters—5-1/2 fluid drams	
0.2 cubic centimeter —3 minims		25 cubic centimeters— 5/6 fluid ounce	
0.25 cubic centimeter —4 minims		30 cubic centimeters—1 fluid ounce	
0.3 cubic centimeter —5 minims		50 cubic centimeters—1-3/4 fluid ounces	
0.5 cubic centimeter —8 minims		60 cubic centimeters—2 fluid ounces	
0.6 cubic centimeter —10 minims		100 cubic centimeters—3-1/2 fluid ounces	
0.75 cubic centimeter —12 minims		120 cubic centimeters—4 fluid ounces	
1 cubic centimeter —15 minims		200 cubic centimeters—7 fluid ounces	
2 cubic centimeters—30 minims		250 cubic centimeters—8 fluid ounces	
3 cubic centimeters—45 minims		360 cubic centimeters—12 fluid ounces	
4 cubic centimeters—1 fluid dram		500 cubic centimeters—1 pint	
5 cubic centimeters—1-1/4 fluid drams		1000 cubic centimeters—1 quart	

* Note: A cubic centimeter (cc.) is the approximate equivalent of a milliliter (ml.). The terms are used interchangeably in general medicine.

TABLES OF HEIGHT AND WEIGHT FOR MEN AND WOMEN*

DESIRABLE WEIGHTS FOR MEN OF AGES 25 AND OVER

Weight in Pounds According to Frame (In Indoor Clothing)

HEIGHT (WITH SHOES ON) 1-INCH HEELS Feet	Inches	SMALL FRAME	MEDIUM FRAME	LARGE FRAME
5	2	112–120	118–129	126–141
5	3	115–123	121–133	129–144
5	4	118–126	124–136	132–148
5	5	121–129	127–139	135–152
5	6	124–133	130–143	138–156
5	7	128–137	134–147	142–161
5	8	132–141	138–152	147–166
5	9	136–145	142–156	151–170
5	10	140–150	146–160	155–174
5	11	144–154	150–165	159–179
6	0	148–158	154–170	164–184
6	1	152–162	158–175	168–189
6	2	156–167	162–180	173–194
6	3	160–171	167–185	178–199
6	4	164–175	172–190	182–204

* Courtesy of the Metropolitan Life Insurance Company.

DESIRABLE WEIGHTS FOR WOMEN OF AGES 25 AND OVER

Weight in Pounds According to Frame (In Indoor Clothing)

HEIGHT (WITH SHOES ON) 2-INCH HEELS Feet	Inches	SMALL FRAME	MEDIUM FRAME	LARGE FRAME
4	10	92– 98	96–107	104–119
4	11	94–101	98–110	106–122
5	0	96–104	101–113	109–125
5	1	99–107	104–116	112–128
5	2	102–110	107–119	115–131
5	3	105–113	110–122	118–134
5	4	108–116	113–126	121–138
5	5	111–119	116–130	125–142
5	6	114–123	120–135	129–146
5	7	118–127	124–139	133–150
5	8	122–131	128–143	137–154
5	9	126–135	132–147	141–158
5	10	130–140	136–151	145–163
5	11	134–144	140–155	149–168
6	0	138–148	144–159	153–173

For girls between 18 and 25, subtract 1 pound for each year under 25.

United States Adopted Name	British Approved or International Nonproprietary Name	United States Adopted Name	British Approved or International Nonproprietary Name
Acenocoumarol	Nicoumalone	Ethylaminobenzoate	Benzocaine
Acetaminophen	Paracetamol	Ethylestrenol	Ethyloestrenol
Acetarsone	Acetarsol	Evans blue	Azovan blue
Actinomycin	Actinomycin C	Fantridone	Fanthridone
Albuterol	Salbutamol	Fibrinolysin, human	Plasmin
Ambuphylline	Bufylline	Floxacillin	Flucloxacillin
Aminitrozole	Acinitrazole	Flucloronide	Fluclorolone acetonide
Amithizone	Thiacetazone	Flurandrenolide	Flurandrenolone
Amobarbital	Amylobarbitone	Flurogestone	Flugestone
Amoxycillin	Amoxycilline	Fonazine	Dimethothiazine
Amphecloral	Amfecloral	Fructose	Levulose
Anazoline	Anoxynaphthonate	Furosemide	Frusemide
Anisotropine	Octatropine	Gestronore	Gestronol
Anthralin	Dithranol	Glyburide	Glibenclamide
Antimony sodium gluconate	Sodium stibogluconate	Glycobiarsol	Bismuth glycolylarsanilate
Antipyrine	Phenazone	Glycopyrrolate	Glycopyrronium
Arylam	Sevin	Heptabarbital	Heptabarbitone
Asparaginase	Colaspase	Hexacarbacholine	Carbolonium
Barbital	Barbitone	Hexachlorophene	Hexachlorophane
Bendazac	Bindazac	Hexamarium	Distigmine
Bendroflumethiazide	Bendrofluazide	Hexestrol	Hexoestrol
Benoxinate	Oxybuprocaine	Hexobarbital	Hexobarbitone
Betazole	Ametazole	Hydralazine	Hydrallazine
Biphenamine	Xenysalate	Hydrocortisone	Cortisol
Bismuth subcarbonate	Bismuth oxycarbonate	Hydroxypropyl methylcellulose	Hypromellose
Bromisovalum	Bromeval	Indigotindisulfonate sodium	Indigo carmine
Bunamiodyl	Buniodyl	Inositol niacinate	Inositol nicotinate
Busulfan	Busulphan	Iodochlorhydroxyquin	Clioquinol
Butabarbital	Secbutabarbitone	Iodopyracet	Diodrast
Butethal	Butobarbitone	Iothiouracil	Iodothiouracil
Butyl aminobenzoate	Butesine	Isoflurophate	Dyflos
Calciferol	Ergosterol	Isoproterenol	Isoprenaline
Calcium benzoylpas	Calcium benzamidosalicylate	Isosorbide dinitrate	Sorbide nitrate
Carbachol	Carbamoylcholine	Leucovorin calcium	Calcium folinate
Carbenoxalone	Carbenoxolone	Lidocaine	Lignocaine
Chaulmoogra oil	Hydnocarpus oil	Mechlorethamine	Mustine
Chloroazodin	Chlorazodin	Meclizine	Meclozine
Chlorobutanol	Chlorbutol	Melanotropin	Intermedin
Chloroguanide	Proguanil	Melphalan	Melfalan
Chlorophenothane	Dicophane	Menadione	Menaphthone
Chlorothen	Chloropyrilene	Menotropins	Follicle-stimulating hormone
Colistimethate	Colistin methanesulphomethate	Meparfynol	Methylpentynol
Corticotropin	Corticotrophin	Mepazine	Pecazine
Cosyntropin	Tetracosactrin	Meperidine	Pethidine
Cromolyn	Cromoglycate	Mephenytoin	Methoin
Cyclobarbital	Cyclobarbitone	Mephobarbital	Methylphenobarbitone
Cyclocumarol	Cyclocoumarol	Metaproterenol	Orciprenaline
Daunomycin	Rubidomycin	Methabarbital	Methabarbitone
Deferoxamine	Desferrioxamine	Methacholine	Acetylmethylcholine
Demeclocycline	Demethylchlortetracycline	Methandrostenolone	Methandienone
Desoxycorticosterone	Deoxycortone	Methantheline	Methanthelinium
Dextroamphetamine	Dexamphetamine	Methenamine hippurate	Hexamine hippurate
Dibucaine	Cinchocaine	Methohexital	Methohexitone
Dichloroisoproterenol	Dichloroisoprenaline	Methopholine	Metofoline
Dicumarol	Dicoumarol	Methscopolamine bromide	Hyoscine methobromide
Diethyl dithiolisophthalate	Ditophal	Methylatropine nitrate	Atropine methyl nitrate
Diethylstilbestrol	Stilboestrol	Methylergonovine	Methylergometrine
Diiodohydroxyquin	Diiodohydroxyquinoline	Methyprylon	Methylprylone
Dinoprost tromethamine	Dinoprostone	Mineral oil	Paraffin, liquid
Disodium-p-melaminylphenyl arsonate	Melarsen	Nequinate	Methyl benzoquate
		Niacin	Nicotinic acid
Dromostanolone	Drostanolone	Niacinamide	Nicotinamide
Dyphylline	Diprophylline	Nikethamide	Nicethamide
Echothiophate	Ecothiopate	Nitroglycerin	Glyceryl trinitrate
Epinephrine	Adrenaline	Norepinephrine	Noradrenaline
Ergocalciferol	Calciferol	Norethindrone	Norethisterone
Ergonovine	Ergometrine	Norethynodrel	Noretynodrel
Estradiol	Oestradiol	Normeperidine	Norpethidine
Estrogen	Oestrogen	Nylidrin	Buphenine
Ethenzamide	Etenzamide	Ouabain	Strophanthin
Ethinyl estradiol	Ethinyloestradiol	Oxtriphylline	Choline theophyllinate

GLOSSARY OF AMERICAN DRUG NAMES AND INTERNATIONAL SYNONYMS* *(Continued)*

United States Adopted Name	British Approved or International Nonproprietary Name	United States Adopted Name	British Approved or International Nonproprietary Name
Peanut oil	Arachis oil	Sulfamethoxypyridazine	Sulphamethoxypyridazine
Penicillin G	Benzylpenicillin	Sulfamoxole	Sulphamoxole
Pentobarbital	Pentobarbitone	Sulfaphenazole	Sulphaphenazole
Pentylenetetrazole	Leptazol	Sulfaproxyline	Sulphaproxyline
Phenobarbital	Phenobarbitone	Sulfasalazine	Sulphasalazine
Physostigmine	Eserine	Sulfasomizole	Sulphasomizole
Phytonadione	Phytomenadione	Sulfathiazole	Sulphathiazole
Polyethylene glycol	Macrogol	Sulfinpyrazone	Sulphinpyrazone
Progestin	Allylestrenol	Sulfisomidine	Sulphasomidine
Proparacaine	Proxymetacaine	Sulfisoxazole	Sulphafurazole
Propoxyphene	Dextropropoxyphene	Sulfomyxin	Sulphomyxin
Pyrilamine	Mepyramine	Tetracaine	Amethocaine
Pyrvinium pamoate	Vipyrnium embonate	Tetramisole	Levamisole
Quinacrine	Mepacrine	Thiabendazole	Mintezol
Riboflavin	Riboflavine	Thialbarbital	Thialbarbitone
Rifampin	Rifampicin	Thiamine	Aneurine
Rolicyprine	Rolicypram	Thimerosal	Thiomersal
Scopolamine	Hyoscine	Thiopental	Thiopentone
Secobarbital	Quinalbarbitone	Thyrotropin	Thyrotrophin
Seperidol	Clofluperol	Thyroxin	Thyroxine
Sodium acetylhydroxyarsanilate	Orsanine	Tilidine	Tilidate
Solasulfone	Solapsone	Triethylenemelamine	Tretamine
Succinylcholine	Suxamethonium	Triflupromazine	Flupromazine
Succinylsulfathiazole	Succinylsulphathiazole	Trihexyphenidyl	Benzhexol
Sulfacetamide	Sulphacetamide	Trimethadione	Troxidone
Sulfadiazine	Sulphadiazine	Trimethaphan	Trimetaphan
Sulfadimethoxine	Sulphadimethoxine	Trimethoprim-sulfamethoxazole	Co-trimoxazole
Sulfaethidole	Sulphaethidole	Troleandomycin	Triacetyloleandomycin
Sulfalene	Sulfametopyrazine	Tromethamine	Trometamol
Sulfameter	Sulphamethoxydiazine	Uracil mustard	Uramustine
Sulfamethazine	Sulfadimidine	Urethan	Urethane
Sulfamethizole	Sulphamethizole	Vinbarbital	Vinbarbitone
Sulfamethoxazole	Sulphamethoxazole	Vitamin A	Retinol

*Modified from Modell, W., Schild, H. O., and Wilson, A.: Applied Pharmacology (American edition). Philadelphia, W. B. Saunders Company, 1976.

LABORATORY REFERENCE VALUES OF CLINICAL IMPORTANCE

prepared by
REX B. CONN, M.D.
Atlanta, Georgia

THE INTERNATIONAL SYSTEM OF UNITS FOR LABORATORY MEASUREMENTS (LE SYSTÈME INTERNATIONAL D'UNITÉS)

Physicians are accustomed to receiving laboratory reports with measurements expressed in metric units such as the gram, liter, or milliliter; however, an extensive modification of the metric system has been adopted by clinical laboratories in many countries, and plans are being formulated to make a similar change in the United States. This adaptation is the International System of Units (Le Système International d'Unités), usually abbreviated S.I. Units. Whereas the metric system utilizes the centimeter, the gram, and the second as basic units, the International System uses the meter, the kilogram, and the second as well as four other basic units.

The overriding consideration for adopting the International System is that it will provide a common language among the various scientific disciplines throughout the world for unambiguous communication regarding all types of measurements. In the medical field, the advantages of conversion are that chemical relationships between various substances will become more readily apparent and there will be an international uniformity in laboratory reporting. The most serious disadvantage in making this conversion is that physicians will have to become accustomed to a new set of figures for almost all laboratory measurements. Because of this inconvenience, as well as a potential for serious misinterpretation of laboratory data, the conversion must be undertaken cautiously and only after a logical plan has been formulated and discussed. There appears to be little question, however, that the International System will be adopted in this country. Clinical laboratories in most western European countries, Canada, and Australia are already using S.I. Units, and American medical journals are adopting the practice of expressing measurements in both conventional and S.I. Units.

The International System

The International System is a coherent approach to all types of measurement which utilizes seven dimensionally independent basic quantities: mass, length, time, thermodynamic temperature, electric current, luminous intensity, and amount of substance. Each of these quantities is expressed in a clearly defined *basic unit* (Table 1).

Two or more basic units may be combined to provide *derived units* (Table 2) for expressing other measurements such as mass concentration (kilograms per cubic meter) and velocity (meters per second). Standardized prefixes (Table 3) for basic and derived units are used to express fractions or multiples of the basic units so that any measurement can be expressed in a value between 0.001 and 1000.

Medical Applications

The most profound change in laboratory reports will result from expressing concentration as amount per volume (moles per liter) rather than mass per volume (milligrams per 100 milliliters). The advantages in the former expression can be seen in the following:

Conventional Units

1.0 gram of hemoglobin
    Combines with 1.37 ml. of oxygen
    Contains 3.4 mg. of iron
    Forms 34.9 mg. of bilirubin

S.I. Units

1.0 mmol of hemoglobin
    Combines with 4.0 mmol of oxygen
    Contains 4.0 mmol of iron
    Forms 4.0 mmol of bilirubin

Chemical relationships between lactic acid and pyruvic acid and the glucose from which both are derived, as well as the relationship between bilirubin and the binding capacity of albumin, are other examples of chemical relationships that will be clarified by using the new system.

There are a number of laboratory and other medical measurements for which the S.I. Units appear to offer little advantage, and some which are disadvantageous because the change would require replacement or revision of instruments such as the sphygmomanometer. The cubic meter is the derived unit for volume; however, it is inappropriately large for medical measurements and the liter has been retained. Thermodynamic

TABLE 1. **Basic Units**

PROPERTY	BASIC UNIT	SYMBOL
Length	metre	m
Mass	kilogram	kg
Amount of substance	mole	mol
Time	second	s
Thermodynamic temperature	kelvin	K
Electric current	ampere	A
Luminous intensity	candela	cd

TABLE 2. Derived Units

DERIVED PROPERTY	DERIVED UNIT	SYMBOL
Area	square metre	m^2
Volume	cubic metre	m^3
	litre	l
Mass concentration	kilogram/cubic metre	kg/m^3
	gram/litre	g/l
Substance concentration	mole/cubic metre	mol/m^3
	mole/litre	mol/l
Temperature	degree Celsius	$C = K - 273.15$

temperature expressed in kelvins is not more informative for medical measurements. Since the Celsius degree is the same as the Kelvin degree, the Celsius scale will be used. Celsius rather than centigrade is the preferred term.

Selection of units for expressing enzyme activity presents certain difficulties. Literally dozens of different units have been used in expressing enzyme activity, and interlaboratory comparison of enzyme results is impossible unless the assay system is precisely defined. In 1964 the International Union of Biochemistry attempted to remedy the situation by proposing the International Unit for enzymes. This unit was defined as the amount of enzyme that will catalyze the conversion of 1 micromole of substrate per minute under standard conditions. Difficulties remain, however, as enzyme activity is affected by the temperature, pH, the type and amount of substrate, the presence of inhibitors, and other factors. Enzyme activity can be expressed in S.I. Units, and the katal has been proposed to express activities of all catalysts, including enzymes. The katal is that amount of enzyme which catalyzes a reaction rate of 1 mole per second. Thus adoption of the katal as the unit of enzyme activity would provide no more information than is obtained when results are expressed in International Units.

TABLE 3. Standard Prefixes

PREFIX	MULTIPLICATION FACTOR	SYMBOL
atto	10^{-18}	a
femto	10^{-15}	f
pico	10^{-12}	p
nano	10^{-9}	n
micro	10^{-6}	μ
milli	10^{-3}	m
centi	10^{-2}	c
deci	10^{-1}	d
deca	10^{1}	da
hecto	10^{2}	h
kilo	10^{3}	k
mega	10^{6}	M
giga	10^{9}	G
tera	10^{12}	T

Hydrogen ion concentration in blood is customarily expressed as pH, but in S.I. Units it would be expressed in nanomoles per liter. It appears unlikely that the very useful pH scale will be discarded.

Pressure measures, such as blood pressure and partial pressures of blood gases, would be expressed in S.I. Units, using the Pascal, a unit that can be derived from the basic units for mass, length, and time. This change probably will not be adopted in the early phases of the conversion to S.I. Units. Similarly, a proposed change in expressing osmolality in terms of the depression of freezing point is inappropriate, because osmolality may be calculated from vapor pressure as well as freezing point measurement.

Conventions

A number of conventions have been adopted to standardize usage of S.I. Units:

1. No periods are used after the symbol for a unit (kg not kg.), and it remains unchanged when used in the plural (70 kg not 70 kgs).

2. A half space rather than a comma is used to divide large numbers into groups of three (5 400 000 not 5,400,000).

3. Compound prefixes should be avoided (nanometer not millimicrometer).

4. Multiples and submultiples are used in steps of 10^3 or 10^{-3}.

5. The degree sign for the temperature scales is omitted (38 C not 38°C).

6. The preferred spelling is metre not meter, litre not liter.

7. Report of a measurement should include information on the system, the component, the kind of quantity, the numerical value, and the unit. For example: *System*, serum. *Component*, glucose. *Kind of quantity*, substance concentration. *Value*, 5.10. *Unit*, mmol/l.

8. The name of the component should be unambiguous; for example, "serum bilirubin" might refer to unconjugated bilirubin or to total bilirubin. For acids and bases, the maximally ionized form is used in naming the component; for example, lactate or urate rather than lactic acid or uric acid.

Tables of Reference Values

Tables accompanying this article indicate "normal values" for most of the commonly performed laboratory tests. The title of the tables has been changed from the "normal values" of previous years to "reference values" to conform to current usage. The reference value is given in conventional units, the conversion factor is indicated when appropriate, and the value in S.I. Units is calculated from these figures. Notes (pp. 924 and 925) are used to provide additional information.

REFERENCE VALUES IN HEMATOLOGY

	CONVENTIONAL UNITS		FACTOR	S.I. UNITS	NOTES
Acid hemolysis test (Ham)	No hemolysis		—	No hemolysis	
Alkaline phosphatase, leukocyte	Total score 14–100		—	Total score 14–100	
Carboxyhemoglobin	Up to 5% of total		0.01	0.05 of total	a
Cell counts					
Erythrocytes					
Males	4.6–6.2 million/cu. mm.		10^6	$4.6\text{–}6.2 \times 10^{12}/l$	
Females	4.2–5.4 million/cu. mm.			$4.2\text{–}5.4 \times 10^{12}/l$	
Children (varies with age)	4.5–5.1 million/cu. mm.			$4.5\text{–}5.1 \times 10^{12}/l$	
Leukocytes					
Total	4500–11,000/cu. mm.		10^6	$4.5\text{–}11.0 \times 10^9/l$	
Differential	*Percentage*	*Absolute*			
Myelocytes	0	0/cu. mm.	10^6	0/1	b
Band neutrophils	3–5	150–400/cu. mm.		$150\text{–}400 \times 10^6/l$	
Segmented neutrophils	54–62	3000–5800/cu. mm.		$3000\text{–}5800 \times 10^6/l$	
Lymphocytes	25–33	1500–3000/cu. mm.		$1500\text{–}3000 \times 10^6/l$	
Monocytes	3–7	300–500/cu. mm.		$300\text{–}500 \times 10^6/l$	
Eosinophils	1–3	50–250/cu. mm.		$50\text{–}250 \times 10^6/l$	
Basophils	0–0.75	15–50/cu. mm.		$15\text{–}50 \times 10^6/l$	
Platelets	150,000–350,000/cu. mm.		10^6	$150\text{–}350 \times 10^9/l$	
Reticulocytes	25,000–75,000/cu. mm.		10^6	$25\text{–}75 \times 10^9/l$	b
	0.5–1.5% of erythrocytes				
Coagulation tests					
Bleeding time (Duke)	1–5 min.		—	1–5 min	
Bleeding time (Ivy)	Less than 5 min.		—	Less than 5 min	
Clot retraction, qualitative	Begins in 30–60 min.		—	Begins in 30–60 min	
	Complete in 24 hrs.		—	Complete in 24 h	
Coagulation time (Lee-White)	5–15 min. (glass tubes)		—	5–15 min (glass tubes)	
	19–60 min. (siliconized tubes)		—	19–60 min (siliconized tubes)	
Fibrinogen	200–400 mg./100 ml.		0.0293	$5.9\text{–}11.7\ \mu\text{mol}/l$	c
Fibrinolysins	0		—	0	
Partial thromboplastin time, activated (APTT)	35–45 sec.		—	35–45 s	
Prothrombin consumption	Over 80% consumed in 1 hr.		0.01	Over 0.80 consumed in 1 h	a
Prothrombin content	100% (calculated from prothrombin time)		0.01	1.0 (calculated from prothrombin time)	a
Prothrombin time (one stage)	12.0–14.0 sec.		—	12.0–14.0 s	
Thromboplastin generation test	Compared to normal control		—	Compared to normal control	
Tourniquet test	Ten or fewer petechiae in a 2.5 cm. circle after 5 min.		—	Ten or fewer petechiae in a 2.5 cm circle after 5 min	
Cold hemolysin test (Donath-Landsteiner)	No hemolysis		—	No hemolysis	
Coombs test					
Direct	Negative		—	Negative	
Indirect	Negative		—	Negative	

Corpuscular values of erythrocytes
(values are for adults; in children, values vary with age)

M.C.H. (mean corpuscular hemoglobin)	27–31 picogm.	0.0155	0.42–0.48 fmol	d
M.C.V. (mean corpuscular volume)	80–105 cu. micra	1.0	80–105 fl	
M.C.H.C. (mean corpuscular hemoglobin concentration)	32–36%	0.01	0.32–0.36	a
Haptoglobin (as hemoglobin binding capacity)	100–200 mg./100 ml.	0.155	16–31 μmol/l	d

Hematocrit

Males	40–54 ml./100 ml.	0.01	0.40–0.54	a
Females	37–47 ml./100 ml.		0.37–0.47	
Newborn	49–54 ml./100 ml.		0.49–0.54	
Children (varies with age)	35–49 ml./100 ml.		0.35–0.49	

Hemoglobin

Males	14.0–18.0 grams/100 ml.	0.155	2.17–2.79 mmol/l	d
Females	12.0–16.0 grams/100 ml.		1.86–2.48 mmol/l	
Newborn	16.5–19.5 grams/100 ml.		2.56–3.02 mmol/l	
Children (varies with age)	11.2–16.5 grams/100 ml.		1.74–2.56 mmol/l	
Hemoglobin, fetal	Less than 1% of total	0.01	Less than 0.01 of total	a
Hemoglobin A$_2$	1.5–3.0% of total	0.01	0.015–0.03 of total	a
Hemoglobin, plasma	0–5.0 mg./100 ml.	0.155	0–0.8 μmol/l	d
Methemoglobin	0–130 mg./100 ml.	0.155	4.7–20 μmol/l	e
Osmotic fragility of erythrocytes	Begins in 0.45–0.39% NaCl	171	Begins in 77–67 mmol/l NaCl	
	Complete in 0.33–0.30% NaCl		Complete in 56–51 mmol/l NaCl	

Sedimentation rate

Wintrobe: Males	0–5 mm. in 1 hr.	—	0–5 mm/h	
Females	0–15 mm. in 1 hr.	—	0–15 mm/h	
Westergren: Males	0–15 mm. in 1 hr.	—	0–15 mm/h	
Females	0–20 mm. in 1 hr.	—	0–20 mm/h	

(May be slightly higher in children and during pregnancy)

Bone marrow, differential cell count

	Range	Average		Range	Average	
Myeloblasts	0.3–5.0%	2.0%	0.01	0.003–0.05	0.02	a
Promyelocytes	1.0–8.0%	5.0%		0.01–0.08	0.05	
Myelocytes: Neutrophilic	5.0–19.0%	12.0%		0.05–0.19	0.12	
Eosinophilic	0.5–3.0%	1.5%		0.005–0.03	0.015	
Basophilic	0.0–0.5%	0.3%		0.00–0.005	0.003	
Metamyelocytes	13.0–32.0%	22.0%		0.13–0.32	0.22	
Polymorphonuclear neutrophils	7.0–30.0%	20.0%		0.07–0.30	0.20	
Polymorphonuclear eosinophils	0.5–4.0%	2.0%		0.005–0.04	0.02	
Polymorphonuclear basophils	0.0–0.7%	0.2%		0.00–0.007	0.002	
Lymphocytes	3.0–17.0%	10.0%		0.03–0.17	0.10	
Plasma cells	0.0–2.0%	0.4%		0.00–0.02	0.004	
Monocytes	0.5–5.0%	2.0%		0.005–0.05	0.02	
Reticulum cells	0.1–2.0%	0.2%		0.001–0.02	0.002	
Megakaryocytes	0.3–3.0%	0.4%		0.003–0.03	0.004	
Pronormoblasts	1.0–8.0%	4.0%		0.01–0.08	0.04	
Normoblasts	7.0–32.0%	18.0%		0.07–0.32	0.18	

REFERENCE VALUES FOR BLOOD, PLASMA AND SERUM

(For some procedures the reference values may vary depending upon the method used)

	CONVENTIONAL UNITS	FACTOR	S.I. UNITS	NOTES
Acetoacetate plus acetone, serum				
Qualitative	Negative	—	Negative	
Quantitative	0.3–2.0 mg./100 ml.	10	3–20 mg/l	
Aldolase, serum	0–11 milliunits/ml. (I.U.) (30°)	1.0	0–11 units/l (30 C)	f
Alpha amino nitrogen, serum	3.0–5.5 mg./100 ml.	0.714	2.1–3.9 mmol/l	
Ammonia, blood	80–110 mcg./100 ml.	0.587	47–65 μmol/l	
Amylase, serum	Less than 160 Caraway units/100 ml.	—	Less than 160 Caraway units/dl	f
Ascorbic acid, blood	0.4–1.5 mg./100 ml.	56.8	23–85 μmol/l	
Base excess, blood	0 ± 2 mEq./liter	1.0	0 ± 2 mmol/l	
Bicarbonate, serum	23–29 mEq./liter	1.0	23–29 mmol/l	
Bilirubin, serum				
Direct	0.1–0.4 mg./100 ml.	17.1	1.7–6.8 μmol/l	
Indirect	0.2–0.7 mg./100 ml. (Total minus direct)	17.1	3.4–12 μmol/l (Total minus direct)	
Total	0.3–1.1 mg./100 ml.	17.1	5.1–19 μmol/l	
Bromsulphalein (BSP)	Less than 5%	0.01	Less than 0.05	a
(Inject 5 mg./kg. body weight, draw sample at 45 min.)				
Calcium, serum	4.5–5.5 mEq./liter	0.50	2.25–2.75 mmol/l	
	9.0–11.0 mg./100 ml.	0.25	2.25–2.75 mmol/l	
	(Slightly higher in children)		(Slightly higher in children)	
	(Varies with protein concentration)		(Varies with protein concentration)	
Calcium, ionized, serum	2.1–2.6 mEq./liter	0.50	1.05–1.30 mmol/l	
	4.25–5.25 mg./100 ml.	0.25	1.05–1.30 mmol/l	
Carbon dioxide content, serum				
Adults	24–30 mEq./liter	1.0	24–30 mmol/l	
Infants	20–28 mEq./liter	1.0	20–28 mmol/l	
Carbon dioxide tension (Pco$_2$), blood	35–45 mm. Hg	—	35–45 mm Hg	g
Carotene, serum	50–300 mcg./100 ml.	0.0186	0.93–5.58 μmol/l	
Ceruloplasmin, serum	23–44 mg./100 ml.	0.0662	1.5–2.9 μmol/l	h
Chloride, serum	96–106 mEq./liter	1.0	96–106 mmol/l	
Cholesterol, serum				
Total	150–250 mg./100 ml.	0.0259	3.9–6.5 mmol/l	
Esters	68–76% of total cholesterol	0.01	0.68–0.76 of total cholesterol	a
Cholinesterase				
Serum	0.5–1.3 pH units	—	0.5–1.3 pH units	f
Erythrocytes	0.5–1.0 pH unit	—	0.5–1.0 pH unit	f
Copper, serum				
Males	70–140 mcg./100 ml.	0.157	11–22 μmol/l	
Females	85–155 mcg./100 ml.	0.157	13–24 μmol/l	
Cortisol, plasma (8 A.M.)	6–16 mcg./100 ml.	27.6	170–440 nmol/l	
Creatine, serum	0.2–0.8 mg./100 ml.	76.3	15–61 μmol/l	

	Conventional	Factor	SI	
Creatine phosphokinase, serum				
Males	0–50 milliunits/ml. (I.U.) (30°)	1.0	0–50 units/l (30 C)	f
Females	0–30 milliunits/ml. (I.U.) (30°) (Oliver-Rosalki)	1.0	0–30 units/l (30 C) (Oliver-Rosalki)	f
Creatine phosphokinase isoenzymes, serum				
CPK-MM	Present	—	Present	
CPK-MB	Absent	—	Absent	
CPK-BB	Absent	—	Absent	
Creatinine, serum	0.7–1.5 mg./100 ml.	88.4	62–133 μmol/l	
Cryoglobulins, serum	0	—	0	
Fatty acids, total, serum	190–420 mg./100 ml.	0.0352	7–15 mmol/l	i
Fibrinogen, plasma	200–400 mg./100 ml.	0.0293	5.9–11.7 μmol/l	c
Folate, serum	5–21 nanogm./ml.	2.27	11–48 nmol/l	
Gamma glutamyltransferase				
Males	6–32 milliunits/ml. (I.U.) (30°)	1.0	6–32 units/l (30 C)	f
Females	4–18 milliunits/ml. (I.U.) (30°)	1.0	4–18 units/l (30 C)	f
Gastrin, serum	0–200 picogm./ml.	1.0	0–200 ng/l	
Glucose (fasting)				
Blood	60–100 mg./100 ml.	0.0555	3.33–5.55 mmol/l	
Plasma or serum	70–115 mg./100 ml.	0.0555	3.89–6.38 mmol/l	
Haptoglobin, serum	100–200 mg./100 ml. (As hemoglobin binding capacity)	0.155	16–31 μmol/l (As hemoglobin binding capacity)	d
Hydroxybutyric dehydrogenase, serum	0–180 milliunits/ml. (I.U.) (30°) (Rosalki-Wilkinson)	1.0	0–180 units/l (30 C) (Rosalki-Wilkinson)	f
	114–290 units/ml. (Wroblewski)	—	114–290 units/ml (Wroblewski)	f
17-Hydroxycorticosteroids, plasma	8–18 mcg./100 ml.	0.0276	0.22–0.50 μmol/l	j
Immunoglobins, serum				
IgG	550–1900 mg./100 ml.	0.01	5.5–19.0 g/l	
IgA	60–333 mg./100 ml.	0.01	0.60–3.3 g/l	
IgM	45–145 mg./100 ml. (Varies with age in children)	0.01	0.45–1.5 g/l (Varies with age in children)	
Insulin, plasma (fasting)	5–25 microunits/ml.	1.0	5–25 milliunits/l	
Iodine, protein bound, serum	3.5–8.0 mcg./100 ml.	0.0788	0.28–0.63 μmol/l	k
Iron, serum	75–175 mcg./100 ml.	0.179	13–31 μmol/l	
Iron binding capacity, serum				
Total	250–410 mcg./100 ml.	0.179	45–73 μmol/l	
Saturation	20–55%	0.01	0.20–0.55	a
17-Ketosteroids, plasma	25–125 mcg./100 ml.	0.0347	0.87–4.34 μmol/l	l
Lactate, blood, venous	0.6–1.8 mEq./liter	1.0	0.6–1.8 mmol/l	
Lactate dehydrogenase, serum	0–300 milliunits/ml. (I.U.) (30°) (Wroblewski modified)	1.0	0–300 units/l (30 C) (Wroblewski modified)	f
	150–450 units/ml. (Wroblewski)	—	150–450 units/ml (Wroblewski)	
	80–120 units/ml. (Wacker)	—	80–120 units/ml (Wacker)	
Lactate dehydrogenase isoenzymes, serum				
LDH₁	22–37% of total	0.01	0.22–0.37 of total	a
LDH₂	30–46% of total		0.30–0.46 of total	
LDH₃	14–29% of total		0.14–0.29 of total	
LDH₄	5–11% of total		0.05–0.11 of total	
LDH₅	2–11% of total		0.02–0.11 of total	

Table continued on the following page

REFERENCE VALUES FOR BLOOD, PLASMA AND SERUM (*Continued*)

(For some procedures the reference values may vary depending upon the method used)

	CONVENTIONAL UNITS	FACTOR	S.I. UNITS	NOTES
Leucine aminopeptidase, serum	14–40 milliunits/ml. (I.U.) (30°)	1.0	14–40 units/l (30 C)	f
Lipase, serum	0–1.5 units (Cherry-Crandall)	—	0–1.5 units (Cherry-Crandall)	f
Lipids, total, serum	450–850 mg./100 ml.	0.01	4.5–8.5 g/l	m
Magnesium, serum	1.5–2.5 mEq./liter	0.50	0.75–1.25 mmol/l	
	1.8–3.0 mg./100 ml.	0.411		
5′-Nucleotidase, serum	Less than 1.6 milliunits/ml. (I.U.) (30°)	1.0	Less than 1.6 units/l (30 C)	f
Nitrogen, nonprotein, serum	15–35 mg./100 ml.	0.714	10.7–25.0 mmol/l	
Osmolality, serum	285–295 mOsm./kg. serum water	—	285–295 mmol/kg serum water	n
Oxygen, blood				
Capacity	16–24 vol.% (varies with hemo-globin)	0.446	7.14–10.7 mmol/l (varies with hemoglobin)	o
Content Arterial	15–23 vol.%	0.446	6.69–10.3 mmol/l	o
Venous	10–16 vol.%	0.446	4.46–7.14 mmol/l	o
Saturation Arterial	94–100% of capacity	0.01	0.94–1.00 of capacity	a
Venous	60–85% of capacity	0.01	0.60–0.85 of capacity	a
Tension, pO_2 Arterial	75–100 mm. Hg	—	75–100 mm Hg	g
P_{50}, blood	26–27 mm. Hg	—	26–27 mm. Hg	g
pH, arterial, blood	7.35–7.45	—	7.35–7.45	p
Phenylalanine, serum	Less than 3 mg./100 ml.	0.0605	Less than 0.18 mmol/l	
Phosphatase, acid, serum	0–7.0 milliunits/ml. (I.U.) (30°)	1.0	0–7.0 units/l (30 C)	f
	1.0–5.0 units (King-Armstrong)	—	1.0–5.0 units (King-Armstrong)	
Phosphatase, alkaline, serum	10–32 milliunits/ml. (I.U.) (30°)	1.0	10–32 units/l (30 C)	f
	5.0–13.0 units (King-Armstrong) (Values are higher in children)	—	5.0–13.0 units (King-Armstrong) (Values are higher in children)	
Phosphate, inorganic, serum				
Adults	3.0–4.5 mg./100 ml.	0.323	1.0–1.5 mmol/l	
Children	4.0–7.0 mg./100 ml.		1.3–2.3 mmol/l	
Phospholipids, serum	6–12 mg./100 ml. (As lipid phosphorus)	0.323	1.9–3.9 mmol/l (As lipid phosphorus)	
Potassium, serum	3.5–5.0 mEq./liter	1.0	3.5–5.0 mmol/l	
Protein, serum				
Total	6.0–8.0 grams/100 ml.	10	60–80 g/l	m
Albumin	3.5–5.5 grams/100 ml.	10	35–55 g/l	q
		0.154	0.54–0.85 mmol/l	
Globulin	2.5–3.5 grams/100 ml.	10	25–35 g/l	
Electrophoresis				
Albumin	3.5–5.5 grams/100 ml.	10	35–55 g/l	q
	52–68% of total	0.01	0.52–0.68 of total	a
Globulin				
Alpha$_1$	0.2–0.4 gram/100 ml.	10	2–4 g/l	m
	2–5% of total	0.01	0.02–0.05 of total	a

Alpha$_2$	0.5–0.9 gram/100 ml.	10	5–9 g/l	m
	7–14% of total	0.01	0.07–0.14 of total	a
Beta	0.6–1.1 grams/100 ml.	10	6–11 g/l	m
	9–15% of total	0.01	0.09–0.15 of total	a
Gamma	0.7–1.7 grams/100 ml.	10	7–17 g/l	m
	11–21% of total	0.01	0.11–0.21 of total	a
Protoporphyrin, erythrocyte	27–61 mcg./100 ml. packed RBC	0.0178	0.48–1.09 μmol/l packed RBC	
Pyruvate, blood	0.01–0.11 mEq./liter	1.0	0.01–0.11 mmol/l	
Sodium, serum	136–145 mEq./liter	1.0	136–145 mmol/l	
Sulfates, inorganic, serum	0.8–1.2 mg./100 ml.	104	83–125 μmol/l	
Testosterone, plasma				
Males	275–875 nanogm./100 ml.	0.0347	9.5–30 nmol/l	
Females	23–75 nanogm./100 ml.	0.0347	0.8–2.6 nmol/l	
Pregnant	38–190 nanogm./100 ml.	0.0347	1.3–6.6 nmol/l	
Thyroid stimulating hormone (TSH), serum	0–7 microunits/ml.	1.0	0–7 milliunits/l	
Thyroxine, free, serum	1.0–2.1 nanogm./100 ml.	12.9	13–27 pmol/l	
Thyroxine (T$_4$), serum	4.4–9.9 mcg./100 ml.	12.9	57–128 nmol/l	
Thyroxine binding globulin (TBG), serum (as thyroxine)	10–26 mcg./100 ml.	12.9	129–335 nmol/l	
Tri-iodothyronine (T$_3$), serum	150–250 nanogm./100 ml.	0.0154	2.3–3.9 nmol/l	
Thyroxine iodine, serum	2.9–6.4 mcg./100 ml.	78.8	229–504 nmol/l	k
Transaminase, serum				
SGOT (aspartate aminotransferase)	0–19 milliunits/ml. (I.U.) (30°) (Karmen modified)	1.0	0–19 units/l (30 C) (Karmen modified)	f
	15–40 units/ml. (Karmen)		15–40 units/ml (Karmen)	
	18–40 units/ml. (Reitman-Frankel)		18–40 units/ml (Reitman-Frankel)	
SGPT (alanine aminotransferase)	0–17 milliunits/ml. (I.U.) (30°) (Karmen modified)	1.0	0–17 units/l (30 C) (Karmen modified)	f
	6–35 units/ml. (Karmen)		6–35 units/ml (Karmen)	
	5–35 units/ml. (Reitman-Frankel)		5–35 units/ml (Reitman-Frankel)	
Triglycerides, serum	40–150 mg./100 ml.	0.01	0.4–1.5 g/l	
		0.0114	0.45–1.71 mmol/l	r
Urate (serum)				
Males	2.5–8.0 mg./100 ml.	0.0595	0.15–0.48 mmol/l	
Females	1.5–7.0 mg./100 ml.	0.0595	0.09–0.42 mmol/l	
Urea				
Blood	21–43 mg./100 ml.	0.167	3.5–7.2 mmol/l	
Plasma or serum	24–49 mg./100 ml.	0.167	4.0–8.2 mmol/l	
Urea nitrogen				
Blood	10–20 mg./100 ml.	0.714	7.1–14.3 mmol/l	k
Plasma or serum	11–23 mg./100 ml.	0.714	7.9–16.4 mmol/l	
Vitamin A, serum	20–80 mcg./100 ml.	0.0349	0.70–2.8 μmol/l	
Vitamin B$_{12}$, serum	300–1000 picogm./ml.	0.738	220–740 pmol/l	

REFERENCE VALUES FOR URINE

(For some procedures the reference values may vary depending upon the method used)

	CONVENTIONAL UNITS	FACTOR	S.I. UNITS	NOTES
Acetone and acetoacetate, qualitative	Negative	—	Negative	
Addis count				
Erythrocytes	0–130,000/24 hrs.	—	0–130 000/24 h	
Leukocytes	0–650,000/24 hrs.	—	0–650 000/24 h	
Casts (hyaline)	0–2000/24 hrs.	—	0–2000/24 h	
Albumin				
Qualitative	Negative	—	Negative	
Quantitative	10–100 mg./24 hrs.	—	10–100 mg/24 h	q
		0.0154	0.15–1.5 μmol/24 h	
Aldosterone	3–20 mcg./24 hrs.	2.77	8.3–55 nmol/24 h	
Alpha amino nitrogen	50–200 mg./24 hrs.	0.0714	3.6–14.3 mmol/24 h	
Ammonia nitrogen	20–70 mEq./24 hrs.	1.0	20–70 mmol/24 h	
Amylase	35–260 Caraway units/hr.	—	35–260 Caraway units/h	f
Bilirubin, qualitative	Negative	—	Negative	
Calcium				
Low Ca diet	Less than 150 mg./24 hrs.	0.025	Less than 3.8 mmol/24 h	
Usual diet	Less than 250 mg./24 hrs.	0.025	Less than 6.3 mmol/24 h	
Catecholamines				
Epinephrine	Less than 10 mcg./24 hrs.	5.46	Less than 55 nmol/24 h	
Norepinephrine	Less than 100 mcg./24 hrs.	5.91	Less than 590 nmol/24 h	
Total free catecholamines	4–126 mcg./24 hrs.	5.91	24–745 nmol/24 h	s
Total metanephrines	0.1–1.6 mg./24 hrs.	5.07	0.5–8.1 μmol/24 h	t
Chloride	110–250 mEq./24 hrs. (Varies with intake)	1.0	110–250 mmol/24 h (Varies with intake)	
Chorionic gonadotropin	0	—	0	
Copper	0–50 mcg./24 hrs.	0.0157	0–0.80 μmol/24 h	
Creatine				
Males	0–40 mg./24 hrs.	0.00762	0–0.30 mmol/24 h	
Females	0–100 mg./24 hrs. (Higher in children and during pregnancy)	0.00762	0–0.76 mmol/24 h (Higher in children and during pregnancy)	
Creatinine	15–25 mg./kg. body weight/24 hrs.	0.00884	0.13–0.22 mmol·kg^{-1} body weight/24 h	
Creatinine clearance				
Males	110–150 ml./min.	—	110–150 ml/min	
Females	105–132 ml./min. (1.73 sq. meter surface area)	—	105–132 ml/min (1.73 m² surface area)	
Cystine or cysteine, qualitative	Negative	—	Negative	
Dehydroepiandrosterone	Less than 15% of total 17-keto-steroids	0.01	Less than 0.15 of total 17-keto-steroids	a
Delta aminolevulinic acid	1.3–7.0 mg./24 hrs.	7.63	10–53 μmol/24 h	

Estrogens				
Males				
Estrone	3–8 μg./24 hrs.	3.70	11–30 nmol/24 h	
Estradiol	0–6 μg./24 hrs.	3.67	0–22 nmol/24 h	
Estriol	1–11 μg./24 hrs.	3.47	3–38 nmol/24 h	
Total	4–25 μg./24 hrs.	3.60	14–90 nmol/24 h	u
Females				
Estrone	4–31 μg./24 hrs.	3.70	15–115 nmol/24 h	
Estradiol	0–14 μg./24 hrs.	3.67	0–51 nmol/24 h	
Estriol	0–72 μg./24 hrs.	3.47	0–250 nmol/24 h	
Total	5–100 μg./24 hrs.	3.60	18–360 nmol/24 h	u
	(Markedly increased during pregnancy)		(Markedly increased during pregnancy)	
Glucose (as reducing substance)	Less than 250 mg./24 hrs.	—	Less than 250 mg/24 h	
Gonadotropins, pituitary	10–50 mouse units/24 hrs.	—	10–50 mouse units/24 h	
Hemoglobin and myoglobin, qualitative	Negative	—	Negative	
Hemogentisic acid, qualitative	Negative	—	Negative	
17-Hydroxycorticosteroids				
Males	3–9 mg./24 hrs.	2.76	8.3–25 μmol/24 h	j
Females	2–8 mg./24 hrs.		5.5–22 μmol/24 h	
5-Hydroxyindoleacetic acid				
Qualitative	Negative	—	Negative	
Quantitative	Less than 9 mg./24 hrs.	5.23	Less than 47 μmol/24 h	
17-Ketosteroids				
Males	6–18 mg./24 hrs.	3.47	21–62 μmol/24 h	l
Females	4–13 mg./24 hrs.		14–45 μmol/24 h	
	(Varies with age)		(Varies with age)	
Magnesium	6.0–8.5 mEq./24 hrs.	0.5	3.0–4.3 mmol/24 h	
Metanephrines (see Catecholamines)				
Osmolality	38–1400 mOsm./kg. water	—	38–1400 mmol/kg water	n
pH	4.6–8.0, average 6.0	—	4.6–8.0, average 6.0	p
	(Depends on diet)		(Depends on diet)	
Phenolsulfonphthalein excretion (PSP)	25% or more in 15 min.	0.01	0.25 or more in 15 min	a
	40% or more in 30 min.		0.40 or more in 30 min	
	55% or more in 2 hrs.		0.55 or more in 2 h	
	(After injection of 1 ml PSP intravenously)		(After injection of 1 ml PSP intravenously)	
Phenylpyruvic acid, qualitative	Negative	—	Negative	
Phosphorus	0.9–1.3 gm./24 hrs.	32.3	29–42 mmol/24 h	
Porphobilinogen				
Qualitative	Negative	—	Negative	
Quantitative	0–0.2 mg./100 ml.	4.42	0–0.9 μmol/l	
	Less than 2.0 mg./24 hrs.		Less than 9 μmol/24 h	
Porphyrins				
Coproporphyrin	50–250 mcg./24 hrs.	1.53	77–380 nmol/24 h	
Uroporphyrin	10–30 mcg./24 hrs.	1.20	12–36 nmol/24 h	
Potassium	25–100 mEq./24 hrs.	1.0	25–100 mmol/24 h	
	(Varies with intake)		(Varies with intake)	

Table continued on the following page

REFERENCE VALUES FOR URINE (*Continued*)

(For some procedures the reference values may vary depending upon the method used)

	CONVENTIONAL UNITS	FACTOR	S.I. UNITS	NOTES
Pregnanediol				
Males	0.4–1.4 mg./24 hrs.	3.12	1.2–4.4 μmol/24 h	
Females				
Proliferative phase	0.5–1.5 mg./24 hrs.		1.6–4.7 μmol/24 h	
Luteal phase	2.0–7.0 mg./24 hrs.		6.2–22 μmol/24 h	
Postmenopausal phase	0.2–1.0 mg./24 hrs.		0.6–3.1 μmol/24 h	
Pregnant 16 weeks	5–21 mg./24 hrs.		16–66 μmol/24 h	
Pregnant 20 weeks	6–26 mg./24 hrs.		19–81 μmol/24 h	
Pregnant 24 weeks	12–32 mg./24 hrs.		37–100 μmol/24 h	
Pregnant 28 weeks	19–51 mg./24 hrs.		59–159 μmol/24 h	
Pregnant 32 weeks	22–66 mg./24 hrs.		69–206 μmol/24 h	
Pregnant 36 weeks	23–77 mg./24 hrs.		72–240 μmol/24 h	
Pregnant 40 weeks	23–63 mg./24 hrs.		72–197 μmol/24 h	
Pregnanetriol	Less than 2.5 mg./24 hrs. in adults	2.97	Less than 7.4 μmol/24 h in adults	
Protein				
Qualitative	Negative	—	Negative	
Quantitative	10–150 mg./24 hrs.		10–150 mg/24 h	m
Sodium	130–260 mEq./24 hrs.	1.0	130–260 mmol/24 h	
	(Varies with intake)		(Varies with intake)	
Specific gravity	1.003–1.030	—	1.003–1.030	
Titratable acidity	20–40 mEq./24 hrs.	1.0	20–40 mmol/24 h	
Urate	200–500 mg./24 hrs.	0.00595	1.2–3.0 mmol/24 h	
	(With normal diet)		(With normal diet)	
Urobilinogen	Up to 1.0 Ehrlich unit/2 hrs.	—	Up to 1.0 Ehrlich unit/2 h	
	(1–3 P.M.)		(1–3 P.M.)	
	0–4.0 mg./24 hrs.	—	0–4.0 mg/24 h	
Vanillylmandelic acid (VMA)	1–8 mg./24 hrs.	5.05	5–40 μmol/24 h	
(4-hydroxy-3-methoxymandelic acid)				

REFERENCE VALUES FOR THERAPEUTIC DRUG MONITORING

	CONVENTIONAL UNITS	FACTOR	S.I. UNITS	NOTES
Carbamazepine, serum	0	4.23	0	
(Tegretol)	Therapeutic levels:		Therapeutic levels:	
	5.0–14.0 mg./liter		21–59 μmol/l	
Digoxin, serum	0	1.28	0	
	Therapeutic levels:		Therapeutic levels:	
With dose of 0.25 mg. per day	0.8–1.6 mcg./liter		1.0–2.3 nmol/l	

With dose of 0.5 mg. per day (Sample obtained 12 to 24 hrs. after last dose)	0.9–2.4 mcg./liter		1.2–3.1 nmol/l
Diphenylhydantoin, serum (Dilantin)	0 Therapeutic levels: 10–20 mg./liter Toxic levels: Above 20 mg./liter	3.65	0 Therapeutic levels: 37–73 μmol/l Toxic levels: Above 73 μmol/l
Ethosuximide, serum (Zarontin)	0 Therapeutic levels: 40–80 mg./liter	7.08	0 Therapeutic levels: 283–566 μmol/l
Lithium, serum	0 Therapeutic levels: 0.8–1.5 mEq./liter Toxic level: Above 2 mEq./liter	1.0	0 Therapeutic levels: 0.8–1.5 mmol/l Toxic level: Above 2 mmol/l
Phenobarbital, serum	0 Therapeutic levels: 10.0–25.0 mg./liter Toxic levels: Vary widely because of developed tolerance	4.31	0 Therapeutic levels: 43–108 μmol/l Toxic levels: Vary widely because of developed tolerance
Primidone, serum (Mysoline)	0 Therapeutic levels: 4.0–10.0 mg./liter	4.58	0 Therapeutic levels: 18–46 μmol/l
Procainamide, serum (Pronestyl)	0 Therapeutic levels: 4.0–8.0 mg./liter	4.24	0 Therapeutic levels: 17–34 μmol/l
Quinidine, serum	0 Therapeutic levels: 2.0–5.0 mg./liter Toxic levels: Over 10 mg./liter	3.08	0 Therapeutic levels: 6.2–15 μmol/l Toxic levels: Over 31 μmol/l
Salicylate, plasma	0 Therapeutic levels: 20–25 mg./100 ml. Toxic levels: Over 30 mg./100 ml. Death 45–75 mg./100 ml.	0.0555	0 Therapeutic levels: 1.0–1.4 mmol/l Toxic levels: Over 1.7 mmol/l Death 2.5–4.2 mmol/l
Theophylline, serum	0 Therapeutic levels: 5.0–20.0 mg./liter Toxic levels: Above 30.0 mg./liter	5.55	0 Therapeutic levels: 28–111 μmol/l Toxic levels: Above 167 μmol/l
Thiocyanate, serum (Metabolite of sodium nitroprusside)	0 Therapeutic levels: 80–120 mg./liter	0.0169	0 Therapeutic levels: 1.4–2.0 mmol/l

REFERENCE VALUES IN TOXICOLOGY

	CONVENTIONAL UNITS	FACTOR	S.I. UNITS	NOTES
Arsenic, blood	3.5–7.2 mcg./100 ml.	0.133	0.47–0.96 μmol/l	
Arsenic, urine	Less than 100 mcg./24 hrs.	0.0133	Less than 1.3 μmol/24 h	
Bromides, serum	0	1.0	0	
	Toxic levels:		Toxic levels:	
	Above 17 mEq./liter		Above 17 mmol/l	
Carbon monoxide, blood	Up to 5% saturation	—	Up to 0.05 saturation	a
	Symptoms occur with 20% saturation		Symptoms occur with 0.20 saturation	
Ethanol, blood	Less than 0.005%	217	Less than 1 mmol/l	
Marked intoxication	0.3–0.4%		65–87 mmol/l	
Alcoholic stupor	0.4–0.5%		87–109 mmol/l	
Coma	Above 0.5%		Above 109 mmol/l	
Lead, blood	0–40 mcg./100 ml.	0.0483	0–2 μmol/l	
Lead, urine	Less than 100 mcg./24 hrs.	0.00483	Less than 0.48 μmol/24 h	
Mercury, urine	Less than 10 mcg./24 hrs.	4.98	Less than 50 nmol/24 h	

REFERENCE VALUES FOR CEREBROSPINAL FLUID

	CONVENTIONAL UNITS	FACTOR	S.I. UNITS	NOTES
Cells	Fewer than 5/cu. mm.; all mononuclear	—	Fewer than 5/μl; all mononuclear	
Chloride	120–130 mEq./liter	1.0	120–130 mmol/l	
	(20 mEq./liter higher than serum)		(20 mmol/l higher than serum)	
Electrophoresis	Predominantly albumin	—	Predominantly albumin	
Glucose	50–75 mg./100 ml.	0.0555	2.8–4.2 mmol/l	
	(20 mg./100 ml. less than serum)		(1.1 mmol/l less than serum)	
IgG				
Children under 14	Less than 8% of total protein	—	Less than 0.08 of total protein	a,m
Adults	Less than 14% of total protein		Less than 0.14 of total protein	
Pressure	70–180 mm. water		70–180 mm water	g
Protein, total	15–45 mg./100 ml.	0.01	0.150–0.450 g/l	m
	(Higher, up to 70 mg./100 ml., in elderly adults and children)		(Higher, up to 0.70 g/l, in elderly adults and children)	

REFERENCE VALUES FOR GASTRIC ANALYSIS

	CONVENTIONAL UNITS	FACTOR	S.I. UNITS	NOTES
Basal gastric secretion (1 hour)				
Concentration	(Mean ± 1 S.D.)		(Mean ± 1 S.D.)	
Males	25.8 ± 1.8 mEq./liter	1.0	25.8 ± 1.8 mmol/l	
Females	20.3 ± 3.0 mEq./liter		20.3 ± 3.0 mmol/l	
Output	(Mean ± 1 S.D.)		(Mean ± 1 S.D.)	
Males	2.57 ± 0.16 mEq./hr.	1.0	2.57 ± 0.16 mmol/h	
Females	1.61 ± 0.18 mEq./hr.		1.61 ± 0.18 mmol/h	
After histamine stimulation				
Normal	Mean output 11.8 mEq./hr.	1.0	Mean output 11.8 mmol/h	
Duodenal ulcer	Mean output 15.2 mEq./hr.		Mean output 15.2 mmol/h	
After maximal histamine stimulation				
Normal	Mean output 22.6 mEq./hr.	1.0	Mean output 22.6 mmol/h	
Duodenal ulcer	Mean output 44.6 mEq./hr.		Mean output 44.6 mmol/h	
Diagnex blue (Squibb): Anacidity	0–0.3 mg. in 2 hrs.	1.0	0–0.3 mg in 2 h	
Doubtful	0.3–0.6 mg. in 2 hrs.		0.3–0.6 mg in 2 h	
Normal	Greater than 0.6 mg. in 2 hrs.		Greater than 0.6 mg in 2 h	
Volume, fasting stomach content	50–100 ml.	—	0.05–0.1 litre	
Emptying time	3–6 hrs.	—	3–6 h	
Color	Opalescent or colorless	—	Opalescent or colorless	
Specific gravity	1.006–1.009	—	1.006–1.009	
pH (adults)	0.9–1.5	—	0.9–1.5	p

GASTROINTESTINAL ABSORPTION TESTS

	CONVENTIONAL UNITS	FACTOR	S.I. UNITS	NOTES
d-Xylose absorption test	After an 8 hour fast, 10 ml./kg. body weight of a 0.05 solution of d-xylose is given by mouth. Nothing further by mouth is given until the test has been completed. All urine voided during the following 5 hours is pooled, and blood samples are taken at 0, 60, and 120 minutes. Normally 0.26 (range 0.16–0.33) of ingested xylose is excreted within 5 hours, and the serum xylose reaches a level between 25 and 40 mg./100 ml. after 1 hour and is maintained at this level for another 60 minutes.		No change	

Table continued on the following page

GASTROINTESTINAL ABSORPTION TESTS (*Continued*)

	CONVENTIONAL UNITS	FACTOR	S.I. UNITS	NOTES
Vitamin A absorption	A fasting blood specimen is obtained and 200,000 units of vitamin A in oil is given by mouth. Serum vitamin A level should rise to twice fasting level in 3 to 5 hours.		No change	

REFERENCE VALUES FOR FECES

	CONVENTIONAL UNITS	FACTOR	S.I. UNITS	NOTES
Bulk	100–200 grams/24 hrs.	—	100–200 g/24 h	
Dry matter	23–32 grams/24 hrs.	—	23–32 g/24 h	
Fat, total	Less than 6.0 grams/24 hrs.	—	Less than 6.0 g/24 h	
Nitrogen, total	Less than 2.0 grams/24 hrs.	—	Less than 2.0 g/24 h	
Urobilinogen	40–280 mg./24 hrs.	—	40–280 mg/24 h	
Water	Approximately 65%	0.01	Approximately 0.65	a

REFERENCE VALUES FOR SEMEN ANALYSIS

	CONVENTIONAL UNITS	FACTOR	S.I. UNITS	NOTES
Volume	2–5 ml.; usually 3–4 ml.	—	2–5 ml; usually 3–4 ml	
Liquefaction	Complete in 15 min.	—	Complete in 15 min	
pH	7.2–8.0; average 7.8	—	7.2–8.0; average 7.8	p
Leukocytes	Occasional or absent	—	Occasional or absent	
Count	60–150 million/ml.	—	60–150 million/ml	
	Below 60 million/ml. is abnormal	—	Below 60 million/ml is abnormal	
Motility	80% or more motile	—	0.80 or more motile	a
Morphology	80–90% normal forms	—	0.80–0.90 normal forms	a

REFERENCE VALUES FOR IMMUNOLOGIC PROCEDURES

	CONVENTIONAL UNITS		FACTOR	S.I. UNITS	NOTES
Syphilis serology (RPR and VDRL)	Negative			No change	
Mono screen	Negative			No change	
R.A. test (latex)	1:40	Negative		No change	
	1:80–1:160	Doubtful			
	1:320	Positive			
Rose test	1:10	Negative		No change	
	1:20–1:40	Doubtful			
	1:80	Positive			
Anti-streptolysin O titer	Normal up to 1:128. Single test usually has little significance. Rise in titer or persistently elevated titer is significant.			No change	
Anti-hyaluronidase titer	Less than 1:200. Significant if rising titer can be demonstrated at weekly intervals.			No change	
C-reactive protein	Negative			No change	
Anti-nuclear antibody	One specimen is sufficient, unless the result is inconsistent with the clinical impression. Most patients with active lupus have high ANA titers (160 or greater); some have lower titers (20–40). Patients with inactive lupus may have a negative test. Antinuclear antibodies are occasionally present in patients with no evidence of systemic lupus, usually in lower titers (20–40).			No change	
Febrile agglutinins	Titers of 1:80 or greater may be significant, particularly if subsequent samples show rise in titer.			No change	
Tularemia agglutinins	1:80	Negative		No change	
	1:160	Doubtful			
	1:320	Positive			
Proteus OX-19 agglutinins	Titers of 1:80 or greater may be significant, particularly if subsequent samples show rise in titer.			No change	
Complement fixation tests	Titers of 1:8 or less are usually not significant. Paired sera showing rise in titer of more than two tubes are usually considered significant.			No change	
C3 Test	80–140 mg./100 ml.		0.01	0.80–1.40 g/l	q
C4 Test	11–75 mg./100 ml.		0.01	0.11–0.75 g/l	

NOTES

a. Percentage is expressed as a decimal fraction.

b. Percentage may be expressed as a decimal fraction; however, when the result expressed is itself a variable fraction of another variable, the absolute value is more meaningful. There is no reason, other than custom, for expressing reticulocyte counts and differential leukocyte counts in percentages or decimal fractions rather than in absolute numbers.

c. Molecular weight of fibrinogen = 341,000.

d. Molecular weight of hemoglobin = 64,500. Because of disagreement as to whether the monomer or tetramer of hemoglobin should be used in the conversion, it has been recommended that the conventional grams per deciliter be retained. The tetramer is used in the table; values given should be multiplied by 4 to obtain concentration of the monomer.

e. Molecular weight of methemoglobin = 64,500. See note d above.

f. Enzyme units have not been changed in these tables because the proposed enzyme unit, the katal, has not been universally adopted (1 International Unit = 16.7 nkat).

g. It has been proposed that pressure be expressed in the Pascal (1 mm Hg = 0.133 kPa); however, this convention has not been universally accepted.

h. Molecular weight of ceruloplasmin = 151,000.

i. "Fatty acids" includes a mixture of different aliphatic acids of varying molecular weight. A mean molecular weight of 284 has been assumed in calculating the conversion factor.

mit direct correlation with hemoglobin content, which is possible when oxygen content and capacity are expressed in molar quantities. One millimole of hemoglobin combines with 4 millimoles of oxygen.

p. Hydrogen ion concentration in S.I. units would be expressed in nanomoles per liter; however, this change has not received general approval. Conversion can be calculated as antilog $(-pH)$.

q. Albumin is expressed in grams per liter to be consistent with units used for other proteins. Concentration of albumin may be expressed in mmol/l also, an expression that permits assessment of binding capacity of albumin for substances such as bilirubin. Molecular weight of albumin is 65,000.

r. Most techniques for quantitating triglycerides measure the glycerol moiety, and the total mass is calculated using an average molecular weight. The factor given assumes a mean molecular weight of 875 for triglycerides.

s. Calculated as norepinephrine, molecular weight 169.18.

t. Calculated as metanephrine, molecular weight 197.23.

u. Conversion factor calculated from molecular weights of estrone, estradiol, and estriol in proportions of 2:1:2.

REFERENCES

1. Baron, D. N., Broughton, P. M. G., Cohen, M., Lansley, T. S., Lewis, S. M., and Shinton, N. K.: J. Clin. Path., 27:590, 1974.

j. Based upon molecular weight of cortisol 362.47.

k. The practice of expressing concentration of an organic molecule in terms of one of its constituent elements originated when measurements included a heterogeneous class of compounds (nonprotein nitrogenous compounds, iodine-containing compounds bound to serum proteins). It was carried over to expressing measurements of specific substances (urea, thyroxine), but the practice should be discarded. For iodine and nitrogen 1 mole is taken as the monoatomic form, although they occur as diatomic molecules.

l. Based upon molecular weight of dehydroepiandrosterone 288.41.

m. Weight per volume is retained as the unit because of the heterogeneous nature of the material measured.

n. The proposal that osmolality be reported as freezing point depression using the millikelvin as the unit has not been received with universal enthusiasm. The milliosmole is not an S.I. unit, and the unit used here is the millimole.

o. Volumes per cent might be converted to a decimal fraction; however, this would not per-

2. Scully, R. E., McNeely, B. U., and Galdabini, J. J.: New Engl. J. Med., *298*:34, 1978.
3. Davidsohn, I., and Henry, J. B.: Clinical Diagnosis by Laboratory Methods, 15th ed. Philadelphia, W. B. Saunders Co., 1974.
4. Dawson, R. M. C., Elliott, D. C., Elliott, W. H., and Jones, K. M.: Data for Biochemical Research, 2nd ed. New York and Oxford, Oxford University Press, 1969.
5. Dybkaer, R.: Amer. J. Clin. Path., *52*:637, 1969.
6. Henry, R. J., Cannon, D. C., and Winkleman, J. W.: Clinical Chemistry—Principles and Techniques, 2nd ed. New York, Harper & Row, 1974.
7. International Committee for Standardization in Hematology, International Federation of Clinical Chemistry and World Association of Pathology Societies: Clin. Chem., *19*:135, 1973.
8. Lehmann, H. P.: Amer. J. Clin. Path., *65*:2, 1976.
9. Miale, J. B.: Laboratory Medicine—Hematology, 5th ed. St. Louis, C. V. Mosby, 1977.
10. Page, C. H., and Vigoureux, P.: The International System of Units (S.I.). U.S. Department of Commerce, National Bureau of Standards, Special Publication 330, 1974.
11. Tietz, N. W.: Fundamentals of Clinical Chemistry, 2nd ed. Philadelphia, W. B. Saunders Co., 1976.
12. Wintrobe, M. D., Lee, G. R., Boggs, D. R., Bithell, T. C., Athens, J. W., and Foerster, J.: Clinical Hematology, 7th ed. Philadelphia, Lea & Febiger, 1974.
13. Young, D. S.: New Engl. J. Med., *292*:795, 1975.

Index

The Right Answers — Right Away!
SAUNDERS CLINICAL LIBRARY

Conn & Conn:
CURRENT DIAGNOSIS 5

This fifth edition is your best source for the latest in medical diagnosis. Completely revised by more than 300 contributors, **Conn & Conn** offers you authoritative, comprehensive information on the diagnosis of both common and rare disorders from chest pain to scleroderma. Order your copy today!
July 1977. 1272 pp. 104 ill. $36.00   **Order #2674-2.**

Gellis & Kagan:
CURRENT PEDIATRIC THERAPY 8

With contributions from 294 experts, **Current Pediatric Therapy 8** is the clinical reference pediatricians turn to most often for useful therapeutic advice. Concise yet detailed information on the latest approaches to the management of childhood disorders fill this time-honored work. New areas of coverage include: accident prevention, breast feeding, sudden infant death syndrome, infant colic, fractures, viral pneumonia and much more.
Feb. 1978. 877 pp. Illustd. $32.00   **Order #4089-3.**

DORLAND'S ILLUSTRATED MEDICAL DICTIONARY,
25th Edition

The "big red" **Dorland**—standard authority for more than 70 years and one of the world's most widely used references—is more indispensable than ever in this totally revised 25th edition. It's a one volume library that gives you immediate access to more than 120,000 terms. Obsolete terms have been deleted and over 14,000 new entries have been included.
June 1974. 1748 pp. Illustd. (23 color plates).
Standard Edition: $24.50.   **Order #3148-7.**
Deluxe Edition: $35.00.   **Order #3149-5.**

Rakel & Conn:
FAMILY MEDICINE, 2nd Edition

For the practitioner who sees it all, **Rakel & Conn** covers it all. It begins with the consideration of social, cultural, psychological and emotional factors that can affect the health of the family. Then it covers epidemiology, etiology, physiology and pathology of commonly encountered diseases and their therapy.
June 1978. 1186 pp. 252 ill. (2 color plates). $38.50
Order #7447-X.

Parsons & Sommers:
GYNECOLOGY, 2nd Edition

For the most current, indispensable information on gynecology available today, this second edition is the one authoritative reference you can't afford to be without! With 95% of the text revised and updated, it covers infertility, contraception, ectopic pregnancy, trophoblastic disease, ovarian carcinoma and much, much more.
May 1978. 1660 pp. 540 ill.
Single Volume $60.00.   **Order #7081-4.**
Two Volume Set: $70.00.   **Order #7084-9.**

Sleisenger & Fordtran:
GASTROINTESTINAL DISEASE, 2nd Edition

All the latest advances in gastroenterology are given the fullest treatment in this landmark volume. The editors have added new material on: endoscopy; nutrition; bile salt metabolism; neuropharmacology; hormone receptors; pediatric considerations of abdominal pain and the acute abdomen; fistulas and abscesses; echography of the abdomen; and scanning techniques including CAT and angiography of the gut.
July 1978. 1977 pp. 1012 ill. (77 in color).
Single Volume: $63.00.   **Order #8362-2.**
Two Volume Set: $68.00.   **Order #8395-9.**

Turn page for more titles ➡

To order, fill in, detach and mail.   No postage required in the U.S.

Office use only. Please don't write here.

TRANS	2
ACT-1	9
ACT-2	
TAX CODE	
TERMS	
SHIP	
PRI	
MSG	

Please send me the following titles on 30-day approval:

☐ **2674-2** Conn & Conn ($36.00)
☐ **4089-3** Gellis & Kagan 8 ($32.00)
☐ **7447-X** Rakel & Conn ($38.50)
☐ **3148-7** Dorland (Standard $24.50)
☐ **3149-5** Dorland (Deluxe $35.00)
☐ **8362-2** Sleisenger & Fordtran (Single Volume $63.00)

☐ **8395-9** Sleisenger & Fordtran (Two Volume Set $68.00)
☐ **7449-6** Halsted ($36.50)
☐ **7868-8** Sabiston (Single Volume $42.50)
☐ **7869-6/0-X** Sabiston (Two Volume Set $53.00)

☐ **5048-I** Eisenberg & Copass ($9.95)
☐ **8034-8** Schwartz et al. ($70.00)
☐ **7498-4** Reece ($15.95)
☐ **8721-0** Taber (About $25.00)
☐ **7081-4** Parsons & Sommers (Single Volume $60.00)
☐ **7084-9** Parsons & Sommers (Two Volume Set $70.00)

☐ Bill me (plus postage & handling)   ☐ Check enclosed (Saunders pays postage and handling)
☐ Credit my salesman

Need extra copies of **Conn '79** *for the hospital, office or friends? Please indicate how many copies and we'll be glad to send them to you on 30-day approval.*
I need _______ copies.

Please Print

Full Name _______________________

Address _______________________

City _______________ State _______ Zip _______

Halsted:

THE LABORATORY IN CLINICAL MEDICINE

To keep up with the advances in laboratory procedures, turn to this fine volume highlighting valuable clinical techniques. It shows you the interface between the pathologic physiology of disease and specific laboratory procedures.
Jan. 1976. 866 pp. 127 ill. $36.50. **Order # 7449-6.**

Sabiston:

Davis-Christopher TEXTBOOK OF SURGERY, 11th Edition

Backed by the expertise and specialized guidance of the Sabiston "surgical team," you'll be able to handle with skill and confidence practically any surgical condition you may face. Rewritten, expanded, and updated, the eleventh edition is virtually a new book. Chapters new to this edition include: surgical problems related to diabetes mellitus; the acute care unit; medullary carcinoma of the thyroid and multiple endocrine neoplasias.
June 1977. 2465 pp. 1805 ill. (l in color).
Single Volume: $42.50. **Order # 7868-8.**
Two Volume Set: $53.00. **Order # 7869-6/0-X.**

NEW Titles in Emergency Medicine...

Eisenberg & Copass:

MANUAL OF EMERGENCY MEDICAL THERAPEUTICS

The first source you'll want to check in a medical emergency is this handy, pocket-sized manual. It provides the quickest, most convenient format for finding critically-needed therapeutic information including: drug therapy for hypertensive emergencies; management of cardiac arrhythmias; drug overdose and its management; differential diagnosis and therapy of cardiac and non-cardiac pulmonary edema; and a guide to 150 drugs commonly prescribed in the emergency room.
Nov. 1978. 311 pp. Illustd. $9.95. **Order # 5048-l.**

Taber:

MANUAL OF GYNECOLOGIC AND OBSTETRIC EMERGENCIES

This concise, soft-bound manual details everything you need to know about urgent female problems routinely seen in the community hospital or in office practice. Among the many outstanding sections are those on spontaneous abortion, ectopic pregnancy, hypertension in pregnancy, coagulation disorders and fluid therapy, and rape.
January 1979. Soft cover. 928 pp. 138 ill.
About $25.00. **Order # 8721-0.**

Reece:

REECE-CHAMBERLAIN MANUAL OF EMERGENCY PEDIATRICS, 2nd Edition

Covering over 200 pediatric injuries and disorders, this edition has been thoroughly revised and updated. You'll find separate sections on true emergencies, presenting complaints, diagnostic entities, and dysfunctions affecting specific organs of the body.
July 1978. 721 pp. Illustd. $15.95. **Order # 7498-4.**

Schwartz, Safar, Stone, Storey & Wagner:

PRINCIPLES AND PRACTICE OF EMERGENCY MEDICINE

This comprehensive two-volume set covers all aspects of traumatic and non-traumatic medical emergencies. With contributions from over 130 top emergency medicine practitioners, it includes basic introductory material; discussions of the pathophysiologic basis of acute illness and injury; clinical considerations; legal and legislative aspects of emergency care; socioeconomic factors and an overview of emergency medicine in other nations.
Aug. 1978. 1535 pp. 409 ill. (5 color plates).
Two Volume Set: $70.00. **Order # 8034-8.**

Printed in USA. Prices shown are US only and subject to change. nlr 1078l

BUSINESS REPLY MAIL

FIRST CLASS   PERMIT NO. 101   PHILADELPHIA, PA

postage will be paid by addressee

W.B. SAUNDERS CO.

west washington square
philadelphia, PA 19105